D1186931

WALTON HOSPITAL — LIVERPOOL
X-RAY DEPARTMENT

Computed Body Tomography
With MRI Correlation
Second Edition

WALTON HOSPITAL — LIVERPOOL
X-RAY DEPARTMENT

COMPUTED BODY TOMOGRAPHY

With MRI Correlation

Second Edition

Editors

Joseph K. T. Lee, M.D.
The Edward Mallinckrodt
Institute of Radiology
Washington University School of Medicine
St. Louis, Missouri

Stuart S. Sagel, M.D.
The Edward Mallinckrodt
Institute of Radiology
Washington University School of Medicine
St. Louis, Missouri

Robert J. Stanley, M.D.
Department of Radiology
The University of Alabama School
of Medicine
University of Alabama at Birmingham
Birmingham, Alabama

Raven Press New York

Raven Press, 1185 Avenue of the Americas, New York, New York 10036

© 1989 by Raven Press, Ltd. All rights reserved. This book is protected by copyright. No part of it may be reproduced, stored in a retrieval system, or transmitted, in any form or by any means, electronic, mechanical, photocopying, or recording, or otherwise, without the prior written permission of the publisher.

Made in the United States of America

Library of Congress Cataloging-in-Publication Data

Computed body tomography with MRI correlation.

    Rev. ed. of: Computed body tomography. c1983.
    Includes bibliographies and index.
    1. Tomography.   2. Magnetic resonance imaging.
I. Lee, Joseph K. T.   II. Sagel, Stuart S., 1940–
III. Stanley, Robert J., 1937–   .   IV. Computed
body tomography. [DNLM: 1. Magnetic Resonance Imaging.
2. Tomography, X-Ray Computed. WN 160 C7365]
RC78.7.T6C6416   1989   616.07'572   87-45368
ISBN 0-88167-331-5

   The material contained in this volume was submitted as previously unpublished material, except in the instances in which credit has been given to the source from which some of the illustrative material was derived.
   Great care has been taken to maintain the accuracy of the information contained in the volume. However, neither Raven Press nor the editors can be held responsible for errors or for any consequences arising from the use of the information contained herein.

9 8 7 6 5 4 3 2

This work is dedicated to our wives,
Christina, Beverlee, and Sally,
and to our children,
Alexander, Betsy, and Catherine,
Scott, Darryl, and Brett,
Ann, Robert, Cathy, and Sara.

Preface

During the six years that have elapsed since the First Edition of our textbook, *Computed Body Tomography,* which was published in 1982, CT has become the screening procedure of choice in evaluating many abdominal and spinal diseases. Improvements in scanning technology have resulted in better spatial resolution and faster data acquisition. This allowed a broader use of CT to areas such as the evaluation of bronchiectasis and articular abnormalities. Furthermore, CT is no longer used exclusively for detection and diagnosis, but to guide biopsy and treatment. To date, the strengths and weaknesses of CT are better defined, and its role in the evaluation of extracranial organs in relationship to other diagnostic techniques is more clearly established.

Concomitant with the maturation of CT technology, magnetic resonance imaging (MRI), described by Paul Lauterbur in 1973, has been introduced into clinical practice. The initial applications of MRI, like CT, focused on the brain because of its size and lack of respiratory or other physiologic motion. Developments of surface coil technology, cardiac triggering, various motion suppression techniques, and fast imaging sequences have made it possible to use MRI for other parts of the body. MRI has replaced CT as the imaging procedure of choice in evaluating many brain and spinal diseases because of its superior soft tissue contrast sensitivity and because of its direct multiplanar imaging capability. In addition, MRI is being used with increasing frequency in evaluating the musculoskeletal and cardiovascular systems. Although MRI also can provide excellent anatomic information about the abdominal and pelvic organs, its role in these areas is less well established and more controversial.

This volume has been prepared to present a comprehensive text on the application of CT and MRI to the extracranial organs of the body. It is intended primarily for use by the radiologist in either clinical practice or training. The internist, pediatrician, and surgeon will also derive helpful information about the relative value and indications for CT and MRI of the body, their patients receiving the ultimate benefits. As in the First Edition, anatomy in each area is stressed initially, since such knowledge is basic to proper interpretation. The CT and MRI findings in a variety of pathologic conditions are described and illustrated. Instruction is provided to optimize the conduct, analysis, and interpretation of CT and MR images. Both technical and interpretative errors can occur in CT and MRI examinations, and, hopefully, the reader will benefit from our previous mistakes.

Logical and cogent discussions of how CT and MRI are properly integrated with other clinical and radiological procedures, as well as with each other, for a variety of problems are included. Both radiologists and referring clinicians often face the dilemma of determining the best radiologic approach toward documenting a specific diagnosis given a set of clinical findings. With the increasing availability of a wide variety of radiologic techniques, there is often a tendency to perform a large number of examinations before drawing a conclusion. This approach is extremely expensive and puts undue constraints on the total resources available for health care, aside from treating the individual patient unfairly by subjecting him to unnecessary discomfort and risk.

The task of deciding which diagnostic test is the most appropriate for a given clinical problem has become a substantial part of medical practice. An adequate understanding of clinical issues, as well as the advantages and limitations of each radiologic technique, is essential for the radiologist to best help the referring clinician. Our recommended uses of CT and MRI have been developed through the cooperative efforts of the diagnostic radiology staffs at the Mallinckrodt Institute and the University of Alabama at Birmingham. Each staff member has established an interest and expertise in a specific anatomic area. The proper sequencing of radiologic tests for a variety of clinical indications has been discussed in countless joint consultations and conferences during the past several years, and from this, our current ideas have evolved. We are well aware that equally valid alternative radiologic approaches to certain clinical problems are possible. Differences in available equipment and personal experience could modify the evaluation of any particular problem. Because of rapid technologic improvements in MRI, our recommendations on the optimal use of CT and MRI are by no means final, and enlightened physicians continually will need to update their ideas about how CT and MRI fit in with other imaging methods.

J. K. T. L.
S. S. S.
R. J. S.

Preface to the First Edition

Computed tomography was first developed for intracranial imaging in the late 1960s by Godfrey Hounsfield at the Central Research Laboratories of EMI Limited. Since that time, major technical advances have resulted in substantial improvements in image quality concomitant with a marked reduction in scanning time. In the past seven years, CT has become gradually accepted as an accurate and practical diagnostic technique, with its clinical applications broadened to include virtually every part of the body. This has occurred despite the initial skepticism of many regarding the value of extracranial CT in comparison to its cost. We have been fortunate to personally witness the germination and development of computed body tomography from its inception, to a technique that now has an enormous impact upon our practice of radiology. This radiological method has fulfilled the expectations of its early users and has proven to be an important and efficacious procedure for the evaluation of a myriad of pathologic problems.

In many cases, the information obtained by CT is unique. On occasion, data derived from CT have enabled reevaluation of traditional concepts of various disease processes. Body CT has supplanted or encroached upon other radiological procedures. Laryngography has been replaced. Lymphangiography for staging lymphoma and other neoplasms has declined drastically. Rapid, sequential, contrast-enhanced CT scans have been successfully substituted for angiography in many patients to diagnose or exclude suspected vascular lesions (e.g., aneurysm, dissection) or to assess the extent of a neoplastic process.

This volume has been prepared to present a comprehensive text on the application of CT to the extracranial regions of the body. It is intended primarily for use by the radiologist either in clinical practice or in training. The internist, pediatrician, and surgeon also will derive beneficial information about the relative value and indications for CT of the body, with their patients as the ultimate beneficiaries. Anatomy in each area is stressed initially, since such knowledge is basic to proper interpretation. Regions often are presented serially to portray the caudad progression of structures. The CT findings in a variety of pathologic conditions are described and illustrated. Instruction is provided to optimize the conduct, analysis, and interpretation of CT scans. Both technical and interpretative errors can occur in CT examinations, and hopefully the reader will benefit from our previous innumerable mistakes.

Comprehensive discussions of how CT is compatible with other clinical and radiological procedures for a variety of problems have been attempted. Both radiologist and referring clinician often are faced with the dilemma of determining the best radiologic approach toward documenting a specific diagnosis given a set of clinical findings. With the burgeoning availability of a wide variety of new radiologic techniques, there is often a tendency to perform a large number of examinations before drawing a conclusion. Such an approach, however, is extremely expensive and puts undue constraints on the total resources available for health care, besides being unfair to the individual patient who is subjected to unnecessary discomfort and risk.

The uses of CT we suggest have been developed through the cooperative efforts of the diagnostic radiology staff at the Mallinckrodt Institute. Each member has established an interest and expertise in a specific area. The proper sequencing of radiologic tests for a variety of clinical indications has been discussed in countless, joint consultations and conferences during the past several years. From this ongoing dialogue, our current ideas have evolved. We are well aware that equally valid alternative radiologic approaches to certain clinical problems are possible. It is obvious that available equipment and personal experience could modify the evaluation of any particular problem. Clearly our recommendations on the optimal use of CT are not final, and the enlightened physician continually will need to update his ideas about how CT fits in with other modalities as clinical research and technology continue to develop.

J. K. T. L.
S. S. S.
R. J. S.
1982

Acknowledgments

Providing recognition to everyone involved in the production of this volume is extremely difficult because of the large number of individuals, both at Washington University and the University of Alabama at Birmingham, who aided immeasurably in forming the final product. We graciously thank the various contributors who kindly provided chapters in their areas of expertise in order to bring depth and completeness to the book.

A special note of gratitude goes to our secretaries, Lynn Losse, Sue Day, Carol Keller, Sheila Wright, and Patty Haring, who spent endless hours typing manuscripts and checking references. Walter Clermont and his staff in the Department of Medical Illustration at Washington University Medical School and Thomas Murry in Mallinckrodt Institute Photography Laboratory were extremely helpful in preparing the illustrative material.

Our thanks go to our residents and the many radiologic technologists who performed and monitored the CT and MRI studies. Their dedication is reflected in the high quality of images used throughout this book.

We also would like to express our appreciation to the publishers, Raven Press, for the professional and sympathetic way they have handled the myriad problems encountered in publication. Most particularly, we would like to thank Mary Rogers and Rita Chabot for their timeless dedication and advice during each stage in the production of this book.

Contents

xiii

Contributors

The Edward Mallinckrodt Institute of Radiology
Washington University School of Medicine
St. Louis, Missouri

Dixie J. Anderson, M.D.
Associate Professor of Radiology

Dennis M. Balfe, M.D.
Associate Professor of Radiology
Director, Gastrointestinal Radiology

Judy M. Destouet, M.D.
Associate Professor of Radiology

W. Thomas Dixon, Ph.D.
Currently, Assistant Professor of Radiology
Emory University
Atlanta, Georgia

Ronald G. Evens, M.D.
Elizabeth Mallinckrodt Professor of Radiology
Director, Mallinckrodt Institute of Radiology

Mohktar Gado, M.D.
Professor of Radiology
Director, Neuroradiology Section

Louis A. Gilula, M.D.
Professor of Radiology
Co-Director, Musculoskeletal Radiology Section

Harvey S. Glazer, M.D.
Associate Professor of Radiology

Fernando Gutierrez, M.D.
Assistant Professor of Radiology

David C. Hardy, M.D.
Currently, Latter Day Saints Hospital
Salt Lake City, Utah

Jay P. Heiken, M.D.
Associate Professor of Radiology
Co-Director, Computed Body Tomography Section

Fred J. Hodges III, M.D.
Professor of Radiology
Co-Director, Neuroradiology Section

Joseph K. T. Lee, M.D.
Professor of Radiology
Director, Magnetic Resonance Imaging Section

Robert G. Levitt, M.D.
Associate Professor of Clinical Radiology

David Ling, M.D.
Currently, Wake Radiology
Raleigh, North Carolina

Mary Victoria Marx, M.D.
Assistant Professor of Radiology

Bruce L. McClennan, M.D.
Professor of Radiology
Director, Abdominal Imaging Section

Barbara S. Monsees, M.D.
Assistant Professor of Radiology

William A. Murphy, M.D.
Professor of Radiology
Co-Director, Musculoskeletal Radiology Section

Roy R. Peterson, Ph.D.
Professor Emeritus of Anatomy
Washington University School of Medicine

Daniel Picus, M.D.
Assistant Professor of Radiology
Director, Vascular and Interventional Radiology Section

Miljenko V. Pilepich, M.D.
Currently, Director, Department of Radiation Oncology
Catherine McCauley Health Center
Ann Arbor, Michigan

David N. Rabin, M.D.
Currently, Assistant Professor of Radiology
Rush Medical College
Chicago, Illinois

William R. Reinus, M.D.
Currently, Ernst Radiology
St. Louis, Missouri

Stuart S. Sagel, M.D.
Professor of Radiology
Director, Chest Radiology Section
Co-Director, Computed Body Tomography Section

Marilyn J. Siegel, M.D.
Associate Professor of Radiology

William G. Totty, M.D.
Associate Professor of Radiology

Todd H. Wasserman, M.D.
Professor of Radiology

Philip J. Weyman, M.D.
Associate Professor of Clinical Radiology

John Wong, M.D.
Assistant Professor of Radiation Physics in Radiology

Department of Radiology
The University of Alabama School of Medicine
University of Alabama at Birmingham
Birmingham, Alabama

Gary T. Barnes, Ph.D.
Professor and Director
Physics Division

Lincoln Berland, M.D.
Associate Professor of Radiology
Chief, Body Computed Tomography and Sonography

Robert E. Koehler, M.D.
Professor and Vice Chairman
Department of Radiology

D. Bradley Koslin, M.D.
Assistant Professor of Radiology

A. V. Lakshminarayanan, Ph.D.
Associate Professor
Physics Division

P. H. Nath, M.D.
Professor of Radiology

Robert J. Stanley, M.D.
Professor and Chairman
Department of Radiology

Jerrold A. van Dyke, M.D.
Currently, Radiology Incorporated
South Bend, Indiana

CHAPTER 1

Computed Tomography: Physical Principles and Image Quality Considerations

Gary T. Barnes and A. V. Lakshminarayanan

FUNDAMENTALS

X-Ray Imaging and Its Limitations

A conventional radiograph is a picture of a patient made with X-rays. Implicit in this definition is that the image is two-dimensional, with its density determined by the projection of the X-ray absorption along the patient's third dimension. As shown schematically in Fig. 1, a patient is a three-dimensional distribution of X-ray linear-attenuation coefficients (μ's), and the projected X-ray image is a two-dimensional function of this distribution, with its gray-scale values related to the attenuation-coefficient integral along a ray or straight-line path in the third direction. This process can be represented mathematically by the expression

$$I(x, y) = I_0 \exp\left[-\int \mu(x, y, z)\, dz\right] \quad [1]$$

where $I(x, y)$ is the X-ray intensity transmitted by the patient at location (x, y), I_0 is the incident intensity, and $\mu(x, y, z)$ is the patient's X-ray linear-attenuation coefficient at point (x, y, z). For simplicity, scatter is neglected, and a parallel, monoenergetic X-ray beam is assumed.

The ability to use an X-ray image to delineate anatomy and convey diagnostic information is related to the fact that different tissues have different linear-attenuation coefficients. These in turn give rise to differences in transmitted X-ray intensities and film densities.

Perception of radiographic detail (i.e., small kidney stones) depends on the presence of contrast, sharpness, noise, and artifacts. A border between two densities is easier to see if the difference in densities is large and abrupt. If the density difference is subtle, it is easier to see if the image is not mottled or grainy in appearance, or if

it is not degraded by artifacts (i.e., spurious densities that will not be present if the image recording, processing, and display stages are functioning correctly). In addition to these factors, *conventional radiography also has the limitation that it is a two-dimensional projection of a three-dimensional object.* As noted in equation (1), the attenuation of X-ray intensity in the projection direction is integrated: There is no spatial resolution in this direction, and anatomic structures are superimposed on top of each other. This "structure noise" often makes interpretation difficult.

Prior to the development of computed tomography (CT), linear and pluridirectional tomography were the only methods for spatially resolving attenuation differences in the projection or third dimension. Utilizing diametrical and synchronous movement of the X-ray tube

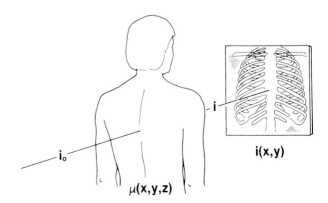

FIG. 1. In conventional projection radiography, the intensity transmitted by the patient at a given point is related to the integral of the patient's linear attenuation coefficients along a ray from the X-ray tube focus to the point.

and image receptor during an exposure, these methods blur structures above and below the fulcrum plane, with the amount of blur increasing with increasing distance from the fulcrum plane. The only structures in the patient that are not blurred lie in a thin section centered at the fulcrum plane, the thickness of which is determined by the tomographic arc and type of movement (i.e., hypocycloidal or linear). Although this improves the spatial resolution in the third dimension, the ability to resolve even moderate contrast differences in the slice is compromised by the superimposition of the blurred overlying and underlying anatomy. Thus, conventional tomography was and is relegated to imaging high-contrast structures such as the lung, inner ear, or kidneys containing contrast material.

The CT Problem and Image Reconstruction

CT, like conventional tomography, images a section or slice of the patient. This is accomplished by obtaining a series of different angular projections or views of the section and reconstructing a two-dimensional image of the slice from this series of one-dimensional projections. However, with CT, in contrast to conventional tomography and radiography, X-rays do not pass through neighboring anatomy, only through the section of interest. Thus, the reconstructed image does not suffer from the superimposition problem and is better able to demonstrate slice anatomy.

Shown in Fig. 2B is a one dimensional projection or view of a slice of the simple phantom whose CT image is shown in Fig. 2A. To reconstruct the image of the slice the first view is edge enhanced (i.e., convolved with an edge enhancing kernel or filter function) and back projected onto the image matrix. These two steps are illustrated in Fig. 2. Fig. 2C is the same view after it was convolved with an appropriate filter function. Figure 2D is the view (Fig. 2C) backprojected onto the image matrix. Note that the view is projected back towards the focal spot, hence the term "backprojection." These two steps are repeated for each subsequent view with the backprojected values being added to the image matrix. The final image is simply the sum of the backprojections of all the different angular views. This adding of views to obtain the final CT image is illustrated in Fig. 3. Of interest is the buildup of the image as more and more views are

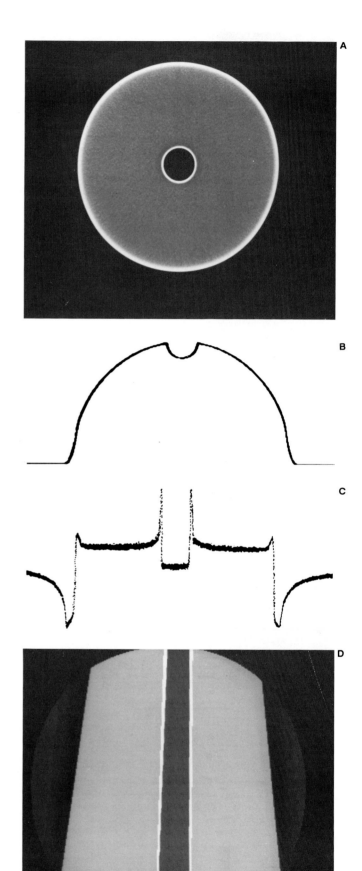

FIG. 2. A: CT image of simple phantom consisting of water between two Lucite cylinders and air in the small central cylinder. **B:** 0° projection of phantom plotted as log attenuation (y axis) versus position (x axis). **C:** Same projection after convolution with edge enhancing filter function. **D:** Backprojection of filtered projection.

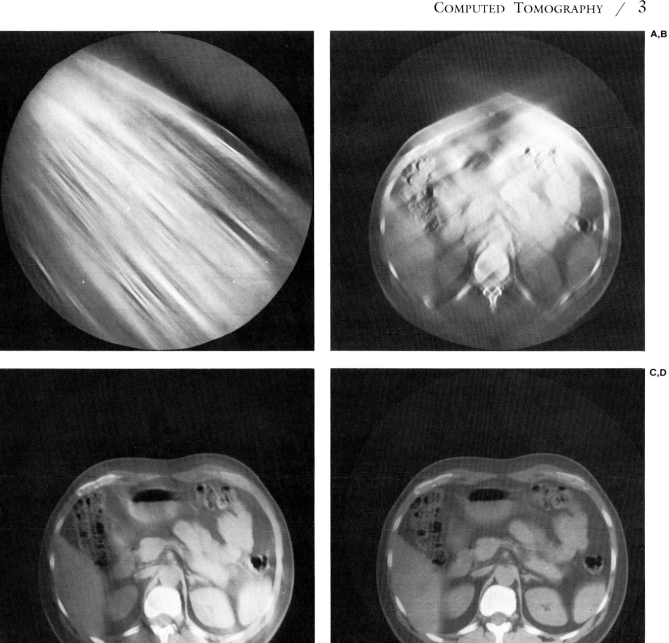

FIG. 3. Images of abdominal scan obtained by summing different number of views. **A:** Views from 0° to 15°. **B:** Views from 0° to 120°. **C:** Views from 0° to 240°. **D:** Views from 0° to 360°. Scan was obtained at 130 kV, 95 mA, 3.6 s.

backprojected onto the image matrix. An accurate reconstruction requires that the views are convolved with an appropriate edge enhancing kernel prior to backprojection.

The image reconstruction methodology described above is known as the filtered backprojection or convolution backprojection algorithm. It was first applied to X-ray image reconstruction from projections in 1971 by Ramachandran and Lakshminarayanan (1). Subsequent improvements in the algorithm included the introduction of the Shepp and Logan kernel (2), which minimized overshoot at abrupt patient attenuation differences, and the extension to divergent X-ray projections (3). Of practical interest is that the first commercial CT scanner (EMI Mark I) did not employ this algorithm initially but used an iterative algorithm. Such algorithms do not perform as well for a given amount of computational time. This along with the ease with which it can be implemented are

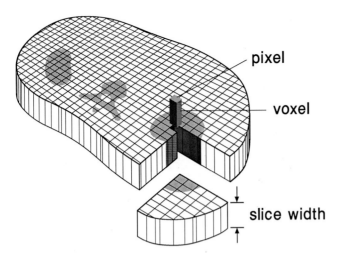

FIG. 4. The pixel value in a CT image represents the linear attenuation coefficient of a right square prism volume element or voxel (i.e., pixel area × slice width).

the reasons why the filtered backprojection algorithm has been employed on all commercial CT scanners since shortly after the EMI Mark I head scanner was introduced.

As illustrated in Fig. 4, the reconstructed image is a two-dimensional array of quantized gray-scale values or picture elements (pixels). These pixel values are directly related to the linear-attenuation coefficients of the corresponding values of the slice:

$$\text{pixel value (Hounsfield units)} = 1,000(\mu/\mu_w - 1) \quad [2]$$

where μ is the average linear-attenuation coefficient of the volume element (voxel) represented by the pixel, and μ_w is the linear-attenuation coefficient of water, where both

are evaluated for the effective energy of the beam exiting the patient. Thus, water has a CT number of zero, and a region with a CT number of 100 Hounsfield units (HU) has a linear-attenuation coefficient that is 10% greater than the linear-attenuation coefficient of water.

Each small volume element or voxel is a right square prism. The height of the voxel is determined by the slice width and the square base by the pixel size. The pixel dimension is in turn related to the display field of view (FOV) and the image matrix size:

$$\text{pixel size} = \text{FOV/matrix size} \quad [3]$$

For example, if one has a 25-cm display FOV or reconstruction circle and a 512 matrix, the pixel size is 0.49 mm. On most scanners, a range of slice widths can be selected between 1 and 10 mm. Likewise, the display FOV is also variable and can be selected so that it is less than or equal to the scan FOV. This allows one to focus the reconstruction on the anatomy of interest. The scan FOV is the region or circle over which data (i.e., projections) are acquired during a scan. The operator selects the scan FOV (typically from a choice of three or more) so that it contains the maximum patient dimension. CT reconstruction algorithms assume that the patient is within the scan FOV and artifacts occur when the patient extends beyond the scan FOV.

CT images typically have 12 bits per pixel, and these bits are used to represent numbers from −1,000 to 3,095, a total of 2^{12} or 4,096 different gray-scale values. Air typically has a CT number of −1,000, whereas fat is in the range of −80 to −100, soft-tissue structures 10 to 80, and bone 400 to 3,000. The number for a given type of tissue

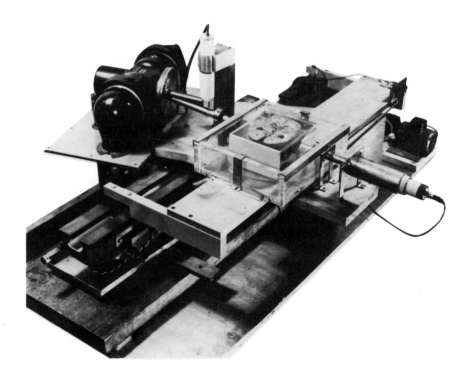

FIG. 5. Godfrey Hounsfield's laboratory CT scanner showing X-ray tube and detector on a lathe bed with a preserved section of the human brain in between (courtesy of G. N. Hounsfield and Thorn EMI).

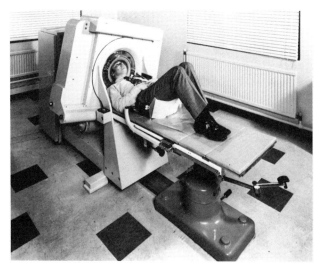

FIG. 6. First clinical prototype EMI brain scanner installed at Atkinson Morley's Hospital, London (courtesy of G. N. Hounsfield and Thorn EMI). Note the water bag surrounding the patient's head.

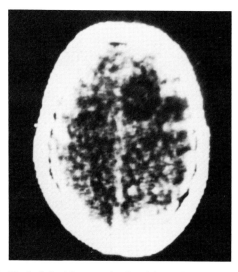

FIG. 7. First clinical image obtained from EMI prototype unit (courtesy of G. N. Hounsfield and Thorn EMI). The patient was a woman with a suspected brain lesion. The scan clearly showed a dark circular cyst.

will vary from scanner manufacturer to manufacturer and for a given scanner is highly dependent on the calibration. If the X-ray-tube voltage (kV) is variable, it is also a function of kV. Because attenuation and differences in attenuation decrease as the effective energy of the X-ray beam increases, the CT number magnitude will be less if the kV is greater, and vice versa.

CT SCANNER EVOLUTION

Early Experimental Systems and Developments

Although Allen M. Cormack published his first experimental results in 1964 in which the attenuation coefficients of a slice of an object were reconstructed from a series of angular projections (4), his publication received little attention at that time.

Some years later, Godfrey N. Hounsfield conducted similar and more extensive experiments using first a γ-ray source and later an X-ray source. In his initial γ-ray experiment, it took nine days to acquire the data (~28,000 measurements) and 2.5 hr to reconstruct the image on a large mainframe computer. Replacing the γ-ray source with an X-ray tube reduced the scanning time to 9 hr. The latter apparatus is shown in Fig. 5 with the X-ray tube and detector mounted on a lathe bed with a preserved cross-sectional specimen of a human brain. At the end of a translational stroke, the brain specimen was rotated 1° and the translational stroke of the X-ray tube and detector repeated. With this apparatus Hounsfield was able to differentiate gray and white matter on the preserved specimen. Mr. Hounsfield was employed at that time at the Central Research Laboratories of EMI in London,

England. His successes led to the development of the EMI head and body scanners and a revolution in the practice of medicine. In 1979 Cormack and Hounsfield received the Nobel prize in medicine for their CT contributions.

First Generation

In early 1972, a clinical prototype EMI head scanner (Mark I) was installed at Atkinson Morley's Hospital, London (Fig. 6) (5), and it proved to be an immediate success (Fig. 7). An improved version was introduced to the U.S. market at the 1972 RSNA meeting. The scanner consisted of a stationary-anode X-ray tube cooled by circulating oil. The X-ray beam was collimated to a pencil beam, and after passing through the patient's head and a water bath, it was detected by a sodium iodide crystal coupled to a photomultiplier tube. Two side-by-side detectors, each with an aperture of 5 mm × 13 mm, were employed to allow two slices to be obtained simultaneously. The X-ray tube and detectors were rigidly coupled by means of a yoke. As illustrated in Fig. 8A, views were obtained by translating the X-ray tube and detector yoke as depicted by the straight arrows and sampling the output of the detectors during this translational scan (160 samples across a 24-cm FOV). The tube and detectors were then rotated 1° (depicted by the curved arrows), followed by another translational scan to obtain a second view. This translate-rotate movement was repeated until 180 attenuation profiles, each 1° apart, were obtained. This took 4.5 min (Fig. 8B shows the ray samples for three views). Another 1.5 min were required to reconstruct the 80 × 80 (3-mm pixel) images of the two slices. The water bag was employed to provide a constant tissue-equivalent path length for the X-ray beam and to mini-

A   B

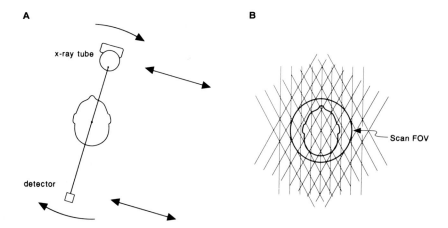

FIG. 8. Principle of the first generation scanner **(A)** and a schematic representation of the ray samples (*parallel lines*) of three views **(B)**.

Scan FOV

mize beam-hardening problems. It also permitted calibration of the detector before and after it scanned across the patient.

Second Generation

Applying these principles to scanning the body as well as the head was the next logical step, and that led to the development of the second-generation EMI 5000 scanner conceptually illustrated in Fig. 9. The pencil beam employed in the Mark I scanner resulted in poor geometrical utilization of the X-ray beam and long scanning times. This was improved in the second-generation EMI 5000 scanner by employing 30 detectors, 3 mm × 13 mm, and a 10° fan beam (i.e., a 13 mm × 177 mm beam at the detectors). As illustrated in Fig. 10, the detectors and the X-ray tube scanned linearly across the patient. Each detector was sampled during the translational tube-and-detector-array movement and resulted in 30 views with 0.33° of angular difference between the views obtained by

neighboring detectors. The X-ray tube and detector array would then rotate 10°, and the translational movement was repeated. Eighteen rotational and translational movements occurred, resulting in a total of 540 projection profiles or views with each view comprised of 600 ray samples. The fastest scanning time was 18 sec. It should be noted that this machine was also of the translate-rotate type and that the views consisted of parallel rays similar to those illustrated in Fig. 8B for the first-generation scanner. However, image quality was markedly improved over the Mark I scanner because of several factors: more views, finer ray sampling, a larger image matrix (i.e., 320 vs. 80), a smaller detector aperture, and reduced scan time. In this and all subsequent CT scanners, the cumbersome water bag was omitted.

Third Generation

In 1975, General Electric (GE) and also Varian Associates announced their third-generation designs. As illustrated in Fig. 10, the X-ray tube and detector array pivot

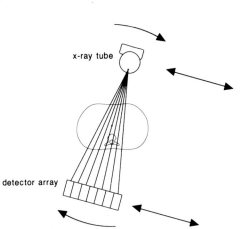

FIG. 9. Principle of second generation scanner. The difference between the first and second generation scanners is that the X-ray beam was collimated to ≃10° fan which encompassed an array of detectors rather than to a pencil beam that encompassed one detector. This permitted fewer translate/rotate movements and shorter scan times.

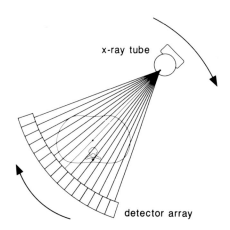

FIG. 10. Principle of third generation scanner. The X-ray tube and detectors are rigidly connected and go through a single rotational movement. Views are acquired by the simultaneous sampling of all detectors during the rotation.

data aquisition and detector assembly

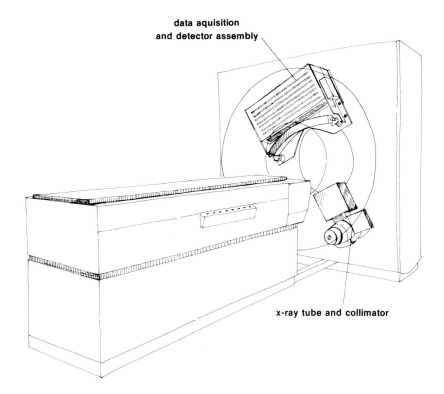

x-ray tube and collimator

FIG. 11. Schematic drawing of a third generation scanner showing the X-ray tube, collimator, detector array and data acquisition system (DAS). The four subsystems are rigidly attached and go through a single rotational movement during a scan. Their weight typically is on the order of 2000 lbs. Also shown are outline drawings of the patient couch and gantry.

around the patient in a single rotational movement during which the views are acquired. In the third-generation geometry, the rays of a view are all acquired simultaneously, and each active detector (the number of active detectors is determined by the scan FOV) is associated with a ray. Also, the views are comprised of divergent rather than parallel ray samples. Depending on the manufacturer, the X-ray tube is either pulsed or on continuously. In the early GE and Varian scanners, the X-ray tube was pulsed to obtain a view. During a 4.8-sec scan on the GE 7800 and 8800 scanners, the tube was pulsed 288 times, and during a 9.6-sec scan, 576 times (60 pulses/second). Thus the 4.8-sec scan was comprised of 288 views and the 9.6-sec scan of 576 views. In both the Varian and GE scanners, the tube and detectors rotated through 360°. The initial Varian design employed slip rings that allowed the X-ray tube and detector array to rotate continuously. The GE scanners utilized a cable take up assembly.

Currently, third-generation scanners are marketed by GE, Philips, Siemens, Toshiba, Elscint, and Shimadzu. Top of the line models typically have approximately 750 detector elements and 360° scan times range from 2 to 4 sec—significantly shorter than the 18 sec scan time obtainable on the first body scanner. Siemens recently introduced a scanner with a 0.75-sec scan time which is achieved by employing slip rings and rotating the tube and detector continuously as was done with the early Varian design. This minimizes the problem of rapidly accelerating and decelerating the large mass of the X-ray tube, collimater, data acquisition system, and associated support structure (Fig. 11).

Fourth Generation

In 1975, Jay Stein of AS&E proposed the fourth-generation geometry, consisting of a stationary detector array and an X-ray tube that rotates through a circle within the array (Fig. 12). An attenuation profile is obtained by sampling a detector as the X-ray tube rotates, and each detector results in a different angular view of the slice of interest. The original AS&E design had 600 detectors and obtained 600 views with 512 rays per view in 5 sec (in a fourth-generation scanner, the number of detectors determines the number of views in a 360° scan). Bismuth germanate crystals coupled to photomultiplier tubes comprised the detector elements. In the late 1970s fourth generation scanners were later marketed by Ohio Nuclear (720 detectors), Pfizer (600 and 2400 detectors), Picker (600 and 1200 detectors), and EMI (1088 detectors). The EMI 7000 scanner was different from the other fourth-generation designs in that it employed a nutating detector ring (Fig. 13). Currently, three companies market fourth-generation or fourth-generation variant designs—Picker, Toshiba, and Imatron. Picker markets a classic fourth-generation design; Toshiba markets a fourth-generating nutating design. Larger fan angles are generally employed with fourth-generation scanners than with most third-generation scanners; this reduces X-ray tube loading. As a result of this and the small inertial mass of the X-ray tube, very short scanning times are possible. The Picker 1200SX scanner, for example, can achieve a scan time of 1.6 sec for a 360° scan and 1.9 sec for the more generally preferred 398° overscan.

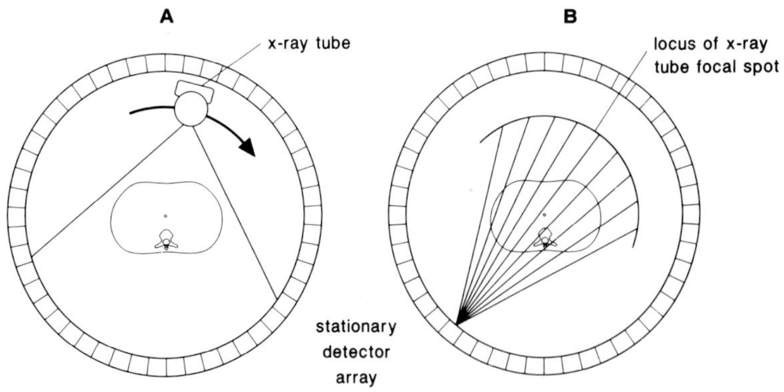

A

x-ray tube

B

locus of x-ray
tube focal spot

stationary
detector
array

FIG. 12. Fourth generation X-ray tube and detector geometry **(A)** and view acquisition **(B)**.

Ultrafast CT Scanner

Imatron markets a fourth-generation variant design, with no moving parts, capable of acquiring an image in 50 msec. The basic design was conceived in the late 1970s by Douglas Boyd and collaborators for the purpose of imaging the heart. The current unit is shown schematically in Fig. 14 and consists of four 216° circular-arc stationary target rings and two 210° circular-arc stationary detector arrays. One detector array has 432 elements, and the other has 864, which are used singly, when gathering data for high-resolution images, or in pairs, when gathering data for cardiac studies. During image acquisition, electromagnetic coils focus a 130-kV electron beam to a small (1 mm × 2 mm) focal-spot size and steer it along one of the four fixed tungsten target rings (Fig. 14A). In the cardiac mode, each detector array acquires a 432-view image in 50 msec, and up to 17 images can be acquired per second. By moving the beam from ring to ring, the heart can be imaged, without moving the patient, virtually free

of motion artifacts. In the high-resolution mode, 864 views can be acquired in 0.1 sec at 130 kV and 60 mAs. The maximum scanning rate with this technique is nine images per second. If the image noise level is too high with this technique, the scanning time (and mAs) can be increased in 0.1-sec increments up to 1.9 sec.

CT SCANNER COMPONENTS

All makes and models of CT scanners are similar in that they have a scanning gantry, X-ray generator, computer system, operator's console, physician's viewing console, and hard-copy camera. These are schematically illustrated in Fig. 15. The scanning gantry in all cases contains an X-ray tube, prepatient collimation system, detector array and associated electronics, and a scanning drive motor. In all but one type of scanner currently being manufactured, high-heat-capacity, rotating-anode X-ray tubes are employed. The anode disk is more massive than

FIG. 13. Schematic drawing of the nutating fourth generation design used in the EMI 7000 and current Toshiba scanners. Even though the detector ring nutates (i.e., moves in and out) during a scan as illustrated in **(A)** through **(D)**, the angular position of each detector is fixed and views are acquired in the same manner as in the standard 4th generation design, i.e., by sampling the detector as the X-ray tube rotates.

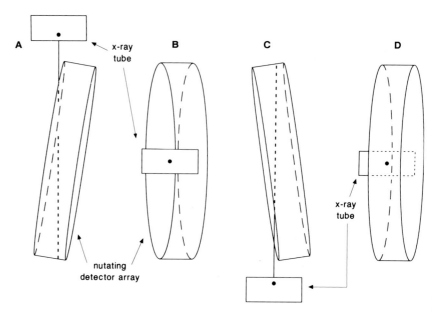

A — x-ray tube

B

C

D

nutating
detector array

x-ray tube

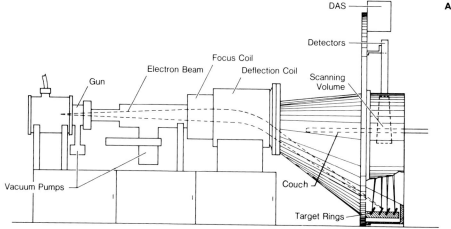

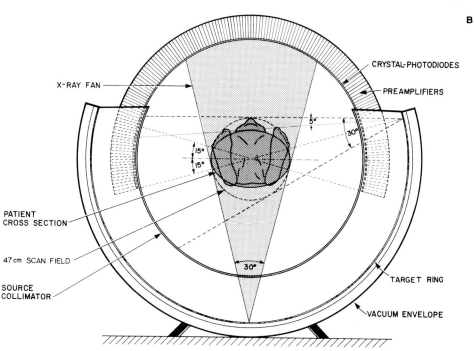

FIG. 14. Longitudinal **(A)** and cross-sectional **(B)** views of electron beam Ultrafast CT scanner (courtesy of D. Boyd and Imatron). The unit employs a stationary detector array and is based on the 4th generation principle. A view is acquired by sampling a detector as the X-ray focus goes through its arc. As with any 4th generation design, the number of views possible is determined by the number of detectors.

is employed for radiographic tubes, and CT scanner tubes typically have heat capacities of the order of 1 million heat units. Also, circulating-oil heat exchangers (or radiators, in some scanners) are routinely employed to enhance the rate at which the housing cools and patients can be scanned. The prepatient collimator, which determines the slice width, usually is multibladed, with the last set of blades positioned close to the patient aperture. Current CT detector arrays employ many (~1,000 or more) small elements (~1 mm × 25 mm). Gas (xenon) ionization chambers or scintillation crystals (CsI or $CdWO_4$) coupled to photodiodes are employed. The signals generated by the detector elements are amplified, digitized, and multiplexed to the computer. The detector and front-end electronics, often referred to as the data-acquisition system (DAS), are housed in the gantry and usually do offset and

gain corrections on the fly on a detector element-by-element basis prior to the multiplexing step.

Highly stable three-phase or constant-potential X-ray generators are employed. During a scan, they are either pulsed or on continuously. The pulsed systems are similar to cine X-ray generators and switch currents of up to 1,000 mA several hundred times per second, employing grid control or tetrode techniques. The peak current outputs of X-ray generators that are on continuously usually are much less, on the order of 100 to 500 mA.

The computer system consists of a CPU/RAM control unit, one or more array processors, magnetic disks, and WORM (write once, read many) optical-disk and/or magnetic-tape archival storage devices. Communication with the system is accommodated through the operator's and the physician's viewing consoles. The CPU control-

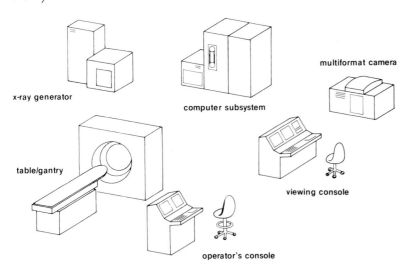

x-ray generator

multiformat camera

computer subsystem

table/gantry

FIG. 15. CT scanner system components.

viewing console

operator's console

unit function usually is that of a multitasking traffic cop. For the most part, image reconstruction takes place in the array processor subsystem. (The exceptions are offset and gain corrections, which are usually handled by the front-end electronics in the gantry.)

Until recently, CT computer systems employed mini-computers. With the advances in microcomputer CPU technology, these have been replaced with single-board computers that are faster, more powerful, and less expensive. The array processors have also become smaller, faster, and cheaper to the customer. State-of-the-art image-reconstruction times are approximately 5 sec for a 512^2 image. It is informative to compute the number of mathematical operations that occur in reconstructing a CT image. Assuming 1,024 views and 1,024 rays or discrete digital samples per view, approximately 200 million mathematical operations occur, i.e., 40 million mathematical operations per second, a most impressive technological achievement.

An important consideration in purchasing a new scanner is that the computer-system architecture support multitasking. That is, background archiving, viewing, and filming activities can be carried on simultaneously with scanning. A desirable feature of the computer software is to do a rapid sequence of scans in which the table is automatically shifted the appropriate distance between slices. The scans are done without waiting for the reconstruction of the first slice to be completed before the second slice is scanned, and so on. This capability markedly improves patient throughput, but is hard on the X-ray tube.

The operator's console and physician's viewing console usually consists of an alphanumeric and an image display. Little variation is evident in the capabilities of the two subsystem components between manufacturers, although some systems are easier to use than others. For reasons of convenience and efficiency, examinations usually are read from multiformatted hard copies rather than from the viewing console. The physician's console generally is reserved for viewing atypical cases and monitoring the

progress of examinations. In the more advanced newer systems, the filming stage is automated. This capability results in considerable time saving. Once the examination is complete, the operator activates a filming protocol, and if the hard-copy camera has a bulk-supply magazine and is directly coupled to a processor, the films automatically drop out of the processor with the proper window and level settings.

TECHNIQUE SELECTION AND RADIATION DOSE

Factors that can be varied in scanning a patient are gantry angulation, slice width, table increment between neighboring slices, milliamperage-second (mAs) per scan, number of scans, interscan delay, scan FOV, and, on some scanners, display FOV, kV, and matrix size. Of these, the slice width, the degree of overlap or separation between slices, the number of slices, and kV and mAs per scan directly affect patient's absorbed radiation dose. If the table-shift increment between adjacent slices is equal to the slice width, the slices are contiguous. If there is overlap, then the average patient radiation dose is higher than if the slices are contiguous. Likewise, if the table-movement distance between two slices is greater than the slice width, then the average patient radiation dose is less. That is,

average patient radiation dose
$$\propto \text{slice width/table-shift increment} \quad [4]$$

where $\propto$ denotes directly proportional to. Implicit in equation (4) is that the absorbed radiation dose to the patient for a series of contiguous slices imaging a given patient volume is independent of slice width. That is, 10 contiguous 10-mm slices will result in the same average skin and axis doses as 20 contiguous 5-mm slices if the same kV and mAs per slice are employed in both cases. As in conventional radiography, the patient radiation dose increases with increasing kV and is directly proportional

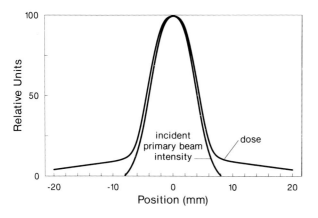

FIG. 16. Plot of the incident (i.e., phantom surface) primary beam intensity across the slice and the associated skin dose profile for a nominal 10 mm slice. The tails and slightly greater breadth of the dose profile are due to scatter.

TABLE 1. *Typical patient skin and axis doses (rad/100 mAs or cGy/100 mAs) for GE 9800 and Picker 1200SX CT scanners[a]*

	GE @ 120 kV	GE @ 140 kV	Picker @ 130 kV
Skin	1.4	1.9	2.6
Axis	1.1	1.6	1.5

[a] Adapted from ref. 7 for a 20 cm × 36 cm phantom and 20 consecutive 10 mm slices.

to mAs. The patient integral dose (i.e., the total radiant energy deposited in the patient) is directly proportional to the number of slices (at given voltage and amperage) and the slice width.

Shown in Fig. 16 are typical incident single slice primary beam and associated skin dose profiles across the slice. The greater width and tails of the dose profile are due to scatter. Within the slice the scatter dose increases and is greatest at the center of the slice where the magnitude of the tails is a significant fraction of the peak value of the dose profile. To understand how the dose to a given point in the patient varies with the number of slices, it is important to realize that a single scan produces a dose profile and that the dose that results from a series of slices is simply the sum of the individual dose profiles. This concept is illustrated in Fig. 17. Because of profile overlap, the dose is greater for a series of contiguous slices than it is for a single slice. How much greater depends on the volume scanned. Once the region scanned exceeds 10 cm, the dose to points in the central region of the scanned volume will not be greatly increased if an additional 5 cm or more is scanned on both sides. Depending on these factors, the skin dose from a series of adjacent slices will be a factor of from 1.2 to 2.0 greater and the central axis dose will be a factor of from 3 to 5 greater than the peak single slice axis dose (6).

In conventional radiography, the dose to the patient is greatest at the skin, where the beam enters the patient; it falls off rapidly through the patient and is least where the beam exits (i.e., ~1%–10% of the entrance dose). In CT, for a series of contiguous slices that is not the case. For a 360° scan, the dose at a point in the center of the slice is only slightly less than the skin dose (how much depends on patient size, kV, and the number of contiguous slices), and the anterior, posterior, and lateral skin doses are about the same. In Table 1, the skin and slice-center doses are tabulated for a typical body habitus. In body CT, 200 to 500 mAs per slice commonly are employed, and the skin doses are quite high compared with those in conventional radiography, typically on the order of 2 to 8 rad for a series of contiguous slices. This, along with the fact that the doses are not significantly less within the patient, results in the average dose to an irradiated volume in CT being much higher (i.e., one or two orders of magnitude greater) than for a single conventional radiograph of the same anatomy.

IMAGE QUALITY

Spatial and Contrast Resolution

The degree to which small, high-contrast detail can be resolved in a CT image depends on the quality of the view data and the reconstruction algorithm. Increasing the algorithm resolution and decreasing the pixel size will improve the resolution up to a point beyond which little or no gain can be realized. This limitation is due to the inherent spatial resolution of the view data, which in turn depends on how finely the views are sampled (ray sampling), and the unsharpness introduced into the projections by the finite size of the focal spot and detector aperture and to a lesser degree, on the number of views (angular sampling) (8).

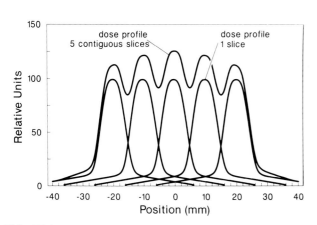

FIG. 17. Individual and total skin dose profiles for five contiguous 10 mm slices. The total dose profile is simply the sum of the doses from the individual slices.

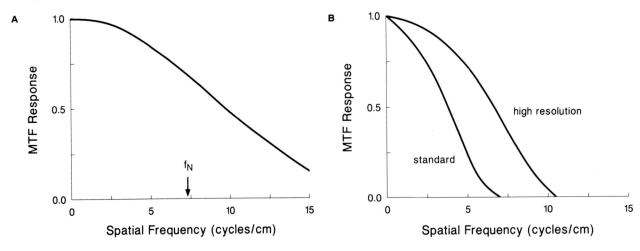

FIG. 18. Geometrical **(A)** and system **(B)** MTFs of GE 9800 scanner (curves derived from published product data and performance specifications for X-3 detector). f_N in **(A)** is the ray sampling Nyquist frequency. The different system MTFs in **(B)** are associated with different kernels and reconstruction algorithms—standard kernel and reconstruction algorithm (984 view) for the standard system MTF and bone detail kernel and target reconstruction (492 view) algorithm for the high resolution system MTF.

The spatial resolution of a CT scanner depends on its geometrical parameters (i.e., focal spot size, detector aperture, and geometrical magnification) and the reconstruction algorithm. A complete description of an imaging system's spatial resolution is given by its modulation transfer function (MTF) which is a plot of the fraction of input subject contrast that is imaged versus spatial frequency. Thus, the system MTF of a scanner is the product of its geometrical MTF and its algorithm MTF (9,10):

$$\text{MTF}_{\text{sys}}(f) = \text{MTF}_{\text{geo}}(f) \cdot \text{MTF}_{\text{alg}}(f) \qquad [5]$$

where f denotes spatial frequency. In general, MTF_{geo} is dominated by a detector term that has a cutoff frequency given by

$$f_c = M/w_a \qquad [6]$$

where w_a is the active width of an element of the detector array, and M is the geometrical magnification factor of the center of the scan FOV. That is the smaller the active width of the detector element and the greater the magnification, the greater the geometrical MTF response. MTF_{alg} is dominated by the reconstruction kernel and also has secondary terms associated with the back-projection interpolation operations. How finely the profile is sampled places an upper limit on the spatial resolution that can be obtained. Likewise, the display-matrix pixel size also places an upper limit on the spatial resolution. These limits are given by the Nyquist frequencies:

$$f_N = 1/(2p) \qquad [7]$$

$$f_N = M/(2d_s) \qquad [8]$$

where d_s is the distance between transmission profile samples (i.e., ray-sampling distance), p is the display pixel size, and M is the geometrical magnification at the center of the scan FOV. Of practical interest is that the spatial

resolution of the reconstructed image cannot exceed the ray sampling Nyquist limit no matter how small the display-matrix pixel size is or the degree of enhancement employed in the reconstruction algorithm. Typically, the kernel is chosen so that the algorithm MTF has a cutoff frequency equal to the limiting resolution (i.e., detector, sampling or display pixel size) of the system.

Shown in Fig. 18 are geometrical, algorithm, and system MTFs of a GE 9800 scanner. Similar curves are shown in Fig. 19 for a Picker 1200SX scanner. Of practical importance is that the sampling Nyquist frequency of the 9800 scanner is less than its detector-aperture cutoff frequency, because the ray-sampling distance is fixed and equal to the detector-to-detector spacing. This spacing is somewhat greater than the active width of the detector element. Spatial-frequency components above the ray-sampling Nyquist frequency will be aliased, i.e., reappear as spatial frequencies at or slightly below the ray-sampling Nyquist frequency. This phenomenon was a source of artifacts in early third-generation scanners (11). Fortunately, it was found that they could be eliminated by offsetting the central ray relative to the X-ray-tube/detector-array center of rotation by one-fourth of the detector-to-detector spacing. As illustrated in Fig. 20, this results in the rays in views 180° apart being shifted by one-half of the detector-to-detector spacing. Aliasing still occurs, but it is 180° out of phase in 180°-apart views and cancels when the back-projections are summed (provided of course that motion does not occur). In a fourth-generation scanner, the ray-sampling distance is arbitrary and usually is chosen so that the sampling Nyquist frequency is equal to or slightly greater than the detector-aperture cutoff frequency.

In cases where spatial resolution is limited by pixel size, depending on the scanner, one or more options are available. The first is to select a display FOV (based on the

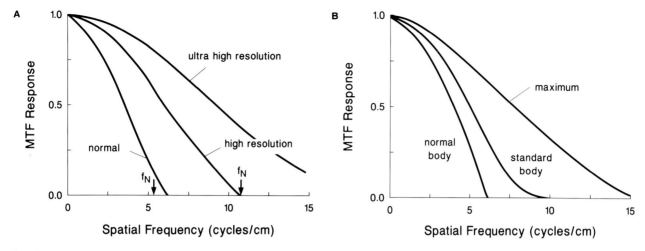

FIG. 19. Geometrical (A) and system (B) MTFs of Picker 1200SX scanner (curves derived from published product data and performance specifications). The lower f_N value in (A) is the 512 ray sampling Nyquist frequency for a 48-cm FOV. The higher f_N value is the 1024 sampling frequency for the same FOV. The different geometrical MTFs are associated with different operator selectable detector apertures (normal: 3.8 mm; high resolution: 2.2 mm; and ultra high resolution: 1.35 mm). The normal and standard body system MTFs in (B) are associated with normal and high resolution geometrical MTFs, bone detail kernels and a 48-cm FOV. The maximum system MTF is associated with the ultra high resolution geometrical MTF and a 12-cm FOV.

maximum patient dimension observed on the scout-scan projection radiograph) that is smaller than the scan FOV. The second is to zoom-reconstruct, either retrospectively or prospectively, on an even smaller FOV for a selected region of interest. In practice, prospective zoom reconstructions using a small display FOV are limited to examining easily localized anatomic regions such as the spine. In either event, these approaches are advantageous because the raw data and a higher-resolution kernel are used to reconstruct the image. They differ from a simple image magnification in which the information from one pixel is spread out over several smaller pixels and interpolation is used to remove the "boxy" appearance of the image.

In addition to using the acquired view information and a higher-resolution kernel to reconstruct the image on a smaller display FOV, on most third-generation scanners it is possible to interleave the data from half of the views with the data from the other half of the views, an idea first suggested by Pelc and Glover in 1979. For example, the ray on the right-hand side of Fig. 20 that samples the patient in between the two rays on the left-hand side can be moved to the left-hand view and placed between these two rays. A ray from some other view can be placed between the next two rays of the view, and so on. The result is that the number of views is reduced by half, and the ray sampling in these views is increased by a factor of two. Provided one has ample views initially and the target reconstruction is confined to the central area of the scan FOV (angular aliasing may occur at the outer regions of the scan FOV), this approach results in improved spatial resolution. The disadvantage is that considerable computer time is required. On fourth-generation scanners, the ray-sampling distance is arbitrary and not limited to the detector-to-detector spacing as it is in third-generation scanners. Because of this, the $\frac{1}{4}-\frac{1}{4}$ offset is not used. Finely sampled views can be acquired initially, and it is not necessary to interleave the data.

Contrast Resolution

Contrast resolution of a CT image, i.e., the ability to resolve large, low-contrast structures in a CT image depends on the inherent CT number differences between

FIG. 20. With the $\frac{1}{4}-\frac{1}{4}$ center line offset, views 180° apart in third generation scanners are shifted by one-half the detector-to-detector (or ray sampling) distance. Ray sampling aliasing occurring in the two views is out of phase and cancels when the views are backprojected and added.

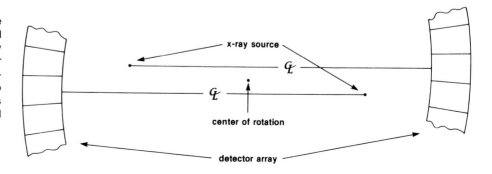

A,B

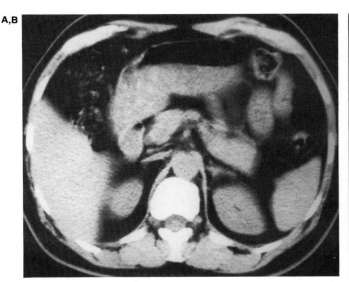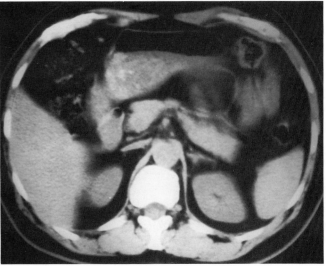

FIG. 21. Comparison of two abdominal images with ≃4X difference in radiation dose. **A:** 130 kV, 50 mA, 3.6 sec (180 mAs). **B:** 130 kV, 185 mA, 3.6 sec (666 mAs). CT number standard deviations for 10 cm² ROIs centered over similar regions of the liver were 9.5 and 5.3 HU, respectively.

the structures and the noise level of the image. CT number differences depend on the X-ray-tube voltage employed during scan acquisition and on whether or not contrast material was administered. Areas with subtle differences will be easier to see in a quiet image than in a grainy or noisy image. The noise level (i.e., the fluctuation in pixel CT number in a uniform region of an image) depends on Poisson statistical fluctuations in the number of X-ray quanta detected (i.e., quantum noise) and algorithm resolution. That is (12, 13)

$$\sigma_{CT}^2 \propto 1/(U_{alg}^3 \cdot N_x) \qquad [9]$$

where σ_{CT} is the standard deviation of the pixel CT number, N_x is the number of detected X-rays associated with the reconstructed image, and U_{alg} is the algorithm blur or unsharpness; σ_{CT} increases when fewer X-rays are detected or when U_{alg} is less, i.e., when a sharper (higher-spatial-frequency content) kernel is employed in the reconstruction algorithm. Likewise, if a less sharp kernel is employed, then there is more algorithm blur, U_{alg} is larger, and the image noise will decrease.

For a given scanner and kV, N_x is directly proportional to the mAs utilized in acquiring the image and the slice width. Because the patient radiation dose is directly proportional to mAs, one can write

$$N_x \propto mAs \cdot h \propto D \cdot h \qquad [10]$$

where D represents the patient radiation absorbed dose, and h the slice thickness. That is, if the mAs/scan is increased, more X-rays are incident on and penetrate the patient, and more X-rays are incident on and are detected by the detector elements. Similarly, if the slice thickness is increased, more X-rays are incident on the patient and are captured by the detector elements. In either event, as indicated by equation (9), the image noise level will be

reduced. Likewise, if the mAs/scan or slice width is decreased, the number of X-rays detected will decrease, and the image noise level increase. The effect of noise on patient images is illustrated in Fig. 21. Here the mAs/scan and patient dose were changed by a factor of 4, and the noise level by a factor of 2. The improved contrast resolution of the higher dose scan is readily apparent.

Contrast–Detail Response

The imaging performance of CT scanners, and radiological equipment in general, often are characterized by contrast–detail curves (14). Such curves plot object contrast on the ordinate and detail size (diameter) on the abscissa. In both cases, logarithmic scales are used. Shown

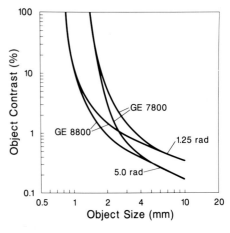

FIG. 22. GE 7800 and 8800 contrast-detail curves for 5 and 1.25 rad skin doses (curves derived from published GE product data and performance specifications for X-1 and X-2 detectors).

in Fig. 22 are typical CT contrast–detail curves. Any object with parameters corresponding to values above a curve can be resolved, and any object with parameter values below the curve cannot. The high-contrast, small object-size limit is determined by the spatial resolution (i.e., MTF) of the scanner and is independent of image noise level. The lower-right low-contrast limit will depend on the image noise level (i.e., the number of X-rays captured by the detectors). It therefore depends on the phantom size and material and, as demonstrated in Fig. 21, on the dose (mAs) and slice thickness. As the mAs is increased, more X-rays are detected, quantum noise is reduced, and lower-contrast objects can be resolved. Likewise, as the slice thickness is increased, more X-rays are detected, quantum noise is reduced, and the ability to resolve large-contrast objects improves.

The fact that the large object low contrast detectability as demonstrated in Fig. 22 is the same for the 7800 and 8800 scanners demonstrates an important point. The 8800 scanners had better spatial resolution (i.e., U_{alg} is less) than 7800 scanners and as a result σ_{CT} levels were higher for a given patient dose. Thus, σ_{CT} within a region of interest by itself is not a good index of contrast resolution, and the spatial resolution of a CT scanner system, which has a very strong effect on σ_{CT}, has little or no effect on contrast sensitivity. Such is not the case for N_x, the number of detected x-rays associated with the reconstructed image.

Artifacts

The complexity of the CT imaging process is such that small inconsistencies in the view data can and often do result in spurious information. In many instances, streaks result. In other cases, the effect may be less obvious, such as superimposition of a noise-like pattern or a subtle distortion in lesion shape. In either event, diagnostic accuracy can suffer. Certain artifacts are inherent to the CT imaging process, and others are due to equipment malfunction. The latter can be corrected. Likewise, many of the former type of artifacts can be suppressed, if not eliminated, by appropriate selection of the scanning parameters and proper scanner calibration. For these reasons, an understanding of the causes of artifacts and how they can be controlled is useful to the practicing radiologist.

Artifacts inherent to the CT imaging process arise because of geometric inconsistencies in the view data, attenuation measurement errors, aliasing, and algorithm effects. Most appear as streaks. The reason for this is that each ray sample is back-projected across the image matrix. If a single ray sample of a view is bad and grossly different from its neighboring ray samples, then it will give rise to a streak on back-projection and in the final image. Likewise, if a view is grossly different from its neighboring views, then streaks will also occur. The CT imaging process is sensitive to changes in the data that vary abruptly from

ray to ray or from view to view. If this occurs, streak artifacts result. It is insensitive to errors that vary gradually from ray to ray or from view to view (15).

As noted in the previous section, aliasing artifacts occur if the projections are sampled too coarsely and are manifest as streaks emanating from high contrast edges. This is rarely a problem with state-of-the-art scanners. Such is not always the case with the artifacts that arise when an insufficient number of views are used to reconstruct the image. As shown earlier (Fig. 3), the accuracy of reconstruction increases as more and more views are included in the reconstruction. When an insufficient number of views are employed, due to incomplete cancellation upon backprojection, radial and tangential streaks appear at points distant to a high contrast edge. The streaks, often referred to as "view insufficiency" streaks, have increasing amplitude as one moves radially out from the center of the image and are most apparent in regions of uniform attenuation. In clinical practice due to patient structure view insufficiency results in the superimposition of a structured noise pattern in the outer region of the field of view. Thus, in order to fully realize the image quality consistent with the radiation dose delivered to the patient and the scanner's system MTF throughout the display FOV, the image has to be reconstructed from a sufficiently large number of views. This number is given by the rule of thumb (16)

$$N_v \approx 3 \cdot \text{FOV}_{dis} \cdot f_{alg} \qquad [11]$$

where FOV_{dis} refers to the display field of view, and f_{alg} to the algorithm (system) limiting spatial resolution in cycles per cm. That is, more views are needed for larger FOVs and higher spatial resolution reconstructions. For example, to achieve a spatial resolution of 8 cy/cm and an artifact-free image across a 35 cm FOV, one needs to utilize approximately 840 views. If significantly fewer than 840 views are employed without degrading the algorithm (and system) resolution, view insufficiency artifacts may appear in the outer regions of the reconstructed image. Also, if more than 840 views and the same dose/scan are employed, the quality of the reconstructed image will not be noticeably improved. Fourth generation scanners generally have a sufficient number of views. Such is not always the case with third generation scanners. Particularly, when faster scans are obtained at the expense of fewer views, and also when target reconstructions are employed. In the latter case the ray data from one-half of the views is interleaved with data from the other one-half of the views. As a result, one-half the original number and higher spatial resolution views are used to reconstruct the image. The high spatial resolution images obtained, however, are susceptible to view insufficiency artifacts if they are not limited to a small, centrally located FOV.

Patient motion is a common problem which results in inconsistencies in the view data. These in turn are manifested as streaks tangent to high-contrast edges that have

A,B

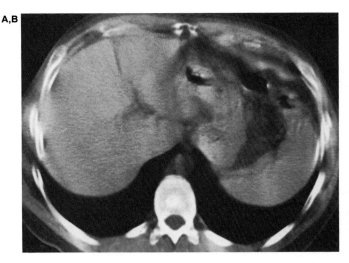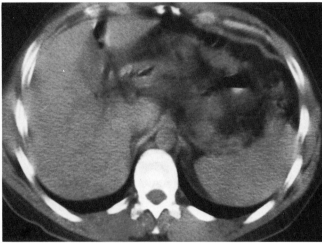

FIG. 23. Comparison of 360° **(A)** and overscanned **(B)** images obtained on a 4th generation scanner at 130 kV and 80 mA and their effect on patient motion artifacts. The respective scan times were 3.2 sec and 3.6 sec.

moved during the scanning. The obvious way to reduce motion artifacts is to employ a short scanning time. In many third-generation scanners this also results in the acquisition of fewer views. One can also overscan (i.e., scan through 400° rather than 360°) and merge the information obtained at the beginning and end of the scanning. Overscanning can be used to good effect in both third- and fourth-generation scanners. In the 360° scan of a fourth-generation scanner, several views will have neighboring rays that were acquired at the beginning and end of the scan. If gross or peristaltic patient motion occurs, inconsistencies result in the adjacent rays obtained at the beginning and end of the scan of several views, and artifacts are present in the reconstructed image. In the overscanned image, ray data from the beginning and end of the scan in the overlap views are merged, resulting in consistent view data and patient-motion artifacts are suppressed. The effect of 360° scanning and over-scanning on a fourth generation scanner and cooperative patient are illustrated in Fig. 23. Streaks associated with patient motion are apparent in several locations in Fig. 23A, particularly in the center and to the right of center. It is of practical interest that the scanning times for the 360° and 398° images were 3.2 and 3.6 sec, respectively, and that the longer scanning time resulted in the image with the least patient-motion artifacts.

In third-generation scanners, the rays in a view are all acquired at essentially the same instant in time. Thus, in a given view, the ray samples vary in a smooth fashion. However, when patient motion occurs during a 360° scan, there can be a discontinuity between the first and last views. This will give rise to streak artifacts oriented along the rays of the first and last views. Because the scan usually starts and stops in the same place each time, these patient-motion artifacts will always have the same orientation in the image. As in the case of fourth-generation scanners,

these patient-motion artifacts can be suppressed by overscanning and merging the initial and final views.

It is often stated (generally because of a limited understanding of CT principles and improper selection of scanning parameters) that fourth-generation scanners are more susceptible to patient-motion artifacts than are third-generation scanners. This is true if one is comparing 360° images of equal time, because patient-motion-related discontinuities in the beginning and final rays of several views (fourth generation) will produce more noticeable streaking

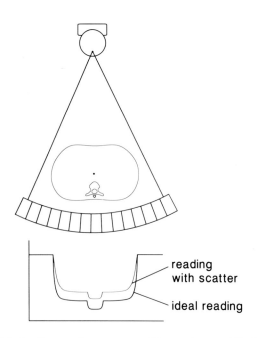

FIG. 24. Scatter produces a smoothly varying contribution to the measured attenuation profile. The measurement error due to scatter is greatest where the maximum attenuation occurs.

than a discontinuity between the first and final views (third generation). However, if one compares underscanned and overscanned images (acquired in the same scanning time), little or no difference will be evident, provided the same number of views are used to reconstruct the image. However, as noted earlier, many third-generation scanners achieve faster scanning times by acquiring fewer views. This can result in an angular-sampling problem and loss in image quality.

Attenuation measurement errors inherent to CT imaging arise from several sources: beam hardening, scattered radiation, patient anatomy outside the scanning FOV, and the partial-volume effect. X-ray beams are polychromatic in nature and contain a spectrum of X-ray energies up to a maximum value determined by the kVp. When such a beam passes through the body, the lower-energy X-rays are preferentially absorbed, and the beam becomes richer in higher-energy photons and more penetrating. As a result, the body appears to be less dense than it would to a monochromatic beam, and a nonlinearity is introduced in the logarithm of the transmitted intensity measurements. If not corrected for, one obtains images with the well-known cupping artifact: lower CT numbers in the center of the image than on the periphery for the same type of tissue. The first-order correction for this phenomenon involves "linearization" of the logarithm of the detector output by making a correction based on the observed attenuation (16). This works well except in body regions where significant bone is present. Because of its higher atomic number, the beam-hardening effect of bone compared to soft tissue is greater than the same

amount of attenuation. This in turn results in streak artifacts between pairs of bones (e.g., the petrous ridges) when only a first-pass correction is employed. This artifact can be minimized by using the initial reconstructed image to determine the amount of bone (and soft tissue) along each ray. This information is then used to provide a more accurate estimate of the linearized data and to reconstruct a second, corrected image. Second-pass beam-hardening corrections are sometimes employed in head scanning, but are not generally used for the body.

Shown in Fig. 24 is a projection of an idealized patient. Even with the highly collimated fan beams employed in CT imaging, the radiation level behind the spine will be somewhat higher because of scatter. This makes the spine look less dense than it actually is and tends to mimic the beam-hardening effect. The problem is more pronounced for thicker body parts and for fourth-generation scanners as compared with third-generation scanners. On third-generation scanners employing gas detectors, the anode/cathode plates are several centimeters deep and act like a high-ratio grid. If solid-state detectors are employed, a grid or collimator is used in front of the detectors. In fourth-generation scanners, the detectors have to detect X-rays from a range of angles and therefore are more susceptible to scatter. Inherent to the fourth-generation design, however, is a substantial air gap between the patient and detector. The other way that scatter is controlled is to employ a beam-shaping or "bow-tie" filter (Fig. 25). Such a filter tends to reduce the X-ray intensity at the sides of a patient where the X-ray beam and scatter production are more intense. This, in turn, reduces radiation

FIG. 25. Attenuation profile without **(A)** and with **(B)** a patient compensating or "bow tie" filter.

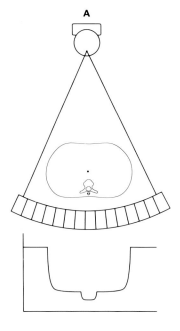

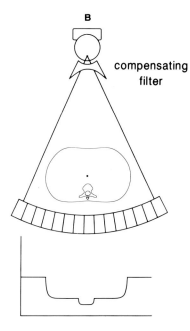

compensating filter

A

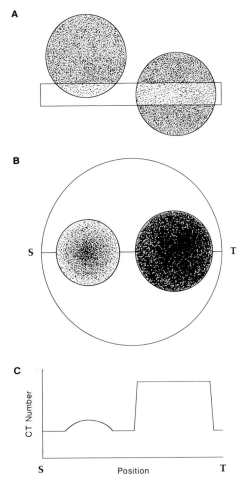

B

S   T

C

CT Number

S   Position   T

FIG. 26. Simple partial volume effect. Illustrated schematically are spherical objects extending partially into and completely into a slice **(A)**, the corresponding CT image **(B)** and a plot **(C)** of the CT numbers along the line ST.

scattered into the central region of a projection. Scatter is not corrected for in the reconstruction process but is taken into account, at least partially, during calibration.

Reconstruction algorithms assume that all the patient's anatomy is within the scan FOV. If that is not the case, the measurements do not represent the attenuation that occurs within the FOV and the reconstruction is in error. This error is manifested by a structured noise pattern in the reconstructed image. The degree of the artifact depends on the amount and anisotropy of the anatomy that is outside the FOV. It goes without saying that the patient should be contained within the scanning FOV.

The assumption is made in CT that the patient has uniform attenuation across the thickness of the slice. If an object extends partially into a ray bundle, then the ray sample underestimates the attenuation. Likewise, if a void is partially encompassed by the ray sample, the attenuation is overestimated. Furthermore, as illustrated schematically in Fig. 26, these errors are not linear functions of the average attenuation. If there is a single-partial-volume object, the errors will cause a local effect, and the average attenuation is reduced (increased) only in the neighborhood of the partial-volume object (void). If there are two or more structures that do not fill the entire beam, the inconsistencies that are created will manifest themselves as streaks connecting the partial-volume objects (19). Local effects will also be present. Both aspects of the problem can be troublesome clinically. Local effects distort borders and yield incorrect quantitative information.

A,B

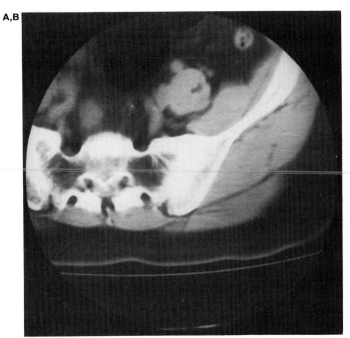
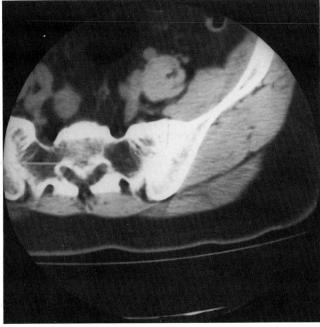

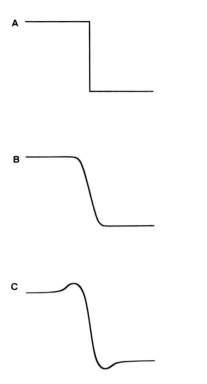

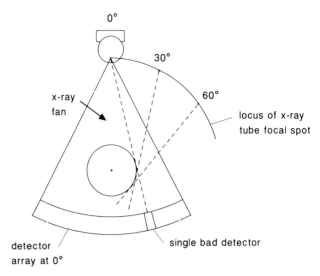

FIG. 29. Origin of ring artifacts on 3rd generation scanners.

FIG. 28. Borders obtained with smoothing **(B)** and edge enhancing **(C)** kernels at an attenuation discontinuity **(A)**.

Streak artifacts often obscure soft-tissue anatomy. Although partial-volume effects can occur in either the axial (craniocaudal) or transverse direction, the most serious effects are due to axial inhomogeneities. The reason for this is that the axial dimension sampled by the ray bundles is much greater than the transverse dimension. Also, because of this, the partial-volume artifacts are more pronounced with thicker slices. This is illustrated in Fig. 27, where the partial-volume streaks are less pronounced in the thinner slice. The effect of simple partial volume averaging is also evident when one compares the differences in the bone detail of the two images. Of note is that since the two scans were obtained at same kV and mAs, fewer X-rays were detected with the thinner slice and more noise is evident (see Eqs. 9 and 10). Another example of simple partial volume averaging is manifest by the merging of the left kidney/liver border in Fig. 21.

The kernel or filter function utilized in the reconstruction algorithm can also introduce artifacts as well as suppress streak artifacts from other sources. If an edge-enhancing kernel is employed, an overshoot will occur at abrupt interfaces between large attenuation differences, such as those for bone and soft tissue (Fig. 28). This over-

shoot is known as the "Gibbs phenomenon," and in CT of the brain it produces a lucency that strongly suggests a subarachnoid space. In body CT the problem can occur when a bone kernel is employed, but it rarely gives rise to clinical problems. However, if a bone or edge-enhancing kernel is employed, the visibility of streak artifacts arising from patient-motion and partial-volume effects is more pronounced. Likewise, if a soft-tissue kernel or less sharp kernel is employed, the streaking will be reduced at the cost of reduced border and small-detail definition. The kernel employed can also affect the CT numbers of small lesions (20) and care should be exercised when one is doing quantitative work.

Artifacts also often arise from equipment malfunctions. For example, if one has a faulty detector or acquisition channel in a third-generation scanner, a ring artifact results. As shown in Fig. 29, the reason for the ring is that during the rotation of the X-ray tube and detector array, the rays measured by a given detector are tangent to a circle. If a detector has an offset or gain difference of 0.1% with the neighboring detectors, a circular artifact will be present in the image (21). Such an artifact indicates that the detector gains need to be calibrated. A faulty detector in a fourth-generation scanner does not give rise to a noticeable artifact, because each detector acquires a view, and the bad data are spread evenly across the image. Also, detector-to-detector channel variations rarely create a problem in a fourth-generation scanner because the detector is calibrated by the raw radiation beam during a scan.

FIG. 27. Comparison of pelvic scans obtained with 10 mm **(A)** and 5 mm **(B)** slice widths (130 kV, 110 mA, 3.6 sec).

X-ray-source fluctuations can also give rise to artifacts in fourth-generation scanners. In third-generation scanners, the rays in a view are all acquired at essentially the same time. Therefore, source fluctuations result in view-to-view variations that are easily corrected by monitoring the X-ray output. Such is not the case in fourth-generation scanners, and Moiré patterns can result if the output variations are synchronized with the data sampling. Because of the spectral variations associated with rotor ripple, this is true even if the tube output is monitored and corrections are made to the data. In practice, rotor-ripple artifacts are minimized by monitoring and correcting for output variations and also by rotating the rotor asynchronously with the data collection.

Calibration and Quality Control

To achieve optimal performance, CT scanners require routine calibrations. The subsystems involved are similar in both the third- and fourth-generation scanners: X-ray generators, detectors, detector electronics, detector location, focal-spot location and alignment, slice width, and corrective factors. The X-ray generator calibration is similar to the calibration of a radiographic generator and involves setting the kV, filament preheat, mAs, pulse duration, etc. The detector-channel gains must be calibrated on third-generation scanners on a weekly or fortnightly basis depending on the manufacturer. As noted earlier, the detector-channel gains on a fourth-generation scanner are calibrated during each scan, because the unattenuated beam is incident on the detectors outside the scan FOV. However, on fourth-generation scanners, one should also do a daily air calibration, which is used to compensate the response of the detector versus X-ray focal-spot position.

Geometrical alignments are extremely important in CT, and the focal spot must be appropriately centered to the scan FOV and also transversely to the center of the detectors. On both third- and fourth-generation scanners, the locations of the focal spot, detectors, and mechanical center of rotation must be accurately determined. Also, the center of the reconstruction FOV may not coincide with the mechanical center of rotation. On third-generation scanners, detector location and focal-spot/detector alignment vary during a scan because of mechanical stresses associated with the large masses of the detector array, DAS assembly, and X-ray tube. All such misalignments result in loss of spatial resolution and losses in X-ray detection efficiency and can, in some instances, introduce streak artifacts.

Finally, the correction to compensate for beam hardening and scatter must be calculated for every scanning condition, i.e., field size, slice width, kV, and spatial-compensating ("bow-tie") filter. Under each circumstance, the CT number of water should be zero. Likewise, in many scanners, air is set at −1,000. This requires that the data be scaled by an appropriate factor before the convolution and back-projection operations.

As noted earlier, spatial resolution and CT numbers can be affected when a scanner is out of calibration. Image noise level can also be affected. These performance parameters should be quantitated when a scanner is installed for each scanning mode to confirm that they meet the manufacturer's specifications. If they do not, particularly the spatial and contrast resolution, it is highly likely that the scanner was not installed or calibrated correctly. Alternatively, there may be a more fundamental problem with one of the subsystems. Presuming the specifications are met, spatial resolution, noise, CT number, and contrast scale for common scanning modes should be monitored on a weekly basis and used to direct preventive-maintenance operations. The patient radiation dose and slice width should be measured at less frequent intervals. The time associated with such monitoring is minimal. Of equal or greater importance is the monitoring of the performance of film processor and multiformat camera. Weekly or fortnightly monitoring of the multiformat camera is generally recommended. The processor, however, should be monitored daily with sensitometric strips. Here, also, one should make sure that base-line data are obtained when the processor temperature, immersion time, developer chemistry, and fixer meet the film manufacturer's recommendations.

ACKNOWLEDGMENT

We thank the CT engineering group of Picker International, Inc. for providing us with software and assistance which made figures 2 and 3 possible, and also for providing to us their measurements of dose profiles and MTF curves.

REFERENCES

1. Ramachandran GN, Lakshminarayanan AV. Three dimensional reconstruction from radiographs and electron micrographs: Application of convolutions instead of Fourier transforms. *Proc Nat Acad Sci* 1971;68:2236–2240.
2. Shepp LA, Logan BF. The Fourier reconstruction of a head section. *IEEE Trans Nuc Sci* 1974;NS21:21–43.
3. Herman GT, Lakshminarayanan AV, Naparstek A. Convolution reconstruction techniques for divergent beams. *Comput Biol Med* 1976;6:259–271.
4. Cormack AM. Representation of a function by its line integrals with some radiological applications, II. *J App Phys* 1964;35:2908–2913.
5. Hounsfield GN. Computerized transverse axial scanning (tomography): Part I. Description of system. *Br J Radiol* 1973;46:1016–1022.
6. Shope TB, Morgan TJ, Showalter CK, et al. Radiation dosimetry survey of computed tomography systems from ten manufacturers. *Br J Radiol* 1982;55:60–69.
7. Wagner LK, Archer BR, Zeck OF. Conceptus dose from two state of-the-art CT scanners. *Radiology* 1986;159:787–792.

8. Yester MV, Barnes GT. Geometrical limitations of computed tomography (CT) scanner resolution. *Proc SPIE* 1977;127:296–303.

9. Glover GH, Eisner RL. Theoretical resolution of computed tomography systems. *J Comput Assist Tomogr* 1979;3:85–91.

10. Barnes GT, Yester MV, King MA. Optimizing computed tomography (CT) scanner geometry. *Proc SPIE* 1979;173:225–237.

11. Brooks RA, Glover GH, Tolbert AJ, et al. Aliasing: A source of streaks in computed tomograms. *J Comput Assist Tomogr* 1979;3: 511–518.

12. Brooks RA, Di Chiro G. Statistical limitations in x-ray reconstructive tomography. *Med Phys* 1976;3:237–240.

13. Riederer SJ, Pelc NJ, Chesler DA. The noise power spectrum in computed x-ray tomography. *Phy Med Biol* 1978;23:446–454.

14. Cohen G. Contrast detail dose analysis of six different computed tomographic scanners. *J Comput Assist Tomogr* 1979;3:197–203.

15. Joseph PM. Artifacts in computed tomography. Chapter 114, vol 5. In: Newton TH, Potts DG, eds. *Radiology of the Skull and Brain: Technical Aspects of Computed Tomography.* St. Louis: C.V. Mosby Co., 1981: 3956–3992.

16. Pelc, NJ, Colsher JG. Principles of x-ray computed tomography Chapter 30, vol 1. In: Taveras JT, Ferrucci JB, eds. *Radiology: Diagnosis-Imaging-Intervention,* Revised Edition. Philadelphia: J.B. Lippincott Co., 1987:1–11.

17. McDavid WD, Waggoner RG, Payne WH, Dennis MJ. Correction for spectral artifacts in cross-sectional reconstruction from x-rays. *Med Phys* 1977;4:54–57.

18. Joseph PM, Spital RD. A method for correcting bone induced artifacts in computed tomography scanners. *J Comput Assist Tomogr* 1978;2:100–108.

19. Glover GH, Pelc NJ. Nonlinear partial volume artifacts in x-ray computed tomography. *Med Phys* 1980;7:238–249.

20. McCullough EC, Morin RL. CT number variability in thoracic geometry. *AJR* 1983;141:135–140.

21. Hounsfield GN. Picture quality of computed tomography. *AJR* 1976;127:3–9.

CHAPTER 2

MRI Physics and Instrumentation

W. Thomas Dixon

Many nuclei in the human body produce magnetic fields. Because magnetic fields easily pass through the body, it is possible to observe the nuclei, and hence the internal contents of the body, from the outside noninvasively. We do not observe single nuclei, but rather the macroscopic *magnetization,* a bulk property of the collection of nuclei within a given voxel. The magnetic fields outside the body, which the imager measures, are produced by the magnetization within the subject. This chapter deals with the origin, manipulation, and measurement of this nuclear magnetization. These concepts are important because the pixel value in an image is proportional to the magnetization in the corresponding voxel in the subject. Equipment and image reconstruction are also discussed.

EQUILIBRIUM NUCLEAR MAGNETIZATION

Nuclear magnetization depends first on the magnetic moments of single nuclei. Magnetic moment is the measure of an object's ability to produce a magnetic field at a distance. It has a magnitude and a direction. Each stable element (except argon and cerium) has a stable isotope with a magnetic nucleus. Hydrogen is the simplest, with a proton for a nucleus. A proton has spin or angular momentum, and it is charged, and so it can be regarded as a current going around a circle. Circular currents and protons both have magnetic moments. In fact, taking the experimentally determined mass, charge, angular momentum, and size, one can calculate a magnetic moment for a proton similar to the observed value. If a nucleus has an even number of protons, the magnetic moments may cancel, as they do in ^{4}He or ^{16}O, but a nucleus containing an odd number of protons is magnetic. Although a neutron has no charge, it has a magnetic moment. Hence, nuclei with odd numbers of neutrons are also magnetic. Throughout the rest of this chapter, the word

"proton" will refer to the hydrogen nucleus, not to elementary particles within complex nuclei.

A magnetic field produces a torque on a magnet that tends to force the magnet to line up with the field; or, equivalently, the energy of a magnet in a field depends on the angle between its magnetic moment and the field, as well as the strength of both the magnet and the field. Lower-energy directions predominate (following Boltzmann) in a large collection of magnets, so the entire collection is at least partially aligned and assumes a magnetization directed along the applied field. This magnetization can produce much larger fields on the outside than any one of the magnets would by itself. In the case of small nuclear magnets, which have magnetic energies much smaller than thermal energies, this magnetization is given by Curie's law:

$$M = N \frac{B}{T} f(\text{nuclear type})$$

where M is the magnetization, N is the number of nuclei, B is the applied field, and T is temperature. The function f is proportional to the square of the magnetic moment of the nuclear magnets, depends slightly on the angular momentum of any one of the (equivalent) magnets, and contains other physical constants. Protons are used for imaging because they are the most abundant magnetic nuclei in the body; the abundant carbon and oxygen isotopes are nonmagnetic. The proton also has the largest magnetic moment of the biologically relevant isotopes and possesses a low spin, which in turn leads to rapid precession and therefore easier detection. Table 1 lists the nuclear properties of different isotopes.

The N and f in Curie's law explain the importance of using protons for imaging, and the B dependence shows the importance of powerful magnets; however, the law does not explain the good natural contrast seen in images, because both N and T are fairly uniform throughout the body. The Curie law applies only at equilibrium, after the

TABLE 1. *Nuclear properties*

Nucleus	Spin ($\hbar$)	Isotopic abundance (%)	Magnetic moment (nuclear magnetons)
^{1}H	1/2	100	2.79
^{2}H	1	0.015	0.86
^{13}C	1/2	1.1	0.70
^{14}N	1	100	0.40
^{17}O	5/2	0.04	−1.89
^{19}F	1/2	100	2.63
^{23}Na	3/2	100	2.22
^{31}P	1/2	100	1.13

"dust has settled" from the last change. However, the behavior of nuclear magnetization before equilibrium is reached varies greatly from tissue to tissue, and this is actually the source of most image contrast.

ANGULAR MOMENTUM AND PRECESSION

A precessing gyroscope that does not fall is a well-known example of the change in behavior produced by angular momentum. Figure 1 is the vector picture of this. Given the direction of rotation of the toy top, the right-hand rule gives the direction of its angular momentum. Given the directions and points of application for the two forces on the top, gravity and the supporting force from the tower, the right-hand rule also gives the direction of the torque on the top (Fig. 1).[1] Torques produce or change existing angular momentum. In the illustration, the torque points out of the plane of the page along the y axis. This turns the angular momentum away from x and toward y. Notice that the torque has no component along z. Therefore, no change in the top's vertical component is produced even though gravity pushes down on the top! The motion of the angular momentum or axis of rotation about the z axis or gravity field is called precession. Nuclei precess about a magnetic field in the same manner. Precession is a completely different motion from the spin that produces angular momentum. The precession rate is independent of the direction of the angular momentum (the angle θ). The precession rate is proportional to field strength and inversely proportional to angular momentum (a disadvantage for high-spin nuclei). In the case of nuclei, the precession rate is called the Larmor frequency and is given by

$$\nu = \frac{\omega}{2\pi} = \frac{\gamma B}{2\pi}$$

The symbols ν, ω, γ, and B refer to frequency (cycles/time), angular frequency (radians/time), gyromagnetic or

magnetogyric ratio, and field strength, respectively. This equation defines the gyromagnetic ratio. For protons, the Larmor frequency is 4.26 kHz/gauss or 42.6 MHz/tesla. Magnet manufacturers specify their products in terms of field strength, but Larmor frequency usually is a much more convenient measure. The Larmor frequency usually is between 1 and 100 MHz in whole-body imagers, with newer machines operating at higher frequencies.

Angular momentum has two important effects for imaging. First, just as a top is not immediately aligned along the field (it precesses about it instead), nuclear dipoles are not immediately aligned, and so Curie's law does not apply immediately. The delay, called relaxation, is responsible for most of the contrast in images. Second, precession makes nuclear magnetization detectable, as will be seen in the section on measuring nuclear magnetization.

MANIPULATING NUCLEAR MAGNETIZATION

Longitudinal magnetization developed in the body must be converted into transverse magnetization before it can be measured. Figure 2 shows how weak radiofrequency (RF) fields can change the direction of magnetization. In Fig. 2A, transverse nuclear magnetization precesses along the solid curve about a strong, steady vertical field. A small field (B_1) applied perpendicular to the main field tips the resultant field along the dotted line, and precession follows the new dotted path. The magnetization moves alternately up and down a slight amount toward the main field. If the small, perpendicular field is removed when the magnetization is at the highest point of the cycle, the gain is preserved, as in Fig. 2B. This process can be repeated (Fig. 2C) until the magnetization points along the main-field axis. This is called a 90° pulse. When repeating the process in Fig. 2B, the magnetization must be in the right orientation every time B_1 is applied, because applying B_1 when the magnetization points the wrong way pushes it down instead of up (Fig. 2A). If B_1 is not applied at the precession frequency of the magnetization, it will push up about half the time, down the other half, and will have little net effect. This ability of a field applied at the precession frequency to produce a large effect, while a field just as strong but with a different frequency has no effect, is called resonance.

Depending on the starting conditions, the magnetization may be moved parallel or antiparallel to the main field. If the initial magnetization starts along the main field (B_0), a 90° pulse will then flip the magnetization to the transverse plane. A 180° pulse, which can invert the longitudinal magnetization from the +z axis to the −z axis, has twice the duration of a 90° pulse or uses a B_1 twice as strong. Smaller flip angles are also possible and useful. In practice, the small perpendicular field, called the RF field, is not abruptly turned on and off, but either oscillates sinusoidally, reversing its direction, or rotates

---

[1] The right-hand rule states that when the fingers of the right hand curl in the direction of the motion (forces), the hitchhiker's thumb points in the direction of angular momentum (torque).

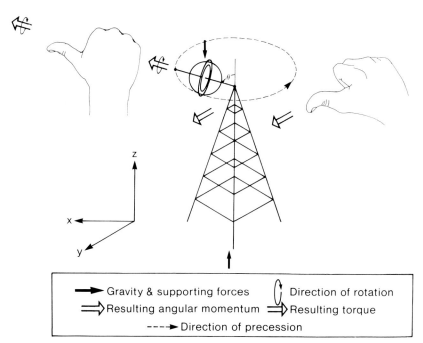

FIG. 1. Precession. Angular momentum causes the top to precess instead of falling. The conventional directions of angular momentum and torque are given by the right-hand rule.

→ Gravity & supporting forces   ↻ Direction of rotation
⇒ Resulting angular momentum   ⇒ Resulting torque
----→ Direction of precession

about the main field fast enough to stay in step with the precessing magnetization while maintaining a constant amplitude. In whole-body imagers, these RF fields typically are strong enough to produce four 90° pulses in about 10 msec. This is described as an RF field strength of 100 Hz.

When we describe a task that takes several days, we speak as if objects around us are stationary. In fact, they all rotate about once every 24 hr. This rotation can complicate instructions greatly; so we simply subtract one revolution per 24 hr from all motions. We describe events in a *rotating frame.* Similarly, all magnetization directions, RF pulses, and whole-body-imaging pulse sequences can be described in a frame rotating at the RF or the Larmor

frequency of the spins (often the same). This simplifies things in two ways, changing Fig. 2C into Fig. 2D. First, magnetization no longer precesses in the rotating frame. Because a main field, conventionally along the z axis, causes precession, there is no field along the z axis in the rotating frame! Second, an RF field rotating about the z axis in the laboratory frame is a steady field in the rotating frame (usually chosen along the x axis). A complicated problem with one constant and one rotating field has been reduced to a simple problem with only a single constant field.

As a more advanced application of the rotating frame, Fig. 3 shows how a 90° pulse followed by a 180° pulse leads to a *spin echo.* Initially the magnetization lies in the

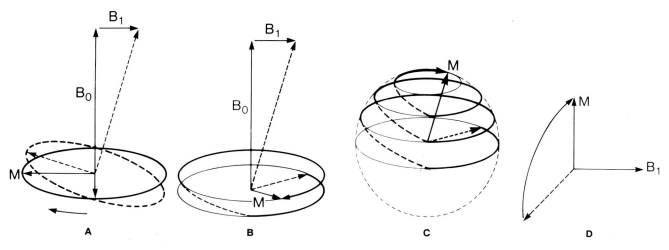

FIG. 2. A weak perpendicular field affects precession. **A:** A steady field tilts the precession axis and path to the dotted lines. **B:** A brief field moves the magnetization permanently closer to B_0. **C:** Repeated brief fields move the magnetization by an arbitrary amount. **D:** A 90° pulse illustrated in the rotating frame. Figure 2C is simplified. The small rotating field, B_1, appears to sit still. M precesses about B_1, when B_1 is present, and is stationary otherwise. B_0 vanishes.

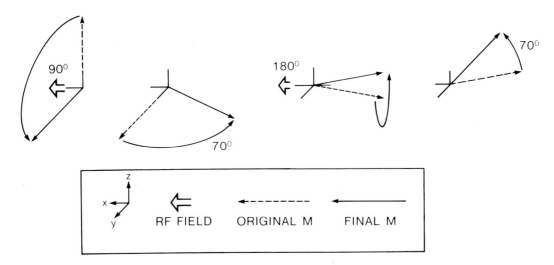

FIG. 3. Generating a Hahn spin echo. **Left** to **right:** A 90° RF pulse moves *M* from *z* to *y* axis. *M* precesses 70° about *z* axis. *M* precesses 180° about *x* axis. *M* precesses another 70° to the −*y* direction; the final position is independent of precession angles before and after the 180° pulse if they are equal.

z direction. A 90° pulse in the *x* direction causes the magnetization to precess 90° about the RF field to the *y* axis. The figure is drawn in a frame rotating at the radio frequency, which is close to but not necessarily equal to the Larmor frequency. If we wait, the magnetization will precess, but very slowly in the rotating frame, about the *z* axis. Suppose we wait long enough for the magnetization to precess 70°, then apply a 180° pulse along the *x* axis as before. The magnetization precesses 180° about the RF field. Before the pulse, it lay 20° (or 160°) to one side of the RF field; after the pulse, it lies 20° to the other side. The magnetization has changed its direction by 40°. If we wait again the same length of time as before, the magnetization will precess another 70°, just as it did before, in the same direction. This will take it to the −*y* direction. If we repeat the experiment with spins having a slightly different Larmor frequency, so that they precess 30° or 60° or 370° during the delays, the result is the same. They end up pointing along the −*y* axis. With a mixture of Larmor frequencies, the signal will decay after the 90° pulse, because total magnetization gets smaller when the contributing magnetizations no longer point in the same direction. After a delay, the second pulse realigns them, and so the signal returns. Additional echoes can be recalled by additional pulses. When Erwin Hahn observed this in 1950, he used the term "spin echo." Another method of producing spin echoes that have different properties is described in the chapter on MRI technique. The term "Hahn echo" can help prevent confusion of the two.

Because resonance is required to convert longitudinal into observable transverse magnetization, a resonant slice can be observed selectively while the rest of a patient is pushed off resonance by a field gradient. The rotating frame lets us see what happens at the edge of a slice that is slightly off resonance.

Let us choose a part of the slice where the gradient has shifted the Larmor frequency 1,200 Hz away from the RF frequency. We shall further suppose an RF field strength of 500 Hz (i.e., resonant spins are flipped 90° in 0.5 msec). Figure 4 illustrates this in a frame rotating at the radio frequency. In this frame, the RF field appears stationary and 500 Hz long. In this case we decided to examine a region where spins precess at 1,200 Hz about the *z* axis in our frame rotating at the radio frequency.

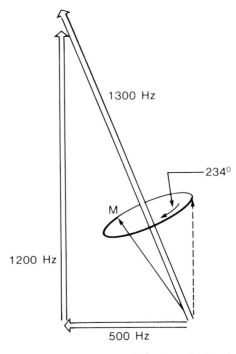

FIG. 4. Effect of an off-resonant 90° pulse. During the pulse, spins precess about an effective field that is the vector sum of the 500-Hz RF field and the 1,200-Hz resonance offset.

This can be caused only by a magnetic field along the z axis having a strength of 1,200 Hz. Figure 4 shows both this 1,200-Hz off-resonant field and the 500-Hz RF field as vectors. These really are vectors, and so they may be replaced by their sum, and the magnetization will behave in the same way. Pythagoras's theorem gives the magnitude of 1,300 Hz; the direction is along the diagonal of the rectangle made by the two fields. The magnetization precesses about this vector, called "the effective field in the rotating frame."

Notice from the figure that we are far enough off resonance that the magnetization will not go all the way down to the xy plane no matter how long the pulse is left on (anything over 500 Hz off resonance assures that). In 0.5 msec at 1,300 Hz, the magnetization precesses 234° about the effective field. In this off-resonant part of the slice, this 90° pulse produces less transverse magnetization than it does in the middle of the slice.

Somewhat farther off resonance, and off center, the effective field is larger, and so 360° precession will occur, which is the same as no pulse at all. Farther off resonance, weak-side lobes occur as precession exceeds 360°, again producing transverse magnetization. Great effort has gone into shaping RF pulses so that their effect falls off abruptly; nevertheless, contiguous slices with perfectly rectangular profiles are an impossible dream.

LONGITUDINAL AND TRANSVERSE RELAXATION

Relaxation, or the gradual return of nuclear magnetization to the value given by the Curie law and to the direction of the applied field, is the source of almost all tissue contrast. Random fields, commonly from other moving protons, cause relaxation. Fields along the applied-field axis cause some spins to precess faster than others, eventually spreading them out in the transverse plane so that transverse magnetization disappears. In other words, the signal (transverse magnetization) produced after the 90° pulse diminishes with time. The time constant that describes the exponential decay of the transverse magnetization following an RF pulse is called "T2." T2 relaxation is also called "spin-spin relaxation," because local magnetic fields from nearby "spins" (nuclei) produce it, or "transverse relaxation," because it involves the loss of magnetization in the transverse (xy) plane. One percent of the magnetization is lost in 1% of a T2; 63% of the initial xy magnetization will be lost in one T2, and 95% will be lost in three T2 periods. Loss of 63% during a relaxation time often is called loss of an "e-fold." Because some tissues relax faster than others (they have shorter T2 values), their signals decay faster than those of others, and contrast may be improved.

Small resonant fields perpendicular to the main field change longitudinal magnetization. It is the resonant component of random fields perpendicular to the main field that causes longitudinal magnetization to relax or grow to follow the Curie law. T1, which has variously been called the longitudinal or spin-lattice relaxation time, is defined as the characteristic time constant for spins to regain their longitudinal magnetization following a 90° RF pulse. In a time T1, longitudinal magnetization will return to 63% of its maximum value, and in three T1 intervals, 95% of the longitudinal magnetization will be reconstituted. T1 also varies from tissue to tissue. If very little time is allowed between measurements, little relaxation occurs, magnetization is small, and the image is dim. Brightness is determined by proton density, T1, and T2. Increasing the time interval between successive 90° pulses allows more longitudinal magnetization to build up, and a brighter image results. However, in the latter case, tissue contrast will be reduced because nearly all tissues will have regained their complete longitudinal magnetizations.

Relaxation rate is the reciprocal of relaxation time. The transverse and longitudinal relaxation rates are more important than proton density in determining tissue contrast, because relaxation rates vary severalfold from one soft tissue to another, whereas proton density varies by only a small fraction. Relaxation rates, rather than times, are used in discussions of tissue relaxation mechanisms and contrast agents because the total relaxation rate is the sum of the rates for all the different relaxation mechanisms. No such rule applies for times. For example, the relaxation rate of a copper solution is just the rate for pure water plus the relaxivity for copper times its concentration. If nickel or iron is added to the solution, another term is added. At low field strengths, many paramagnetic agents increase transverse and longitudinal relaxation rates by about the same amount (at higher fields, the longitudinal relaxation becomes less effective). Because the normal longitudinal relaxation rate of tissue (1/T1) is considerably smaller than its transverse rate (1/T2), these substances increase the tissue longitudinal rate by a larger fraction than the transverse rate, accounting for the need to use a T1-weighted, rather than a T2-weighted, sequence after administration of contrast material.

MEASURING NUCLEAR MAGNETIZATION

A receiver coil is used to detect an MR signal. A coil consists of single or multiple loops of copper wire (or tubing or sheet) designed to detect a change in magnetic field as indicated by the voltage induced in the wire. Figure 5 shows magnetic-field lines emanating from a magnetized sample. Some of these lines pass through a nearby single-turn coil. The number of these lines passing through the coil is called the flux linked to the coil. If this flux changes, an electromotive force (EMF) will appear across the coil. The EMF is proportional to the rate of change of this flux. Precessing nuclear magnetization produces a flux that

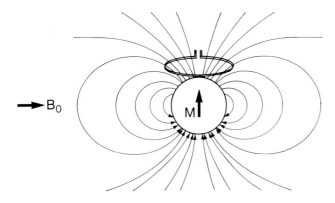

FIG. 5. Flux produced by a magnetized object. *M* is the magnetization vector. Some of the flux lines pass through the single-turn coil over the object.

changes back and forth between plus and minus a value that depends on geometry and the amount of precessing magnetization. Thus, the EMF that is measured electronically is a measure of the nuclear magnetization, the quantity we wish to image.

Notice that the magnetization in the illustration is perpendicular to the main applied field and therefore precesses. Were it along the main field, as called for by Curie's law, it could still induce a flux in a coil, but the flux would not change, and so no EMF would be induced. Any general magnetization can be arbitrarily divided into a longitudinal component (which lies along the field and is silent) and a signal-producing, precessing component transverse to the field. Only the transverse magnetization should be considered in the following coil discussion.

Coil Size

A coil of the proper size close to the target maximizes flux linkage and hence signal. Most flux lines will not reach a very large coil. Very few flux lines find their way through a coil that is too small. In general, the target size should bear a relationship to coil size and proximity based on certain physical principles. A coil radius $\sqrt{2}$ times the distance from the coil center to the target maximizes flux. The coil axis should be perpendicular to the field in most practical cases.

Signal strength is not the only consideration in the choice of the size and placement of the coil. Larger coils give uniform sensitivity over a larger region; small coils do not detect undesirable signal outside the area of interest. If the moving abdominal wall and the heart can be kept out of range of a coil, motion artifacts will not degrade images of the spine. Coil selection also affects the "noise" seen in an image, because noise depends on the square root of the coil resistance measured at the proton Larmor frequency. Resistance is defined as power loss when a unit of current is pushed through the coil. Power is lost three ways: The copper heats up because it is resistive; the coil's

varying magnetic field induces currents in the patient, and so the patient is heated; the coil voltage produces electric fields that also heat the patient. Leaving a small space between the coil and the patient usually keeps the third factor, electrostatic loss, to a fairly small fraction of the total. Most coils have built-in spacers. Power loss due to heating of copper wire (copper loss) is minimized by using thick, large-caliber conductors, sometimes silver-plated. Hollow tubes often are used because RF electricity flows only near the surface. Very little can be done, in terms of coil construction, about electromagnetic losses, because magnetic coupling is essential to receiving the signal. However, by choosing a small coil that is not sensitive outside the region of interest, noise will be reduced because outlying regions will not be heated.

Coil Geometry

The center of the head can be imaged by a single-loop coil placed behind or in front of the head or, more desirably, by using both coils simultaneously. The usual arrangement, called a saddle coil, consists of two rectangular loops bent around a cylinder, rather than of two flat, circular loops. Saddle coils give more uniform images with higher signal-to-noise ratios (at the center) than does a single-loop coil. The field of view is more uniform with saddle coils because one coil is most sensitive where the other is least sensitive. Two independent measurements taken sequentially with a single-loop surface coil can be combined to improve the signal-to-noise ratio by $\sqrt{2}$. The loops in the saddle coil produce two (nearly) independent measurements simultaneously to give the same benefit. These measurements may be combined by wiring the loops in series to double the signal voltage, or by wiring them in parallel to halve the resistance.

These principles have been extended to the point that new designs are difficult to recognize as coils. More than two coils can be combined, as, for example, in quadrature coils or the birdcage resonator. Pieces of the coil may be left out in high-frequency coils. In the latter case, the coil current does not have time to move much charge, and small charges can simply move back and forth from one end of the wire to the other.

Other coil geometries are appropriate when the long axis of the subject lies perpendicular rather than along the field. Such designs also are appropriate for breasts in superconducting magnets. A solenoid, which looks like a spring, can be used with its axis perpendicular to the field. These often have four or five turns and can be treated as four or five single loops electrically in series. In contrast, a cylinder with a slot cut down its length is similar to a one-turn loop; with two slots it behaves like a half-turn coil, etc. These are called loop-gap resonators. All of these modifications are designed to provide good sensitivity, appropriate field of view, easy tuning, rapid setup, and patient comfort.

IMAGE RECONSTRUCTION

A two-dimensional slice can be selected from a three-dimensional patient by applying a field gradient during the RF pulses. Only spins resonant with the RF will be observed (Fig. 6). These will lie in a slice perpendicular to the so-called slice-selection gradient. Slice thickness is determined by the strength of both the gradient and the RF. Slice position along the gradient direction is determined by the pulse frequency.

Field gradients along the three axes are produced by three separate coils and their accompanying power supplies. Oblique views are generated by using more than one coil at a time. The gradients can be considered small adjustments to the field, because they usually produce less than a 1% change in field from one end of the magnet to the other. Nevertheless, the gradient power supplies require many kilowatts. Inadequate gradient power can limit the minimum pixel size and slice thickness. Forces on the gradient coils produce the repetitive knocking or pinging sound of an imager.

The transverse magnetization in the slice must be assigned to pixels in the image. The EMF generated in the receiver coil has the same frequency as the precession frequency of the spins that produced it. With a gradient in the head-to-foot direction, tissues will produce EMFs with frequencies that depend on the z coordinate of the tissue (Fig. 6B). A spectrum or signal-versus-frequency plot (Fig. 6C) looks just like an X-ray projection with the beam directed left-to-right, except that nuclear magnetization replaces X-ray density. It is possible to repeat the experiment while incrementing the gradient orientation, hence projection angle. This method is still used in X-ray computed tomography (CT) and was used in Lauterbur's first experiments, but it is seldom used today.

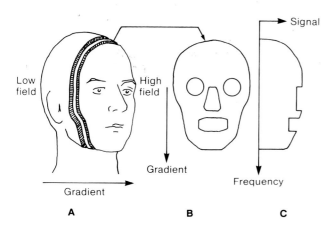

FIG. 6. Image formation. **A:** A 90° RF pulse in the presence of an anterior–posterior gradient produces transverse magnetization restricted to a coronal slice. **B:** A head-to-foot gradient produces different Larmor frequencies at chin and top of head. **C:** Signal intensity versus frequency is a projection of the slice.

The reconstruction method in general use now is called two-dimensional Fourier-transform (2-D FT) imaging or *spin-warp imaging.* With this method, the selective pulse keeps magnetization from behind the eyes out of the projection in Fig. 6B. Signal from above and below the eyes can be excluded on the basis of frequency. In order to separate the right eye from the left eye, two sets of signals are obtained: one with a right-to-left gradient on, and the other with the gradient off. This third gradient in the right-to-left direction is applied after the selective RF pulse, but before the signal is observed. The gradient strength and duration are chosen to force magnetization in the right eye to precess 180° farther than that in the left, which is not affected. With the right-to-left gradient on, the total magnetization in the two eyes is zero, because the two magnetizations point in opposite directions, and no signal is seen from the eye region. By comparing the signals received with this gradient on and then off, the contribution from each eye can be determined. If the subject has no right eye, the two experiments will give the same signal, and if instead he has no left eye, the signal will be the same except for a 180° phase change. Using two values of the left–right gradient (zero and one other), an image that is only 2 pixels wide is produced by solving two equations in two unknowns. To get more resolution, more measurements are made using more values of the left–right gradient, and a larger set of equations is solved. The initial gradient during the RF pulse is called the slice-selection gradient. The next one to be applied is called the phase-encoding or warp gradient, and the gradient that is used during signal measurement (in this example, the head-to-foot gradient) is called the read gradient (occasionally called the frequency-encoding gradient). Their orientation determines the orientation of the image and artifacts. The number and strength of gradients used determine slice thickness, matrix size, field of view, and pixel size. A common value is the 256 square matrix, with a 20- to 50-cm field of view and a 3- to 15-mm slice thickness. The imaging technique described here has largely replaced the older back-projection technique because it is less troubled by the star-type artifacts seen in CT.

This 2-D spin-warp technique (2-D FT) is easily modified for direct 3-D imaging: The RF pulses can select a very thick slice that will be reduced to a stack of thinner slices during reconstruction; alternatively, nonselective RF pulses that use no gradient can be used. The same phase-encoding technique that was used for one dimension in 2-D imaging must now be used for two dimensions. The number of acquisitions needed to finish the task is therefore increased by a factor equal to the number of slices in the stack. There is some argument about the quality of this technique for numbers of slices less than about 32; so this increased time requirement has been a stumbling block. Recently, rapid imaging techniques have become popular, and this is likely to rekindle interest in 3-D imaging.

MAGNETS

Doubling the field strength doubles the nuclear magnetization and halves the time for it to precess. Together, these effects make the signal proportional to the square of the field strength. The field strength is therefore an important property of a magnet. Field uniformity is also important, because the position of a spin is determined by its frequency. Field gradients or adjustments used intentionally in imaging must be larger than those accidentally present in an inhomogeneous, poorly shimmed magnet in order to prevent severe distortion of position and intensity. Stronger gradients can overcome increased magnet inhomogeneities, but this increases the gradient amplifier cost, and the image noise increases with the square root of gradient strength. The magnetic susceptibility of the average patient introduces inhomogeneities of a couple parts per million; so there is little point in producing a magnet better than that.

Field homogeneity, along with size, is what makes imaging magnets unique. Although much is made of their strength, they are no stronger or larger than scrap-yard magnets.

Early imaging magnets consisted of four or six resistive current loops attached to an open frame. These were relatively cheap, but the power required to operate one increases with the square of its field. This took tens of kilowatts at fields over 0.1 T. This design has been replaced with more expensive superconducting solenoids having a 1-m bore diameter. These magnets consume no power, but require liquid helium to keep them cold enough to operate. Superconducting magnets produce higher fields than do resistive magnets. A field homogeneity within tens of parts per million is usual inside a 50-cm-diameter sphere, although some magnets have been made much better, and all are much better in a smaller region near the center. Because superconducting magnets are not connected to a power supply, but are simply short-circuited and allowed to run, they are temporally stable without complicated regulation hardware.

The magnet problem could be considered solved were it not for fringe fields. The return path for the flux lines extends well outside superconducting or resistive magnets. These fringe fields interfere with pacemakers, video terminals, and other devices; conversely, steel beams in the fringe field degrade the field uniformity within the magnet. Special construction and restricted access in the fringe-field area around an imager usually cost as much as the imager itself. Fringe fields are much smaller around ferromagnet imagers, with either permanent magnets or electromagnets, and so siting is easier. Initial capitalization and operating costs sometimes are less than those for superconducting systems. However, weight, field homogeneity, and temporal drift can be drawbacks.

Shielding, in the form of iron return paths, can reduce the fringe fields of superconducting magnets, but is costly and heavy. Superconducting return paths are being developed as an alternative to iron return paths for shielding. These also will add costs and weight to the system.

REFERENCES

1. Chen C-N, Hoult DI, Sank VJ. Quadrature detection coils—a further $\sqrt{2}$ improvement in sensitivity. *J Magn Reson* 1983;54:324–327.
2. Hayes CE, Edelstein WA, Schenck JF, Mueller OM, Eash M. An efficient, highly homogeneous radiofrequency coil for whole-body NMR imaging at 1.5 T. *J Magn Reson* 1985;63:622–628.
3. Grist TM, Hyde JS. Resonators for *in vivo* ^{31}P NMR at 1.5 T. *J Magn Reson* 1985;61:571.
4. Kneeland JB, Jesmanowicz A, Froncisz W, Grist TM, Hyde JS. High resolution localized magnetic resonance imaging using loop-gap resonators. *Radiology* 1986;158:247.
5. Hahn EL. Spin echoes. *Phys Rev* 1950;80:580.
6. Edelstein WA, Hutchison JMS, Johnson G, Redpath T. Spin-warp NMR imaging and applications to human whole-body imaging. *Phys Med Biol* 1980;25:751–756.
7. Hutchison JMS. NMR scanning: the spin warp method. In: Witcofski RL, Karstaedt N, Partain CL, eds. *Proceedings of an international symposium on nuclear resonance imaging.* Winston-Salem, NC: Bowman Gray School of Medicine, 1982.
8. Lauterbur PC. Image formation by induced local interactions: examples employing nuclear magnetic resonance. *Nature (Lond)* 1973;247:190.
9. Budinger TF, Margulis AR, eds. *Medical magnetic resonance imaging and spectroscopy: a primer.* Berkeley, CA: Society of Magnetic Resonance in Medicine, 1986.
10. Morgan CJ, Hendee WR. *Introduction to magnetic resonance imaging.* Denver: Multi-Media Publishing, 1984:13–42.
11. Morris PG. *Nuclear magnetic resonance imaging in medicine and biology.* Oxford University Press, 1986.

CHAPTER 3

CT Techniques

Dixie J. Anderson and Lincoln Berland

Computed tomography (CT) has become the initial imaging procedure for evaluating many clinical problems, as well as a noninvasive, efficacious means for assessing and monitoring patients with a wide variety of cancers and other chronic illnesses. More than 12 years of experience have documented the value of body CT, such that CT has become readily accessible and a vital part of quality medical care (21). As the numbers of CT examinations have substantially increased, it has become ever more important to conduct CT in a way that maximizes diagnostic information and minimizes risks and cost. Our goals for this chapter are to define a working knowledge of the technical aspects of the CT unit, to discuss and illustrate technique modifications that can optimize CT images, and to highlight practical differences among several CT scanners. Sections on the CT scanner (with a special section on radiation dose), the CT image, the CT patient, and CT contrast agents are included. The chapter will conclude with CT protocols established at our institutions for various imaging situations. Our hope is that this information will be easily and often accessed.

Although our personal experience is with the Siemens Somatom DR3, the General Electric 8800 and 9800, the Philips T350, and the Picker 1200, we have largely avoided referring to specific scanners, except for illustrations of generally applicable points. Comments regarding these specific scanners are not intended to support or criticize them exclusively.

CT SCANNERS: DESIGN, VARIABLES, AND OPTIONS

The physical principles of CT are detailed in Chapter 1. A review of the unique qualities of CT, however, is in order. CT, an X-ray-generated imaging study, requires roughly the same photon density as conventional radiography (approximately 10^7 photons/cm^2), but is designed to focus X-rays on a limited cross-sectional tissue plane and to utilize those X-rays more efficiently. The efficiency of this imaging method results in excellent contrast sensitivity. The capability of resolving subtle attenuation differences on the order of 0.25% to 0.5% is far superior to that for conventional radiography, which requires approximately a 10% difference in density for detection. The reasons for the improved contrast sensitivity include (a) reduction in scatter, (b) removal of superimposed information, (c) sophisticated detection systems, and (d) sensitive display technique. Scatter reduction is accomplished primarily by use of a narrowly collimated X-ray beam and, to a lesser extent, by the configuration of the detector array. Overlapping information is successfully removed in the image display through the combination of transverse scanning and computer reconstruction techniques. The detecting systems employ a high signal-to-noise ratio with a wide dynamic range and are coupled with image processing that makes use of virtually all of the available data.

CT Generations and Designs

CT scanners currently utilize one of two designs (Fig. 1), referred to as third-generation or fourth-generation, reflecting an evolution from earlier and slower tube-detector arrangements. Neither of these later designs has proved to be clearly better than the other, though each has its unique advantages and deficiencies that may make some difference in selected instances.

The first-generation CT scanners, called translate-rotate scanners, utilized a pencil-thin X-ray beam passed linearly over a small increment of the patient while a detector on the far side of the patient mechanically followed the X-ray source. After a single pass, the tube and detector were rotated a small increment, typically 1°, and the process was repeated until 180° were covered. First-generation equipment is no longer built.

A,B

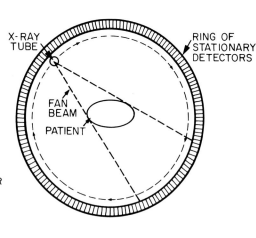

FIG. 1. Third-generation versus fourth-generation CT. In a third-generation CT unit (**A**), the X-ray tube moves synchronously with the opposed detector arc. In a fourth-generation unit (**B**), the X-ray tube moves independently within the stationary circular detector array.

The second-generation tube-detector design used a fan-shaped X-ray beam that otherwise employed the same translate-rotate geometry. This has also been abandoned.

The third-generation design, currently used by Elscint, General Electric, Siemens, and Philips, has advanced to the "rotate-rotate" scanner, in which the tube and detector array are directly opposite each other, and both move in a circle around the patient. Because of this design, there is no opportunity for monitoring an unattenuated X-ray beam during an examination. Thus, third-generation machines are prone to detector imbalance and detector-related artifacts. However, third-generation units tend to have a lower axial dose distribution (Fig. 2) and produce fewer artifacts related to patient motion than do fourth-generation machines.

The fourth-generation systems, presently used by Picker and Thompson-CGR, rotate the X-ray tube, but keep the detector array stable, the so-called rotate-stationary or rotate-only scanner. The tube travels within a circular detector arrangement. In certain fourth-generation scanners, e.g., Toshiba, a detector ring is placed inside the ring of travel of the X-ray tube such that the detector array must "wobble" out of the X-ray-beam path in a motion termed "nutation."

Though neither is inherently superior to the other, both the third- and fourth-generation designs are far superior to the earlier CT units. These improved designs have resulted in much faster imaging.

In another totally different design, the Imatron, the X-ray source consists of a large stationary electron gun, with a massive anode target oriented in a semicircular ring around the patient. This allows extremely short imaging times, on the order of 50 msec. Originally intended as a cardiac imaging device, the Imatron has now been adapted for general-purpose imaging.

X-Ray Source

All X-ray sources for CT (and conventional radiography) are polychromatic, emitting X-rays over a broad spectrum of energies. This is particularly important in CT because the detector systems translate the received X-rays into a single numerical value without evaluating the relative contribution of the number of photons (photon fluence) and the strength of each photon in kilovolts (kV).

Most CT units utilize a modified-rotating-anode, large-heat-capacity X-ray tube. Several variables in the operation of the CT X-ray tube can be defined: the mode (continuous or pulsed) of the X-ray beam, the energy (kV/mA), and the arc or length of tube travel. The mode of the X-ray beam, part of the CT-unit design, cannot be altered. The energy of the X-ray beam is usually determined by using a set voltage, with the amperage dictated by the thickness and physical density of the part to be examined. Most units will allow selection of a variable scanning arc inscribed by the X-ray tube during scanning. This may be defined by the number of degrees in the arc or by the number of sections or sectors included in a single scan. The standard scan is usually based on a 270 to 360° arc, whereas an "overscan" consists of more than a 360° arc.

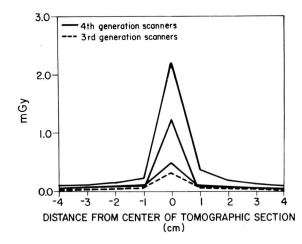

FIG. 2. Radiation dose versus CT imaging design. Axial dose distributions recorded at 1-cm intervals from a central, single CT slice vary considerably depending on the CT scanner model. The three solid lines show representative dose distributions recorded by four fourth-generation scanning units. The dashed line represents approximate dose distributions recorded among three third-generation CT units. (Adapted from ref. 10.)

Whereas angiographic X-ray tubes are called on for series of exposures about two to five times during a procedure, CT scanners may perform 30 or more exposures per patient for 15 to 30 examinations per day at high tube output. Consequently, the life of a CT X-ray tube may be short compared with other X-ray tubes. The usual CT scanner tube warranty is for 20,000 to 50,000 slices. However, the average operating output will influence the longevity of the CT-unit X-ray tube. A CT-unit X-ray tube that is operated constantly at the maximal milliamperage setting or is often used for dynamic scanning without decreasing the output will need to endure even greater stress (or be replaced more often) than an X-ray source that is infrequently called on to operate at or near maximum output.

Detectors

Among the different CT units there are many variations in the detector systems. Differences involve the type of detector as well as the size, number, and spatial arrangement of the detectors within the detector array. In general, the greater the efficiency of each detector and the greater the number of detectors, the better the resolution, both contrast sensitivity and spatial discrimination. The quality of a detector array is determined by the composition of the detectors and the spatial arrangement of the detector array. Each detector is composed of solid-state crystals or pressurized xenon. Crystal detectors often absorb nearly 100% of the incident photons, whereas xenon detectors absorb 60% to 80% of the incoming photons. Despite this marked difference in sensitivity, xenon is still used in some systems because of its low cost and because gas detectors are easier to calibrate against one another. The trend, however, has been toward the solid-state systems.

Scatter reduction, a major reason for the excellent contrast resolution of CT imaging, is accomplished primarily by narrow-beam collimation. The scattered X-rays available to the detectors are filtered by some combination of collimation at the detector array (a grid fixed to the detector array, and/or the use of long, slender detectors) or an air gap.

Couch and Gantry

CT scanners use a cantilever design for the patient-support table that can handle large forces. Specifications for current CT couches will include a rating for the maximum weight of a patient, typically 300 to 450 lb maximum. The gantry aperture is large enough (usually 54–70 cm) to accommodate even very large individuals and to permit CT-guided biopsy and nonaxial direct scanning, as well as to allow scanning, if necessary, with the patient's arms comfortably within the gantry rather than extended overhead.

State-of-the-art tables will increment in 1-mm steps and require less than 3 sec to accommodate rapid-sequence imaging at several levels.

Gantry angulation is another feature important for specialized applications, especially imaging the spine and head. The entire assembly housing the tube and detector array may be moved in either direction 15° to 30°.

Imaging Variables

Several machine variables are controlled by the operator. These include voltage, amperage, scanning speed, collimation, scanning interval, field of view, pixel size, gantry tilt, and the arc of the X-ray tube travel or number of sector scans.

The voltage is maintained at a set level except in unusual circumstances. At our institutions, 120 to 130 kV, depending on the CT scanner, is used for all body CT examinations. If voltage is varied, for whatever reason, it is important to remember that such a change will affect attenuation values (85).

The amperage is adjusted for the size and composition of the part of the body being examined. This may vary from low values (20 mA) for an examination of the larynx to maximal output for an examination of the pelvis in a large patient. Photon deficiency (Fig. 3) may result from an inappropriately low amperage, whereas unnecessary radiation exposure is delivered to the patient if the amperage is too high.

Optimal scanning speed is, in general, the fastest speed available within the limitation of achieving adequate photon flux. Current scanners typically acquire data for one image in less than 5 sec. Fast scanning virtually eliminates motion artifacts due to peristalsis, dramatically decreases respiratory-motion artifacts, and has been shown to significantly improve diagnostic accuracy (58). Fast scanning speeds qualitatively improve images, especially where physiological motion is a problem, such as in the upper abdomen or lower thorax. Short scanning times also allow "dynamic" imaging (rapid sequential images), important for CT evaluation of blood vessels and organ or lesion perfusion. Dynamic imaging involves rapid, sequential images at one level (usually 4–16/min), usually obtained without interscan image processing.

Slice-collimation selection depends on the purpose of the examination. If one is concerned with imaging very complex anatomic regions, such as the larynx, or extremely small anatomic structures, such as distal pulmonary airways in a search for bronchiectasis, or small adrenal masses, thin slices from 1 to 4 mm are needed. For most examinations, however, 5- to 10-mm collimation is used; 1- to 4-mm slice widths are reserved for detailed examinations, sometimes as a supplement to an initial study in which a small lesion is identified or suspected. Thick slices may result in misleading attenuation

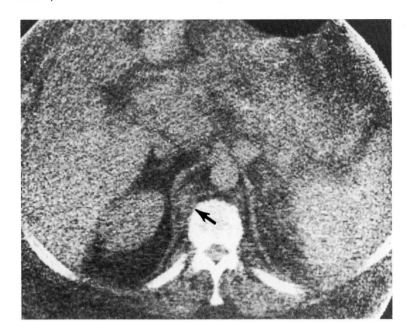

FIG. 3. Effect of photopenia. Coarse mottling of the image is caused by a paucity of X-rays reaching the detectors in this obese patient. The enlarged retrocrural lymph node (*arrow*) is partially obscured by the photopenia artifact.

values because of partial-volume averaging of small structures. Contrariwise, a CT examination with very narrow collimation requires more slices to cover the same longitudinal area, thereby increasing examination time. As slice collimation is decreased, there is a concomitant decrease in signal and an increase in image "noise" (Fig. 4). This will be more dramatic in larger individuals, in whom a decrease in slice width will lead to visible photon deficiency. An increase in amperage will maintain image quality (Fig. 5); however, the radiation dose may be markedly increased.

The scanning interval, or the distance between adjacent images, is closely related to slice collimation as well as to the clinical problem. Contiguous images or nearly contiguous images are most frequently used. In certain instances, it is more practical to use 2 cm of spacing; e.g., in abdominopelvic surveys for possible neoplastic disease, 2-cm intervals have been shown to produce results nearly as accurate as those for contiguous images (28).

The field of view or "zoom" factor is selected to match the cross-sectional size of the part to be examined. The zoom factor will determine the pixel size, typically varying from 0.1 to 2.0 mm. Selecting an inappropriately large field of view will compromise spatial resolution, because resolution is partially related to pixel size. Even more important, an inordinately large field of view introduces uncertainties in the attenuation values, because the computer algorithm is designed from and based on examination of a volume of tissue density without the extreme variations in attenuation introduced by including a large volume of surrounding air. Using a field of view smaller than the cross-section being examined, sometimes called a target scan, is appropriate in selected instances to improve spatial resolution. The field-of-view options are quite varied on a state-of-the-art scanner, permitting selection of centered or off-center specific field sizes, as well as a display of a cursor-specified region of an image. These small-field reconstructions can be selected either prior to imaging or

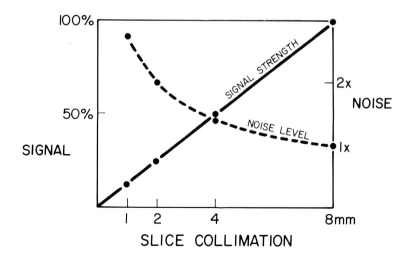

FIG. 4. Slice collimation, signal, and noise. A relative representation of the effect of slice collimation on signal-to-noise ratio. To compensate the loss of signal strength due to narrow collimation, amperage may be increased, realizing that the dose will be increased concomitantly.

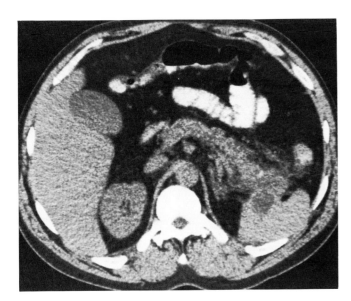 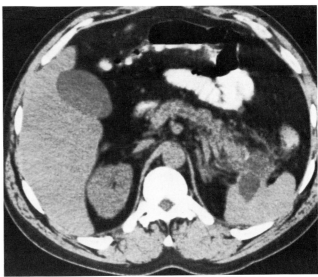

FIG. 5. Thin collimation, varying amperage. **A:** CT image through the upper abdomen was performed with 2-mm collimation and 280 mA. **B:** CT image at the same level used 2-mm collimation and 1,240 mA for only a small gain in image quality.

as a secondary choice subsequent to an initial standard reconstruction. Although the former option may exclude important findings in the periphery, reprocessing the raw data at the larger field size can demonstrate the entire image.

Spatial Resolution

Spatial resolution has to do with the ability to define structures in an image that are only slightly separated in the imaged object. With high subject contrast and good precision, spatial resolution is approximately 1.5 times the pixel size, or, using standard CT systems, about 0.5 to 1.5 mm. Although this compares poorly with the results on mammography studies (resolution of approximately 0.1 mm) or conventional film/screen imaging (0.2–0.4 mm), it is important to remember that spatial resolution does not represent the smallest-size object that is detectable on a CT image. The imaging advantage of CT is more directly influenced by subject contrast than by spatial resolution. That is, the contrast of the object often is more important than size in determining whether or not a specific lesion will be distinguishable. "Contrast sensitivity" has to do with the ability to define subtle alterations in attenuation values reflecting small differences in the transmission of X-rays through the imaged object. For example, gas bubbles or surgical staples too small to be detected with the rated spatial resolution may be easily visible if they are quite different in attenuation value from their surroundings, whereas larger structures that are similar in attenuation to adjacent tissues may not be detected. Also, the locations of small objects relative to the positions of the pixels in which they are seen may affect visualization. If a tiny object falls on the border between two pixels,

its density will be averaged between the adjacent pixels, and it may go undetected, whereas if it falls squarely within a pixel, it is more likely to be seen.

Spatial resolution is directly related to signal strength and indirectly related to quantum mottle. Therefore, voltage, amperage, and collimation, the variables that control photon fluence or signal, will change spatial resolution. The more radiation available as signal at the detector, the better the spatial resolution. The size of the patient, therefore, is another variable that influences image quality. The greater the thickness of the patient, the more radiation will be absorbed, and the less signal will be seen at the detectors. It has been shown that at 125 kV, the signal will diminish by about 50% for each 4 cm of patient thickness. Resolution is similarly affected by the number of projections used to generate an image. If the number of projections is maintained at 750 to 1,000 or more, the resolution will not be limited by this parameter.

Motion interferes with optimal spatial resolution. Consequently, as the time required to produce an image has decreased, CT image resolution has dramatically improved (Fig. 6).

Imaging Options

Digital Radiograph

An image-projection radiograph (topogram, scanogram, scout view, localizer image, or pilot scan), analogous to a plain film, can be generated on virtually all CT units. This is accomplished by moving the scanning couch through the gantry aperture while the stationary CT X-ray tube is rapidly pulsed, producing many contiguous narrow image bands. This series of thin slit sections 1 to 1.5 mm in

A,B

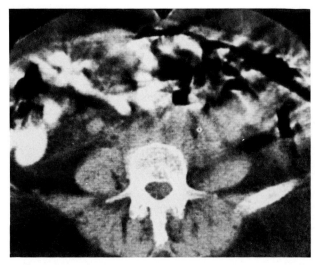 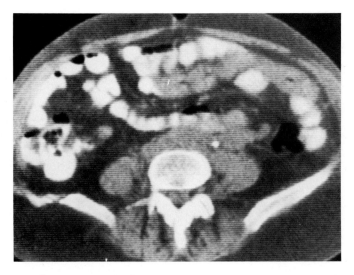

FIG. 6. Spatial resolution, motion artifact, and scanning speed. An 18-sec image (**A**) of the mid-abdomen is compared with a 3-sec image in the same patient (**B**). The effect of respiratory and bowel motion on resolution is dramatic.

thickness is then reconstructed in a plain-film format. Any of four views (posteroanterior, anteroposterior, lateral, and oblique) may be obtained by positioning the X-ray tube appropriately. Different CT units have different limits on the scout-film length, varying from 256 to 512 mm, depending on the manufacturer. The entire procedure, including reconstruction time, is accomplished in a few seconds.

The digital radiographic image often is of sufficient detail and quality to be used as a preliminary plain radiographic film and frequently helps to guide or, later, correlate selection of the scanning level. As a scout film for the abdomen, it allows identification of excessive amounts of retained barium prior to obtaining cross-sectional images. It also demonstrates extraneous high-density objects, such as snaps and EKG leads, that could produce unnecessary image-degrading artifacts. It may be used to localize appropriate scanning levels, e.g., a pulmonary nodule or a particular disc space, which may then be marked on the viewing console by a line cursor and entered into the computer to initiate imaging at those precisely defined levels (Fig. 7). Further, if plain films are unavailable, the digital image may be critical for interpreting certain CT images. For example, evaluating catheters and differentiating between abnormal calcifications and surgical clips may be facilitated by a digital radiograph. As compared with conventional radiography, however, these studies have poor spatial resolution. Although this is not a major problem for CT imaging purposes, it does limit the use of the scout image as a substitute for conventional roentgenography. Nevertheless, the digital study has been recommended by some for CT pelvimetry because of the low radiation dose as compared with a conventional abdominal film (20).

Other advantages of the CT digital radiograph are that it provides the ability to quickly localize a lesion for a CT-guided biopsy procedure and the capability of displaying the imaging levels at the end of a CT examination. The record of the conduct of a particular examination is especially useful to the radiation oncologist, who often needs to correlate tumor extent with surface and bony landmarks used for radiation-port planning. The development of software programs to display tumor margins on CT-generated digital radiographs from cross-sectional images has facilitated the transfer of CT information for treatment planning (34,66,67).

Using the CT-generated radiograph to guide radiation therapy requires working closely with radiation therapy personnel. Patient positioning must closely simulate the therapy position, including positioning the patient's arms as they will be during therapy (55). The usually curved CT couch must be replaced with a flat couch insert. Customized positioning devices are also valuable (61). If the patient is to be treated in two positions, then both positions should be simulated, because significant changes in organ–tumor relationships can occur, especially when the region of interest is near the diaphragm. Optimally, because the radiation therapy will be delivered during quiet respiration, the CT images needed solely for therapy planning can also be obtained during quiet respiration.

Volumetric calculations, potentially helpful for tumor-mass follow-up, can be performed with CT (57) and displayed on the scanogram. Consistent and reliable measurements have been obtained. Single determinations have been shown to vary from about 2% to 4% from the mean when measuring areas greater than 8 cm^2. However, for smaller areas, more significant variation can occur (69).

Digital radiographs have some utility in certain orthopedic evaluations. Leg-length discrepancy analysis (27) is one example. The capability of obtaining two perpendicular views without changing the patient's position is extremely helpful.

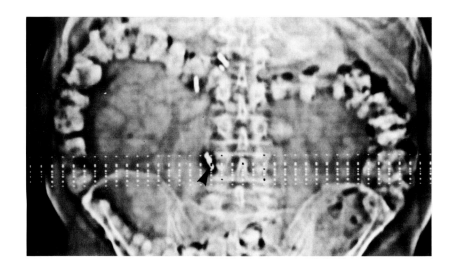

FIG. 7. Digital radiograph. A preliminary CT digital film accomplishes dual purposes: (a) allows monitoring for radiodense materials such as retained barium or surgical clips, (b) allows targeting a certain region for imaging, such as in this prone patient prior to biopsy of a paraspinal mass known to be located near the most caudad surgical clip (*arrowhead*).

Dynamic Imaging

Dynamic imaging refers to rapid, repetitive image acquisition, usually without image processing between scans. There are two basic types of dynamic imaging. The first is rapid sequential imaging, with table incrementation between each scan (survey or incremental dynamic imaging), and the second is rapid sequential imaging at a single level (single-level dynamic imaging). The dynamic imaging program may permit up to 12 scans per minute before tube cooling delays are encountered, as compared with the rate for routine imaging of about 3 to 4 per minute. For most clinical applications, 6 to 8 images per minute are sufficient.

Among different scanners there are differences with respect to the possible number of scans per minute, the interscan delay, the potential number of scans in a dynamic sequence, and the X-ray tube heat limits. For some units, amperage settings must be decreased significantly to achieve a standard dynamic series. As a guideline, the amperage should have to be lowered no less than about one-half to two-thirds of the standard recommended amperage to achieve a satisfactory 15-scan dynamic sequence. After the raw data are accumulated, the reconstruction process is performed to generate the series of dynamic images.

The ability to program a variable interscan delay is also a standard capability for modern scanners. A 3-sec scan delay is commonly used, permitting as many as 12 scans per minute, and allowing patients to breathe between scans. Increasing the interscan delay often allows higher amperage settings and even better patient cooperation with regard to breath holding.

Multiplanar Reconstruction

Multiplanar reconstruction will reorient the CT data in other planes, typically coronal or sagittal. These alternate images have many potential uses, especially in complex anatomic regions such as the spine, the appendicular skeleton, the pelvis, and the regions adjacent to the diaphragm. These reformatted images are optimized as contiguous, or even overlapping, narrowly collimated images. Commonly, contiguous 2.0- to 5.0-mm slices are utilized. In addition, optimally, the ratio of scan interval to pixel size should be about 3:1 or less to achieve high-quality images. For example, in CT evaluations for disc disease, contiguous scans at 3-mm intervals with a pixel size of 1 mm will produce diagnostic-quality sagittal images. A 10-mm scan interval coupled with a pixel size of 1 mm, on the other hand, common to many body CT studies, results in partial-volume-averaging image degradation, often to an unacceptable degree.

Three-Dimensional Reformatting

Three-dimensional (3-D) CT imaging has become feasible and is of considerable benefit in certain clinical situations (54,72,73,81). The most useful applications have been in complex anatomic regions such as the face. Surgical reconstruction of complex facial anomalies has been facilitated by the addition of the third dimension and by the ability to observe complex anatomy in various planes and from various perspectives. Other clinical situations believed to have benefited from 3-D CT imaging have involved (a) complex fractures of the spine, osseous pelvis, shoulder, and face, (b) articular disorders of the hip, and (c) spinal stenosis. It is possible to construct plastic models of these anatomic regions by computer-coupling the CT data with a milling machine. Among other benefits, these models create the opportunity to perform rehearsal surgery. Finally, 3-D imaging has an obvious attraction for anyone involved in teaching complex anatomy.

The imaging requirements for 3-D CT studies are thinly collimated (2-mm) contiguous or overlapping (5-mm slices with 3-mm spacing) images acquired with minimal patient motion. Image-processing programs are available requiring region- and tissue-specific 3-D filters.

The advantages of this technique are partly offset by the disadvantages of the high cost of the software system and the additional time, on the order of an hour, required to generate these image displays. The radiation dose usually is a definite disadvantage of this technique, though in selected bone reconstructions, by dramatically decreasing the exposure factors, the radiation dose may be identical with the dose incurred during routine CT imaging (2).

Direct Nonaxial Imaging

Direct coronal and sagittal CT imaging has been advocated for detailed evaluation of extensive and complex tumors. Such studies can be achieved with equipment modifications available commercially. Body-support devices and bicycle-type seats can be attached to the scanning unit so that direct images can be obtained in many patients (74,75). The main disadvantage of this approach, however, is the additional time needed to make the necessary couch modifications. In addition, these techniques are best applied when imaging young, agile patients who can more easily assume the positions necessary. These practical considerations, plus the development of magnetic-resonance imaging (MRI), have curtailed our application of these techniques.

Dual-Energy Imaging

Although a certain set voltage is utilized for routine CT studies, imaging with two different voltages is an attractive option that allows more specific tissue characterization. The technique of dual-energy imaging has been applied to bone densitometry and would be valuable in other situations, such as pulmonary nodule evaluations. Rapidly alternating between two different energies is most easily accomplished with a CT unit that has the capability of delivering a pulsed X-ray beam. A CT scanner that depends on a continuous X-ray beam will generate two separate images made at different energies. Often this latter approach is limited by motion artifacts.

Magnification

In CT studies, "magnification" may refer to a simple photographic enlargement, i.e., displaying the same information over a larger field made up of larger pixels. However, some CT units allow one to select a magnification factor by moving the tube and detector array relative to the center of the scanning field. If such a magnification factor is used, oftentimes a lower amperage with a smaller focal spot must be selected. This variable tube–detector geometry often will necessitate use of a longer scanning time.

The nomenclature for magnification and focal-spot size selection includes terms such as "precision," "high-precision," "high-detail," and "high-resolution" imaging. The terminology and choices are confusing, and the high-resolution mode on some scanners may limit one to longer scanning times or poorer contrast detectability without that being clearly specified. Additionally, as will be reemphasized, "high-resolution" imaging usually entails a higher radiation dose. It is often necessary to critically analyze the method of attaining better resolution and the radiation dose required to achieve it before using a particular program specified by the manufacturer.

Radiation Dose

General Population and Patients

Because CT is now widely available in the United States and in many parts of the world, the contribution of CT to the radiation dose delivered to the general population is a matter for serious consideration. Although the radiation doses from individual CT studies have decreased over the past several years (10), the collective radiation dose from all diagnostic examinations to the general population has dramatically increased. It is estimated that CT imaging currently contributes 7% to 8% of the active bone-marrow dose delivered via diagnostic radiology to the adult American population (16). Surface doses range from 10 to 70 milligray (mGy) (1 mGy = 0.1 rad) for most examinations, with the more common CT studies involving the lower exposures. Even so, high-resolution techniques necessitating narrowly collimated and overlapping images and single-level dynamic imaging can result in extremely high radiation doses (47). Although such doses are not excessive when compared with those for certain other radiographic procedures, such as angiography, every effort should be made to minimize this radiation exposure. By far the most important consideration is to be sure that the information being provided by the CT examination is of sufficient importance to the health of the person being imaged to justify the exposure. Attention must also be directed toward using the lowest acceptable amperage and limiting the number of repeat scans at one level.

Whereas variations in amperage can influence the radiation dose rather dramatically, other scanning variables usually affect the dose in a relatively minor way. Scan collimation, for example, will affect the radiation dose (Fig. 8). The thinner the slice thickness, the smaller the dose. However, to counterbalance the decreased photon fluence of a thinner slice, the amperage often is increased to improve image quality, thus increasing the radiation

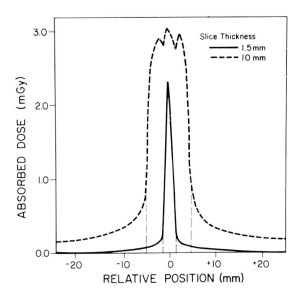

FIG. 8. Effect of scan collimation on radiation dose. The radiation dose imparted during a 10-mm collimated scan (*dashed line*) is much larger than the dose delivered with a 1.5-mm thin scan (*solid line*). Even when multiple thin adjacent slices are used, the dose will not exceed that used for a thick slice, provided the technique is not varied in other ways and provided that overlapping slices are not involved.

dose. Often, the improved image quality is not sufficient to warrant the higher dose (Fig. 5).

One often overlooked source of increased radiation dose is gantry angulation and inadvertent slice overlap. At 25° of angulation, a 10-mm slice intersects almost 12 mm of the table; therefore, table incrementation must be altered appropriately when using gantry angulation.

Scanning parameters often can be optimized to produce quality images with a significant reduction in radiation dose (59). These considerations are even more important in pediatric CT examinations. The longer life expectancy of children and the probable higher sensitivity to radiation both dictate greater potential risks in children.

Determination of the radiation dose for CT studies is more complicated than dose determinations for many other radiographic studies. Because the CT X-ray beam is traversing the circumference (or a portion of the circumference) of the scanned volume, the dose distribution will be more homogeneous than the dose distribution for a volume exposed by an X-ray beam in a single direction. It is more appropriate, then, to speak of representative depth dose than to use surface doses for describing CT exposures. However, even a representative depth dose will not reflect the actual dose distribution. Nonuniformity of the dose distribution in a scanned volume is the rule rather than the exception in CT studies (65). This is because of a variety of influences on the absorbed dose, including the scanning motion, beam collimation, and beam geometry.

A CT dose descriptor, the CT dose index or CTDI (64), has been required of CT equipment manufacturers by the

Food and Drug Administration since 1984. The CTDI is equal to an average dose at specified locations within a phantom, e.g., central axis, 1 cm from the surface. The CTDI denotes the central dose at that point due to a series of scans and includes both primary and scattered radiation. This index has been shown to be an excellent predictor of absorbed dose (within ±5% of patient doses) for chest and abdominal CT studies; however, it is somewhat less accurate for head CT examinations (18).

Most of the concern regarding body CT radiation doses in adults is based on the risk of somatic effects, primarily the risk of inducing cancer. An important concept in dose considerations is the *somatically effective dose equivalent.* The concept assumes that the health detriment associated with a dose to a given organ can be expressed as the product of the dose and a weighting factor that denotes the susceptibility of that tissue to radiogenic damage. The weighting factor is the product of the probability of occurrence of a detrimental effect and the severity of the induced effect. For example, the weighting factor for the thyroid would be higher if thyroid cancer were less medically manageable. The computed effective dose equivalent yields a single indicator of risk for a given nonuniform exposure of the body, e.g., a CT examination, that is numerically equal to the uniform radiation dose equivalent that would impart the same health detriment. Weighting factors have been derived from the data of the Beir III report (6,37). The female breast is relatively sensitive to radiation exposure, as evidenced by a high weighting factor. Consequently, chest CT performed in young women carries a theoretical risk not seen in men.

Unfortunately, there have been few studies addressing CT effective doses. However, several sources (17,35) provide sufficient organ doses due to CT examinations to permit the computation of effective doses using the existing weighting factors. Absorbed doses, carefully measured both with phantoms and during patient imaging (10,24,59), for a usual abdominal examination have been documented at 0.14 to 1.01 mGy (59). Technical factors such as the scanning arc will dictate the dose distribution (48).

Personnel

The radiation dose to a person in the CT examination room is unique in radiology, because the radiation exposure comes from a concentric moving source encased in a protective gantry. The patterns of stray radiation are therefore different from those with conventional radiography. Because there is no fixed point source, but rather a moving source, the inverse-square rule is not applicable at short distances from the scanner. The extraaxial field of radiation produced by scatter radiation, either direct scatter or scatter from the patient, is highest in the horizontal plane of the patient and will have an hourglass shape because of the shielding effect of the gantry and associated housing (Fig. 9). At longer distances from the CT unit, stray radiation more closely resembles that from a point source, and the inverse-square rule is better approximated. The actual dose to a person in the scanning room is low (based on a representative abdominal study using 125 kV and 16- × 8-mm slices), on the order of 0.04 mGy (4 mrad) per hour of tube operation at a distance of 1 m from the scanned subject. This level of personnel exposure, due almost entirely to scattered radiation from the patient, is comparable to that incurred at a similar distance in 1 to 2 min of fluoroscopy of the abdomen. Thus, it is possible, if there is poor attention to radiation precautions, to exceed allowed personnel exposure limits. However, the dose may be minimized to a person in the room by standing as far from the scanner and the patient as is feasible. If standing in the room to inject intravenous contrast material, a person can best be protected by standing in the shadow of the gantry cladding and by using extension tubing to increase the distance from the unit, or by using a power injector. The time of exposure can be minimized by stepping from the room as soon as the injection is completed. In addition, shields such as standard lead aprons or movable lead shields reduce exposure to negligible levels and are strongly advocated.

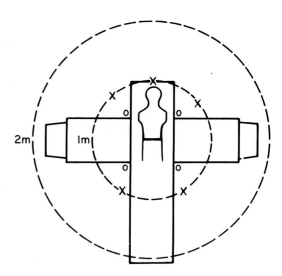

FIG. 9. Radiation exposure in CT rooms. Radiation exposures in a plane at the height of the table top were measured using a torso phantom and the following technique: 125 kV, 310 mA, 8-mm collimation. The highest radiation levels were at points 0, with measurements of 6.7 to 8.9 μGy/slice (0.67–0.89 millirad/slice). At 1 m from the center point (1 m), measurements varied from 1.3 to 4.7 μGy/slice (0.13–0.47 millirad/slice). At 2 m from the center point, the radiation exposure was 0.8 μGy/slice (0.08 millirad/slice).

Fetus

Another practical concern is the conceptus dose. Pregnancy is a relative contraindication to CT imaging; however, occasionally a woman undergoes a CT examination and is later discovered to have been pregnant at the time of the study. Phantom studies performed with two common CT units (80) have shown the conceptus dose to vary considerably depending on the scanning conditions. However, for an abdominal examination that encompasses the fetus, consisting of 25 scans at 1-cm intervals, the conceptus dose is approximately 60 mGy (80), but may vary from 30 to 100 mGy depending on voltage, patient size, and depth of the fetus. A dose of 100 mGy (10 rad) or more is thought by some to carry a high risk of inducing serious deleterious fetal effects, especially in the first trimester.

CT IMAGES

Pixels, Voxels, Attenuation Values

The CT image is a mosaic of individual picture elements or pixels in a matrix, usually of 512 rows and columns. Each pixel represents a variably sized (most often 1 × 1 × 10 mm) volume element or voxel within the scanning field, depending on the zoom factor. The depth of this tissue block is determined by the scan collimation or scan thickness. Voxel size is directly coupled to spatial resolution, because structures smaller than the voxel, unless they are quite different in attenuation from the surrounding tissues, will not be seen. In most current systems, the display is well matched to resolution, and the detail is limited only by the X-ray geometry, rather than by the method chosen for display.

CT imaging allows attenuation values to be assigned to various organs and anatomic regions. However, there is considerable variation in these numbers, such that CT attenuation values cannot be regarded as absolute (43). The most important factors affecting CT numbers include the processing algorithm of the CT unit, the exposure factors, the patient's body habitus, the configuration of the image, the presence of adjacent artifact-inducing structures, the height of the examining couch, partial-volume averaging, and individual CT machine variations. Because of these many variables, quantitative applications of CT imaging, such as bone mineral analysis and pulmonary nodule calcium determinations, demand great attention to detail (13).

Image Processing

CT images are created by "filtered back-projection" of the raw data. Each CT system has a unique process for managing the numerical information, although the processes are similar. The operator may alter the display of the CT image by employing reconstruction filters or "kernels" to best represent the clinically relevant detail. This process involves superimposing a mathematical curve or function on the actual detector response curve to modify pixel values based on the difference in density between adjacent voxels. These filtering functions usually are nonlinear and often are quite complex. Many such kernels or algorithms are available (7). A few of these filters are used relatively often in clinical practice: (a) a sharp or high-pass spatial filter, (b) an edge-enhancement kernel, and (c) a smoothing function.

The sharp filter enhances higher spatial frequencies and sacrifices the display of lower spatial frequencies, producing better-defined edges, but slightly noisier images. In general, sharp kernels are preferred for looking at high-contrast areas such as bone.

An edge-enhancement kernel, simply described, emphasizes regional borders of differing attenuation values.

A smoothing function alters voxel values by mathematically averaging adjacent voxels to diminish variations that might be due to statistical noise.

These filters may be variously combined to form other kernels. One must become familiar with the algorithm choices of the available CT machine to be able to choose among them knowledgeably. For example, high-resolution lung images may be achieved by employing a high spatial filter with edge enhancement in addition to narrow collimation, often referred to as a "bone algorithm" (62,71).

Reconstruction speed will vary among CT units, and depending on the level of image quality desired, variations are also available on any individual CT unit. Though acceptable reconstruction times are highly subjective, a reconstruction time longer than about 15 sec may significantly hamper examination efficiency.

CT images are viewed by utilizing preselected windows or by manually selecting a window width and window center. The window width determines the number of attenuation values to be displayed over the 20 available shades of gray. That number may be very large, including 2,000 CT numbers, or very small, such as 100 CT attenuation values. The window center determines where that range of CT numbers will be centered. For example, a narrow window width of 100 and a window center at zero will specify that all CT values less than −50 be displayed as black, and all CT numbers greater than +50 be displayed as white, with the CT numbers between −50 and +50 being displayed over the available shades of gray. One image may require several different window settings to demonstrate the available information (Fig. 10).

Manually manipulating window widths or routinely requesting narrow window widths with window levels of 30 to 100 is mandatory when searching for subtle attenuation differences. One excellent and dramatic example of that point is seen in the CT evaluation for aortic dissection. The differential contrast enhancement between true and false lumens or an intimal flap may be seen as isolated signs of dissection. Unless narrow-window-width

displays are reviewed, such subtle evidence of a dissection may be overlooked (76).

Filming is a critical link in the diagnostic process, because films are the primary method of diagnosis in most institutions. We prefer a format with 12 to 15 images on a 14 × 17 film. Although this potentially diminishes the perceptibility of detail by making images relatively small, this is believed to be a reasonable pragmatic compromise.

A camera option worth considering is a bulk-loaded or auto-loaded film capacity in which films are automatically fed into the camera, rather than individually loaded by cassette. Because filming requires a great deal of time, the use of a bulk-loaded system can significantly decrease personnel overtime or even eliminate the need for a partial or full-time position in a busy institution. Direct connection to an automatic processor is also desirable.

Artifacts

Artifacts are common in CT, even with state-of-the-art scanners. Many of the common CT artifacts are related to the exposure time, which, relative to conventional radiography, is quite long. Patient motion, patient breathing, bowel motion, blood vessel pulsations, and cardiac motion all contribute artifacts to the CT image even when 3- to 5-sec scan times are used. Residual barium in bowel, moving air–fluid levels in the abdominal viscera, and the radiopaque markers of various tubes and catheters virtually always produce artifacts on CT images (Fig. 11). However, these artifacts rarely are extensive enough to prevent a diagnostic examination.

High-density objects, such as surgical ligation clips, are other common sources of CT artifacts. The degree of image degradation, to a large extent, depends on the type of surgical clip. Four commonly used clip materials, tantalum, stainless steel, titanium, and polydioxanone, have been studied in vitro (31). Tantalum, with its very high radiodensity, produced severe artifacts that tended to obscure virtually the entire image. Stainless steel also produced artifacts, but these were limited to the region near the staple, preserving the rest of the image. The titanium clip and the nonmetallic resorbable polydioxanone clip caused almost no artifact. (These latter surgical devices also only minimally degraded MR images.)

Other metallic objects, such as femoral prostheses, usually seriously degrade the CT image. There are computer techniques available that allow linear interpolation of the missing data (38). This algorithm requires that the operator use a light pen to identify margins of the artifact source. The image data are then recalculated, and a new image is reconstructed. This process, requiring approximately 2 min per image, is very successful when the metallic object is structurally simple. For more complex objects, this method works less well.

Another common artifact in CT, especially in the pelvis

A,B

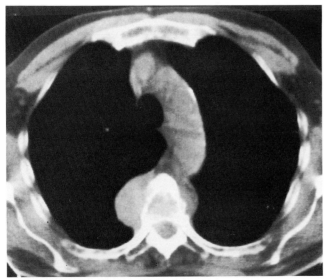

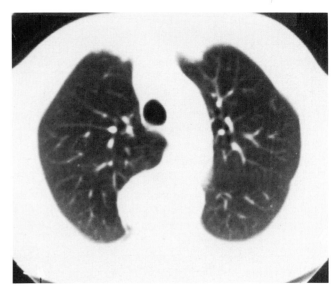

C

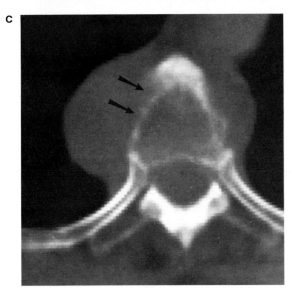

FIG. 10. Window manipulation. Three different window settings for otherwise identical images allow specific evaluation of (**A**) soft tissue of the mediastinum and chest wall, (**B**) the lungs, and (**C**) bone in this patient with a plasmacytoma originating from and eroding a thoracic vertebral body (*arrows*).

FIG. 11. Computer-generated artifacts. Previously administered conventional barium retained in the splenic flexure compromises image quality only slightly in this instance. However, more extensive collections can seriously degrade the image and preclude or delay CT examination.

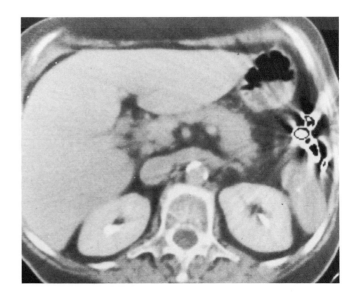

and shoulder regions, results from what is termed the "beam-hardening effect." Lower-energy components of the polychromatic X-ray beam are preferentially absorbed in the patient, leaving the transmitted beam with photons of higher average voltage. Thus, the greater the thickness and/or the greater the physical density of tissue traversed by the X-ray beam, the higher the average energy of the beam becomes. Tissues exposed to this higher average energy will appear to have lower attenuation values than would be seen if the beam-hardening effect were not present. Beam hardening may be alleviated somewhat by filtering the X-ray beam with a metal filter as it leaves the tube, thus narrowing the X-ray spectrum before it is affected by the patient. X-rays are then attenuated exponentially in the patient, and standard computed corrections are made for beam hardening. These corrections are imperfect, however, and are affected by numerous factors, including the size of the patient, the positions of dense structures within the field, the presence of contrast material that alters the overall tissue density, and the immediate surroundings of the region of interest.

Most types of artifacts (e.g., streaks, density changes, beam-hardening artifact) have multiple physical causes, and most physical sources of artifacts (e.g., motion) have several different types of effects on images (7). Therefore, when acting to minimize an artifact, one should realize that total elimination of the artifact may be impossible. However, simple changes such as taking external lines and cables out of the scanner gantry may vastly improve an image. In the case of beam hardening, the multiple effects include a cupping artifact and a shift in CT attenuation number. The cupping artifact consists of a low-density streak between or adjacent to high-density structures. The CT number shift of beam hardening usually is linear or "streaked" across an image, extending from a high-density region. These are particularly noticeable near dense areas such as the femoral heads or ribs or metallic prostheses.

Flow artifacts after intravenous administration of contrast material are extremely common and may simulate intraluminal abnormalities (29,79). Such a "pseudothrombus" most often occurs in large venous structures such as the superior vena cava or the suprarenal inferior vena cava. Laminar flow or the effect of unopacified venous effluent leads to the appearance of an irregular and poorly defined region of relative lack of contrast enhancement. One can often distinguish the pseudothrombus simply by observing higher attenuation values than would be expected for a true thrombus and noticing its relative lack of margination. If these observations are not conclusive, a dynamic imaging sequence should be carried out. The appearance of a pseudothrombus will change on successive images and will disappear completely on images obtained at peak contrast enhancement.

Vertebral body pseudofractures have been described as

CT image artifacts seen in severe spinal curvature (9). A coronally oriented fracture will be simulated in severe kyphosis, and a sagittally oriented fracture will be seen in severe scoliosis. A CT digital radiograph in the same plane as the deformity will define this type of artifact and should prevent misinterpretation.

Different CT scanners have different sensitivities to artifact formation, affecting the incidence, intensity, and types of artifacts. Third-generation CT units, for example, often demonstrate ring artifacts due to detector imbalance. These may simulate abnormalities.

Unique artifacts related to the digital imaging techniques involved in obtaining a preliminary CT digital film have been described. The best-defined artifact of scanogram systems is the image alteration secondary to motion during a scanogram utilizing a narrow scanning beam (11). Angled contours, pseudofractures of bone, image shortening or lengthening, and simulated soft-tissue masses may all occur as a result of subject motion during image acquisition.

CT PATIENTS

Preparation

The person being scanned is, of course, central to a CT examination. Most patients are more than willing to cooperate, but they need to know what they can expect and what is expected of them. It is important to explain how long an examination is likely to take and how long patients will need to hold their breath. Likewise, informing patients of the need to hold still and the need for each breath holding to be of approximately the same depth can greatly facilitate efficient imaging. It is advisable to rehearse a sequence before beginning the examination.

There are times when it is helpful to ask a patient to hyperventilate slightly prior to imaging to increase the length of a breath holding. Occasionally there is such difficulty in suspending respiration that fewer artifacts will be encountered if the patient is asked to breathe quietly.

Patient preparation unique to the region being examined will be dealt with in more detail in the section on imaging protocols at the end of this chapter. We prefer that oral intake be restricted, or that only clear liquids be administered, prior to an abdominal CT study or any study that is likely to require intravenous contrast material. The reasons for this approach are to decrease the chance of aspiration, to allow the patient to tolerate larger amounts of oral contrast material, and to minimize the chance that there will be filling defects in the stomach. When imaging the abdomen, large volumes of oral contrast material should be given to obtain adequate bowel opacification.

Respiratory Commands

The optimal phase of respiration during which to image varies by region, recommendations are in the examination protocols later in this chapter. Asking the patient to practice the following respiratory commands prior to imaging is effective in achieving patient cooperation. Most patients are able, with minimal coaching, to follow the respiratory commands for CT examinations. Repetitive imaging is more demanding, however, and patient cooperation is necessary for studies that include more than one body region, such as the chest and abdomen.

Variations in image appearance due to respiratory-phase differences are not trivial, especially in the lower chest and upper abdomen. In this region, it is more critical to have complete patient cooperation. For example, interscan variations in the degree of inspiration may make it difficult to completely examine a pulmonary nodule. Failure to detect a 1.5-cm pulmonary nodule has been reported and attributed to interscan respiratory variation (42). Imaging at end tidal volume has been used to avoid this possible pitfall, because more consistent respiratory cycles can be expected when respiration is suspended in expiration rather than in inspiration. However, this latter technique has limited utility because it results in suboptimal images for evaluating lung interstitium and mediastinum.

Feedback monitoring has been advocated by some (60) to improve the patient's respiratory control. This technique, requiring placement of a strain gauge around the lower thorax, has not been generally adopted, because it is cumbersome and time-consuming.

In addition to varying the imaging level for both normal organs and pathologic findings, the phase of respiration may determine the appearances of certain structures. The configuration and thickness of the diaphragmatic crura may change depending on the phase of respiration and the degree of muscular contraction of the diaphragm (1,82). In expiration, or with a Valsalva maneuver, the diaphragm may appear thickened and irregular.

Positioning

Supine positioning is routinely used for most CT studies. The patient position for body imaging usually is not critical, therefore comfort may dictate the imaging position. Other positions are helpful at times for differentiating between normal variation and pathologic abnormalities. For example, a prominent gastroesophageal junction may be differentiated from a mass by use of left lateral decubitus or prone images (Fig. 12).

Certain anatomic structures change their relative locations according to the imaging position (4). The descending aorta and the kidneys show dramatic caudal and ventral displacement on prone views, as compared with supine. The heart, pulmonary nodules, pulmonary hila, liver, spleen, stomach, and transverse colon also move caudally and ventrally in the prone position. Other structures, such as the gastroesophageal junction, duodenum, and pelvic structures, show minimal or no change.

CT CONTRAST ENHANCEMENT

Contrast enhancement using both oral and intravenous material is valuable in CT. Oral contrast material is used in virtually all abdominal CT studies and is used in chest examinations when it is important to define the esophagus more precisely. The utility of intravenous contrast material is not in question; all agree that it is extremely useful. However, there is no consensus on a "best approach" for using intravenous contrast material to tailor the CT examination to answer specific questions. At the Mallinckrodt Institute, intravenous contrast material is used in approximately 35% of abdominal studies and in about 20% of chest studies in a tailored fashion to answer specific questions. At the University of Alabama at Birmingham, more than 80% of CT studies are performed with intravenous contrast material. The advantages of "routine" intravenous administration of contrast material are to decrease the time required to do a study by dispensing with

A,B

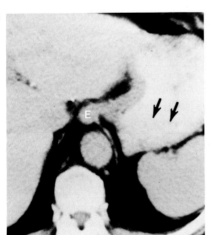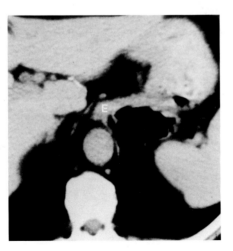

FIG. 12. Patient position. A: With the patient supine, the posterior gastric fundus is incompletely opacified even after administration of additional contrast material, suggesting a possible gastric-wall mass (arrows). B: Image after prone positioning demonstrates a normal posterior gastric fundus. (A left lateral decubitus position is helpful when the medial aspect of the posterior fundus is suspected to be abnormal.)

the noncontrast images and to reduce the need to closely monitor studies. In addition, normal or anomalous vascular structures are immediately identified.

The disadvantages are that substantial numbers of individuals are subjected to intravenous contrast material unnecessarily, and the subsequent administration of contrast material is limited by the routine dose. In addition, it may be more difficult to obtain optimal and consistent enhancement with the infusion technique. Suboptimal contrast enhancement may not allow sufficient definition to distinguish vascular structures and may even obscure pathologic lesions.

Gastrointestinal Contrast Enhancement

Bowel opacification is mandatory in almost all abdominal CT examinations, because unopacified bowel may simulate pathologic abnormalities (Fig. 13). The two commonly used oral contrast agents are dilute barium (e.g., Readi Cat, E-Z-EM Co.) and dilute water-soluble iodine (e.g., Gastroview, Mallinckrodt). Either will provide quite satisfactory bowel opacification. Barium has the advantages of being inert and, according to some, of being more palatable to more patients. There does not appear to be sufficient evidence to attribute superiority of any of these agents for all oral contrast indications. Guidelines already established for oral contrast material in conventional radiology apply in CT as well: A suspicion of bowel perforation mandates a water-soluble agent, whereas the possibility of aspiration dictates use of dilute barium. Another contrast material, a 12.5% corn oil emulsion (COE) has been recommended, though not yet tested in a large series, for use in asthenic individuals and for more careful evaluation of the stomach and duodenum (56). It can also be used in those situations in which conventional oral contrast material would obscure adjacent calcifications. Because use of the fat-density agent results in bowel loops with low-density centers, COE should be avoided in CT examinations performed to search for an abscess. It should also be avoided when there is a potential for aspiration. Because of these latter drawbacks and the limited advan-

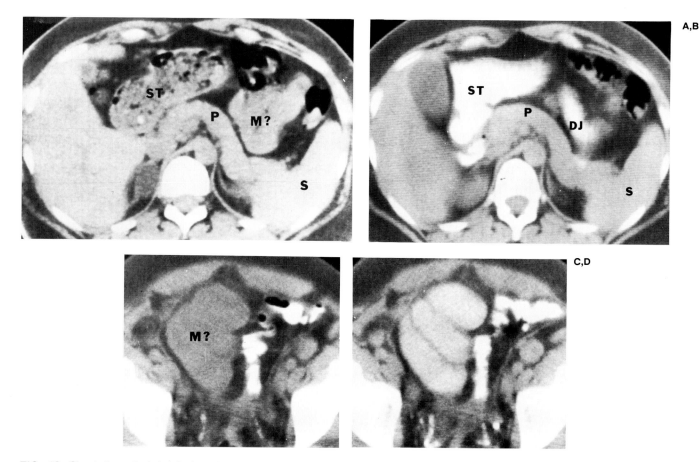

FIG. 13. Simulation of abdominal and pelvic masses by unopacified bowel. **A:** Image through the upper abdomen shows a questionable soft-tissue mass (M?); P, pancreas; S, spleen; ST, stomach. **B:** Subsequent image after oral administration of contrast agent demonstrates opacification as well as a change in the configuration of the suspected mass consistent with a small-bowel loop at the duodenal-jejunal junction (DJ). **C:** Image of the pelvis in another patient shows a questionable large mass (M?). **D:** Image after additional administration of low-density barium and a suitable delay shows the suspected mass to be some mildly dilated ileal loops.

tages of this agent, it has not yet received widespread acceptance.

Beyond the considerations of what contrast material is to be used, there are some variations in how one may achieve adequate or optimal opacification of various enteric regions. Gastric distension, necessary for evaluation of gastric-wall thickness, can be accomplished by administering oral contrast material immediately prior to imaging. An alternative approach is to administer gas granules (e.g., E-Z-EM Co.) with the contrast material, thus distending the stomach better than with contrast material alone (Fig. 14). Rapid distension of the stomach tends to stimulate peristalsis, leading to a greater number of artifacts generated from moving air–fluid levels; however, these artifacts usually do not interfere with the diagnostic value of the image. Whereas 0.1 mg glucagon intravenously has been advocated to reduce peristalsis, this is rarely, if ever, necessary when 3- to 5-sec imaging times are used.

Colonic opacification may be achieved in several ways. Large volumes (600–800 ml) of dilute barium administered orally at least several hours prior to the examination usually are successful. However, a small volume (30 ml) of iodinated water-soluble contrast material given the night before the examination also produces excellent distal bowel opacification (46). When colonic opacification is incomplete, rectal insufflation of air or radiopaque contrast material may be helpful.

Vascular Contrast Enhancement

Indications

Specific indications for intravenous contrast material in CT include determining the relative vascularity and the vascular characteristics of a mass, distinguishing vessels or differentiating a vascular anomaly or abnormality from a neoplastic mass, maximizing anatomic and lesion detectability, and opacifying the urinary tract. Iodinated intravenous contrast agents aid in the search for subtle findings or occult lesions (8,51). Often the attenuation-value difference between normal and abnormal will increase after administration of contrast material. This is particularly true in the liver, where minimally dilated intrahepatic and extrahepatic bile ducts sometimes are recognized confidently only on postcontrast images. Intravenous administration of contrast material clearly increases the sensitivity of CT and should therefore always be used, unless contraindicated, when the liver and biliary tract are regions of primary interest.

Intravascular Contrast Agents

Iodinated intravenous contrast material, first introduced for urography in 1929, is used extensively in CT. Among the many available iodinated contrast agents, three characteristics (iodine content, viscosity, and osmolality) are important in regard to their use in CT because they determine the ability to inject a maximum amount of iodine in a small volume and to deliver that volume quickly, and, to some degree, they determine the number and extent of adverse reactions. These features for the commonly used contrast agents are listed in Table 1 (22). The pharmacologic parameters of these urographic contrast agents are otherwise similar; there are no significant differences in tissue dynamics or distribution. In general, all these agents share a low risk of reaction or serious complication. The technique of administration of contrast material does not affect the incidence of adverse reactions (32). The total amount of iodine delivered, however, does seem to be important; patients receiving less than 20 g of iodine have been shown to have fewer

A,B

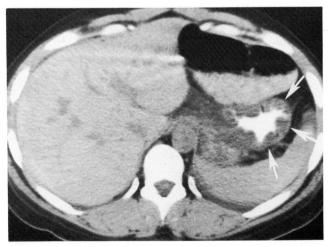 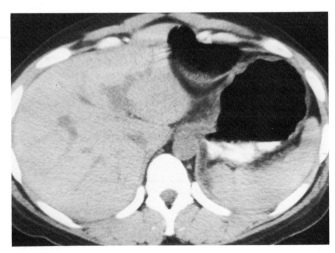

FIG. 14. Bowel distension. A: Gastric-wall thickening in the fundus is suggested (*arrows*) on initial image. However, after more oral contrast material and effervescent tablets were administered (B), the gastric wall appears normal.

TABLE 1. *Parameters for intravenous contrast agents*

Agent	Iodine content (mg/ml)	Viscosity (in cP) at 37°C	Osmolality
Conray-400	400	4.1	2348
Isovue	370	9.4	796
Renografin-76	370	9.0	2188
Hypaque-76	370	9.0	2016
Hexabrix	320	7.5	600
Hypaque-50	300	2.3	1515
Renografin-60	288	3.9	1549
Conray-60	282	4.0	1539
Conray-43	202	2.0	1000

adverse reactions (3). Unfortunately, most indications require more than 20 g of iodine.

We have preferred to use iothalamate meglumine (Conray-400) in the majority of CT studies and have used it almost exclusively for bolus injection. The substantially more expensive nonionic agents are reserved for elderly patients or individuals, diabetic or not, with compromised renal function who are at high risk for developing adverse reactions. Though high cost has been a deterrent to widespread use, it has been suggested that low-osmolality agents may be indicated in high-risk patients, specifically for CT studies requiring large doses of intravenous contrast material (45).

Techniques of Administration

Studies of bolus geometry for contrast agents have shown that the injection speed and volume are both important factors in maximizing contrast enhancement (14). The vascular opacification achieved by bolus technique can be compared with that achieved via infusion by observing the arteriovenous iodine difference as measured on CT images. Three phases of intravascular contrast enhancement can be defined: a bolus-effect phase, a nonequilibrium phase, and an equilibrium phase (12). Maximum vascular enhancement, the bolus effect, occurs only with rapid injection of contrast medium (52) (Fig. 15). This phase is transient, lasting only about 40 to 60 sec. The second or nonequilibrium phase occurs about 1 min after bolus administration or during rapid infusion of a relatively large volume of contrast material. The final phase, or equilibrium, occurs when there is a negligible arteriovenous iodine difference. This phase corresponds to approximately 2 min post bolus and persists until the end of the infusion. Based on these types of observations, it is apparent that a bolus of contrast material produces maximal opacification of both vessels and parenchyma (12,84). It is during the bolus effect and nonequilibrium phase that clinically useful information is provided, when lesions are least likely to be isodense because of slow infusion of contrast material into them.

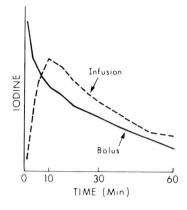

FIG. 15. Bolus versus infusion. The bolus technique of administering intravenous iodinated contrast material results in a higher concentration of intravascular iodine than infusion methods can achieve when equal amounts of contrast material are injected. A bolus of contrast material combined with sequential or dynamic imaging is the optimal method for administering intravenous contrast material when high intravascular levels are desired. (Adapted from ref. 52.)

Following vascular enhancement, there is enhancement of the soft tissues, corresponding to phases two and three. Dependent on diffusion, this characteristic is more variable than vascular opacification. Diffusion of the contrast material from vessels begins almost immediately following injection, so that after one pass through the body, 50% to 75% of the material has diffused from the vascular space, and approximately 45 min after injection the CT numbers return to base-line values (83). Pragmatically, soft-tissue enhancement has some value in improving lesion detectability, e.g., in kidney and liver, and in distinguishing between normal organs and pathologic processes. For example, a soft-tissue mass in a nephrectomy bed that is enhanced to the same degree as the pancreas becomes less suspicious for recurrent renal carcinoma and more likely to be a normal pancreatic tail (Fig. 16).

Many approaches to intravenous administration of contrast material have been used, reflecting the inadequacies of any one method. However, the major techniques are (a) simple, hand-delivered bolus injection, (b) variations of the bolus method, (c) infusion, (d) mechanical injection, and (e) CT angiography.

A small-volume (25–50 ml) bolus technique at one or a few scanning levels is used to achieve vessel opacification (Fig. 17) and to determine the vascular characteristics of a specific lesion (Fig. 18). The injection of contrast material containing 10 to 20 g of iodine, performed quickly (within 2 min) to ensure a well-defined bolus, should be delivered into a large vein through an 18- or 19-gauge needle. A medially directed antecubital vein that enters the basilic system should be chosen, if possible, because it has a more direct route to the superior vena cava and will not be obstructed by the over-the-head arm position usually adopted during CT with intravenous contrast ma-

A,B

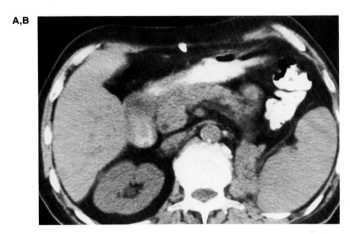
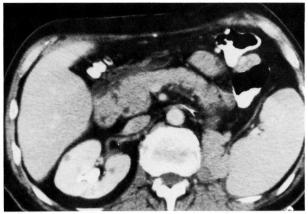

FIG. 16. Intravenous contrast enhancement. **A:** A soft-tissue mass in the left nephrectomy site, appearing discontinuous with the pancreas, was suspicious for recurrent neoplasm. However, after intravenous contrast material was administered (**B**), the "mass," enhancing to the same degree as the body of the pancreas, was shown to be the tail of the pancreas.

terial. To delineate specific vessels, e.g., suspected aortic dissection or renal vein thrombosis, the bolus technique combined with dynamic imaging i.e., serial images at a predetermined level, is required for optimal evaluation (39,83). One or more of these serial images may clarify a confusing finding, e.g., demonstrate tortuous or anomalous vessels simulating a mass. Time–density curves have been obtained using this technique; however, they appear to have limited practical value.

Although bolus administration is the most effective method of achieving excellent vascular enhancement, usually it is difficult or impossible to obtain a sufficient number of images after a single injection to assess more than one plane of interest, because the effect lasts less than a minute. Repeating small-volume bolus injections at a few selected levels is possible, but because of limita-

tions on the amount of urographic contrast material that may be safely administered (a total dose less than or equal to 1 g iodine/kg has been recommended), evaluating large regions such as the entire liver is not feasible. Another practical approach is to combine a small bolus injection followed in quick succession by a rapid infusion. Initially, a small-volume (25–50 ml) bolus is given, followed by prompt infusion of 150 ml of 60% iodine solution through an 18- or 19-gauge needle. This usually allows 12 to 18 images to be obtained while infusing contrast material.

Infusion flow rates of 20 to 50 ml/min usually will achieve medium- and large-vessel enhancement and are clinically effective in many instances, such as when evaluating both kidneys or the intrahepatic and extrahepatic biliary tree. If reconstruction times are relatively long, delayed processing may be appropriate. This method al-

A,B

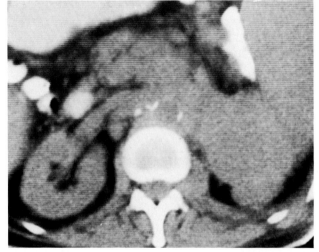
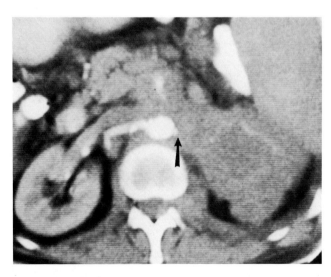

FIG. 17. Vascular enhancement. **A:** A bulky lymphomatous mass occupies the left renal fossa and merges with paraaortic lymph nodes surrounding the aorta on a precontrast image. **B:** Image after a bolus injection of contrast material shows an opacified normal right renal artery, but the left renal artery is totally obstructed near its origin (*arrow*).

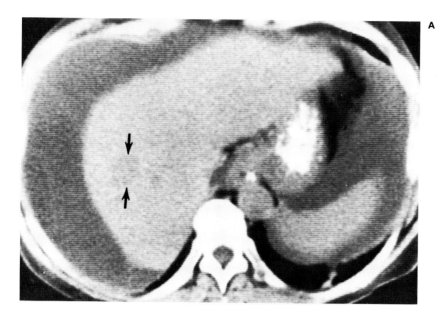

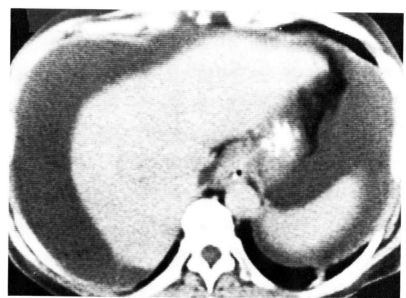

FIG. 18. Bolus versus infusion techniques. A: A low-attenuation-value hepatic lesion (*arrows*) is seen in this precontrast image from a patient with cirrhosis and ascites. B: After intravenous administration of contrast material by rapid infusion, there is subtle enhancement of the lesion as compared with surrounding normal liver parenchyma rendering the lesion indistinguishable. C: Subsequent CT after a bolus injection of contrast material clearly demonstrates marked enhancement of the lesion, consistent with an arteriovenous fistula, presumably due to a prior liver biopsy.

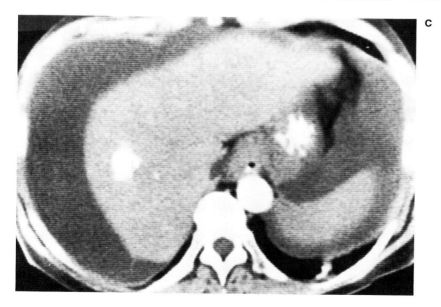

lows more flexibility in imaging because it ensures effective contrast enhancement with the convenience of obtaining multiple images at different levels. In addition, infusion may be superior to the bolus technique for opacifying certain organs such as the uterus (41). However, infusions of contrast material are sometimes more difficult to monitor, especially if imaging times are lengthy. Relative venous obstruction due to arm position may produce poor enhancement; thus, the advantages of contrast material may be lost while still exposing the patient to the risk of contrast-related reactions. Furthermore, in some cases, diagnostic information may be diminished by the infusion technique because of the tendency of some parenchymal lesions to become isodense with surrounding tissue (Fig. 18).

It has been shown that the speed of the injection definitely influences contrast enhancement (14). Injection speed can be maximized and best controlled by using a mechanical injector. Power injectors coupled with at least a 20-gauge venous catheter have proved safe with injection rates up to 5 ml/sec (23,44,53). Extensive extravasation, however, is a potential complication of mechanical injection of contrast material. Careful preparatory patient instruction, close monitoring of the injection, and a remote-control capability to stop the injection are all necessary to prevent untoward results. Mechanical injection is most effectively utilized in combination with table indexing to examine several different levels. Alternatively, administering 100 to 150 ml of contrast material through an 18- or 19-gauge needle will accomplish the same purpose (39). This "large-volume bolus" requires someone in the examination room to inject the contrast agent continuously while the examination is in progress. Different levels are selected by moving the couch between scans. This technique has proved successful in several situations, including evaluations of the pulmonary hila (63).

Hepatic CT angiography performed in conjunction with selective catheterization of celiac or mesenteric arteries has contributed important information in patients with known tumor involvement of the liver (49). Specifically, it is more sensitive than either conventional contrast-enhanced CT or conventional angiography for detection of additional foci of primary or metastatic liver involvement. Selective CT angiography is particularly helpful in detecting small tumors in the left lateral segment (49). In addition, it successfully demonstrates portal vein involvement and establishes the blood flow distribution of hepatic arterial branches. All of these findings can be important to the surgeon contemplating lobectomy or arterial embolization therapy.

The appearance of a lesion after injection of contrast material can be crucial in making a specific diagnosis. For example, a cavernous hemangioma of the liver or an arteriovenous malformation has unique enhancement characteristics (5,36). The dose and type of injection and the timing of the study are critical in obtaining maximum information following administration of contrast material for this purpose. The optimal volume of contrast agent depends somewhat on the size of the lesion relative to the anticipated vascular supply, with larger lesions requiring larger doses. In general, however, 25 to 50 ml of contrast material will suffice, administered as a bolus injection, followed by immediate serial imaging, with a minimum of three images obtained in the first minute. If a hepatic cavernous hemangioma, which typically demonstrates delayed central contrast enhancement, is suspected, larger doses, e.g., 100 ml, often are required, combined with delayed imaging at 1- to 5-min intervals up to 10 min.

Contrast Enhancement of Other Regions

Rarely it may be useful to opacify the thoracic duct, e.g., in suspected thoracic duct laceration. Oral ingestion of 50% ethiodized oil (Ethiodol) and a fat emulsion (Magnacal) has been shown to enhance the thoracic duct after a few hours delay (15).

Direct enhancement of the bile ducts with conventional cholangiographic agents has very limited, if any, application, because even mildly elevated bilirubin levels preclude duct opacification. Gallbladder opacification can be achieved in more than 80% of patients by giving oral cholangiographic contrast material the night prior to the CT examination; however, the indication for performing such a study is exceedingly rare.

Other Contrast Agents

Although water-soluble contrast agents are readily available, widely accepted, and relatively risk-free, the tissue dynamics of these agents are far from ideal (25). The iodinated compounds, extensively studied long before the advent of CT, are not specifically metabolized or concentrated except in the kidney, and even more important, as has been described, they are quickly equilibrated with the extravascular space (49,50). These characteristics limit the specificity of today's intravenous contrast agents. Research has been directed toward developing organ- or lesion-targeted compounds (32). Contrast agents specifically designed for hepatic CT are being developed. Contrast agents primarily taken up by the reticuloendothelial system are attractive alternatives to the water-soluble agents. The advantages are (a) greater sensitivity, (b) greater organ selectivity, and (c) longer duration of contrast enhancement. One such agent, a liposoluble organ-specific contrast agent (EOE-13) (70,78), is an ethiodized oil emulsion injected intravenously. Selective uptake by the reticuloendothelial system results in contrast enhancement of the liver and spleen. Though this agent improves the capability for detecting small hepatic and splenic lesions (70,77) and allows greater specificity in evaluating upper-quadrant masses (78) when normal splenic tissue is a consideration, it remains an experimental drug with numerous problems. Modified, but chemically closely related, products are under development. Several other hepatic contrast agents are also being investigated, including radiopaque liposomes, iodinated starch particles, perfluorocytylbromide, iodipamide ethyl ester, and cholesteryl iopanoate.

CT TECHNIQUES UNIQUE TO SPECIFIC REGIONS AND INDICATIONS

Conduct of Posttraumatic CT Examinations

Posttraumatic abdominal CT examinations are best performed utilizing intravenous contrast material. Except in unusual circumstances, only postcontrast imaging is done, because these images virtually always contain more precise information than those without contrast enhancement. There are some theoretical advantages to imaging prior to intravenous administration of contrast material. For example, an isodense or hyperdense hematoma may be seen best without intravenous contrast material. However, the potential benefits of obtaining images with and without the use of intravenous contrast material have not been found to be worth the additional time and effort. Expeditious conduct of the CT examination is very important in these patients, who often have multiple serious injuries. The approach used by us and by others (19) has been to administer a bolus of contrast medium, followed by a rapid infusion. Intravenous contrast material makes identification of nonenhancing collections easier by enhancing the adjacent tissues. Hematomas, for example, are more obvious after administration of contrast material.

Posttraumatic abdominal CT images should be obtained at 10-mm intervals with 10-mm collimation through the upper abdomen, including both kidneys. Imaging the pelvis has also been found to be mandatory, because fluid collections may pool in the pelvis and otherwise not be appreciated. Images through the pelvis with 10-mm collimation and at 2-cm intervals generally are sufficient.

Though the lower thorax is included on abdominal CT images, it is easy to miss abnormalities such as pneumothorax and lung contusions if the pertinent images are not viewed with lung window settings. As a guideline, if lung is included in the study, then images at lung window settings should be obtained for review.

Finally, artifacts can be minimized if one takes the time to remove as many tubes and other foreign objects from the scanning field as possible prior to imaging. Decompressing the stomach just prior to imaging also helps decrease the artifacts, presumably by diminishing peristalsis.

Imaging Protocols

There is a common and understandable aversion to cookbook medicine. None of us wants to monitor CT or any other imaging study by rote or reflex. However, to agree on a standard method for evaluating a given region and specific indication not only is acceptable but should be encouraged. It provides a model against which other methods can be compared. It allows organized analysis of results. It also affords the practical advantage of delegating responsibility to trainees or technologists in some rational and predictable manner. Arranged by region of interest and indications, Tables 2 to 22 present some of the common protocols used for body CT examinations. (CT examinations of the spine, as well as pediatric CT, are addressed in their respective sections.) Kept in the CT examination room, these protocols can serve as an immediate reference and as a teaching tool for technologists and radiologists being introduced to CT. These guidelines are not designed to avoid all thought processes, but rather to provide a consistent approach that may be further tailored according to the clinical question to be answered and the initial image findings. There may be a relatively large number of cases that cannot be neatly categorized according to the following protocols. Also, some examinations will overlap two or more regions of interest. Modifications will be required in each instance.

TABLE 2. *Region of interest: larynx*

Oral contrast:	None
Digital scout film:	Lateral
Phase of respiration:	During slow inspiration[a]
Slice thickness:	3–5 mm
Slice interval:	3–5 mm
Superior extent:	Base of tongue
Inferior extent:	Proximal trachea
Intravenous contrast:	All patients with prior neck surgery should receive 30 ml Conray-400 by bolus, followed by rapid infusion of 150 ml Conray-60; also useful at times in assessing for lymphadenopathy.
Comments:	(1) The neck should be hyperextended. (2) The patient should be instructed not to swallow during imaging. (3) A small field of view (120–250 cm) affords the best resolution. (4) Metallic tracheostomy tubes should be replaced by a plastic tracheostomy appliance.

[a] Various laryngography maneuvers may be used to better define problem areas: *phonation* (''e'') used for distending the pyriform sinuses, supraglottic tumors around the sinuses, and aryepiglottic folds; *reverse* ''e'' for laryngeal ventricles (very difficult for most patients to accomplish in supine position).

TABLE 3. *Region of interest: neck and mediastinum. Indication: search for parathyroid adenoma*

Oral contrast:	None
Digital scout film:	Anteroposterior from thyroid notch to carina
Phase of respiration:	During slow inspiration
Slice thickness:	3–5 mm to left innominate vein, then 8–10 mm to carina
Slice interval:	3–5 mm to left innominate vein, then 8–10 mm to carina
Superior extent:	Thyroid cartilage
Inferior extent:	Carina
Intravenous contrast:	30 ml Conray-400 by bolus, followed by rapid infusion of 150 ml Conray-60
Comments:	(1) The neck should be hyperextended. (2) Images should be reconstructed on a small field of view to optimize resolution.

TABLE 4. *Region of interest: neck and mediastinum. Indication: brachial plexus evaluation*

Oral contrast:	None
Digital scout film:	Anteroposterior of the neck and upper chest, with arms at side[a]
Phase of respiration:	Suspended inspiration
Slice thickness:	2–5 mm
Slice interval:	2–5 mm
Superior extent:	Cricoid ring or C4
Inferior extent:	Horizontal course of left innominate vein or T4
Intravenous contrast:	Contrast infusion may be used to clarify confusing areas. The contralateral side should be infused to prevent contrast-induced artifacts related to undiluted contrast material; bolus injections often cause artifacts (26).
Comments:	Filming at bone windows as well as at lung and mediastinal settings should be considered.

[a] With some CT scanners, fewer artifacts may result if the arms are elevated overhead.

TABLE 5. *Region of interest: chest. Indication: survey*

Oral contrast:	None
Digital scout film:	Anteroposterior
Phase of respiration:	Suspended inspiration
Slice thickness:	8–10 mm 4–5-mm collimation may improve spatial resolution and should be considered to define fissures, airways, and other confusing areas
Slice interval:	10 mm[a]
Superior extent:	Superior margin of clavicles
Inferior extent:	Through adrenals
Intravenous contrast:	Used routinely at University of Alabama at Birmingham, but is used only when necessary to define the mediastinum and/or determine the relationship of a mass to mediastinal vessels at Mallinckrodt Institute of Radiology.
Comments:	To achieve optimal opacification of the hila, mechanical injection of 75–100 ml at a rate of 2 ml/sec for 15 sec, followed by 1 ml/sec, has been effective. Automatic table indexing during injection allows survey of the entire hilar regions.

[a] 5-mm intervals if 5-mm collimation is used.

TABLE 6. *Region of interest: chest. Indication: characterization of a pulmonary nodule*

Oral contrast:	None
Digital scout film:	Orientation to depend on chest radiographic visualization of the nodule
Patient position:	Supine[a]
Phase of respiration:	End tidal volume ("Breathe in, breathe out, relax, hold your breath")
Slice thickness:	1–2 mm
Slice interval:	Contiguous
Superior extent:	Relative to site of lesion
Inferior extent:	Relative to site of lesion
Intravenous contrast:	Usually not necessary unless a vascular malformation is suspected
Comments:	(1) It is important to specify the machine and processing filter to be used uniformly for all pulmonary nodule evaluations. A sharp filter has produced the best results. (2) 8–10-mm collimation is used to localize the nodule; then 2-mm collimation at 2-mm increments is used to scan through the nodule. (3) At completion of clinical study, if the nodule is at least 6 mm in diameter and remains indeterminate (regular border, no obvious diffuse calcification), a chest phantom (Computerized Imaging Reference Systems, Norfolk, Va.) with the appropriate simulated nodule in a comparable position should then be scanned, and attenuation values between the patient's nodule and that of the phantom compared. (4) It is imperative that the reference nodule never be smaller than the patient's nodule. (5) The image of the patient used for CT-number determination should be through the center of the nodule, i.e., the image that shows the nodule to be the largest. (6) If an arteriovenous malformation is suspected, then rapid rescanning after a 50-ml intravenous contrast bolus is recommended.

[a] Prone position may be useful to distinguish between a suspected pulmonary nodule and a pulmonary vessel (68).

TABLE 7. *Region of interest: chest. Indication: suspect aortic dissection*

Oral contrast:	None
Digital scout film:	Anteroposterior
Phase of respiration:	Suspended inspiration
Slice thickness:	8–10 mm
Slice interval:	10 mm
Superior extent:	Superior to arch of aorta
Inferior extent:	Through mid-ventricular level
Intravenous contrast:	After initial noncontrast survey of thoracic aorta, bolus injections of approximately 30–50 ml each at the level of the mid-ascending aorta (so that ascending aorta and descending aorta are seen simultaneously) and again at the arch level. (1) If no dissection, examination complete. (2) If type B dissection is demonstrated, start rapid infusion, and survey entire thorax (can do at 20-mm intervals) to determine extent of dissection, down to its caudal level (may need to go into abdomen). (3) If type A dissection is demonstrated, generally can stop and proceed to surgery or, sometimes, to angiography.
Comment:	Should stop the examination if noncontrast images show fresh blood in the mediastinum, pleural space, or pericardium.

TABLE 8. *Region of interest: chest.*
Indication: evaluate for bronchiectasis

Oral contrast:	None
Digital scout film:	Anteroposterior
Phase of respiration:	Suspended inspiration
Slice thickness:	2–4 mm (30)
Slice interval:	10 mm
Superior extent:	Lung apex
Inferior extent:	Diaphragm
Intravenous contrast:	None

TABLE 9. *Region of interest: abdomen-pelvis. Indication: survey*

Oral contrast:	600–900 ml oral contrast at least 1 hr before scanning, plus 300 ml oral contrast agent 15 min before scan begins
Digital scout film:	Anteroposterior
Phase of respiration:	Suspended expiration
Slice thickness:	8–10 mm
Slice interval:	15–20 mm
Superior extent:	Xiphoid (to include all of the retrocrural area)
Inferior extent:	Symphysis (or lower if inferior inguinal nodes need to be studied)
Intravenous contrast:	To evaluate vascularity of a mass or to define suspected lesions

TABLE 10. *Region of interest: pancreas. Indications: survey*

Oral contrast:	300–600 ml oral contrast agent 15 min before scanning
Digital scout film:	Anteroposterior
Phase of respiration:	Suspended expiration
Slice thickness:	8–10 mm (occasionally 4–5 mm in areas of special interest)
Slice interval:	10 mm
Superior extent:	Approximately 20 mm below xiphoid (or mid-L1)
Inferior extent:	Through third duodenum (or L2–3 interspace)
Intravenous contrast:	Enhancement of pancreatic parenchyma and surrounding vessels is exceedingly helpful in defining an observed or suspected abnormality.
Comments:	(1) Intravenous contrast agent is administered to visualize the pancreas and distinguish tortuous splenic vessels that may simulate a pancreatic mass. Aneurysms or pseudoaneurysms about the pancreas or dilated pancreatic duct may be documented as well. (2) In thin patients, a study of the entire pancreas may be optimized by scanning during an infusion of contrast material; however, a suspicious area in or near the pancreas usually is best evaluated using bolus technique. (3) Small or ductal lesions may be detected using 150 ml 60% intravenous contrast, with scanning begun 30 sec after the start of the injection.

TABLE 11. *Region of interest: liver-pancreas. Indication: suspected obstructive jaundice*

Oral contrast:	300 ml contrast agent 15 min before imaging, unless a common bile duct stone is strongly suspected
Digital scout film:	Anteroposterior
Patient position:	Supine
Phase of respiration:	Suspended expiration
Slice thickness:	10 mm; 4–5 mm collimation for improved spatial resolution should be considered, especially when (a) a point of transition from a dilated biliary system to a more normal biliary duct is seen and (b) common bile duct stones are suspected
Slice interval:	10 mm; 5-mm intervals should be used if 5-mm collimation is selected
Superior extent:	Dome of liver
Inferior extent:	Through third duodenum
Intravenous contrast:	Rapid infusion of contrast medium should begin once the appropriate level through the cephalad extent of the liver parenchyma is established. Bolus injections (25–50 ml) may be used to clarify a selected view.

TABLE 12. *Region of interest: abdomen. Indication: survey following acute trauma*

Oral contrast:	600 ml oral contrast at least 1 hr before imaging, plus 300 ml oral contrast 15 min before imaging begins; use water-soluble contrast material if bowel perforation is suspected
Digital scout film:	Anteroposterior
Phase of respiration:	Suspended expiration
Slice thickness:	8–10 mm
Slice interval:	10–20 mm, depending on clinical situation
Superior extent:	Top of diaphragm
Inferior extent:	Variable, depending on clinical situation
Intravenous contrast:	Should be used in *all* patients who have *no* contraindications to iodinated contrast: 50 ml Conray-400 as a bolus, followed by a rapid infusion of 150 ml of Conray-60. If a power injector is available, load the syringe with 200 ml Conray-60. Inject 1 ml/sec for 50 sec, then reduce injection rate to 0.5 ml/sec for the remainder. Begin imaging 50 sec after the initiation of contrast administration. Precontrast images usually are not necessary in acutely injured patients.

TABLE 13. *Region of interest: abdomen. Indication: suspect aortic aneurysm rupture or dissection*

Oral contrast:	None if acute rupture is suspected; otherwise, 600 ml oral contrast at least 1 hr before imaging; 300 ml oral contrast 15 min before imaging begins.
Digital scout film:	Anteroposterior
Phase of respiration:	Suspended expiration
Slice thickness:	8–10 mm
Slice interval:	10 mm at level of renal arteries; 20 mm for rest of abdomen
Superior extent:	Xiphoid
Inferior extent:	Aortic bifurcation (or lower if the status of iliac arteries is in question)
Intravenous contrast:	If aortic leak is suspected, precontrast images will help define fresh hemorrhage. Intravenous contrast material will be necessary in most, if not all, cases.

TABLE 14. *Region of interest: liver. Indications: survey for focal liver lesions (metastases)*

Oral contrast:	300 ml oral contrast material 15 min before imaging
Digital scout film:	Anteroposterior
Phase of respiration:	Suspended expiration
Slice thickness:	8–10 mm
Slice interval:	8–10 mm
Superior extent:	Dome of liver (approximately 20 mm above xiphoid)
Inferior extent:	Through the inferior tip of right lobe
Intravenous contrast:	(1) Localize dome of liver using the preliminary digital radiograph. (2) 18–20-gauge angiocatheter (18 preferred) into a medial antecubital vein. A mechanical injector is preferred if an appropriate intravenous route is available. The catheter should be monitored closely to ensure proper function of the injector. (Contrast extravasation is not uncommon with the use of automatic injectors and may lead to serious complications.) If there is any indication of malfunction, specifically extravasation, the injection should be terminated. (3) With the injector syringe loaded with 200 ml Conray-60, use an injection rate of 2 ml/sec for 15 sec, then a rate of 1 ml/sec for the duration of the imaging. (4) Start imaging 15 sec after injection is begun. (5) At least 8 images per minute should be obtained using the dynamic mode. Imaging of the entire liver should be completed in less than 3 min. (6) If there is a strong clinical suspicion of liver metastases and findings on conventional postcontrast images are either negative or equivocal, the liver should be reexamined at 1-cm intervals, 4–6 hr later. In these cases, a minimum of 150 ml of Conray-60 (90 g I) should be delivered before the needle is removed. The delayed imaging technique will not be beneficial unless the patient has received at least 50 g of iodine intravenously.

TABLE 15. *Region of interest: liver. Indication: characterization of a known focal mass*

Oral contrast:	Optional
Phase of respiration:	Suspended expiration
Slice thickness:	8–10 mm
Slice interval:	10 mm
Technique:	Precontrast images are obtained to locate the lesion. Bolus injection of 50–100 ml Conray-400, depending on the size of the lesion. Obtain 3–5 images during the first 60 sec following bolus injection, followed by an image at 2 min. If a cavernous hemangioma is suspected, additional images through the lesion should be obtained at 4, 6, 10, and 15 min, if necessary.

TABLE 16. *Region of interest: adrenal*

Oral contrast:	300–600 ml oral contrast material 30 min before imaging
Phase of respiration:	Suspended expiration
Slice thickness:	8–10 mm collimation (see Comments)
Slice interval:	10 mm (4–5-mm intervals to be used when collimation is reduced to 4–5 mm)
Superior extent:	Dome of diaphragm
Inferior extent:	To lower poles of kidneys (see Comments)
Intravenous contrast:	Occasionally helpful, e.g., to differentiate tortuous splenic artery or a venous varix from an adrenal mass or to accentuate the difference between a small nonenhancing mass and surrounding structures.
Comments:	(1) 10-mm collimation is usually adequate if screening for pheochromocytoma or adenoma in Cushing syndrome. For aldosteronoma (Conn syndrome), however, 4–5-mm collimation is essential to exclude a small adenoma. If screening for pheochromocytoma in an adult, and the adrenal area is normal, images to include the aortic bifurcation are necessary in order to detect involvement of the organ of Zuckerkandl. Images of the pelvis and mediastinum may also be obtained if there is biochemical or strong clinical support for the diagnosis of extraadrenal pheochromocytoma. (2) Glucagon should not be used in patients suspected of having pheochromocytoma, because it may precipitate a hypertensive crisis.

TABLE 17. *Region of interest: kidney*

Oral contrast:	300–600 ml oral contrast material 30–60 min before imaging
Phase of respiration:	Suspended expiration
Slice thickness:	8–10 mm
Slice interval:	10 mm
Superior extent:	Just above upper poles
Inferior extent:	Through lower poles
Intravenous contrast:	To define the vascular enhancement characteristics of a mass, a bolus injection of 50 ml of contrast material will suffice in most instances.
Comments:	(1) Precontrast images usually are of minimal value unless renal calculi, perinephric hematoma, or calcified masses are suspected. When the need for dynamic imaging is anticipated, precontrast images are obtained to select the appropriate level(s) for evaluation. Otherwise, the precontrast images may be bypassed completely. (2) A repeat bolus of 25–50 ml may be necessary to evaluate lesions at different levels. (3) If transitional cell carcinoma is suspected, smaller doses, i.e., 10–25 ml, should be used so as not to obscure caliceal or ureteral lesions.

TABLE 18. *Region of interest: pelvis. Indication: survey*

Oral contrast:	600 ml oral contrast material at least 1 hr before imaging; if possible, 300 ml dilute barium suspension the evening before imaging to identify the colon
Phase of respiration:	Suspended expiration or normal respiration
Slice thickness:	8–10 mm
Slice interval:	10–20 mm
Superior extent:	Iliac crest
Inferior extent:	Symphysis pubis
Intravenous contrast:	20 ml Conray-400 15–20 min before the examination to define the bladder and ureters; to define vascular characteristics of pelvic masses or to detect myometrial invasion in endometrial cancer, a larger volume of intravenous contrast material (50–100 ml) is needed
Comments:	(1) In females, insertion of a vaginal tampon prior to the exam is desirable. (2) If oral contrast material has not progressed to the colon, a contrast enema or rectal catheter may be helpful in defining the rectosigmoid colon.

TABLE 19. *Region of interest: pelvis. Indications: search for undescended testicle*

Oral contrast:	600 ml oral contrast material at least 1 hr before imaging; if possible, 300 ml dilute barium suspension the evening before imaging to identify the colon
Phase of respiration:	Suspended expiration or normal respiration
Slice thickness:	8–10 mm (see Comments)
Slice interval:	10 mm
Inferior extent:	Begin at level of inferior pubic symphysis and proceed superiorly.
Superior extent:	If the testis or mass is not defined in the inguinal ring or true pelvis, the abdomen should be imaged to the level of the renal hilus.
Comments:	In pediatric patients, contiguous images using 5-mm slice thickness often are required.

TABLE 20. *Region of interest: shoulder joint arthrogram*

Patient position:	Supine, with arms at sides in neutral position
Digital scout film:	Anteroposterior
Oral contrast:	None
Phase of respiration:	Suspended respiration
Slice thickness:	4 mm
Scan interval:	Contiguous
Superior extent:	Mid-acromioclavicular joint
Inferior extent:	Inferior surface of glenoid
Intravenous contrast:	None
Comments:	For very large individuals, imaging with the contralateral arm extended over the head may be necessary to avoid artifacts.
	The hip joint is best evaluated by contiguous 5-mm images. Occasionally, 3-mm or 1.5-mm images may be helpful in special circumstances, e.g., when looking for subtle changes of aseptic necrosis. No gantry angulation. Region of interest is from the roof of acetabulum to the greater trochanter.

TABLE 21. *Region of interest: forefoot and midfoot*

Digital scout film:	Anteroposterior
Slice thickness:	2–4 mm
Slice interval:	2–4 mm
Anterior extent:	Just distal to the region of interest
Posterior extent:	Just proximal to the region of interest
Intravenous contrast:	None (unless there is a question of a vascular lesion or a soft-tissue lesion whose margins are not well defined without contrast material)
Comments:	(1) Ideally, the feet should be positioned so that the CT sections will be at right angles to the plane of interest. Optimally, the feet should be flat on the table and as symmetric as possible, with the patient supine and the knees flexed. Pillows underneath the knees will allow the legs and knees to be relaxed. The knees and feet should be taped to the table so that no motion will occur. If necessary, a towel or sponge may be placed under the forefoot for sufficient dorsiflexion to enable the knees to clear the gantry. (2) An alternative position may be selected if optimal positioning cannot be achieved or if the region of interest would be parallel to the CT sections, e.g., transverse fracture of the calcaneus or suspected abnormality at one of the intertarsal joints. With the patient supine, the legs may be extended, with feet and toes vertical. The feet should be secured to the table as symmetrically as possible. (3) Narrower sections should be used for detailed anatomy, and longer slice intervals can be utilized for determining the extent of a larger process.
Additional comments:	The history should be elicited for these patients, and the site of point tenderness should be identified. Often, there may be a need to look both at soft-tissue and bone windows, as some symptoms can be related to the tendon and tendon sheaths.

TABLE 22. *Region of interest: subtalar joint*

Digital scout film:	Anteroposterior
Slice thickness:	2 mm
Slice interval:	2 mm
Zoom:	Full integer, 2–5 (usually 3), to fill the screen with both feet
Anterior extent:	Talonavicular joint
Posterior extent:	Posterior aspect of subtalar joint
Intravenous contrast:	None
Comments:	(1) Ideally, the feet should be positioned so that the CT sections will be at right angles to the plane of interest. Optimally, the feet should be flat on the table and as symmetric as possible, with the patient supine and the knees flexed. Pillows underneath the knees will allow the legs and knees to be relaxed. The knees and feet should be taped to the table so that no motion will occur. If necessary, a towel or sponge may be placed under the forefoot for sufficient dorsiflexion to enable the knees to clear the gantry. (2) An alternative position may be selected if optimal positioning cannot be achieved or if the region of interest would be parallel to the CT sections, e.g., transverse fracture of the calcaneus or suspected abnormality at one of the intertarsal joints. With the patient supine, the legs may be extended with feet and toes vertical. The feet should be secured to the table as symmetrically as possible. (3) Narrower sections should be used for detailed anatomy, and longer section intervals can be utilized for determining the extent of a larger process.

REFERENCES

1. Anda S, Roysland P, Fougner R, Stovring J. CT appearance of the diaphragm varying with respiratory phase and muscular tension. *J Comput Assist Tomogr* 1986;10:744–745.
2. Andre MP, Horn RA, Bielecki D, Dev P, Resnick D. Patient dose considerations for three-dimensional CT displays. *Radiology* 1985;157(P):177.
3. Ansell G, Tweedle MCK, West CR, Evans P, Couch L. The current status of reactions to intravenous contrast media. *Invest Radiol* 1980;15:532–539.
4. Ball WS, Wicks JD, Mettler FA Jr. Prone-supine change in organ position: CT demonstration. *AJR* 1980;135:815–820.
5. Barnett PH, Zerhouni EA, White RI, Siegelman SS. Computed tomography in the diagnosis of cavernous hemangioma. *AJR* 1980;134:439–447.
6. Beir III. The effects on populations of exposure to low levels of ionizing radiation. Report of the Advisory Committee on the Biological Effects of Ionizing Radiations. Washington, DC, Division of Medical Science, National Academy of Sciences, National Research Council, 1980.
7. Berland LL. *Practical CT: technology and techniques.* New York: Raven Press, 1987.
8. Berland LL, Lawson TL, Foley WD, Melrose BL, Chintapalli KN, Taylor AJ. Comparison of pre- and postcontrast CT in hepatic masses. *AJR* 1982;138:853–858.
9. Boechat MI. Spinal deformities and pseudofractures. *AJR* 1987;148:97–98.
10. Brasch RC, Cann CE. Computed tomographic scanning in children. II. An updated comparison of radiation dose and resolving power of commercial scanners. *AJR* 1982;138:127–133.
11. Brody AS, Saks BJ, Field DR, Skinner SR, Capra RE. Artifacts seen during CT pelvimetry: implications for digital systems with scanning beams. *Radiology* 1986;160:269–271.

12. Burgener FA, Hamlin DJ. Contrast enhancement in abdominal CT: bolus vs. infusion. *AJR* 1981;137:351–358.
13. Cann CE. Quantitative CT applications: comparison of current scanners. *Radiology* 1987;162:257–261.
14. Claussen CD, Banzer D, Pfretzschner C, Kalender WA, Schorner W. Bolus geometry and dynamics after intravenous contrast medium injection. *Radiology* 1984;153:365–368.
15. Day DL, Warwick WJ. Thoracic duct opacification for CT scanning. *AJR* 1985;144:403–404.
16. Evens RG, Mettler FA. National CT use and radiation exposure: United States 1983. *AJR* 1985;144:1077–1081.
17. Fearon T, Vucich J. Normalized pediatric organ-absorbed doses from CT examinations. *AJR* 1987;148:171–174.
18. Fearon T, Vucich J. Pediatric patient exposures from CT examinations: GE CT/T 9800 scanners. *AJR* 1985;144:805–809.
19. Federle MP. CT of upper abdominal trauma. *Semin Roentgenol* 1984;19:269–280.
20. Federle MP, Cohen HA, Rosenwein MF, Brant-Zawadzki MN, Cann CE. Pelvimetry by digital radiography: a low-dose examination. *Radiology* 1982;143:733–735.
21. Fineberg HV, Wittenberg J, Ferrucci JT, Mueller PR, Simeone JF, Goldman J. The clinical value of body computed tomography over time and technologic change. *AJR* 1983;141:1067–1072.
22. Fischer HW. Catalog of intravascular contrast media. *Radiology* 1986;159:561–563.
23. Foley WD, Gleysteen JJ, Lawson TL, et al. Dynamic computed tomography and pulsed Doppler ultrasonography in the evaluation of splenorenal shunt patency. *J Comput Assist Tomogr* 1983;7:106–112.
24. Fuld IL, Matalan TA, Vogelzang RL, et al. Dynamic CT in the evaluation of physiologic status of renal transplants. *AJR* 1984;142:1157–1160.
25. Gardeur D, Lautrau J, Millard JC, Berger N, Metzger J. Pharmacokinetics of contrast media: experimental results in dog and man with CT implications. *J Comput Assist Tomogr* 1980;4:178–185.
26. Gebarski KS, Glazer GM, Gebarski SS. Brachial plexus: anatomic, radiologic, and pathologic correlation using computed tomography. *J Comput Assist Tomogr* 1982;6:1058–1063.
27. Glass RBJ, Posnanski AK. Leg-length determination with biplanar CT scanograms. *Radiology* 1985;156:833–834.
28. Glazer GM, Goldberg HI, Moss AA, Axel L. Computed tomographic detection of retroperitoneal adenopathy. *Radiology* 1982;143:147–149.
29. Godwin JD, Webb WR. Contrast-related flow phenomena mimicking pathology on thoracic computed tomography. *J Comput Assist Tomogr* 1982;6:460–464.
30. Grenier P, Maurice F, Musset D, Menu Y, Nahum H. Bronchiectasis: assessment by thin-section CT. *Radiology* 1986;161:95–99.
31. Gross SC, Kowalski JB, Lee S-HH, Terry B, Honickman SJ. Surgical ligation clip artifacts on CT scans. *Radiology* 1985;156:831–832.
32. Hagman LA, Evans RA, Fahr LM, Hinick VA. Renal consequences of rapid high dose contrast CT. *AJR* 1980;134:553.
33. Havron A, Seltzer SE, Davis MA, Shulkin P. Radiopaque liposomes: a promising new contrast material for computed tomography of the spleen. *Radiology* 1981;140:507–511.
34. Haynor DR, Borning AW, Griffin BA, Jacky JP, Kalet IJ, Shuman WP. Radiotherapy planning: direct tumor location on simulation and port films using CT. Part I. Principles. *Radiology* 1986;158:537–540.
35. Huda W. Is energy imparted a good measure of the radiation risk associated with CT examinations? *Phys Med Biol* 1984;29:1137–1142.
36. Itai Y, Furui S, Araki T, Tasaka A. Computed tomography of cavernous hemangioma of the liver. *Radiology* 1980;137:149–155.
37. Johansson L, Mattsson S. *Proceedings of an international symposium on the assessment of radioactive contamination in man.* Vienna: IAEA, 1985.
38. Kalender WA, Hebel R, Ebersberger J. Reduction of CT artifacts caused by metallic implants. *Radiology* 1987;164:576–577.
39. Koehler PR, Anderson RE. Computed angiotomography. *Radiology* 1980;137:843–845.
40. Kormano M, Dean PB. Extravascular contrast material: the major component of contrast enhancement. *Radiology* 1976;121:379–382.
41. Kormano MJ, Goske MJ, Hamlin DJ. Attenuation and contrast enhancement of gynecologic organs and tumors in CT. *Eur J Radiol* 1981;1:307–311.
42. Krudy AG, Doppman JL, Herdt JR. Failure to detect a 1.5 centimeter lung nodule by chest computed tomography. *J Comput Assist Tomogr* 1982;6:1178–1180.
43. Levi C, Gray JE, McCullough EC, Hattery RR. The unreliability of CT numbers as absolute values. *AJR* 1982;139:443–447.
44. McCarthy S, Moss AA. The use of a flow rate injector for contrast-enhanced computed tomography. *Radiology* 1984;151:800.
45. McClennan BL. Low osmolality contrast media: premises and promises. *Radiology* 1987;162:1–8.
46. Mitchell DG, Bjorgvinsson E, ter Meulen D, Lane P, Greberman M, Friedman AC. Gastrografin versus dilute barium for colonic CT examinations: a blind, randomized study. *J Comput Assist Tomogr* 1985;9:451–453.
47. Mosely RD, Linton OW. 1984 conference on CT dosimetry (editorial). *AJR* 1985;144:1087–1088.
48. Murphy F, Heaton B. Patient doses received during whole body scanning using an Elscint 905 CT scanner. *Br J Radiol* 1985;58:1197–1205.
49. Nakao N, Miura K, Takayasu Y, Wada Y, Miura T. CT angiography in hepatocellular carcinoma. *J Comput Assist Tomogr* 1983;7:780–787.
50. Newhouse JH, Murphy RX. Tissue distribution of soluble contrast: effect of dose variation and changes with time. *AJR* 1981;136:463–467.
51. Oppenheimer DA, Young SW. Diatrizoate CT distribution kinetics: a study of human tissue characterization. *J Comput Assist Tomogr* 1983;7:274–277.
52. Ono N, Martinez CR, Fara JW, Hodges FJ III. Diatrizoate distribution in dogs as a function of administration rate and time following intravenous injection. *J Comput Assist Tomogr* 1980;4:174–177.
53. Parvey LS, Grizzard M, Coburn TP. Use of infusion pump for intravenous enhanced computed tomography. *J Comput Assist Tomogr* 1983;7:175–176.
54. Pate D, Resnick D, Andre M, et al. Perspective: three-dimensional imaging of the musculoskeletal system. *AJR* 1986;147:545–551.
55. Purdy JA, Prasad SC. Computed tomography applied to radiation therapy treatment planning. Medical physics of CT and ultrasound: tissue imaging and characteristics. *Med Phys* 1980;(monograph 6):224.
56. Raptopoulos V, Davis MA, Davidoff A, et al. Fat-density oral contrast agent for abdominal CT. *Radiology* 1987;164:653–656.
57. Reid MH. Organ and lesion volume measurements with computed tomography. *J Comput Assist Tomogr* 1983;7:268–273.
58. Robbins AH, Pugatch RD, Gerzof SG, Spira R, Rankin SC, Gale DR. An assessment of the role of scan speed in perceived image quality of body computed tomography. *Radiology* 1981;139:139–146.
59. Robinson AE, Hill EP, Harpen MD. Radiation dose reduction in pediatric CT. *Pediatr Radiol* 1986;16:53–54.
60. Robinson PJ, Jones KR. Improved control of respiration during computed tomography by feedback monitoring. *J Comput Assist Tomogr* 1982;6:802–806.
61. Sewchand W, Aygun C, Micholsa G, Salazar OM. Patient immobilization during CT for treatment planning of head and neck cancer. *Radiology* 1986;158:251–252.
62. Shaffer KA. Bone algorithm for high resolution. *Radiology* 1980;137:825–829.
63. Shepard JAO, Dedrick CG, Spizarny DL, McLoud TC. Dynamic incremental computed tomography of the pulmonary hila using a flow-rate injector. *J Comput Assist Tomogr* 1986;10:369–371.
64. Shope TB, Gagne RM, Johnson GC. A method of describing the doses delivered by transmission x-ray computed tomography. *Med Phys* 1981;8:488–495.
65. Shope TB, Morgan TJ, Showalter CK. Radiation dosimetry survey of computed tomography systems from ten manufacturers. *Br J Radiol* 1982;55:60–69.
66. Shuman WP, Griffin BW, Luk KH, Mack LA, Hanson JA. CT and radiation therapy planning: impact of LOCATE scoutview images. *AJR* 1982;139:985–989.
67. Shuman WP, Griffin BW, Yosky CS, et al. The impact of CT CORRELATE scoutview images on radiation therapy planning. *AJR* 1985;145:633–638.
68. Spirt BA. Value of the prone position in detecting pulmonary nodules

by computed tomography. *J Comput Assist Tomogr* 1980;4:871–873.

69. Staron RB, Ford E. Computed tomographic volumetric calculation reproducibility. *Invest Radiol* 1985;21:272–274.

70. Sugarbaker PH, Vermess M, Doppman JL, Miller DL, Simon R. Improved detection of focal lesions with computed tomographic examination of the liver using ethiodized oil emulsion (EOE-13) liver contrast. *Cancer* 1984;54:1489–1495.

71. Todo H. Lung anatomy in the pig. *Invest Radiol* 1986;21:689–696.

72. Totty WG, Vannier MW. Complex musculoskeletal anatomy: analysis using three dimensional surface reconstruction. *Radiology* 1984;150:173–177.

73. Vannier MW, Marsh JL, Warren JO. Three dimensional CT reconstruction images for craniofacial surgical planning and evaluation. *Radiology* 1984;150:179–184.

74. van Waes PFGM, Feldberg MAM, Goldberg HI, et al. Direct coronal and direct sagittal CT of abdomen and pelvis: an approach to staging malignancies. *Radiographics* 1986;6:213–244.

75. van Waes PFGM, Zonneveld FW. Direct coronal body computed tomography. *J Comput Assist Tomogr* 1982;6:58–66.

76. Vasile N, Mathiew D, Keita K, Lellouche D, Block G, Cachera JP. Computed tomography of thoracic aortic dissection: accuracy and pitfalls. *J Comput Assist Tomogr* 1986;10:211–215.

77. Vermess M, Bernardino ME, Doppman JL, et al. Use of intravenous liposoluble contrast material for the examination of the liver and spleen in lymphoma. *J Comput Assist Tomogr* 1981;5:709–713.

78. Vermess M, Inscoe S, Sugarbaker P. Use of liposoluble contrast material to separate left renal and splenic parenchyma on computed tomography. *J Comput Assist Tomogr* 1980;4:540–542.

79. Vogelzang RL, Gore RM, Neiman HL, Smith SJ, Deschler TW, Vrla RF. Inferior vena cava CT pseudothrombus produced by rapid arm-vein contrast infusion. *AJR* 1985;144:843–846.

80. Wagner LK, Archer BR, Zeck OF. Conceptus dose from two state-of-the-art CT scanners. *Radiology* 1986;159:787–792.

81. Weeks PM, Vannier MW, Stevens WG, Gayou D, Gilula LA. Three-dimensional imaging of the wrist. *J Hand Surg* [Am] 1985;10A:32–39.

82. Williamson BRJ, Gouse JC, Rohrer DG, Teates CD. Variation in the thickness of the diaphragmatic crura with respiration. *Radiology* 1987;163:683–684.

83. Young SW, Noon MA, Nassi M, Castellino RA. Dynamic computed tomography body scanning. *J Comput Assist Tomogr* 1980;4:168–173.

84. Young SW, Turner RJ, Castellino RA. A strategy for contrast enhancement of malignant tumor using dynamic CT and intravascular pharmacokinetics. *Radiology* 1980;137:137–147.

85. Zatz LM. The effect of the kVp level on EMI values. *Radiology* 1976;119:683–688.

CHAPTER 4

MR Imaging Techniques

Joseph K. T. Lee, Robert E. Koehler, and Jay P. Heiken

Magnetic resonance (MR) imaging is a new imaging technique capable of producing thin tomographic sections. In contrast to computed tomography (CT), which requires ionizing radiation, MR imaging is based on the interaction between radio waves and atomic nuclei in the presence of a strong magnetic field. Whereas the pixel intensity in CT reflects electron density, in MR imaging it reflects the density of mobile nuclei modified by their magnetic relaxation times, T1 and T2. Because the hydrogen atom, which consists of a single proton in its nucleus, is the most abundant element in the body and because it has a strong magnetic moment, it is the nucleus used most commonly for *in vivo* imaging.

As with CT, certain parameters in MR imaging are fixed by the manufacturer, and other parameters are under operator control. Parameters that are generally fixed by the manufacturer include field strength and acquisition technique (projection reconstruction vs. Fourier transform). Parameters under operator control include the type of radiofrequency (RF) coil, imaging planes, matrix size, section thickness, section gap, pulse sequences, total number of sections, number of data averages, and field of view. The availability of such a large number of operator-controlled parameters poses a real challenge to the practicing radiologist, because even large lesions can go undetected if inappropriate techniques (e.g., pulse sequences) are used. But proper selection of these factors will result in images of high quality that will show appropriate tissues to best advantage with a reasonable expenditure of time.

This chapter is intended to provide readers with a practical guide to conducting MR imaging examinations of the extracranial organs. Basic physical principles and the rationale for various imaging sequences will be discussed first. This will be followed by a list of specific imaging protocols useful for various organ systems. Because the conduct of MR examinations is partially influenced by hardware features and software capabilities that vary from one manufacturer to another, the guidelines in this chapter may need to be modified for different types of MR imagers. However, the fundamental bases from which these guidelines are derived should be applicable to all MR systems.

PHYSICAL PRINCIPLES

It is well established that a nucleus with an odd number of nucleons (protons and neutrons) possesses angular momentum or spin. Because the hydrogen proton is the nucleus most commonly used for imaging, it will be used as an example in the following discussion. Because the proton bears an electric charge, its spinning produces a tiny, local magnetic field comparable to that of a small bar magnet. The strength and direction of the magnetic field surrounding each proton are described by a vector quantity known as magnetic moment. In the absence of a strong external magnetic field, the protons are randomly oriented. When immersed in a strong static magnetic field, the randomly oriented protons have to align either with or against the field. More protons align with the external field than against the field because their energy state is more favorable (Fig. 1). Because more protons align with the external field than against it, a net magnetization, called longitudinal magnetization, exists in the direction of the magnetic field (z axis). A more detailed analysis will show that protons do not align perfectly with the magnetic field, but rather are tilted at an angle. Thus, the externally applied magnetic field exerts a torque on the proton's nuclear magnetic moment, causing it to precess about the direction of the external field in the same way as the earth's gravitational field causes a gyroscope to precess about the vertical axis. The frequency of precession, called the resonant frequency, is proportional to the strength of the external magnetic field.

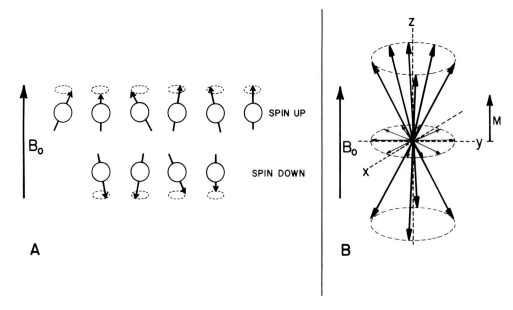

FIG. 1. Net magnetization in a static external magnetic field. **A:** At equilibrium, more protons are aligned with the field (spin up) than against the field (spin down) because the energy state for spin-up orientation is more favorable. Thus, a net magnetization vector is present in the direction of the external magnetic field (B_0). **B:** The protons precess about the z axis at the same frequency, but they do not precess coherently (i.e., in phase). Therefore, the various magnetization components in the x–y plane cancel out. (M) net magnetization vector.

At equilibrium in a static, external magnetic field, the net magnetization vector of the protons lies in the z axis. Although the protons precess about the z axis at the same frequency, they do not precess coherently. Therefore, the magnetization components of the various protons in the x–y plane (transverse magnetization) cancel out (Fig. 1B), and no net transverse magnetization is detectable.

Transverse magnetization is produced by applying a short burst of RF energy (i.e., radio waves) at the resonant frequency in a direction perpendicular to the main field (z axis). The degree to which the net magnetization is displaced from the z axis depends on the strength and duration of the applied RF pulse (Fig. 2). A 90° RF pulse causes the longitudinal magnetization to rotate 90° from

the z axis into the transverse x–y plane. Immediately after a 90° RF pulse is discontinued, the net magnetization vector precesses in the x–y plane (around the z axis) and gradually returns to its equilibrium state of alignment along the z axis, a process called free precession. Oscillation of the magnetization vector in the x–y plane induces a voltage that is amplified and detected as an RF signal at the precessional frequency. This signal, which rapidly decays to zero and appears as an exponentially diminishing sinusoidal oscillation, is called free-induction decay (FID). The rate of regrowth of the longitudinal magnetization and the decay of the signal are determined by two time constants called T1 and T2, both of which will be discussed in more detail in subsequent sections.

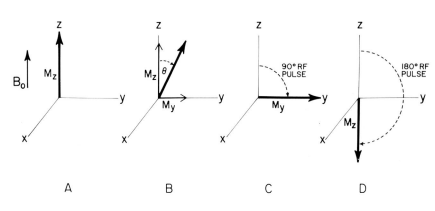

FIG. 2. Establishment of transverse magnetization. **A:** At equilibrium in the static external magnetic field (B_0), the net magnetization vector (M_z) lies entirely along the z axis. **B:** An RF pulse at the Larmor frequency (resonant frequency), oriented perpendicular to the external magnetic field, tips the net magnetization vector away from the z axis toward the x–y plane. This produces a net transverse magnetization vector M_y. The angle of the deflection θ depends on the strength and duration of the applied RF pulse. **C:** An RF pulse that tips the net magnetization 90° from the z axis into the x–y plane is called a 90° pulse. **D:** A 180° pulse inverts the net magnetization vector (M_z) from the positive z direction to the negative z direction.

Spatial information can be derived by analyzing the frequency of the emitted RF signals. As discussed previously, the precessional frequency of protons depends on the strength of the local magnetic field in which they lie. Although the main magnetic field is designed to be uniform, additional magnetic fields can be superimposed on the main static field. Each superimposition creates spatial variations in the net magnetic field, resulting in a magnetic-field gradient. At each point along this gradient, protons precess at slightly different resonant frequencies. By applying gradient fields along all three axes, the precise location of a proton can thus be determined. The three gradients that are used in two-dimensional Fourier-transform image-reconstruction techniques are called the *slice-selection gradient,* the *phase-encoding gradient,* and the *read* or *frequency gradient.* Depending on the direction of the slice-selection gradient, transverse, coronal, and sagittal sections can be obtained. A more detailed discussion of image reconstruction techniques can be found in Chapter 2.

BASIS OF MR SIGNAL INTENSITY

In contradistinction to CT, in which the pixel intensity reflects a single parameter (electron density), the pixel intensity in proton MR imaging depends on four parameters: density of mobile protons, T1, T2, and flow. The effect of proton density, also called spin density, on the appearance of a tissue on an MR image is relatively straightforward. High proton density increases MR signal intensity and tends to brighten the image. However, tissues with few mobile protons (low proton density), such as cortical bone or the dense fibrous tissue of ligaments and tendons, appear dark on MR images. The effects of T1 and T2 on pixel intensity are not so fixed and can be altered by using different imaging techniques. Blood flow is another complex phenomenon with variable effects on pixel intensity.

T1 Relaxation

T1, which has variously been called the longitudinal, thermal, or spin-lattice relaxation time, is a measure of the time required for the protons in a substance to become magnetized after being placed in a magnetic field, or, alternatively, the time required to regain longitudinal magnetization (z axis) following a 90° RF pulse (Fig. 3). In a time T1, longitudinal magnetization will return to 63% of its maximum value, and in three T1 intervals, 95% of the longitudinal magnetization will be reconstituted. If a second 90° RF pulse is applied before the entire longitudinal magnetization is regained, the resultant signal will be reduced. Thus, differences in T1 relaxation values for various tissues can be emphasized in an MR image by adjusting the interval between successive RF pulses.

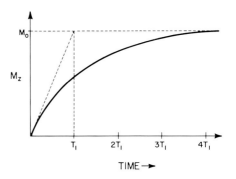

FIG. 3. Spin-lattice relaxation (T1). After an RF pulse is discontinued, the net magnetization (M_z) gradually returns to its equilibrium level (M_0) in the z axis. The time constant that describes the rate of recovery of the z magnetization is the spin-lattice (longitudinal) relaxation time, T1. T1 can also be defined as the time it would take for the linear extrapolation (*slanted-dotted line*) of the longitudinal relaxation curve's initial slope to reach the equilibrium magnetization (M_0).

T1 is determined by the rate of dispersion of energy from the resonating protons to their local environment or "lattice." All molecules have natural motions due to vibration, rotation, and translation. Small molecules, like water, generally move rapidly, whereas larger molecules like proteins move more slowly. When the frequency of molecular motions and precessional frequency are similar, T1 relaxation is efficient and rapid; when the two are different, T1 relaxation is more prolonged. Cholesterol, a medium-sized molecule, has natural frequencies close to those used for proton MR imaging and thus has a short T1. The water molecule is small and moves too rapidly; large proteins move too slowly. Both have natural frequencies significantly different from the proton resonant frequency and thus have long T1 values. Water in the bulk phase, like urine, has a long T1, whereas water held in hydration layers, like proteinaceous solutions, has a much shorter T1. T1 values for most biological tissues are in the range of 200 to 2,000 msec.

T2 Relaxation

T2 is the exponential time constant for decay of the transverse magnetization following an RF pulse (Fig. 4). This decay is due to dephasing or loss of coherence among the protons in the excited region. The dephasing of protons is caused by the effects of interactions between neighboring nuclei. In most substances, individual protons experience slightly different local magnetic environments because of varying interactions with neighboring nuclei. These local fields are strongest when the protons are held in fixed positions, such as in a solid. In a liquid, the local magnetic fields from neighboring molecules fluctuate rapidly as the molecules move about and contribute little to the net magnetic field at any point. Thus, solids lose their transverse magnetization more quickly than liquids and have short T2 values.

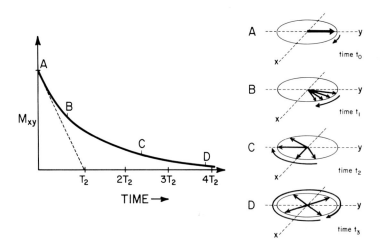

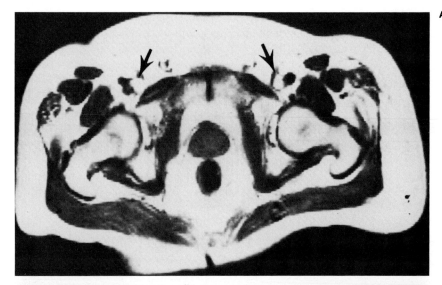

FIG. 4. Spin–spin relaxation (T2). After an RF pulse is discontinued, the net transverse magnetization (M_{xy}) decreases exponentially with a time constant T2. T2 can be defined as the time it would take for the linear extrapolation (*dotted line*) of the transverse relaxation curve's initial slope to reach equilibrium (i.e., zero). **A:** Immediately after an RF pulse, all protons point in the same direction (are "in phase"), producing a single net magnetization vector in the x–y plane. **B:** Shortly afterward, the protons quickly dephase because of slight differences in precessional frequencies caused by interactions with neighboring nuclei. As a result, the individual magnetization vectors of the protons begin to fan out in the x–y plane. **C:** At a slightly later time (t_2), the individual protons are spread farther apart in the x–y plane. **D:** At time t_3, complete dephasing has occurred. The individual x–y magnetization vectors cancel each other, resulting in zero net magnetization in the x–y plane.

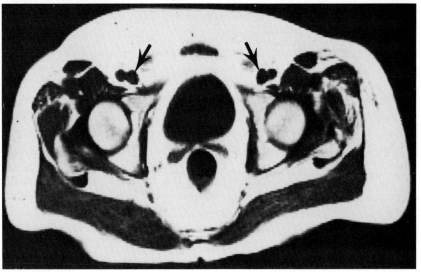

FIG. 5. Flow-related enhancement in the femoral veins. **A:** Transverse MR image (TR = 500 msec, TE = 35 msec). This is the most caudad section in a multisection imaging volume. The high signal noted within both femoral veins (*arrows*) is related to the entry-slice phenomenon and is not due to thrombi. **B:** Two centimeters cephalad to **A.** Note that both femoral veins (*arrows*) appear as areas of "signal void."

The time constant that characterizes the actual, observed decay of transverse magnetization is termed T2* ("T2-star"). T2* is caused by the combined effects of interactions between neighboring nuclei and inhomogeneity of the applied magnetic field. The inhomogeneity of the applied magnetic field results primarily from the intentional linear grading of the magnetic field used for spatial localization and to a lesser degree from unintentional inhomogeneity secondary to imperfect engineering. These imperfections in the applied magnetic field are great in magnitude compared with the subtle, intrinsic, local magnetic variations in the tissue sample being imaged.

T2* is considerably shorter than T2, which represents only the intrinsic, sample-dependent component of the signal decay. T2 relaxation is sometimes called spin-spin relaxation because it results from exchange of energy between neighboring nuclei. In a time T2, 63% of the transverse $(x–y)$ magnetization will be lost; in three T2 intervals, 95% will be lost. For most biologic tissues, T2 falls in the range of 20 to 300 msec.

Blood Flow

Flowing blood can have a variable signal intensity depending on the imaging sequence and the velocity and direction of flow. At high velocities, i.e., greater than 10 cm/sec, blood may flow through an imaging plane before formation of a spin echo and therefore produce no signal at all. Turbulent flow may also appear dark because the random motion of the fluid elements causes rapid loss of coherence. Contrarily, slowly flowing blood produces a high signal because of flow-related enhancement and even-echo rephasing. In flow-related enhancement, the increased signal is due to the replacement in the imaged

plane of some of the demagnetized protons by fully magnetized protons that produce comparatively higher signal intensities. When multisection imaging is used, flow-related enhancement can be seen in the aorta in the most cephalad section and in the inferior vena cava in the most caudad section (Fig. 5). Flow-related enhancement is maximal when low-velocity flow is imaged at short repetition times (TR). As flow velocity increases, the magnitude of flow-related enhancement decreases, but the effect may be seen in several sections of a multisection imaging volume.

When multiple echoes are acquired by applying repetitive 180° pulses, the intensity of the even echoes can exceed that of the odd echoes. The effect is due to rephasing of "isochromats" (small groups of protons that precess in phase throughout an imaging sequence), which occurs after each full 360° rotation, i.e., all even echoes, following an initial 90° pulse. This phenomenon is particularly prominent in slow laminar flow and accounts for the high signal intensities of venous structures on even-echo images (Fig. 6).

IMAGING TECHNIQUES

The most unusual feature of MR imaging is that tissue contrast can be radically altered by using different signal-acquisition techniques. In other words, contrast between lesions and adjacent normal tissues, as well as contrast between various normal tissues and organs, can be increased or decreased depending on the particular imaging sequence used. The following is a description of the imaging techniques now in common use in the clinical setting.

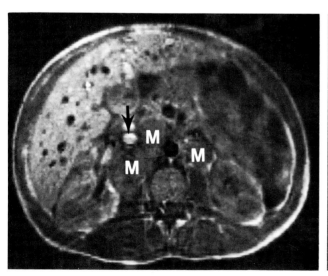 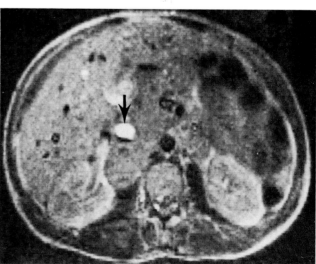

A,B

FIG. 6. Even-echo rephasing phenomenon. Images were obtained with (A) TR = 500 msec, TE = 35 msec; (B) TR = 500 msec, TE = 70 msec. A: Signal is noted in the inferior vena cava (*arrow*). Extensive retroperitoneal lymphadenopathy (M) is present. B: The signal in the inferior vena cava (*arrow*) is higher on this even-echo image than that in A, indicating that the caval signal is due to slow laminar flow, not to a thrombus.

Spin Echo

The spin-echo (SE) technique is currently the most frequently employed sequence in clinical imaging. It is sensitive to T1 and T2 as well as to hydrogen density and flow.

The SE pulse sequence consists of a 90° RF pulse followed by a 180° RF pulse (Fig. 7). The 90° pulse tips the net magnetization vector from the z axis to the y axis. Immediately after the 90° RF pulse, the magnetization precesses in the x–y plane about the z axis at the precessional frequency. The protons, which are initially in phase, begin to dephase largely because of the application of the read gradient. This is because protons that lie in an area of higher magnetic-field strength precess at a slightly faster rate than protons in a region of lower field strength. Spin-spin interactions, i.e., T2 relaxation, also contribute to the dephasing process. After a given time interval, the faster protons will have moved ahead of the slower protons in the x–y plane. Loss of transverse magnetization (dephasing) due to the external-field inhomogeneity can be partially offset by applying a 180° pulse, which causes the protons to flip 180° about the x axis, so that the faster protons are then "behind" the slower ones. However, because of the precessional-frequency differences created by the read gradient, the faster protons continue to precess at a more rapid rate and eventually catch up with the slower ones, resulting in the reconvergence of transverse magnetization. This rephasing produces a signal, called a spin echo[1] (Fig. 8).

The time interval between the 90° pulses and the resulting echo is called the echo delay or the echo time (TE). The number of echoes received depends on the number of 180° pulses applied. The repetition time, TR, is the time between the beginning of the initial 90° pulse and the beginning of the following 90° pulse, which reinitiates the entire SE sequence again.

The intensity (I) of the SE signal can be approximated mathematically:

$$I = N(H)f(v)(1 - e^{-TR/T1})e^{-TE/T2}$$

where $N(H)$ is the mobile proton density, and $f(v)$ is a function of flow. This equation indicates that the intensity of the MR signal increases as hydrogen density and T2 increase and as T1 decreases. It should also be noted that the intensity of the MR signal changes with TR and TE. Both TR and TE are user-selectable parameters. T1 and T2 values between tissues can be emphasized or deemphasized by varying TR and TE values.

---

[1] "Spin echo" is a generic term referring to the reappearance of an MR signal after an FID has apparently died away, as a result of the effective reversal of the dephasing of the spins (refocusing) by different techniques. An echo produced following 90°–180° RF pulses is called a Hahn echo; an echo produced by reversal of the magnetic-field gradient is called a gradient echo. However, the term "spin echo" is now generally used to denote the echo produced by the combination of a refocusing 180° RF pulse and the reversal of the read gradient.

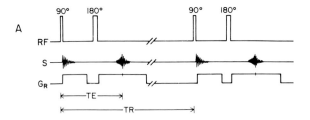

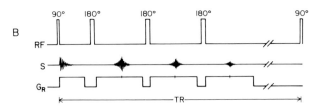

FIG. 7. SE pulse sequence. **A:** This sequence begins with a 90° RF pulse. A read gradient (G_R) is turned on to create a linear gradation in the frequencies of the protons in the x–y plane. G_R is then turned off, and a 180° pulse given. G_R is then turned back on, producing a rephasing of protons, and an RF signal (S) is measured at the time of an echo. The echo time (TE) is a time interval between the 90° pulse and the subsequent echo. The repetition time (TR) is the interval between successive 90° pulses. **B:** If the 90° pulse is followed by multiple 180° pulses before another 90° pulse is given, multiple echoes will result with each successive echo decreasing in signal amplitude.

After the SE, the MR signal again diminishes to zero, with a rate constant determined by T2 and field nonuniformity. Realignment with the external field (longitudinal magnetization) grows exponentially at a rate T1. After several T1 periods, longitudinal magnetization is reestablished, and a second SE sequence can be performed. In clinical MR imaging, several SEs are averaged together to increase the signal. If the second 90° pulse is started before full longitudinal magnetization is reestablished, the resultant SE will be weaker. Because recovery of longitudinal magnetization depends on T1, the time between successive 90° pulses (TR) can be used to discriminate among T1 values for various tissues. When the TR is shortened, substances with longer T1 values recover less longitudinal magnetization between successive 90° pulses than do short-T1 substances. Thus, the MR signal decays from an initial value that is less than maximal. In other words, as TR is shortened, the amount of T1 weighting increases. However, if a relatively long TR is used, allowing complete recovery of longitudinal magnetization by all substances between successive 90° pulses, then the amplitude of the MR signal will be independent of T1.

As stated previously, the amplitude of the MR signal, a function of T2, decreases with longer TE. When the SE is acquired soon after the 90° pulse (short TE), there is little time for decay and thus minimal T2 effect on the image. When TE is prolonged, T2 weighting increases.

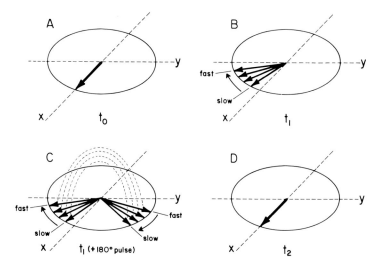

FIG. 8. Formation of an echo. **A:** Immediately after a 90° RF pulse, the protons are in phase and point in the same direction in the x-y plane (in this example, along the x axis). **B:** At time t_1, the protons start to spread out over the x-y plane because of slight differences in their precessional frequencies caused mainly by application of the read gradient (G_R). The protons with faster precessional rates will have moved farther from the initial axis of alignment (i.e., the x axis) than those with slower rates. **C:** If a 180° pulse is applied, the protons will be flipped 180° such that the slower protons are now "ahead" of the faster protons. **D:** At time t_2, the faster protons have caught up with the slower protons, so that the net x-y magnetization vectors of the protons are once again aligned. This refocusing of the protons results in an echo at time t_2.

Substances with longer T2 values will generate stronger signals than substances with shorter T2 values if both are acquired with a long TE and if proton density and T1 values are comparable.

The importance of choosing the proper pulse-sequence parameters can be illustrated by imaging two substances: one with short T1 and T2 values and the other with long T1 and T2 values. At short TR, the signal from a substance with a long T2 and long T1 will start to decay from a lower initial value, but will persist longer than that from a substance with shorter T1 and T2 values. The two signals will become isointense at a particular value of TE, and thereafter the long-T2 substance will be more intense at longer values of TE. If inappropriate values of TR and TE were chosen, the two substances would be isoin-tense and would be indistinguishable from one another (Fig. 9).

Short TR and TE values produce T1-weighted images; long TR and TE values result in T2-weighted images. A long TR and a short TE produce a proton-density-weighted image, with mixed T1 and T2 weighting. A TR less than 500 msec is considered to be short, and a TR greater than 1,500 msec is considered to be long. A TE less than 30 msec is considered to be short, and more than 80 msec to be long. Both T1- and T2-weighted sequences are necessary to detect and characterize many lesions.

Table 1 is a summary of relative relaxation values for different structures in the body and their relative brightnesses (signal intensities) on T1- and T2-weighted SE images.

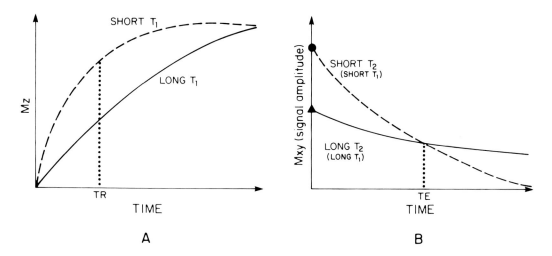

FIG. 9. Relationship between tissue contrast and pulsing time. **A:** After an RF pulse is discontinued, the tissue having a short T1 reconstitutes its longitudinal magnetization (M_z) more quickly than the tissue having a long T1. If a short TR is chosen, as indicated by the *dotted line,* the T1 difference between these two tissues will be accentuated. **B:** Using a short TR, as indicated in **A,** the tissue with a long T1 can recover only a portion of its total magnetization between successive 90° pulses and thus starts to decay from a lower amplitude than the tissue with a short T1. Because of the shorter T2 of the latter tissue, its signal decays at a much faster rate than for tissue with a long T2. If an inappropriate TE is chosen, as indicated by the *dotted line,* these two tissues will emit similar-intensity signals and become indistinguishable from each other.

TABLE 1. *Signal intensities in MRI of the body (0.3–0.6 tesla)*

TISSUE	T_1	T_2	Spin Density	Image Brightness* T1-weighted TR=300-500 ms TE=15-35 ms	Image Brightness* T2-weighted TR=1500+ ms TE=80-90 ms
Muscle	4+	2+	3+	██	██
Liver	3+	3+	3+	░░	▓▓
Spleen	4+	4+	3+	▒▒	░░
Kidneys	4+ **	4+	3+	▓▓	░░
Abscess, Infarct, many tumors	5+	5+	3+	██	░░
Hematoma 1-6 days				Varies with age	
Weeks	2+	5+	4+	░░	▢
Red marrow	4+	3+	3+	▒▒	▒▒
Yellow marrow	1+	4+	4+	▢	░░
Fat	1+	4+	5+	▢	░░
Urine, cysts, edema	6+	6+	5+	▓▓	▢
Cortical bone, ligaments			1+	██	██
Metal, air			0	██	██
Flowing blood				Variable due to motion effects	

*Long T1 darkens tissue image on T1-weighted image. Long T2 brightens tissue image on T2-weighted image. High spin density always brightens image.

**Renal medulla has longer T1 than cortex and appears darker on T1-weighted images.

Inversion Recovery

Another method for obtaining images that reflect T1 differences is inversion recovery (IR) (Fig. 10). In this technique, a 180° pulse (inverting pulse) is first applied to flip the net magnetization vector from the positive z axis to the negative z axis. After the 180° pulse is discontinued, T1 relaxation begins to take place. In order to tip the magnetization vector into the x–y plane so that it can be measured, a 90° pulse is then applied. The time interval between the 180° pulse (inverting pulse) and the 90° pulse is called the inversion time (TI). Although a signal can be detected after the 90° pulse, it is generally not measured until a second 180° pulse (refocusing pulse) is applied. In other words, the IR technique actually consists of a 180° inverting pulse followed by a standard SE sequence. The pixel intensity of IR images depends on TI as well as TR and TE (Fig. 11).

The MR signal derived from the IR sequence may be positive or negative, depending on the direction of the net magnetization vector at the time the 90° pulse is applied. If the net magnetization vector has relaxed little and remains near the $-z$ axis at the onset of the 90° pulse, either because a short TI was used or because of a long tissue T1, the resultant signal will be negative. In contrast, if the magnetization vector has realigned with the $+z$ axis when the 90° is applied, either because of a long TI or a short T1, the generated signal will be positive. However,

most current imagers detect the magnitude, but not the sign, of the MR signal. Hence, large negative signals are displayed with signal reversal as large positive signals to

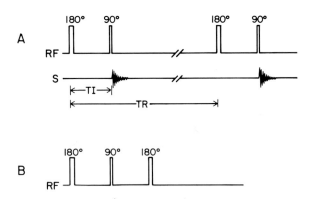

FIG. 10. IR pulse sequence. **A:** A 180° RF pulse first inverts the net magnetization from the positive z axis onto the negative z axis. After a time interval TI, a 90° pulse tips the magnetization vector into the x–y plane so that it can be detected. **B:** In practice, when using the IR technique, the 90° pulse is generally followed by a second 180° pulse, and the signal is measured during SE. (TR) time interval between successive 180° pulses; (TE) time interval between the 90° pulse and the subsequent SE; (S) RF signal; (G_R) read gradient.

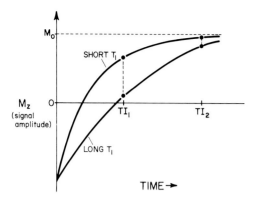

FIG. 11. Relationship between tissue contrast and inversion time in IR. After a 180° inverting pulse, tissues with a short T1 recover their equilibrium magnetization in the z axis (M_0) more quickly than do those with a long T1. Initial inversion of the net magnetization vector accentuates the difference between tissues with rapid and slow T1 relaxation because, compared with other pulse sequences, it allows twice the magnetization change during TI. If an appropriate TI is chosen (e.g., TI_1), tissue differences in T1 will be accentuated. However, if a longer TI such as TI_2 is chosen, image contrast based on T1 differences will be diminished.

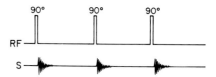

FIG. 12. Partial saturation. This sequence consists of a series of equally spaced 90° RF pulses. An echo is produced by reversal of the imaging gradient without a refocusing 180° pulse. A reduced RF pulse angle (<90°) is now being used to obtain images within a few seconds.

yield greater image brightness; lower-amplitude negative signals are displayed as smaller positive signals with reduced image brightness. Thus, the magnitude of the signal initially decreases as the magnetization recovers and becomes less negative. After the magnetization passes through zero, the magnitude of the signal starts to increase as the net magnetization becomes more positive. The time at which the magnetization passes through zero is called the null point. If the 90° pulse is applied at this time, there will be no signal.

Although the IR sequence provides excellent soft-tissue contrast (e.g., white–gray matter differentiation in the brain), it requires a longer data-acquisition time for a given spatial resolution and signal-to-noise ratio than the SE technique. Therefore, the IR sequence has now largely been abandoned by the users of medium- and high-field-strength imagers.

Partial Saturation

The partial-saturation (PS) sequence is equivalent to an SE sequence without a refocusing 180° RF pulse. It consists of a series of equally spaced 90° pulses (Fig. 12). The term "saturation" refers to the reduction of the longitudinal magnetization vector to zero by the 90° pulses. After application of a single RF pulse, an echo of the FID is formed by reversal of the imaging gradients. If the first 90° pulse is followed by a second, the starting value of the second FID is determined by the amount of longitudinal relaxation that has occurred in the interval between the two 90° pulses. If this interval is significantly less than four times T1, then the longitudinal magnetization will not have recovered to its initial value, and

each subsequent 90° pulse will have a smaller magnetization vector to tip into the x–y plane. Thus, using the PS technique, a tissue with a short T1 will yield a stronger signal than a tissue with a long T1 if the repetition time is short.

If the repetition time between successive 90° pulses is sufficiently long to allow total recovery of longitudinal magnetization by all tissues, then the amplitudes of the MR signals from different tissues will be based solely on differences in proton density among those tissues, not on their T1 values. This type of PS pulse sequence is called "saturation recovery" (SR). Although SR yields a stronger signal than the PS technique, the latter sequence provides better tissue contrast because it offers T1 information as well. Because there is no refocusing 180° RF pulse, this technique is very sensitive to the effects of magnetic-field inhomogeneities and thus has not received widespread acceptance in clinical imaging.

Recently, there has been renewed interest in PS techniques that use reduced RF-pulse angles in conjunction with a very short TR for rapid imaging (single-breath-holding imaging). This technique has been variously called FLASH, GRASS, SRPS, etc. In this technique, a very short TR (15–50 msec) is used—about a factor of 10 lower than what is used conventionally for PS imaging. Because imaging time is proportional to TR, this leads directly to a corresponding reduction in imaging time. In order to avoid fully saturating the magnetization with a short TR, a flip angle of less than 90° is substituted for the standard excitation pulse. An echo is generated by gradient reversal rather than by a 180° refocusing pulse. Because of the absence of a 180° refocusing pulse, a shorter TE can be chosen with this technique than with the SE method. The tissue contrast varies with the flip angle used. Using this technique, a single section can be imaged in as little as 2 sec, certainly within the single-breath-holding period for most patients. Although this technique shows great promise for eliminating artifacts related to respiratory motion, for providing cine views of the heart, and for evaluating dynamic contrast enhancement, its clinical applications have not yet been fully evaluated.

Proton Spectroscopic Imaging (Chemical-Shift Imaging)

There are three different ways to perform chemical-shift imaging. The first type involves selective excitation or selective saturation of a particular resonant frequency and requires MR imagers with excellent field homogeneity. The second type employs phase-encoding gradients in two dimensions and is too time-consuming for routine clinical imaging. The third type, called the phase-contrast technique, is a modification of the conventional SE technique. It can produce separate water and fat images with good spatial resolution within a reasonable imaging time (less than 30 min) using commercially available MR imagers. This technique exploits the difference in rate of precession between protons in water molecules and protons in fatty acid molecules. Because there is a difference in resonant frequency of 3 parts per million (50 Hz in a 0.3-tesla field) between water and fat protons, the MR signal can be considered to be a vector sum of the magnetizations of fat protons precessing at one frequency and water protons precessing at a slightly higher frequency. Conventional MR imaging data are obtained, with both sets of protons contributing to the SE. The magnetization vectors of water and fat are pointing in the same direction (i.e., are in phase), and this image is called the in-phase image or a water-plus-fat image. A second set of data is acquired with the time of the read gradient or the 180° pulse modified so that the signal is acquired when the water and fat magnetizations point in opposite directions (i.e., are out of phase). The resulting image is called an opposed image or a water-minus-fat image. These two images can be added to produce a water image or subtracted to yield a fat image. Figure 13 is a schematic diagram illustrating the difference between the in-phase and the opposed-phase sequences at a 0.35-tesla field strength. Several studies have shown that this technique is useful for detecting fatty infiltration of the liver and is superior to conventional SE methods for detecting liver metastases in selected patients. Clinical application of this technique in other areas of the body has been less rewarding.

MACHINE VARIABLES AND OPTIONS (OTHER IMAGING PARAMETERS)

The detectability of a lesion depends on tissue contrast and spatial resolution. Optimal contrast between normal tissue and a lesion can be achieved by selecting a proper imaging sequence and its pulsing times (i.e., TR, TE) as described in the previous section. In order to obtain high spatial resolution, other machine variables have to be chosen. These include the type of receiver coil, section thickness, matrix size, and number of data averages. Because the acquisition of a series of MR images is a time-consuming process, the time required to complete such an examination also needs to be considered. The imaging time is related not only to the number of imaging sequences performed but also to the specific imaging parameters chosen for each of these sequences, particularly the TR and TE, the number of views (matrix size), and

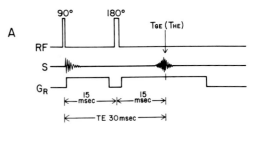

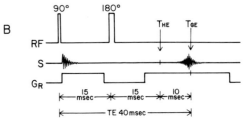

FIG. 13. Pulse sequence in proton spectroscopic imaging. **A:** In the conventional SE technique, water and fat magnetizations are pointing in the same direction at the time of the echo (TE = 30 msec). This echo time corresponds to that for either a Hahn SE (T$_{HE}$) or a gradient echo (T$_{GE}$). Whereas the time interval between a 180° pulse and a Hahn SE is always equal to the time interval between the 90° and 180° pulses, the gradient echo does not have a fixed relationship to the timing of the two RF pulses. **B:** In the proton spectroscopic imaging technique, the onset of the read gradient (G$_R$) is delayed by 10 msec after the 180° pulse. As a result, the water and fat magnetizations are no longer pointing in the same direction at the time of the gradient echo (T$_{GE}$) because water protons precess faster than fat protons. At T$_{GE}$ (TE = 40 msec) the water and fat magnetizations point in opposite directions. Consequently, in the resulting image, pixel intensity is the difference between the water signal and fat signal. T$_{HE}$ is equal to the time of the Hahn SE (30 msec).

the number of acquisitions averaged. Slice thickness also indirectly affects imaging time, because thin (5 mm or less) slices require the use of a greater number of averages. The data-acquisition time for a single sequence can be computed using the following formula:

Data acquisition time (min)

$$= \frac{TR \text{ (sec)} \times \begin{array}{c}\text{No. of matrix elements}\\\text{along phase-encoding axis}\end{array} \times \begin{array}{c}\text{No. of}\\\text{acquisitions}\end{array}}{60}$$

For example, the time required to complete a T1-weighted sequence using a TR of 0.3 sec, two acquisitions, and 256 views along the phase-encoding axis will be 0.3 × 256 × 2 ÷ 60 = 2.56 min. Assuming that the number of views along the phase-encoding axis and the number of acquisitions remain the same, the use of a TR of 3 sec for a T2-weighted sequence will then take 3 × 256 × 2 ÷ 60 = 25.6 min.

Because only a small fraction of imaging time is used for actual data collection, and the rest is used to allow recovery of longitudinal magnetization by the excited protons, more than one section can be imaged during a single imaging sequence. The maximum number of sections that can be obtained in a pulsing sequence can be determined by the TR and the longest TE of that sequence. In general, data acquisition from one section can be completed in 100 msec, unless TEs longer than 70 msec are used. Assuming that TEs of 35 msec and 70 msec are used, a TR of 500 msec will yield a maximum of 5 sections per sequence, whereas a TR of 1,500 msec will yield a maximum of 15 sections per sequence.

In addition to the data-acquisition time, image reconstruction (about 5–15 sec/section) and the time required for the technologist to program, scout, position, and tune each sequence (2–4 min each) must be added to estimate the total examination time. In general, the total examination time for a patient will be 1.5 to 2 times the data-acquisition time.

Receiver Coil

In order to improve the signal-to-noise ratio, the smallest possible receiver coil that will accommodate the organ of interest should be used and applied closely to the body part being imaged. When small or relatively superficial body parts, such as the orbit, neck, breast, scrotum and extremities, are imaged with a large body coil, the signal-to-noise ratio suffers because of a low filling factor. The use of surface coils in these areas improves spatial resolution. With most equipment, the body coil is still used as the transmitter coil in order to achieve a more uniform RF irradiation. Disadvantages of surface coils include rapid drop-off of signal strength with increasing distance from the coil and a limited imaging volume.

Voxel Size

The voxel size is determined by the section thickness and the number of views per unit area. Thinner sections and larger numbers of views per unit area result in smaller voxel size and therefore better spatial resolution. Similarly, better spatial resolution can be achieved by decreasing the imaged volume while maintaining the number of views constant. This process is called "zoom imaging" and is accomplished by increasing the strength of the magnetic-field gradients. However, smaller voxel sizes may not lead to greater lesion detectability, because they have poorer signal-to-noise ratio. In order to improve the signal-to-noise ratio when a smaller voxel size is used, the number of data averages must be increased, which in turn results in longer imaging time. For examination of large body parts, such as the liver, a section thickness of 10 mm usually suffices; for smaller anatomic regions, such as the temporomandibular joint, a section thickness of 3 mm or less is preferred. At present, satisfactory images of most areas require 256 views along the phase-encoding axis.

Number of Averages

This represents the number of times each data observation is repeated. As in the case of the number of views, doubling the number of averages doubles the imaging time. Image quality improves with increasing number of averages. This is especially true because motion artifact and noise are both less noticeable in images obtained with 8 or 16 averages than in those obtained with one average. Unfortunately, routine use of 16 averages is prohibitive because of the imaging time required. In general, one average is used for a section thickness of 10 mm when TR is longer than 2,000 msec. Multiple averages are used when shorter TRs are used or when thinner sections are desirable.

Cardiac Triggering

Several techniques have been developed to minimize artifacts caused by cardiac motion in order to allow clear depiction of intracardiac and nearby structures. These techniques restrict data acquisition to specific phases of the cardiac cycle. The three techniques that have been used for cardiac triggering are pressure-cuff plethysmography, laser-Doppler velocimetry, and electrocardiography (EKG).

In cuff plethysmography, a cuff placed around the patient's arm detects changes in limb dimension with arterial pulsation. The output of this signal is used to initiate the data-acquisition sequence. Laser-Doppler velocimetry uses a flow-meter transducer that detects a signal that is generated in relation to changes in capillary blood volume and velocity during systole. Laser light is directed to a portion of the body that has a rich superficial capillary bed (e.g., the earlobe); the light is reflected by tissue and carried out of the image through fiberoptic light cables. With both of these techniques there is a delay in the onset of signal acquisition caused by the distance between the heart and the sampling site, i.e., the arm or earlobe. This delay ranges from 200 to 400 msec and precludes imaging during the first third of the cardiac cycle.

EKG triggering is now the preferred technique for obtaining cardiac images. Most systems use low-resistance electrodes and short leads. The electrical signals from the leads are converted into light pulses that are transmitted out of the imaging room over fiberoptic light guides.

Cardiac triggering of the pulse sequence prolongs the MR examination time to some degree. With this technique, the TR is determined by the patient's heart rate, i.e., the R-R interval. For example, TR varies from 1,000 msec to 600 msec when the heart rate is 60 to 100 beats per minute. If a longer TR is desired, data acquisition can be triggered on alternate heart beats. The time delay between the triggering signal (R wave) and initiation of the imaging sequence can be varied. Short time delays (e.g.,

100 msec) produce the most satisfactory images. Images obtained during late diastole tend to have less anatomic resolution. Furthermore, images obtained at the cardiac apex often have poor spatial resolution, possibly as a result of diaphragmatic motion. Cardiac arrhythmia will lead to inconstant triggering, which in turn will result in degraded anatomic resolution.

Respiratory Triggering

Artifacts due to respiratory motion cause blurring of MR images of the chest and abdomen. At least two basic techniques have been developed in an attempt to reduce artifacts caused by respiratory motion.

In the conventional respiratory triggering technique, only data from a certain segment of the respiratory cycle, usually between end expiration and beginning inspiration, are used for image reconstruction. This effect can be achieved in two ways. In the first method, sometimes called non-spin-conditioned gating, a respiration-sensing device, usually consisting of a belt and fiberoptic system to sense stretching of the belt with breathing, turns the imaging sequence on and off at appropriate times in the respiratory cycle. As a result, data are acquired only during the selected phase of the respiratory cycle. Because of the intermittent interruptions in pulsing, with resultant tissue relaxation, T1 measurements are inaccurate. A different approach is to acquire data continuously at a preset TR, but to use only the data from a certain phase of the respiratory cycle for image reconstruction. This technique, called spin-conditioned gating, does not cause errors in T1 values because tissues are not subjected to long periods of relaxation.

If the conventional respiratory gating technique is used with tidal breathing, it will require two to four times more imaging time than nongated studies when a TR of 500 msec is used. The time penalty will be proportionately less either for studies with longer TRs or for studies in which patients are instructed to lengthen the time between each breath. Such modified breathing patterns can be used only in cooperative patients.

The other approaches to reduction of respiratory-motion artifact are referred to as respiratory-ordered phase encoding (ROPE) or centrally ordered phase encoding (COPE). Both of these newly developed techniques are designed to reduce motion artifacts without prolonging the imaging time. They differ from the conventional gating technique in that all data collected throughout the respiratory cycle are used for image reconstruction. They differ from the nongated technique in the order in which data in a section are collected. Whereas the data in a section are acquired sequentially with the nongated technique, the order in which each line of data is collected in ROPE or COPE is determined by the phase of respiration. These techniques are most successful in reducing respiratory-

motion artifact if the patient's respiration is monotonic. Irregular respiration will decrease the efficacy of these two techniques.

PRACTICAL CONSIDERATIONS (PATIENT PREPARATION AND SAFETY)

The duties of a radiologist overseeing MR imaging examinations go beyond the selection of pulsing parameters. A high-quality, diagnostic MR imaging examination, which often takes 30 to 60 min to complete, cannot be achieved without the cooperation of the patient being examined. In order to assure patient cooperation and safety, a brief description of the examination and a list of contraindications should be given before the examination. Such instructions usually are given by the technologist involved. All metal objects worn or carried by the patient should be removed before the patient enters the imaging room. Because the imaging time is long, every effort should be made to maximize patient comfort. These include placing pillows beneath the patient's knees to prevent back pain, providing sheets to keep the patient warm, and providing earplugs for reducing the noise level. Patients are instructed to breath normally and to remain as still as possible during data acquisition. Children less than 6 years of age usually require sedation; older children generally will cooperate after verbal assurance.

Several theoretical biological effects are associated with exposure of humans to the types of magnetic fields employed in MR imaging. These effects include changes in chemical kinetics and membrane permeability as well as reduction in nerve conduction velocity. However, studies to date suggest that these effects are not detectable at the field strengths used for imaging. The principal concerns with MR imaging at present are possible tissue heating effects associated with large metallic prostheses, influences on the operation of cardiac pacemakers, and the remote possibility that the fetus may somehow be more sensitive to magnetic or RF fields. Currently, we do not examine patients with intracranial aneurysm clips, because the magnetic fields used in MR imaging are capable of exerting significant torque on aneurysm clips having a high nickel content. In addition, we recommend that patients with pacemakers and electrical neurostimulators be excluded from MR examinations. Medically unstable patients requiring life-support equipment are also excluded from MR studies. Because of limited data available concerning possible effects of MR on the fetus of less than 3 months gestational age, we do not examine women during the first trimester of pregnancy. However, we have successfully examined patients with a variety of intrathoracic and intraabdominal surgical clips, patients with hip prostheses, and pregnant women in the second and third trimesters.

ARTIFACTS

An understanding of MR imaging artifacts is important lest they be misinterpreted as pathologic conditions. New artifacts, unfamiliar to most practicing radiologists, have emerged with MR imaging. The following is a brief description of some of the more commonly encountered artifacts. The underlying mechanisms for such artifacts and methods to minimize them are also presented.

Motion

Physiologic motions, which include cardiac pulsations, respiratory excursions, and intestinal peristalsis, are the causes of the most frequent artifacts encountered in MR imaging of the thorax and abdomen. Motion causes ghost images to occur in the phase-encoding direction (Fig. 14). It also leads to image blurring in the direction of motion. In addition, respiratory-motion artifacts affect T1 and T2 measurements because of volume averaging and the spurious areas of high signal intensity produced by the ghost images.

Artifacts produced by cardiac motion can be minimized with EKG triggering, which does not significantly prolong data-acquisition time. Respiratory triggering using the conventional methods increases imaging time by a factor of 2 to 4. The more recently developed techniques (e.g., ROPE and COPE), which use phase reordering in data collection, can reduce respiratory-motion artifacts without increasing the imaging time. Motion-induced artifacts can also be reduced by using a short-TR and -TE sequence or fewer matrix elements along the phase-encoding axis (e.g., 128 elements instead of 256 elements).

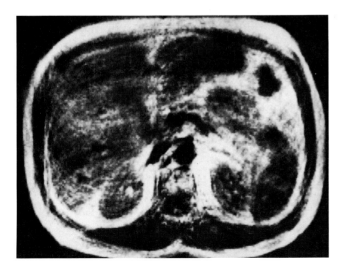

FIG. 14. Respiratory-motion artifact. A transaxial MR image of the upper abdomen shows marked blurring of intraabdominal structures due to overlapping ghost images.

Aliasing (Wraparound Artifact)

Aliasing occurs when the diameter of the imaged object exceeds the field of view. It can occur in both the frequency- and the phase-encoding directions. In the frequency axis, wraparound artifacts are due to a low rate of data sampling. Because of a low sampling rate, the high-frequency signal masquerades as a low-frequency signal (Fig. 15). The missed assignment of frequency results in an artifact in which the portion of the object extending beyond the field of view appears within the imaged volume, but on the side opposite the actual body part. Wraparound artifact occurring in the frequency axis can be eliminated by using filters in that direction.

In the phase-encoding direction, location is determined by the amount of phase shift occurring during multiple applications of the phase-encoding gradient. Within the field of view, the amount of phase shift can vary from 1° to 360° (one cycle). Aliasing occurs when the phase shift from the area immediately outside the field of view has accumulated more than one cycle of shift (i.e., greater than 360°) and mimics the signal from a location with a small accumulation of phase shift. The resultant artifact appears on the side opposite the actual body part. It has the same orientation and is of the same intensity as the true image (Fig. 16). Wraparound artifact along the phase-encoding axis can be eliminated by increasing the field of view.

Chemical Shift Artifact

Artifacts produced by chemical-shift misregistration occur along the frequency axis as a result of the difference in the precessional frequency between protons in fat and those in water. Because of the location of a proton is deter-

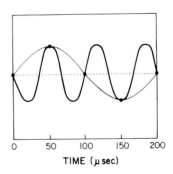

FIG. 15. Genesis of wraparound artifact in the frequency axis. Because of a low sampling rate, the high-frequency signal masquerades as a low-frequency signal. This frequency ambiguity is responsible for the production of wraparound artifacts in the frequency axis. A higher sampling rate would correctly represent the peaks and valleys of the high-frequency signal.

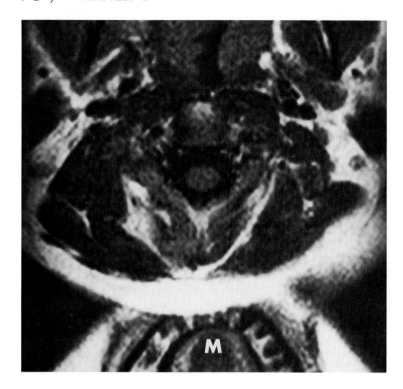

FIG. 16. Wraparound artifact in the phase-encoding direction. Transverse MR image of the neck. The mandible (M), which lies outside the anterior limit of the field of view, appears within the imaged volume, but at the opposite side of the image. The artifact has the same orientation and the same intensity as the true image.

mined by its precessional frequency, fat and water protons will be assigned to different locations in the image even when they originate from the same pixel, because fat protons precess more slowly than water protons. The resultant artifact appears as a low intensity band on one side of the water–fat interface and as a high-intensity band on the opposite (Fig. 17). Chemical-shift artifact is more pro-

nounced with high magnetic field strength and can be reduced by increasing the steepness of the frequency encoding gradient.

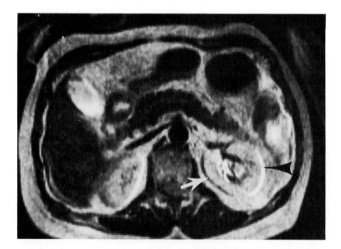

FIG. 17. Chemical-shift artifact. Transaxial MR image of the middle abdomen shows a high-intensity band (*arrowhead*) along the lateral aspect of the left kidney and a low-intensity band (*arrow*) along the medial aspect of the left kidney. These two bands represent chemical-shift misregistration artifacts and occur at the water–fat interface along the frequency axis. A similar artifact can be seen in the right kidney, but is less obvious in this image.

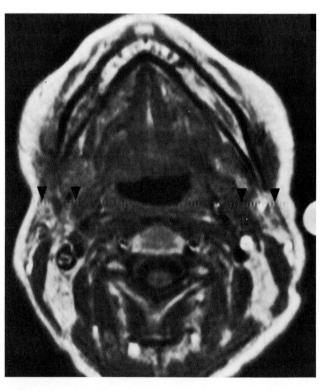

FIG. 18. Zero-line artifact. Transverse MR image through the mandible demonstrates a zero-line artifact with a zipper-like appearance along the frequency axis (*arrowheads*). (From ref. 31.)

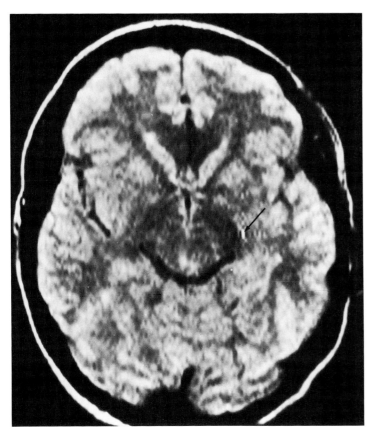

FIG. 19. Zero-line artifact. In other MR imaging systems, the zero-line artifact appears along both the frequency and phase axes, creating a cross-like appearance. A central bright dot (*arrow*) appears at the junction of these two zero-line artifacts and should not be taken as a multiple sclerosis plaque. (From ref. 31.)

Zero Line Artifact

A zero-line artifact usually has a zipper-like appearance and is due to system noise. In MR imaging, the signal from each point in the selected slice is represented by a sinc function (sine X/X) that drops off rapidly about a given center point. For signals in the normal range of amplitude, the side lobes are minimal, and each point is displayed as a single pixel of appropriate grade level. Noise appears as a high-amplitude point with persistent side lobes of the sinc function. The side lobes account for the zipper-like appearance of the artifact in the final image.

Because of differences in signal processing, the zero-line artifact occurs only along the frequency axis in some MR systems (Fig. 18). In other systems, this artifact is seen along both the frequency and phase axes, creating a cross-like appearance (Fig. 19).

Truncation Artifact

This is an edge artifact that consists of alternating high- and low-intensity bands that parallel zones of abrupt change in signal intensity (Fig. 20). It is most evident as

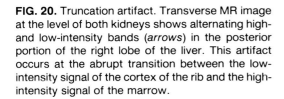

FIG. 20. Truncation artifact. Transverse MR image at the level of both kidneys shows alternating high- and low-intensity bands (*arrows*) in the posterior portion of the right lobe of the liver. This artifact occurs at the abrupt transition between the low-intensity signal of the cortex of the rib and the high-intensity signal of the marrow.

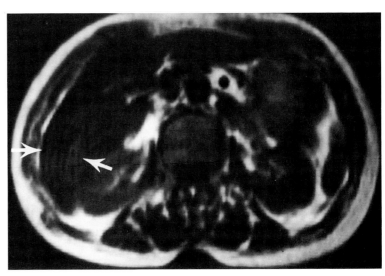

slight periodic "ringing" or duplication of the interface between high-intensity signals of bone marrow and low-intensity signals of bone in the skull. This artifact is due to the inability of a finite number of sine waves to perfectly describe a square wave, resulting in "overshooting" and "undershooting" about the corners of the wave. It can occur along both the phase and frequency axes and can be reduced by increasing the number of acquisition matrix elements.

Gradient-Power Drop-off

A drop-off in power of the gradient will result in compression of the image along the affected axis (Fig. 21). Correction requires returning the amplitude of the faulty gradient amplifier to its proper level.

Metallic Artifacts

Metallic artifacts usually appear as foci of low signal intensity surrounded by a high-intensity rim (Fig. 22). They may occasionally appear as foci of low signal intensity alone or as multiple high-intensity rings. Spatial distortion also may occur with metallic artifacts. Extraneous

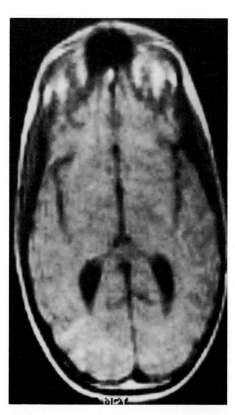

FIG. 21. Gradient-power drop-off. Compression of the image along the left-to-right axis is due to a drop-off in power of this gradient. (Courtesy of Murray A. Solomon, M.D., San Jose, California.)

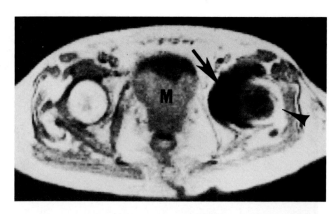

FIG. 22. Metallic artifact. Transaxial MR image shows an area of signal void surrounded by a rim of high signal intensity (*arrowhead*) in the region of the left hip prosthesis. In addition, there is also distortion of the signal medially (*arrow*). (M) bladder neoplasm.

metallic objects such as hair pins and rings must be removed before the patient enters the imaging room.

Static Electricity

Static electricity produces a characteristic artifact consisting of alternating bands of varying intensity that cover the entire image (Fig. 23). This artifact is observed most commonly when a wool blanket is used to cover the patient and when the humidity of the room is low. Occasionally a static discharge is caused by a cotton shirt or by nylon stockings. This problem can be avoided by using sheets rather than blankets to cover patients and by asking all patients to change into hospital gowns. Furthermore, the humidity of the room should be kept at an optimal level (55% at 68°F).

PROTOCOLS UNIQUE TO SPECIFIC REGIONS

Tables 2 to 26 summarize our general approach to the conduct of MR imaging by region of interest. These protocols are meant to serve as a general reference for radiologists and technologists performing MR imaging. These guidelines provide a basic approach that may be tailored according to the clinical problems and the hardware and software capabilities available. Definitions of some of the terms used in these tables are given in the following paragraphs.

Zero Reference

An effort is made to place the region of interest in the center of the magnetic field, where field intensity and homogeneity are maximal. This is achieved with the aid of

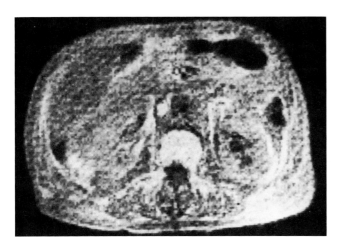

FIG. 23. Static-electricity artifact. A transaxial MR image of the abdomen is degraded by uniform pattern of alternating bands of varying signal intensity. This artifact was caused by a wool blanket used to cover the patient.

laser lights mounted on the front of the gantry. The part of the body localized by the crossing of the light beams oriented in the transverse, sagittal, and coronal planes will be at the center of the magnetic field when the patient is advanced a specified distance into the magnet. Whereas the zero reference in the transverse and sagittal planes can be adjusted by changing the position of the patient, the zero reference in the coronal plane is more difficult to adjust because of the fixed height of the table. The section at the plane of the transverse beam is considered to be at the zero transaxial level. Sections cephalad and caudad are referred to by the plus or minus distance from the zero level. The longitudinal light beam is ideally placed in the midsagittal plane of the body. This is the zero sagittal plane. Other sagittal sections are referred to by their distance from the zero plane, as in the case of the transverse plane.

Center Section

Most imagers now in use are capable of producing multiple sections of images during one sequence. The position of the center section for each sequence is determined in relation to the zero reference of the plane being imaged.

In general, the zero reference used in positioning the patient is also used as the center section if the first imaging sequence is transaxial. If the first imaging sequence is sagittal or coronal, we recommend a "scout image" to select a center section. Three scout images can be obtained in less than 1 min when a short TR (0.3 sec), a 128×128 matrix, and a single data acquisition are used. The transaxial or sagittal scout image is used to determine the center position in the coronal plane, whereas a transaxial or coronal scout image is used to select the center section in the sagittal plane.

After the first imaging sequence, center sections for subsequent sequences may be selected by using a pertinent image from a preceding sequence. This is done by electronically superimposing the coordinates of the other two orthogonal planes on the image and choosing the appropriate offset on the cathode-ray tube (CRT) monitor.

Interleaving

Although most MR imagers have a multisection imaging capability, some lack the ability to produce a series of contiguous sections. When this is the case, the operator is required to conduct two imaging sequences one after the other, with the center section of the second sequence offset by a distance equal to the thickness of the sections. The second sequence thus fills the gaps between the sections of the first sequence. This maneuver is called interleaving. Because interleaving requires additional imaging time, it should be performed only when information from contiguous sections is crucial.

TABLE 2. *Neck (0.3–0.6 T)*

Parameter	First sequence	Second sequence
Receiver coil	Surface coil	
Patient position	Supine	
Zero reference	Transverse, area of interest; sagittal, midline	Same as first sequence
Imaging plane	Transaxial	
Center section	Zero reference	
Section thickness	5 mm	
Section gap	5 mm (interleave if necessary)[a]	5 mm (interleave if necessary)[a]
Pulse parameters	SE, TR 1,500–2,100, TE 28–35, 56–90	SE, TR 500, TE 28–35, 56–70
Number of sections	15–21	5
Zoom factor	1	1
Data acquisitions	1–2	2–4

[a] Interleaving usually is necessary when searching for a parathyroid adenoma.

TABLE 3. *Thorax (0.3–0.6 T)*

Parameter	First sequence	Second sequence
Receiver coil	Body coil	
Patient position	Supine	
Zero reference	Transverse[a]; sagittal, midline	
Imaging plane	Transaxial	
Center section	Zero reference	
Section thickness	10 mm	
Section gap	0–10 mm	0–3 mm (interleave if necessary)
Pulse parameters	SE, TR 500–700, TE 28–35, 56–70	SE, TR 1,500–2,100, TE 28–35, 56–90
Number of sections	5–7	5–15
Zoom factor	1	
Data acquisitions	2	1–2

[a] When examining mediastinum or hilum, center 5–6 cm below sternal notch; can also use chest radiograph or CT as guide; When examining lung parenchyma or pleura, center over region of interest, as determined by chest radiographs or CT.

TABLE 4. *Cardiac/thoracic aorta (0.3–0.6 T)[a]*

Parameter	First sequence
Receiver coil	Body coil[b]
Patient position	Supine
Zero reference	Transverse;[c] sagittal, midline
Imaging plane	Transaxial[d]
Center section	Determined from coronal scout image
Section thickness	10 mm
Section gap	0–10 mm (interleave if necessary)
Pulse parameters	SE, TR–determined by heart rate,[e] TE 28–35, 56–70
Number of sections	5
Zoom factor	1
Data acquisitions	2

[a] The anatomic resolution of cardiac structures on MR images is significantly improved with EKG triggering. The operator selects the time delay (generally 100 msec) between the triggering signal (R wave) and the initiation of the imaging sequence. Five images are obtained from the cardiac base to apex. Each image is delayed 100 msec from the previous image. Therefore, each section through the heart is obtained at a different point in the cardiac cycle.

[b] For infants and small children, the head coil is used.

[c] Center 2–4 cm above PMI for cardiac imaging. Center over region of interest, as determined by chest radiographs, for imaging of thoracic aorta. Involvement of the abdominal aorta can be assessed, if necessary, by recentering midway between the xiphoid and umbilicus. These images can be obtained without EKG triggering with TR 1,500–2,100, TE 28–35, 56–70 (15–21 sections) (see Table 8).

[d] The transverse images usually are sufficient for demonstrating most cardiac/aortic anatomy and pathology. Coronal or sagittal images can also be obtained and may be helpful in showing portions of the heart that lie parallel to the transaxial plane (e.g., inferior wall of the left ventricle). Images similar to the angiographic left anterior oblique (LAO) or right anterior oblique (RAO) views may be helpful in patients with complex congenital heart disease. The angiographic LAO view also may be helpful in showing the relationship of an arch aneurysm or intimal flap to arch vessels. To obtain these views, the patient is placed on the examination table with the right shoulder rotated approximately 30° anteriorly. A non-gated survey image (TR 300 msec/TE 30 msec, 1 signal average) is obtained in the transaxial plane. A grid is then superimposed, and plane offsets are electronically chosen for sagittal or coronal EKG-triggered SE pulse sequences. The sagittal views are equivalent to the conventional angiographic LAO view (short axis of left ventricle), whereas the coronal view is equivalent to the conventional angiographic RAO view (long axis of left ventricle). Oblique images can also be obtained with the patient in the supine position by electronic rotation of the imaging axis.

[e] The repetition time (TR) is dependent on the patient's heart rate (e.g., effective TR is 750 msec for a heart rate of 80 beats per minute). Although not generally performed, data can be acquired on alternate heart beats in order to obtain images with a longer repetition time. However, triggering data acquisition on alternate heart beats doubles the imaging time.

TABLE 5. *Pancreas/spleen (0.3–0.6 T)*

Parameter	First sequence	Second sequence	Third sequence
Receiver coil	Body coil		
Patient position	Supine or prone		
Zero reference	Transverse, 4–6 cm below xiphoid for imaging the pancreas, 2–4 cm below xiphoid for imaging the spleen; sagittal, midline		
Imaging plane	Transaxial		
Center section	Determined from sagittal scout image	Area of interest as determined by first sequence	
Section thickness	10 mm	10–15 mm	Repeat second sequence with 10–15-mm offset to interleave, if necessary
Section gap	0–3 mm	10–15 mm	
Pulse parameters	SE, TR 1,500–2,100, TE 28–35, 56–90	SE, TR 300–500, TE 15–20	
Number of sections	5–21	7–14	
Zoom factor	1		
Data acquisitions	1–2	2–6	

TABLE 6. *Liver: search for metastases or characterization of hepatic mass detected by another imaging technique (0.3–0.6 T)*

Parameter	First sequence	Second sequence	Third sequence
Receiver coil	Body coil		
Patient position	Supine or prone		
Zero reference	Transverse, 3–5 cm below xiphoid; sagittal, midline		
Imaging plane	Transaxial		
Center section	Determined from coronal scout image		Repeat second sequence with 5–10-mm offset, if necessary
Section thickness	10 mm		
Section gap	0–5 mm	5–10 mm	
Pulse parameters	SE, TR 1,500–2,100, TE 28–35, 56–90	SE, TR 300–500, TE 15–20	
Number of sections	15–21	7–14	
Zoom factor	1		
Data acquisitions	1–2	2–6	

TABLE 7. *Liver: distinction between focal fatty infiltration and metastasis (0.3–0.6 T)*

Parameter	First sequence	Second sequence
Receiver coil	Body coil	
Patient position	Supine or prone	
Zero reference	Transverse, variable, depending on the location of the lesion; sagittal, midline	
Imaging plane	Transaxial	
Center section	Zero reference	
Section thickness	10 mm	Repeat first sequence with 10-mm offset to interleave if first sequence is performed with a section gap of 10 mm and if it misses the lesion
Section gap	0–10 mm	
Pulse parameters	Proton spectroscopic imaging[a] (opposed image), TR 1,500, TE 38, 70[b]	
Number of sections	5–15	
Zoom factor	1	
Data acquisitions	2	

[a] Distinction between focal fatty infiltration and hepatic metastasis may be difficult, if not impossible, on CT. Such a distinction is easily made with proton spectroscopic imaging using the opposed image. While the signal intensity of fatty infiltration is equal to or less than that of paraspinal muscles on the opposed image, the signal intensity of a hepatic metastasis is at least two times that of paraspinal muscles.

[b] The TEs of 38 and 70 msec are optimal for a magnetic-field strength of 0.5 T. The appropriate TEs will increase with increasing magnetic-field strength.

TABLE 8. *Retroperitoneum–aorta (0.3–0.6 T)*

Parameter	First sequence	Second sequence
Receiver coil	Body coil	
Patient position	Supine or prone	
Zero reference	Transverse, midpoint between xiphoid and umbilicus; sagittal, midline	
Imaging plane	Transaxial	Sagittal
Center section	Zero reference	Region of interest as determined from first sequence
Section thickness	10 mm	
Section gap	0–10 mm	0–3 mm
Pulse parameters	SE, TR 1,500–2,100, TE 28–35, 56–70	SE, TR 500, TE 28–35, 35–70
Number of sections	15–21	5
Zoom factor	1	
Data acquisitions	1–2	2–4

TABLE 9. *Retroperitoneum: screening for lymphadenopathy (0.3–0.6 T)*

Parameter	First sequence	Second sequence
Receiver coil	Body coil	
Patient position	Supine or prone	
Zero reference	Transverse, midpoint between xiphoid and umbilicus; sagittal, midline	Transverse, midpoint between umbilicus and pubic symphysis;[a] sagittal, midline
Imaging plane	Transaxial	
Center section	Zero reference	Zero reference
Section thickness	10 mm	
Section gap	10 mm	
Pulse parameters	SE, TR 300–1,000, TE 15–20	Same as first sequence
Number of sections	7–14	
Zoom factor	1	
Data acquisitions	2–4	

[a] For best results, the patient should be recentered by adjusting the table position rather than by electronic means, because large electronic adjustments in centering place the imaged volume out of the center of the magnetic field.

TABLE 10. *Retroperitoneum: differentiation between fibrosis and recurrent tumor (0.3–0.6 T)*

Parameter	First sequence	Second sequence
Receiver coil	Body coil	
Patient position	Supine or prone	
Zero reference	Transverse, region of interest; sagittal, midline	
Imaging plane	Transaxial	Transaxial
Center section	Determined from coronal scout image	
Section thickness	10 mm	10–15 mm
Section gap	0–3 mm	10–15 mm
Pulse parameters	SE, TR 1,500–2,100, TE 28–35, 80–90	SE, TR 300–500, TE 15–20
Number of sections	5–21	7–14
Zoom factor	1	
Data acquisitions	1–2	2–4

TABLE 11. *Kidney: staging for renal neoplasms (0.3–0.6 T)*

Parameter	First sequence	Second sequence	Third sequence	Fourth sequence
Receiver coil	Body coil			
Patient position	Supine or prone			
Zero reference	Transverse, midpoint between xiphoid and lower costal margins; sagittal, midline			
Imaging plane	Transaxial or coronal[a]		Transaxial	Sagittal or coronal[c]
Center section	Determined from sagittal scout image	Repeat first sequence with 10-mm[b] offset to interleave, if necessary	Region of interest as determined from first two sequences	Region of interest as determined from first three sequences
Section thickness	10–15 mm		10 mm	
Section gap	10–15 mm[b]		0–3 mm	0–10 mm
Pulse parameters	SE, TR 300–500, TE 15–20		SE, TR 1,500–2,100, TE 28–35, 56–90	SE, TR 500, TE 28–35, 56–70
Number of sections	7–14		15–21	5
Zoom factor	1			
Data acquisitions	2–4		1–2	2

[a] If the lesion is small or located in the upper or lower pole, the first sequence should be performed in the coronal plane instead of the transaxial plane.

[b] If equipment allows no gap between sections (i.e., contiguous sections), no offset or interleaving is required.

[c] Sagittal images (fourth sequence) usually are unnecessary, but occasionally help in evaluating tumor extension into adjacent structures and in assessing the extent of tumor thrombus in the inferior vena cava.

TABLE 12. *Adrenal (0.3–0.6 T)*

Parameter	First sequence	Second sequence	Third sequence
Receiver coil	Body coil		
Patient position	Supine or prone		
Zero reference	Transverse, 2–4 cm below xiphoid; sagittal, midline		
Imaging plane	Transaxial	Transaxial	Sagittal or coronal[a]
Center section	Determined from coronal scout image	Region of interest as determined from first sequence	Region of interest as determined from prior sequences
Section thickness	10 mm		
Section gap	0–3 mm	0–10 mm	0–10 mm
Pulse parameters	SE, TR 1,500–2,100, TE 28–35, 56–90	SE, TR 300–500, TE 15–20	SE, TR 300–500, TE 15–20
Number of sections	15–21	5	5
Zoom factor	1		
Data acquisitions	1–2	2–6	2–6

[a] Sagittal or coronal images usually are unnecessary, but occasionally may be helpful in demonstrating the relationship of an adrenal mass to adjacent structures.

TABLE 13. *Pelvis: staging of bladder, prostate, and gynecologic neoplasms (0.3–0.6 T)*

Parameter	First sequence	Second sequence	Third sequence	Fourth sequence
Receiver coil	Body coil			
Patient position	Supine or prone			
Zero reference	Transverse, 4–6 cm above pubic symphysis or midpoint between pubic symphysis and iliac crest; sagittal, midline			
Imaging plane	Transaxial	Transaxial	Transaxial	Sagittal or coronal[b]
Center section	Zero reference	Region of interest as determined by first sequence		Region of interest as determined from prior sequences
Section thickness	5–10 mm[a]	5–15 mm[a]	Repeat first sequence with 5–15-mm offset to interleave, if necessary	
Section gap	0–3 mm	10–15 mm		0–5 mm
Pulse parameters	SE, TR 1,500–2,100, TE 28–35, 56–90	SE, TR 300–500, TE 15–20		SE, TR 1,500–2,100, TE 28–35, 56–90
Number of sections	15–21	7–14		9–21[c]
Zoom factor	1			
Data acquisitions	1–2	2–4		1–2

Note: The first three sequences can be used for general pelvic imaging.

[a] A 5-mm slice thickness is used for imaging the prostate, 10–15-mm for bladder and gynecologic neoplasms.

[b] The choice of a sagittal or coronal view depends on the location of the neoplasm. In bladder imaging, if the neoplasm involves the lateral wall of the bladder, a coronal section is optimal. However, if the bladder neoplasm is located in the anterior or posterior wall, sagittal sections are much more helpful. In staging gynecologic neoplasms, we prefer sagittal images. In contradistinction, we prefer coronal to sagittal images in staging prostatic carcinoma because both seminal vesicles can be displayed in a single section. If time permits, images in all three orthogonal planes should be obtained.

[c] Number of slices determined by the size of the patient.

TABLE 14. *Renal transplantation (0.3–0.6 T)*

Parameter	First sequence	Second sequence
Receiver coil	Surface coil	
Patient position	Supine	
Zero reference	Center of surgical scar	
Imaging plane	Coronal	
Center section	Determined from sagittal scout image	
Section thickness	10–15 mm	
Section gap	10–15 mm	0–3 mm
Pulse parameters	SE, TR 300–500, TE 15–20	SE, TR 1,500–2,100, TE 28–35, 56–90
Number of sections	7–14	
Zoom factor	1	1
Data acquisitions	2–4	1–2

TABLE 15. *Scrotum (0.3–0.6 T)*

Parameter	First sequence	Second sequence
Receiver coil	Surface coil	
Patient position	Supine	
Zero reference	Center of scrotum[a]	
Imaging plane	Coronal	
Center section	Determined from transverse scout image	
Section thickness	5 mm	5 mm
Section gap	5 mm (interleave with 5-mm offset if necessary)	5 mm (interleave with 5-mm offset if necessary)
Pulse parameters	SE, TR 300–500, TE 15–20	SE, TR 1,500–2,100, TE 28–35, 56–90
Number of sections	7–14	
Zoom factor	1.5	1.5
Data acquisitions	2–4	2

[a] The scrotum should be elevated with sheets, and the receiver coil should be placed 1–2 cm above the scrotum.

TABLE 16. *Temporomandibular joint (TMJ) for disc position (0.3–1.5 T)*

Parameter	First sequence	Second sequence	Third sequence
Receiver coil	Appropriate surface coil with 1-coil or 2-coil array		
Patient position	Variable[a]		Repeat first and second sequences with mouth opened to maximize disc deformity or document recapture of disc
Zero reference	2–2.5 cm deep to skin in coronal plane; transverse, center of receiver coil; sagittal, center of receiver coil		
Imaging plane	Coronal (corresponds to lateral radiographic projection)		
Center section	Zero reference		
Section thickness	3 mm (or thinner)		
Section gap	3 mm (interleave)	Repeat first sequence with 3–5-mm offset to interleave	
Pulse parameters	SE, TR 700,[b] TE 15–20		
Number of sections	3–5		
Zoom factor	3.5		
Data acquisitions	2		

[a] Much of the patient positioning relates to system and coil parameters that determine the geometrical relationships between the transmitter (body) and receiver (surface) coils. If only one relationship is possible, this will determine the patient's head position. For example, if the surface coil must be in the coronal plane, the patient's head will of necessity be turned to the left or right, and the "lateral" image of the disc acquired through the coronal plane. If a 2-coil array is used, the head is held straight up, and both sides are examined simultaneously. For successful TMJ imaging, the patient must be comfortable and stable. When the mouth is held in an open or partially open position, the sequence must be short enough to be tolerated. A bite block makes the patient more comfortable and stable.

[b] T1-weighted (short-TR, short-TE) sequences provide adequate spatial resolution and contrast among fat (high signal), bone marrow (high signal), muscle (intermediate signal), compact bone (low signal), and TMJ disc (low signal).

TABLE 17. *Femoral head for ischemic necrosis (0.3–1.5 T)*

Parameter	First sequence	Second sequence	Third sequence
Receiver coil	Body coil		
Patient position	Supine		
Zero reference	Transverse, femoral artery pulse in groin; sagittal, midline of body		
Imaging plane	Transaxial	Coronal	Coronal
Center section	Zero reference	Determined from transaxial image	
Section thickness	10 mm		
Section gap	10 mm (interleave if necessary)	10 mm	0 mm
Pulse parameters	SE, TR 300–500, TE 15–20	SE, TR 300–500, TE 15–20	SE, TR 3,000, TE 90
Number of sections	3–5	3–9	3–9
Zoom factor	1–1.2		
Data acquisitions	1	2–4	1

Note: Pulse sequence 1 is used to provide localization for choice of the single best coronal plane through the femoral head showing the central weight-bearing region. It can be accomplished rapidly and also serves to help localize infarcts dorsally or ventrally. Pulse sequence 2 (coronal plane) optimally shows the important subchondral/subcortical cancellous region. A short-TR, short-TE (T1-weighted) sequence emphasizes contrast differences between devascularized and normal bone marrow. A T2-weighted sequence serves to differentiate ischemic necrosis from other pathologic processes.

TABLE 18. *Extremity for soft-tissue mass/bone tumor (0.3–1.5 T)*

Parameter	First sequence[a]	Second sequence[b]	Third sequence[c]
Receiver coil	Body coil or appropriate surface coil if small or superficial part		
Patient position	Supine or other comfortable position		
Zero reference	Transverse, center of mass as determined by physical examination or estimated from conventional radiographs; sagittal, midline of extremity or estimated midline of mass		
Imaging plane	Transaxial	Sagittal or coronal	Sagittal or coronal
Center section	Zero reference	Center of mass as determined from transaxial image	Center long axis of bone or as determined from transaxial image
Section thickness	10 mm		
Section gap	0 mm		
Pulse parameters	SE, TR 2,100–3,000, TE 35–90	Same	SE, TR 300–700, TE 15–20
Number of sections	6–15		3–5
Zoom factor	1–1.2		
Data acquisitions	2 (only 1 average required at 0.5 T or above)		1–2

[a] The first pulse sequence provides a survey in the transaxial plane that confirms tumor localization and provides information regarding local relationships. It is a dual-echo examination, with the short echo emphasizing anatomic information and the longer echo providing T2-weighted images. The latter images optimize contrast between muscle and mass.

[b] Sequence 2 provides direct definition of proximal and distal extents of the tumor mass.

[c] Sequence 3 is T1-weighted and provides excellent differentiation of tumor from bone marrow. It is also used to help differentiate lipoma and hematoma (both having high signal on T1-weighted sequences) from other masses. It should also show contrast between mass and muscle in the unlikely event that the two were isointense on pulse sequence 1. The sagittal or coronal plane is employed to determine intramedullary spread of the tumor.

TABLE 19. *Any bone for osteomyelitis/infarct/metastasis (0.3–1.5 T)*

Parameter	First sequence[a]	Second sequence[b]
Receiver coil	Body coil or appropriate surface coil if small or superficial part	
Patient position	Supine, prone, or other comfortable position	
Zero reference	Transverse, centered on region of interest as estimated by combination of physical findings, conventional radiographs, radionuclide bone scans, or CT; sagittal, centered on region of interest	
Imaging plane	Transaxial, sagittal, or coronal, whichever optimally displays marrow cavity (e.g., coronal for the distal femur or proximal tibia)	Same as first sequence
Center section	Zero reference	
Section thickness	3–10 mm (wrist 3 mm; knee, ankle 5 mm; hip 10 mm)	
Section gap	3–10 mm (interleave if necessary)	
Pulse parameters	SE, TR 300–500, TE 15–20	SE, TR 2,100–3,000, TE 90
Number of sections	3–9, depending on thickness of bone to be examined	
Zoom factor	1 or greater if necessary	
Data acquisitions	1–2 (only 1 average required at 1.5 T)	1

[a] MR imaging can detect and localize infection, ischemia, and tumor in bone marrow. T1-weighted (short-TR, short-TE) sequences provide anatomic information and emphasize contrast differences between abnormal and normal marrow.

[b] A T2-weighted sequence is used to differentiate bone infarct (short T2) from infection and tumor (long T2).

TABLE 20. *Ligaments and tendons (0.3–1.5 T)*

Parameter	First sequence
Receiver coil	Appropriate limited-field-of-view coil
Patient position	Long axis of tendon in one of the orthogonal planes
Zero reference	Central axis of tendon or ligament sought
Imaging plane	Parallel to long axis of tendon
Center section	Zero reference or appropriate offset in *x* or *y* axis as determined from transaxial section
Section thickness	3–5 mm
Section gap	3–5 mm (interleave as necessary)
Pulse parameters	SE, TR 300–500, TE 15–20
Number of sections	5 or less
Zoom factor	1–1.5
Data acquisitions	2–4

Note: T1-weighted (short-TR, short-TE) sequences provide sufficient signal and contrast between fat (high signal) and ligaments or tendons (low signal) for detection of normal and abnormal structures.

TABLE 21. *Cartilage (0.3–1.5 T)*

Parameter	First sequence	Second sequence
Receiver coil	Appropriate limited-field-of-view coil	
Patient position	Long axis of bone in one of the orthogonal planes	
Zero reference	Joint surface of bone	
Imaging plane	Perpendicular to joint surface[a] (sagittal or coronal)	Select[a]
Center section	Zero reference	
Section thickness	3–5 mm	
Section gap	3–5 mm (interleave)	
Pulse parameters	SE, TR 900, TE 15–20[b]	SE TR 3000, TE 28–35, 70–90
Number of sections	11 or less	19 or less
Zoom factor	1–2.5	
Data acquisitions	2	1

[a] For imaging the knee joint, the first sequence is in coronal plane and the second sequence is in sagittal plane.

[b] A mixed (balanced) pulse sequence provides better separation of articular cartilage, fibrocartilage, and joint fluid than T1- or T2-weighted sequences.

TABLE 22. *Muscle diseases (0.3–1.5 T)*

Parameter	First sequence
Receiver coil	Body coil for thighs, head coil for legs, surface coil for arms
Patient position	Supine or any comfortable position
Zero reference	Transverse, middle of muscle mass or middle of long bone; sagittal, central long axis of extremity or midline between extremities
Imaging plane	Transaxial
Center section	Zero reference
Section thickness	10 mm
Section gap	10 mm (interleave if necessary)
Pulse parameters	SE, TR 300–500, TE 15–20
Number of sections	3–9, depending on volume for survey
Zoom factor	1
Data acquisitions	2

Note: Muscle diseases cause fatty replacement of muscles. Short-TR, short-TE (T1-weighted) sequences optimize contrast differences between normal and infiltrated muscle masses. Sagittal or coronal planes can be added if direct display of longitudinal muscle anatomy is required.

TABLE 23. *Breast (0.3–1.5 T)*

Parameter	First sequence[a]	Second sequence[b]	Third sequence
Receiver coil	Surface coil designed to accommodate a single breast or both breasts simultaneously		
Patient position	Prone with breast(s) suspended in center of receiver coil		
Zero reference	Determined by surface-coil configuration; for a single-breast design with breast centered; transverse, center of coil; sagittal, center of coil		
Imaging plane	Transaxial, corresponds to mammographic craniocaudal view		As necessary to provide a second plane of view
Center section	Zero reference		
Section thickness	3–5 mm		
Section gap	0 if contiguous slices; 3–5 mm if conventional multislice		
Pulse parameters	SE, TR 2,100–3,000, TE 90	SE, TR 300–500, TE 15–20	As necessary to provide further tissue characterization
Number of sections	11–15	1 (single most informative site)	
Zoom factor	1–1.7		
Data acquisitions	2 (only 1 average required at 0.5 T or above)	2–4	

[a] For breast imaging, it is necessary to optimize signal strength and spatial resolution. In order to survey breast tissue, contiguous slices are required through as much of the breast's volume as possible. For the patient's comfort, and to reduce motion unsharpness, the sequence should be as short as possible. The first sequence recommended here meets these goals and provides T2 contrast, which is important for detection of certain pathologic conditions.

[b] The second sequence provides T1 contrast.

TABLE 24. *Cervical spine and cord (0.3–1.5 T)*

Parameter	First sequence	Second sequence	Third sequence	Fourth sequence	Fifth sequence
Receiver coil	Head or surface coil				
Patient position	Supine				
Zero reference	Transverse, thyroid prominence; sagittal, midline				
Imaging plane	Sagittal				Transaxial[e]
Center section	Zero reference[a]	Offset by 5 mm to interleave[b]	Same as first sequence	Offset by 5 mm to interleave[b]	Select[e]
Section thickness	5 mm				
Section gap	0–5 mm[b]				Select[e]
Pulse parameters	SE, TR 300–500,[c] TE 15–35		SE, TR 1,500–2,100,[d] TE 28–35, 90–120		
Number of sections	5–7		7		
Zoom factor	1				
Data acquisitions	0.5 T, 2–4; 1.5 T, 2		0.5 T, 2; 1.5 T, 1		0.5 T, 2; 1.5 T, 1

[a] For precise midline imaging, one may start with a scout image in coronal plane and use the "grid" to find the midline of the spine.

[b] If equipment allows no gap between sections (i.e., contiguous sections), no offset or interleaving is required.

[c] When using contiguous sections, one may increase TR to 700 msec to provide for enough sections across the spine in a single sequence. Ideal for (a) cord swelling, atrophy, cavitation, or blood clot, (b) compression of the cord by spondylosis or tumor; (c) involvement of bone by tumor or inflammation.

[d] Ideal for showing (a) disc herniation, (b) some cases of bone tumor, (c) some cases of parenchymal disease in the cord, e.g., tumor, demyelination.

[e] This transaxial series may be needed in some cases to show anatomic relationships, particularly in laterally located lesions. Select the section level using the "grid" on one of the images of the preceding sequences that shows the lesion(s) to best advantage.

TABLE 25. *Thoracic spine and cord (0.3–1.5 T)*

Parameter	First sequence	Second sequence	Third sequence	Fourth sequence	Fifth sequence
Receiver coil	Surface coil				
Patient position	Supine				
Zero reference	Transverse, middle of sternum,[a] xiphoid notch;[b] sagittal, midline				
Imaging plane	Sagittal				Transaxial
Center section	Zero reference[c]	Offset by 5 mm to interleave[d]	Same as first sequence	Offset by 5 mm to interleave[d]	Select[g]
Section thickness	5 mm				
Section gap	0–5 mm[d]				
Pulse parameters	SE, TR 300–500,[e] TE 15–35		SE, TR 1,500–2,100,[f] TE 28–35, 90–120		Select[g]
Number of sections	5–7		7		
Zoom factor	1.5				
Data acquisitions	0.5 T, 2–4; 1.5 T, 2		0.5 T, 2; 1.5 T, 1		

[a] For upper and middle thoracic region, including cervicothoracic junction.

[b] For middle and lower thoracic region, including thoracolumbar junction.

[c] Obtain a coronal scout image and use the "grid" to find the midline of the spine. In cases of scoliosis, one may find it necessary to select several midline planes for different segments of the region examined.

[d] If equipment allows no gap between sections (i.e., contiguous sections), no offset or interleaving is required.

[e] Ideal for (a) swelling, atrophy, cavitation, or tethering of the cord, (b) involvement of bone by tumor or inflammation. When using contiguous sections, one may increase TR to 700 msec to provide for enough sections across the spine in a single sequence.

[f] Ideal for showing (a) disc herniation, (b) some cases of tumor, (c) some cases of parenchymal disease of the cord.

[g] This transaxial series may be needed in some cases to show anatomic relationships, particularly in laterally located lesions. Select the section level using the "grid" on one of the images of the preceding sequences that shows the lesion(s) to best advantage.

TABLE 26. *Lumbar spine (0.3–1.5 T)*

Parameter	First sequence	Second sequence	Third sequence	Fourth sequence	Fifth sequence
Receiver coil	Surface coil				
Patient position	Supine				
Zero reference	Transverse, umbilicus (L3); sagittal, midline				
Imaging plane	Sagittal		Sagittal		Transaxial
Center section	Zero reference[a]	Offset by 5 or 10 mm to interleave[b]	Same as first sequence	Offset by 5 mm to interleave[b]	Select[f]
Section thickness	5 mm				
Section gap	0–5 mm[b]				
Pulse parameters	SE, TR 300–500,[c,d] TE 15–35		SE, TR 1,500–2,100,[e] TE 28–35, 90–120		Select[f]
Number of sections	5–7		7		
Zoom factor	1.5				
Data acquisitions	0.5 T, 2–4; 1.5 T, 2		0.5 T, 2; 1.5 T, 1		

[a] For precise midline imaging, usually it is necessary to obtain a scout image in the coronal plane and use the "grid" to find the midline of the lumbar spine. In cases of scoliosis, it may be necessary to select several midline planes for different "segments" of the lumbar spine.

[b] If equipment allows no gap between sections (i.e., contiguous sections), no offset or interleaving is required.

[c] Ideal for evaluating (a) status of bone, CSF space (dural sac), and epidural fat, (b) encroachment on the dural sac by spondylosis, (c) intradural masses. When using contiguous sections, one may increase TR to 700 msec to provide for enough sections across the spine in a single sequence.

[d] When using contiguous sections, one may increase TR to 700 msec to provide for enough sections across the spine in a single sequence.

[e] Ideal for demonstrating (a) disc herniation, (b) involvement of bone by tumor or inflammation; (c) intradural masses.

[f] Use the grid on the sagittal section that shows the lesion to best advantage. The center section should be through the lesion. The pulse parameter and number of sections depend on which pulse sequence in the sagittal series showed the lesion best.

SELECTED REFERENCES

General

1. Bradley WG, Adey WR, Hasso AN. *Magnetic resonance imaging of the brain, head, and neck: a text atlas.* Rockville, Maryland: Aspen Publications, 1985.
2. Heiken JP, Glazer HS, Lee JKT, Murphy WA, Gado M. *Manual of clinical magnetic resonance imaging.* New York: Raven Press, 1986.
3. Kaufman L, Crooks LE, Margulis AR. *Nuclear magnetic resonance in medicine.* Tokyo: Igaku-Shoin, 1981.
4. Morgan CJ, Hendee WR. *Introduction to magnetic resonance imaging,* Denver: Multi-Media Publishing, 1984.
5. Partain CL, Price RR, Patton JA, et al. *Magnetic resonance (MR) imaging,* Philadelphia: WB Saunders, 1983.

Physical Principles

6. Bradley WG, Newton TH, Crooks LE. Physical principles of nuclear magnetic resonance. In: Newton TH, Potts DG, (eds.) *Modern neuroradiology: advanced imaging techniques.* San Anselmo, California: Clavadel Press, 1983:15–62.
7. Bradley WG, Waluch V. Blood flow: magnetic resonance imaging. *Radiology* 1985;154:443–450.
8. Bradley WG, Kortman KE, Crues JV. Central nervous system high resolution magnetic resonance imaging: effect of increasing spatial resolution on resolving power. *Radiology* 1985;156:93–98.
9. Bradley WG, Waluch V, Lai KS, Fernandez EJ, Spalter C. The appearance of rapidly flowing blood on magnetic resonance images. *AJR* 1984;143:1167–1174.
10. Fullerton GD, Cameron IL, Ord VA. Frequency dependence of magnetic resonance spin-lattice relaxation of protons in biological materials. *Radiology* 1984;151:135–138.
11. Kumar A, Welti D, Ernst R. NMR zeugmatography. *J Magn Reson* 1985;18:69–85.
12. Lauterbur PC. Image formation by induced local interactions: Examples employing nuclear magnetic resonance. *Nature* 1973;242:190–191.
13. Mills CM, Brant-Zawadski M, Crooks LE, Kaufman L, Sheldon P, Norman D, Bank W, Newton TW. Nuclear magnetic resonance: Principles of blood flow imaging. *AJR* 1983;142:165–170.
14. Pykett IL, Newhouse JH, Buonanno FS, et al. Principles of nuclear magnetic resonance imaging. *Radiology* 1982;143:157–168.
15. Waluch V, Bradley WG. NMR even echo rephasing in slow laminar flow. *J Comput Assist Tomogr* 1984;8:594–598.
16. Wehrli FW, MacFall JR, Newton TH. Parameters determining the appearance of NMR images. In: Newton TH, Potts, DG, eds. *Modern neuroradiology: advanced imaging techniques,* San Anselmo, California: Clavadel Press, 1983:15–61.

Imaging Techniques

17. Axel L. Surface coil magnetic resonance imaging. *J Comput Assist Tomogr* 1984;8:381–384.
18. Bailes DR, Gilderdale GM, Bydder GM, Collins AG, Firmin DN. Respiratory ordered phase encoding (ROPE): a method for reducing respiratory motion artifacts in MR imaging. *J Comput Assist Tomogr* 1985;9:835–838.
19. Brateman L. Chemical shift imaging: a review. *AJR* 1986;146:971–980.
20. Bydder GM, Young IR. Clinical use of the partial saturation and saturation recovery sequences in MR imaging. *J Comput Assist Tomogr* 1985;9:1020–1032.
21. Bydder GM, Young IR. MR imaging: clinical use of the inversion recovery sequence. *J Comput Assist Tomogr* 1985;9:659–675.
22. Crooks LE, Barker B, Chang H, Feinberg D, Hoenninger JC, Watts JC, Arakawa M, Kaufman L, Sheldon PE, Botvinick E, Higgins CB. Magnetic resonance imaging strategies for heart studies. *Radiology* 1984;153:459–465.
23. Dixon WT. Simple proton spectroscopic imaging. *Radiology* 1984;153:189–194.
24. Edelman RR, Hahn PF, Buxton R, Wittenberg J, Ferrucci JT, Brady TJ. Rapid magnetic resonance imaging with suspended respiration: Initial clinical application in the abdomen. *Radiology* 1986;161:125–131.
25. Ehman RL, McNamara MT, Pallack M, Hricak H, Higgins CB. Magnetic resonance imaging with respiratory gating: techniques and advantages. *AJR* 1984;143:1175–1182.
26. Feiglin DH, George CR, MacIntyre WJ, O'Donnell JK, Go RT, Pavlicek W, Meaney TF. Gated cardiac magnetic resonance structural imaging: optimization by electronic axial rotation. *Radiology* 1985;154:129–132.
27. Lanzer P, Barta C, Botvinick EH, Wiesendanger HUD, Modin G, Higgins CB. ECG-Synchronized cardiac MR imaging: Methods and evaluation. *Radiology* 1985;155:681–686.
28. Murphy WA, Gutierrez FR, Levitt RG, Glazer HS, Lee JKT. Oblique views of the heart by magnetic resonance imaging. *Radiology* 1985;154:225–226.
29. Runge VM, Clanton JA, Partain CL, James AE. Respiratory gating in magnetic resonance imaging at 0.5 Tesla. *Radiology* 1984;151:521–523.
30. Sepponen RE, Sipponen JT, Tanttu JI. A method for chemical shift imaging: demonstration of bone marrow involvement with proton chemical shift imaging. *J Comput Assist Tomogr* 1984;8:585–587.

Artifacts

31. Bellon EM, Haacke EM, Coleman PE, Sacco DC, Steiger DA, Gangarosa RE. MR artifacts: a review. *AJR* 1986;147:1271–1281.
32. Mechlin M, Thickman D, Kressel HY, Gefter W, Joseph P. Magnetic resonance imaging of postoperative patients with metallic implants. *AJR* 1984;143:1281–1284.
33. Pusey E, Lufkin RB, Brown RKJ, Solomon MA, Stark DD, Taqrr RW, Hanafee WN. Magnetic resonance imaging artifacts: Mechanism and clinical significance. *Radiographics* 1986;6:891–911.
34. Schultz CL, Alfidi RJ, Nelson AD, Kopiwoda SY, Clampitt ME. The effect of motion on two-dimensional Fourier transformation magnetic resonance images. *Radiology* 1984;152:117–121.
35. Soila KP, Viamonte M, Starewicz PM. Chemical shift misregistration effect in magnetic resonance imaging. *Radiology* 1984;153:819–820.
36. Weinreb JC, Brateman L, Babcock EE, Maravilla KR, Cohen JM, Horner SD. Chemical shift artifact in clinical magnetic resonance imaging at 0.35 T. *AJR* 1985;145:183–185.

Safety

37. Budinger TF. Potential medical effects and hazards of human NMR studies. In: Kaufman L, Crooks LE, Margulis AR (eds.) *Nuclear magnetic resonance in medicine,* New York and Tokyo: Igaku-Shoin, 1981:207–231.
38. Davis PL, Crooks LE, Arakawa M, McRee R, Kaufman L, Margulis AR. Potential hazards in NMR imaging: heating effects of changing magnetic fields and RF fields on small metallic implants. *AJR* 1981;137:857–860.
39. Geard CR, Osmak RS, Hall EJ, Simon HE, Maudsley AA, Hilal SK. Magnetic resonance and ionizing radiation. A comparative evaluation in vitro of oncogenic and gevotoxic potential. *Radiology* 1984;152:199–202.
40. New PFJ, Rosen BR, Brady TJ, Bounanno FS, Kistler JP, Burt CT, Hinshaw WS, Newhouse JH, Pohost GM, Taveras JM. Potential hazards and artifacts of ferromagnetic and nonferromagnetic in surgical and dental materials and devices in nuclear magnetic resonance imaging. *Radiology* 1983;147:139–148.
41. Pavlicek W, Geisinger M, Castle L, Borkowski GP, Meaney TF, Bream BL, Gallagher JH. The effects of nuclear magnetic resonance on patients with cardiac pacemakers. *Radiology* 1983;147:149–153.
42. Schwartz JL, Crooks LE. NMR imaging produces no observable mutations or cytotoxicity in mammalian cells. *AJR* 1980;139:583–585.
43. Soulen RL, Budinger TF, Higgins CB. Magnetic resonance imaging of prosthetic heart valves. *Radiology* 1985;154:705–707.
44. Wolff S, Crooks LE, Brown P, Howard R, Painter RB. Tests for DNA and chromosomal damage induced by nuclear magnetic resonance imaging. *Radiology* 1980;136:707–710.

CHAPTER 5

Interventional Computed Tomography

Daniel Picus, Philip J. Weyman, and Dixie J. Anderson

Percutaneous procedures using radiologic guidance have become common over the past 10 years. Increasingly, these procedures are accepted as primary methods of both diagnosis and treatment. Radiologists use a variety of modalities to guide these procedures, primarily fluoroscopy, ultrasound, and computed tomography (CT). Fluoroscopy is relatively inexpensive and readily available, but has poor contrast resolution and shows structures in only two dimensions. Ultrasound is relatively inexpensive and portable and additionally allows cross-sectional imaging. However, ultrasound is limited to relatively superficial structures, has marked difficulty with overlying bowel gas and bone, and has limited applicability in patients with surgical dressings and draining wounds (62).

Computed tomography offers precise, three-dimensional localization of lesions for biopsy and/or drainage. This provides detailed depiction of the relationships of vital structures surrounding the lesion in question and allows precise planning of a percutaneous access route. The superior contrast resolution of CT allows imaging of bowel (air), visceral organs, and bone, as well as orally and intravenously administered contrast agents. In the abdomen, the use of oral contrast material is essential to distinguish between abscess cavities and normal bowel. The enhancement provided by intravenous contrast material can yield information regarding tumor vascularity prior to biopsy and the relationships of surrounding major vascular structures.

Perhaps the greatest impact of CT as a guide for interventional procedures is its ability to define the exact location of the needle tip within a lesion. This allows small structures to be biopsied or aspirated with a high degree of accuracy and therefore with less risk of complications.

Finally, CT is extremely versatile. Postsurgical patients with overlying dressings, draining wounds, and ostomies can be imaged easily. CT delineates bone and bowel gas without the difficulties inherent in ultrasound imaging. Patients can be placed in a wide variety of positions and approached from any angle.

Although CT provides excellent images, there are disadvantages in performing CT-guided procedures. CT is a relatively expensive technology. These procedures often are time-consuming, and CT has limited availability because of competition within an always busy diagnostic schedule. In addition, when performing CT-guided procedures, passage of guide wires and catheters cannot be monitored as easily as it can with fluoroscopy. Finally, access to the patient may be limited secondary to the CT gantry.

Our policy is that CT is used to guide interventional procedures only when fluoroscopy or ultrasound guidance is unsatisfactory. Superficial lesions that are seen easily with conventional radiographs (e.g., lung lesions, bone lesions. gas-filled abscess cavities) should be approached with fluoroscopic guidance. Ultrasound guidance should be used when the lesion can be imaged with ultrasound (e.g., cystic lesions, liver metastases) and when a simple, safe access route is available.

Computed tomography is most useful in the areas of the retroperitoneum (e.g., lymph nodes, adrenal glands, pancreas), pelvis (e.g., lymph nodes, abscess drainage, tumor biopsy), and mediastinum and for the following types of masses: small lesions or collections less than 3 cm in diameter, masses close to major vascular structures, intraabdominal lesions surrounded by loops of bowel, and any lesion that is not easily demonstrated by either ultrasound or fluoroscopy.

PERCUTANEOUS BIOPSY

Percutaneous biopsy is the most frequently performed CT-guided procedure. Its most common indication is to document neoplastic disease (primary, metastatic, or recurrent), differentiating neoplastic disease from inflammatory disease, postoperative changes, post-therapy changes, or normal structure (Fig. 1). By providing histologic diagnosis, percutaneous biopsy may obviate sur-

A,B

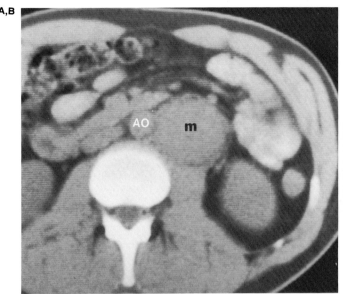

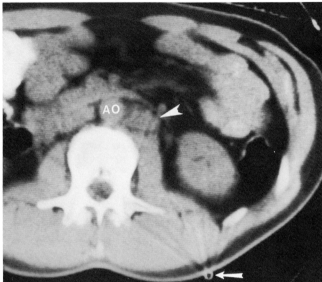

C

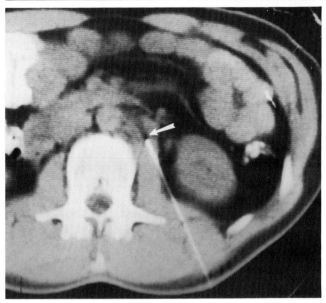

FIG. 1. CT-guided biopsy. **A:** CT scan demonstrates a large mass (m) due to metastatic seminoma lateral to the aorta (AO). **B:** Scan obtained after 6 months of chemotherapy shows that the paraaortic mass had markedly diminished in size (*arrowhead*). To determine whether this mass represented residual tumor or fibrotic tissue, a percutaneous biopsy under CT guidance was elected. On a scan performed in the prone position, a metallic marker (*arrow*) was placed on the skin surface to mark the proposed entry site. **C:** After advancing the biopsy needle, a CT scan confirms that the tip is in the paraaortic mass. Shadowing (*arrow*) of the needle distally confirms that the needle tip is within the scan plane.

gery and dictate appropriate palliative therapy in a patient with an incurable malignancy. In other patients, it may allow more precise pretherapy planning.

Needle Selection

There is wide variety among the needles available for percutaneous biopsy (Table 1, Fig. 2). The particular gauge and tip configuration selected depend on the type of lesion to be biopsied, the amount of tissue necessary for a diagnosis, what normal structures surround the lesion (e.g., bowel, vessels), and, perhaps most important, the individual preference of the radiologist and the pathologist. For instance, it does little good to obtain a cytologic specimen if the pathologist is unfamiliar with cytopathology (6,67).

Aspirating Needles

The smallest-gauge needles used are the so-called aspirating needles (20 or 22 gauge). These are simple beveled needles that are used to obtain cytologic specimens. Occasionally, chunks of tissue also are aspirated with these fine-gauge needles and can be spun down and processed as a cell block for histology. Perhaps the best known of these aspirating needles is the thin-walled Chiba needle (Fig. 2). These needles are particularly useful when normal organs (especially bowel) must be crossed in order to obtain a biopsy. Puncture of either bowel or vascular structures with a 22-gauge needle is safe and frequently unavoidable for deep-seated lesions (*vide infra*) (6,37).

Excellent results have been reported using fine-needle aspiration biopsy. Harter et al. (37) reported an overall accuracy of 90% using fine-needle aspiration with im-

TABLE 1. *Needles*

Needle	Gauge	Comments
Aspiration		
Chiba (Cook)	20, 22	Very flexible, difficult to steer; cytologic specimen only
Modified aspiration		
Turner (Cook)	18, 20, 22	Potential for obtaining tissue core
Greene (Cook)	18, 20, 22	Potential for obtaining tissue core
Madayag (Waters Instruments)	22	Potential for obtaining tissue core
Franseen (Cook)	18, 20	Potential for obtaining tissue core
Rotex (Surgimed)	21	Potential for obtaining tissue fragments
Cutting		
Trucut (Cook)	14, 16	Tissue core obtained
Lee (Cook)	20	Tissue core obtained
Westcott (Becton-Dickinson)	20	Tissue core obtained

mediate review of the cytologic material by a cytopathologist. Similar accuracy rates of 80% to 100% have been reported in the literature (6,22,47,67). However, the availability of an experienced cytopathologist is necessary for consistent, accurate diagnoses.

The major disadvantage of these thin-walled needles is the difficulty in directing the needle to the lesion, especially with deep-seated lesions in obese patients. These needles are extremely flexible and may be difficult to steer in a straight line (*vide infra*). In addition, the beveled tip may cause the needle to bend. Multiple passes may be required. However, with practice, accuracy can be increased (37). In addition, CT allows precise localization of the needle tip, and thus confirmation of correct placement.

Modified Aspirating Needles

Modified aspirating needles combine the safety of a "skinny" needle with the ability to obtain a tissue core for histologic diagnosis (Table 1). These needles are available in 18, 20, and 22 gauge. Andriole et al. (3) have shown that with needles of progressively larger bores, more tissue can be obtained for histologic analysis. The larger-gauge needles are generally reserved for cases in which the lesion can be reached without traversing bowel or major vascular structures. These larger-gauge needles should not be used if the lesion is hypervascular. Modified aspirating needles are available with a variety of tip configurations (Fig. 2).

The Turner needle has a 45° bevel with a sharp cutting edge on the cannula. This allows a small core of tissue to be obtained. The Madayag and Greene needles both have 90° bevels, each with a different type of pencil-point stylet (41). These needles theoretically are easier to steer because of their pencil-point tips, but they may yield less tissue than a needle with a more acute bevel (3).

The Franseen needle has a trephine tip with three cutting teeth. This needle is easy to steer and yields excellent cores of tissue (3). The Franseen needle is our needle of choice for biopsies of liver and soft-tissue masses.

The Rotex needle has a stylet with a screw tip designed to hold tissue fragments. An outer cannula then slides over the stylet, trapping the tissue specimen. Some believe that this needle results in significant crush artifact (3). However, the Rotex needle has been recommended specifically for lung biopsies, and excellent results with tissue retrieved from both malignant and benign lesions have been reported (58).

Cutting Needles

Cutting needles are available in a variety of sizes: 14 to 20 gauge (Table 1). These needles actually cut a core of

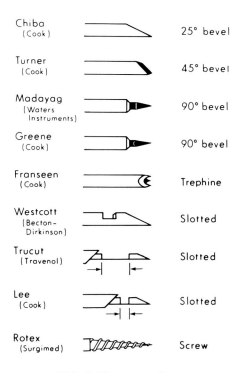

FIG. 2. Biopsy needles.

tissue, yielding an excellent histologic specimen. The larger cutting needles are generally reserved for large, easily accessible lesions (e.g., liver, soft tissue).

The Trucut needle is a typical cutting needle (Fig. 2). It consists of a slotted needle and a cutting cannula. The specimen is held in the slot of the needle and sliced off with the overlying cannula. The cannula also prevents loss of the specimen during withdrawal. Both the Lee and Westcott needles are of a similar design, but are available in 20 gauge.

Because of potential bleeding risks, cutting-needle biopsies should be performed only on hospitalized patients. We generally prefer to use a modified aspirating needle first, reserving the cutting needle for repeat biopsies of appropriate lesions.

Technique

A list of the basic equipment required for CT-guided procedures is shown in Table 2. The technique of CT-guided biopsy is straightforward. Patient preparation consists of discussing the procedure with the patient and obtaining standard informed consent. The only preprocedural laboratory values that we obtain routinely are a prothrombin time, partial thromboplastin time, and platelet count. Because of the very low complication rate, we routinely perform many biopsies as outpatient procedures. Outpatients remain in the department for 2 to 3 hr following the biopsy for observation.

The first step in CT-guided biopsy is a careful review of the patient's history and previous diagnostic studies, including a complete CT scan of the area to be biopsied. After reviewing the previous CT scan, optimal patient positioning can be determined (e.g., prone, supine, decubitus), as well as the appropriate level to biopsy.

When prebiopsy planning is complete, the appropriate level is located and scanned. This can be done relatively quickly by referring to normal anatomic landmarks such as the xiphoid or the top of the kidney. When the lesion to be biopsied is near the hemidiaphragm, either above or below, the phase of respiration is crucial. End tidal volume ("breath in, breath out, relax, and stop breathing") seems to be the most reproducible respiratory pattern and best tolerated by the patient.

Once the appropriate level is found, the needle entry site is selected by placing a metallic marker (e.g., buckshot) on the skin (Fig. 1). Placing the metal marker is facilitated by using the laser localizing light available on most CT scanners. The scan is repeated to confirm the marker location as ideal for needle entry. The distance to the lesion and the angle of entry are planned using the line cursor function to simulate the needle path. Ideally, the shortest vertical line from skin to lesion is chosen, although a longer needle path may be selected to avoid critical structures.

The skin is prepared with povidine-iodine solution (Betadine) and sterilely draped. Lidocaine (1%) is used for local anesthesia. If necessary, diazepam or other anxiolytics can be given intravenously. Occasionally, it may be useful to repeat the scan with the anesthesia needle in place to confirm correct entry site and angle.

The biopsy needle then is advanced to the correct depth. A variety of depth markers can be used, including a needle stop, sterile tape, or even the protective plastic needle sheath cut to the correct length (13). When advancing the needle (especially the thin-walled 20- and 22-gauge needles), it is critical to maintain a straight course in order to achieve accurate placement of the needle into the lesion. One hand should be placed at the skin and used to stabilize and steer the needle, while the other hand is placed on the needle hub and used to advance the needle. During the passage of the needle, the patient is instructed to suspend respiration in the same phase as that used for scanning (*vide supra*). Usually a gritty sensation or hard mass will be felt when a solid lesion is entered.

When the needle is in place, a scan may be obtained to confirm the location of the needle tip. Several CT scans may be required to document the exact location of the needle tip, especially if the tract is angled. A topogram may be performed to rapidly locate the appropriate scan plane for the needle tip. A shadowing artifact (Fig. 3) confirms that the needle tip is indeed within the scan plane. If the tip of the needle is not within the lesion, it cannot be easily redirected. It is generally best to remove the nee-

TABLE 2. *Biopsy and/or drainage procedure supplies*

Gloves
Scalpel blade
"BB" for skin marker
Transparent centimeter rule
Marking pen
Betadine
1% lidocaine
Sterile 4 × 4
Sterile drape
Sterile needles (18, 21, 23 gauge)
Sterile syringes
Sterile tape (or needle stop)
Needles
    Spinal needles (18, 20, 22 gauge)
    Chiba (20, 22 gauge; 15, 20 cm lengths)
    Trucut and Lee (14, 16, 18 gauge)
    Franseen (18, 20 gauge)
Catheters
    Pigtail catheter (8, 10 French)
    Sump catheter (12, 14 French)
Fascial dilators (6, 8, 10 French)
Guide wires (0.025, 0.038 J-tipped)
Aerobic and anaerobic culture tubes
Tubes for chemistries
Formalin or nonbacteriostatic saline
Albuminized glass slides
Suture (nylon or prolene)
Drainage bag and connecting tubing

dle entirely and reintroduce it. Although usually unnecessary, it is possible to inject a small amount of contrast material or air if there is difficulty in locating the needle tip. Stephenson et al. (66) have shown that such contrast injection does not affect the diagnostic quality of the biopsy material.

Once the needle tip is documented to be in the lesion, material is sampled by the appropriate technique, depending on the type of needle used. Negative pressure on the attached syringe while advancing the needle is sufficient to obtain material through an aspirating needle. A twisting motion combined with suction is required for the modified aspirating and cutting needles. It is important to release suction and allow the pressure to equalize before removing the needle from the body. This maneuver makes retrieval of the tissue sample much easier because it allows the specimen to remain in the needle, rather than being sucked into the syringe.

Diagnostic yield is enhanced by close cooperation with the pathologist. Optimally, the cytopathologist or a skilled cytopathology technologist is available to come to the radiology department to process the specimen immediately and provide a preliminary reading similar to the service provided to the surgeon (i.e., frozen section). This guides the decision as to whether or not additional samples are needed and decreases the rate of false-negative and inadequate biopsies. Because this service sometimes is not available, and because it is difficult to predict the adequacy of an aspirate from its gross appearance, most radiologists empirically obtain two to six samples, especially when using an aspirating needle (22).

Cytologic specimens can be smeared on glass slides and immediately fixed in 95% alcohol. These slides then can be rapidly stained with toluidine blue and examined by the cytopathologist. Histologic material is placed directly in formalin or in a balanced salt solution and delivered to the pathology laboratory to be processed in the standard fashion. If indicated, specimens also can be sent for routine microbiology studies.

Postbiopsy monitoring usually is continued for 2 to 3 hr and should include an expiration chest radiograph if upper abdomen or chest lesions have been biopsied.

Double-Needle and Tandem-Needle Techniques

To eliminate repetition of the time-consuming localization process for each pass, two different methods have been developed. The first is a double-needle technique. A large-gauge needle (18 or 19 gauge) is used as a sleeve for a smaller-gauge (21 or 22 gauge) biopsy needle. The first needle may be either a short (3.8 cm) needle used to cross the abdominal musculature or a longer needle of sufficient length to reach the lesion (18,35). The smaller-gauge needle then is passed through the larger-gauge "introducing" needle to obtain the biopsy. The introducing needle, although it may be helpful in crossing the superficial musculature, takes away one big advantage of the thin needle—its flexibility. The safety of a thin-gauge needle is due to both its size and its flexibility. Therefore, for example, respiratory motion with the needle in place is less likely to cause significant damage to internal organs.

The second method, which has largely replaced the double-needle technique, is the tandem-needle approach (20) (Fig. 4). A thin needle is advanced to the margin of the lesion and is left in place to act as a guide for the actual biopsy needle. Subsequent needle passes are made immediately adjacent to the guide needle. The first needle is not withdrawn until the final sample is obtained. Thus,

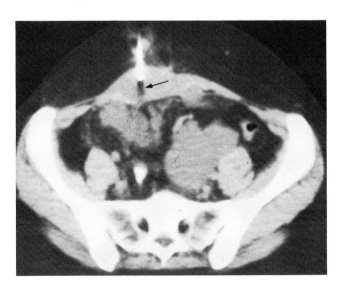

FIG. 3. Biopsy of nonpalpable rectus muscle mass in an obese woman. The needle enters the mass at a slight angle and therefore is not entirely displayed on a single scan. However, the position of the needle tip is known to be in the lesion by virtue of the shadowing artifact (*arrow*). Diagnosis: metastatic lung adenocarcinoma.

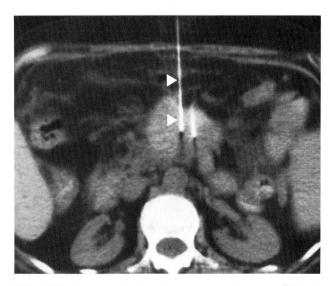

FIG. 4. Tandem-needle technique, pancreatic mass. Second needle (*arrowheads*) is passed parallel to the guide needle.

reproducibility of the needle path, angle, and depth is assured without having to scan repeatedly patients after each needle pass.

Angled Biopsy

It is generally preferable to keep the needle track perpendicular to the axis of the patient and thus in a single CT scan plane. This simplifies needle placement as well as CT documentation of the needle tip in the lesion. Occasionally, an angled approach is necessary in order to avoid crossing the pleura, lung, vital organs, or major vascular structures.

Determination of the correct depth and angle with multiple axial scans is difficult. A geometric approach can simplify the problem (20,25,73). This method applies the fundamentals of geometry to calculate the length and angle of the needle path needed to get to the lesion X from a safe skin site Y (Figs. 5 and 6). The first step is to determine the straight vertical distance from the skin surface to the lesion. The point on the skin directly overlying the lesion is labeled Z, and the lesion is designated X. The distance from Z to X is measured using the computer software and is labeled B. Thus far, the method is no different from the usual perpendicular approach. The second step is to review serial scans and determine a safe skin entry point Y for the needle insertion site in the same sagittal plane as the lesion. The distance from Z to Y is labeled A. A right triangle is then constructed. Using the Pythagorean Theorem ($A^2 + B^2 = C^2$), the length of the third side C—representing the path of the needle—can be calculated. Finally, the angle of entry a can be calculated using trigonometry. The tangent of angle a is equal to the ratio of the opposite side B over the adjacent side A. The angle of the needle to the horizontal will be equal to angle a. Once the needle length and the angle are calculated, the biopsy procedure is performed as any other. It is mandatory that the needle stay in the intended sagittal plane and that a goniometer be available to allow the operator to obtain the proper needle angle.

A simpler application of this approach (25) is to transfer the full-scale distances A (measured directly from the patient) and B (measured by CT software) onto two edges of a large index card. Connecting these two lines, a triangle can be completed with C representing the length of the desired needle path. The angle of the approach also can be measured directly from the index card by measuring a using a goniometer. Alternatively, the triangle can be cut out, turned over, and held by the side of the patient to directly guide the needle path length and angle (Fig. 7). This method circumvents the need to use trigonometric tables and is less likely to lead to mistakes.

Complications

Based on a vast collective experience, skinny-needle biopsies can be performed without undue concern of puncturing vascular structures, vital organs, or bowel loops (4,6,32,40,55,67). Inadvertent punctures of the bowel, urinary bladder, gallbladder, ureter, and even large vessels are almost always without clinical sequelae (43,67). However, it is prudent to avoid these structures when an alternative path is conveniently available.

Theoretically, the risk from needle biopsy increases as the diameter of the needle increases. In addition, there is a significant increase in risk when a cutting needle is employed. Still, complications from large-bore and cutting needles are minimal when adequate precautions are taken and CT guidance is available (33).

The primary complication of percutaneous biopsy procedures is bleeding. The incidence of significant bleeding (i.e., requiring transfusion) is extremely low—less than 1% (19,21). Highly vascularized lesions impose an increased risk from percutaneous biopsy. But even in these cases, skinny-needle biopsies can be performed in the routine manner and are almost always well tolerated. A relative contraindication to percutaneous biopsy is a bleeding disorder. However, frequently this can be remedied by administering appropriate blood products or medications (e.g., vitamin K) to reverse the clotting disorder.

Other complications have been reported, and the overall complication rate is approximately 2% (6,9,20,21,67). Bacterial contamination, bowel perforation, sepsis, and pancreatitis are all extremely rare events—less than 1%. Other, less serious complications include vasovagal reactions, transient fever, and asymptomatic pneumothorax. Complications associated with biopsies of specific anatomic sites are discussed later.

SELECTED BIOPSY SITES

Chest, Lung, and Mediastinum

The use of fluoroscopic guidance for biopsy of lung lesions is a well-established procedure. Because of its sim-

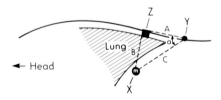

FIG. 5. Prone patient, triangulation method: construction of a right triangle (X, Y, Z), with Z at a point directly above the mass (X) to be biopsied. Y is the prospective needle entry site. The needle path length C and angle a can be calculated according to the Pythagorean Theorem.

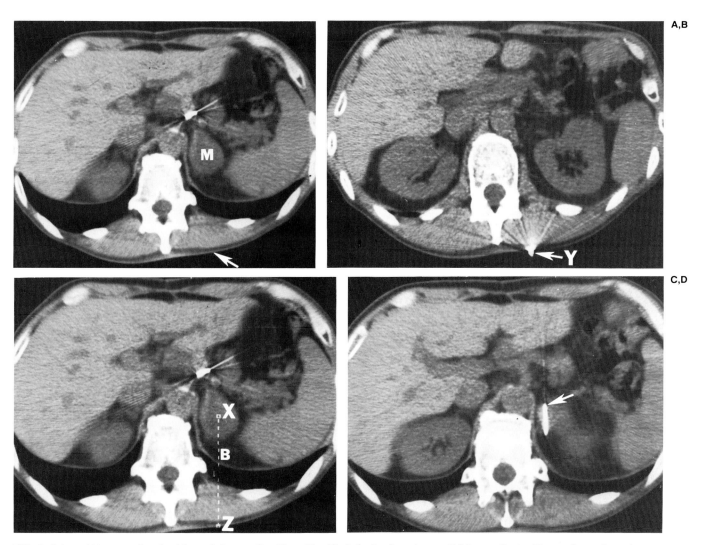

FIG. 6. Adrenal biopsy using the triangulation method (see Fig. 5). **A:** Left adrenal mass (M) in a patient with esophageal carcinoma. Patient scanned prone. A directly perpendicular needle track would necessitate crossing the lung (*arrow* = skin site, *Z*, above mass). **B:** Therefore, a safe skin entry site (*Y*) is selected 6 cm lower (*A* = 6 cm). A metallic marker indicates the proposed skin entry site (*arrow*). **C:** The distance (*B*) from the skin (*Z*) to the mass (*X*) is calculated using computer software. This allows both the length of the needle path (*C*) and the angle of entry (*a*) to be calculated. **D:** Scan documenting position of the needle tip in the mass (*arrow*). Diagnosis: metastatic esophageal carcinoma.

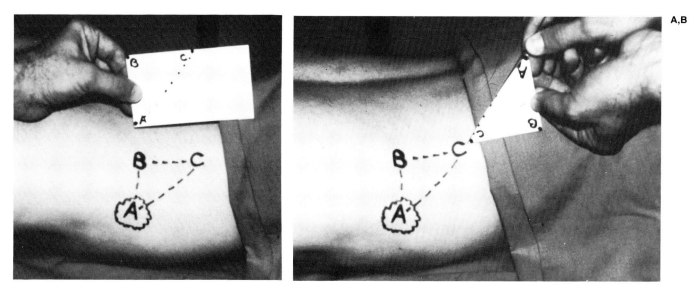

FIG. 7. Triangulation method, direct guidance. **A:** The mass (*A*), skin site above the mass (*B*), and skin entry site (*C*) are measured from the CT scan and transferred to an index card. **B:** The card is then turned over and held by the side of the patient to directly guide the angle and depth of biopsy.

plicity and accuracy, it is the method of choice for biopsy of most chest lesions. In less than 10% of patients, however, CT guidance is useful. These cases include mediastinal lesions, lesions not easily seen with fluoroscopy (e.g., small, ill-defined apical), and lesions adjacent to major vascular structures (Fig. 8) (1,15,23,24,29,30). Because CT allows more accurate placement of the needle within the lesion, CT guidance increases the reliability of a negative biopsy (6). Reported accuracy rates for CT-guided biopsies in the chest range from 80% to 95% (1,23,30).

The CT-guided biopsy technique is similar to that used with fluoroscopic guidance. Because of respiratory motion, it is critical that the patient suspend respiration in the identical phase used for the localizing scan. In general, small-gauge aspirating needles (20 or 22 gauge) are preferred, although large-bore and cutting needles can be used for accessible mediastinal and chest-wall lesions. van-Sonnenberg et al. (69) have recently described a coaxial technique (similar to the double-needle technique described earlier) for biopsy of pulmonary lesions. This allows multiple biopsies with only one needle track through the pleura.

Pneumothorax is the major complication of chest biopsies and occurs in approximately 10% to 15% of patients. However, only 10% to 20% of these patients require chest tube placement (1,23,30,69). Once a pneumothorax occurs, additional biopsies become much more difficult and probably should not be attempted (Fig. 9). Equipment for immediate chest tube placement should be available any time a chest biopsy is performed.

Liver

"Blind" percutaneous liver biopsy is the method of choice for diagnosis of diffuse liver disease. The accuracy of this procedure is 80% to 100%. However, for focal hepatic lesions, the accuracy of blind biopsy is much lower— 20% to 60% (78). Using either ultrasound or CT guidance, focal hepatic lesions can be sampled with an accuracy of 85% to 95% (6,51,61,78,80). Both of these methods allow precise placement of the needle tip within even small focal hepatic masses. In general, we prefer ultrasound guidance, when possible, because of its ready availability and lower cost. However, CT guidance often is necessary when the lesion cannot be seen by ultrasound because of size, depth, overlying rib, or echo characteristics. CT also is preferred for lesions close to the hemidiaphragm when an angled approach may be necessary (vide supra).

We generally use an 18-gauge Franseen needle for liver biopsies (both ultrasound- and CT-guided). With this needle we consistently obtain a tissue core for histology. The yield with 18-gauge needles is higher (90–95%) than with smaller-gauge aspirating needles (80–85%) (51,61,80).

Significant complications are rare (approximately 1%), consisting mainly of hemorrhage (51,61,78). When highly

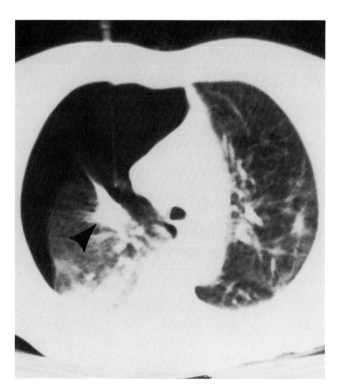

FIG. 9. Lung biopsy complicated by pneumothorax. This patient suspected of having brain metastases had a right-lung mass (*arrowhead*) that was not visible with fluoroscopy. On the first needle pass with CT guidance, a large pneumothorax developed. Subsequent attempts at needle placement were unsuccessful, as the collapsed lung continually moved away from the advancing needle tip. The patient was asymptomatic, and no chest tube was required.

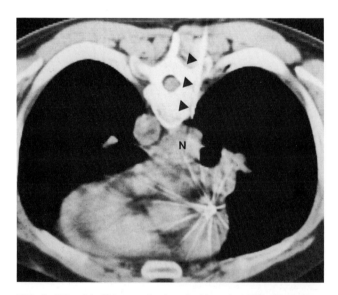

FIG. 8. CT-guided biopsy of subcarinal lymph nodes (N). Patient prone. Mediastinal lesions such as this are difficult to see with fluoroscopy. In addition, major vascular structures (e.g., aorta, heart) are directly adjacent, necessitating accurate needle placement (*arrowheads*). The tip of the needle was in the mass and was seen on next contiguous scan. Diagnosis: metastatic renal cell carcinoma.

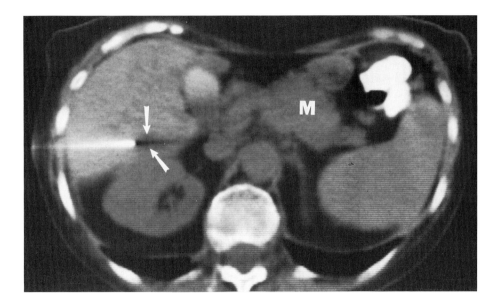

FIG. 10. CT-guided biopsy of a 1-cm liver lesion (*arrows*) in a patient with a pancreatic mas (M). The liver lesion is partially obscured by the artifact from the needle tip. The liver lesion was approached first because our diagnostic yield is higher with liver biopsies (histology) than with pancreatic biopsies (cytology). Diagnosis: metastatic adenocarcinoma consistent with a pancreatic primary.

vascular lesions are avoided, there does not appear to be an increased risk for bleeding complications for 18-gauge needle biopsies versus 22-gauge needle biopsies (61,78).

Pancreas

A CT-guided biopsy of the pancreas usually is performed to establish a definitive diagnosis of pancreatic carcinoma and sometimes to differentiate between it and subacute or chronic pancreatitis. CT-guided biopsy is helpful in two groups of patients. Most candidates are patients who have a mass in either the body or tail of the pancreas along with CT or clinical findings indicating that the tumor is unresectable (e.g., liver metastases). In these patients, we prefer first to try biopsy of potential metastatic lesions in the liver, because there is a higher diagnostic yield over pancreatic biopsy (Fig. 10). The second group of patients includes those with a recurrent mass following surgical resection of a pancreatic tumor. CT-guided biopsies generally are not done in patients with a mass in the head of the pancreas. In these individuals, surgery may be performed for biliary and/or gastric diversion. Open surgical biopsy generally is done at that time. If these patients are to be managed with percutaneous biliary drainage, CT-guided or fluoroscopically guided biopsy can be performed after the drainage tube has been placed.

We use 20- or 22-gauge aspirating needles for pancreatic biopsies and obtain material for cytologic analysis (56). The needle is directed vertically, generally through the overlying stomach and bowel (Fig. 11). The tandem-needle technique (*vide supra*) may be useful in these patients because accuracy increases with multiple passes (22,31). Accuracy rates for cytologic diagnosis with fine-needle aspiration biopsy in pancreatic carcinoma range from 65% to 95% (6,22,31,67).

Complications of percutaneous pancreatic biopsy are extremely rare (6,31). Ferrucci et al. (21) have reported a single case of needle-track seeding by pancreatic carcinoma, as well as a case of transient sepsis following pancreatic biopsy (22). Neither complication affected the patient's overall course. Goldstein et al. (31) performed multiple abdominal biopsies on dogs using 22-gauge needles. Subsequent laparotomies failed to reveal any abnormality except rare tiny spots of blood on the serosal surface of the bowel. Bowel contents were not seen free in the peritoneal cavity and could not be expressed through the needle holes, even with manual compression of the bowel.

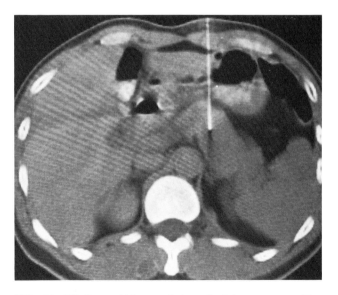

FIG. 11. CT-directed biopsy of the tail of the pancreas. The 20-gauge Chiba needle is routinely passed directly through overlying bowel.

Adrenal Gland and Kidneys

The adrenal gland is a common site for metastatic lesions. However, an adrenal mass in a patient with cancer has only a 40% to 50% chance of being a metastasis (5,7,46,60). Just as commonly, an adrenal mass will represent a nonfunctioning adenoma. CT-guided percutaneous biopsy of the adrenal gland is a valuable tool to help diagnose the cause of an adrenal mass. Accuracy rates using 18- to 22-gauge needles range from 80% to 90% (5,7,38,46,60).

Generally, these patients are biopsied in the prone position, using a posterior approach (Fig. 6). When using this approach, the needle track may cross the pleura and result in a pneumothorax. Therefore, an angled approach may be necessary (*vide supra*). Alternatively, the right adrenal gland can be simply and safely biopsied from a lateral transhepatic approach, thus avoiding the pleura without necessitating an angled approach (63).

Hemorrhage is a rare complication following biopsy of the adrenal gland (7). An additional potential complication is inadvertent biopsy of a pheochromocytoma, with resultant hypertensive crisis and possible hemorrhage (11,54). If a pheochromocytoma seems a possibility on the basis of clinical findings, catecholamine levels should be determined prior to biopsy.

CT guidance for biopsy of renal lesions seldom is required. In almost all cases, ultrasound guidance is sufficient and is preferred. CT guidance may be indicated for lesions that are small or are poorly delineated by ultrasonography (Fig. 12) (76).

Retroperitoneum and Pelvis

Computed tomography is the guidance method of choice for percutaneous retroperitoneal and pelvic biopsies. No other modality shows these structures as clearly. CT allows very accurate needle placement so that periaortic and paracaval masses can be safely sampled. Indications for retroperitoneal and pelvic biopsies include diagnoses of (a) metastatic disease in lymph nodes, (b) lymphoma, (c) recurrent tumor following surgery or chemotherapy/radiation therapy, and (d) primary retroperitoneal sarcomas.

Retroperitoneal masses generally are approached posteriorly with the patient lying prone. Occasionally, a direct anterior approach is used (Fig. 13). Larger-gauge needles are preferred, particularly for diagnosis of lymphoma, because histologic architecture is important in arriving at a specific diagnosis (79). Accuracy rates for lymph node biopsies generally are higher with metastatic carcinoma (80–90%) than with lymphoma (50–70%) (6,58,79).

Pelvic masses usually are approached directly anteriorly with the patient supine, because the bony pelvis prevents a posterior approach (Fig. 14). Occasionally, an oblique

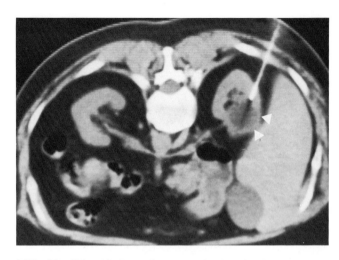

FIG. 12. CT-guided renal cyst aspiration. Patient scanned prone. Aspiration was requested because the cyst had a perceptible wall (*arrowheads*). Ultrasound could not adequately image the cyst because of the overlying ribs.

course along the iliopsoas muscle is helpful, particularly when using larger-gauge needles. For perirectal masses, a posterior approach through the greater sciatic notch has been shown to be useful. CT-guided biopsy can be helpful in diagnosing recurrent carcinoma following abdominoperineal resection (43).

Serious complications are rare after retroperitoneal or pelvic biopsies. Although the major potential complication is hemorrhage, no significant hemorrhagic episode has been reported (6,43,79).

Parathyroid Glands

Computed tomography may be helpful in locating ectopic parathyroid glands, but the CT appearance of para-

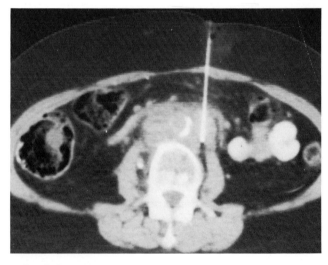

FIG. 13. Retroperitoneal lymph node biopsy. Absence of overlying bowel allowed an anterior approach using an 18-gauge Franseen needle. Diagnosis: metastatic cervical carcinoma.

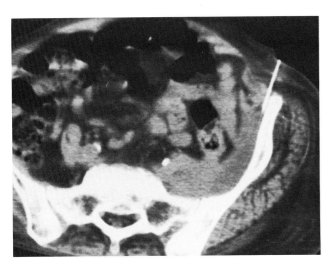

FIG. 14. Iliopsoas biopsy. Needle is angled along the left iliac bone. Diagnosis: abscess.

thyroid tissue is not specific. Differential diagnosis of a soft-tissue mass in the neck or mediastinum includes consideration of thyroid tissue, lymph nodes, and occasionally a normal structure. In order to improve this specificity, CT-guided aspiration of the mass, with assay for parathyroid hormone, has been shown to be useful (17).

The mass generally is approached directly anteriorly with a 22-gauge needle (Fig. 15). CT provides unequivocal documentation of the needle tip within the lesion. If material cannot be aspirated, gentle irrigation with 1 or 2 ml of saline may be helpful.

Doppman et al. (17) reported excellent results of CT-guided parathyroid aspiration in seven patients. A diag-

nosis of ectopic parathyroid gland was made in all seven cases. They experienced no complications using a 22-gauge needle.

THERAPEUTIC PROCEDURES

Drainage Procedures

Computed tomographic guidance for percutaneous aspiration and drainage is a logical extension of the techniques used for CT-guided biopsy. The most common collections aspirated and/or drained are abscess cavities. However, CT guidance also is useful to treat a wide variety of other fluid collections, including bilomas, pancreatic pseudocysts, urinomas, and lymphoceles.

Abscess Drainage

Computed tomography is a highly accurate method for detection of abdominal abscesses and generally is the imaging technique of choice for their diagnosis. CT provides a detailed three-dimensional display of the collection and surrounding structures. This allows precise planning of a safe access route for percutaneous drainage. Often, with large, superficial collections, ultrasound can provide similar information. As discussed earlier, we prefer to use ultrasound guidance (in conjunction with fluoroscopy) when collections can be easily imaged with this technique. However, ultrasound frequently is limited by overlying bowel gas, bone, or surgical wounds and drains. CT is our

A,B

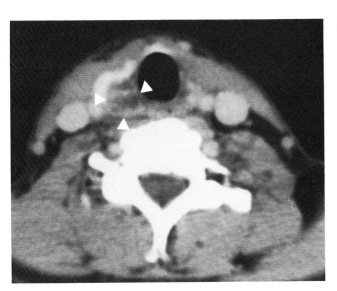
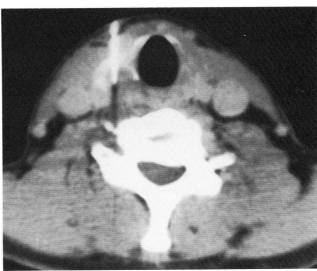

FIG. 15. Parathyroid aspiration. Patient with persistently elevated serum levels of calcium and parathyroid hormone following neck exploration and subtotal parathyroidectomy. **A:** CT scan shows right paratracheal mass (*arrowheads*) just behind the right lobe of the thyroid. **B:** CT-guided aspiration with assay for parathyroid hormone allowed definitive diagnosis of a parathyroid adenoma. Surgical removal restored normal serum calcium levels.

A,B

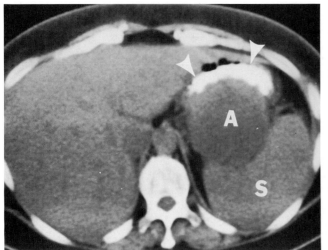 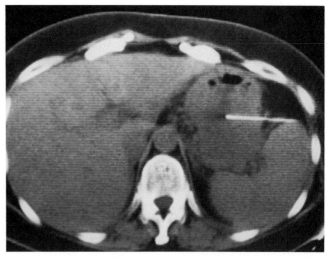

FIG. 16. Difficult access route. **A:** Retrogastric fluid collection (A). Difficult access secondary to surrounding stomach (*arrowheads*) and spleen (S). **B:** Catheter placed successfully using CT guidance. Pus was drained.

primary guidance technique for percutaneous abscess drainage, particularly for small deep collections and those surrounded by bowel loops.

Indications and patient selection.

Percutaneous abscess drainage (PAD) is most successful if the collection is (a) well defined, (b) unilocular, (c) free-flowing, and (d) accessible via an extraperitoneal-dependent approach (2,14,27,28,44,48,50,57,68,70,72). These criteria include more than 90% of intraabdominal abscesses (27). Many unfavorable situations (e.g., multiloculated, necrotic tissue, poorly defined) may be amenable to percutaneous drainage, particularly if the patient is a high-risk surgical candidate or not a surgical candidate at all (72). Frequently, in these cases, the patient's condition can be improved so that, if necessary, definitive surgical drainage eventually can be performed. We consider the only absolute contraindication to PAD to be lack of a safe access route. With CT guidance, this is rarely a problem (Fig. 16).

Technique.

Access Route. Each patient should have a complete diagnostic CT scan performed before PAD. In general, the shortest, straightest route to the collection is preferred. However, the track should clearly avoid bowel loops, major vessels, and the pleural space. This may require using the angled approach discussed earlier (Fig. 17).

Diagnostic Aspiration. Although CT is a very sensitive method for detecting abscesses, its specificity is low. A wide variety of other collections can produce similar CT findings. These include hematomas, necrotic tumors, loculated ascites, urinomas, bilomas, and lymphoceles.

Therefore, prior to drainage of an abscess, a diagnostic aspiration should be performed (Fig. 18).

Generally, diagnostic aspiration is done with a 20- or 22-gauge Chiba needle. This is particularly helpful when the collection is in a difficult location requiring needle passage through normal structures. Passage through bowel, though safe, should be avoided for fear of infecting a potentially sterile collection. Aspiration of viscous material often is difficult through the fine 22-gauge needle. Therefore, when necessary, a larger-gauge (18-gauge) needle can be used.

The technique of needle placement is identical with that used for percutaneous biopsy (*vide supra*). If the material is obviously purulent, placement of the drainage catheter can begin immediately. However, if the collection is not clearly infected, a Gram stain can be quickly performed. Generally, drainage catheters are not placed in sterile collections.

Catheter Selection. Adequate drainage requires a catheter with a large enough lumen to drain the material freely and multiple side holes to minimize occlusion. Two systems are generally used: pigtail catheter or sump catheter (26,28,35,52,57,68,70,71) (Fig. 19).

Pigtail catheters are modeled after angiographic catheters, except that their side holes are on the inner curve of the pigtail portion of the catheter. This helps drainage to be maintained even as the cavity collapses. These catheters come in sizes ranging from 8 to 14 French. The curled distal tip is relatively atraumatic to the cavity walls and helps provide stability within the lesion. The major disadvantage of these catheters is the relatively small lumen and side holes. Therefore, pigtail catheters mainly are useful for draining collections of low viscosity.

The system that generally is more effective and the one we prefer is the sump catheter. The vanSonnenberg sump

A,B

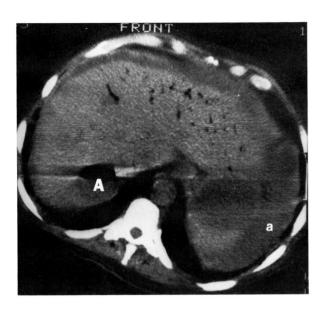

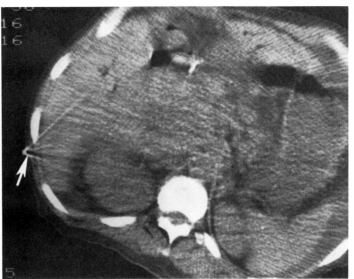

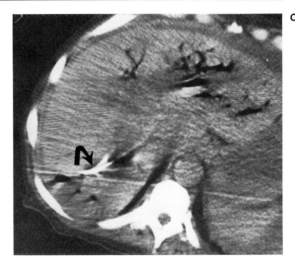

C

FIG. 17. Angled approach to abscess drainage. **A:** Septic patient suspected of having liver abscess (A) high in the right posterior lobe of the liver. Note surrounding lung, as well as air in the bile ducts (a = ascites). **B:** To avoid crossing the lung, a skin site was selected 7 cm lower, and a metallic marker was placed on the proposed skin entry site (*arrow*). **C:** Using the technique shown in Fig. 7, an 8.3 French pigtail catheter (*arrow*) was placed in the collection, and 50 ml of pus was drained.

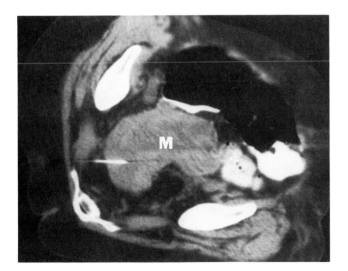

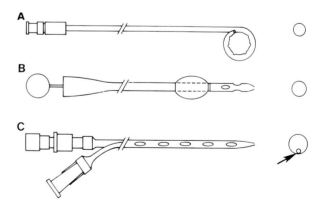

FIG. 18. Diagnostic aspiration. Patient with widely metastatic breast cancer and a distal colonic obstruction. CT scan demonstrated a pelvic mass (M). A diverticular abscess was suspected. Diagnostic aspiration with an 18-gauge needle found a hard, gritty mass. No fluid could be aspirated. Biopsy showed metastatic adenocarcinoma.

FIG. 19. Drainage catheters. Pigtail (**A**), trocar (**B**), and sump (**C**) catheters are shown diagrammatically. The cross-sectional view to the right of each catheter demonstrates the single lumen for the pigtail and trocar catheters and the double lumen of the sump catheter. The air-vent lumen of the sump catheter is indicated (*arrow*).

catheter (Meditech, Inc.) is a flexible, double-lumen tube with large oval side holes (45,50,71). The double-lumen design allows for concomitant irrigation and drainage. Perhaps even more important, this design allows continuous withdrawal of fluid under suction (usually low, intermittent suction). Suction applied to pigtail catheters tends to collapse the cavity wall around the catheter, occluding the drain holes. Therefore, pigtail catheters usually are left to dependent drainage only. The sump catheter, however, prevents tissue encroachment on the side holes by allowing air to enter through the sump lumen, while suction is applied to the primary lumen. In addition, the large caliber (12 or 14 French) of this catheter and its large side holes are helpful when draining thick, viscous material. Other similar sump catheters are available.

Catheter Placement. Placement of both types of drainage catheters is performed primarily by the Seldinger technique. Occasionally the trocar technique is used.

The Seldinger technique uses standard angiographic methods (Fig. 20). Using CT guidance, an 18-gauge needle (plain or sheathed) is placed in the collection, usually along the same track used for diagnostic aspiration. After material is freely aspirated, a 0.038-inch-diameter J-tipped guide wire is passed into the collection through the outer portion of the needle/sheath. A scan obtained at that time assures that the guide wire is coiled in the collection.

The needle then is removed, and, if necessary, an 8 French dilator is passed to enlarge the track. Finally, the appropriate-size catheter is threaded over the guide wire and into the lesion. The guide wire is removed, and the position of the pigtail is confirmed with repeat scanning.

If desired, once the guide wire is in place, the remaining steps may be performed under fluoroscopic guidance. Generally, the needle/sheath is removed and the patient is transferred to the fluoroscopy room with the wire taped in place.

When the collection is large and superficial (i.e., simple access route), the drainage catheter may be placed directly by using the trocar technique (Fig. 21). In this method, the catheter is mounted on a sharp metal introducer, and the entire apparatus is placed through the front wall of the collection in one step, similar to placement of a chest tube. The catheter then is advanced over the metal stylet into the cavity, and the stylet is removed.

Management.

After the catheter is in place, the collection is aspirated as completely as possible. Following this, *gentle* saline ir-

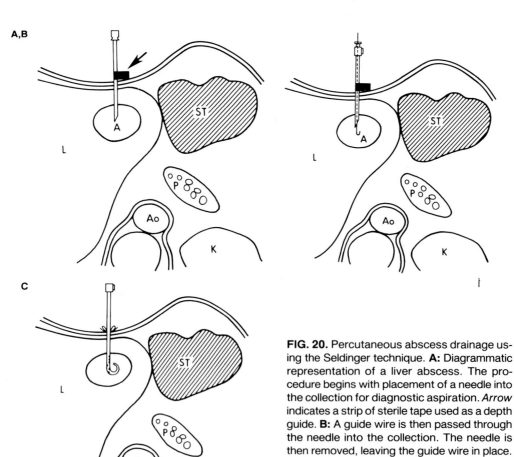

FIG. 20. Percutaneous abscess drainage using the Seldinger technique. **A:** Diagrammatic representation of a liver abscess. The procedure begins with placement of a needle into the collection for diagnostic aspiration. *Arrow* indicates a strip of sterile tape used as a depth guide. **B:** A guide wire is then passed through the needle into the collection. The needle is then removed, leaving the guide wire in place. **C:** A catheter is then threaded over the guide wire, and the guide wire is removed. The catheter is secured in place with suture material. (Adapted from ref. 28.)

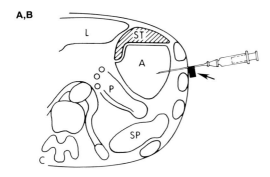

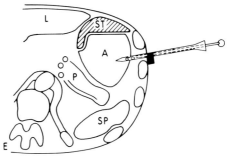

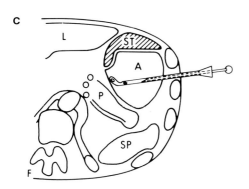

FIG. 21. Percutaneous abscess drainage using trocar technique. **A:** Aspiration of this diagrammatic retrogastric collection with a thin needle is done as an initial confirmatory procedure. The needle stop is indicated (*arrow*). **B:** The trocar unit is advanced to a previously determined distance, with a needle stop in place to prevent puncture of the back wall of the abscess. **C:** Keeping the stylet in place, the catheter is advanced over the stylet until the drainage tube is well seated in the cavity. The trocar is removed, and dependent drainage is begun. (Adapted from ref. 28.)

rigation may be performed until the drainage is clear. A major therapeutic benefit occurs with the initial drainage, and frequently the clinical response is immediate. A full course of the appropriate systemic antibiotic therapy always is given.

Catheters are left to gravity drainage or to low, intermittent suction. Frequent irrigation may be helpful in small volumes both to keep the catheter patent and to reduce the viscosity of the retained material. The catheter is left in place as long as it continues to drain. This usually requires 3 to 10 days (2,57,70). When drainage ceases, the catheter is withdrawn gradually—several centimeters per day. A final scan may be helpful to assure complete resolution of the collection before catheter removal (Fig. 22).

Several points should be emphasized. If the patient re-

A,B,C

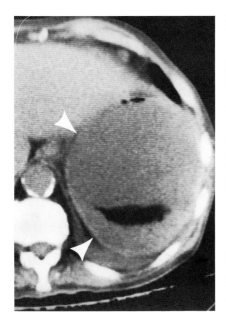
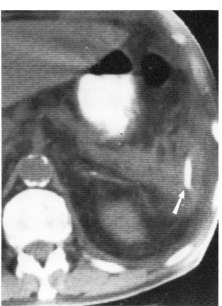
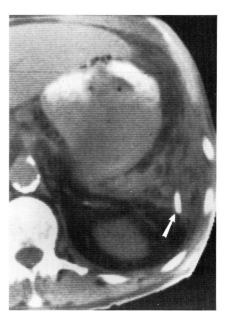

FIG. 22. Successful percutaneous abscess drainage. **A:** Febrile patient 1 month following splenectomy. CT scan demonstrates a large splenic bed fluid collection (*arrowheads*). **B:** CT scan following placement of the tube and aspiration of 500 ml of gross pus. The collection has diminished in size. Drainage catheter is seen (*arrow*). **C:** Two weeks later, drainage had ceased, and repeat outpatient CT shows no residual collection. The catheter (*arrow*) was then withdrawn slowly over the next several days.

mains febrile after the procedure, incomplete drainage should be suspected. Repeat CT should be performed promptly and additional catheters placed into undrained locules. If drainage tapers and then dramatically increases, a fistulous communication (usually enteric or biliary) may be present (Fig. 23). This can be confirmed with sinography. If a fistulous tract is present, percutaneous drainage still can succeed. However, this may require extended drainage with complete bowel rest (48,57,70).

Results and complications.

PAD minimizes manipulation of the abscess cavity. In theory, this should decrease the risk of sepsis. In addition, PAD has the advantages of (a) avoiding the risks of surgery and anesthesia, (b) saving considerable time and expense, and (c) making nursing care easier because of the closed drainage system.

PAD compares favorably with operative treatment in

A,B

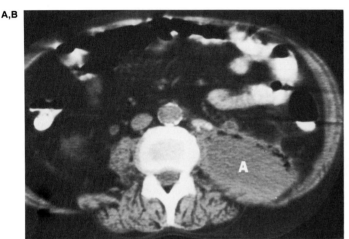
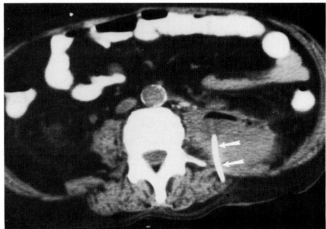

C

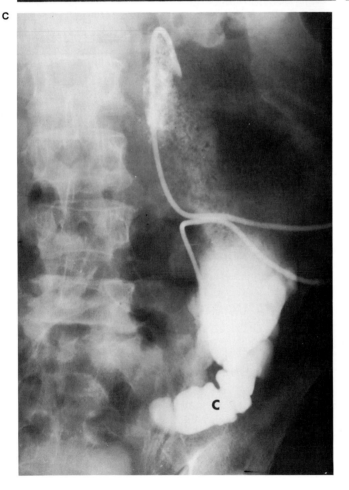

FIG. 23. A: Febrile patient with left flank pain. CT scan shows a left psoas fluid collection (A) with gas bubbles. Two 14 French sump catheters were placed, and pus was drained. **B:** Ten days later, the patient had persistent feculent drainage. Repeat CT showed a persistent collection that should have been well drained by the sump catheter (*arrows*). **C:** Injection of the drainage catheter demonstrates fistulous communication with the colon (C). A diverticular abscess was the cause.

terms of overall clinical success, duration of drainage, and recurrence rate. Success rates of 80% to 90% are widely reported with PAD (2,8,14,28,44,48,57,70). These favorable results for PAD may be related to the high diagnostic accuracy of CT, which facilitates complete delineation of the extent of the collection (27). In addition, vigorous follow-up with repeat CT scans, along with aggressive catheter repositioning and additional catheter placement, is critical to achieving successful drainage. Failure of PAD is most often due to failure to recognize loculations or septations, fistulous communication with the bowel, premature catheter withdrawal, or an attempt to drain a relatively solid collection (e.g., pancreatic phlegmon, necrotic tumor) (48,70).

Complication rates for PAD range from 10% to 15%, with serious complications occurring in less than 5% of cases (2,27,44,48,68,70). Minor complications include mild bleeding, skin infection, and transient bacteremia. Major complications include serious hemorrhage, sepsis, empyema, and bowel perforation. These latter complications occur in less than 5% of cases and result in death in less than 1%. Recurrence rates after successful PAD are approximately 5% in most reported series (2,44,48,70). These figures compare favorably with those for surgical management of abscesses, which is associated with mortality of approximately 10% to 20% and a recurrence rate of 15% to 30% (2,8,44). In addition, the overall length of hospitalization is consistently less with PAD (11 days) than with open surgical drainage (21 days) (8).

Specific sites.

Subphrenic Space. The left and right subphrenic spaces are common sites for abscesses following abdominal surgery. Generally these are treated easily by PAD, but they require extra planning for access routes. It is important to avoid transgressing the pleural space to prevent potential empyema formation. The angled approach described earlier for percutaneous biopsy is most useful (Fig. 17).

Pancreas. Pancreatic abscesses are, in reality, often semisolid phlegmon, and their percutaneous management is controversial (30,33,34,38,41). The surgical mortality among patients with pancreatic abscesses approaches 80%. Some authors have reported moderate success in draining these collections percutaneously (38,41). We have had only limited experience and prefer surgical drainage if the patient can tolerate it. When percutaneous drainage of a pancreatic abscess is attempted, multiple catheters of very large bore are necessary in order to adequately drain this semisolid material. Frequent irrigation may also be helpful (41).

Pelvis. For pelvic abscess drainage, the anterior approach often is not available because of overlying bladder, bowel, and bone. Consequently, two alternative approaches—transgluteal and transrectal—are used. We prefer to drain pelvic abscesses transgluteally through the greater sciatic foramen (Fig. 18). Butch et al. (9) reported successful PAD by this route in 17 of 21 patients (81%). The most common complication with this approach is pain, which usually disappears in the initial 24 hr. However, in approximately 20% of cases this pain persists and may be caused by neural plexus irritation. Because of this, others advocate pelvic PAD by the transrectal route when possible (42,53).

Pancreatic Pseudocysts

Percutaneous treatment of pancreatic pseudocysts remains controversial. Traditional surgical therapy consists of internal drainage with marsupialization into either the stomach or bowel (65). In certain cases, however, percutaneous therapy may be helpful, and surgery can be avoided.

The primary indication for percutaneous intervention is infection. If there is a question of an infected pseudocyst, percutaneous aspiration with CT guidance can easily be accomplished to provide a diagnosis. PAD can follow if indicated (45,74). In patients with infected pseudocysts, surgical drainage often may be difficult, particularly if the pseudocyst wall has not matured.

In patients with mature pseudocysts (4–6 weeks old) and severe abdominal pain, CT-guided drainage can be offered as an alternative to surgical drainage (39,45,59,74). Percutaneous drainage is performed in a manner identical with that described for PAD. Recently, drainage directly through the stomach has been described in an attempt to perform a percutaneous cystogastrostomy (39,59). Although the tract to the stomach probably does not remain patent permanently following catheter removal, there has been success with this technique.

The true recurrence rate for percutaneous pseudocyst drainage is unknown, but may range from 10% to 30% (39,45,59,74). Surgical recurrence rates are approximately 10% (65).

Miscellaneous Drainage Procedures

Theoretically, any fluid collection in the body can be drained percutaneously with CT guidance. Examples include lymphoceles, bilomas, urinomas, and hematomas (75,77). The technique is identical with that described earlier for PAD.

Percutaneous Nephrostomy. Percutaneous nephrostomy is best performed with a combination of ultrasound and fluoroscopic guidance. CT guidance may be helpful in rare cases (36). Haaga et al. (36) used CT guidance for percutaneous nephrostomy in renal transplant patients. They stated that CT guidance may be helpful in these patients to avoid both the peritoneum and inadvertent bowel puncture. The procedure can be done in conjunction with fluoroscopy for nephrostomy tube placement

A,B

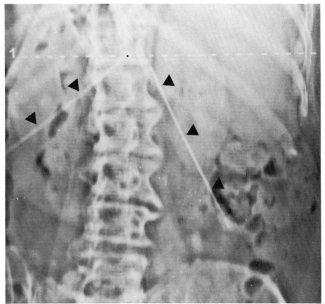 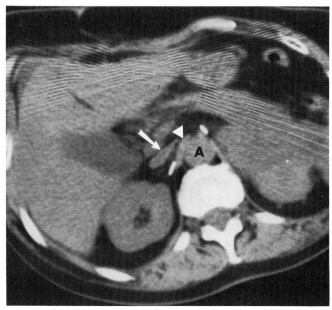

FIG. 24. CT-guided percutaneous neurolysis in a patient with pancreatic carcinoma. **A:** Anteroposterior topogram demonstrating angled course of both 22-gauge Chiba needles (*arrowheads*). The needle path is usually angled to avoid lung and pleura. **B:** CT scan showing the tips of the needles adjacent to the aorta (A) and the right diaphragmatic crus (*arrowhead*). Inferior vena cava is seen (*arrow*).

once the guide wire is inserted. We have not had occasion to use this technique, and we perform percutaneous nephrostomy in renal transplant patients using ultrasound and fluoroscopic guidance.

Cecostomy. CT guidance also has been used successfully to place percutaneous cecostomy tubes for cecal decompression in Ogilvie syndrome (12,16). This can be done from either an anterior or a posterior approach. The posterior retroperitoneal route may be preferred to avoid crossing the peritoneum. The advantage of percutaneous cecal decompression is that surgery can be avoided in these high-risk patients.

Neurolysis

Celiac nerve block has been performed for many years to treat intractable pain, usually secondary to pancreatic carcinoma. Routinely, this procedure is done either with fluoroscopic guidance or blindly with reference to bony landmarks. However, CT guidance has been shown to be helpful (10,34,64).

The celiac plexus is located immediately inferior to the celiac artery and wraps around the anterior surface of the aorta. The technique for CT-guided percutaneous neurolysis is similar to that for percutaneous biopsy. The patient is scanned prone, locating the appropriate level. Chiba needles (22 gauge) are then placed from the back on both sides of the spine. The needle tips are located anterior and lateral to the aorta, as well as medial to the adrenal glands, just below the celiac artery. The access route must be selected carefully to avoid the pleura, kid-

ney, renal vein, aorta, and, on the right side, the inferior vena cava (Fig. 24).

When the CT scan shows the needle tip in the appropriate location, 10 ml of 1% lidocaine may be injected to assess pain relief (34). If the patient has subjective pain relief following injection of lidocaine, 10 to 20 ml of absolute ethanol is injected through both needles. Either air or contrast material can be mixed with the alcohol to serve as a marker. Follow-up scans are obtained to trace the spread of the alcohol.

Pain relief has been reported in 30% to 90% of cases, but this is difficult to grade, because one must rely on the subjective impression of the patient (10,34,64). Complications of the procedure include weakness and numbness in the T-10–L-2 distribution, impotence, voiding difficulties, and postural hypotension. The reported complication rate using fluoroscopic guidance is less than 5%. Although it is too early to tell if the complication rate with CT-guided neurolysis will be lower, early studies reported no serious complications (10,34).

REFERENCES

1. Adler OB, Rosenberger A, Peleg H. Fine-needle aspiration biopsy of mediastinal masses: evaluation of 136 experiences. *AJR* 1983;140:893–896.
2. Aeder MI, Wellman JL, Haaga JR, Hau T. Role of surgical and percutaneous drainage in the treatment of abdominal abscesses. *Arch Surg* 1983;118:273–280.
3. Andriole JG, Haaga JR, Adams AB, Nunez C. Biopsy needle characteristics assessed in the laboratory. *Radiology* 1983;148:659–662.
4. Berg JW, Robbins GF. A late look at the safety of aspiration biopsy. *Cancer* 1962;15:826–827.

5. Berkman WA, Bernardino ME, Sewell CW, Price RB, Sones PJ Jr. The computed tomography-guided adrenal biopsy. An alternative to surgery in adrenal mass diagnosis. *Cancer* 1984;53:2098–2103.
6. Bernardino ME. Percutaneous biopsy. *AJR* 1984;142:41–45.
7. Bernardino ME, Walther MM, Phillips VM, et al. CT-guided adrenal biopsy: accuracy, safety, and indications. *AJR* 1985;144:67–69.
8. Brolin RE, Nosher JL, Leiman S, Lee WS, Greco RS. Percutaneous catheter versus open surgical drainage in the treatment of abdominal abscesses. *Am Surg* 1984;50(2):102–108.
9. Butch RJ, Mueller PR, Ferrucci JT Jr, et al. Drainage of pelvic abscesses through the greater sciatic foramen. *Radiology* 1986;158:487–491.
10. Buy J-N, Moss AA, Singler RC. CT guided celiac plexus and splanchnic nerve neurolysis. *J Comput Assist Tomogr* 1982;6(2):315–319.
11. Casola G, Nicolet V, vanSonnenberg E, et al. Unsuspected pheochromocytoma: risk of blood-pressure alterations during percutaneous adrenal biopsy. *Radiology* 1986;159:733–735.
12. Casola G, Withers C, vanSonnenberg E, Herba MJ, Saba RM, Brown RA. Percutaneous cecostomy for decompression of the massively distended cecum. *Radiology* 1986;158:793–794.
13. Chen SM. A single method of limiting needle depth during percutaneous biopsy. *Radiology* 1982;143:269.
14. Clark RA, Towbin R. Abscess drainage with CT and ultrasound guidance. *Radiol Clin North Am* 1983;21(3):445–459.
15. Cohan RH, Newman GE, Braun SD, Dunnick NR. CT assistance for fluoroscopically guided transthoracic needle aspiration biopsy. *J Comput Assist Tomogr* 1984;8(6):1093–1098.
16. Crass JR, Simmons RL, Frick MP, Maile CW. Percutaneous decompression of the colon using CT guidance in Ogilvie syndrome. *AJR* 1985;144:475–476.
17. Doppman JL, Krudy AG, Marx SJ, et al. Aspiration of enlarged parathyroid glands for parathyroid hormone assay. *Radiology* 1983;148:31–35.
18. Dunnick NR, Fisher RI, Chu EW, Young RC. Percutaneous aspiration of retroperitoneal lymph nodes in ovarian cancer. *AJR* 1980;135:109–113.
19. Evans WK, Ho C, McLoughlin MJ, Tao L. Fatal necrotizing pancreatitis following fine-needle aspiration biopsy of the pancreas. *Radiology* 1981;141:61–62.
20. Ferrucci JT Jr, Wittenberg J. CT biopsy of abdominal tumors: aids for lesion localization. *Radiology* 1978;129:739–744.
21. Ferrucci JT Jr, Wittenberg J, Margolies MN, Carey RW. Malignant seeding of the tract after thin-needle aspiration biopsy. *Radiology* 1979;130:345–346.
22. Ferrucci JT Jr, Wittenberg J, Mueller PR, Simeone JF, Kirkpatrick RH, Taft PD. Diagnosis of abdominal malignancy by radiologic fine-needle aspiration. *AJR* 1980;134:323–330.
23. Fink I, Gamsu G, Harter LP. CT-guided aspiration biopsy of the thorax. *J Comput Assist Tomogr* 1982;6(5):958–962.
24. Gatenby AA, Mulhern CB, Broder GJ, Moldofsky PJ. Computed tomography-guided biopsy of small apical and peripheral upper-lobe lung masses. *Radiology* 1984;150:591–592.
25. Gerzof SG. Triangulation: indirect CT guidance for abscess drainage. *AJR* 1981;137:1080–1081.
26. Gerzof SG, Robbins AH, Birkett DH, Johnson WC, Pugatch RD, Vincent ME. Percutaneous catheter drainage of abdominal abscesses guided by ultrasound and computed tomography. *AJR* 1979;133:1–8.
27. Gerzof SG, Robbins AH, Johnson WC, Birkett DH, Nabseth DC. Percutaneous catheter drainage of abdominal abscesses. *N Engl J Med* 1981;305:653–657.
28. Gerzof SG, Spira R, Robbins AH. Percutaneous abscess drainage. *Semin Roentgenol* 1981;16:62–71.
29. Gobien RP, Skucas J, Paris BS. CT-assisted fluoroscopically guided aspiration biopsy of central hilar and mediastinal masses. *Radiology* 1981;141:443–447.
30. Gobien RP, Stanley JH, Vukic I, Gobien BS. Thoracic biopsy: CT guidance of thin-needle aspiration. *AJR* 1984;142:827–830.
31. Goldstein HM, Zornoza J, Wallace S, et al. Percutaneous fine needle aspiration biopsy of pancreatic and other abdominal masses. *Radiology* 1977;123:319–322.
32. Gothlin JH. Post-lymphographic percutaneous fine needle biopsy of lymph nodes guided by fluoroscopy. *Radiology* 1976;120:205–207.
33. Haaga JR. New techniques for CT-guided biopsies. *AJR* 1979;133:633–641.
34. Haaga JR, Kori SH, Eastwood DW, Borkowski GP. Improved technique for CT-guided celiac ganglia block. *AJR* 1984;142:1201–1204.
35. Haaga JR, Reich NE, Havrilla TR, Alfidi RJ. Interventional CT scanning. *Radiol Clin North Am* 1977;15:449–456.
36. Haaga JR, Zelch MG, Alfidi RJ, Stewart BH, Daugherty JD. CT-guided antegrade pyelography and percutaneous nephrostomy. *AJR* 1977;128:621–624.
37. Harter LP, Moss AA, Goldberg HI, Gross BH. CT-guided fine-needle aspirations for diagnosis of benign and malignant disease. *AJR* 1983;140:363–367.
38. Heaston DK, Handel DB, Ashton PR, Korobkin M. Narrow gauge needle aspiration of solid adrenal masses. *AJR* 1982;138:1143–1148.
39. Ho CS, Taylor B. Percutaneous transgastric drainage for pancreatic pseudocyst. *AJR* 1984;143:623–625.
40. Holm HH, Als O, Gammelgaard J. Percutaneous aspiration biopsy procedures under ultrasonic visualization. In: Taylor KJW, ed. *Diagnostic ultrasound in gastrointestinal disease.* New York: Churchill Livingstone, 1978:137–149 (Clinics in diagnostic ultrasound; vol 1).
41. Isler RJ, Ferrucci JT Jr, Wittenberg J, et al. Tissue core biopsy of abdominal tumors with a 22 gauge cutting needle. *AJR* 1981;136:725–728.
42. Jacques PF, Mauro M. Drainage of pelvic abscesses through the greater sciatic foramen (letter to the editor). *Radiology* 1986;160:278–279.
43. Jacques PF, Staab EV, Richey W, Photopoulos G, Swanton M. CT-assisted pelvic and abdominal aspiration biopsies in gynecological malignancy. *Radiology* 1978;128:651.
44. Johnson WC, Gerzof SG, Robbins AH, Nabseth DC. Treatment of abdominal abscesses. Comparative evaluation of operative drainage versus percutaneous catheter drainage guided by computed tomography or ultrasound. *Ann Surg* 1981;194(4):510–520.
45. Karlson KB, Martin EC, Fankuchen EI, Mattern RF, Schultz RW, Cassarella WJ. Percutaneous drainage of pancreatic pseudocysts and abscesses. *Radiology* 1982;142:619–624.
46. Katz RL, Shirkhoda A. Diagnostic approach to incidental adrenal nodules in the cancer patient. *Cancer* 1985;55:1995–2000.
47. Kline TS, Neal HS. Needle aspiration biopsy: a critical appraisal eight years and 3,267 specimens later. *JAMA* 1978;239:36–39.
48. Lang EK, Springer RM, Glorioso LW, Cammarata CA. Abdominal abscess drainage under radiologic guidance: causes of failure. *Radiology* 1986;159:329–336.
49. Lieberman RP, Hafez GR, Crummy AB. Histology from aspiration biopsy: Turner needle experience. *AJR* 1982;138:561–564.
50. Martin EC, Karlson KB, Fankuchen EI, Cooperman A, Casarella WJ. Percutaneous drainage of postoperative intraabdominal abscesses. *AJR* 1982;138:13–15.
51. Martino CR, Haaga JR, Bryan PJ, LiPuma JP, El Yousef SJ, Alfidi RJ. CT-guided liver biopsies: eight years' experience. Work in progress. *Radiology* 1984;152:755–757.
52. Mauro MA, Jacques PF. Modified trocar-cannula system for percutaneous pancreatic abscess drainage. *Radiology* 1981;139:227–228.
53. Mauro MA, Jacques PF, Mandell VS, Mandel SR. Pelvic abscess drainage by the transrectal catheter approach in men. *AJR* 1985;144:477–479.
54. McCorkell SJ, Niles NL. Fine-needle aspiration of catecholamine-producing adrenal masses: a possibly fatal mistake. *AJR* 1985;145:113–114.
55. McLoughlin MJ, Ho CS, Langar B, McHattie J, Tao LC. Fine needle aspiration biopsy of malignant lesions in and around the pancreas. *Cancer* 1978;41:2413–2419.
56. Mitchell ML, Carney CN. Cytologic criteria for the diagnosis of pancreatic carcinoma. *Am J Clin Pathol* 1985;83:171–176.
57. Mueller PR, vanSonnenberg E, Ferrucci JT Jr. Percutaneous drainage of 250 abdominal abscesses and fluid collections. Part II: Current procedural concepts. *Radiology* 1984;151:343–347.
58. Nahman BJ, Van Aman ME, McLemore WE, O'Toole RV. Use of the Rotex needle in percutaneous biopsy of pulmonary malignancy. *AJR* 1985;145:97–99.
59. Nunez D, Yrizarry JM, Russell E, et al. Transgastric drainage of pancreatic fluid collections. *AJR* 1985;145:815–818.
60. Pagani JJ. Normal adrenal glands in small cell lung carcinoma: CT-guided biopsy. *AJR* 1983;140:949–951.

61. Pagani JJ. Biopsy of focal hepatic lesions. Comparison of 18 and 22 gauge needles. *Radiology* 1983;147:673–675.
62. Pelaez JC, Hill MC, Dach JL, Isikoff MB, Morse B. Abdominal aspiration biopsies. Sonographic v computed tomographic guidance. *JAMA* 1983;250(19):2663–2666.
63. Price RB, Bernardino ME, Berkman WA, Sones PJ Jr, Torres WE. Biopsy of the right adrenal gland by the transhepatic approach. *Radiology* 1983;148:566.
64. Rosen RJ, Miller DL, Imparato AM, Riles TS. Percutaneous phenol sympathectomy in advanced vascular disease. *AJR* 1983;141:597–600.
65. Rosenberg IK, Kahn JA, Walt AJ. Surgical experience with pancreatic pseudocysts. *Am J Surg* 1969;117:11–17.
66. Stephenson TF, Mehnert PJ, Marx AJ, et al. Evaluation of contrast markers for CT aspiration biopsy. *AJR* 1979;133:1097–1100.
67. Sundaram M, Wolverson MK, Heiberg E, Pilla T, Vas WG, Shields JB. Utility of CT-guided abdominal aspiration procedures. *AJR* 1982;139:1111–1115.
68. vanSonnenberg E, Ferrucci JT Jr, Mueller PR, Wittenberg J, Simeone JF. Percutaneous drainage of abscesses and fluid collections: technique, results, and applications. *Radiology* 1982;142:1–10.
69. vanSonnenberg E, Lin AS, Deutsch AL, Mattrey RF. Percutaneous biopsy of difficult mediastinal, hilar, and pulmonary lesions by computed-tomographic guidance and a modified coaxial technique. *Radiology* 1983;148:300–302.
70. vanSonnenberg E, Mueller PR, Ferrucci JT Jr. Percutaneous drainage of 250 abdominal abscesses and fluid collections. Part I: Results, failures, and complications. *Radiology* 1984;151:337–341.
71. vanSonnenberg E, Mueller PR, Ferrucci JT Jr, Neff CC, Simeone JF, Wittenberg J. Sump catheters for percutaneous abscess and fluid drainage by trocar or Seldinger technique. *AJR* 1982;139:613–614.
72. vanSonnenberg E, Wing VW, Casola G, et al. Temporizing effect of percutaneous drainage of complicated abscesses in critically ill patients. *AJR* 1984;142:821–826.
73. vanSonnenberg E, Wittenberg J, Ferrucci JT Jr, Mueller PR, Simeone JF. Triangulation method for percutaneous needle guidance: the angled approach to upper abdominal masses. *AJR* 1981;137:757–761.
74. vanSonnenberg E, Wittich GR, Casola G, et al. Complicated pancreatic inflammatory disease: diagnostic and therapeutic role of interventional radiology. *Radiology* 1985;155:335–340.
75. Vazquez JL, Thorsen MK, Dodds WJ, et al. Evaluation and treatment of intraabdominal bilomas. *AJR* 1985;144:933–938.
76. Whelan TV, Healy GF, Patel TG. Renal biopsy: localization using computed tomography. *Urol Radiol* 1985;7:94–96.
77. White M, Mueller PR, Ferrucci JT Jr, et al. Percutaneous drainage of postoperative abdominal and pelvic lymphoceles. *AJR* 1985;145:1065–1069.
78. Whitmire LF, Galambos JT, Phillips VM, et al. Imaging guided percutaneous hepatic biopsy: diagnostic accuracy and safety. *J Clin Gastroenterol* 1985;7(6):511–515.
79. Zornoza J, Cabanillas FF, Altoff TM, Ordoñez N, Cohen MA. Percutaneous needle biopsy in abdominal lymphoma. *AJR* 1981;136:97–103.
80. Zornoza J, Wallace S, Ordoñez N, Lukeman J. Fine-needle aspiration biopsy of the liver. *AJR* 1980;134:331–334.

CHAPTER 6

Neck

Harvey S. Glazer, Dennis M. Balfe, and Stuart S. Sagel

The development of cross-sectional imaging has improved the ability of the radiologist to provide useful information for evaluation of the larynx and soft-tissue structures of the neck. Computed tomography (CT) has been shown to be a sensitive technique in defining the locations and relationships of masses to adjacent structures (65,89). It is not only helpful in confirming the clinical impression of a neck or laryngeal mass (sometimes providing a definitive diagnosis) but also occasionally will demonstrate a lesion that is not apparent on physical examination. Moreover, CT often provides information complementary to the clinical examination with respect to deep extension of masses as well as evaluation of other areas that are not accessible to palpation or laryngoscopy. Although most studies are performed for suspected mass lesions, CT is also helpful for assessment of patients following trauma.

Magnetic resonance imaging (MRI) is a newer cross-sectional imaging technique for evaluating the larynx and neck that provides anatomic information comparable to that from CT in most cases (13,39,57,65,114–116,125). The high contrast among blood vessels, masses, and adjacent soft tissues it provides makes MRI an alternative to CT. MRI is particularly helpful in those patients in whom intravenous contrast material cannot be administered or in whom there is poor separation on CT between a mass and surrounding soft-tissue structures of similar density.

CT TECHNIQUE

Optimal demonstration of neck and laryngeal anatomy is achieved with CT scanners with rapid imaging times (less than 5 sec) and the capability to obtain narrowly collimated sections. The patient is examined supine with the neck slightly extended to make the larynx perpendic-

ular to the imaging plane. Lowering the shoulders will help reduce the shoulder artifacts that can degrade images in the lower neck. Hyperextension of the neck is not needed and should be avoided in patients with large supraglottic tumors, because it may increase the patient's airway obstruction (65). A lateral digital-projection radiograph (topogram, scanogram) may be helpful in planning the study, but in most cases superficial anatomic landmarks will suffice.

Contiguous 4- or 5-mm-thick sections are obtained during slow inspiration, generally starting at the angle of the mandible to just above the thoracic inlet. Of course, the extent of the examination may be altered depending on the clinical circumstances or the initial CT findings. If images are obtained during suspended inspiration, the airway may appear falsely narrowed because of adduction of the true and false vocal cords and collapse of the hypopharynx. It is important to tell the patient to avoid coughing, swallowing, or moving during imaging.

In some cases, very thin (1.0–2.0 mm) and/or overlapping sections may be helpful in further evaluating subtle abnormalities, for example, in the larynx around the ventricle between the true and false vocal cords (93,103). Multiplanar reconstruction can also be performed (102). However, it usually does not provide significant additional information.

Images obtained while the patient phonates the letter "e" will provide distension of the pyriform sinuses and improve visualization of the apex of the pyriform sinus, posterior pharyngeal wall, and aryepiglottic folds (29,30). A modified Valsalva maneuver is also helpful in distending the pyriform sinus.

Iodinated contrast material generally is administered intravenously using a bolus of 50 ml of 60% iodinated solution, followed by a rapid infusion of 100–150 ml of 60% iodinated solution. It is most useful in distinguishing masses, especially lymph nodes, from adjacent vascular structures. It is particularly helpful in postoperative patients, in whom normal anatomic landmarks may be distorted. In selected cases (e.g., evaluation of paragangliomas), dynamic imaging at a single level may be helpful in characterizing the vascularity of a lesion.

MRI TECHNIQUE

Neck masses above the level of the cricoid cartilage can be imaged using a head coil. However, a malleable surface coil that conforms to the contour of the neck is valuable for imaging lower-neck masses that cannot fit within the imaging volume of the head coil. Image quality is significantly improved using surface coils, especially if thin sections (5 mm or less) of the larynx are to be obtained. A body coil may be used for masses that arise in the thoracic inlet and extend into the superior mediastinum. The center section is chosen according to the region of interest, as determined by physical findings or other radiologic studies. A spin-echo pulse sequence with very short TR and short TE (e.g., TR = 300 msec, TE = 15 msec) can be used initially for localization. Patients are instructed to breathe shallowly and to avoid moving or swallowing, to minimize motion-related artifacts. Images of the larynx generally are obtained using 5-mm-thick sections. Larger masses in the extralaryngeal soft tissues usually can be studied using a section thickness of 1 cm.

Transaxial images alone are performed in most cases. Coronal and sagittal views will demonstrate anatomy with equal clarity and may provide additional information in selected cases. For example, sagittal images may be helpful in demonstrating extension of a supraglottic tumor into the base of the tongue, whereas coronal images may better show the relationship of an intralaryngeal mass to the laryngeal ventricle or a supraclavicular mass to the lung apex and/or superior mediastinal structures.

Most laryngeal and neck masses are optimally demonstrated using a relatively T1-weighted (short-TR/short-TE) spin-echo pulse sequence (39,57,65). With this pulse sequence, low-intensity tumors (long T1) are easily separated from high-intensity fat (short T1) in the preepiglottic, paralaryngeal, and perivascular spaces. In addition, there is less image degradation from motion-related artifacts on T1-weighted images than on T2-weighted images because of the shorter imaging time required. However, T2-weighted images may be crucial to precisely distinguish between tumors (long T2) and muscle (short T2). T2-weighted images may also be helpful in demonstrating cystic components of masses, in detecting parathyroid adenomas, and in distinguishing between posttreatment fibrosis and recurrent tumor (37,40,50,52,110). However, in most cases, T1-weighted images are satisfactory for demonstrating laryngeal and neck abnormalities.

A,B

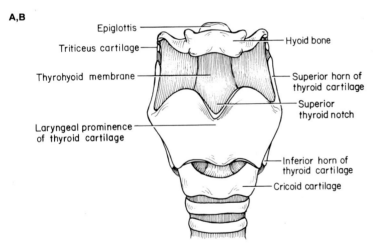

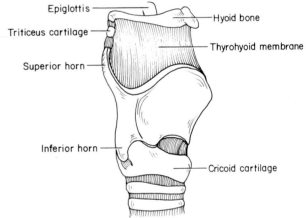

C

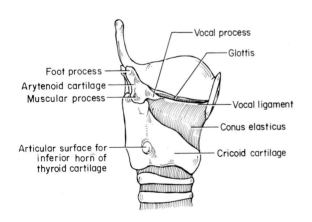

FIG. 1. Schematic drawings of laryngeal skeleton. **A:** Frontal view. **B:** Lateral view. **C:** Lateral view after removal of right thyroid lamina.

NORMAL ANATOMY

CT

The normal symmetry of the larynx and neck is extremely helpful in evaluating patients suspected of having abnormalities. However, normal degrees of asymmetry must be recognized to avoid misinterpretation. Discussion of the normal anatomy of the neck as seen with CT can be divided into considerations of the laryngeal skeleton, superficial and deep soft tissues of the larynx, the airway, and the soft tissues of the neck.

Laryngeal Skeleton

The laryngeal skeleton, consisting of the hyoid bone and the epiglottic, thyroid, arytenoid, and cricoid cartilages, protects the airway and supports the soft-tissue structures (true and false vocal cords, aryepiglottic folds) within the larynx (Figs. 1 and 2). Each of these individual bone and cartilaginous structures has a characteristic appearance that allows for easy orientation of individual CT images (Figs. 3, 5, and 9). The amount of cartilaginous mineralization varies widely among patients, but is generally most extensive in older men (3).

The hyoid bone is tripartite, consisting of a central body and two greater cornua; it surrounds the upper (free) portion of the epiglottis and superior aspect of the preepiglottic space (Fig. 3B–D). The paired greater cornua extend posterolaterally from the anterior central body. A normal linear lucency may be seen between the body and greater cornua. This represents a fibrous connection and should not be confused with a fracture (Fig. 3C). The hyoid bone is attached to the thyroid cartilage by the thyrohyoid membrane and to the epiglottis by the hyoepiglottic ligament. It is suspended in the neck between the suprahyoid and infrahyoid strap muscles.

The air-containing valleculae, which frequently are asymmetrical in size, lie posterior to the hyoid bone and anterior to the free margin of the epiglottis (Fig. 3A–C). They are separated by the median glossoepiglottic fold, which attaches the epiglottis to the base of the tongue.

The epiglottis is seen on CT as a thin curved band of soft-tissue density posterior to the valleculae and anterior to the air-containing laryngeal vestibule (Fig. 3). The epiglottis is broadest at its free portion just above the hyoid bone. The body or fixed portion of the epiglottis tapers below the level of the hyoid to a point at its caudal margin, the petiole. At this level it attaches to the thyroid lamina just below the thyroid notch via the thyroepiglottic ligament. The epiglottis consists of elastic cartilage and therefore only rarely calcifies (Fig. 4).

The thyroid cartilage is the largest of the laryngeal cartilages (Figs. 5 and 6). It is open posteriorly and consists of two laminae that join anteriorly in the midline at the laryngeal prominence. Normal paramedian thinning may be seen anteriorly (Fig. 6C). The superior thyroid notch is a normal midline separation between the two laminae just above the glottis and should not be mistaken for cartilaginous destruction. The thyroid cartilage has an anterior V-shaped contour at the level of the true vocal cords, whereas it is more rounded caudally. The superior and inferior cornua project off the posterior borders of the lamina (Fig. 1). The superior cornua attach to the hyoid bone by the lateral thyrohyoid ligament. If calcified, small triticeus cartilages may be seen within the ligament. The inferior cornua articulate with the posterolateral margin of the cricoid cartilage forming the cricothyroid joint. There is a normal separation of approximately 1.5 mm between the two. More important, the two joints are normally symmetrical in appearance. The infrahyoid strap muscles are seen as soft-tissue bands anterior and parallel to the thyroid lamina (Fig. 5A).

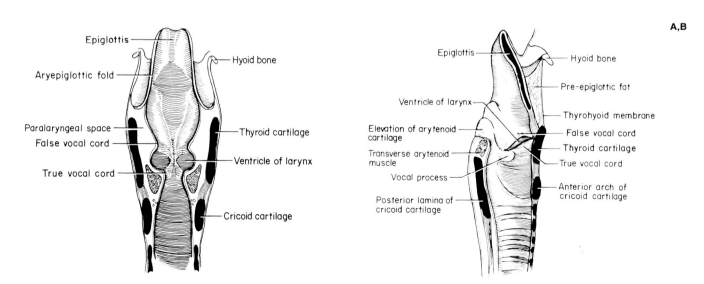

A,B

FIG. 2. Section through laryngeal skeleton and surrounding soft tissues. **A:** Coronal view. **B:** Sagittal view.

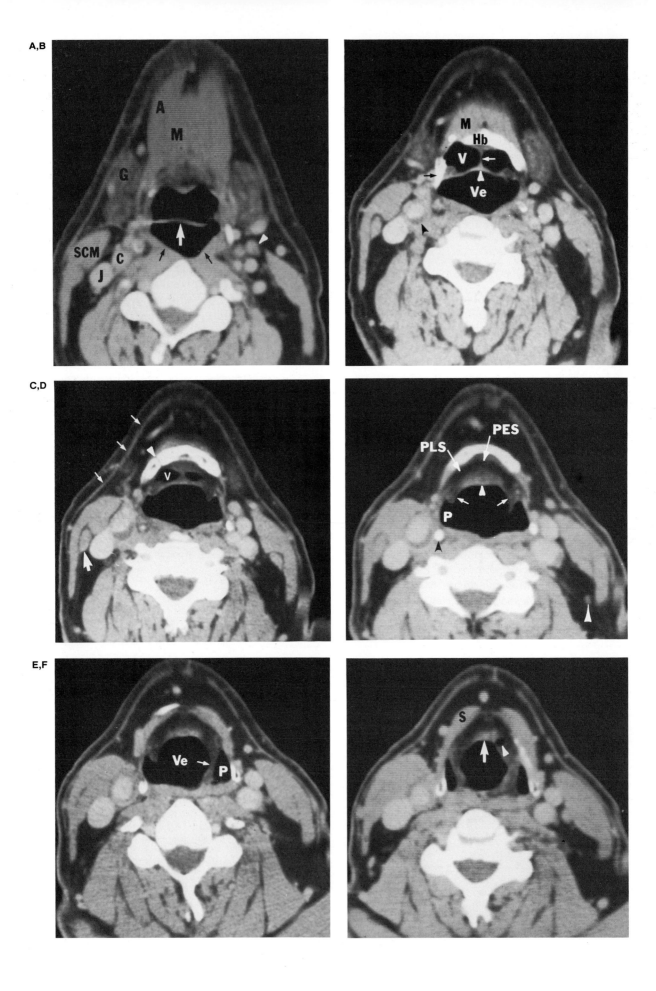

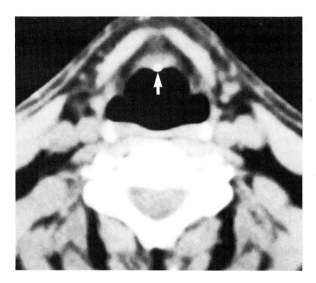

FIG. 4. Calcification in epiglottic cartilage (*arrow*).

A large amount of variation in the degree of thyroid cartilage mineralization can occur normally (Figs. 5 and 6) (3,65,127). Cartilages may be uniformly calcified or have a rim of cortical calcification, or there may be peripheral ossification surrounding a low-density medullary space. However, the pattern of mineralization often is irregular or incomplete, with segmental interruptions that may simulate neoplastic invasion. The inner surface of the thyroid cartilage may also be less mineralized than the outer surface. Although the two thyroid laminae tend to be relatively symmetrical in appearance in each individual patient, asymmetric mineralization is not unusual.

The arytenoid cartilages are paired, usually densely calcified, triangular structures that are positioned laterally on the superior surface of the cricoid cartilage (Fig. 5). The small, tapering vocal processes project anteriorly from the base of the arytenoids to attach to the vocalis muscle

A,B

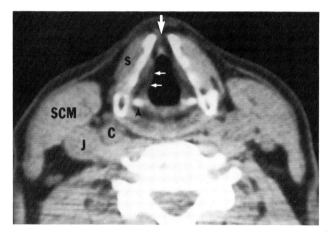
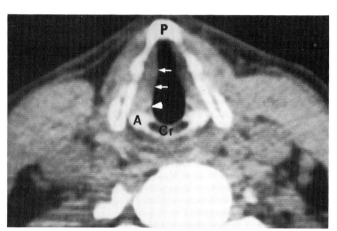

FIG. 5. Normal anatomy: level of false and true vocal cords. **A:** The false vocal cord (*small arrows*), which lies medial to the fat-containing paralaryngeal space, is seen at the level of the foot process (*arrowhead*) of the arytenoid cartilage and the thyroid notch (*large arrow*). Incomplete mineralization of the thyroid lamina is a normal variation and should not be mistaken for cartilage destruction; (C) common carotid artery, (J) internal jugular vein; (S) infrahyoid strap muscles; (SCM) sternocleidomastoid muscle. **B:** The anteromedially projecting vocal process (*small arrowhead*) of the arytenoid cartilage (A), which articulates with the cricoid cartilage (Cr), demarcates the level of the true vocal cord (*small arrows*). The thyroid lamina have fused anteriorly to form the laryngeal prominence (P). The soft tissues at the anterior commissure just posterior to the prominence should normally be less than 2 mm in thickness. The laryngeal airway is elliptical in shape, with a long anteroposterior axis, and also closely abuts the cricoid cartilage posteriorly.

←——————————————————————————————

FIG. 3. Normal anatomy: supraglottic larynx (serial caudal 4-mm images at 4-mm intervals). **A:** The suprahyoid portion of the epiglottis (*white arrow*) is seen posterior to the valleculae and anterior to the laryngeal vestibule; (C) internal carotid artery; (J) internal jugular vein; (G) submandibular gland; (A) anterior belly of digastric muscle; (M) mylohyoid and geniohyoid muscles; (SCM) sternocleidomastoid muscle; (*black arrows*) posterior pharyngeal wall; (*arrowhead*) normal high internal jugular lymph nodes. **B:** The body (Hb) and a portion of the right greater cornu (*black arrow*) of the hyoid bone are visible. The two air-filled valleculae (V), which can normally be asymmetric, are separated by the median glossoepiglottic fold (*white arrow*). The low-attenuation zone posteriorly within the right carotid artery represents atherosclerotic plaque (*black arrowhead*); (*white arrowhead*) epiglottis; (Ve) vestibule, (M) mylohyoid and geniohyoid muscles (suprahyoid strap muscles). **C:** The valleculae (v) are smaller in size. Normal lucency (*white arrowhead*) between the body and greater cornus of the hyoid bone is seen; (*large arrow*) omohyoid muscle; (*small arrows*) platysma muscle. **D:** The fat-containing preepiglottic space (PES) is seen anterior to the soft-tissue-density epiglottis (*small white arrowhead*) and extends laterally into the paralaryngeal space (PLS) and then posteriorly into the aryepiglottic folds (*arrows*); (P) pyriform sinus; (*black arrowhead*) superior cornus of thyroid cartilage; (*large white arrowhead*) normal spinal accessory lymph node. **E:** The left aryepiglottic fold (*arrow*) is more clearly seen separating the laryngeal vestibule (Ve) and left pyriform sinus (P). The aryepiglottic folds may normally be asymmetric in thickness. **F:** Just above the thyroid notch, the epiglottis (*large arrow*) has tapered and is not nearly as broad as its suprahyoid portion. A small amount of air (*arrowhead*) is seen within a minimally dilated left saccule of the laryngeal ventricle; (S) infrahyoid strap muscles.

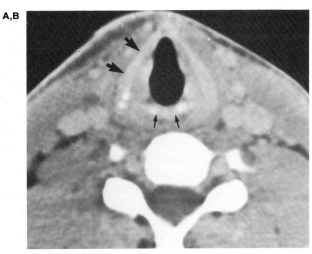

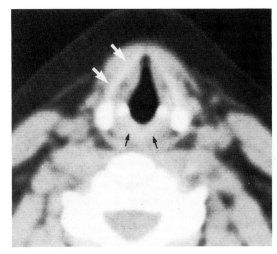

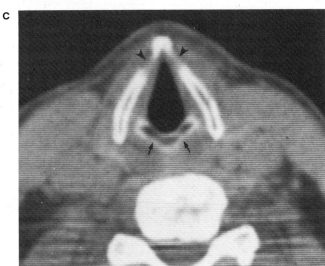

FIG. 6. Variations in thyroid (*large arrows*) and cricoid (*small arrows*) cartilage mineralization in (**A**) 18-year-old male, (**B**) 21-year-old female, and (**C**) 50-year-old male. Paramedian thinning (*arrowheads*) normally can be seen.

and are the best landmarks for defining the level of the true vocal cords. The top of the cricoid cartilage can be seen between the arytenoids at this level. The foot processes of the arytenoid cartilage project superiorly at the level of the false vocal cords, whereas the muscular processes extend posterolaterally toward the thyroid lamina. There is normally 2 mm or less separation between the thyroid cartilage and muscular processes of the arytenoid. The corniculate cartilages lie atop the arytenoids and usually cannot be separated from the foot processes of the arytenoid. The small paired cuneiform cartilages, if calcified, can barely be seen slightly anterior to the foot processes within the aryepiglottic folds (Fig. 7). With quiet breathing during slow inspiration, the arytenoid cartilages are in an abducted position. During phonation or a modified Valsalva maneuver, the arytenoid cartilages adduct and rotate symmetrically toward the midline to oppose each other (Fig. 8).

The cricoid cartilage rests on the first tracheal ring and provides the major foundation for the larynx (Fig. 9). It represents the most caudal portion of the laryngeal skeleton and is the only circumferential cartilaginous ring in the airway. The cricoid cartilage is signet-ring-shaped and slopes inferiorly from the posterior to the anterior arch (Fig. 1C). The wider posterior lamina measures 2 to 3 cm in height, whereas the narrower anterior arch is 5 to 7 mm in height. Below the level of the true vocal cords, the cricoid cartilage moves progressively more anteriorly, eventually forming a complete ring in the low subglottis. In adults, the cricoid cartilage usually is completely mineralized and has a well-defined outer cortical rim with a low-density center, which may represent a medullary space or noncalcified cartilage. Normally, no soft tissue should be visible between the airway and the inner margin of the cricoid cartilage below the level of the true vocal cords.

Superficial Soft Tissues of the Larynx

The intrinsic superficial soft-tissue structures of the larynx consist of the aryepiglottic folds, false vocal cords, and true vocal cords. The aryepiglottic folds are obliquely

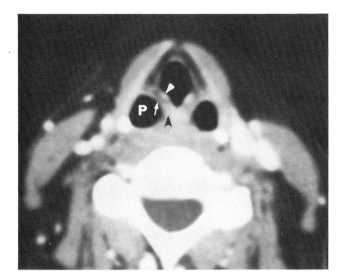

FIG. 7. Cuneiform cartilage (*white arrowhead*); (*black arrowhead*) faintly visible corniculate cartilage just cephalad to foot process of arytenoid cartilage; (*arrow*) aryepiglottic fold; (P) pyriform sinus.

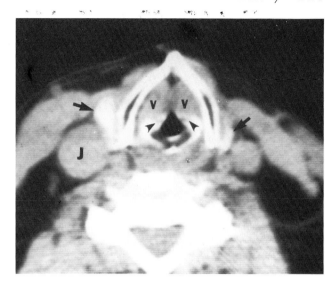

FIG. 8. Adduction of true vocal cords. During phonation, the true vocal cords (v) and vocal processes of the arytenoid cartilages (*arrowheads*) are adducted; (*arrows*) upper pole of thyroid gland; (J) normal right internal jugular vein.

oriented paired structures that separate the laryngeal vestibule from the pyriform sinuses (Fig. 3D–F). They first extend laterally from the superior margin of the epiglottis, then pass medially and inferiorly toward the false vocal cords. Fibro-fatty tissue in the paralaryngeal space extends posteromedially into each aryepiglottic fold, accounting for their relatively low attenuation value on CT. Each fold is approximately 2 to 3 mm thick superiorly and thickens gradually to approximately 5 mm inferiorly. The

aryepiglottic folds may normally be asymmetric during inspiration, but appear more symmetrical and are more easily visualized with distension of the pyriform sinuses during phonation or a modified Valsalva maneuver (Fig. 10).

Although the pyriform sinuses are intrinsically part of the hypopharynx, they are closely related to laryngeal structures and lie within the borders of the laryngeal skeleton (Fig. 3D and 3E). These bilateral structures, which

A,B

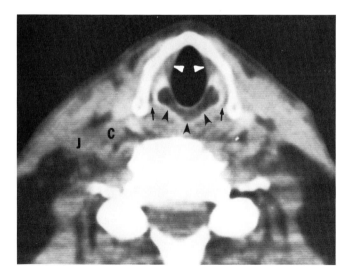 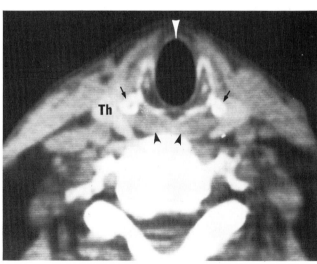

FIG. 9. Normal anatomy: subglottic level. **A:** The cricoid cartilage (*black arrowheads*), consisting of a dense cortical rim with a lower-density medullary space, is seen. The cricothyroid joints (*arrows*) are symmetric bilaterally. The undersurfaces of the true vocal cords (*white arrowheads*) are seen anterolaterally; (C) common carotid artery; (J) internal jugular vein. **B:** On the next caudal image, the cricoid ring is about two-thirds complete, except anteriorly at the cricothyroid membrane (*white arrowhead*). The subglottic airway is more circular than at the true-vocal-cord level and is closely apposed to the cricoid cartilage; (*arrows*) inferior cornua of thyroid cartilage; (*black arrowheads*) cricopharyngeus–cervical esophagus; (Th) thyroid gland.

A,B

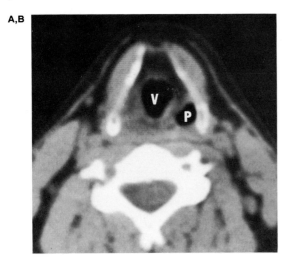
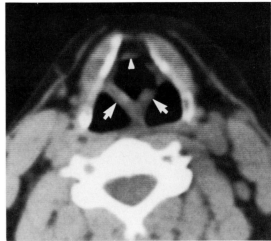

FIG. 10. Value of modified Valsalva maneuver. **A:** The right pyriform sinus is not seen; (P) left pyriform sinus; (V) laryngeal vestibule. **B:** Image obtained during a modified Valsalva maneuver distends the pyriform sinuses. The aryepiglottic folds (*arrows*), which separate the laryngeal vestibule from the pyriform sinuses, also are better seen; (*arrowhead*) epiglottis.

usually contain some air during quiet inspiration, lie lateral to the aryepiglottic folds, medial to the thyrohyoid membrane or thyroid cartilage, and posterior to the paralaryngeal space. The apex of the pyriform sinus is seen just lateral to the cricoarytenoid joint near the level of the true vocal cords. The two pyriform sinuses join in the postcricoid region and merge with the cervical esophagus. Frequently they are partially collapsed during quiet breathing, but become well distended during a modified Valsalva maneuver or phonation (Fig. 10). Asymmetry in size and inferior extent of the pyriform sinuses is not unusual.

The false vocal cords appear as two parallel bands of soft tissue that attach to the inner surface of the thyroid cartilage (Fig. 5A). The foot processes of the arytenoid cartilage usually are visible posteriorly. In comparison with the true vocal cords, the false vocal cords contain fewer muscle fibers and more fat and are therefore of lower density on CT. Soft-tissue thickening is normally seen anteriorly behind the thyroid lamina at the level of the false vocal cords. This is partially related to the insertion of the thyroepiglottic ligament.

The laryngeal ventricle separates the false and true vocal cords and is only occasionally seen on CT (Fig. 11). On transaxial images, it appears as a crescent-shaped, air-filled space. Thinner sections performed with a reverse "e" maneuver may result in improved demonstration (93).

The ventricular saccule represents an upward extension of the laryngeal ventricle and may be seen as a small collection of air anterolateral to the false vocal cords or aryepiglottic fold (Fig. 3F). It is more frequently seen on images obtained during phonation or a modified Valsalva maneuver, which increases intralaryngeal pressure and distends the saccule.

The true vocal cords enclose two bands of elastic tissue,

the vocal ligaments, that attach anteriorly to the laryngeal prominence, forming the anterior commissure, and posteriorly to the vocal processes of the arytenoid cartilage (Fig. 5B). The posterior commissure lies between the vocal processes on the anterior surface of the cricoid lamina. The vocalis muscle lies lateral and parallel to the vocal ligament. The attenuation value of the true vocal cords is similar to that for surrounding skeletal muscle. On CT, the true vocal cords are normally seen in an abducted position during slow inspiration. They are triangular in shape and taper from posterior (where they measure approximately 9 mm in thickness) to anterior (where they measure about 2 mm in thickness). The undersurface of the true vocal cords extends approximately 5 mm below the midportion of the true vocal cords. The thyroid lamina

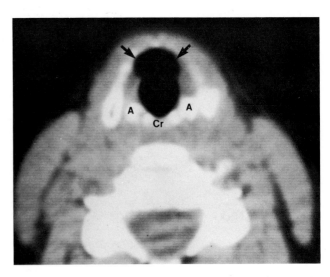

FIG. 11. Laryngeal ventricle (*arrows*); (A) arytenoid cartilages; (Cr) cricoid cartilage.

usually has a rounded contour at this level. With the vocal cords in abduction, the soft tissues at the anterior commissure immediately posterior to the fused thyroid lamina usually are less than 2 mm in thickness. Similarly, only minuscule soft tissue should be seen just in front of the posterior commissure. If the vocal cords are adducted, the soft tissues may appear falsely thickened at both the anterior and posterior commissures (Fig. 8). Apparent thickening of the anterior commissure also may result if the neck is not positioned properly and images are not obtained parallel to the vocal cords. As a result, the posterior portion of the true vocal cord may be in the plane of section, but the anterior plane may be through the false-vocal-cord level. Careful attention to patient positioning, and, if necessary, obtaining thin sections at the level of the true vocal cords, should clarify most problems.

Deep Soft Tissues of the Larynx

In the supraglottic portion of the larynx there are three adjacent deep compartments: the preepiglottic space and the paired lateral paralaryngeal spaces (Figs. 2 and 3). The preepiglottic space is a triangularly shaped area that is bordered superiorly by the valleculae and base of the tongue, posteriorly by the epiglottis, anteriorly by the hyoid bone, and laterally by the paralaryngeal space, thyrohyoid membrane, and thyroid cartilage. The preepiglottic space extends caudally from the hyoid bone to just above the anterior commissure. Because it is composed primarily of fat, it has a homogeneous, near-fat attenuation value on CT. However, an area of higher attenuation may be seen at the level of the hyoid bone. This is secondary to the hyoepiglottic ligament and/or glandular structures and should not be confused with neoplasm (Fig. 12).

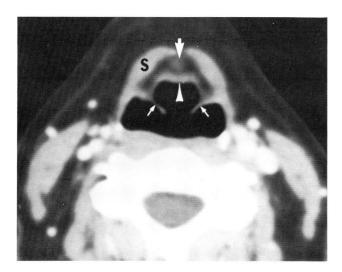

FIG. 12. Hyoepiglottic ligament (*large arrow*) is seen within the preepiglottic space; (S) infrahyoid strap muscles; (*arrowhead*) epiglottis; (*small arrows*) aryepiglottic folds.

The preepiglottic space appears continuous laterally with the paralaryngeal space, although histologically the quadrangular membrane may separate the two spaces (Fig. 3D) (51). It also has a relatively low density on CT because of its fat content, but may contain small areas of higher attenuation value. The paralaryngeal spaces are bordered medially by the aryepiglottic folds, laterally by the thyrohyoid membrane and thyroid cartilage, and posteriorly by the pyriform sinuses. The paralaryngeal space is well seen at the false-vocal-cord level, but narrows toward the level of the true vocal cord. Occasionally, a thin low-density zone can be seen between the true vocal cord and thyroid lamina, representing the inferior extension of the paralaryngeal space.

The conus elasticus or cricothyroid membrane separates the deep soft-tissue spaces of the infraglottis into an anterior and two lateral compartments, which are continuous with one another (65). The lateral compartments are continuous superiorly with the paralaryngeal space and undersurface of the true vocal cords, whereas the anterior compartment abuts the cricothyroid ligament. The conus elasticus is not seen on CT and is so closely adherent to the cricoid cartilage that no soft-tissue density is seen between the inner surface of the cricoid cartilage and the airway (Fig. 9).

Airway

The shape of the laryngeal airway varies depending on the level imaged (28). The supraglottic portion of the airway, the laryngeal vestibule, is bordered by the epiglottis anteriorly, the aryepiglottic folds laterally, and the apices of the arytenoid cartilages posteriorly (Fig. 3C). It is elliptical in shape, with a longer lateral axis. The vestibule is widest superiorly and narrows inferiorly to become more triangular or pear-shaped at the level of the false vocal cords. At the true-vocal-cord level, the airway is elliptical, with a long anteroposterior axis (Fig. 5B). The subglottic region has a more circular shape and is closely apposed to the cricoid cartilage (Fig. 9B). Below the cricoid, the tracheal air column may be circular or horseshoe-shaped, with a flat posterior border. However, a smooth posterior impression on the airway due to the esophagus may be seen.

Soft Tissues of the Neck

The neck extends from the mylohyoid muscle, which separates the neck from the floor of the mouth, to the first rib, which marks the level of the thoracic inlet. The neck traditionally has been divided into two paired symmetric triangular spaces, the anterior and posterior triangles (Fig. 13) (65,89,91).

The anterior triangles meet in the midline and are bor-

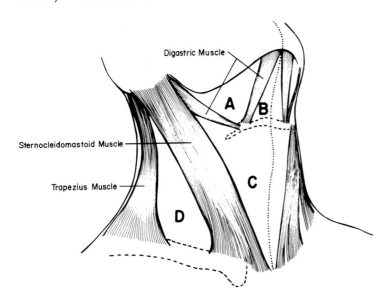

Digastric Muscle

Sternocleidomastoid Muscle

Trapezius Muscle

FIG. 13. Triangles of the neck; (A) submandibular triangle; (B) submental triangle; (C) infrahyoid division of anterior triangle; (D) posterior triangle. (Note: A and B represent the suprahyoid division of the anterior triangle.) (Adapted from ref. 87.)

dered by the sternocleidomastoid muscle posterolaterally, the mandible superiorly, and the midline medially (Fig. 13). The hyoid bone separates each anterior triangle into a suprahyoid division and infrahyoid division (89,91). The suprahyoid division (submental and submandibular triangles) is separated from the floor of the mouth by the mylohyoid muscle. The submental triangle, formed by the anterior bellies of the digastric muscles and the hyoid bone, contains only a few lymph nodes and branches of the facial artery and vein. The submandibular triangle, bordered by the anterior and posterior bellies of the digastric muscles and the mandibular rami, contains lymph nodes and the submandibular gland, which often are asymmetric in size (Fig. 3A).

The infrahyoid division of the anterior triangle contains many of the major structures of the neck, including the hypopharynx, larynx, trachea, esophagus, thyroid and parathyroid glands, and the structures of the carotid sheath and lymph nodes (Fig. 14). The carotid sheath structures (common carotid artery medially, internal jugular vein laterally, and vagus nerve posteriorly) lie deep to the sternocleidomastoid muscle and form the posterior border of the anterior triangle. The internal jugular vein is seen more anteriorly on images through the lower neck. The right internal jugular vein, which frequently is larger than the left, can simulate a neck mass on physical examination and non-contrast-enhanced CT images (Fig. 15) (41).

The normal thyroid gland is routinely seen, appearing on non-contrast-enhanced CT images as a soft-tissue structure with attenuation values higher than those for normal muscle; this reflects its high iodine content and is particularly noticeable in young patients (Fig. 16) (47). Because of its abundant vascular supply, it is enhanced after intravenous administration of contrast material. The upper pole of the thyroid gland can be seen between the thyroid lamina and the infrahyoid strap muscles, whereas the body of the thyroid gland lies lateral to the cricoid

cartilage and trachea, and anterior and medial to the carotid artery and jugular vein. The thyroid isthmus usually can be seen connecting the two lobes anterior to the trachea. The normal parathyroid glands usually are not seen on CT. However, the inferior thyroid artery and veins, sometimes identified in the fat posterior to the carotid artery, anterior to the longus colli muscles, and lateral to the esophagus, mark the location of the normal parathyroid glands, as well as the recurrent laryngeal nerves (65). The expected course of each recurrent laryngeal nerve can be traced. The right recurrent laryngeal nerve branches from the vagus nerve at the anterior border of the right subclavian artery and passes caudally, looping around the vessel, before ascending medially in the tracheoesophageal

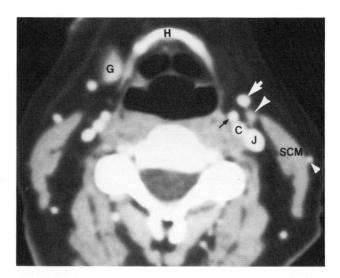

FIG. 14. Normal neck anatomy; (C) internal carotid artery; (J) internal jugular vein; (G) submandibular gland; (H) hyoid bone; (SCM) sternocleidomastoid muscle; (*small arrow*) external carotid artery; (*large arrow*) anterior jugular vein; (*small arrowhead*) external jugular vein; (*large arrowhead*) normal internal jugular lymph node.

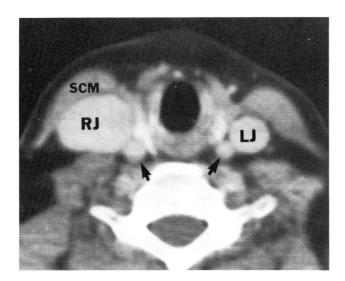

FIG. 15. Dilatation of right internal jugular vein. The right internal jugular vein (RJ) is very large, and the sternocleidomastoid muscle (SCM) is draped over it anteriorly. More caudal scans demonstrated a normal course of the jugular vein and no obstructing mass; (*arrows*) common carotid artery; (LJ) left internal jugular vein.

groove. The left recurrent laryngeal nerve leaves the vagus nerve adjacent to the anterior surface of the aortic arch and passes around the arch through the aortopulmonary window to ascend in the tracheoesophageal groove. Both nerves enter the larynx under the lower border of the cricopharyngeal muscle.

The posterior triangle is composed primarily of fat, but also contains lymph nodes, small vessels, and the spinal accessory and many small cutaneous nerves. It is bordered by the sternocleidomastoid muscle anterolaterally, the cervical spine and paraspinal musculature medially, and the trapezius muscle posteriorly, with the clavicle as its base. The inferior belly of the omohyoid muscle, occasionally seen as a soft-tissue-density structure underneath the sternocleidomastoid muscle, should not be confused with an enlarged lymph node (Fig. 3C).

CT provides accurate delineation of the lymph nodes in the neck. Normal lymph nodes usually are homogeneous and of soft-tissue density, similar in attenuation value to muscle on both precontrast and postcontrast images (Figs. 3A and D and 14). Peripheral enhancement

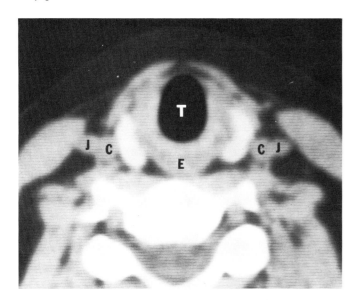

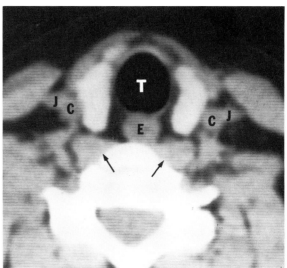

A,B

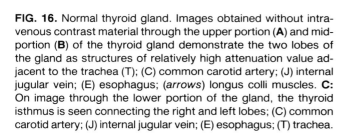

FIG. 16. Normal thyroid gland. Images obtained without intravenous contrast material through the upper portion (**A**) and midportion (**B**) of the thyroid gland demonstrate the two lobes of the gland as structures of relatively high attenuation value adjacent to the trachea (T); (C) common carotid artery; (J) internal jugular vein; (E) esophagus; (*arrows*) longus colli muscles. **C:** On image through the lower portion of the gland, the thyroid isthmus is seen connecting the right and left lobes; (C) common carotid artery; (J) internal jugular vein; (E) esophagus; (T) trachea.

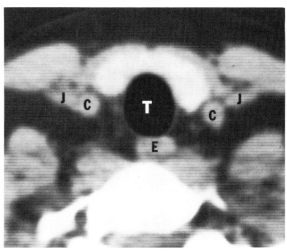

C

of the lymph node normally is not seen. Occasionally, fatty replacement of a portion of the lymph node, a benign reactive process, may be observed and should not be confused with central necrosis. Fatty foci usually occur in a peripheral or noncentral portion of the lymph node.

Normal lymph nodes usually range in size from 3 to 5 mm in diameter. However, they may be up to 1.5 cm in diameter in the upper neck (e.g., jugulodigastric, submandibular nodes) (65).

The lymph nodes in the head and neck generally are divided into 10 major groups (65,89,91,94). The first six groups (occipital, mastoid, parotid, submandibular, facial, and submental) form a lymphoid ring at the junction between the head and neck and usually are easily palpable. Sublingual and retropharyngeal nodes (groups 7 and 8) lie deep to these lymph nodes and may be difficult to assess clinically. Identification of retropharyngeal nodes, which are most frequently located along the lateral borders of the longus capitis muscle at C1-C2, is particularly important for tumors of the nasal cavity, nasopharynx, and hard and soft palate (66,67).

The anterior cervical group of lymph nodes (group 9) is located below the level of the hyoid bone between the two carotid sheaths (65,89,91). It consists of a superficial group along the course of the anterior jugular vein and a deep group (juxtavisceral) adjacent to the thyroid, trachea, and esophagus.

The lymph nodes of the lateral cervical group (group 10) are divided into superficial (external jugular) and deep (internal jugular, spinal accessory, and transverse cervical) groups (Figs. 17 and 18) (65,89,91). The superficial group follows the course of the external jugular vein. The three chains of the deep group form a triangle of lymph nodes that are the major sites of metastases from laryngeal and hypopharyngeal carcinoma. The nodes of the internal jugular chain are located in the anterior triangle deep to the sternocleidomastoid muscle and follow the course of the internal jugular vein. They normally tend to be largest in the upper neck. The jugulodigastric node is the largest node in the upper portion of the internal jugular chain and usually is seen slightly above the hyoid bone near the junction between the internal jugular vein and posterior belly of the digastric muscle.

The lymph nodes of the spinal accessory chain are located lateral and posterior to the spinal accessory nerve between the sternocleidomastoid and trapezius muscles (Fig. 18A and B). They join the internal jugular vein group above the hyoid bone. Lymph nodes immediately posterior to the jugular vein are anterior and medial to the nerve and are considered internal-jugular-vein lymph nodes (65).

The transverse cervical chain forms the base of the deep group of the lateral cervical nodes and joins the inferior jugular and spinal accessory chains (65,89,91). These nodes are seen in the supraclavicular area and the inferior aspect of the posterior triangle (Fig. 18C).

MRI

The normal anatomy of the larynx and neck as seen on MR images is similar to that demonstrated on CT (Figs. 19 to 24) (12,56,58,115). The signal from the laryngeal skeleton varies depending on the degrees of calcification and ossification and the fat content. Calcified or ossified cartilage is seen as an area of low signal intensity on MR images, whereas the fatty, medullary portion is higher in signal intensity. In some cases it may be more difficult with MRI than with CT to identify and distinguish the laryngeal cartilages from paralaryngeal soft tissues and the infrahyoid strap muscles. This is especially true in younger patients, in whom the cartilage is only beginning to calcify. The epiglottis, which is fibroelastic cartilage, yields an intermediate signal intensity, similar to that for skeletal muscle, and is easily distinguished from the adjacent high-intensity fat in the preepiglottic and paralaryngeal spaces.

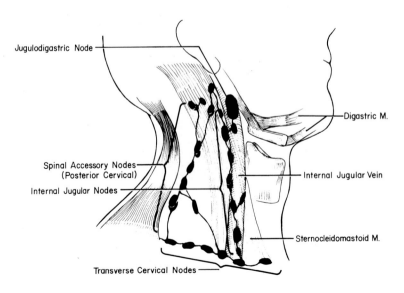

FIG. 17. Groups of deep lateral cervical lymph nodes. The jugulodigastric node is the largest node in the upper portion of the internal jugular chain. (Adapted from ref. 94.)

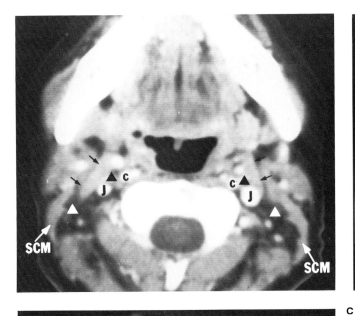

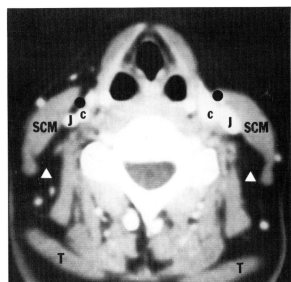

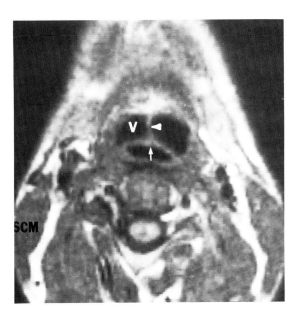

FIG. 18. Locations of major groups of cervical lymph nodes on CT images. **A:** Upper neck. **B:** Middle neck. **C:** Lower neck; (*black triangle*) jugulodigastric nodes (upper node of internal jugular chain); (*black dot*) internal jugular nodes; (*white triangle*) spinal accessory (posterior cervical) nodes; (*asterisk*) transverse cervical nodes; (C) common carotid artery; (c) internal carotid artery; (J) internal jugular vein; (T) trapezius muscle; (Th) thyroid gland; (*black arrows*) posterior belly of digastric muscle; (*white arrow*) scalenus anterior muscle.

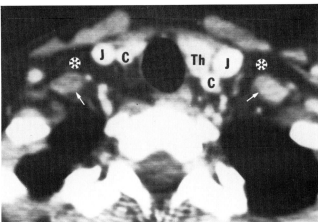

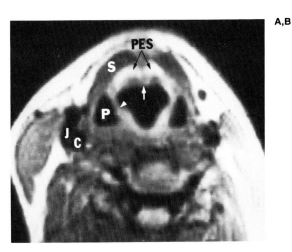

FIG. 19. Normal anatomy: high supraglottic larynx (T1-weighted images). **A:** The medium-signal-intensity epiglottis (*arrow*) seen posterior to the air-containing valleculae (V), is slightly higher in signal intensity than the sternocleidomastoid muscle (SCM); (*arrowhead*) glossoepiglottic fold. **B:** On a more caudal image in another patient, the high-signal-intensity preepiglottic space (PES) is well seen adjacent to the medium-signal-intensity infrahyoid strap muscles (S). The aryepiglottic folds (*arrowhead*) are slightly higher in signal intensity than the epiglottis (*arrow*) because of their fat content; (C) common carotid artery; (J) internal jugular vein; (P) pyriform sinus.

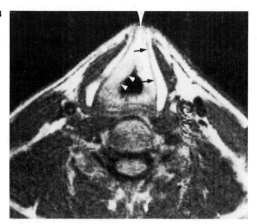

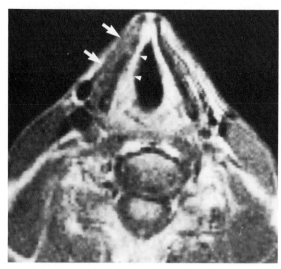

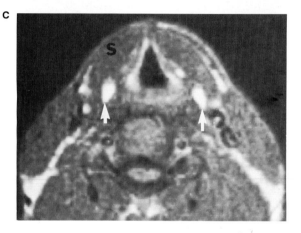

FIG. 20. Normal anatomy: level of false vocal cords (T1-weighted images). **A:** The paralaryngeal space and false vocal cords (*small arrowheads*) are relatively high in signal intensity, because of loose areolar and glandular tissue. The calcified portion of the thyroid lamina is seen as a low-signal-intensity zone (*arrows*) adjacent to the high-intensity medullary fat; (*large arrowhead*) thyroid notch. (From ref. 39, reprinted with permission.) **B:** In another patient at the same level, a more substantially calcified thyroid cartilage appears as a black strip separating the medium-signal-intensity infrahyoid strap muscles (*arrows*) and high-intensity paralaryngeal space and false vocal cord (*arrowheads*). **C:** High signal intensity from medullary fat within portions of the thyroid lamina (*arrows*) is seen in a different patient. Note how other areas of the thyroid cartilage blend in with the infrahyoid strap muscles (S).

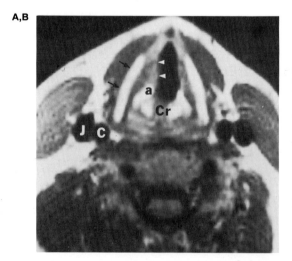

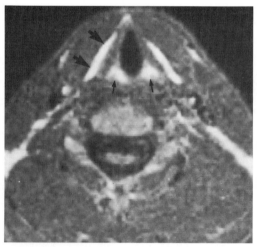

FIG. 21. Normal anatomy; level of the true vocal cords (T1-weighted images). **A:** The signal intensity of the true vocal cords (*arrowheads*) is slightly higher than that of the strap muscles; (a) vocal process of arytenoid cartilage; (Cr) top of cricoid cartilage; (C) common carotid artery; (J) internal jugular vein; (*arrows*) thyroid lamina. **B:** In another patient, high signal intensity from fatty marrow within the thyroid cartilage (*large arrows*), arytenoid cartilage, and cricoid cartilage (*small arrows*) sharply contrasts with the lower signal intensity of the strap muscles and true vocal cords.

A,B

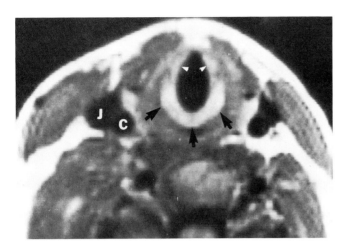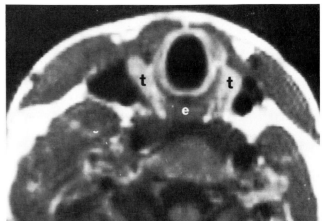

FIG. 22. Normal anatomy: subglottic level. **A:** On T1-weighted MR image, the cricoid cartilage (*arrows*) is well visualized secondary to fat within its medullary cavity; (*small arrowheads*) undersurfaces of the vocal cords; (C) common carotid artery; (J) internal jugular vein. **B:** On image 1 cm caudal, the airway is closely apposed to the cricoid ring. The thyroid gland (t) is intermediate in signal intensity between muscle and fat; (e) esophagus.

The intrinsic soft-tissue structures of the larynx usually are easily identified on MRI (Figs. 19–21). However, image degradation from swallowing, as well as motion-related artifacts because of prolonged imaging time, may impair their demonstration. The aryepiglottic folds are higher in signal intensity than the adjacent epiglottis because of their fat content. Similarly, the false vocal cords are of relatively high signal intensity because of loose areolar tissue and glands in the submucosa. In comparison, low signal intensity from the vocalis muscle results in the true vocal cords being similar or slightly higher in signal intensity to the strap muscles. Whereas the laryngeal ventricle frequently is not visualized on CT, it is frequently seen on coronal or sagittal MR images (Fig. 23).

Because the deep soft-tissue spaces of the larynx are composed primarily of fat, they are high in signal intensity on MR images and are easily distinguished from the true vocal cords and calcified thyroid cartilage (Figs. 19 to 21). An area of decreased signal may be seen within the pre-epiglottic space, secondary to the hyoepiglottic ligament.

Normal-size lymph nodes are easily seen as intermediate-signal-intensity structures in the neck on T1-weighted MR images (Fig. 25). The normal vascular structures are identified as distinct areas of signal void. Intraluminal signal from slowly flowing blood could conceivably be confused with an enlarged lymph node. However, demonstration of an increase in intensity on second-echo images (even-echo rephasing), as well as review of sequential images, usually is sufficient to confirm that a blood vessel is being imaged.

The normal thyroid gland yields a signal intensity intermediate between those of fat and strap muscles on T1-

A,B

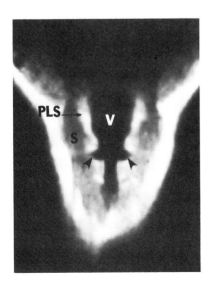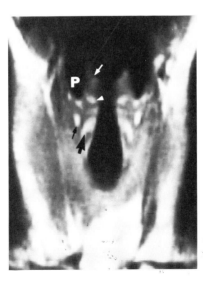

FIG. 23. Coronal T1-weighted MR images of larynx. **A–B:** Successive dorsal images; (*large black arrow*) cricoid cartilage; (*small black arrow*) thyroid cartilage; (*small black arrowheads*) laryngeal ventricle; (*small white arrowhead*) arytenoid cartilage; (*small white arrow*) aryepiglottic fold; (P) pyriform sinus, (PLS) paralaryngeal space; (V) vestibule; (S) strap muscles.

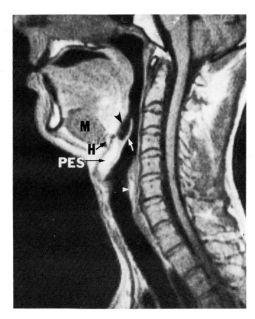

FIG. 24. Sagittal T1-weighted MR image of larynx; (*white arrow*) epiglottis; (*white arrowhead*) cricoid cartilage; (*black arrowhead*) vallecula; (H) hyoid bone; (M) mylohyoid and geniohyoid muscles; (PES) preepiglottic space.

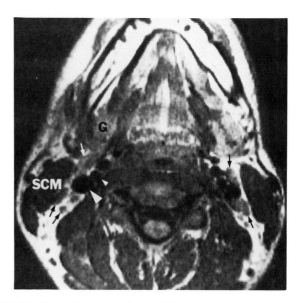

FIG. 25. Normal lymph nodes on T1-weighted image. Multiple intermediate-signal-intensity internal jugular and spinal accessory lymph nodes are seen (*arrows*); (*small arrowhead*) internal carotid artery; (*large arrowhead*) internal jugular vein; (G) submandibular gland; (SCM) sternocleidomastoid muscle.

weighted images (Fig. 22) (45,114). The signal-intensity difference between thyroid and muscle is accentuated on T2-weighted images. Although the thyroid gland usually is homogeneous on T1-weighted images, small areas of very high signal intensity may be seen on T2-weighted images, presumably representing incidental areas of nodular hyperplasia or cystic degeneration. As with CT, the normal parathyroid glands cannot be visualized reliably with MRI and distinguished from adjacent lymph nodes and nerves.

PATHOLOGY

Malignant Neoplasms

Laryngeal and Hypopharyngeal Neoplasms

For purposes of staging, the larynx is divided into the glottic, supraglottic, and infraglottic larynx. Although pyriform sinus neoplasms arise from the alimentary tract and are considered part of the hypopharynx, they lie within the laryngeal skeleton and therefore will be included in this discussion. The pattern of spread and biological aggressiveness of tumors depends in part on the primary site of origin. Tumors tend to be progressively more aggressive proceeding from the glottis to the supraglottis to the hypopharynx (5,119).

More than 90% of epithelial malignant neoplasms of the larynx are squamous cell carcinomas (5). Carcinosarcoma, adenocarcinoma, adenoid cystic carcinoma, oat-cell carcinoma, and metastases are much less common.

Malignant neoplasms may rarely arise from the supporting tissues of the larynx, and they include chondrosarcoma, fibrosarcoma, and lymphoma.

CT has replaced contrast laryngography, conventional tomography, and plain-film radiography for the staging of most patients with malignant laryngeal and hypopharyngeal neoplasms (2,61,64,65,95). The latter techniques give information similar to that provided by laryngoscopy, primarily showing mucosal abnormalities and alterations of the airway. The cross-sectional imaging provided by CT allows evaluation of the intrinsic and deep soft-tissue structures of the larynx, as well as the cartilaginous skeleton and adjacent soft tissues of the neck. More recently, MRI has also been used for evaluation of laryngeal and hypopharyngeal neoplasms and provides similar information in many cases (13,39,57,125).

Laryngoscopy is the most accurate method for examining the laryngeal mucosa and glottic function. However, deep spread of tumor often is only suggested by tumor size and abnormal vocal cord mobility. Extension of neoplasm into the preepiglottic and paralaryngeal spaces or invasion of the adjacent cartilaginous skeleton is not directly assessed and may be difficult to detect even with deep biopsy. The decision among radiation therapy, conservation surgery, or total laryngectomy requires a very accurate delineation of tumor extent to provide the simplest, least invasive form of therapy while avoiding treatment failures (79–81). CT complements laryngoscopy by evaluating those portions of the larynx and hypopharynx that are difficult to examine with laryngoscopy. CT can confirm that a tumor is limited or show that there is submucosal extension with cartilaginous destruction. This additional information can be helpful in making appropriate therapeutic decisions.

On CT, tumors are seen as areas of soft-tissue thickening that alter the normal symmetric anatomy. This finding, however, is nonspecific and may also be secondary to hemorrhage, edema, inflammation, or fibrosis (65,93, 101). The CT findings must therefore be interpreted in conjunction with the clinical history. Moreover, the examination should be performed prior to laryngoscopic biopsy in order to prevent confusion of postbiopsy hemorrhage and edema with tumor.

Glottic tumors.

Approximately 50% to 60% of laryngeal carcinomas arise from the glottis, and 75% of these originate on the anterior half of the true vocal cord (28,100). Tumors that are localized to a normal mobile true vocal cord generally do not need to be evaluated with CT. These tumors may be treated by radiation therapy or vertical hemilaryngectomy (15,73). However, radiation is generally preferred because voice quality post treatment usually is superior. If performed, CT may show focal or diffuse thickening of the true vocal cord (Fig. 26). However, subtle asymmetry may also fall within the normal range. Moreover, images may appear normal when laryngoscopy demonstrates a small tumor. This finding almost always indicates localized disease. A paralyzed true vocal cord may have a CT appearance identical with that of a cord thickened by neoplasm. In most cases, laryngoscopy can distinguish between the two conditions. CT (or MRI) may also be helpful in detecting extralaryngeal masses that involve the recurrent laryngeal nerve and result in vocal cord paralysis (35,48).

Most glottic tumors are localized lesions that spread along the intrinsic laryngeal musculature, but may extend to involve other parts of the larynx (51). The primary role of CT in patients with glottic tumors is for evaluation of the anterior and posterior commissures, the paralaryngeal and subglottic spaces, and the thyroid and cricoid cartilages. Anterior extension of tumor is via the anterior commissure, where the soft tissue is normally less than 2 mm thick (Figs. 27 and 28). Any increase in thickness in this area should be considered abnormal and suspicious for tumor extension, although it also may be secondary to hemorrhage or reactive edema. Once tumor has spread to the anterior commissure, it can extend to the contralateral true vocal cord. Generally, involvement of more than 30% of the contralateral true vocal cord precludes successful vertical hemilaryngectomy, although "extended" surgery may be possible (6). The tumor can also extend directly into the thyroid cartilage, inferiorly into the subglottic space, or superiorly into the false vocal cord and low preepiglottic space.

True-vocal-cord tumors also may spread to the posterior commissure and result in thickening of the soft tissues over the arytenoid cartilage (Fig. 28). Rotation or displacement of the arytenoid cartilages may be seen in association with such spread, which usually is seen only with more advanced tumors (65).

The paralaryngeal space provides a pathway for vertical extension of laryngeal carcinoma. A thin line of fat density representing the paralaryngeal space may be seen medial to the thyroid cartilage adjacent to the true vocal cord. This space is wider at the level of the false vocal cords. Therefore, extension into the paralaryngeal space at the false-vocal-cord level is easier to demonstrate. It frequently may be difficult with CT to determine extension into the

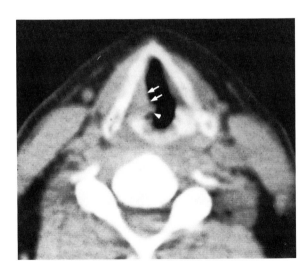

FIG. 26. Localized true-vocal-cord carcinoma. Tumor thickens the posterior aspect of the right true vocal cord (*arrows*); (*arrowhead*) vocal process of arytenoid cartilage.

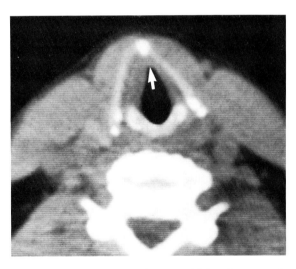

FIG. 27. True-vocal-cord carcinoma, with involvement of anterior commissure. Tumor of right true vocal cord extends anteriorly and thickens tissues at the anterior commissure (*arrow*). The left true vocal cord is normal.

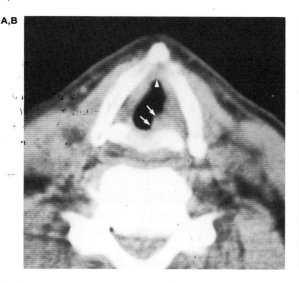
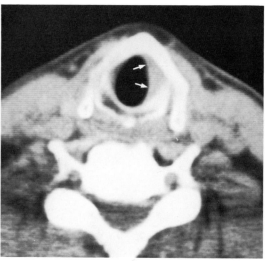

FIG. 28. True-vocal-cord carcinoma, with involvement of anterior and posterior commissures with subglottic extension. **A:** Left-true-vocal-cord tumor extends posteromedially over the arytenoid cartilage toward the posterior commissure (*arrows*) and anteriorly across the anterior commissure (*arrowhead*). **B:** Subglottic extension of tumor (*arrows*) separates the airway from the cricoid cartilage.

false vocal cord itself, because larger tumors can deform the false vocal cord without actually invading it. This distinction usually is more easily made at laryngoscopy.

Subglottic extension of a true-vocal-cord tumor greater than 8 to 9 mm anteriorly and 5 to 6 mm posteriorly usually is an indication for total laryngectomy (51,81). The different measurements relate to the cricoid arch sloping inferiorly from posterior to anterior. However, the relationship between the tumor and the cricoid ring, which provides the major support for the larynx, is more important than specific measurements. This relationship is easily demonstrated by CT, because normally there is no soft-tissue thickening between the cricoid cartilage and the airway below the undersurface of the true vocal cords (Fig. 28). Extension into the soft tissues of the neck may occur anteriorly through the cricothyroid membrane or posterolaterally between the cricoid and thyroid cartilages. Subglottic extension deep to the conus elasticus may not be apparent on the laryngoscopic examination.

Laryngoscopic demonstration of vocal cord fixation in patients with laryngeal carcinoma is thought to be highly suggestive of deep infiltration by tumor (51). Although phonation images also can demonstrate cord fixation, CT is most helpful in distinguishing the possible causes of a fixed cord prior to surgery, as well as in showing deep extension of tumor in those patients with normally mobile true vocal cords (69). Causes of vocal cord fixation include tumor invasion of the thyroid cartilage, cricoarytenoid joint, or vocalis muscle and paralaryngeal space. Subglottic extension of tumor, with fixation of the cord to the cricoid cartilage or tumor involvement of the recurrent laryngeal nerve, can also lead to vocal cord fixation. Occasionally, CT will prove helpful by showing that vocal cord fixation

is related to previous occult trauma and that the laryngeal tumor is less extensive than suspected clinically.

If cartilage destruction is present, the tumor cannot be cured by conservation surgery or radiation therapy alone (79). Although CT may be helpful in demonstrating cartilaginous invasion, there are certain limitations and pitfalls (Fig. 29) (3,46,59,60,97,101,126). The thyroid cartilage normally may have an irregular pattern of

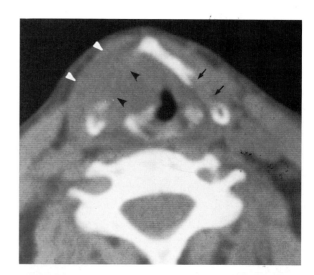

FIG. 29. Thyroid cartilage destruction. A large carcinoma of the right true vocal cord that involves the anterior commissure also destroys the right thyroid lamina (*black arrowheads*) and extends into the adjacent soft tissues (*white arrowheads*). Cortical thinning of the posterior aspect of the left thyroid lamina (*arrows*) is a normal variation and should not be interpreted as cartilage destruction.

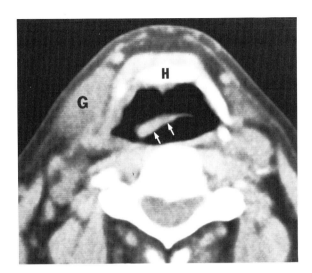

FIG. 30. Epiglottic carcinoma. Image at the level of the hyoid bone (H) demonstrates thickening of the right side of the free margin of the epiglottis (*arrows*); (G) submandibular gland.

calcification and ossification (Figs. 5 and 6). Moreover, if the patient is rotated slightly, images through the superior or inferior portion of the cartilage may simulate invasion. Therefore, in most cases, only moderately or far-advanced involvement can be confidently diagnosed. Conversely, subtle cartilage invasion will frequently be missed. Fragmentation of the normal cartilage, with tumor extension into the adjacent soft tissues, may be seen with extensive cartilaginous destruction. Cartilage involvement may also be suggested by distortion without obvious destruction (e.g., focal bowing of the thyroid cartilage adjacent to the tumor). More limited cases may show defects in the car-

tilage adjacent to the tumor with or without abnormal soft tissue in the central medullary cavity. However, proximity of the tumor to the cartilage does not equate with invasion. Therefore, when the CT findings are equivocal, biopsy of the cartilage should be recommended to confirm the need for possible radical surgery.

Supraglottic tumors.

The supraglottis is bounded superiorly by the top of the epiglottis and inferiorly by the laryngeal ventricle. Approximately 20% to 30% of all laryngeal carcinomas arise in the supraglottic region and are classified as anterior supraglottic (epiglottis), marginal (aryepiglottic fold), laryngeal ventricle, or false-vocal-cord lesions (100).

Anterior supraglottic or epiglottic carcinoma may be seen on CT as a thickening of one of the margins of the epiglottis or as a bulky mass (Figs. 30–33). The preepiglottic and paralaryngeal spaces serve as pathways for tumor spread in both circumferential and cephalocaudad directions. Tumor may also spread along the aryepiglottic fold. Lesions that involve the infrahyoid portion of the epiglottis have an increased tendency to invade the preepiglottic space. Extralaryngeal spread or thyroid cartilage invasion is unusual except in very aggressive tumors; if present, a total laryngectomy is necessary. In this circumstance, cartilage invasion usually is at the level of the anterior commissure (65).

Early epiglottic lesions may be treated with radiation therapy or supraglottic laryngectomy. However, extension into the preepiglottic space usually precludes successful treatment by radiation therapy alone (15). The determi-

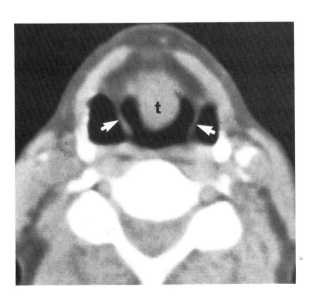

FIG. 31. Epiglottic carcinoma. Polypoid tumor (t) of the laryngeal surface of the epiglottis projects into the laryngeal vestibule; (*arrows*) aryepiglottic folds.

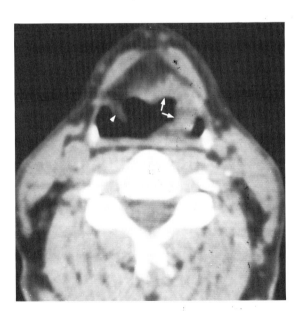

FIG. 32. Epiglottic carcinoma. Tumor thickens the left side of the epiglottis and extends into the paralaryngeal space and left aryepiglottic fold (*arrows*); (*arrowhead*) normal right aryepiglottic fold.

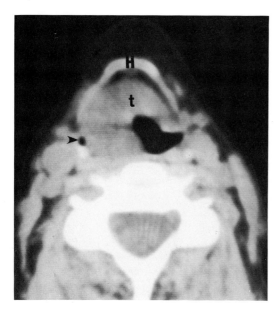

FIG. 33. Epiglottic carcinoma. A large epiglottic tumor (t) extends into the preepiglottic space and right aryepiglottic fold, almost totally obliterating the right pyriform sinus (*arrowhead*); (H) hyoid bone.

anteriorly at the false-vocal-cord level on CT should not be misinterpreted as tumor.

Normal asymmetry of the valleculae on CT may make evaluation of superior extension of epiglottic tumors into the valleculae or base of the tongue difficult. However, in most cases, physical examination is adequate. In some patients, CT may show spread into the tongue base when the physical examination is negative (65).

Marginal supraglottic tumors arise on the aryepiglottic fold and extend primarily into the paralaryngeal space. These lesions result in thickening of the aryepiglottic fold and often are better demonstrated on images performed during phonation or a modified Valsalva maneuver (Fig. 34). These tumors are more aggressive than anterior supraglottic tumors. Extension into the preepiglottic space and occasionally across the midline can occur. In these cases, it may be difficult to determine whether the mass arose in the aryepiglottic fold or epiglottis. In patients with marginal supraglottic tumors, CT may be helpful in selecting patients for partial laryngopharyngectomy, because deep spread across the midline would require a total laryngopharyngectomy (62).

Tumors of the false vocal cord and laryngeal ventricle involve the paralaryngeal space early and, from there, may spread to the lower epiglottis and preepiglottic space (Fig. 35). More inferior extension to the glottis is a relatively late finding. As with anterior and marginal supraglottic tumors, CT is helpful in demonstrating submucosal extension of tumor that may not be apparent at laryngoscopy.

nation of preepiglottic involvement usually is difficult or impossible to make clinically. High contrast between the tumor mass and adjacent fat in the preepiglottic space allows excellent delineation of tumor extension on CT (Fig. 33). CT is also helpful in evaluating the region of the anterior commissure. A tumor-free margin of 3 to 5 mm above the level of the anterior commissure usually is necessary to perform a supraglottic laryngectomy (80). This may be difficult to assess on physical examination if the tumor is bulky. The normal soft-tissue thickening seen

Pyriform sinus tumors.

Tumors of the pyriform sinus account for 10% to 20% of laryngeal carcinomas and are more aggressive than le-

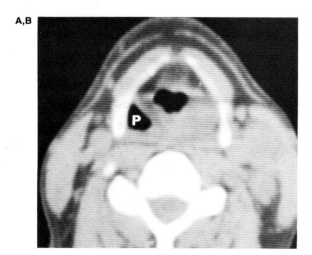
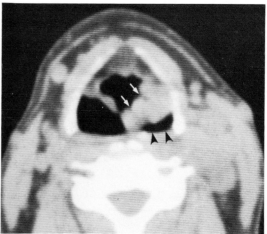

FIG. 34. Carcinoma of left aryepiglottic fold: value of modified Valsalva maneuver. **A:** Left aryepiglottic fold and pyriform sinus are not seen. Lymphadenopathy is present in the left internal jugular chain beneath the sternocleidomastoid muscle; (P) right pyriform sinus. **B:** Image obtained during modified Valsalva maneuver clearly demonstrates tumor of the left aryepiglottic fold (*arrows*) compressing the left pyriform sinus (*arrowheads*).

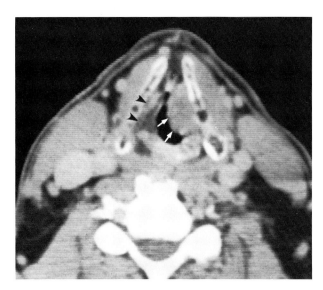

FIG. 35. Localized false-vocal-cord tumor. Carcinoma involving the left false vocal cord (*white arrows*) obliterates the normal low-attenuation paralaryngeal space and bulges into the airway; (*arrowheads*) normal right paralaryngeal space.

ryngeal space (Fig. 37). When the tumor reaches the cricothyroid space, it characteristically widens this space and can extend out into the soft tissues of the neck or into the postcricoid region (Fig. 37) (55). This finding is helpful in distinguishing pyriform sinus from supraglottic neoplasms. Tumor can occasionally extend into the lateral soft tissues of the neck through the thyrohyoid membrane. Pyriform sinus tumors are also more commonly associated with thyroid cartilage destruction. Cricoarytenoid joint involvement may be seen because of its proximity to the inferior tip of the pyriform sinus.

Although limited lesions may be treated by radiation, or partial pharyngectomy or laryngopharyngectomy, cartilage destruction or tumor extension across the midline, into the cricothyroid space, into the postcricoid region, or into the extralaryngeal soft tissues precludes a limited surgical approach or radiation therapy alone (62). CT is helpful in demonstrating these findings and assisting the clinician in planning the appropriate therapy. Because the pyriform sinuses normally may be asymmetrical on CT images, images obtained during phonation or modified Valsalva maneuver may be helpful in distending the pyriform sinus and improving visualization of the tumor (30).

sions that arise within the endolarynx (28). They tend to spread submucosally and frequently are more extensive than is apparent on endoscopy. Tumors may extend to the posterior pharyngeal wall and along the pharyngoepiglottic fold to involve the base of the tongue (Fig. 36). They may also invade the aryepiglottic fold or preepiglottic space and mimic supraglottic tumors. Pyriform sinus carcinoma frequently extends vertically within the parala-

Subglottic tumors.

Primary subglottic tumors are rare and account for less than 5% of all malignant laryngeal tumors (28,65). They usually are advanced lesions at presentation and because of their proximity to the cricoid cartilage and cricothyroid space usually are treated with total laryngectomy and postoperative radiation. More frequently, the subglottic

A,B

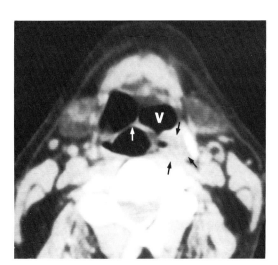 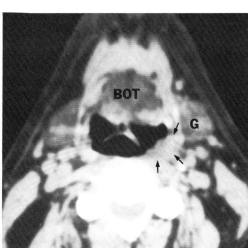

FIG. 36. Pyriform sinus carcinoma, with extension along posterolateral pharyngeal wall. **A:** Tumor (*black arrows*) fills the left pyriform sinus; (*white arrow*) epiglottis; (V) vallecula. **B:** Tumor (*black arrows*) extends cephalad along the left posterolateral pharyngeal wall; (BOT) base of tongue; (G) submandibular gland.

A,B

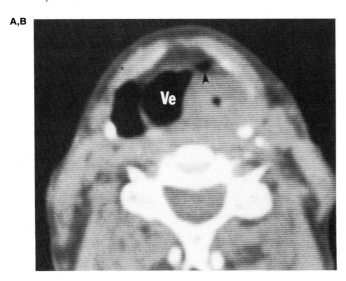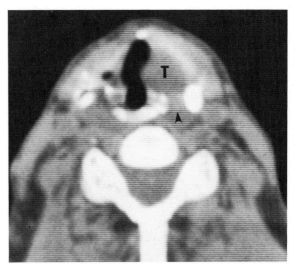

FIG. 37. Transglottic pyriform sinus carcinoma. **A:** Large tumor almost totally obliterates the left pyriform sinus and compresses the laryngeal vestibule (Ve). A dilated saccule (*arrowhead*) of the laryngeal ventricle is also seen. **B:** Tumor (T) extends caudally to involve the left true vocal cord and widen the space (*arrowhead*) between the arytenoid cartilage and left thyroid ala.

region is involved as a result of extension from glottic or supraglottic carcinoma (Fig. 28).

In contradistinction to laryngeal carcinoma, chondrosarcoma of the larynx commonly arises in the subglottic region (Fig. 38) (5). Approximately 70% arise from the cricoid cartilage, usually from the posterior lamina. The thyroid cartilage is involved in approximately 20% of patients. Both chondrosarcomas and benign chondromas contain cartilaginous matrix calcification and, in the absence of metastases, cannot be differentiated radiographically.

Transglottic tumors.

Transglottic tumors extend across the laryngeal ventricle to involve the supraglottic, glottic, and often the subglottic compartments (Fig. 37). Because transglottic extension may be deep within the paralaryngeal space, patients may be understaged clinically (119). Moreover, these tumors are associated with very high incidences of thyroid cartilage destruction, extralaryngeal spread, and lymph node metastases. Patients usually are treated with total laryngectomy, frequently combined with radiation therapy.

A,B

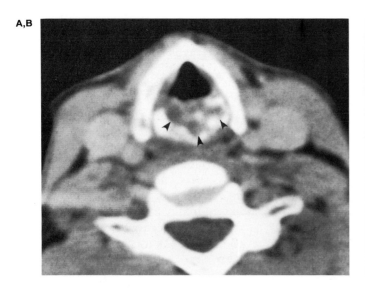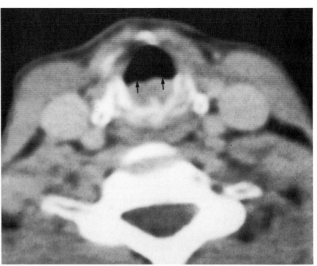

FIG. 38. Chondrosarcoma of the cricoid cartilage. Serial images show a large mass (*arrowheads*) (**A**) containing punctate and curvilinear calcifications arising from the cricoid cartilage, with subsequent narrowing of the subglottic airway (*arrows*) (**B**).

A,B

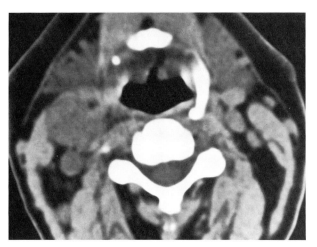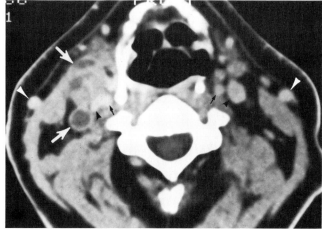

FIG. 39. Lymph node metastases: effect of intravenous contrast material. **A:** Precontrast CT image demonstrates multiple soft-tissue masses that are difficult to distinguish from adjacent vessels. **B:** Vessels are well seen on postcontrast image. Several of the lymph nodes contain areas of necrosis (*large white arrows*); (*small black arrow*) internal carotid artery; (*black arrowhead*) internal jugular vein; (*white arrowhead*) external jugular vein.

Lymph node metastases.

Identification of lymph node metastases affects both the management and survival of patients with hypopharyngeal and laryngeal carcinoma. In general, the 5-year survival is decreased by approximately 50% when local lymph node metastases are present (5). The incidence of regional metastases depends on the site and size of the primary tumor. Whereas supraglottic and pyriform sinus tumors have a high incidence (25–50%) of nodal metastases at the time of clinical presentation because of the abundant lymphatics draining this area, small tumors of the glottis have a substantially lower incidence of metastases (0–2%) (28). Midline tumors (e.g., epiglottic carcinoma) may metastasize to both sides of the neck.

Prior to the availability of cross-sectional imaging techniques, the staging of lymph node disease in the neck was done only with the clinical examination. CT has been shown to be helpful in demonstrating the presence and extent of cervical lymph node metastases (Figs. 39 and 40) (27,61,68,118). Diagnostic criteria based on CT findings have been established for staging the neck (Table 1) (67). Lymph nodes 1.5 cm or greater in diameter are considered abnormal. A nodal mass of any size with central lucency and peripheral enhancement (indicating central necrosis) is also considered abnormal. Fatty foci within normal lymph nodes may rarely mimic central necrosis. False-positive diagnoses may result from reactive lymph nodes that attain a size larger than 1.5 cm, whereas false-negative diagnoses may result from microscopic or small macroscopic deposits in normal-size lymph nodes. Although enlarged reactive lymph nodes usually cannot be distinguished from neoplastic lymph nodes, demonstra-

tion of central necrosis is highly suggestive of neoplastic involvement. Obliteration of fascial planes around enlarged lymph nodes in the nonoperated or nonirradiated neck generally is indicative of extranodal spread of tumor or extension of tumor into adjacent soft tissues. In most circumstances, CT cannot reliably distinguish between abutment, adherence, and fixation of a lymph node mass to adjacent vessels. Because the foregoing findings are not specific for metastatic disease, the CT findings must be correlated with the patient's history and other clinical findings. In some cases, benign cystic masses as well as inflammatory lymph node disease may be difficult to differentiate from cystic metastases (108).

In a patient with clinically normal findings on examination of the neck, CT may be helpful in confirming the clinical impression. Moreover, in some patients, CT may show that suspicious findings on the physical examination are secondary to normal anatomic structures, resulting in downgrading possible N_1 necks to N_0. In approximately 5% to 6% of patients with clinically normal findings on physical examination, CT will correctly upstage the neck to N_1 (67,68). Contralateral lymph node involvement may be detected that can upstage an N_1 or N_2 neck to N_3.

The information provided by CT can be used by the clinician in planning surgery and/or radiation therapy. Although the approach to the patient will vary among institutions, some generalizations can be made (61,65). The N_0 neck may be treated effectively with surgery or radiation therapy. Neck dissection usually is preferred for patients with N_1 and N_2 necks, although radiation can be used, especially when it is the method for treating the primary tumor. In patients in whom a neck dissection is planned, CT may be helpful in deciding whether a radical

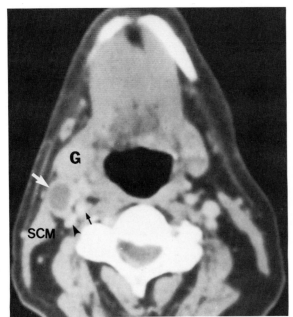

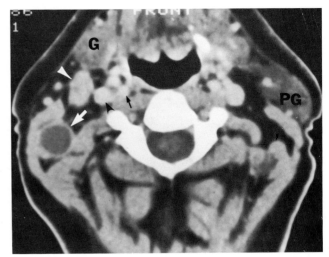

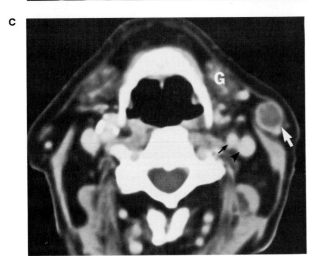

FIG. 40. Lymph node metastases. Postcontrast CT images in three different patients demonstrating necrotic lymph node metastases (*large white arrows*); (*small black arrow*) internal carotid artery; (*small black arrowhead*) internal jugular vein; (G) submandibular gland; (SCM) sternocleidomastoid muscle. **A:** High internal jugular vein lymph node. **B:** Spinal accessory (posterior triangle) lymph node; (*large white arrowhead*) enlarged internal jugular node without necrosis; (PG) parotid gland. **C:** External jugular lymph node.

TABLE 1. *Criteria for staging lymph node metastases in the neck[a,b]*

N₀	Nodes less than 15 mm in size and of homogeneous density
N₁	Nodes 15–29 mm in size in largest diameter, or node of any size with evidence of necrosis clearly demonstrated
N₂	Single homolateral node 3–6 cm in size; more than one positive homolateral node 15 mm or greater, or less than 15 mm with necrosis; conglomerate homolateral nodal mass 3–6 cm in size
N₃	Homolateral nodal mass greater than 6 cm; bilateral nodes or contralateral nodes

[a] Adapted from the American Joint Committee for Cancer Staging and End-Results Reporting. *Manual for Staging of Cancer 1983.*
[b] In bilateral adenopathy, each side of the neck should be staged separately.
From Mancuso et al. (67), reprinted with permission.

or modified-radical neck dissection (preservation of the spinal accessory nerve) should be performed by showing whether or not the course of the spinal accessory nerve is free of tumor. Postoperative radiation is given if extranodal extension of tumor is present. N_3 necks often are unresectable because of fixation to the carotid artery and therefore are treated with radiation with or without adjunctive chemotherapy, followed, in some cases, by surgery.

MRI

With the introduction of surface-coil technology, MRI is comparable to CT for demonstrating most intralaryngeal neoplasms and showing their relationships to adjacent structures (13,57). Using T1-weighted spin-echo pulse sequences, most laryngeal neoplasms are of intermediate to

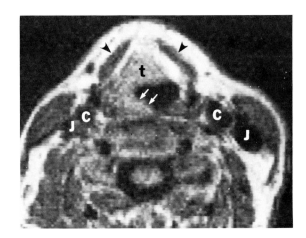

FIG. 41. Epiglottic carcinoma, with invasion of preepiglottic space. A large tumor (t) of the epiglottis is seen extending into the preepiglottic space and right aryepiglottic fold (*arrows*) on T1-weighted MR image; (C) internal carotid artery; (J) internal jugular vein; (*arrowheads*) strap muscle.

low signal intensity (Figs. 41–43). Contrast between tumor and the preepiglottic or paralaryngeal spaces is optimized using this pulse sequence. On T2-weighted images, the signal intensity of the mass relative to that for muscle increases. Extension of relatively higher-intensity tumor into the adjacent lower-intensity base of the tongue, strap muscles, or pharyngeal constrictor muscles, therefore, would be more easily seen using this pulse sequence (Fig. 42). However, contrast between the tumor and adjacent fat is decreased.

Cartilage destruction on MR images is identified either as a defect in the normal low-signal-intensity cartilage or as infiltration of the normal high-intensity medullary fat by lower-intensity tumor on T1-weighted images (Fig. 42). As with CT, normal variations in the degree of cartilage mineralization can be confused with cartilage destruction. However, incompletely ossified cartilage may not be as well identified by MRI and may blend in with adjacent strap muscles.

Delineation of the airway is degraded by respiratory and swallowing motion. This is currently more of a problem with MRI than with CT because of the longer imaging time. In some cases, the degree of airway compromise by masses may be overestimated by MRI. Moreover, images obtained during phonation or with a modified Valsalva maneuver have been shown to be helpful when evaluating the larynx with CT. Such images cannot currently be obtained with MRI.

Most lymph node metastases are intermediate in signal intensity (similar to or slightly greater than muscle) on T1-weighted images (Fig. 44). They increase in relative signal intensity on more heavily T2-weighted images and therefore may become more difficult to define as discrete masses separate from fat (Fig. 45). Central necrosis, a useful sign of metastatic involvement of normal-size nodes, may be seen as high-signal-intensity foci on T2-weighted images, although the sensitivity of MRI in displaying such an abnormality is as yet unknown (Fig. 46). However, in most circumstances, MRI relies on size as the major criterion for distinguishing normal and abnormal lymph nodes. Similar to CT, enlarged granulomatous, hyperplastic, or neoplastic lymph nodes cannot be distinguished by virtue of their signal intensity (Fig. 47) (18,39).

A,B

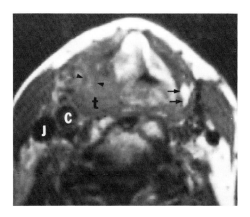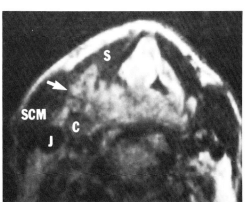

FIG. 42. Pyriform sinus carcinoma, with thyroid cartilage destruction and extralaryngeal extension. **A:** On T1-weighted MR image, a large tumor (t) is seen in the region of the right pyriform sinus. Fat within the medullary cavity in the posterior portion of the left thyroid lamina (*small arrows*) is high in signal intensity, whereas the right thyroid lamina is destroyed and its medullary cavity is replaced by low-intensity tumor (*arrowheads*). Distinction between the tumor and strap muscles is poor; (C) common carotid artery; (J) internal jugular vein. **B:** On T2-weighted image, the extralaryngeal extension of tumor (*large arrow*) and the strap muscles (S) are better delineated. Contrast between the tumor and fat within the paralaryngeal space is decreased; (C) carotid artery; (J) jugular vein; (SCM) sternocleidomastoid muscle.

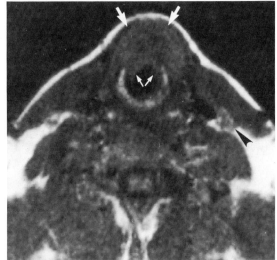

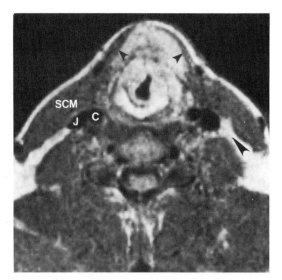

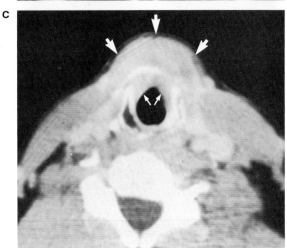

FIG. 43. Subglottic extension of tumor, with spread into the extralaryngeal soft tissues. **A:** On T1-weighted MR image, tumor is seen in the subglottic space (*small arrows*) adjacent to the cricoid cartilage. Extension through the cricothyroid membrane anteriorly into the extralaryngeal soft tissues (*large arrows*) is also demonstrated; (*large arrowhead*) lymph node metastasis. **B:** On a balanced (long TR, short TE) MR image at a slightly higher level, contrast between tumor and adjacent strap muscles (*small arrowheads*) is accentuated. The lymph node metastasis (*large arrowhead*), however, is poorly seen; (C) common carotid artery; (J) internal jugular vein; (SCM) stenocleidomastoid muscle. **C:** On CT image, subglottic (*small arrows*) and extralaryngeal (*large arrows*) extensions of tumor are also seen.

Clinical Application

MRI and CT are equivalent in patients in whom identification of the tumor depends on distinguishing between the tumor and adjacent fat. Therefore, deep extension of tumor into the preepiglottic or paralaryngeal spaces is equally well demonstrated by both techniques. However, T2-weighted images usually are superior in those cases in which CT cannot distinguish between the tumor and adjacent musculature.

In selected cases, the multiplanar capabilities of MRI may be helpful in demonstrating the extent of laryngeal tumors (e.g., sagittal images for showing extension into the base of the tongue, or coronal images for showing the relationships of the tumor to the ventricle or subglottic space) (57). However, in our experience, transaxial images alone are sufficient in most cases.

MRI and CT share certain limitations for evaluation of laryngeal neoplasms and lymph node metastases. Neither examination is histologically specific, and in most cases edema, inflammation, and tumor can have similar signal intensities or attenuation values (13,40,46,101). Currently, both examinations rely on changes in morphology to identify abnormalities. Contiguity of neoplasm with adjacent structures is not equivalent to definite in-

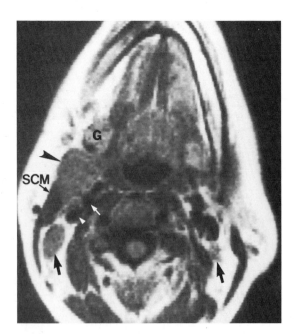

FIG. 44. Lymph node metastases. On T1-weighted MR image, enlarged spinal accessory (*large arrows*) and high internal jugular lymph nodes (*large arrowhead*) are well seen; (G) submandibular gland; (SCM) sternocleidomastoid muscle; (*small arrow*) internal carotid artery; (*small arrowhead*) internal jugular vein.

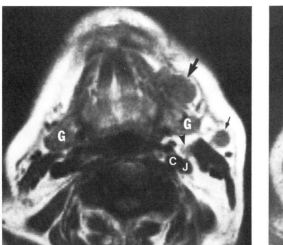
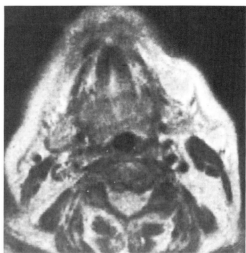

FIG. 45. Lymph node detection: effect of pulse sequence. **A:** On a T1-weighted MR image, intermediate-signal-intensity submandibular (*large arrow*), external (*small arrow*), and internal (*arrowhead*) jugular lymph nodes are seen; (C) internal carotid artery; (J) internal jugular vein; (G) submandibular gland. **B:** On a T2-weighted image, the lymph nodes are more difficult to distinguish from adjacent fat.

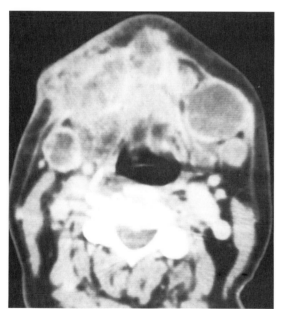
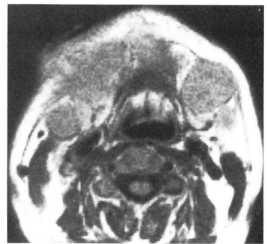

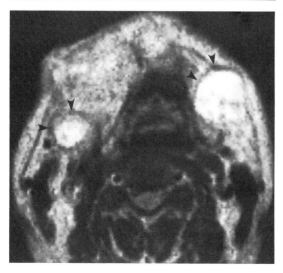

FIG. 46. Necrotic lymph node metastases. **A:** On CT image just above the level of the hyoid bone, multiple enlarged, partially necrotic lymph nodes are seen. **B:** On T1-weighted image at approximately the same level, the lymph nodes are of intermediate signal intensity. **C:** Areas of necrosis are high in signal intensity on T2-weighted image; (*arrowheads*) outer wall of necrotic lymph nodes.

A,B

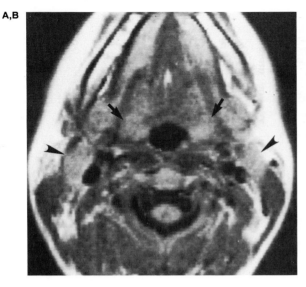 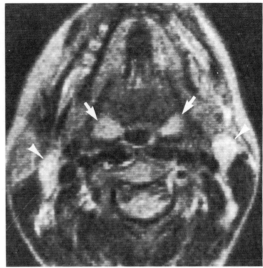

FIG. 47. Lymphoid tissue in normal volunteer. **A:** On T1-weighted MR image, tonsillar lymphoid tissue (*arrows*) and enlarged (probably hyperplastic) high internal jugular lymph nodes (*arrowheads*) are intermediate in signal intensity. **B:** On T2-weighted image, the lymphoid tissue increases in relative signal intensity and is more easily distinguished from adjacent muscle. Neoplastic tissue may exhibit a similar relative increase in signal intensity. (From ref. 39.)

vasion on either examination. Moreover, subtle invasion, such as into cartilage, usually will be missed on both examinations.

Because CT currently can be performed more expeditiously in most circumstances, it remains our primary examination for evaluating patients with laryngeal carcinoma. MRI is reserved for those patients to whom intravenous contrast material cannot be given or for whom the CT examination is equivocal in defining tumor extent. As imaging times become faster and new techniques develop, the role of MRI for these patients may change.

Cervical Nodal Metastases From Unknown Primary

Occasionally, a patient will present with a cervical nodal metastasis from an unknown primary. In many of these patients, clinical examination will demonstrate the site of the primary tumor, most frequently squamous cell carcinoma of the upper aerodigestive tract. If the history and physical examination are unrevealing, needle-aspiration biopsy of the mass is performed. The general approach to these patients, as outlined by Mancuso, depends on the histology of the tumor and location of the lymph nodes (61,65). Patients with squamous cell carcinoma (especially if the node is in the jugulodigastric region) should undergo CT of the nasopharynx, oropharynx, and hypopharynx, followed by endoscopy and biopsy of the suspicious sites. In some of these patients, CT will demonstrate an unsuspected tumor (75). If the node is low in the neck, bronchogenic or esophageal carcinoma should also be considered as possible primaries. Metastatic adenocarcinoma to

the middle to lower neck nodes may be secondary to thyroid carcinoma, as well as a primary tumor below the clavicles. If the biopsy reveals lymphoma, an appropriate staging work-up can be performed.

Other Malignant Neoplasms

Lymphoma.

Lymphoma is the most common primary malignancy in the extralaryngeal portion of the neck and is the most frequent cause of a unilateral neck mass in the 20- to 40-year age group (89). Involvement of all nodal groups can be seen, especially the internal jugular and spinal accessory groups. In contrast to squamous cell carcinoma, lymph nodes involved by lymphoma usually do not show central necrosis (Fig. 48). However, central necrosis may be seen after treatment. Lymphoma may also involve extranodal sites in the neck, including the thyroid (Fig. 49).

Thyroid malignant neoplasms.

CT is not routinely used for initial evaluation of patients suspected of having thyroid malignant neoplasms, but it may be helpful in demonstrating the extent of the tumor, specifically extracapsular spread and nodal involvement (Figs. 50–53) (65). The relationships of the tumor to the trachea and esophagus are also well shown. MRI may provide similar information (Figs. 49 and 51).

Up to 25% of patients can present with cervical lymph node metastases from an occult thyroid carcinoma (109).

A,B

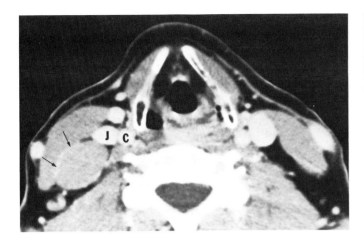

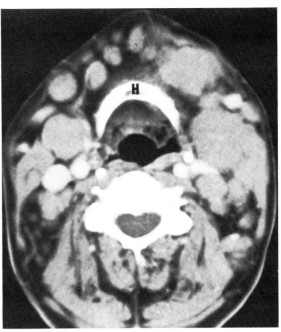

FIG. 48. Lymphoma. A: An enlarged lymph node (*arrows*) is seen posterior to the right internal jugular vein (J); (C) common carotid artery. B: In another patient, multiple enlarged lymph nodes are seen. In neither image is central necrosis seen; (H) hyoid bone.

Metastases from papillary adenocarcinoma may undergo cystic degeneration (Fig. 52). Contrast enhancement may also be seen, reflecting their vascularity. Occasionally, CT may suggest the correct diagnosis by demonstrating this appearance in conjunction with a thyroid mass (Fig. 53). If the lymph node is solitary and almost completely replaced by tumor, it may clinically and radiographically mimic a parenchymal cyst.

Posttreatment Larynx and Neck

The anatomy of the larynx and soft tissues of the neck is altered after surgery and/or radiation therapy. Although most patients with recurrent disease have symptoms that are highly suggestive of recurrence, the physical examination may be difficult. CT has been helpful in confirming the clinical impression of recurrent disease and showing the extent of tumor (19,20,44,76). In particular, it may be beneficial in patients with pain who show negative or equivocal findings on clinical examination. The information provided by CT can help the clinician select the appropriate biopsy site. CT-directed biopsy of suspicious areas can also be performed (31). MRI has also proved helpful in evaluating the posttreatment neck, especially in those patients in whom normal anatomical landmarks are obliterated on CT or to whom intravenous contrast material cannot be administered (40).

A,B

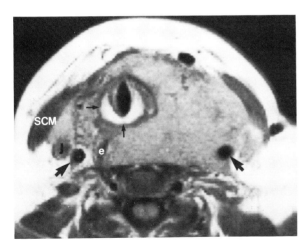

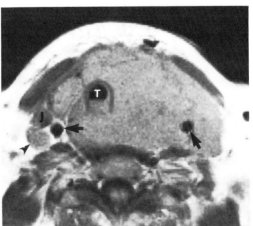

FIG. 49. Thyroid lymphoma. A,B: Balanced MR images demonstrate an extensive tumor infiltrating the left and right neck and displacing the common carotid arteries posterolaterally (*large arrows*). The left internal jugular vein is not visualized and is most likely occluded. The cricoid cartilage (*small arrows*) is well visualized because of the high signal from medullary fat; (J) right jugular vein; (e) esophagus; (SCM) stenocleidomastoid muscle; (T) trachea; (*arrowhead*) enlarged lymph node.

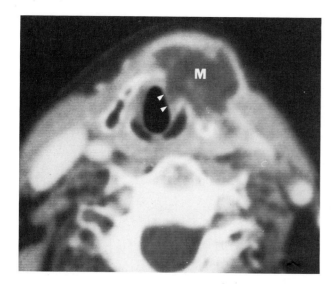

FIG. 50. Thyroid carcinoma. Postcontrast CT image shows a large, irregular, low-density mass (M) destroying the left thyroid lamina and invading the left true vocal cord (*arrowheads*). More caudal images showed the mass arising from the left lobe of the thyroid.

A,B

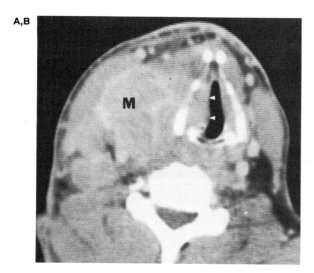
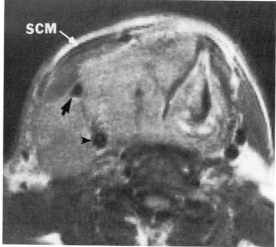

FIG. 51. Thyroid carcinoma. **A:** Postcontrast CT image demonstrates a large mass (M) infiltrating the right side of the neck and involving the right recurrent laryngeal nerve, resulting in right-true-vocal-cord paralysis (*white arrowheads*). **B:** Similar findings are seen on T1-weighted MR image; (*black arrowhead*) common carotid artery; (*arrow*) internal jugular vein; (SCM) sternocleidomastoid muscle.

FIG. 52. Cystic metastasis from thyroid carcinoma. A multiloculated, inhomogeneous low-density mass (*arrows*) is seen posterior to the left internal jugular vein (J) and sternocleidomastoid muscle (SCM); (C) common carotid artery; (*arrowheads*) clinically unsuspected thyroid carcinoma. (Courtesy of Dr. Jagan Ailinani, Carbondale, Illinois.)

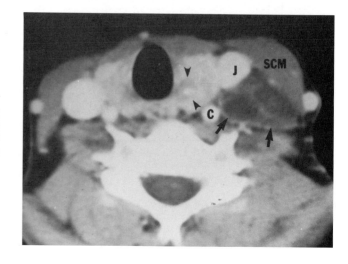

A,B

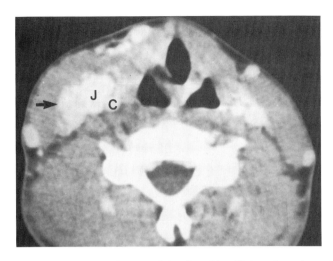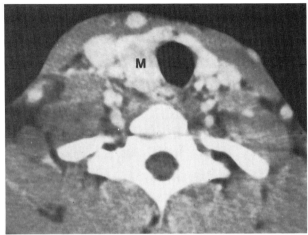

FIG. 53. Papillary carcinoma of the thyroid, with lymph node metastases. **A:** An enlarged, contrast-enhanced lymph node (*arrow*) is seen in the right side of the neck; (C) common carotid artery; (J) internal jugular vein. **B:** CT image through the level of thyroid gland demonstrates a low-density mass (M) enlarging the right lobe of the thyroid gland.

Post surgery.

In the immediate postoperative period, the fat planes usually are obliterated secondary to hemorrhage and edema, but later are replaced by fibrosis. The extent of these changes depends on the bulk of the initial tumor, the type of surgical procedure, the amount of radiation given, and whether or not any postoperative complications, such as infection, develop (65). Because the amount of alteration of soft-tissue planes varies, a base-line CT image 6 to 8 weeks following therapy may be helpful, especially in those patients with a greater likelihood of tumor recurrence.

Although most patients with localized true-vocal-cord carcinomas are treated with radiation therapy, a *vertical hemilaryngectomy* is also an effective treatment. The true

vocal cord, the laryngeal ventricle, the false vocal cord, and ipsilateral thyroid lamina are removed. If the anterior commissure is involved, up to one-third of the contralateral true vocal cord can be removed. The resection site is closed using the perichondrium of the resected thyroid cartilage, which acts as a "pseudocord" to allow phonation and maintain glottic competence (20).

The normal CT appearance of the larynx following vertical hemilaryngectomy has been described (Fig. 54) (20). In the high supraglottic region, the ipsilateral aryepiglottic fold is absent, and on the same side there is decreased fat in the preepiglottic space. More inferiorly, the surgically formed pseudocord is seen contiguous with the regenerated thyroid lamina. The long axis of the glottis is tilted toward the operated side. The pseudocord is straight or

A,B

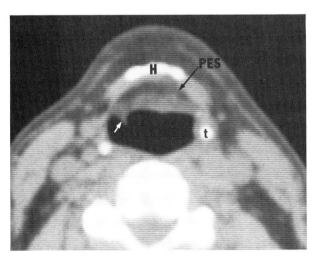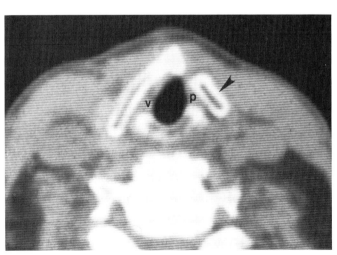

FIG. 54. Normal anatomy after left vertical hemilaryngectomy. **A:** Level of superior cornua of thyroid cartilage (t); (PES) preepiglottic space, with diminution in fat content; (H) hyoid bone; (*arrow*) residual aryepiglottic fold on nonoperated side. **B:** Level of glottis. Note tilt of airway toward the operated side; (*arrowhead*) residual left thyroid lamina; (p) surgically created pseudocord; (v) undersurface of residual right true vocal cord.

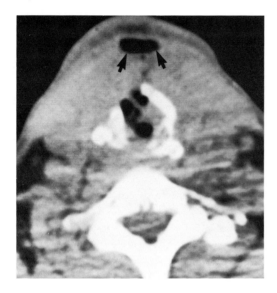

FIG. 55. Abscess post right vertical hemilaryngectomy. Extensive soft-tissue swelling, with an air–fluid level (*arrows*), is seen anterior to the larynx. Several smaller air bubbles extend to the larynx.

slightly concave, whereas the residual true vocal cord is partly convex. The thickness of the anterior commissure is generally greater than in the nonoperated patient, usually measuring 3 to 5 mm. The subglottic airway remains symmetric.

Signs of recurrent intralaryngeal tumor following vertical hemilaryngectomy include convexity of the pseudocord at the glottic level, increased width of the residual true vocal cord, subglottic tumor, or extralaryngeal masses (20). Granulation tissue, a postoperative inclusion cyst, or irregular calcification of the regenerating thyroid cartilage can mimic tumor recurrence. The extent of inflammatory processes following surgery also can be demonstrated by CT (Fig. 55).

Supraglottic laryngectomy is a form of conservation surgery used for selected lesions of the epiglottis, single arytenoid, aryepiglottic fold, and false vocal cord. The structures removed include the epiglottis, aryepiglottic folds, false vocal cords, preepiglottic space, the superior portion of the thyroid cartilage, and a portion or all of the hyoid bone. The procedure may be extended to re-

A,B

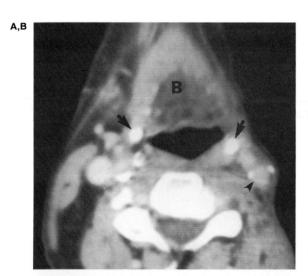

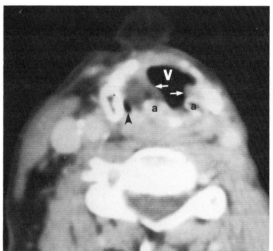

C

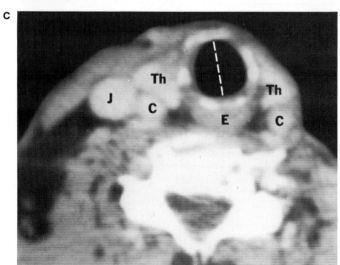

FIG. 56. Normal anatomy after supraglottic subtotal laryngectomy and left radical neck dissection. **A:** Base-of-tongue level; (*arrows*) residual hyoid bone; (B) base of tongue; (*arrowhead*) left internal carotid artery. **B:** Mid-neck level. A portion of the thyroid cartilage has been removed. The pseudo–false cords (*arrows*) are seen extending anterolaterally from the arytenoid cartilages (a); (V) laryngeal vestibule; (*small arrowhead*) pyriform sinus. **C:** Low-neck level. The axis of the airway (*dotted line*) is tilted slightly away from the side of the radical neck dissection; (C) common carotid artery; (J) right internal jugular vein; (Th) thyroid gland; (E) esophagus.

move the superior portion of the arytenoid cartilage or a portion of the medial wall of the pyriform sinus, if these structures are involved. The free margin of the pyriform sinus is sutured to the mucosal margin of the laryngeal ventricle, creating a fold of tissue that resembles the false vocal cords ("pseudo–false cords") (76).

On images through the supraglottic region, the epiglottis, aryepiglottic folds, and preepiglottic space are absent (Fig. 56) (76). The mucosal folds (pseudo–false cords) that separate the laryngeal vestibule from the pyriform sinus are seen extending anterolaterally and superiorly from the arytenoid cartilages to the anterior pharyngeal wall. They are symmetric, may have a convex medial border, and are low in density centrally. Images at the level of the true vocal cords appear normal except for slight tilting of the laryngeal axis away from the side of the neck dissection. As in other postoperative patients, findings of tumor recurrence include a soft-tissue mass, obliteration of fat planes, cartilage destruction, and lymphadenopathy.

Laryngeal tumors that are not amenable to conservation surgery or radiation therapy or have recurrence after these treatments usually are managed with *total laryngectomy.* This surgical procedure involves removal of the entire larynx and preepiglottic space, with placement of a permanent tracheostomy. The hyoid bone, strap muscles, and a portion of the thyroid gland are also removed. A conical passageway, the neopharynx, is created using mucosal, muscular, and connective-tissue layers and extends from the base of the tongue to the proximal esophagus (19).

At the level of the base of the tongue, the neopharynx is seen as a round or oval soft-tissue mass anterior to the vertebral body (Fig. 57) (19). It may contain a small amount of air either within its lumen or within an anastomotic diverticulum. More caudally, the neopharynx has a more rounded configuration. The fat planes surrounding the neopharynx and neurovascular bundle may be slightly indistinct secondary to postsurgical or postradiation fibrosis (19).

Tumor recurrence may occur in lymph nodes adjacent

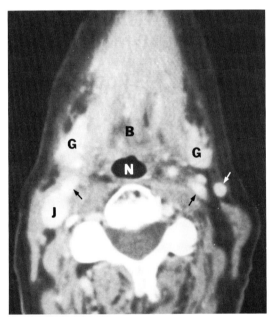

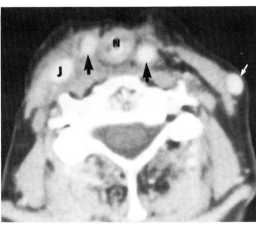

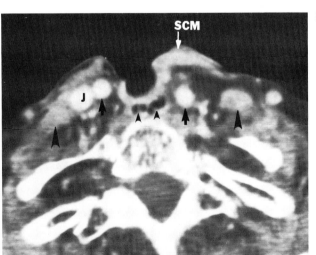

FIG. 57. Normal anatomy after total laryngectomy and modified left neck dissection. **A:** Base-of-tongue level. **B:** Midneck level. **C:** Tracheostomy level. Appearance of multiple lumina in the esophagus (*small arrowheads*) is secondary to apposition of anterior and posterior walls by mucus threads; (B) base of tongue; (G) submandibular gland; (J) right internal jugular vein; (N) neopharynx; (SCM) sternocleidomastoid muscle; (*small black arrow*) internal carotid artery; (*large black arrow*) common carotid artery; (*small arrow*) external jugular vein; (*large arrowhead*) scalenus anterior muscle.

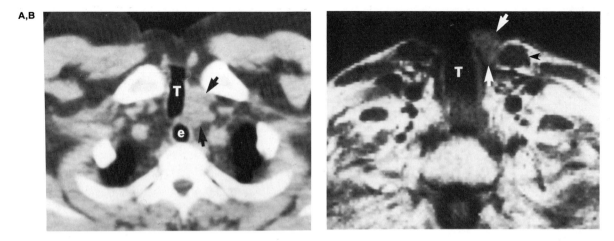

FIG. 58. Recurrence post total laryngectomy. **A:** CT image delineates extent of tumor recurrence (*arrows*) adjacent to tracheostomy (T) and esophagus (e). **B:** T1-weighted MR image in another patient demonstrates depth of recurrent tumor (*arrows*) adjacent to tracheostomy (T) and sternal head of sternocleidomastoid muscle (*arrowhead*).

to the neopharynx or neurovascular bundle or within the mediastinum (Fig. 58) (19). Thickening of the tracheal wall or peristomal soft tissues is suspicious for tumor recurrence. Localized inflammatory processes, such as abscess, may mimic tumor recurrence.

The standard *radical neck dissection* includes surgical lymphadenectomy, with resection of the sternocleidomastoid muscle, internal jugular vein, spinal accessory nerve, and submandibular salivary gland. On CT or MR images there will be flattening of the ipsilateral neck surface and absence of these normal structures (Figs. 59 and 60). Because most of the venous drainage of the neck is

now to the other side of the neck, the contralateral internal jugular vein is frequently enlarged (106).

Modifications of the standard neck dissection have been developed that differ depending on which anatomic structures are preserved. For example, with a functional (Bocca) neck dissection, which is used when no or only small clinically positive nodes are present, a lymphadenectomy is performed without removing other normal structures. The CT images appear relatively normal except for slight obscuration of tissue planes around the internal jugular vein (106).

Myocutaneous flaps have been used for repair of large

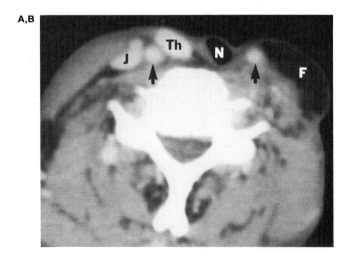
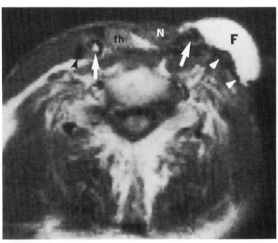

FIG. 59. Pectoralis flap post total laryngectomy and left neck dissection. **A:** Normal anatomic structures are well seen on this contrast-enhanced CT image; (*arrows*) common carotid artery; (J) right internal jugular vein; (Th) right lobe of thyroid gland; (F) pectoralis flap; (N) neopharynx. **B:** Similar findings are seen on balanced MR image at the same level. The fatty portion of the flap (F) is very high in signal intensity, whereas the muscular and fibrous portions (*white arrowheads*) are much lower in signal intensity; (*arrows*) common carotid artery; (*black arrowhead*) right internal jugular vein; (N) neopharynx; (th) right lobe of thyroid gland.

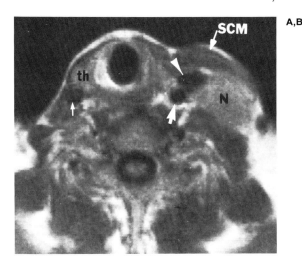

FIG. 60. Recurrent tumor post right radical neck dissection. **A:** Postcontrast CT image demonstrates lymph node metastasis (N) posterior to the left internal carotid artery (*large arrow*) and internal jugular vein (*large arrowhead*); (*small arrow*) right internal carotid artery; (*small arrowhead*) left external jugular vein; (G) submandibular gland; (SCM) sternocleidomastoid muscle. **B:** Similar findings are seen on a T1-weighted MR image from a different patient; (N) lymph node metastasis; (SCM) sternocleidomastoid muscle; (th) thyroid gland; (*large arrow*) left common carotid artery; (*arrowhead*) left internal jugular vein; (*small arrow*) right common carotid artery.

surgical defects. Because the nerve supply is interrupted, the muscle atrophies and is seen as a large fatty mass with scattered strands of atrophic muscle (Fig. 59) (106). Nodular masses or infiltrations of fat are unusual and may be secondary to inflammation or recurrent tumor.

Post radiation therapy.

Surprisingly, after radiation therapy the tumor site may often return to a near-normal appearance (65). There may be slight thickening of the platysma muscle, and linear strands may be seen within the subcutaneous fat. Above 6,800 to 7,000 rads, changes may be more extensive and may include thickening of the pharyngeal wall, epiglottis, and aryepiglottic folds and increased density in the paralaryngeal and preepiglottic space. Most of these changes resolve in 8 to 12 weeks after completion of radiation. However, intralaryngeal edema may persist secondary to lymphedema. These changes tend to be symmetric; when asymmetric, they may represent residual or recurrent tumor. However, edema may also be asymmetric, especially when the primary tumor is lateralized (Fig. 61). In patients with extensive fibrosis as a result of radiation therapy, the true vocal cords may remain in a paramedian position, with adduction of the arytenoid cartilages.

If the primary tumor or nodal mass was large, residual

soft-tissue thickening may be present even after successful treatment. Similarly, focal areas of increased density may remain within the deep-tissue planes. CT cannot reliably

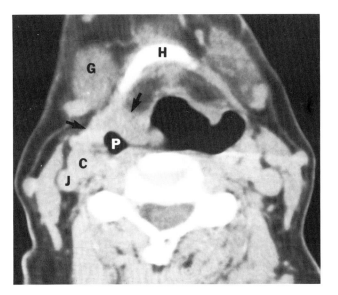

FIG. 61. Postradiation edema mimicking tumor. Marked thickening of the soft tissues (*arrows*) is seen in the right side of the supraglottis, with partial obliteration of the pyriform sinus (P). Slightly increased attenuation of the preepiglottic space reflects prior irradiation; (H) hyoid bone; (G) submandibular gland; (C) internal carotid artery; (J) internal jugular vein.

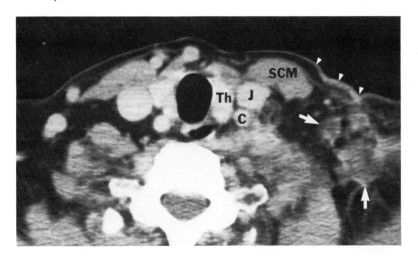

FIG. 62. Recurrent tumor post radiation therapy for breast carcinoma. The skin overlying the left supraclavicular fossa is thickened (*arrowheads*), and multiple linear septae are noted within the subcutaneous fat, probably as a result of previous irradiation. In addition, multiple metastatic transverse cervical (supraclavicular) nodes (*arrows*) are seen; (C) common carotid artery; (J) internal jugular vein; (SCM) sternocleidomastoid muscle; (Th) thyroid gland.

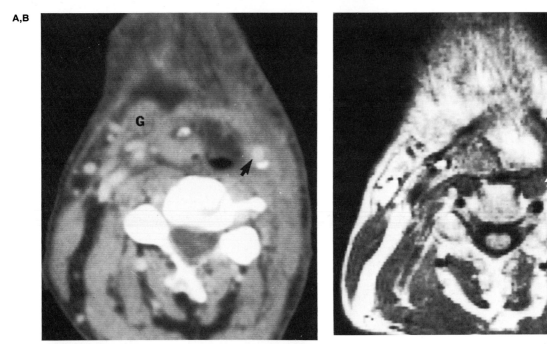

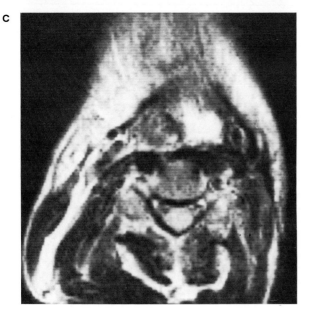

FIG. 63. Normal neck after laryngopharyngectomy, left neck dissection, pectoralis flap, and radiation therapy: value of MRI. **A:** On contrast-enhanced CT image, muscular landmarks are difficult to define, and lymphadenopathy is difficult to exclude; (*arrow*) left internal carotid artery; (G) submandibular gland. **B:** On T1-weighted MR image, the left internal carotid artery (*arrow*) is seen anterior to adjacent musculature. Areas of very low signal (*arrowheads*) presumably represent fibrous tissue. **C:** On T2-weighted image, the areas of presumed fibrosis remain very low in signal intensity. (From ref. 40.)

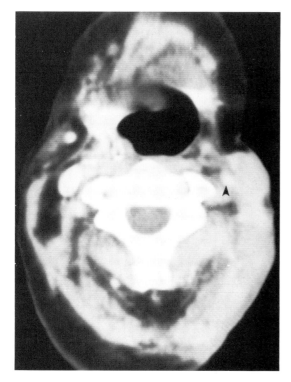

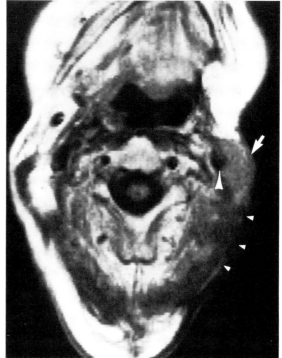

A,B

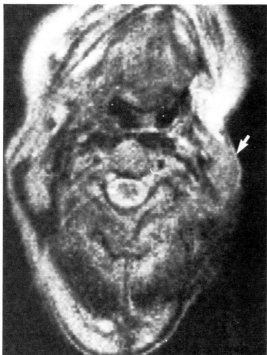

C

FIG. 64. Recurrent epidermoid carcinoma of left side of neck after radiation therapy and left neck dissection: value of MRI. **A:** On CT image after intravenous administration of contrast material, there is thickening of the soft tissues along the left side of the neck, with obscuration of the normal landmarks; (*black arrowhead*) left internal carotid artery. **B:** On T1-weighted MR image at approximately the same level, an intermediate-signal-intensity mass (*arrow*) is seen that corresponded to a new mass felt on physical examination. The posterior, lower-signal-intensity area (*small white arrowheads*) corresponded to chronically thickened, fibrotic soft tissues; (*large white arrowhead*) left internal carotid artery. **C:** On T2-weighted image, the recurrent tumor (*arrow*) remains higher in signal intensity than the posterior fibrotic area. The mass regressed after radiation therapy. (From ref. 40.)

distinguish between posttreatment fibrosis and residual tumor, focal inflammation, or edema (Fig. 61) (46,65). A progressive increase in size of the mass, or development of a new mass, especially when associated with new symptoms, is highly suggestive of recurrent or persistent tumor (Fig. 62).

Clinically evident chondronecrosis is rare after radiation therapy (65). CT findings include inward bowing of the thyroid cartilage, which may progress to fragmentation,

with airway narrowing. The cricoid and thyroid cartilages may collapse on one another, and the arytenoid cartilages may be displaced. The intralaryngeal soft tissues are diffusely thickened, making it difficult to exclude recurrent tumor. Patients frequently require laryngectomy.

On MR images, the signal intensity of tumor decreases after radiation therapy and approaches that of skeletal muscle (65). This change in signal intensity is most noticeable on T2-weighted images. Posttreatment fibrosis or

A,B

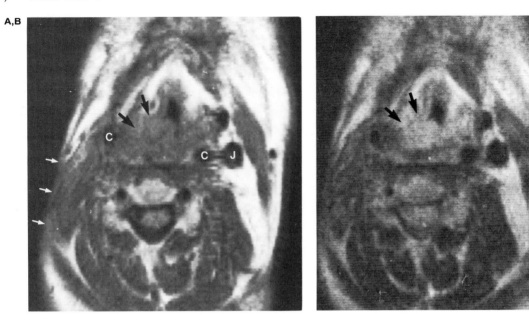

FIG. 65. Posttreatment edema mimicking tumor recurrence after neck dissection, with pectoralis flap and radiation therapy. **A:** On T1-weighted MR image through the supraglottic area, thickened soft tissue (*black arrows*) over the right arytenoid is intermediate in signal intensity; (*white arrows*) pectoralis flap; (C) common carotid artery; (J) left internal jugular vein. **B:** On T2-weighted image, this area (*arrows*) is increased in relative signal intensity; it corresponded to chronically edematous tissues. (From ref. 40.)

scarring also has been described as being low in signal intensity on T2-weighted images (Figs. 63 and 64) (37,40). In comparison, the signal intensity of tumor is much higher on T2-weighted images. Although this finding may be helpful in some patients for distinguishing between recurrent or persistent tumor and posttreatment fibrosis, the demonstration of relatively high signal intensity is not specific for tumor recurrence. Postradiation edema, hy-

perplastic lymphadenopathy, infection, and hemorrhage can yield signal intensities similar to that for recurrent tumor (Fig. 65) (13,40,125). Moreover, small nests of residual tumor may be present in a predominantly fibrotic mass (65). Because responses to radiation will vary depending on the organ system treated, tumor size, and individual patient response and histology, the MRI appearance post treatment will also vary.

A,B

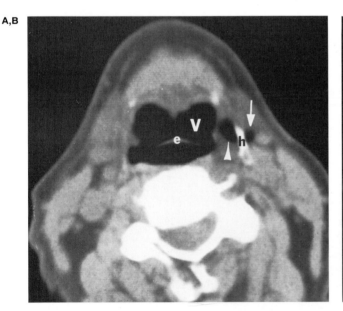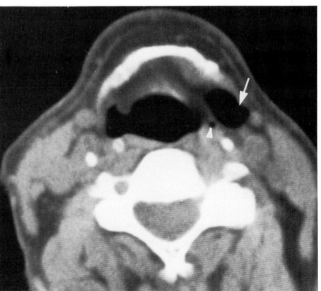

FIG. 66. Air-filled mixed laryngocele. **A:** Small air-filled external component of laryngocele (*arrow*) is seen just lateral to the posterior cornua of the hyoid bone (h). Larger internal component (*large arrowhead*) is adjacent to medial aspect of hyoid; (V) vallecula; (e) epiglottis. **B:** Communication between the two components of the laryngocele (*arrow*) is seen on a more caudal image. Left pyriform sinus (*small arrowhead*) is compressed by internal component of the laryngocele. (From ref. 38.)

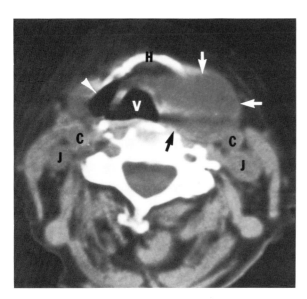

FIG. 67. Bilateral laryngoceles. A fluid-filled, mixed laryngocele (*arrows*) fills the left paralaryngeal space and extends through the thyrohyoid membrane into the left neck. An air-filled, mixed laryngocele (*arrowhead*) is seen on the right; (V) laryngeal vestibule; (H) hyoid bone; (C) internal carotid artery; (J) internal jugular vein.

Benign Disorders

Larynx

A variety of benign lesions can involve the larynx, most of which do not require CT (or MRI) for clinical management. In some patients, CT may be helpful in showing the extent of the process.

Benign mucosal and saccular disorders.

Vocal cord polyps are the most common benign lesions in the larynx and usually are secondary to excessive or incorrect use of the voice. CT usually is not used to evaluate these patients. The CT findings may appear normal or show only a slight bulge of the true vocal cord, indistinguishable from a small cancer (65).

A *laryngocele* is an abnormal dilatation of the saccule of the laryngeal ventricle. Laryngoceles may be confined to the larynx and extend superiorly within the paralaryngeal space or extend through the thyrohyoid membrane into the neck. Although the clinical diagnosis may be straightforward, occasionally a laryngocele may mimic a submucosal neoplasm on laryngoscopy. CT is accurate in establishing the diagnosis of laryngocele and demonstrating its total extent (Figs. 66–69) (38). Uncomplicated laryngoceles usually appear on CT as air-filled structures in the paralaryngeal space (internal) or lateral neck (external) or in both locations (mixed). If the neck of the laryngocele is obstructed by tumor or chronic inflammation, a well-circumscribed fluid-filled mass may result that is either of near-water density or of soft-tissue density, depending on its composition. When the mass is of soft-tissue density because it contains mucoid or purulent material, its location and smooth surface, in the absence of a mucosal abnormality on laryngoscopy, should suggest a laryngocele (Fig. 68). However, a small neoplasm near the origin of the saccule may not be apparent on CT.

A cyst arising from the second branchial cleft may have a CT appearance similar to that for a fluid-filled external laryngocele. However, branchial cleft cysts usually are seen anterior to the sternocleidomastoid muscle and are separate from the thyrohyoid membrane. The diagnosis of the laryngocele is also more obvious if an internal component is seen. A postoperative inclusion cyst can look identical with a fluid-filled laryngocele (38). Pharyngoceles and Zenker's diverticula should not be confused with air-filled external laryngoceles, because they can be traced directly to the pyriform sinus or postcricoid region, respectively.

Benign laryngeal neoplasms.

Benign tumors of the larynx are rare and are most commonly secondary to squamous papillomas and hemangiomas. Lipomas, rhabdomyomas, pleomorphic adenomas, fibromas, chondromas, and neuromas of the larynx may also be seen (5). Most of these lesions have a nonspecific but typically smooth appearance on CT. Lipomas can be diagnosed by their negative CT numbers. Chondromas usually exhibit a pattern of punctate and ring-shaped calcifications (93).

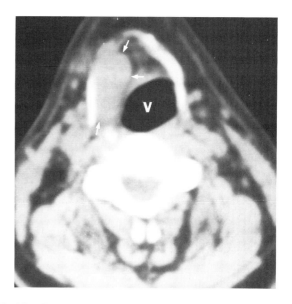

FIG. 68. Infected internal laryngocele. Soft-tissue-density mass (*arrows*) with smooth borders fills the right paralaryngeal space. Overlying mucosa was normal at laryngoscopy; (V) laryngeal vestibule.

A,B

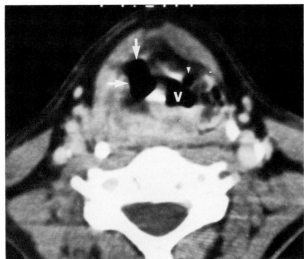
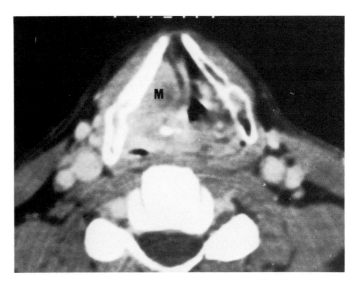

FIG. 69. Laryngeal carcinoma, with secondary laryngocele. A: Air-filled internal laryngocele (*arrow*) fills the right paralaryngeal space and displaces the laryngeal vestibule (V) to the left; (*arrowhead*) mildly dilated saccule of left laryngeal ventricle. B: A large tumor mass (M) involves the right false vocal cord, with deep extension into the right paralaryngeal space between the thyroid lamina and the arytenoid cartilage. More caudal images demonstrated subglottic extension of tumor.

Inflammation.

The CT findings of laryngeal involvement by rheumatoid arthritis have been described (10). Subluxation and/or ankylosis of the cricoarytenoid joint can result from chronic involvement by rheumatoid arthritis. Some authors believe that CT provides important complementary information to laryngoscopy regarding the structural

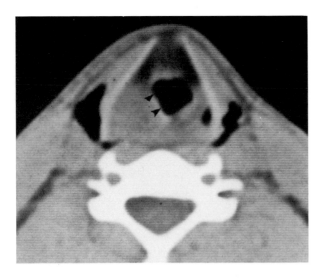

FIG. 70. Posttraumatic soft-tissue swelling, with intact cartilage. The right aryepiglottic fold and pyriform sinus are obliterated by soft-tissue thickening. The airway (*arrowheads*) is slightly compressed. Both thyroid lamina are intact. Subcutaneous air external to the lamina is secondary to tracheostomy.

integrity of the larynx in these patients. CT findings include erosions or sclerosis of the cricoarytenoid joint and glottic narrowing. Anteromedial displacement of the arytenoid cartilage and decreased vocal cord mobility or absence thereof may also be seen.

Both infectious (e.g., tuberculosis) and noninfectious granulomatous disease (e.g., sarcoid, Wegener's granulomatosis) can involve the larynx. Focal or diffuse thickening of the laryngeal soft tissues, sometimes with marked airway narrowing, may be seen on CT (117). These findings alone are nonspecific and may mimic those for a malignant neoplasm.

Trauma.

Conventional frontal and lateral radiographs frequently are the first radiologic studies performed to evaluate the injured larynx. Although they may provide useful information regarding airway narrowing, prevertebral soft-tissue swelling, and subcutaneous air, laryngeal fractures often are difficult or impossible to demonstrate. The cross-sectional display of CT allows rapid and accurate evaluation of cartilaginous injuries, adjacent soft-tissue changes, and airway compromise (Figs. 70–74) (28,32,63,65). CT is especially useful in patients with extensive supraglottic or anterior cervical soft-tissue swelling that prevents adequate laryngoscopic and physical examination.

Blunt trauma to the larynx usually is secondary to a force applied in an anteroposterior direction, pushing the larynx against the cervical spine. This may injure the soft tissues as well as the laryngeal skeleton. Injury to the in-

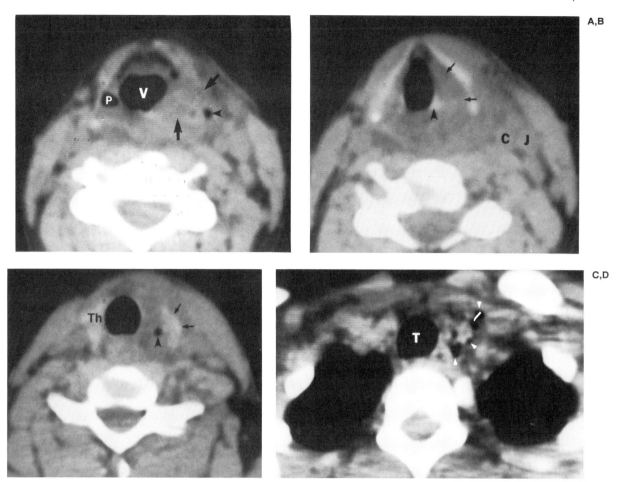

A,B

C,D

FIG. 71. Traumatic perforation of pyriform sinus, with abscess formation secondary to tracheal intubation. **A:** Image at the level of the pyriform sinus demonstrates a soft-tissue mass (*arrows*) obliterating the left pyriform sinus and deforming the left posterolateral aspect of the laryngeal vestibule (V); (P) right pyriform sinus; (*arrowhead*) gas bubble in adjacent soft tissues. **B:** At the false-vocal-cord level there is widening of the left paralaryngeal space (*arrows*) and increased distance between the foot process of the arytenoid cartilage (*arrowhead*) and the left thyroid lamina. Mildly enlarged lymph nodes are also present behind the left internal jugular vein (J); (C) common carotid artery. **C:** The left lobe of the thyroid gland (*arrows*) is displaced laterally by a soft-tissue mass containing a small gas bubble (*arrowhead*); (Th) right lobe of thyroid. **D:** Image through the lung apices demonstrates multiple gas bubbles (*arrowheads*) in the superior mediastinum; (T) trachea. (From ref. 121.)

tralaryngeal soft tissues may also occur during intubation (Fig. 71). Blood or edema can spread through the deep soft-tissue spaces of the larynx in a pattern similar to that of tumor and inflammation (65,121). Hematoma and edema can extend superiorly and inferiorly in the paralaryngeal space, as well as anteriorly into the preepiglottic space.

When the thyroid cartilage is compressed against the cervical spine, the normal posterior separation of the lamina may be increased (65). Vertical or oblique fractures of the thyroid lamina may result (Fig. 72). The superior thyroid notch or normal areas of incomplete ossification should not be confused with a fracture. Soft-tissue swelling usually is present in association with a fracture. Dislocation of the arytenoid cartilage at the cricoarytenoid joint

may occur in conjunction with thyroid cartilage injury or may be seen as an isolated injury, possibly related to intubation. The dislocated arytenoid cartilage usually lies more anterior and medial than normal, with foreshortening of the ipsilateral cord. However, subtle changes may be difficult to distinguish from vocal cord paralysis alone.

Avulsion of the epiglottis may be difficult to detect because the epiglottis usually is not calcified (65). However, extensive swelling in the region of the anterior commissure and preepiglottic space, associated with an altered orientation of the epiglottis, should suggest the diagnosis.

True-vocal-cord dysfunction may be secondary to direct injury to the cords, extensive hematoma or edema in the deep soft tissues of the larynx or at the commissures, or damage to the recurrent laryngeal nerve (65). CT is helpful

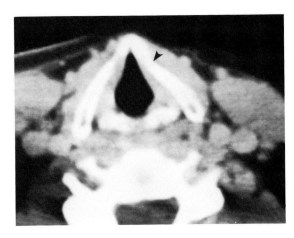

FIG. 72. Fracture of thyroid cartilage. A minimally depressed fracture of the left thyroid lamina (*arrowhead*) is seen. The adjacent strap muscles are slightly thickened secondary to hemorrhage or edema. The true vocal cords and cricoid cartilage are normal.

in distinguishing these causes from vocal cord dysfunction resulting from dislocation of the cricoarytenoid or cricothyroid joint or other cartilaginous injuries.

Fractures of the cricoid cartilage usually occur in two or more places, because the cricoid is a complete ring (65). Separation of the posterior portion of the cricoid can actually widen the airway. Vocal cord dysfunction may occur because the cricoid supports the arytenoid cartilage.

Distortion of the laryngeal skeleton and/or airway narrowing may result from prior laryngeal trauma (65). Minimally displaced fractures usually heal without deformity. Fibrotic webs may form and thicken the soft tissues adjacent to the airway. Inward bowing of the thyroid cartilage and, in some cases, more severe distortion, with nonunion or malunion of cartilaginous fragments, may be seen. The true vocal cords may remain in a paramedian position secondary to arytenoid dislocation, fibrotic webs, or injury to the recurrent laryngeal nerve. Occasionally, CT will reveal an old occult fracture that distorts the normal laryngeal airway and mimics a laryngeal mass on laryngoscopy.

Most cases of chronic laryngeal and subglottic stenosis are related to prior intubation. Fluoroscopic and conventional tomography remains the initial radiologic procedure for evaluation of most of these patients. CT can demonstrate the site and degree of airway narrowing, but short segmental stenoses may be missed because of partial-volume averaging with air in the adjacent trachea or larynx. Narrow collimation (1.0–2.0-mm slice thickness) can be used to minimize this problem. Shoulder artifacts may also limit accurate evaluation of the lower extent of stenosis and may interfere with image reformatting (65). Sagittal and coronal MR images may prove useful in delineating the vertical extent of stenoses and, in addition, are not limited by shoulder artifacts. However, neither

conventional CT nor MRI can demonstrate segments of tracheomalacia. Although the use of cine CT for dynamic evaluation of the extrathoracic airway has been described, this technique is limited to a few institutions (24).

Soft Tissues of the Neck

Congenital and developmental abnormalities.

Second-branchial-cleft cyst is one of the most common congenital cystic neck masses. Although the clinical diagnosis is often obvious, other neck masses (e.g., deep neck abscess, jugular vein thrombosis, neoplasm) can mimic branchial cleft cysts. CT may be helpful in confirming the clinical impression and showing the extent of the cyst, but more important, it may suggest a different diagnosis that will alter the patient's management (43,104). Fistulograms are recommended for a patient with a cutaneous sinus tract arising from the second branchial apparatus.

Branchial cleft cysts can occur anywhere from the tonsillar fossa to the supraclavicular area, but most are located in the upper neck anterior to the sternocleidomastoid muscle (SCM). On CT, they usually appear as a well-defined, near-water-density mass displacing the SCM posterolaterally or posteriorly, the carotid artery and jugular vein posteromedially or medially, and the submandibular gland anteriorly (Fig. 75) (43). When they are large, they can extend more posteriorly under the SCM. Extension of the cyst between the internal and external carotid arteries may be a helpful sign in distinguishing between branchial cleft cysts and other cystic neck masses, especially when the location is atypical (96).

The density of the mass and the thickness and enhancement of its wall may increase depending on the de-

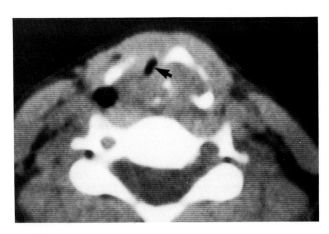

FIG. 73. Comminuted fracture of thyroid cartilage. Multiple fractures of the thyroid cartilage are seen, with extensive hemorrhage and edema severely compressing the airway (*arrow*).

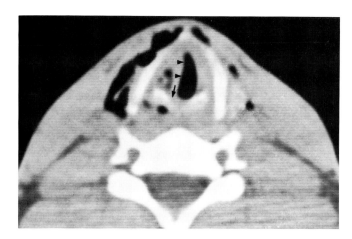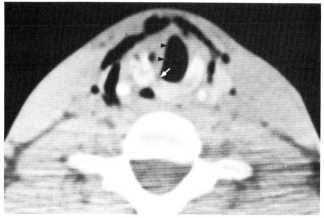

FIG. 74. Fracture of cricoid cartilage. **A,B:** A fracture (*arrow*) through the right side of the cricoid cartilage is seen. Edema/hemorrhage thicken the right true vocal cord and narrow the airway (*arrowheads*). Extensive soft-tissue air is also present.

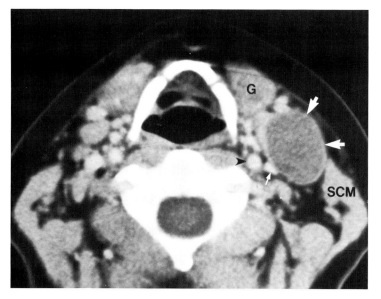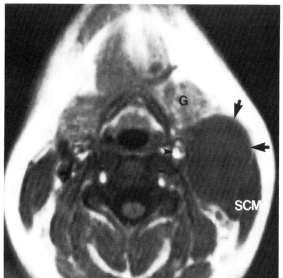

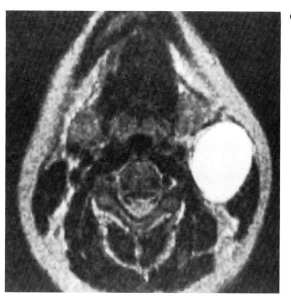

FIG. 75. Branchial cleft cyst. **A:** A thin-wall, homogeneous, water-density mass (*large arrows*) is seen lateral to the left internal carotid artery (*arrowhead*) and internal jugular vein (*small arrow*) and anterior to the sternocleidomastoid muscle (SCM); (G) submandibular gland. **B:** On T1-weighted MR image, the mass (*large arrows*) is homogeneous and similar in signal intensity to adjacent sternocleidomastoid muscle (SCM) (note that the mass has increased in size during the 1-month interval between the CT and MRI examinations); (*arrowhead*) flow artifact within left internal carotid artery; (G) submandibular gland. **C:** On T2-weighted MR image, the cyst is increased in relative signal intensity, becoming much brighter than all surrounding tissues.

A,B

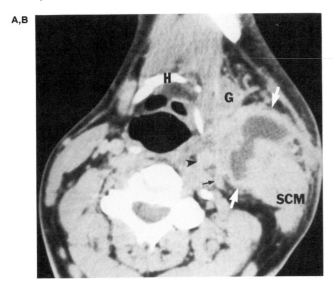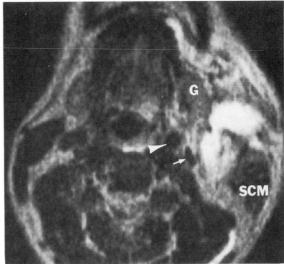

FIG. 76. Infected branchial cleft cyst. **A:** CT image at the level of the hyoid bone (H) demonstrates a thick-wall, partially cystic mass (*large arrows*) anterior to the sternocleidomastoid muscle (SCM). The surrounding fascial planes are thickened; (*arrowhead*) left internal carotid artery; (*small arrow*) left internal jugular vein; (G) submandibular gland. **B:** On T2-weighted MR image at approximately the same level, the central fluid component of the mass is much higher in signal intensity than the thickened wall; (*arrowhead*) left carotid artery; (*small arrow*) left jugular vein; (SCM) sternocleidomastoid muscle; (G) submandibular gland.

gree and chronicity of associated inflammation (Fig. 76). However, a very thick irregular wall is unusual. The surrounding fascial planes usually are preserved unless the cyst is infected. Clinical history and physical examination are very helpful, because the CT appearance may be atypical and mimic necrotic neoplastic lymph nodes or an abscess.

Most cystic neck masses are very high in signal intensity on T2-weighted MR images because of the long T2 of fluid (Figs. 75 and 76) (17). Simple cysts have thin or imperceptible walls and frequently are low in signal intensity on T1-weighted images, reflecting the long T1 of fluid. However, hemorrhagic cysts may be higher in signal intensity on T1-weighted images, presumably secondary to T1 shortening from methemoglobin (7). Similarly, cysts with a high protein content (e.g., infected cysts) have a higher signal intensity than simple cysts on T1-weighted images. As with CT, necrotic lymph node metastases may be indistinguishable from a complicated cyst on MR images.

Cystic hygromas arise from lymphoid tissue and most frequently present before 2 years of age as a mass posterior to the SCM. If they are large, they may demonstrate extension into the superior mediastinum or into the anterior neck. CT images usually show a thin-walled, generally multiloculated, homogeneous, near-water-density mass, although occasionally they may appear as solitary cysts (Fig. 77) (89,104,108). Because they may infiltrate the adjacent soft tissues, the surrounding fascial planes may be obliterated. Depending on their lipid content, com-

ponents of cystic hygromas may be relatively high in signal intensity on T1-weighted MR images (Fig. 78).

Thyroglossal duct cysts arise from remnants of the thyroglossal duct and are secondary to secretions from its epithelial lining. They usually present in young patients as an asymptomatic mass in the anterior neck in the midline or slightly off midline. They may develop anywhere along the course of the duct from the foramen cecum of the tongue to the pyramidal lobe of the thyroid gland. Sixty-five percent of these cysts are located below the hyoid bone, 20% suprahyoid, and 15% at the level of the hyoid

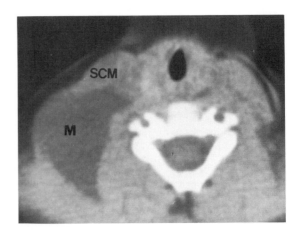

FIG. 77. Cystic hygroma. A large, low-attenuation mass (M) is seen in the right posterior triangle; (SCM) sternocleidomastoid muscle.

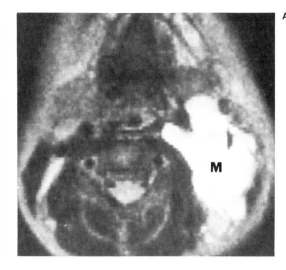

A,B

FIG. 78. Cystic hygroma. A: On T1-weighted MR image, a multiloculated mass (M), slightly lower in signal intensity than fat, is seen in the posterior triangle, displacing the sternocleidomastoid muscle laterally (*small arrowheads*). The mass infiltrates between adjacent soft tissues and separates the internal carotid artery (*large arrowhead*) and internal jugular vein (*arrow*). B: The mass (M) is very high in signal intensity on the T2-weighted MR image, reflecting its fluid nature.

(5). Although cysts that arise in the region of the hyoid bone usually are seen anterior to it, they may be located within or posterior to the hyoid bone (87). Infrahyoid thyroglossal duct cysts usually are embedded within the strap muscles. The diagnosis usually is apparent on clinical examination, but may be confusing in adults, especially if the cyst is lateral to the midline.

On CT, thyroglossal duct cysts usually are of low density, are occasionally septated, are well circumscribed, and may demonstrate peripheral-rim enhancement (Fig. 79) (90). Increased attenuation of the cyst usually is associated with increased protein content and coexistent or prior inflammation. Rarely, solid areas may be seen that represent a complicating papillary carcinoma (Fig. 80).

Cervical thymic cysts are rare causes of a cystic neck mass (108). They are believed to arise from remnants of the thymopharyngeal duct and are most frequently seen between the ages of 2 and 13 years. Thymic cysts usually are located in the low neck, off midline, and anterior to the carotid artery and internal jugular vein. They may simulate thyroid cysts on CT.

Cysts can also occur within the parathyroid gland (108). Microscopic cysts are discovered in the parathyroid glands at pathologic examination of normal glands, but rarely are large enough to present as clinically palpable neck masses. Most are associated with inferior parathyroid glands and usually are located caudal to the inferior thyroid border. Approximately 20% of the cysts are functioning and produce elevated serum concentrations of parathyroid hormone. Because of their intimate relationship to the thyroid, *parathyroid cysts* cannot be distinguished radiographically from thyroid cysts (Fig. 81).

However, analysis of the fluid obtained from cyst aspiration usually demonstrates elevated parathyroid hormone levels compared with serum levels. This finding may be seen with hyperfunctioning and nonhyperfunctioning cysts. In comparison, thyroid cysts will have elevated T3 and T4 levels.

Dermoid cyst is the most common form of a teratomatous cyst, and it is composed of two germ-cell layers, ectoderm and mesoderm (108). Those arising in the head and neck account for only 7% of all dermoid cysts, with most of these located in the orbit, nasal cavity, or floor of the mouth. Although they are rare in the neck, demonstration of a midline or near-midline mass that contains fat and fluid in a young child should suggest the diagnosis.

Teratomas contain elements of all three germ-cell layers and are most frequently seen in infants (108). They originate in or are adjacent to the thyroid gland and have been reported to have an inhomogeneous cystic appearance on CT. Malignant teratomas of the neck are uncommon and almost always are seen in adults.

Hemangiomas are congenital vascular abnormalities that usually are evident clinically by 6 months of age and frequently regress spontaneously by age 7 years. The two major types of hemangiomas are capillary and cavernous. Capillary hemangiomas are composed of capillary-size vessels, whereas cavernous hemangiomas consist of larger, dilated vascular channels. Hemangiomas may be localized to the skin or involve the deeper soft tissues of the neck. CT may be useful in defining the extent of deeper lesions, which frequently displace or infiltrate normal structures and may encroach on the airway (70,92,99). Hemangiomas may become enhanced inhomogeneously or

A,B

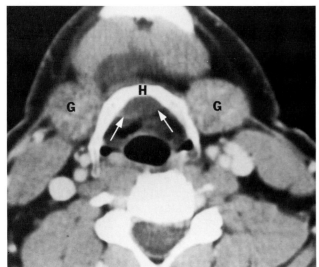
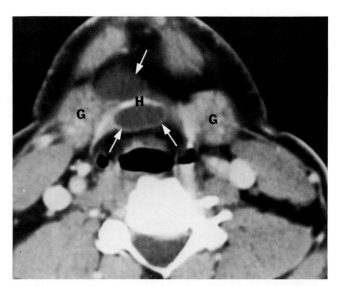

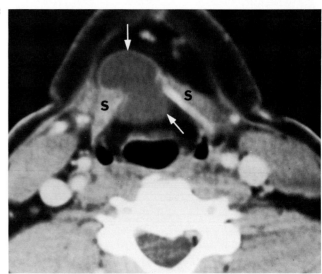

FIG. 79. Thyroglossal duct cyst. **A,B:** A homogeneous, low-attenuation mass (*arrows*) is seen, with components anterior and posterior to the hyoid bone (H); (G) submandibular gland. **C:** The infrahyoid portion of the mass (*arrows*) is seen on a more caudal image; (S) infrahyoid strap muscles.

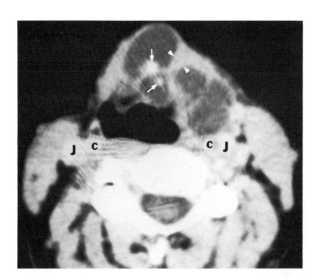

FIG. 80. Papillary carcinoma arising in thyroglossal duct cyst. A multiloculated cystic mass is seen anterior to the supraglottic portion of the larynx. Focal areas of calcification (*arrows*) and thickened soft-tissue septa (*arrowheads*) are seen within the mass; (c) common carotid artery; (J) internal jugular vein. (Courtesy of Dr. Edward Ragsdale, Alton, Illinois.)

demonstrate early peripheral enhancement, with a gradual centripetally advancing border of opacification. Thrombosed and fibrosed portions of the mass will not be enhanced. Occasionally, phleboliths will be present and suggest the diagnosis. Angiography usually is necessary if surgery is contemplated.

Hemangiomas of the neck have an MRI appearance similar to that for hemangiomas in other parts of the body (49,107,111) (Fig. 82). On T2-weighted images, they are characteristically very high in signal intensity. In addition, areas of low signal intensity may be seen secondary to fibrosis or phleboliths within the lesion. Serpiginous areas of low signal intensity, representing a feeding or draining vessel, may also be seen. Although simple parenchymal cysts may also be very high in signal intensity on T2-weighted images, they usually are lower than hemangiomas in signal intensity on T1-weighted images, reflecting the long T1 of fluid. However, as stated earlier, complicated parenchymal cysts may have a varied appearance and can be expected to mimic hemangiomas in some circumstances.

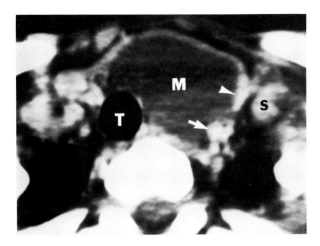

FIG. 81. Parathyroid cyst. A large, low-attenuation mass (M) displaces the trachea (T) to the right and the left common carotid artery (*arrow*) and internal jugular vein (*arrowhead*) to the left; (S) scalenus anterior muscle. Preoperative diagnosis was a thyroid cyst. No clinical manifestations of parathyroid hyperfunction were present.

Benign neoplasms.

Benign neoplasms are relatively uncommon in the extralaryngeal portion of the neck and usually are secondary to paragangliomas, neural lesions, or lipomas. On CT, carotid *paragangliomas* appear as lobulated, well-circumscribed masses that displace the internal carotid artery posterolaterally and the external carotid artery anteromedially (Fig. 83). They become enhanced, markedly and homogeneously, sometimes to the same extent as the surrounding vasculature. Angiography usually is necessary for surgical planning (65,92).

Paragangliomas are similar to other tumors on MR images in that they usually are of the same or slightly greater signal intensity than muscle on T1-weighted images and much greater in signal intensity on T2-weighted images. However, many of these lesions will also demonstrate multiple serpiginous and punctate areas of signal void on both T1- and T2-weighted images, secondary to rapid flow in the tumor vessels (Fig. 84) (82). Similar findings have been described in other vascular lesions, such as hemangiomas (49,107). Foci of even-echo rephasing reflecting relatively slowly flowing blood may also be seen. Although calcification within other tumors may also produce focal areas of signal void, this is not usually in a serpiginous pattern, nor will even-echo rephasing be demonstrated.

Neural tumors (e.g., neurofibromas, Schwannomas) can occur anywhere along the course of the cranial or cervical nerve roots. Vagal tumors, for example, are seen between the internal jugular vein and carotid artery. Smooth expansion of a vertebral foramen may be seen secondary to tumors arising from cervical nerve roots. The attenuation value of a neural tumor depends on the relative proportions of neural tissue and fibrous elements and the degree of cystic degeneration. The lower density of some neural tumors has been attributed to the high lipid content of neural tissue (Fig. 85) (54,99). Varying degrees of contrast enhancement may be seen. Although malignant nerve sheath tumors are more frequently infiltrative and have a heterogeneous appearance, benign tumors may look similar. MRI may be helpful in evaluating paraspinal neurogenic tumors by showing their intraspinal extension (11,98). Central areas of decreased signal intensity, possibly due to fibrous tissue, have been described in some neurofibromas.

A,B

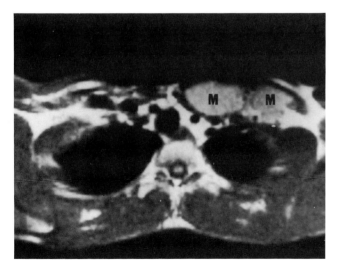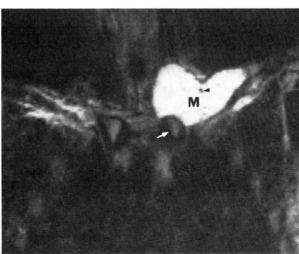

FIG. 82. Cavernous hemangioma. **A:** On this T1-weighted MR image, a multilobulated mass (M) is seen in the left supraclavicular fossa. **B:** On T2-weighted coronal MR image, the mass (M) is very high in signal intensity. The coronal view nicely demonstrates the relationship of the mass to the medial head of the clavicle (*arrow*) and the left lung apex. Low-signal-intensity focus within the mass (*arrowhead*) may represent a calcified phlebolith or area of fibrosis.

A,B

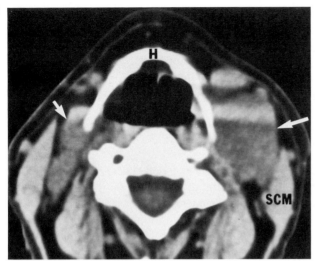 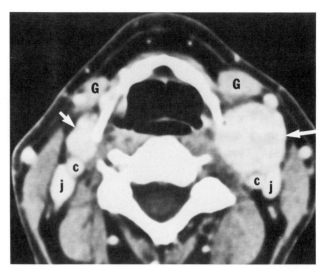

FIG. 83. Bilateral paragangliomas: CT. **A:** Precontrast CT image at the level of the hyoid bone (H) demonstrates a large mass (*large arrow*) anteromedial to the left sternocleidomastoid muscle (SCM). A smaller mass (*small arrow*) is seen on the right. **B:** Both masses (*arrows*) are enhanced homogeneously and markedly after intravenous administration of contrast material; (c) internal carotid artery; (j) internal jugular vein; (G) submandibular gland.

Lipomas are the most common neck tumors arising from connective tissue and are easily diagnosed with CT or MRI, being homogeneous and similar in attenuation value or signal intensity to subcutaneous fat (Fig. 86). Thin fibrous septa may sometimes be seen within the mass. Most lipomas are localized and occur in the subcutaneous tissue, but they can be seen in any neck compartment. Adjacent structures usually are displaced and sometimes compressed, but not infiltrated. If the mass is inhomogeneous, contains areas of soft-tissue density, or is poorly defined, a liposarcoma should be suspected.

Inflammation.

The major diagnostic considerations in patients suspected of having inflammatory masses in the neck include abscess, inflammatory or malignant lymphadenopathy, jugular thrombophlebitis, and an infected branchial cleft cyst. Although the CT findings may help in determining the cause of the neck mass, aspiration biopsy is sometimes needed.

CT is most useful in showing the extent of the inflammatory process and its relationship to the airway and dis-

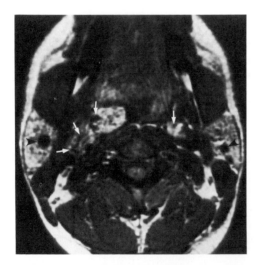

FIG. 84. Bilateral carotid body paragangliomas: MRI. Multiple punctate and serpiginous areas of signal void (*arrows*) secondary to high-velocity flow in tumor vessels are noted on a balanced (long TR, short TE) MR image; (*arrowheads*) retromandibular vein within the parotid gland. (From ref. 82.)

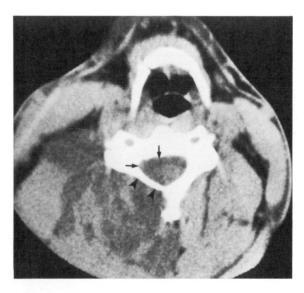

FIG. 85. Neurofibroma. A large, low-attenuation mass infiltrates the right paraspinal muscles, thins the adjacent vertebral lamina (*arrowheads*), and extends into the cervical spinal canal (*arrows*).

A,B

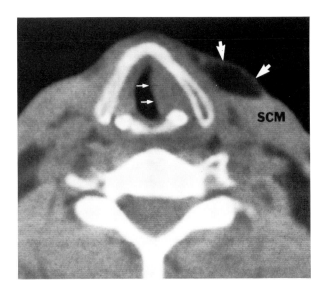

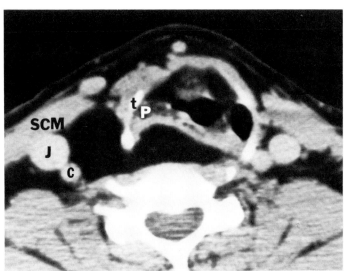

FIG. 86. Lipoma. A: A homogeneous mass (*large arrows*), similar in attenuation to adipose tissue, is seen anterior to the sternocleidomastoid muscle (SCM); (*small arrows*) left-true-vocal-cord carcinoma. B: In another patient, a lipoma is identified posterior to the right sternocleidomastoid muscle (SCM) and medial to the right common carotid artery (C) and internal jugular vein (J). It extends behind the right thyroid lamina (t) and compresses the right pyriform sinus (P). C: Similar findings are seen on T1-weighted MR image.

C

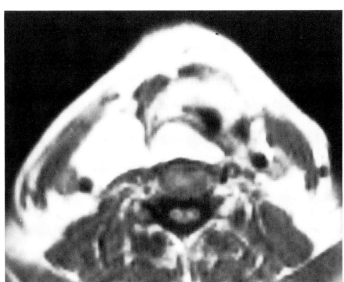

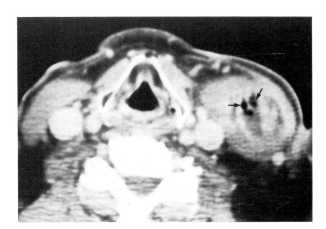

FIG. 87. Abscess of left sternocleidomastoid muscle. The left sternocleidomastoid muscle is enlarged and contains central areas of low attenuation, with gas bubbles (*arrows*).

tinguishing cellulitis from abscess (Fig. 87) (78). Whereas cellulitis appears as soft-tissue swelling, with obliteration of adjacent fascial planes, an abscess usually appears as a well-defined low-attenuation mass that may contain gas bubbles. A thick wall that is enhanced after intravenous injection of contrast material also may be seen. This finding, however, is nonspecific and can be seen with neoplasms and tuberculous adenitis (88,92). Therefore, the CT findings need to be correlated with clinical and laboratory information. Neck abscesses may be treated in some patients with antibiotics and CT-directed catheter drainage (16).

Jugular vein thrombosis.

Jugular vein thrombosis may result from indwelling catheters, intravenous drug abuse, infections, or compression by tumor. Occasionally, postoperative venous

A,B

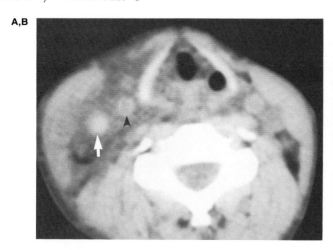 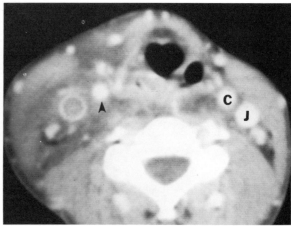

FIG. 88. Jugular vein thrombosis. **A:** On image obtained prior to intravenous administration of iodinated contrast material, the right internal jugular vein (*arrow*) has a high attenuation value. Adjacent soft-tissue swelling is seen; (*arrowhead*) right internal carotid artery. **B:** On the postcontrast image, the wall of the right internal jugular vein is enhanced. The lumen is now relatively low in attenuation value because the thrombus is not enhanced; (*arrowhead*) right internal carotid artery; (C) left internal carotid artery; (J) left internal jugular vein.

thrombosis will be clinically confused with hematoma, abscess, or residual tumor.

CT findings include enlargement of the jugular vein, a nonenhancing defect within the vessel lumen, enhancement of the vessel wall (presumably via flow through the arterially supplied vasa vasorum), and opacification of venous collaterals (Fig. 88) (1,26,83). If the thrombosis is acute, it may be relatively high in attenuation value on precontrast CT images. There may be soft-tissue swelling, with obliteration of fascial planes around the vessel from local inflammation. On a single section, a thrombosed vein may mimic a metastasis because of the enhancing

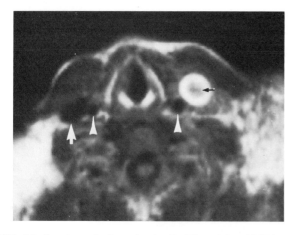

FIG. 89. Jugular vein thrombosis. On T1-weighted MR image, a central, low-intensity area (*small arrow*) is seen within the left internal jugular vein corresponding to the retracted clot. The more liquid, peripheral portion of the thrombus is high in signal intensity; (*arrowheads*) left and right common carotid arteries; (*large arrow*) normal right internal jugular vein.

periphery and lower-attenuation center; however, a correct diagnosis can be achieved by careful review of consecutive images.

MRI may also be helpful in detecting jugular vein thrombosis (9,25) (Fig. 89). In this condition, the normal signal void within the jugular vein is replaced by relatively bright intraluminal signal on both T1- and T2-weighted images. In some cases, the thrombus may demonstrate a high-signal-intensity peripheral ring that corresponds to the more liquid portion of the thrombus and a central lower-intensity area corresponding to the retracted clot.

Although the demonstration of signal void within the jugular vein is indicative of patency, intraluminal signal is not specific for jugular vein thrombosis and may be seen with slowly flowing blood. In a multisection sequence of the neck, venous blood may demonstrate flow-related signal enhancement in the most cephalad image (8). Arterial blood will show the opposite pattern, reflecting the opposite directions of venous and arterial blood flow. Decreasing intraluminal signal may be noted over several slices into the imaging volume. Moreover, slowly flowing blood may demonstrate an absolute increase in signal intensity on the second-echo images (even-echo rephasing). Although the appearance of slowly flowing blood may be confusing, recognition of flow-related enhancement patterns and even-echo rephasing usually allows distinction between intraluminal thrombosis and slowly flowing blood. Phase-image reconstruction and other flow-sensitive imaging techniques may allow distinction between intraluminal thrombus and flow-related artifacts in more confusing cases (25).

Ultrasound is also a reliable technique for diagnosing jugular vein thrombosis and provides adequate infor-

A,B

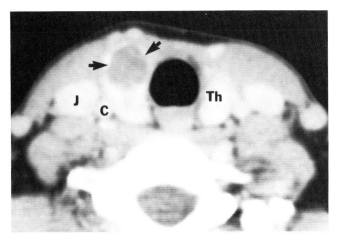 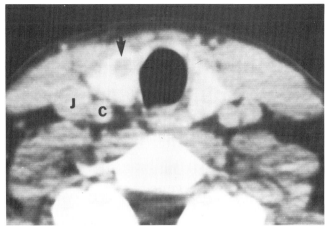

FIG. 90. Nonspecificity of CT appearance of thyroid nodules. **A:** A relatively low-attenuation mass (*arrows*), due to nodular hyperplasia, is seen in the right lobe of the thyroid gland; (C) common carotid artery; (J) internal jugular vein; (Th) left lobe of thyroid. **B:** A smaller, relatively low-attenuation nodule (*arrow*), due to metastatic adenocarcinoma, is present in the right lobe of the thyroid gland of another patient; (C) carotid artery; (J) jugular vein.

mation in most cases (122). Its main advantages are that it is noninvasive, inexpensive, and portable. Visualization of the vein beneath the mandible and clavicle is limited. However, determination of the total extent of jugular vein thrombosis infrequently influences therapeutic decisions.

Thyroid disease.

Radionuclide scintigraphy and ultrasound are the primary imaging techniques for evaluating suspected thyroid disease. CT currently has a limited role in evaluating most of these patients. Nevertheless, it is important to recognize the CT appearance of various gland abnormalities, be-

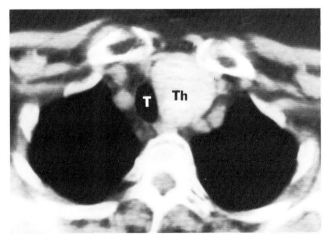

FIG. 91. Intrathoracic goiter. The goiter (Th) is higher in attenuation value than adjacent mediastinal structures, secondary to its high iodine content. The trachea (T) is mildly compressed and displaced to the right.

cause the thyroid is routinely seen on images of the neck. Occasionally, an unsuspected thyroid mass may be seen in a patient examined for cervical metastases of an unknown primary. In addition, CT may be useful for evaluation of intrathoracic goiter.

Alterations in density, homogeneity, and size of the thyroid gland are CT signs of thyroid disease (85). Several authors have found a correlation between the attenuation of the thyroid on CT and its iodine concentration (47). The attenuation value of abnormal thyroid glands usually is lower than that for normal controls. Thyroid diseases may be diffuse (e.g., thyroiditis), focal (e.g., cysts, adenoma, carcinoma), or multifocal (e.g., multinodular goiter). The difference between normal and abnormal regions of thyroid usually is accentuated after administration of iodinated contrast material. Unfortunately, the size of the lesion, the presence or absence of calcification, and the enhancement pattern are not sufficiently reliable in distinguishing benign and malignant disease (Fig. 90). Sonography is more accurate than CT in detecting smaller nodules within the thyroid and differentiating cystic and solid masses, but it likewise is limited by its lack of specificity. The findings of lymph node masses, vocal cord paralysis, and/or tracheal invasion are highly suggestive of malignant neoplasm (Figs. 50–53).

In the past, radionuclide scintigraphy has been the primary method for evaluating suspected intrathoracic goiter. However, the thyroid image may be negative if the goiter contains little or no functioning tissue. In most cases, CT can accurately diagnose an intrathoracic goiter and distinguish it from numerous other causes of superior mediastinal masses (Figs. 91–94) (4,34,36,105). CT is also very helpful preoperatively in showing the location and extent of the goiter and its relationship to normal me-

A,B

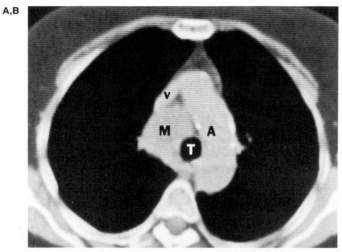

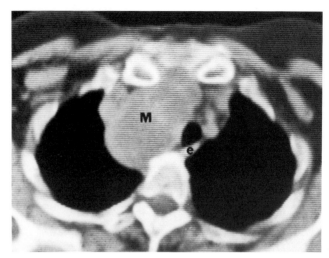

C

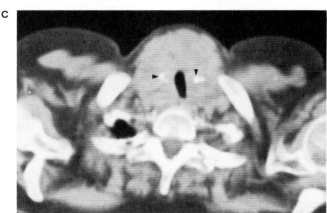

FIG. 92. Intrathoracic goiter mimicking right paratracheal lymphadenopathy. **A:** CT image at level of aortic arch (A) demonstrates a soft-tissue mass (M) anterolateral to trachea (T) and displacing the superior vena cava (v) anteriorly. **B:** At the level of the sternal notch, the mass (M) is enlarged, appears inhomogeneous, and displaces the trachea, esophagus (e), and great vessels laterally. **C:** On a more cephalad image, the mass is continuous with diffusely enlarged cervical thyroid gland that contains several coarse calcifications (*arrowheads*) and compresses the trachea. (From ref. 36.)

A,B

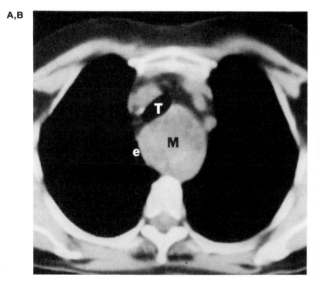

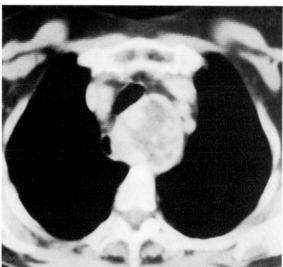

FIG. 93. Intrathoracic goiter: effect of intravenous administration of contrast material. **A:** A large mass (M) displaces the trachea (T) anteriorly and the esophagus (e) laterally. **B:** Portions of the mass are enhanced markedly after intravenous administration of contrast material. Lower-attenuation areas presumably represent areas of cystic degeneration within the goiter. The mass was continuous with the cervical thyroid on more cephalad images.

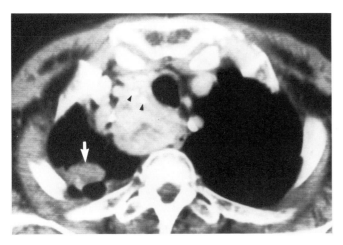

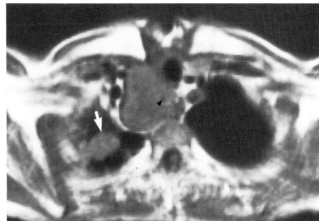

A,B

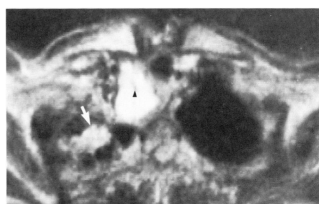

C

FIG. 94. Intrathoracic goiter in patient with bronchogenic carcinoma. **A:** Postcontrast CT image demonstrates a large intrathoracic goiter containing several areas of calcification (*arrowheads*) and low-attenuation areas of cystic degeneration. More cephalad images showed continuity with cervical thyroid; (*arrow*) bronchogenic carcinoma. On T1-weighted (**B**) and T2-weighted (**C**) MR images, the goiter and bronchogenic carcinoma (*arrow*) are similar in signal intensity, emphasizing the nonspecificity of signal intensity. Focal areas of low signal intensity (*arrowheads*) within the goiter represent calcification and cannot be recognized as such.

diastinal vessels. This information is useful in deciding the surgical approach, especially in those lesions with large posterior components that may require a thoracotomy in addition to a neck exploration.

On CT, intrathoracic goiter almost always is continuous with a cervical thyroid on serial images (Fig. 92). Extension to the neck may not be present if there has been prior thyroid surgery, if the gland is ectopic, or if the connection between the cervical and mediastinal components is only a narrow fibrous or vascular pedicle (4). The goiter usually is located in the anterior mediastinum in front of the great vessels. Larger masses displace the mediastinal vessels anterolaterally. Interdigitation between the trachea and esophagus and extension into the posterior mediastinum can also be seen.

Intrathoracic goiters usually are well defined and often contain focal areas of calcification and low-attenuation areas of cystic degeneration (Figs. 92–94). The attenuation of the intrathoracic component frequently is less than that of the cervical thyroid, but greater than that of muscle (Fig. 91). This appearance, however, is highly variable and relates to the iodine content of the goiter. If the iodine content is very low, the CT density may be similar to that for surrounding soft tissue. Though generally unnecessary for diagnosis, intravenous administration of contrast ma-

terial may result in marked enhancement, reflecting the vascularity of the mass (Figs. 93 and 94). Prolonged enhancement, more than 2 min after injection, may also be seen and is believed to be related to iodine uptake by the gland (34). Because of the multinodularity of intrathoracic goiters and their variable iodine content, the enhancement pattern is frequently inhomogeneous. Thyroid carcinoma with mediastinal extension may be indistinguishable from a goiter, but its margins with the mediastinal vessels and fat usually are obliterated. Invasion of adjacent structures may also be present in association with cervical/mediastinal lymphadenopathy and pulmonary nodules.

MRI may play a role similar to that of CT in evaluating the thyroid, specifically in showing the extent of large thyroid masses (45). Intrathoracic extension of goiters, for example, can be demonstrated on axial, coronal, or sagittal images (Fig. 94). Currently, specific tissue characterization of thyroid masses is not possible with MRI (33,45,74,77). Benign and malignant lesions can have similar signal intensities. The contrast between most thyroid masses and normal thyroid tissue is optimal on T2-weighted images (Fig. 95). Thyroid nodules may be of varying signal intensities relative to normal thyroid on T1-weighted images. High signal intensity on T1-weighted images may reflect hemorrhage or highly proteinaceous material

A,B

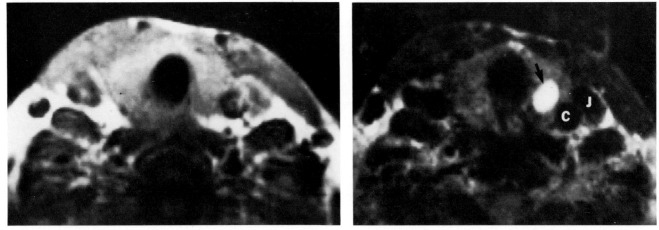

FIG. 95. Thyroid nodule: nodular hyperplasia. **A:** On T1-weighted MR image, the left thyroid nodule is isointense with the remainder of the thyroid. **B:** On T2-weighted image, the nodule (*arrow*) markedly increases in signal intensity relative to surrounding tissues; (C) common carotid artery; (J) internal jugular vein.

within the nodule. Most masses are hyperintense on T2-weighted images. Multinodular goiters may be heterogeneous on T2-weighted images. Calcification cannot be identified as such with MRI and appears as areas of low or no signal intensity (Fig. 94). Diffuse increase in signal intensity on T1- and T2-weighted images has been described in Graves disease and correlated with serum thyroxin levels and 24-hr radioactive-iodine uptake (14). It is uncertain whether or not MRI will have any clinical role in these patients.

Parathyroid disease.

Various radiologic techniques have been used for preoperative localization of parathyroid abnormalities in patients with primary hyperparathyroidism. Several noninvasive imaging procedures are available: high-resolution sonography, CT, and parathyroid scintigraphy using a subtraction technique with technetium 99m and thallium 201 (21,53,72,86,112,113,123,124). MRI also has been used for evaluation of these patients, but experience is

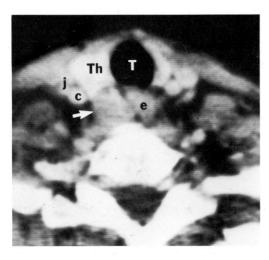

FIG. 96. Parathyroid adenoma. Adenoma (*arrow*) is seen in right tracheoesophageal groove; (c) common carotid artery; (j) internal jugular vein; (e) esophagus; (Th) right lobe of thyroid gland; (T) trachea.

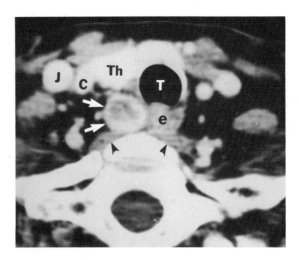

FIG. 97. Partially necrotic parathyroid adenoma. An oval mass with a low-density center (*arrows*) is seen posterior to the right lobe of the thyroid gland (Th) and adjacent to the right side of the esophagus (e); (C) common carotid artery; (J) internal jugular vein; (*arrowheads*) longus colli muscle; (T) trachea. (Courtesy of Dr. Naris Rujanavech, St. Louis, Missouri.)

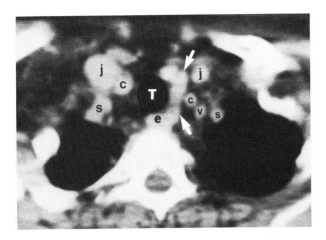

FIG. 98. Parathyroid adenoma in superior mediastinum. An elliptical mass (*arrows*) is seen adjacent to the left side of the trachea (T); (e) esophagus; (c) common carotid artery; (j) internal jugular vein; (s) subclavian artery; (v) vertebral artery.

limited (50,52,84,110). The decision to use preoperative imaging depends not only on the availability and accuracy of each technique but also on the expertise and operative approach of individual surgeons.

Benign parathyroid adenomas account for approximately 80% to 85% of cases of primary hyperparathyroidism, with multiglandular hyperplasia occurring in most of the remaining patients. Rarely, parathyroid carcinoma is the cause of primary hyperparathyroidism. An experienced surgeon can permanently cure 90% to 95% of patients undergoing initial neck exploration without using any preoperative imaging procedure. However, preoperative localization may be useful if the surgeon is willing to perform a unilateral neck exploration (i.e., removal of adenoma and one normal ipsilateral gland) and does not insist on identifying all four glands (120).

Much less controversial is the use of preoperative radiologic imaging of parathyroid glands in postoperative patients with persistent and recurrent hyperparathyroidism. In these patients, surgical landmarks may be obscured by scarring and adhesions, resulting in greater morbidity during surgical reexploration. Although most parathyroid adenomas will still be accessible from the neck, approximately 20% are located in the anterior or superior mediastinum and require mediastinotomy for resection (120).

CT has been most helpful in detecting such mediastinal parathyroid adenomas in these postoperative patients. Although the initial experience with CT in detecting cervical adenomas was less encouraging because of shoulder streak artifacts and poorer spatial resolution, more recent studies using improved equipment and more rigorous technique have resulted in improved sensitivity (113). Narrowly collimated images (e.g., 4-mm images obtained at 4–5-mm intervals) from the hyoid bone to the manu-

brium and 8- to 10-mm images at 10-mm intervals to the carina, with rapid scanning during bolus/drip intravenous administration of contrast material, allow distinction between the parathyroid mass and adjacent vessels (Fig. 96). Approximately 25% of adenomas show contrast enhancement, but usually to a lesser degree than vessels or the adjacent thyroid gland (112). Central necrosis may occasionally be seen (Fig. 97). Calcification is only rarely seen. In the absence of invasion of adjacent structures, there are no reliable imaging findings that allow distinction between parathyroid adenoma and carcinoma.

Parathyroid adenomas may be seen posterior to the superior or inferior pole of the thyroid gland. An adenoma in the posterior superior mediastinum usually lies in the tracheoesophageal groove caudal to the thyroid gland at the level of the cervicothoracic junction and usually is flattened along its margin with the trachea (Fig. 98). Because the esophagus usually deviates to the left at the thoracic inlet, it may obscure a left-side adenoma. In these situations, administration of thick barium paste is helpful. Parathyroid adenomas may also be seen behind the sternothyroid muscle at the level of the thoracic inlet. More caudal tumors usually are seen anterior to the arch and great vessels (Fig. 99). Rarely, intrathyroidal parathyroid adenomas may be seen and are difficult to distinguish from thyroid masses. Parathyroid glands have also been described adjacent to the carotid bifurcation at the level of the hyoid bone (23). In equivocal cases, percutaneous aspiration under CT (or ultrasound) guidance to obtain samples for parathyroid hormone assay may be helpful for confirmation of an adenoma in an ectopic location (22,42).

Initial reports from several authors have shown that MRI can detect parathyroid gland enlargement in the neck, as well as ectopic parathyroid tissue in the mediastinum (50,52,84,110). Contrast between adenomas and surrounding tissues, especially the thyroid gland, is optimal on T2-weighted images because of the long T2 of parathyroid adenomas (Fig. 100). However, the degree of increase on T2-weighted images is variable. Moreover, it may be less apparent at lower field strengths (0.35–0.5 T) than at higher field strengths (1.5 T) or if images less heavily T2-weighted are used (84). T1-weighted images provide better anatomic resolution, as well as better distinction between the adenoma and adjacent fat. As with CT, intrathyroidal masses or lymph nodes may be difficult to distinguish from a parathyroid adenoma. Experience with imaging hyperplastic glands is even more limited. Although they may have signal characteristics similar to those for adenomas, individual hyperplastic glands in a given patient may have different signal intensities.

Other imaging techniques also have been used for preoperative localization of parathyroid abnormalities. High-frequency (10-MHz) real-time sonography can detect up to 82% of cervical glands in postoperative patients with

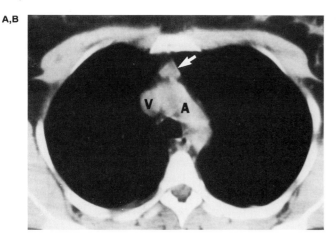
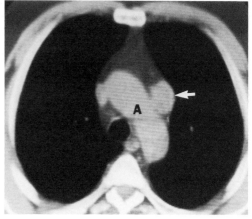

FIG. 99. Parathyroid adenoma in anterior mediastinum. **A:** An intrathymic parathyroid adenoma (*arrow*) is seen anterior to the aortic arch (A); (V) superior vena cava. **B:** A larger adenoma (*arrow*), in another patient, is seen just lateral to the aortic arch (A).

persistent or recurrent hyperparathyroidism (86). Sensitivity is related to the size and location of the adenoma, as well as the technique used and the experience of the operator, and has been reported to vary widely in the literature. Acoustic shadows may obscure adenomas located behind the trachea or esophagus. Mediastinal tumors cannot be detected by sonography because of the overlying bony thoracic cage.

Subtraction scintigraphy with technetium 99m and thallium 201 has been shown to be an accurate technique for identification of parathyroid adenomas (123,124). Both neck and mediastinal glands can be identified. Thyroid nodules can result in false-positive diagnoses. Al-

though this technique cannot show the relationships of the adenoma to other structures, in several cases we have found it to be very useful prior to and in the interpretation of a subsequent CT examination.

Whether ultrasound or double-tracer scintigraphy should be used initially depends on the availability and local experience with these techniques. If the results of either examination are negative or equivocal, or if additional confirmation is required, CT or MRI can be performed. More invasive localizing tests (angiography or selective venous sampling) may be reserved for patients in whom the findings on noninvasive techniques are negative or equivocal (71).

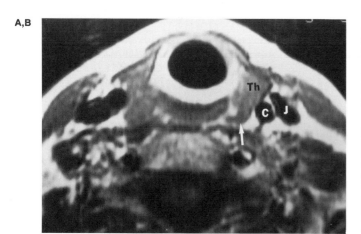
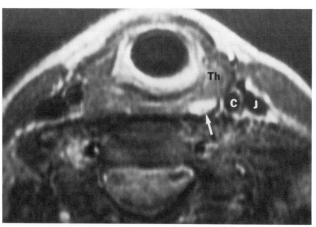

FIG. 100. Parathyroid adenoma. **A:** On a T1-weighted MR image, a small mass (*white arrow*) is present posterior to the left lobe of the thyroid (Th). It is similar in signal intensity to the thyroid gland; (C) common carotid artery; (J) internal jugular vein. **B:** On a T2-weighted image, the adenoma (*arrow*) is high in signal intensity and easily distinguishable from the adjacent thyroid gland (Th). (From ref. 110.)

REFERENCES

1. Albertyn LE, Alcock MK. Diagnosis of internal jugular vein thrombosis. *Radiology* 1987;162:505–508.
2. Archer CR, Sagel SS, Yeager VL, Martin S, Friedman WH. Staging of carcinoma of the larynx: comparative accuracy of computed tomography and laryngography. *AJR* 1981;136:571–575.
3. Archer CR, Yeager VL. Evaluation of laryngeal cartilages by computed tomography. *J Comput Assist Tomogr* 1979;3:604–611.
4. Bashist B, Ellis K, Gold RP. Computed tomography of intrathoracic goiters. *AJR* 1983;140:450–460.
5. Batsakis JG: *Tumors of the head and neck: clinical and pathologic considerations,* 2nd ed. Baltimore: Williams & Wilkins, 1979.
6. Biller HF, Ogura JF, Pratt LL. Hemilaryngectomy for T_2 glottic cancers. Arch Otolaryngol 1971;93:238–243.
7. Bradley WG Jr, Schmidt PG. Effect of methemoglobin formation on the MR appearance of subarachnoid hemorrhage. *Radiology* 1985;156:99–103.
8. Bradley WG Jr, Waluch V, Lai K-S, Fernandez EJ, Spalter C. The appearance of rapidly flowing blood on magnetic resonance images. *AJR* 1984;143:1167–1174.
9. Braun IF, Hoffman JC Jr, Malko JA, Pettigrew RI, Dannels W, Davis PC. Jugular venous thrombosis: MR imaging. *Radiology* 1985;157:357–360.
10. Brazeau-Lamontagne L, Charlin B, Levesque R-Y, Lussier A. Cricoarytenoiditis: CT assessment in rheumatoid arthritis. *Radiology* 1986;158:463–466.
11. Burk DL, Brunberg JA, Kanal E, Latchaw RE, Wolf AL. Spinal and paraspinal neurofibromatosis: surface coil MR imaging at 1.5T. *Radiology* 1987;162:797–801.
12. Castelijns JA, Doornbos J, Verbeeten B Jr, Vielvoye GJ, Bloem JL. MR imaging of the normal larynx. *J Comput Assist Tomogr* 1985;9:919–925.
13. Castelijns JA, Kaiser MC, Valk J, Gerristen GJ, van Hattum AH, Snow GB. MR imaging of laryngeal cancer. *J Comput Assist Tomogr* 1987;11:134–140.
14. Charkes ND, Maurer AH, Siegel JA, Radecki PD, Malmud LS. MR imaging in thyroid disorders: correlation of signal intensity with Graves disease activity. *Radiology* 1987;164:491–494.
15. Cocke EW, Wang CC. Cancer of the larynx selecting optimum treatment. Part 1. *CA* 1976;26:194–200.
16. Cole DR, Bankoff M, Carter BL. Percutaneous catheter drainage of deep neck infections guided by CT. *Radiology* 1984;152:224.
17. Dietrich RB, Lufkin RB, Kangarloo H, Hanafee WN, Wilson GH. Head and neck MR imaging in the pediatric patient. *Radiology* 1986;159:769–776.
18. Dillon WP, Mills CM, Kjos B, De Groot J, Brant-Zawadzki M. Magnetic resonance imaging of the nasopharynx. *Radiology* 1984;152:731–738.
19. DiSantis DJ, Balfe DM, Hayden RE, Sagel SS, Sessions D, Lee JKT. The neck after total laryngectomy: CT study. *Radiology* 1984;153:713–717.
20. DiSantis DJ, Balfe DM, Hayden R, Sessions D, Sagel SS. The neck after vertical hemilaryngectomy: computed tomographic study. *Radiology* 1984;151:683–687.
21. Doppman JL, Krudy AG, Brennan MF, Schneider P, Lasker RD, Marx SJ. CT appearance of enlarged parathyroid glands in posterior superior mediastinum. *J Comput Assist Tomogr* 1982;6:1099–1102.
22. Doppman JL, Krudy AG, Marx SJ, et al. Aspiration of enlarged parathyroid glands for parathyroid assay. *Radiology* 1983;148:31–35.
23. Doppman JL, Shawker TH, Krudy AG. Parathymic parathyroid: CT, US, and angiographic findings. *Radiology* 1985;157:419–423.
24. Ell SR, Jolles H, Keyes WD, Galvin JR. Cine CT technique for dynamic airway studies. *AJR* 1985;145:35–36.
25. Erdman WA, Weinreb JC, Cohen JM, Buja LM, Chaney C, Peshock RM. Venous thrombosis: clinical and experimental MR imaging. *Radiology* 1986;161:233–238.
26. Fishman EK, Pakter RL, Gayler BW, Wheeler PS, Siegelman SS. Jugular venous thrombosis: diagnosis by computed tomography. *J Comput Assist Tomogr* 1984;8:963–968.
27. Friedman M, Shelton VK, Mafee M, Bellity P, Grybauskas V, Skolnik E. Metastatic neck disease: evaluation by computed tomography. *Arch Otolaryngol* 1984;110:443–447.
28. Gamsu G. Computed tomography of the larynx and piriform sinuses. In: Moss AA, Gamsu G, Genant H, eds. *Computed tomography of the body.* Philadelphia: WB Saunders, 1983:65–143.
29. Gamsu G, Mark AS, Webb WR. Computed tomography of the normal larynx during quiet breathing and phonation. *J Comput Assist Tomogr* 1981;5:353–360.
30. Gamsu G, Webb WR, Shallit JB, Moss AA. Computed tomography in carcinoma of the larynx and pyriform sinus—the value of phonation CT. *AJR* 1981;136:577–584.
31. Gatenby RA, Mulhern CB, Strawitz J. CT-guided percutaneous biopsies of head and neck masses. *Radiology* 1983;146:717–719.
32. Gayler BW, Kashima HK, Martinez CR. Computed tomography of the neck. *CRC Crit Rev Diagn Imaging* 1985;23:319–374.
33. Gefter WB, Spritzer CE, Eisenberg B, et al. Thyroid imaging with high-field strength surface-coil MR. *Radiology* 1987;164:483–490.
34. Glazer GM, Axel L, Moss AA. CT diagnosis of mediastinal thyroid. *AJR* 1982;138:495–498.
35. Glazer HS, Aronberg DJ, Lee JKT, Sagel SS. Extralaryngeal causes of vocal cord paralysis: CT evaluation. *AJR* 1983;141:527–531.
36. Glazer HS, Aronberg DJ, Sagel SS. Pitfalls in CT recognition of mediastinal lymphadenopathy. *AJR* 1985;144:267–274.
37. Glazer HS, Lee JKT, Levitt RG, et al. Radiation fibrosis: differentiation from recurrent tumor by MR imaging. *Radiology* 1985;156:721–726.
38. Glazer HS, Mauro MA, Aronberg DJ, Lee JKT, Johnston DE, Sagel SS. Computed tomography of laryngocoeles. *AJR* 1983;140:549–552.
39. Glazer HS, Niemeyer JH, Balfe DM, et al. Neck neoplasms: MR imaging. Part I. Initial evaluation. *Radiology* 1986;160:343–348.
40. Glazer HS, Niemeyer JH, Balfe DM, et al. Neck neoplasms: MR imaging. Part II. Posttreatment evaluation. *Radiology* 1986;160:349–354.
41. Glazer HS, Sagel SS. The larynx and hypopharynx. In: Carter BL, ed. *Computed tomography of the head and neck.* New York: Churchill Livingstone, 1985:1–30.
42. Gooding GAW, Clark OH, Stark DD, Moss AA, Montgomery CK. Parathyroid aspiration biopsy under ultrasound guidance in the postoperative hyperparathyroid patient. *Radiology* 1985;155:193–196.
43. Harnsberger HR, Mancuso AA, Byrd S, Muraki AS, Johnson L, Hanafee WN. Branchial cleft anomalies and their mimics: the role of CT. *Radiology* 1984;152:739–748.
44. Harnsberger HR, Mancuso AA, Muraki AS, Parkin JL. The upper aerodigestive tract and neck: CT evaluation of recurrent tumor. *Radiology* 1983;149:503–510.
45. Higgins CB, McNamara MT, Fisher MR, Clark OH. MR imaging of the thyroid. *AJR* 1986;147:1255–1261.
46. Hoover LA, Calcaterra TC, Walter GA, Larrson SG. Preoperative CT scan evaluation for laryngeal carcinoma: correlation with pathologic findings. *Laryngoscope* 1984;94:310–315.
47. Iida Y, Konishi J, Harioka T, Misake T, Endo K, Torizuka K. Thyroid CT number and its relationship to iodine concentration. *Radiology* 1983;147:793–795.
48. Jacobs CJM, Harnsberger HR, Lufkin RB, Osborn AG, Smoker WRK, Parkin JL. Vagal neuropathy: evaluation with CT and MR imaging. *Radiology* 1987;164:97–102.
49. Kaplan PA, Williams SM. Mucocutaneous and peripheral soft-tissue hemangiomas: MR imaging. *Radiology* 1987;163:163–166.
50. Kier R, Blinder RA, Herfkens RJ, Leight GS, Spritzer CE, Carroll BA. MR imaging with surface coils in primary hyperparathyroidism. *J Comput Assist Tomogr* 1987;11:863–868.
51. Kirchner JA. Two hundred laryngeal cancers: patterns of growth and spread as seen in serial section. *Laryngoscope* 1977;87:474–482.
52. Kneeland JB, Krubsack AJ, Lawson TL, et al. Enlarged parathyroid glands: high-resolution local coil MR imaging. *Radiology* 1987;162:143–146.
53. Krudy AG, Doppman JL, Brennan MF, et al. The detection of mediastinal parathyroid glands by computed tomography, selective arteriography, and venous sampling: an analysis of 17 cases. *Radiology* 1981;140:739–744.

54. Kumar AJ, Kuhajda FP, Martinez CR, Fishman EK, Jezic DV, Siegelman SS. Computed tomography of extracranial nerve sheath tumors with pathological correlation. *J Comput Assist Tomogr* 1983;7:857–865.

55. Larsson S, Mancuso AA, Hoover L, Hanafee WN. Differentiation of pyriform sinus cancer from supraglottic laryngeal cancer by computed tomography. *Radiology* 1981;141:427–432.

56. Lufkin R, Hanafee W. Application of surface coils to MRI anatomy of the larynx. *AJR* 1985;145:483–489.

57. Lufkin RB, Hanafee WN, Wortham D, Hoover L. Larynx and hypopharynx: MR imaging with surface coils. *Radiology* 1986;158:747–754.

58. Lufkin RB, Larsson SG, Hanafee WN. NMR anatomy of the larynx and tongue base. *Radiology* 1983;148:173–175.

59. Mafee MF, Schild JA, Michael AS, Choi KH, Capek V. Cartilage involvement in laryngeal carcinoma: correlation of CT and pathologic macrosection studies. *J Comput Assist Tomogr* 1984;8:969–973.

60. Mafee MF, Schild JA, Valvassori GE, Capek V. Computed tomography of the larynx: correlation with anatomic and pathologic studies in cases of laryngeal carcinoma. *Radiology* 1983;147:123–128.

61. Mancuso AA. Cervical lymph node metastases. In: Bragg DG, Rubin P, Youker JE, eds. *Oncologic imaging.* New York: Pergamon Press, 1985:47–61.

62. Mancuso AA. Larynx and hypopharynx. In: Bragg DG, Rubin P, Youker JE, eds. *Oncologic imaging.* New York: Pergamon Press, 1985:103–123.

63. Mancuso AA, Hanafee WN. Computed tomography of the injured larynx. *Radiology* 1979;133:139–144.

64. Mancuso AA, Hanafee WN. A comparative evaluation of computed tomography and laryngography. *Radiology* 1979;133:131–138.

65. Mancuso AA, Hanafee WN. *Computed tomography and magnetic resonance imaging of the head and neck.* Baltimore: Williams & Wilkins, 1985.

66. Mancuso AA, Harnsberger HR, Muraki AS, Stevens MH. Computed tomography of cervical and retropharyngeal lymph nodes: normal anatomy, variants of normal and applications in staging head and neck cancer. Part I: Normal anatomy. *Radiology* 1983;148:709–714.

67. Mancuso AA, Harnsberger HR, Muraki AS, Stevens MH. Computed tomography of cervical and retropharyngeal lymph nodes: normal anatomy, variants of normal and applications in staging head and neck cancer. Part II: Pathology. *Radiology* 1983;148:715–723.

68. Mancuso AA, Maceri D, Rice D, Hanafee WN. CT of cervical lymph node cancer. *AJR* 1981;136:381–385.

69. Mancuso AA, Tamakawa Y, Hanafee WN. CT of the fixed vocal cord. *AJR* 1980;135:429–434.

70. Michael AS, Mafee MF, Valvassori G, Tan WS. Dynamic computed tomography of the head and neck: differential diagnostic value. *Radiology* 1985;154:413–419.

71. Miller DL, Doppman JL, Krudy AG, et al. Localization of parathyroid adenomas in patients who have undergone surgery. Part II. Invasive procedures. *Radiology* 1987;162:138–141.

72. Miller DL, Doppman JL, Shawker TH, et al. Localization of parathyroid adenomas in patients who have undergone surgery. Part I. Noninvasive imaging methods. *Radiology* 1987;162:133–137.

73. Million RR, Cassisi NJ: Larynx. In: *Management of head and neck cancer. A multidisciplinary approach.* Philadelphia: Lippincott, 1984:315–364.

74. Mountz JM, Glazer GM, Dmuchowski C, Sisson JC. MR imaging of the thyroid: comparison with scintigraphy in the normal and diseased gland. *J Comput Assist Tomogr* 1987;11:612–619.

75. Muraki AS, Mancuso AA, Harnsberger HR. Metastatic cervical adenopathy from tumors of unknown origin: the role of CT. *Radiology* 1984;152:749–753.

76. Niemeyer JH, Balfe DM, Hayden RE. Barium and CT evaluation of the neck following supraglottic subtotal laryngectomy. *Radiology* 1987;162:493–498.

77. Noma S, Nishimura K, Togashi K, et al. Thyroid gland: MR imaging. *Radiology* 1987;164:495–499.

78. Nyberg DA, Jeffrey RB, Brant-Zawadzki M, Federle M, Dillon W. Computed tomography of cervical infections. *J Comput Assist Tomogr* 1985;9:288–296.

79. Ogura JH, Biller HF. Conservation surgery in cancer of the head and neck. *Otolaryngol Clin North Am* 1969;2:641–665.

80. Ogura JH, Sessions DG, Spector GJ. Conservation surgery for epidermoid carcinoma of the supraglottic larynx. *Laryngoscope* 1975;85:1808–1815.

81. Ogura JH, Henneman H. Conservation surgery of the larynx and hypopharynx—selection of patients and results. *Can J Otolaryngol* 1973;2:11–16.

82. Olsen WL, Dillon WP, Kelly WM, Norman D, Brant-Zawadzki M, Newton TH. MR imaging of paragangliomas. *AJR* 1987;148:201–204.

83. Patel S, Brennan J. Diagnosis of internal jugular vein thrombosis by computed tomography. *J Comput Assist Tomogr* 1981;5:197–200.

84. Peck WW, Higgins CB, Fisher MR, Ling M, Okerlund MD, Clark OH. Hyperparathyroidism: comparison of MR imaging with radionuclide scanning. *Radiology* 1987;163:415–420.

85. Radecki PD, Arger PH, Arenson RL, et al. Thyroid imaging: comparison of high-resolution real-time ultrasound and computed tomography. *Radiology* 1984;153:145–147.

86. Reading CC, Charboneau JW, James EM, et al. Postoperative parathyroid high-frequency sonography: evaluation of persistent or recurrent hyperparathyroidism. *AJR* 1985;144:399–402.

87. Reede DL. The neck—thyroid and parathyroid glands. In: Carter BL, ed. *Computed tomography of the head and neck.* New York: Churchill Livingstone, 1985:31–57.

88. Reede DL, Bergeron RT. Cervical tuberculous adenitis: CT manifestations. *Radiology* 1985;154:701–704.

89. Reede DL, Bergeron RT, Osborn AG. CT of the soft tissues of the neck. In: Bergeron RT, Osborn AG, Som PM, eds. *Head and neck imaging excluding the brain.* St. Louis: Mosby, 1984:491–530.

90. Reede DL, Bergeron RT, Som PM. CT of thyroglossal duct cysts. *Radiology* 1985;157:121–125.

91. Reede DL, Whelan MA, Bergeron RT. Computed tomography of the infrahyoid neck. Part I: Normal anatomy. *Radiology* 1982;145:389–395.

92. Reede DL, Whelan MA, Bergeron RT. Computed tomography of the infrahyoid neck. Part II. Pathology. *Radiology* 1982;145:397–402.

93. Reid MH. Laryngeal carcinoma: high-resolution computed tomography and thick anatomic sections. *Radiology* 1984;151:689–696.

94. Rouvier H. *Anatomy of the human lymphatic system.* Ann Arbor, Michigan: Edwards Brothers, 1938:1–82.

95. Sagel SS, Aufderheide JF, Aronberg DJ, Stanley RJ, Archer C. High resolution computed tomography in the staging of carcinoma of the larynx. *Laryngoscope* 1981;91:292–300.

96. Salazar JE, Duke RA, Ellis JV. Second branchial cleft cyst: unusual location and a new CT diagnostic sign. *AJR* 1985;145:965–966.

97. Schild JA, Mafee MF, Valvassori GE, Bardawil WA. Laryngeal malignancies and computerized tomography: a correlation of tomographic and histopathologic findings. *Ann Otol Rhinol Laryngol* 1982;91:571–575.

98. Jamroz GA, Siegel MJ, Glazer HS, Abramson CL. Intraspinal extension of neuroblastoma imaged by MRI. *J Comput Assist Tomogr* 1986;10:593–595.

99. Silver AJ, Mawad ME, Hilal SK, Ascherl GF Jr, Chynn KY, Baredes S. Computed tomography of the carotid space and related cervical spaces. Part II. Neurogenic tumors. *Radiology* 1984;150:729–735.

100. Silverman PM. CT staging of laryngeal and hypopharyngeal carcinoma. In: Glazer GM, ed. *Staging of neoplasms.* New York: Churchill Livingstone, 1986:55–77.

101. Silverman PM, Bossen EH, Fisher SR, Cole TB, Korobkin M, Halvorsen RA. Carcinoma of the larynx and hypopharynx: computed tomographic-histopathologic correlations. *Radiology* 1984;151:697–702.

102. Silverman PM, Johnson GA, Korobkin M. High resolution sagittal and coronal reformatted CT images of the larynx. *AJR* 1983;140:819–822.

103. Silverman FM, Korobkin M. High-resolution computed tomography of the normal larynx. *AJR* 1983;140:875–879.

104. Silverman PM, Korobkin M, Moore AV. Computed tomography of cystic neck masses. *J Comput Assist Tomogr* 1983;7:498–502.

105. Silverman PM, Newman GE, Korobkin M, Workman JB, Moore

AV, Coleman RE. Computed tomography in the evaluation of thyroid disease. *AJR* 1984;141:897–902.

106. Som PM, Biller HF. Computed tomography of the neck in the postoperative patient: radical neck dissection and the myocutaneous flap. *Radiology* 1983;148:157–160.

107. Som PM, Braun IF, Shapiro MD, Reede DL, Curtin HD, Zimmerman RA. Tumors of the parapharyngeal space and upper neck: MR imaging characteristics. *Radiology* 1987;164:823–829.

108. Som PM, Sacher M, Lanzieri CF, et al. Parenchymal cysts of the lower neck. *Radiology* 1985;157:399–406.

109. Som PM, Sacher M, Lanzieri CF, Shugar JMA, Biller HF. Two benign CT presentations of thyroid-related papillary adenocarcinoma. *J Comput Assist Tomogr* 1985;9:162–166.

110. Spritzer CE, Gefter WB, Hamilton R, Greenberg BM, Axel L, Kressel HY. Abnormal parathyroid glands: high-resolution MR imaging. *Radiology* 1987;162:487–491.

111. Stark DD, Felder RC, Wittenberg J, et al. Magnetic resonance imaging of cavernous hemangioma of the liver: tissue-specific characterization. *AJR* 1985;145:213–222.

112. Stark DD, Gooding GAW, Clark OH. Noninvasive parathyroid imaging. *Semin Ultrasound Comput Tomogr Magn Reson* 1985;6:310–320.

113. Stark DD, Gooding GAW, Moss AA, Clark OH, Ovenfors CO. Parathyroid imaging: comparison of high-resolution CT and high-resolution sonography. *AJR* 1983;141:633–638.

114. Stark DD, Lufkin RB, Hanafee WN. The neck. In: Brant-Zawadzki M, Norman D, eds. *Magnetic resonance imaging of the central nervous system.* New York: Raven Press, 1987:359–390.

115. Stark DD, Moss AA, Gamsu G, et al. Magnetic resonance imaging of the neck. Part I. Normal anatomy. *Radiology* 1983;150:447–454.

116. Stark DD, Moss AA, Gamsu G, et al. Magnetic resonance imaging of the neck. Part II. Pathologic findings. *Radiology* 1983;150:455–461.

117. Stein MG, Gamsu G, Webb WR, Stulbarg MS. Computed tomography of diffuse tracheal stenosis in Wegener granulomatosis. *J Comput Assist Tomogr* 1986;10:868–870.

118. Stevens MH, Harnsberger HR, Mancuso AA, Davis RK, Johnson LP, Parkin JL. Computed tomography of cervical lymph nodes: staging and management of head and neck cancer. *Arch Otolaryngol* 1985;111:735–739.

119. Tucker GF Jr. The anatomy of laryngeal cancer. *Can J Otolaryngol* 1974;3:417–427.

120. Wang C. Surgical management of parathyroid disorders. In: Cummings CW, Fredrickson JM, Harker LA, Krause CJ, Schiller DE, eds. *Otolaryngology—head and neck surgery.* St. Louis: Mosby, 1986:2525–2542.

121. Ward MP, Glazer HS, Heiken JP, Spector JG. Traumatic perforation of the pyriform sinus: CT demonstration. *J Comput Assist Tomogr* 1985;9:982–984.

122. Wing V, Scheible W. Sonography of jugular vein thrombosis. *AJR* 1983;140:333–336.

123. Winzelberg GG, Hydovitz JD. Radionuclide imaging of parathyroid tumors: historical perspectives and newer techniques. *Semin Nucl Med* 1985;15:161–170.

124. Winzelberg GG, Hydovitz JD, O'Hara KR, et al. Parathyroid adenomas evaluated by Tl-201/Tc-99m pertechnetate subtraction scintigraphy and high-resolution ultrasonography. *Radiology* 1985;155:231–235.

125. Wortham DG, Hoover LA, Lufkin RB, Fu YS. Magnetic resonance imaging of the larynx: a correlation with histologic sections. *Otolaryngol Head Neck Surg* 1986;94:123–133.

126. Yeager VL, Archer CR. Anatomical routes for cancer invasion of laryngeal cartilages. *Laryngoscope* 1982;92:449–452.

127. Yeager VL, Lawson C, Archer CR. Ossification of the laryngeal cartilages as it relates to computed tomography. *Invest Radiol* 1982;1:11–19.

CHAPTER 7

Thorax: Technique and Normal Anatomy

Stuart S. Sagel and Harvey S. Glazer

The plain chest radiograph remains the primary radiologic technique to evaluate the thorax, mainly because it is simple to obtain, comparatively inexpensive, and relatively sensitive in providing information about the lungs, pleura, and bones. Particular clinical advantages of computed tomography (CT) in assessing the thorax include its cross-sectional imaging format (allowing distinction between structures that are superimposed on conventional radiography), superior contrast sensitivity (permitting distinction of much smaller differences in electron densities than with conventional roentgenography, by a factor of approximately 10), and wide dynamic range (capturing the entire spectrum of densities within the thorax, including the lungs, soft tissues, and bones, with a single exposure) (76,106,121,137).

The cross-sectional depiction of anatomy achieved with CT provides an additional dimension to conventional radiology and can help to clarify or detect suspected abnormalities in locations where overlapping structures would otherwise prevent a full three-dimensional evaluation. This is particularly true in the mediastinum (11,27,68,72), in the subpleural areas of the lung, and in the peridiaphragmatic region. The format, however, means that only a small part of the thorax is demonstrated on each slice. The inability of the patient to accurately reproduce the same lung volume for each sequential scan can lead to some missed areas between slices, introducing the possibility of failure to detect a small pulmonary lesion (82). In addition, the transaxial imaging plane may be disadvantageous for displaying longitudinally oriented structures, such as the aorta, or for evaluating structures that largely fall in the same plane of section, such as the diaphragm. Such limitations may be overcome by appropriately utilized direct sagittal or coronal imaging with magnetic resonance imaging (MRI).

The naturally high contrast that is observed within the aerated lungs has always made conventional radiographic techniques extremely effective for evaluation of pulmo-

nary parenchymal abnormalities. The superior contrast sensitivity of CT is a critical asset in the thorax for evaluation of the individual elements composing the mediastinum and chest wall profiled by their surrounding fat, and sometimes in determining the density of pulmonary nodules. The better contrast sensitivity and wider dynamic range of CT as compared with conventional roentgenography reflect the superiority of electronic detectors over film-screen combinations, as well as the extremely efficient scatter rejection inherent in generating a CT image (15). The improved density discrimination of CT aids in distinguishing among the vascular, lipomatous, water, and soft-tissue densities of various thoracic lesions (116). Such tissue characterization may be crucial in differentiating between a benign process and malignant disease and, in some patients, obviates further invasive diagnostic evaluation. It cannot be overemphasized, however, that CT is incapable of providing a histologic diagnosis for the overwhelming majority of largely soft-tissue-density masses, and some tissue sampling technique is generally required for such distinction. Unfortunately, in most instances, MRI has failed to fulfill its promise as being a more specific discriminator of the type of pathologic process than CT.

Computed tomography is inferior to standard radiography in terms of spatial and temporal resolution (12). The former deficit results mainly from the larger size of the CT X-ray detector as compared with the rare-earth or calcium tungstate crystals of intensifying screens. Although spatial resolution in the longitudinal axis can be improved somewhat by narrow collimation, this decreases the number of photons reaching the detector (thus increasing quantum noise and decreasing contrast sensitivity) (20,92,144) and also necessitates a larger number of scans to cover a given area. The latter results not only in increased examination time but also in some increase in absorbed radiation dose. Temporal resolution is limited by the time required to produce a scan. Only one commercially available scanner, designed primarily for cardiac studies, has a scan time short enough to stop cardiac motion (141).

TECHNIQUE

Almost all adults, except the rare writhing patient, can be satisfactorily studied with CT. Because of the expanding indications for CT (and MRI) in solving problems related to the thorax, plus the myriad and sometimes unpredictable forms in which a pathologic process may become manifest, no single technique is optimal for all studies. An eclectic approach to the examination is recommended. After review of the already available clinical and radiologic data, each study should be tailored to the particular primary clinical problem to be resolved. It is optimal that studies be monitored, while in progress, by the radiologist, who might intervene and modify the protocol at any stage because of evolving findings. All examinations should be reviewed, ideally before the patient is removed from the scanner, but at least while the patient is still in the scanning area. The short image reconstruction times available with almost all modern scanners should make this feasible.

The CT examination of the thorax generally is begun with a digital localization radiograph ("topogram," "scout view," etc.), usually in the anteroposterior projection. The levels selected for scanning can be determined from this radiograph and ultimately displayed on it. After photography with the completed CT examination, it can be used for correlation with the transverse CT images, which may be of value in planning radiation therapy or in deciding on an approach to biopsy.

Computed tomography of the thorax usually is performed in the supine position with the patient's arms elevated above the head to minimize artifacts from the shoulders and upper extremities. The patient is asked to suspend respiration in full inspiration during the brief time of scanning, which provides optimal assessment of the pulmonary parenchyma. In expiration, the pulmonary vessels are crowded together, lung density is increased, and the mediastinum appears wider (122). In the supine position, the attenuation values of the posterior portions of the lungs are higher than those of the anterior areas, because pulmonary perfusion is greater and lung inflation is slightly diminished in the dependent zones. These gradients are reversed with the patient prone. Consequently, on rare occasion, when the posterior lung base is the region of primary concern, prone scans that increase the aeration in this area can help better define the vessels and distinguish them from nodules or infiltrates. Similarly, a patient scanned supine infrequently shows a curvilinear band of increased density posteriorly in the lungs adjacent to the pleural surface; this almost certainly represents transient subsegmental atelectasis, because it disappears promptly when the patient is scanned in the prone position. Lateral decubitus scans may rarely be of value in distinguishing between a complex pleural process and pulmonary abnormality (e.g., empyema from lung abscess); they also can be helpful in directing an interventional biopsy or drainage procedure.

Scan Thickness and Time

Initially, contiguous scans 8 to 10 mm thick generally are obtained from the lung apex through the caudal costophrenic angles. In patients known to have or suspected of having bronchogenic carcinoma, scanning should be extended into the upper abdomen to include the adrenals and liver, because the former is a relatively common site of metastasis. Narrower collimation (2–5 mm) may be advantageous or necessary in selected cases when partial-volume averaging needs to be reduced. Thin slices can be valuable in areas of complex anatomy, such as the hila or aortopulmonary window (Fig. 1), where little fat may be present, for detection of small mediastinal masses (e.g., thymoma or parathyroid adenoma), especially in thin patients, for precise depiction of bronchial anatomy and documentation of bronchiectasis, and for quantitative densitometric analysis of a small pulmonary nodule. In selecting the optimal slice thickness, several variables must be considered: the depicted size of the abnormality to be detected or demonstrated, the range of density of the suspected lesion relative to that of surrounding anatomy (subject contrast), and the anatomy of the area relative to the orientation of the scan plane (19). In general, it is true that the greater the slice thickness, the more likely that an individual anatomic detail will be lost through the phenomenon of partial-volume averaging. However, as emphasized previously, the constant trade-off between improved spatial resolution in the cephalocaudal axis with narrow collimation must be balanced against the increased image "noise" and longer examination time. In the low-density lung parenchyma, a large slice thickness is advantageous, because most pathologic pulmonary processes are of much higher density than the normal lung and thus are visible if only a small portion of the abnormality is included in the slice thickness. Pulmonary nodules as small as 1 mm in diameter can be depicted on a 10-mm-thick CT section. Thick sections of the lung also make it easier to distinguish between normal structures, such as pulmonary vessels, which may be obliquely oriented through the plane of section, and pathologic processes. In the mediastinum, where generally enough profiling fat is present, 10-mm sections permit detection of lesions as small as 3 mm.

Short scanning times (4 or 5 sec) are particularly important in the thorax to eliminate artifacts related to respiration. The vast majority of patients can sustain breath holding for such periods if they are instructed properly before scanning commences. The few additional moments

A,B

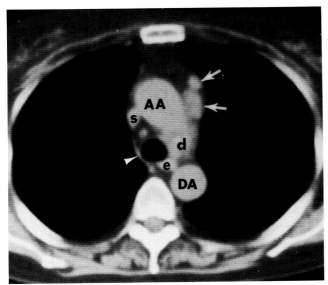 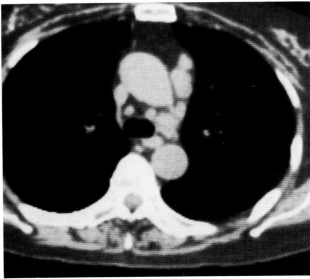

FIG. 1. Value of narrow collimation. **A:** Scan with 8-mm collimation at level of aortopulmonary window demonstrates a soft-tissue density (d) in the subaortic window between the ascending aorta (AA) and descending aorta (DA). Is this due to lymphadenopathy or partial-volume averaging with the top of the pulmonary artery? Enlarged lymph nodes in the paraaortic area (*arrows*) would favor the former possibility. A normal-size pretracheal (azygos) lymph node is seen medial to the azygos vein arch (*arrowhead*). (s) superior vena cava; (e) esophagus. **B:** Scan with 4-mm collimation demonstrates that the mass in subaortic window is composed of discretely enlarged lymph nodes.

required to provide breathing instructions and for rehearsal are quickly rewarded in terms of study quality. Shorter scan times (1–2 sec) are selected only if it is apparent that longer breath holding may be a problem in a given patient.

Window Settings

The scale of CT numbers generated by the reconstruction process is greatest in the thorax, ranging from the almost air density of the lungs to the substantially higher bone density of the vertebral bodies. Such disparate densities cannot be effectively displayed in a single image because of the limited number of shades of gray that can be electronically depicted or appreciated by the human retina (12). Each thoracic CT examination should have each scan level viewed with at least two and sometimes three different window settings. There should be one optimized for the mediastinum and chest wall, and one for the lungs; whenever necessary, an additional setting for the bones should be used. The "double-window" technique showing the mediastinum and lung simultaneously is not advocated; false images are created at interfaces, and anatomy is sometimes distorted. Whereas the images generated may be interesting to show in a conference, they are unsatisfactory for routine clinical diagnosis.

The precise settings often are a matter of subjective preference or are related to specific equipment variabilities. Narrow window width settings are rarely needed in the thorax because of the high natural contrast present. If accurate size measurements are sought, the window level should be placed at the midpoint between the average CT number of the structure to be measured and the average CT number of the surrounding tissue (13,80). For example, the size of a pulmonary nodule having an attenuation value of 100 Hounsfield units (HU) surrounded by lung with an average value of −700 HU will be most accurately determined at a window level of −300 HU.

Multiplanar Reconstruction

Coronal, sagittal, and/or oblique images may be generated from the data provided by a series of consecutive transaxial scans. Such rearrangement achieved by computer manipulations can be useful in regions of complex anatomy, such as in the peridiaphragmatic areas (34). The quality of these reformatted views improves with thinner and more closely spaced transverse sections, which necessarily requires a far greater number of scans to cover a given area and is thus quite time-consuming. For practical purposes, it is rare that such reformatted images provide clinically relevant information in addition to that obtained from the transverse images. Most experienced interpreters of CT images can visually reconstruct three-dimensional anatomy by mentally integrating successive CT slices. On occasion, these reconstructions can be helpful in conveying three-dimensional information to less experienced clinicians or for teaching purposes.

A,B

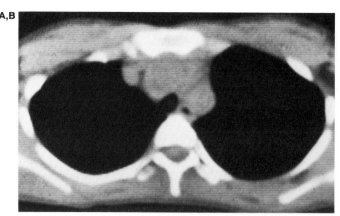
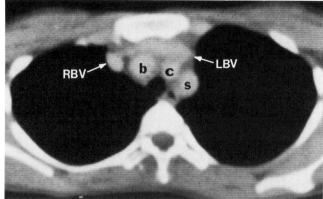

FIG. 2. Intravenous administration of contrast material, modified infusion, manual technique. Normal superior mediastinum in patient with a paucity of mediastinal fat. **A:** The mediastinal vessels are not well delineated, making exclusion of lymphadenopathy difficult. **B:** On scan after contrast enhancement, the mediastinal arteries and veins are well demonstrated; no abnormal mass is present. (RBV) right brachiocephalic vein; (LBV) left brachiocephalic vein; (b) brachiocephalic artery; (c) left common carotid artery; (s) left subclavian artery.

Intravenous Contrast Enhancement

The thorax has the highest intrinsic natural contrast of any body part. The pulmonary vessels and ribs have markedly different densities than the adjacent aerated lung. In the majority of adults, the mediastinal vessels and lymph nodes are embedded in sufficient amounts of surrounding fat that they can be readily distinguished. Therefore, provided normal anatomy is known in detail and sequential scans are carefully analyzed, routine use of intravenous contrast material is unnecessary in most patients. However, in properly selected cases, intravenous administration of contrast material may be not only beneficial but also essential to arrive at the proper diagnosis.

Use of intravenous contrast agents generally should be reserved for cases in which (a) insufficient mediastinal fat is present, making identification of normal vascular structures difficult, (b) confusion arises concerning differentiation of a normal variant or congenital anomaly involving a mediastinal vessel from a pathologic process, either a vascular abnormality (e.g., aneurysm) or a soft-tissue mass, or (c) characterization of a lesion by observing its enhancement pattern is desired (e.g., separation of complex pleuroparenchymal abnormality).

Intravenous contrast material should preferentially be injected through an 18- or 19-gauge needle into a medially directed antecubital vein, because drainage is directly to the basilic system and the superior vena cava. If a laterally

A,B

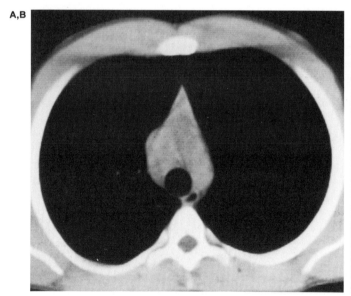
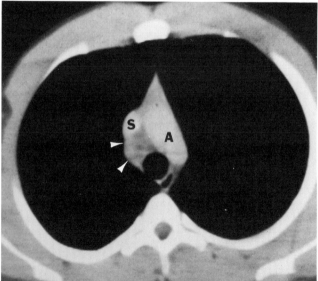

FIG. 3. Intravenous administration of contrast material, modified infusion, manual technique. Right paratracheal lymphadenopathy in thin patient. **A:** The normal mediastinal vessels are not well defined. **B:** On scan after contrast enhancement, an enlarged 3-cm right paratracheal lymph node mass (*arrowheads*) is depicted; (S) superior vena cava; (A) aortic arch.

directed antecubital vein is chosen, because these drain into the cephalic system, flow of contrast material into the cava often is impeded because of multiple interposed valves and the circuitous course resulting from placing the arms above the head in the usual position for scanning.

Several different methods of intravenous contrast enhancement can be used for body CT scanning, each having a particular advantage depending on the clinical situation. These techniques can be separated into two categories: "modified" infusion or "dynamic" scanning.

When a large area of the thorax requires evaluation during intravenous administration of contrast material (e.g., the entire mediastinum in a thin patient), sustained enhancement of the major vessels may be accomplished manually (Figs. 2 and 3) or with a power injector (Fig. 4) by using a "modified" infusion technique. This continuous type of infusion provides a relatively constant level of intravenous contrast material that can be maintained for the relatively long periods required to complete scanning of large areas. The simple rapid infusion of intravenous contrast material advocated in the early days of body CT scanning has become obsolete; a bolus injection

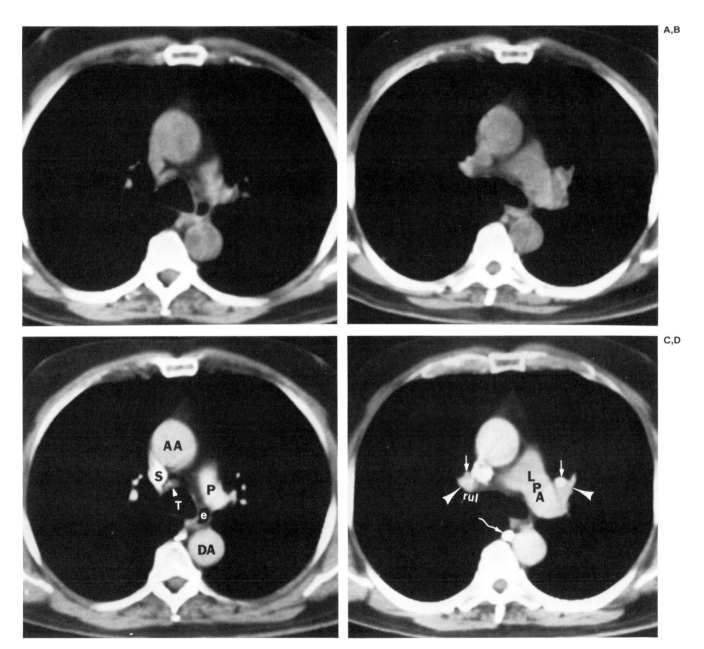

FIG. 4. Intravenous administration of contrast material, modified infusion, power injector. Normal anatomy. **A,B:** Non-contrast-enhanced scans at level of distal trachea and carina, respectively. **C,D:** Same levels after contrast enhancement; (AA) ascending aorta; (DA) descending aorta; (P) top of left pulmonary artery; (LPA) left pulmonary artery; (S) superior vena cava; (T) trachea; (e) esophagus; (rul) right-upper-lobe bronchus; (*straight arrows*) superior pulmonary veins; (*large arrowheads*) upper-lobe pulmonary arteries; (*small arrowhead*) normal pretracheal lymph node; (*curved arrow*) azygos vein.

A,B

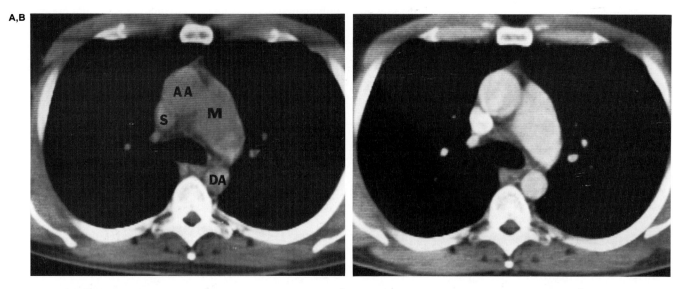

FIG. 5. Intravenous administration of contrast material, bolus technique. **A:** A soft-tissue-density "mass" (M) is seen in the aortopulmonary window; (AA) ascending aorta; (DA) descending aorta; (S) superior vena cava. **B:** Scan after contrast enhancement shows that apparent mass is clearly an enlarged main and left pulmonary artery.

should always precede the infusion to obtain an initial relatively high level of intravenous contrast material.

Following a bolus of 35 to 50 ml of 60% iodinated contrast material, a rapid infusion of 150 ml of 60% contrast material is started. Such an infusion through an 18-gauge needle usually takes 6 to 8 min to accomplish. If scanning is begun coincident with the initiation of the infusion, at least 20 to 25 scans can be obtained on almost all modern scanners during this time period, thus easily encompassing the large area of interest. Use of a mechanical flow-rate injector (e.g., Medrad Mark IV) also allows a sustained but more reproducible level of contrast enhancement (112,113,130). However, it requires the insertion of an

"Intracath" into a medially directed antecubital vein to markedly diminish the risk of extravasation of contrast material into the soft tissues. A communicative, cooperative patient is essential if a power injector is used, because the injection must be terminated immediately if local "burning" (pain) occurs, to prevent substantial tissue damage. The injector is loaded with 150 ml of 60% contrast material. Contrast material is injected at a rate of 2 ml/sec for 15 sec (to "prime the pump," similar to the manual technique just described), and then at 1 ml/sec for whatever time is necessary to complete scanning. Scanning is commenced 16 sec after initiation of the injection.

A,B

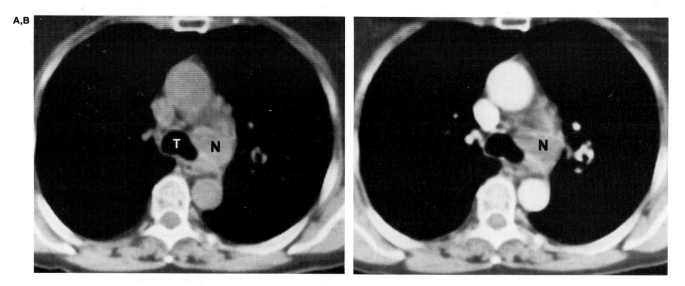

FIG. 6. Intravenous administration of contrast material, bolus technique. **A:** A soft-tissue-density mass (N) is seen in the aortopulmonary window, flattening the left side of the distal trachea (T). **B:** Scan after administration of contrast material demonstrates no notable enhancement of markedly enlarged subaortic lymph nodes (N).

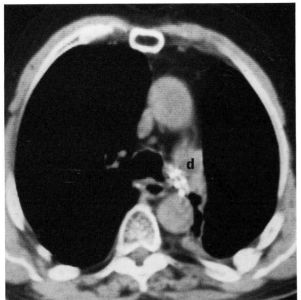 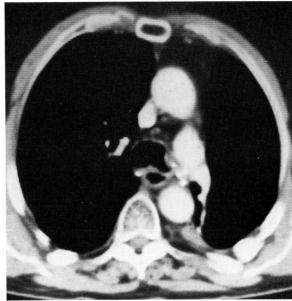

FIG. 7. Intravenous administration of contrast material, bolus technique, in a 73-year-old man 2 years following left upper lobectomy for bronchogenic carcinoma. **A:** Soft-tissue density (d) seen in aortopulmonary window just lateral to metallic clips. Does this represent recurrent carcinoma? **B:** Scan after contrast enhancement demonstrates that the density in question is the normal remaining left main and lower-lobe artery displaced cephalad by the previous surgery.

The major drawbacks of the "modified" infusion techniques are the use of a high total volume of contrast material (up to 200 ml of 60% solution) and the generally lower level of vascular enhancement than can be achieved using "dynamic" techniques.

Dynamic scanning is defined simply as the ability to acquire a series of scans in a short period of time. A short scan time (5 sec or less) with a minimal delay (3 sec or less) between them is presumed. Combined with a rapid bolus injection of intravenous contrast material, it can be performed at a single level after a relatively small bolus (25–50 ml) or at sequential levels during the administration of a larger and more sustained bolus (100 ml).

Dynamic scanning at a single level after a bolus injection of contrast material provides phasic information regarding blood flow and the "vascularity" of a lesion or structure at that level (Figs. 5–7). It ensures dense opacification of any potential vascular structure under investigation on at least one of the serial images (Fig. 8). Guesswork that otherwise might be necessary because of individual variations in circulation times is eliminated, and consequently the volume of contrast material required for a diagnostic study is often reduced. Four scans at approximately 8, 15, 22, and 30 sec after initiation of the bolus injection usually suffice to see the peripherally injected contrast material progressing through the mediastinal veins and arteries. The peak enhancement of a structure reveals whether it is supplied by a systemic or pulmonary artery or vein (Fig. 9). This generally enables clear depiction of all major vessels at that level and can

permit diagnosis of such entities as pulmonary arteriovenous malformation (Fig. 10) and sequestration (58,118).

Incomplete mixing of unopacified and opacified blood in the superior vena cava after a bolus injection occasionally can create a "filling defect" simulating a thrombus (57). Such flow-related artifacts may be central or peripheral. Dynamic scanning should always show that the apparent filling defect is inconsistent (e.g., seen only on the first or last scan) and is therefore artifactual (Fig. 11).

A small amount of air occasionally is seen in a central vein after intravenous injection of contrast material (Fig. 12). Whereas this has been described in association with a mass obstructing the superior vena cava, it certainly can occur without vascular obstruction and probably is due to some air present in the syringe or tubing that is inadvertently injected (32).

Reports of previous studies using older equipment and infusions of contrast material have described nonvascular structures, such as lymph nodes (e.g., angiofollicular lymph node hyperplasia) or masses (e.g., goiter), that have been enhanced sufficiently to be confused with a large vascular structure, or perhaps a thrombus-filled aneurysm might simulate a neoplasm by not filling with contrast material. Such occurrences rarely, if ever, happen today if proper bolus technique and modern equipment are used.

Rapid serial scanning at contiguous levels during a bolus injection of contrast material, often called "dynamic incremental scanning," provides anatomic information about a larger area and is valuable for confidently distinguishing blood vessels from nonvascular structures or

Text continues on page 179.

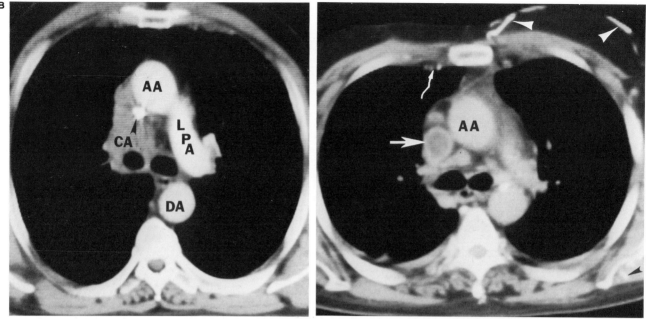

FIG. 8. Intravenous administration of contrast material, assessment of the status of the superior vena cava. **A:** Marked narrowing of superior vena cava (*arrowhead*) in patient with bronchogenic carcinoma (CA) infiltrating the mediastinum; (AA) ascending aorta; (LPA) left pulmonary artery; (DA) descending aorta. **B:** Large thrombus (*straight arrow*) in superior vena cava in patient with lymphoma (and Raaf catheter in right brachiocephalic vein). Note the large venous collaterals in the left anterior chest wall and around the left scapula (*arrowheads*) following injection of contrast material into a left medial antecubital vein; (AA) ascending aorta; (*curved arrow*) enhanced internal mammary vessels.

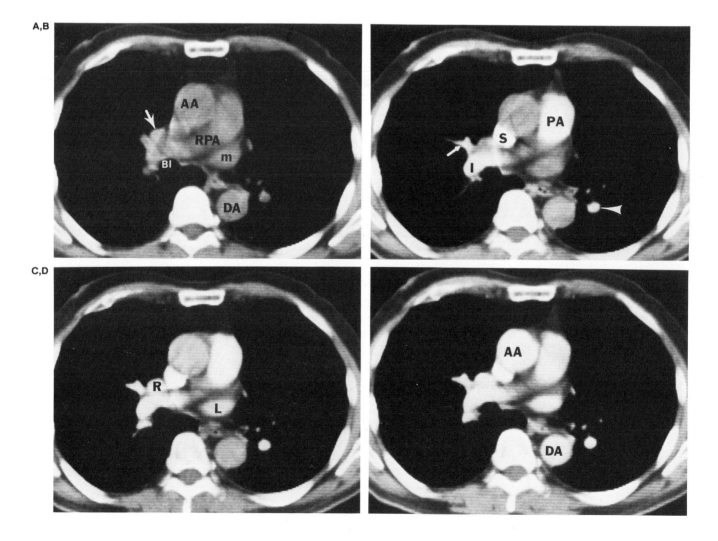

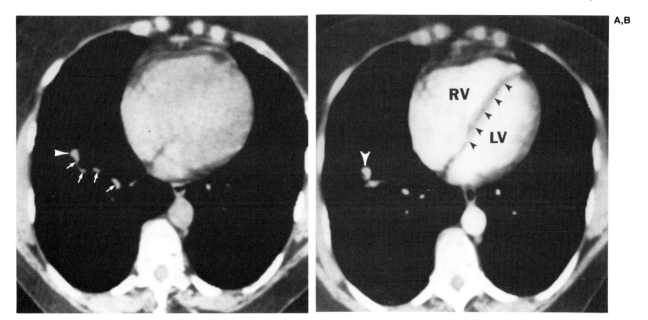

FIG. 10. Pulmonary arteriovenous malformation in a 51-year-old woman referred for evaluation of a right-lower-lobe "nodule" detected on plain chest roentgenogram; on CT scan with standard collimation, a noncalcified right-lower-lobe nodular density was seen. **A:** This 2-mm collimated scan shows the noncalcified nodule (*arrowhead*) to be contiguous with an enlarged right-lower-lobe vessel (*arrows*). **B:** Scan following bolus injection of intravenous contrast material shows enhancement of nodular lesion (*white arrowhead*) to same degree as contiguous enlarged vessel; (RV) right ventricle; (LV) left ventricle; (*black arrowheads*) interventricular septum.

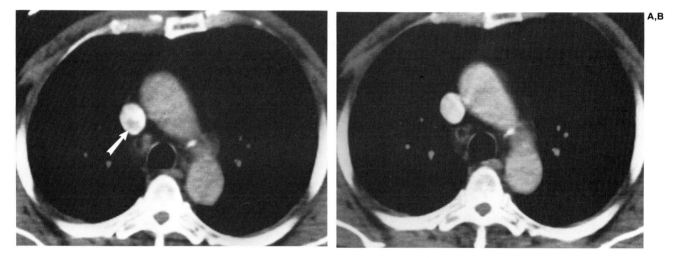

FIG. 11. Flow defect in superior vena cava following bolus intravenous injection of contrast material. **A:** Filling defect (*arrow*) posteriorly within the superior vena cava is seen on the initial scan. **B:** Scan 8 sec later shows that the defect has disappeared and simply represented a flow-related artifact (compare with Fig. 8B).

FIG. 9. Pulmonary hila, dynamic single-level scanning. **A:** Non-contrast-enhanced CT scan shows a slightly lobulated density (*arrow*) anteriorly in the right hilum and a questionable ovoid mass (m) in the left hilum posterior to the origin of the right pulmonary artery (RPA); (AA) ascending aorta; (DA) descending aorta; (BI) bronchus intermedius. **B:** Initial scan immediately after bolus injection of contrast material. The superior vena cava (S) is densely opacified, and there is enhancement of the main pulmonary artery (PA), the right interlobar pulmonary artery (I), the truncus anterior branch (*arrow*), and the left-lower-lobe pulmonary artery (*arrowhead*). **C:** Scan at same level 8 sec later shows enhancement of the structures in question, which represent, respectively, the right superior pulmonary vein (R) and the junction of the left pulmonary vein with the left atrial appendage (L). **D:** Scan 8 sec later optimally opacifies the ascending (AA) and descending (DA) aorta.

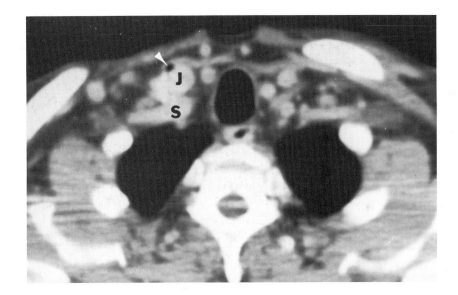

FIG. 12. A small amount of air (*arrowhead*) is seen in the right internal jugular vein (J) on scan performed during infusion of contrast material into a right medial antecubital vein. The air has refluxed anteriorly from the right subclavian vein (S).

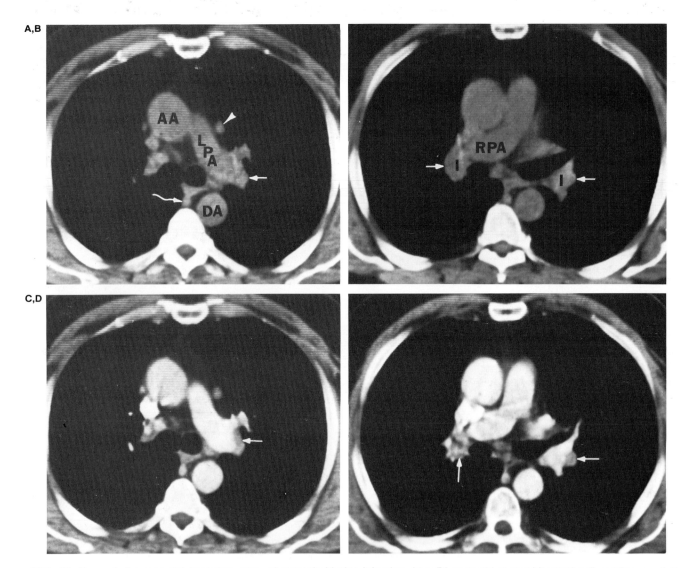

FIG. 13. Dynamic incremental scanning, manual extended bolus injection, in a 51-year-old man with renal cell carcinoma. **A,B:** Sequential caudal non-contrast-enhanced scans through the hila demonstrate mild lobularity (*straight arrows*) bilaterally, especially around the interlobar pulmonary arteries (I). A mildly enlarged left subaortic node (*arrowhead*) is also noted; (AA) ascending aorta; (DA) descending aorta; (LPA) left pulmonary artery; (RPA) right pulmonary artery; (*curved arrow*) azygos vein. **C,D:** Contrast-enhanced scans demonstrate bilateral hilar lymphadenopathy (*arrows*) surrounding the hilar arteries.

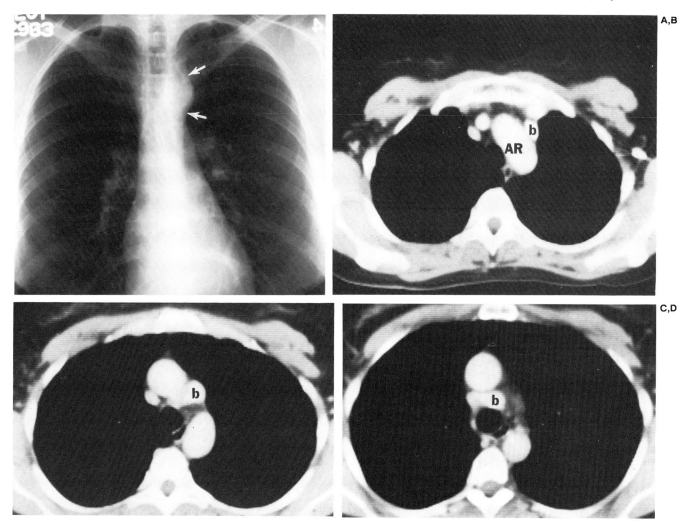

FIG. 14. Dynamic incremental scanning, power injector. **A:** Posteroanterior chest radiograph in a 38-year-old woman demonstrates widening of the mediastinum (*arrows*) superimposed on the aortic knob. **B–D:** Serial caudal scans during sustained intravenous bolus injection of contrast material demonstrate an anomalous left brachiocephalic vein (b) coursing underneath the aortic arch (AR), to join the right brachiocephalic vein, accounting for extra density seen on plain chest radiograph.

masses within the area (e.g., the entire pulmonary hila) (Fig. 13) (47,79,120). The technique is best accomplished with a more extended bolus injection. Scanning commences after about 50 ml of the 100-ml total is injected, and the table is moved during the interscan delay. The mechanical flow-rate injector previously described for use in the modified infusion technique can also be used to deliver a sustained bolus (a constant rate of 2 ml/sec, with scanning begun 20 sec after the start of the injection, is optimal) (Fig. 14). This serves to eliminate scattered radiation exposure to radiologic personnel; the previously described caveats regarding the use of this injector still apply.

CT Numbers

The use of CT numbers for *in vivo* tissue characterization is compromised by a variety of technical and geo-metric factors. Such numbers cannot be taken as absolute values; they are semiquantitative at best (86). These attenuation values are influenced by patient geometry, the specific scanner, the reconstruction filter and scan time, the size and position of the object to be measured, and the composition of surrounding tissues (156).

The X-ray beam used is not monochromatic, and its lower-energy components are selectively attenuated as it passes through the body, making the beam "harder" with depth. Because the harder beam experiences less attenuation, the CT numbers are lower in the center of the body. Some compensations are possible, but simple corrections are not feasible because of the heterogeneity of the thorax and the variable thicknesses of the chest wall and mediastinum, the aeration of the lung, and the presence of any interposed bone (93). In interpreting dynamic scans after intravenous injection of contrast material, some of the changes in the object under study may be artifactual, relating to the changing iodine concentrations in surrounding tissues. Although time–density curves may look impressive in articles or presentations, their true scientific basis is somewhat suspect (119), and they almost never add critical information to that which can be extracted from careful visual inspection of serial images.

The CT number calculated for a voxel is the average attenuation of all of its contents (15). When the object of interest does not completely fill a given voxel, the number, in part, will reflect the attenuation value of whatever extraneous material fills the rest of the voxel. Such partial-volume effects are particularly troublesome in assessing pulmonary nodules because of the large difference in density between the soft tissue of the nodule and the surrounding aerated lung. Although narrow collimation can reduce such partial-volume artifacts in the longitudinal (z) axis, some artifact will persist at the edges of a nodule in the transverse plane (x and y axes). Voxels at the edges are also subject to artifacts introduced during the mathematical reconstruction process, especially when edge enhancement or smoothing algorithms are used.

Motion not only degrades spatial resolution but also can create streaks in the reconstructed image tangent to the moving surface. This problem may occur in even fully cooperative patients along the free wall of the left ventricle because of its vigorous motion and the high degree of contrast between it and the adjacent lung. Respiratory motion may sometimes cause doubling of an image, in addition to blurring; a thickened dilated bronchus might be simulated. Radiating patterns of streak artifacts can arise from surgical clips, pacemaker wires and electrodes, and prosthetic valves; motion of these metallic objects aggravates the streaking.

MRI

Although MRI has a completely different physical basis than CT for generation of thin tomographic sections, current (proton) imaging is predominantly an anatomic study. In most instances, as with X-ray CT, tissue-specific diagnosis remains impossible. Because in these circumstances CT and MRI provide relatively comparable data, prevailing technical and economic factors militate against MRI being considered the procedure of choice for tomographic imaging of the thorax (4). Generally, it is reserved for answering specific questions raised by prior CT studies that were equivocal or confusing. However, in a patient in whom vascular abnormality is suspected, especially when the patient is allergic to iodinated contrast material or has severe renal disease, or when venous access for injection is extremely difficult, MRI generally will be the preferred technique. Usually there is no difficulty in readily recognizing vascular variants or anomalies that might cause confusion on non-contrast-enhanced CT studies (Fig. 15). Although MRI obviates intravenous contrast material, most CT studies of the thorax are diagnostic without the necessity for its use, so that this is not a major advantage.

Because of the substantial imaging times required to generate both T1- and T2-weighted sequences, most MRI studies are tailored to a particular clinical problem, and the whole thorax is not imaged. Even then, the study requires 30 to 45 min to accomplish, compared with about 20 min for the usual CT examination. Prior to the study, the procedure should be carefully explained to the patient. This will greatly aid in decreasing any claustrophobic tendencies and almost always will preclude premature ter-

A,B

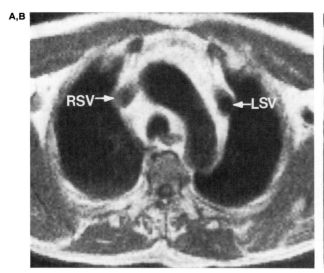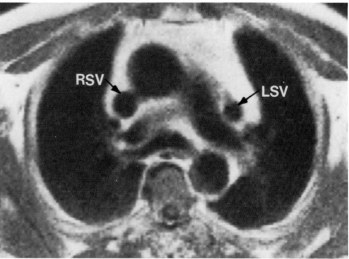

FIG. 15. Right (RSV) and left (LSV) superior vena cavae easily identified as vessels with absence of signal on MR images at two different levels.

mination of the examination before it is completed. Instructing the patient to inspire shallowly, while mainly using the diaphragm ("abdominal breathing") and attempting to hold the thorax relatively rigid, can improve anatomic definition in the mediastinum and anterior chest wall (Fig. 16).

MRI of the thorax is optimally accomplished using relatively T1-weighted (short TR, such as 500 msec; short TE, such as 15–30 msec) spin-echo pulse sequences (Fig. 17) (43,87,151). On T1-weighted images, tissues with shorter T1 values, such as mediastinal or axillary fat, are easily distinguished from masses of relatively lower intensities that usually have longer T1 values. On balanced images (long TR, short TE), signal intensities for most tissues are increased, improving the overall signal-to-noise ratio and image quality. Although in some cases this may be helpful in better demonstrating parenchymal and pleural disease, the contrast between most mediastinal masses and fat is decreased, sometimes making delineation of discrete masses more difficult. On T2-weighted images (long TR, long TE), tissues with longer T2 values, such

as fluid, have the most intense signal. Therefore, a pulse sequence that is more T2-weighted allows separation of higher-intensity cystic components of masses because of the long T2 value of fluid. Pleural fluid is also more easily seen (154). Contrast between chest-wall masses and muscle, of relatively low intensity, is also improved. However, in general, the contrast between most masses and mediastinal fat is decreased on T2-weighted images because of overlap in their T2 values. Scans usually are obtained at 1-cm intervals, with a thickness of 1 cm.

Although inherent cardiac motion does impair the spatial resolution of MR images of the chest, diagnostic studies of the mediastinum can be performed without cardiac triggering in most patients. Cardiac triggering does improve image quality, especially in the evaluation of hilar and juxtacardiac abnormalities and in the evaluation of the thoracic aorta. Advantages, however, are less obvious in the upper mediastinum and in patients with extensive mediastinal disease (Fig. 18). The disadvantages of cardiac triggering include slightly longer setup and imaging times. In addition, the radiologist has less control over the rep-

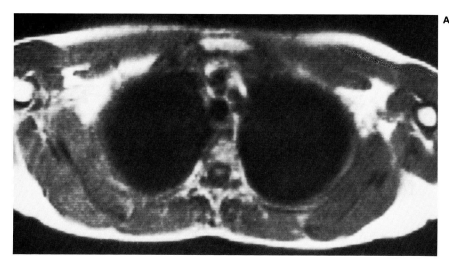

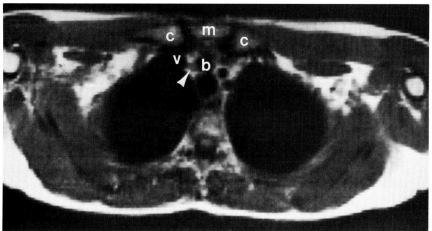

FIG. 16. MRI, effect of breathing. **A:** On T1-weighted spin-echo (SE) sequence with patient breathing "normally" there is some obscuration of the anatomic structures of the anterior chest wall and the great vessels in the mediastinum. **B:** After patient was instructed to breath shallowly and try to use just the diaphragm for respiration, the anatomy is more distinct. A small normal lymph node (*arrowhead*) can be seen between the right brachiocephalic vein (v) and the brachiocephalic artery (b). The manubrium (m) and clavicular heads (c) are well defined.

A

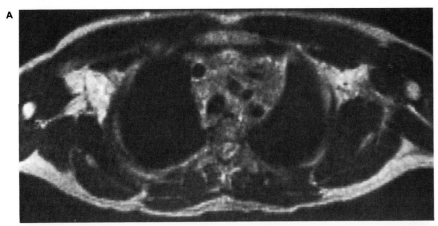

B

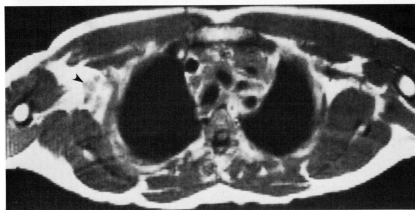

FIG. 17. MRI, dependence on pulse sequence selection. **A:** T2-weighted SE sequence (TR = 2,100 msec, TE = 90 msec) demonstrates mediastinal widening. **B:** T1-weighted SE sequence (TR = 500 msec, TE = 30 msec) shows multiple enlarged lymph nodes of intermediate signal intensity (higher than muscle, lower than subcutaneous fat) accounting for the widening. In addition, lymphadenopathy in the right axilla (*arrowhead*) is now visible. There is absence of signal in the great vessels and trachea.

etition time, because it is determined by the patient's heart rate. For example, a heart rate of 75 beats per minute translates to an effective TR of 800 msec. Images can be obtained with a longer TR by triggering data acquisition to alternate heart beats. An irregular cardiac rhythm will result in inconstant triggering. Potential confusion also can arise from intravascular signal during diastole.

Respiratory motion degrades MR images by increasing "noise" from ghost artifacts as well as from spatial blurring. The ghost artifacts propagate along the direction of the phase-encoding gradient and may obscure underlying normal or abnormal anatomy. Various techniques have been investigated to reduce image degradation. Using the respiratory cycle to control data collection (respiratory gating or triggering in which signal acquisition is limited to periods of apnea between breaths) may improve image quality, but imaging time is substantially prolonged. Several software strategies have been used to diminish respiratory artifacts without increasing scan time. Respiratory-ordered phase encoding (ROPE) diminishes ghost artifacts, but degradation from spatial blurring is not corrected. Recent attempts to reduce imaging time by using shorter echo delays with smaller flip angles may allow images to be obtained during breath holding (64). How-

ever, experience has been limited, especially in applying these techniques to the chest, and it is uncertain whether or not overall image quality will be sufficient.

Depending on the site and nature of any suspected or detected abnormality on the initial transaxial series of images, additional series, with or without EKG gating, can be obtained in the coronal, sagittal, or oblique plane (148). Such direct imaging in these orthogonal planes is fairly easy to accomplish with MRI and can be obtained without degradation in spatial resolution, as occurs with reformatted CT scans (Fig. 19). For practical purposes, transaxial MR images suffice to solve most clinical problems. However, these alternative planes may be valuable or critical in selected patients. Structures oriented cephalocaudally in the sagittal (e.g., aorta or trachea) (Figs. 20 and 21) or the coronal (e.g., superior vena cava) planes may be best imaged in this format (52,148). Theoretically, at least, these additional planes can provide an additional perspective and may be beneficial in defining anatomic relationships in complex areas and avoiding misinterpretation problems related to partial-volume averaging. For example, coronal imaging may be optimal for assessing the aortopulmonary window (Fig. 22), clearly distinguishing between the bottom of the aortic arch and the

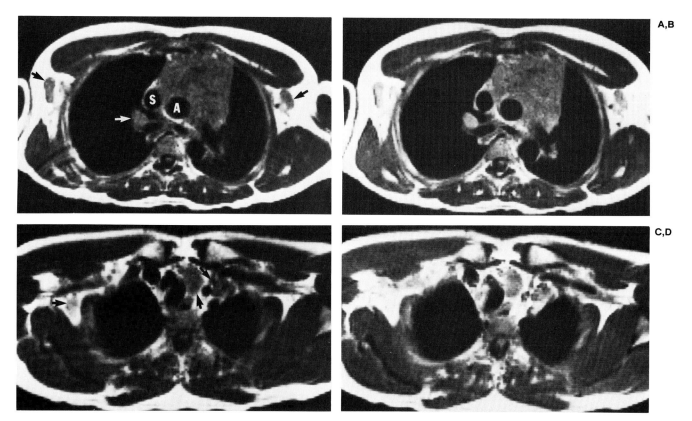

FIG. 18. MRI, effect of cardiac triggering. **A:** Nontriggered (TR = 500 msec, TE = 30 msec) image demonstrates right hilar and axillary lymphadenopathy (*arrows*) as well as extensive infiltration of the thymus in patient with lymphoma; (A) aorta; (S) superior vena cava. **B:** Similar findings are seen on the triggered image (TR = 850 msec, TE = 30 msec). The vascular structures are more sharply defined. Because the TR is longer, the overall signal is increased. However, mass/fat contrast is decreased, most noticeably in the axilla. **C:** On a more cephalad nontriggered image in the same patient, superior mediastinal and right axillary lymphadenopathy (*arrows*) is seen. **D:** Intraluminal signal within the arch vessels on a cardiac triggered image at the same level makes identification of these vessels more difficult than on the nontriggered image.

FIG. 19. MRI, oblique sagittal imaging. **A:** Standard transaxial image obtained initially to calculate angle between ascending and descending aorta. **B:** Oblique sagittal image demonstrating entire thoracic aorta in patient without atherosclerotic tortuosity; (AA) ascending aorta; (DA) descending aorta; (*arrowhead*) origin of left carotid artery; (*arrow*) origin of left subclavian artery.

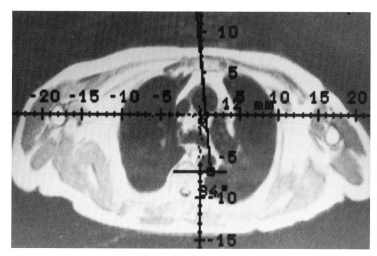

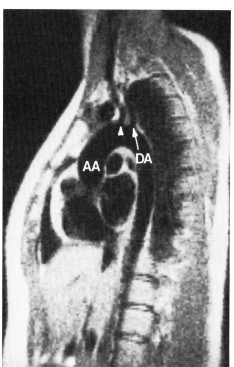

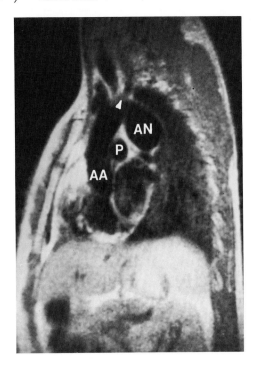

FIG. 20. MRI, oblique sagittal imaging. A posttraumatic aneurysm (AN) of the proximal descending aorta, originating just distal to the left subclavian artery (*arrowhead*), is seen; (AA) ascending aorta; (P) right pulmonary artery. (From ref. 52.)

top of the pulmonary artery and determining whether or not any mass is present, as well as best defining the relationship between a mass and the spinal canal. Similarly, sagittal imaging may optimally depict the extent of a mass near the pulmonary apex or the diaphragm.

Certain restrictions limit the application of MRI. Patients with cardiac pacemakers or ferromagnetic clips on medium- or large-size arteries and patients who are extremely ill (especially if mechanical ventilation or electronic monitoring is required) are not candidates for MRI.

CT-Guided Needle Biopsy

Fluoroscopy remains the radiologic procedure of choice to guide most percutaneous needle biopsies of thoracic lesions. It is readily available and relatively inexpensive to use, and it permits real-time depiction of the needle tip and the lesion throughout the course of the biopsy procedure. Most lung lesions can be biopsied quicker and easier using fluoroscopic guidance rather than CT guidance. In addition, because the radiologist is close to the patient throughout the procedure, the likelihood of complications probably is lessened. The patient is less likely to suddenly move, because of surprise or confusion, than if left alone in the CT scanner while needle position is being confirmed. Criteria for determining which lesions require direct needle guidance by CT vary somewhat and

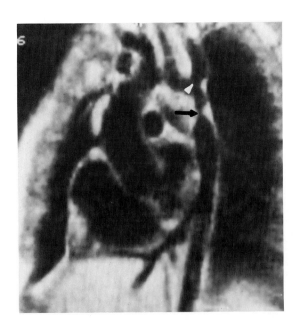

FIG. 21. MRI, oblique sagittal imaging. A coarctation of the aorta (*arrow*) is seen distal to the left subclavian artery (*arrowhead*).

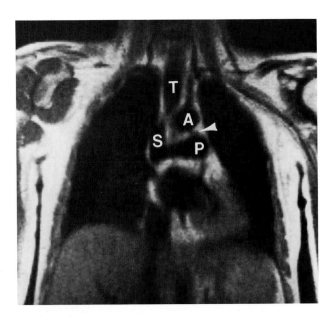

FIG. 22. MRI, coronal imaging. The fat and a normal lymph node (*arrowhead*) are clearly depicted within the aortopulmonary window. (A) aortic knob; (P) main pulmonary artery; (S) superior vena cava; (T) trachea.

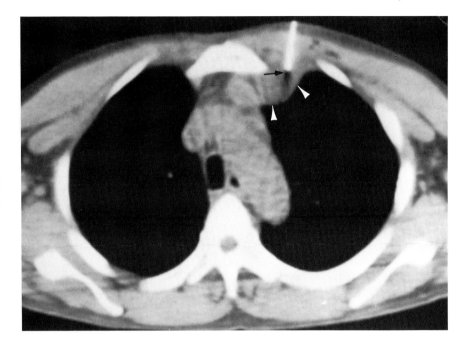

FIG. 23. CT-guided percutaneous needle biopsy. Pleural-based mass (*arrowheads*) that was difficult to define and localize on fluoroscopy was easily biopsied with an 18-gauge cutting-type (Franseen) needle. Low-density artifact (*arrow*) demarcates correct position of needle tip within the mass. Diagnosis: recurrent Hodgkin disease.

depend in part on the experience of the radiologist responsible for the procedure. In our institution, only about 10% of transthoracic needle biopsies are done under CT guidance. Such CT guidance is required only when the mass to be biopsied is not well seen or localized during fluoroscopy (Fig. 23), or when precise needle tip direction and/or placement are critical to avoid puncture of a major vessel (Fig. 24).

It should be emphasized, however, that in our practice, CT scans are almost always available to provide information about a thoracic lesion prior to any contemplated percutaneous biopsy. CT can precisely define the lesion and its extent prior to the biopsy procedure (using any technique), and it accurately depicts surrounding structures that must be traversed using a percutaneous approach (24,53). Adjunctive data regarding the relation-

A,B

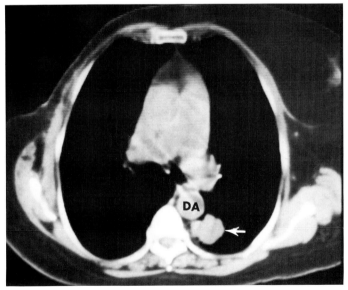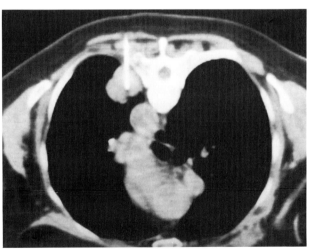

FIG. 24. CT-guided percutaneous needle biopsy. **A:** Scan in 59-year-old woman following right mastectomy demonstrates a lobulated 3-cm mass (*arrow*) in the superior segment of the left lower lobe. At fluoroscopy, the lesion could not be confidently distinguished from the descending aorta (DA). **B:** Aspiration biopsy of mass performed with CT guidance with patient in the prone position. Diagnosis: bronchogenic carcinoma.

ships of the mass to large vessels, to the pulmonary fissures, and to nearby bullae can be obtained. Such preinterventional information can be invaluable in planning the simplest and most appropriate biopsy approach and in facilitating a safe route for any needle placement. The use of cursors and grids with CT scans allows depth and angulation measurements to be exact. In most patients, the major vascular structures can be avoided during manipulation of the needle. Although in the pre-CT era these vessels were sometimes traversed with a thin aspirating needle, it seems judicious to avoid them whenever possible. If CT identifies a large necrotic component to the mass, the biopsy needle preferably will be directed toward the periphery of the lesion. With this information, most pulmonary lesions and many mediastinal masses can be biopsied percutaneously without the need for direct CT guidance. Even with central lesions that may be obscured on the lateral chest radiograph or on lateral fluoroscopy, the use of preliminary CT scanning, which is much more informative than conventional tomography, will reveal the relationships of the lesion to familiar fluoroscopically recognizable landmarks, such as the spine, trachea, or aortic arch.

Sometimes, preliminary CT examination may identify other unsuspected sites of disease that may be more rewarding for biopsy in terms of clinical management. For example, an enlarged mediastinal lymph node or an occult adrenal mass, which might represent metastasis, might more profitably be biopsied than a pulmonary lesion. A positive result not only would solidify a diagnosis of primary bronchogenic carcinoma but also would prove that it had extended beyond the realm of surgical cure. Of perhaps even more importance, occasionally the prebiopsy information provided by CT obviates the procedure entirely, such as when unsuspected lipoid pneumonia, hamartoma, sequestration, or pulmonary arteriovenous malformation is diagnosed or strongly suspected. Sometimes an alternative procedure, such as an angiogram, may be substituted.

Direct CT guidance for percutaneous needle biopsy is advantageous for certain thoracic lesions or specific clinical circumstances (1,36,44). Optimal direction can be provided to relatively small mediastinal masses, chest-wall lesions, pleural-based disease beneath a rib, and some pulmonary nodules in the lung apex or paraspinally above the medial diaphragmatic sulcus, all of which can be difficult or impossible to see fluoroscopically. Virtually any needle approach may be chosen to avoid or minimize traversing a lung, thus eliminating or greatly reducing the risk of a pneumothorax (65). An axillary entry may be used for upper-lobe masses, or an extrapleural paravertebral route for access to lesions in the paraesophageal area (155). Upper-lobe masses can be biopsied much easier under direct CT guidance than lower-lung-field lesions. The latter exhibit marked excursion with respiration and can be very difficult to impale under CT guidance.

As with fluoroscopically directed percutaneous needle biopsy, premedication of the patient generally is unnecessary. Once direct guidance by CT has been decided on, the patient is positioned appropriately within the gantry, depending on the location of the lesion to be biopsied as determined by the prior CT study and/or chest radiographs. Equipment with a large gantry opening (e.g., 70 cm) and very short scan and reconstruction times greatly facilitates the subsequent procedure. Supine or prone positioning usually is preferred because these are the most stable and comfortable for the patient. Anterior or lateral lesions are most often approached with the patient supine in the conventional position for CT scanning. The prone position is used for posteriorly located lesions. Lateral or oblique positions may be needed occasionally to bring lesions into favorable position for needle access (Fig. 25). This need, however, generally is much less with CT guidance than with fluoroscopy. When the shortest route to the lesion through the chest wall is not possible because of interposed bone, cartilage, breast tissue, or a large vessel or neural plexus, then an angled approach, sometimes with triangulation, can be readily calculated and accomplished (Fig. 26). Because there is no magnification or geometric distortion on CT scans, precise measurements from the point of entry on the skin to the lesion can be determined.

The preliminary localization "radiograph" (topogram) usually helps to quickly determine at which level(s) to obtain the necessary transverse CT scan(s). A marker (or grid) placed on the skin can assist in subsequent guidance of the needle and selection of the best puncture site. The latter determination can be made from the combined findings on the topogram and the CT images.

The needle chosen for the biopsy procedure often depends on the requirements for specimen analysis. Material from an 18- or 20-gauge aspirating needle almost always suffices for cytologic diagnosis, whereas a larger-bore cutting-type needle (e.g., Franseen) may be required to provide sufficient tissue for diagnosis of lymphoma from an enlarged lymph node, chest-wall mass, or an infiltrated thymus.

The needle is advanced at increments of 2 to 3 cm, with the patient always suspending respiration during this short period (as well as when the needle is withdrawn). A scan of the needle tip can be obtained at any time to ensure proper direction and placement. The position of the needle tip can be determined quickly and easily from a repeat topogram, from which the exact level for a transaxial CT scan may be established. The depth of the needle tip and its relation to the target lesion can be ascertained. Generally, scanning to corroborate needle position is most reproducible at resting lung volumes (relaxed expiration). As with fluoroscopic-directed biopsies, to reduce the number of pleural punctures it is advisable to verify that the needle path is correct while the tip is still within the chest wall, because the risk of pneumothorax generally

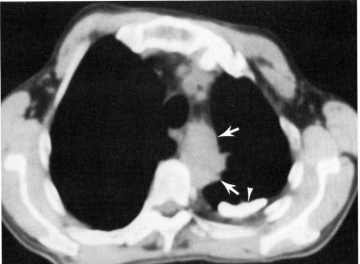

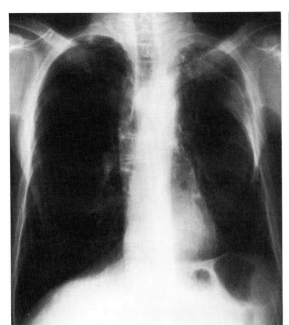

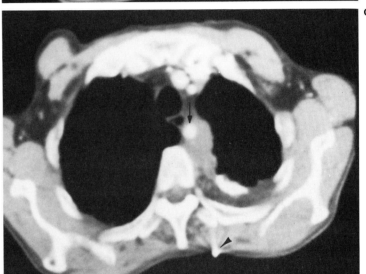

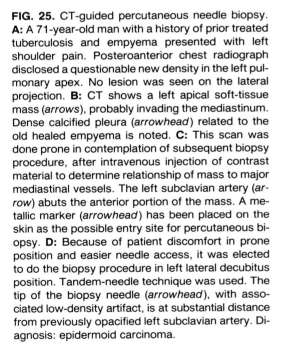

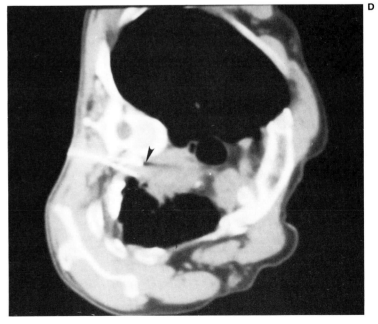

FIG. 25. CT-guided percutaneous needle biopsy. **A:** A 71-year-old man with a history of prior treated tuberculosis and empyema presented with left shoulder pain. Posteroanterior chest radiograph disclosed a questionable new density in the left pulmonary apex. No lesion was seen on the lateral projection. **B:** CT shows a left apical soft-tissue mass (*arrows*), probably invading the mediastinum. Dense calcified pleura (*arrowhead*) related to the old healed empyema is noted. **C:** This scan was done prone in contemplation of subsequent biopsy procedure, after intravenous injection of contrast material to determine relationship of mass to major mediastinal vessels. The left subclavian artery (*arrow*) abuts the anterior portion of the mass. A metallic marker (*arrowhead*) has been placed on the skin as the possible entry site for percutaneous biopsy. **D:** Because of patient discomfort in prone position and easier needle access, it was elected to do the biopsy procedure in left lateral decubitus position. Tandem-needle technique was used. The tip of the biopsy needle (*arrowhead*), with associated low-density artifact, is at substantial distance from previously opacified left subclavian artery. Diagnosis: epidermoid carcinoma.

A

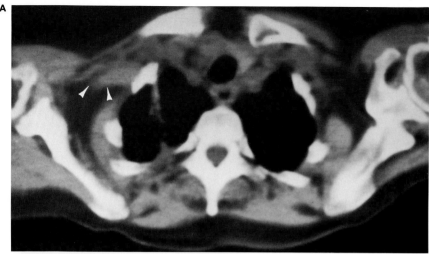

B

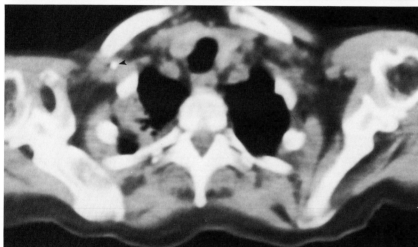

FIG. 26. CT-guided percutaneous needle biopsy. **A:** Scan in 73-year-old woman following right mastectomy with new right shoulder pain shows a vague soft-tissue density (*arrowheads*) in the region of the right brachial plexus, around the axillary sheath. Radiation fibrosis is noted in the right pulmonary apex. **B:** Tip of needle (*arrowhead*) guided into mass through supraclavicular approach using triangulation. Diagnosis: recurrent adenocarcinoma.

increases with the number of times the pleura is crossed. In thin patients, it may be difficult to stabilize the needle with the soft tissues of the chest wall; in such cases, a shorter, larger-gauge needle may be placed first, through which the biopsy needle is subsequently passed.

A quick needle thrust through the pleura seems to help prevent pleural tears. When the needle tip has been verified to reach into the periphery of the target, the cannula is removed, and a 30-ml syringe is attached to the needle hub. Strong suction is then applied while the syringe and needle are simultaneously advanced forward and backward for 1 to 2 cm a few times into the lesion while rotating them in a clockwise and counterclockwise direction, before needle withdrawal. To avoid having to repeat the procedure, "wet prep" specimens are immediately checked by a cytopathology technologist to determine their adequacy.

Because a pneumothorax is the most common complication, a CT scan through the chest, usually at the site of biopsy (Fig. 27), or an upright chest radiograph, must be obtained at the completion of the procedure. If a notable pneumothorax is encountered, it may be evacuated

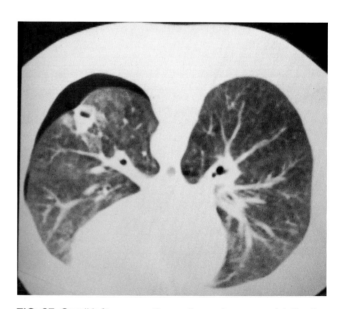

FIG. 27. Small left pneumothorax (scan done prone) following CT-guided needle aspiration of small cavitary left-lower-lobe lesion.

via a catheter inserted using the Seldinger technique; the catheter may be attached to a suction device or a Heimlich valve for sustained drainage.

NORMAL THORACIC ANATOMY

Virtually all gross anatomic structures within the thorax can be graphically demonstrated by CT. Normal fat, which always can be recognized by its characteristic low CT number (usually ranging from −80 to −120 HU), is present in sufficient amounts in most adults to depict clearly and sort out the various adjacent complex anatomic structures in the mediastinum and chest wall that cannot be distinguished by conventional radiographic techniques.

Although the transverse axial anatomy has a different appearance on MRI, the normal morphologic relationships are the same, and similar anatomic information is supplied by both techniques. Whereas the image displays of CT are based on X-ray attenuation values, they reflect magnetic tissue signal intensity with MRI. Mediastinal and hilar vascular structures are always easily visible on MRI because their blood-filled lumina usually do not produce a signal, in contrast to the higher-intensity mediastinal fat. Air-containing structures (trachea, bronchi, and lung) are devoid of signal because of their low proton density. Therefore, hilar vessels and bronchi are distinguished primarily by location rather than signal intensity. In areas where a vessel or bronchus contacts the lung, their wall is seen as a white stripe slightly less intense than fat. Segmental bronchi are much more easily seen by CT. Muscle, mediastinal lymph nodes, and the collapsed esophagus are intermediate in signal intensity. Because cortical bone yields a very low signal intensity, because of its low proton density, osseous structures, especially the ribs, may be more difficult to demonstrate. However, the central medullary portions of bones are well seen because of their fat content.

As is true throughout diagnostic radiology, accurate interpretation of abnormalities requires a detailed knowledge of normal anatomy, as well as an awareness of the wide range of anatomic variants and congenital anomalies that may occur. The thoracic anatomy will be described and depicted in two separate forms. Initially, important anatomic relationships will be stressed via representative levels throughout the entire thorax. Then details will be given about specific and important anatomic structures that commonly are seen on multiple cephalocaudal scans (e.g., the pulmonary hila, which extend from the level of the aortopulmonary window caudally to the left atrium).

Characteristic Transaxial Sections

The cross-sectional anatomy of the thorax can be conceptualized through a series of characteristic sections. Though somewhat arbitrary, a series of nine basic levels

has been selected for illustration and discussion to provide an orderly demonstration of major structural associations. These levels, in caudad order, have been named for the most consistent or dominant anatomic structure; common deviations from these most typical CT patterns will be shown:

1. Sternoclavicular joint
2. Crossing left brachiocephalic vein
3. Aortic arch
4. Aortopulmonary window
5. Left pulmonary artery
6. Main and right pulmonary arteries
7. Left atrium
8. Cardiac ventricles
9. Retrocrural space

Sternoclavicular Junction

The thoracic inlet joins the superior mediastinum to the neck, characteristically at a level parallel to the first rib (Figs. 28 and 29). The transaxial plane of CT displays the myriad anatomic structures in this area without superimposition (145,157). Just above the sternoclavicular articulation, at the level of the sternal notch, the inferior lobes of the thyroid may surround the upper trachea (Fig. 30). The esophagus, the other major visceral mediastinal structure at this level, frequently contains some air. Through the level of the manubrium and its articulation with the clavicular heads, five major mediastinal vessels usually are noted anterior and lateral to the trachea. These include the three major branches of the aortic arch (the brachiocephalic, left common carotid, and left subclavian arteries) and the two brachiocephalic veins. The brachiocephalic (innominate) veins, located just posterior to the clavicular heads, are formed near the first ribs where the subclavian veins join the internal jugular veins. The brachiocephalic artery, the largest vessel, lies directly in front of or just to the right of the trachea. The exact position of the bifurcation of the brachiocephalic artery is variable, depending on its length and tortuosity. Cephalad to the bifurcation, six major mediastinal vessels will be present, as the right subclavian and right common carotid arteries are seen as discrete structures. The left common carotid artery lies to the left and slightly posterolateral to the brachiocephalic artery; it has the smallest diameter of the three major arterial branches from the aorta. The left subclavian artery, which throughout its course is a relatively posterior structure, commonly comes in contact with the mediastinal pleural reflection of the left upper lobe and sometimes indents it in a convex fashion. The right brachiocephalic vein usually abuts the right upper lobe. The subclavian arteries and veins exit and enter the mediastinum by crossing over the first rib, behind the proximal portions of the clavicles. The subclavian vein commonly can be followed as it crosses the first rib to become the

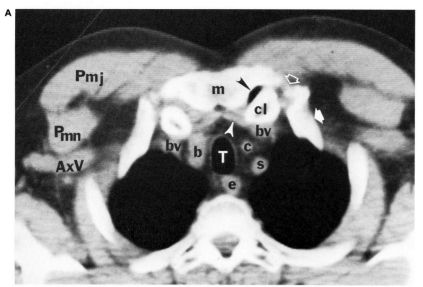

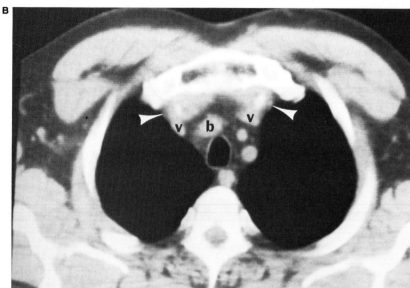

FIG. 28. Sternoclavicular junction. **A:** Through the manubrium (m) and its articulation with the heads of the clavicles (cl), five major vessels are noted surrounding the trachea (T). The brachiocephalic veins (bv) lie immediately posterior to the clavicular heads. The brachiocephalic artery (b) is the largest of the vessels off the aortic arch; the left carotid artery (c) is the smallest, and the left subclavian artery (s), which commonly indents the left upper lobe, is intermediate in size. Air within the sternoclavicular joint (*black arrowhead*) is common with the arms positioned above the head; (*closed arrow*) first rib; (*open arrow*) first costal cartilage; (Pmj) pectoralis major muscle; (Pmn) pectoralis minor muscle; (AxV) axillary vein; (*white arrowhead*) sternothyroid muscle; (e) esophagus. **B:** Caudad 1 cm, the brachiocephalic artery (b) has moved anterior to the trachea. Soft tissue (*arrowheads*) surrounding the inferior portion of the clavicular head should not be confused with a mass anterior to the brachiocephalic veins (v).

FIG. 29. Sternoclavicular junction. The brachiocephalic artery has divided into the right subclavian artery (s) and the right carotid artery (c) at the sternoclavicular level, which is located relatively cephalad in this patient. The left subclavian vein can be seen coursing over the left first rib to become the left axillary vein (vein), just in front of the anterior scalene muscle (M). The axillary artery, seen well on the right (*arrow*), courses behind both the anterior scalene and then the pectoralis minor muscles.

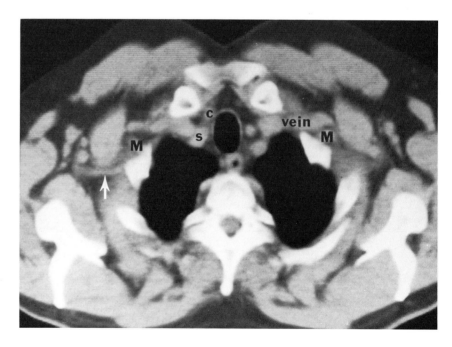

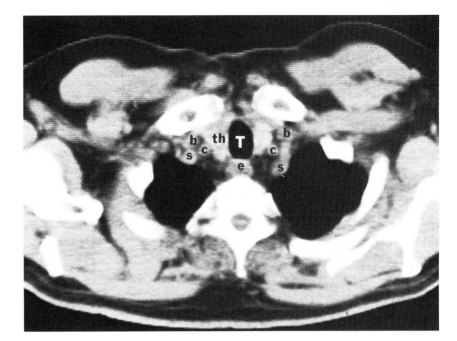

FIG. 30. At a level above the sternal notch, the inferior lobes of the thyroid (th) are seen lateral to the trachea (T); (c) common carotid arteries; (s) subclavian arteries; (b) brachiocephalic veins; (e) esophagus.

axillary vein where it lies behind the pectoralis muscles. The axillary vein lies anterior and the axillary artery posterior to the anterior scalene muscle. The subclavian arteries, however, are much more difficult to trace because of sharper degrees of angulation as these vessels arch over the apex of the lung slightly cranial and posterior to the subclavian veins. The subclavian and axillary arteries are accompanied by branches of the brachial plexus, which are rarely visible on CT because of their small size (and slightly lower density). Although the great vessels generally can be recognized with confidence by noting their characteristic configurations on serial scans, tortuosity and/or ectasia of these vessels may cause confusion, similar to that encountered on conventional radiographs (127).

The use of intravenous contrast material for vascular enhancement will almost always resolve the problem (Figs. 31 and 32).

Crossing Left Brachiocephalic Vein

The two brachiocephalic veins have two fundamentally different courses (Fig. 33). The right vein has a nearly vertical path throughout its length. The left brachiocephalic vein has a longer route, and usually at the level of the bottom of the manubrium and upper body of the sternum it is oriented horizontally as it crosses from left to right in the anterior mediastinum to join its mate on

A,B

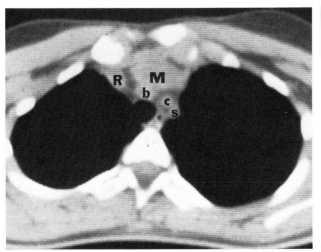 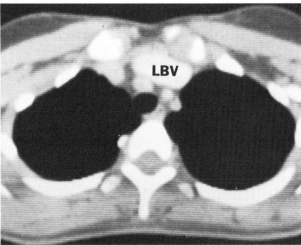

FIG. 31. Prominent left brachiocephalic vein. **A:** A suspicious soft-tissue mass (M) is seen anterior to the great vessels; (R) right brachiocephalic vein; (b) brachiocephalic artery; (c) left carotid artery; (s) left subclavian artery. **B:** After intravenous administration of contrast material into a left antecubital vein, a distended left brachiocephalic vein (LBV) can be seen accounting for the apparent soft-tissue mass. (From ref. 50.)

A

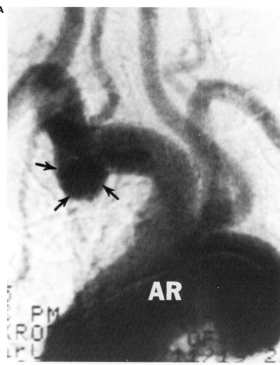

FIG. 32. Tortuous brachiocephalic artery. **A:** Digital aortic arch (AR) arteriogram demonstrating a tortuous brachiocephalic artery (*arrows*). **B:** A soft-tissue density (*arrowheads*) is seen adjacent to the trachea (T); (b) brachiocephalic artery; (c) left carotid artery; (s) left subclavian artery; (v) brachiocephalic veins. **C:** Scan after bolus injection of contrast material demonstrates that a mildly dilated tortuous brachiocephalic artery (b) accounts for the paratracheal density.

B,C

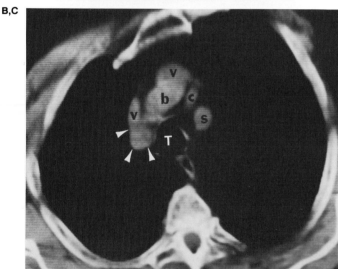

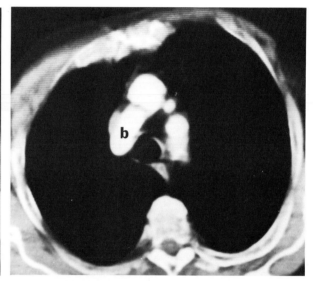

the opposite side to form the superior vena cava. The precise position of this traversing vein is highly variable; it can be found at virtually any level of the superior mediastinum and may cross over as low as in front of the aortic arch (Fig. 34). This may occur in patients with atherosclerosis and a tortuous, relatively high aortic arch; such an anatomic relationship could simulate an aortic dissection. Sometimes the course of the left brachiocephalic vein is quite vertical (Fig. 35). In both of these situations, careful scrutiny of multiple contiguous scans usually allows the correct interpretation. There is also considerable variability in the size of the left brachiocephalic vein. Mild distension may be a normal variant. If it is desired to maximally enhance the left brachiocephalic vein after intravenous contrast administration, the injec-

tion should be in a left medial antecubital vein (Fig. 31). The right internal mammary vein may be quite prominent and easily seen (Fig. 36); normal thymic veins also may be demonstrated (Fig. 37). Rarely, the left vertebral artery may arise separate from the aortic arch, and an additional great vessel will be seen at this level (Fig. 38).

Aortic Arch

The aortic arch (Fig. 39) usually has an oblique course, extending posteriorly and to the left. The anterior portion of the arch lies in front of the trachea and is intimately related to the anteromedial aspect of the superior vena cava on the latter's left side. The midportion of the arch typically lies just to the left of the trachea, and its posterior portion at the junction of the aortic knob and the de-

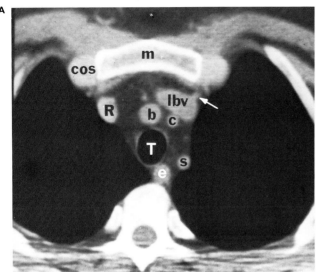

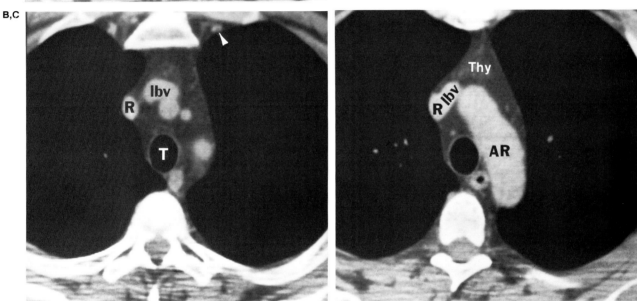

FIG. 33. Crossing left brachiocephalic vein. **A–C:** Sequential caudal scans demonstrate the left brachiocephalic vein (lbv) moving across the anterior mediastinum from the patient's left to his right to join the right brachiocephalic vein (R), subsequently forming the superior vena cava; (T) trachea; (e) esophagus; (b) brachiocephalic artery; (c) left carotid artery; (s) left subclavian artery; (*arrow*) left internal mammary vein; (m) manubrium; (cos) costal cartilage of the first rib; (*arrowhead*) internal mammary vessels; (AR) aortic arch; (Thy) thymus.

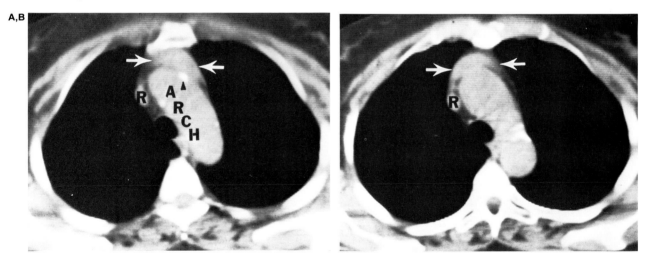

FIG. 34. Crossing left brachiocephalic vein. **A,B:** Sequential caudal scans in elderly woman with atherosclerosis show the horizontal portion of the left brachiocephalic vein (*arrows*) in front of the anterior aspect of the aortic arch (ARCH), before joining the right brachiocephalic vein (R). Mediastinal fat plane between the left brachiocephalic vein and the intimal calcification (*arrowhead*) of the aorta could simulate an aortic dissection.

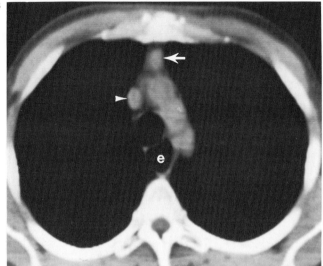

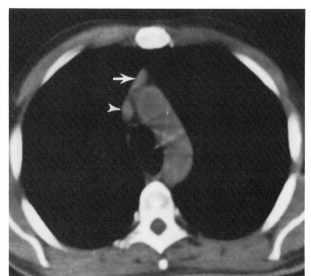

A,B

C

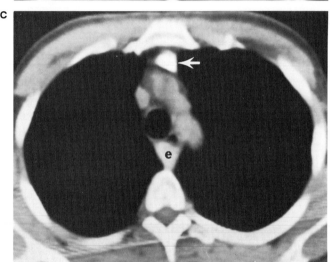

FIG. 35. Vertical left brachiocephalic vein. **A,B:** Sequential caudal scans show left brachiocephalic vein (*arrow*) approaching the right brachiocephalic vein (*arrowhead*). Esophagus (e) is dilated because of distal obstructing carcinoma. **C:** Early dynamic scan after intravenous injection of contrast material in left antecubital vein demonstrates enhancement of left brachiocephalic vein (*arrow*). Esophagus (e) opacified by oral contrast material. (From ref. 4.)

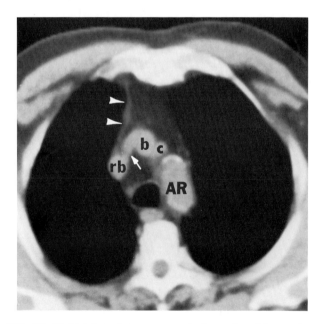

FIG. 36. Right internal mammary vein (*arrowheads*) coursing toward right brachiocephalic vein (rb); (*arrow*) left brachiocephalic vein; (b) brachiocephalic artery; (c) left carotid artery; (AR) top of posterior portion of aortic arch.

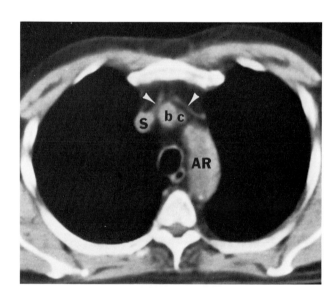

FIG. 37. Prominent thymic veins (*arrowheads*); (S) superior vena cava at confluence of brachiocephalic veins; (b) brachiocephalic artery; (c) left carotid artery; (AR) top of aortic arch.

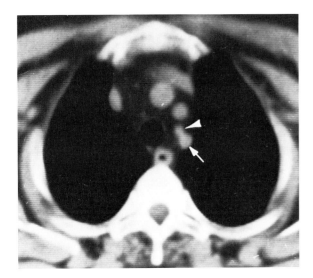

FIG. 38. Left vertebral artery (*arrowhead*) arising separately from left subclavian artery (*arrow*).

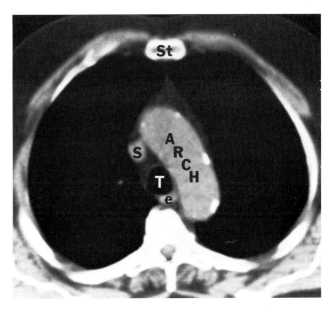

FIG. 39. Aortic arch (ARCH); (S) superior vena cava; (T) trachea; (e) esophagus; (St) body of sternum.

scending aorta is just lateral to the esophagus. In the elderly population with arteriosclerosis, the aortic arch frequently is not a horizontal structure, but rather has a cephaloposterior course, with the three great arteries arising sequentially at slightly different levels (Fig. 40). The brachiocephalic artery tends to originate first at the most caudal level, followed by the left common carotid artery, and finally by the left subclavian artery from the most

cephaloposterior portion of the knob. The top of such a tortuous aortic arch may be partially contained within one of the slices and can simulate an abnormal lung mass (115). Sections at this level may occasionally contain the arch of the azygos vein as it crosses over the right-upper-lobe bronchus, moving anteriorly along the right lateral

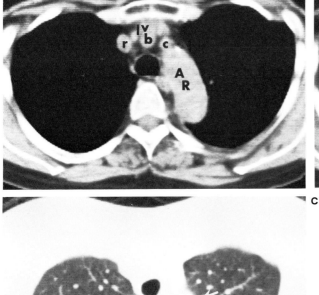

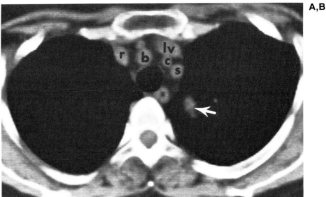

A,B

C

FIG. 40. Tortuous aortic arch. **A:** The great vessels may arise at different levels; here the brachiocephalic artery (b) and the left carotid artery (c) are seen distinct from the top of the middle and posterior portions of the aortic arch (AR); (r) right brachiocephalic vein; (lv) left brachiocephalic vein. **B:** On scan 1 cm cephalad, the left subclavian artery (s) is now seen. The very top of the aortic arch (*arrow*), only partially contained in this slice, may simulate an abnormal lung mass. **C:** Same level, lung window setting, the top of the aortic arch (*arrows*) again simulates a lung mass. Analyzing the sequential scans should allow proper interpretation.

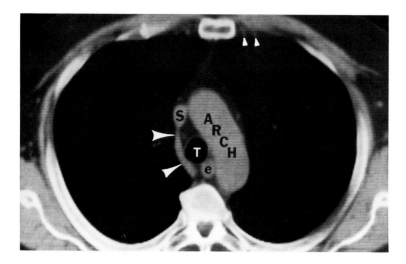

FIG. 41. Aortic arch (ARCH) and azygos vein arch (*large arrowheads*); (S) superior vena cava; (T) trachea; (e) esophagus; (*small arrowheads*) internal mammary vessels.

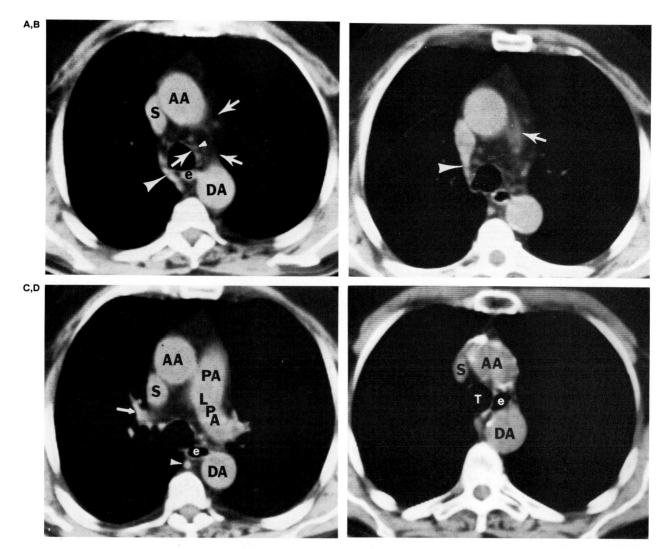

FIG. 42. Aortopulmonary window. **A:** The window (*arrows*) is largely filled with fat and small lymph nodes (*small arrowhead*); (AA) ascending aorta; (DA) descending aorta; (S) superior vena cava; (e) esophagus; (*large arrowhead*) posterior portion of azygos vein arch. **B:** On scan 1 cm caudad, the top of the main pulmonary artery (*arrow*) could be confused with mass in the window; (*arrowhead*) anterior portion of azygos vein arch. **C:** Section 1 cm caudad through top of main (PA) and left pulmonary arteries (LPA); (AA) ascending aorta; (DA) descending aorta; (S) superior vena cava; (*arrow*) truncus anterior; (*arrowhead*) azygos vein; (e) esophagus. **D:** In another patient, the esophagus (e), filled with air, is positioned in the aortopulmonary window because of adhesions with the descending aorta; (T) trachea; (AA) ascending aorta; (DA) descending aorta; (S) superior vena cava.

wall of the distal trachea to enter the posterior aspect of the superior vena cava (Fig. 41). In about 90% of the population, the azygos arch is positioned more caudally at the aortopulmonary level (136). The anterior mediastinum in front of the aortic arch typically has a triangular configuration, with the apex pointing anteriorly. In older adults, the anterior mediastinum is composed almost entirely of fat, which is the residual of the normal thymus.

Aortopulmonary Window

This level usually corresponds to the region of the distal trachea (Fig. 42). In most adults this area is filled with fat, and perhaps a few small lymph nodes. However, the cephalocaudal dimensions of the aortopulmonary window are quite variable, and the cephalad portion of the left pulmonary artery may lie just beneath the aortic arch and may be mistaken for a mass or enlarged lymph nodes. Careful examination of adjacent slices almost always leads to the proper interpretation. In the elderly population, the esophagus may be displaced into the aortopulmonary window because of adhesions with a tortuous descending aorta. Air within its lumen should permit distinction on CT (Fig. 42D); this can be a potential pitfall on MRI, because the air is not as easily recognized, and an abnormal mass may be simulated. The range of normal diameters for the ascending and descending aorta for adults is rather broad. The ascending aorta is always larger than the descending portion at the same level. The ratio can vary from 2.2 in young adults down to 1.1 in older individuals (5). The azygos vein arch is most commonly located at this level; its characteristic course can be traced from its initial prevertebral location as it courses anteriorly in intimate contact with the right lateral wall of the trachea to enter the posterior aspect of the superior vena cava. The area medial to the junction of the azygos arch and the superior vena cava (sometimes called the pretracheal retrocaval space) usually contains some lymph nodes (often referred to as the azygos nodes), up to 10 mm in diameter, in addition to fat and some connective tissue (128). The clinical importance of this region derives from the critical role of these pretracheal (azygos) lymph nodes. They drain the bronchopulmonary (hilar) and subcarinal lymph nodes efferently and are afferent links with the more cephalic middle mediastinal paratracheal nodes.

Left Pulmonary Artery

The posterior extension of the main pulmonary artery, the left pulmonary artery (Fig. 43), lies just to the left and lateral to the carina or left main-stem bronchus. The left superior pulmonary vein often is visible lateral to the posterior portion of the left pulmonary artery. Typically, the origin of the right-upper-lobe bronchus from the right main-stem bronchus is seen at this same level, as is the right-upper-lobe pulmonary artery (truncus anterior). On rare occasion, the main and left pulmonary arteries are positioned at an unusually high level relative to the aortic arch and can mimic a mass in the left side of the mediastinum on CT or plain chest radiographs (96). Careful evaluation of sequential scans, and, if necessary, intravenous administration of iodinated contrast material (Fig. 44), should allow the proper interpretation to be made.

A,B

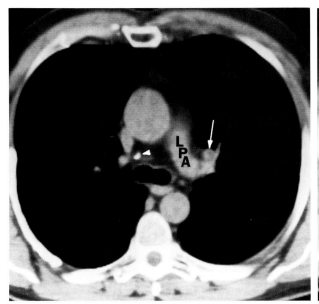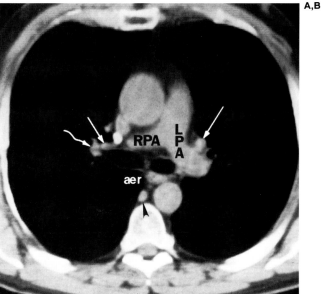

FIG. 43. Left pulmonary artery. A,B: The left pulmonary artery (LPA) is imaged on two sequential caudal scans. (In another patient, in Fig. 42C, the left pulmonary artery is imaged on a single scan.) (RPA) origin of right pulmonary artery; (*white arrowhead*) calcified pretracheal lymph node; (*straight arrows*) superior pulmonary veins; (*curved arrow*) truncus anterior; (aer) azygoesophageal recess; (*black arrowhead*) azygos vein.

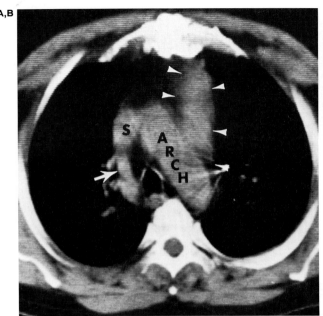
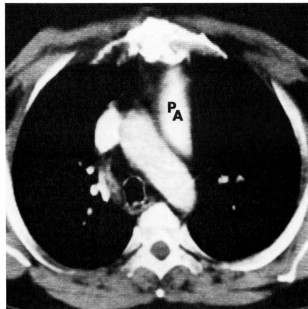

FIG. 44. High pulmonary artery. **A:** An oblong soft-tissue density (*arrowheads*) is seen anterior to the aortic arch (ARCH); (S) superior vena cava; (*arrow*) azygos vein arch. **B:** Scan after intravenous administration of contrast material demonstrates that the density is a cephalad-positioned main and left pulmonary artery (PA).

Main and Right Pulmonary Arteries

The right pulmonary artery extends posteriorly and to the right from the main pulmonary artery (Fig. 45), coursing posterior to the superior vena cava and anterior to the bronchus intermedius. The intrapericardial portion of the right pulmonary artery should be visible in all patients and normally measures 12 to 15 mm in diameter in adults (107). The normal diameter of the main pulmonary artery should not exceed 29 mm (83). The left interlobar pulmonary artery usually is present just posterolateral to the left-upper-lobe bronchus. The right and left superior pulmonary veins generally are seen respectively just anterior to the lateral aspect of the right pulmonary artery and the left-upper-lobe bronchus. The medial part of the right lower lobe is seen immediately behind the bronchus intermedius as it insinuates itself into the azygoesophageal recess. Similarly, lung frequently inserts into a small notch between the left interlobar pulmonary artery and the descending aorta.

Left Atrium

Lying between the aortic root and right atrium anteriorly, and the azygos vein, esophagus, and descending aorta posteriorly, the left atrium (Figs. 46 and 47) has anteroposterior measurements through its midportion of about 3 to 4.5 cm (63). The inferior pulmonary veins course into its posterolateral aspects. The aortic root lies to the right and posterior to the main pulmonary artery

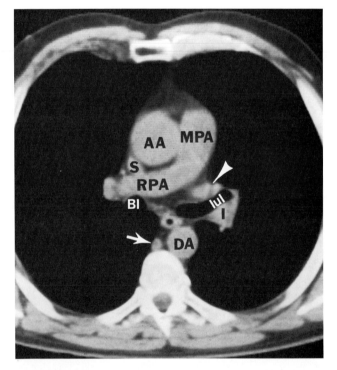

FIG. 45. Main and right pulmonary arteries. The right pulmonary artery (RPA) extends posteriorly and to the right from the main pulmonary artery (MPA), coursing behind the superior vena cava (S) and anterior to the bronchus intermedius (BI). Lung inserts into a notch between the left interlobar pulmonary artery (I) and the descending aorta (DA); (AA) ascending aorta; (lul) left-upper-lobe bronchus; (*arrowhead*) left superior pulmonary vein; (*arrow*) azygos vein.

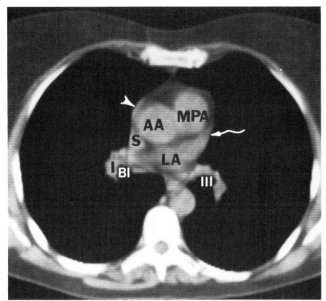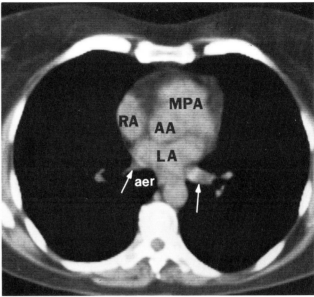

A,B

FIG. 46. Left atrium. A,B: Sequential caudal scans through the upper portion and midportion of the left atrium (LA). The main pulmonary artery and pulmonary outflow tract (MPA) lie somewhat anterior to the root of the ascending aorta (AA); (S) superior vena cava; (I) right interlobar pulmonary artery; (BI) bronchus intermedius; (III) left-lower-lobe bronchus; (*arrowhead*) right atrial appendage; (*curved arrow*) junction of left superior pulmonary vein and left atrial appendage; (RA) right atrium; (*straight arrows*) inferior pulmonary veins; (aer) azygoesophageal recess.

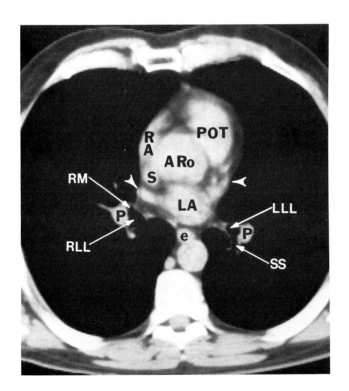

FIG. 47. Left atrium (LA); (ARo) aortic root; (POT) pulmonary outflow tract; (RA) right atrial appendage; (S) superior vena cava; (P) lower-lobe pulmonary arteries; (*arrowhead*) superior pulmonary veins; (e) esophagus; (RM) right-middle-lobe bronchus; (RLL) right-lower-lobe bronchus; (LLL) left-lower-lobe bronchus; (SS) superior-segment bronchus of left lower lobe.

and right ventricular outflow tract. Because the pulmonary valve is not visible on CT, clear distinction between the latter two anatomic structures is not possible. The pulmonary valve typically lies at the level of the right atrial appendage and is more cephalad than the aortic valve. The aortic sinuses may give the aortic root an ovoid configuration, where it is slightly larger in diameter than the more cephalad ascending aorta. The coronary arteries often are visible in the mediastinal fat at their origins from the sinuses. Calcification of the coronary arteries or the valves permits their clear depiction on CT (Fig. 48). Subepicardial fat may be abundant within and demarcate the interatrial and atrioventricular grooves. The azygoesophageal recess is also seen at this level and is almost always concave in adults; it becomes deeper and more medial with increasing age and the presence of emphysema (Fig. 49) (90). In children and in adults with a narrow anteroposterior diameter of the thorax, the normal deep lung concavity of the recess may display a medial convexity due to bulging of the esophagus (Fig. 50) (109).

Cardiac Ventricles

The right ventricle (Fig. 51) forms the right and anterior portions of the heart at this level and is separated from the left ventricle by the interventricular septum, which usually is visible only when intravenous contrast material opacifies the blood (Fig. 10B). Contrast material also is required to predict the internal chambers and the thickness

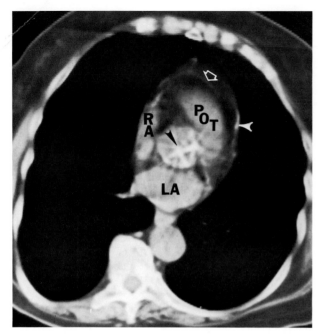

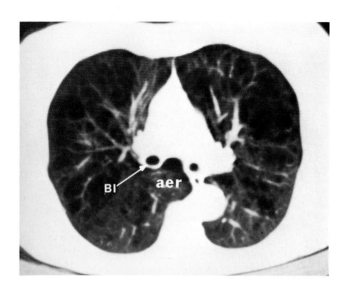

FIG. 49. Deep, wide azygoesophageal recess (aer) in patient with severe emphysema, at level of bronchus intermedius (BI).

FIG. 48. Calcification of aortic valve (*black arrowhead*) and left anterior descending coronary artery (*white arrowhead*); (RA) right atrial appendage; (POT) pulmonary outflow tract; (LA) left atrium; (*open arrow*) pericardium.

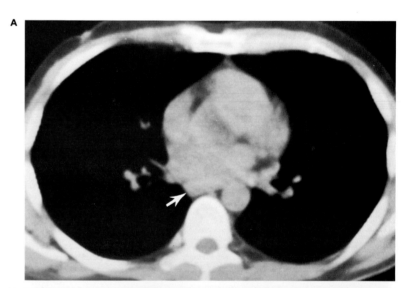

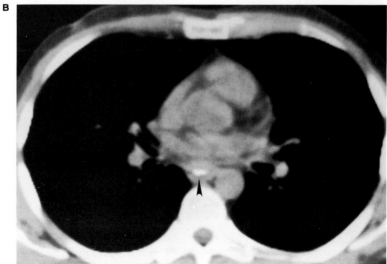

FIG. 50. A: Soft-tissue density (*arrow*) bulging into the azygoesophageal recess in patient with narrow anteroposterior diameter of thorax. B: Repeat scan after oral administration of contrast material demonstrates that the esophagus (*arrowhead*) is responsible for the density.

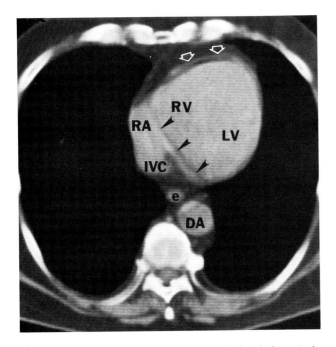

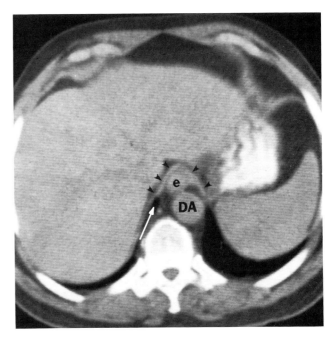

FIG. 51. Cardiac ventricles. At the ventricular level, the anterior pericardium (*open arrows*) is identified as a thin line of soft-tissue density between the pericardial (mediastinal) fat anteriorly and the underlying epicardial fat posteriorly. The coronary sinus (*arrowheads*) is seen posterolateral to the right ventricle (RV), and medial to the right atrium (RA) and inferior vena cava (IVC); (LV) left ventricle; (e) esophagus; (DA) descending aorta.

FIG. 52. Retrocrural space. The right and left diaphragmatic crura (*arrowheads*) surround the distal thoracic esophagus (e) and descending aorta (DA). Air in the right lower lobe is seen extending medial (*arrow*) to the upper portion of the right crus just lateral to the azygos vein.

of the myocardium. Sometimes there is a shallow impression on the anterior surface of the heart over the area of the interventricular groove; the left anterior descending coronary artery may be visible within the fat in the indentation. The pericardium overlying the anterolateral aspect of the heart is almost always seen in adults. Caudally, the horizontal portion of the coronary sinus, the main venous drainage of the cardiac muscle, may appear as a tongue-like structure posterior to the right ventricle and medial to the inferior vena cava. Occasionally, on more cephalad scans the vertical portion of the coronary sinus may be seen along the left posterolateral aspect of the left atrium (97).

Retrocrural Space

The caudal extent of the posterior mediastinum is enclosed by the diaphragmatic crura (Fig. 52). The space posteromedial to the crura serves as the major connecting route between the thorax and abdomen. The retrocrural space, at the level of the aponeurotic hiatus in the diaphragm for passage of the esophagus and the descending aorta, also includes fat, the azygos and hemiazygos veins, the thoracic duct, and associated lymph nodes (Fig. 53) (131). The normal nodes in this area probably do not exceed 6 mm in cross-sectional diameter (Fig. 54) (17). Rarely, it may appear that there is gas within the retro-

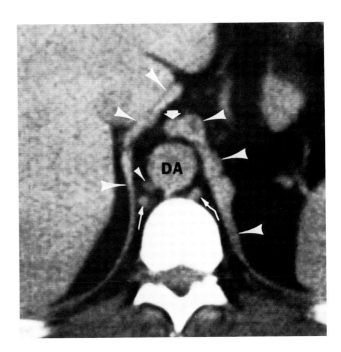

FIG. 53. Retrocrural space. The distal esophagus (*thick arrow*) is seen in an opening between the diaphragmatic crura (*large arrowheads*); the lobulations of the left crus are a normal variation. In the retrocrural space lie the descending aorta (DA), azygos vein (*thin arrow*), hemiazygos vein (*curved arrow*), thoracic duct (*small arrowhead*), and surrounding fat.

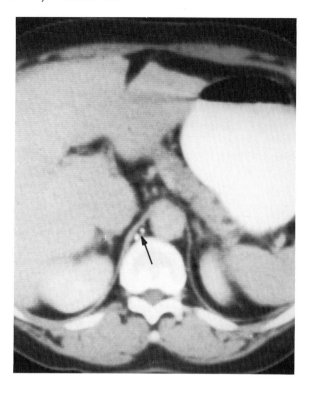

FIG. 54. Retrocrural space. In a scan obtained after a previous lymphangiogram, opacified lymph nodes (*arrow*) are seen medial to the right diaphragmatic crus.

crural space (134), because of the most caudal portion of a normal right lower lobe extending especially deep into the posterior costophrenic sulcus; because of partial-volume averaging, a single scan may show the aerated lung insinuating medial to the decussating right diaphragmatic crus (Fig. 55). With lung window settings, vessels may be seen within this air, which should not be confused with a mediastinal or retroperitoneal abscess.

Specific Anatomic Structures

Mediastinal Lymph Nodes

The ability to recognize normal lymph nodes on CT is directly related to the amount of mediastinal fat present. Lymph nodes appear as round or oval soft-tissue densities within the lower-density background of the mediastinal fat (Figs. 4C, 42A, and 56). They often are found in clusters of two or three. Normal lymph nodes can be seen in about 90% of adults, especially in the middle mediastinum. Viewing of serial contiguous scans can be crucial in differentiating lymph nodes and vessels.

In autopsy dissections, the average number of mediastinal lymph nodes found has been 64; the majority of these nodes, which drain the lung, are located adjacent to the tracheobronchial tree (46,117). Several systems of anatomic classification exist, based on the locations of these nodes (49). We and others have found a minor modification (Fig. 57) (Table 1) of the American Thoracic Society classification most applicable clinically to the CT findings (49,51). This system allows easy categorization

A,B

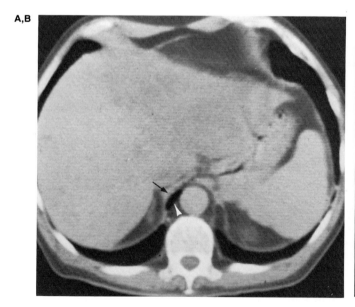
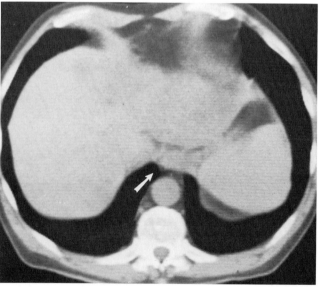

FIG. 55. A: Gas (*arrowhead*) medial to the right diaphragmatic crus (*arrow*) appears to be within the retrocrural space. **B:** Scan 1 cm cephalad shows that this is just partial-volume averaging of the right lower lobe extending medially in the costophrenic sulcus (*arrow*). Scans caudal to **A** showed no air in the retrocrural space.

(Fig. 58) of any enlarged lymph nodes according to their accessibility to various tissue-sampling techniques currently available (Table 2). Lymph nodes in the pretracheal and paratracheal area are accessible to biopsy through a transcervically inserted mediastinoscope (Carlens procedure). Surgical sampling, short of a formal thoracotomy, of the prevascular anterior mediastinal, aortopulmonary-window, or hilar lymph nodes requires a limited anterior parasternal approach (mediastinotomy or Chamberlain procedure). Extensive and complex intercommunications exist among these myriad groups of lymph nodes, and the classification serves no useful purpose in predicting the specific cause of any pathologic process based on the location of affected nodes.

There has been wide variation, ranging from 6 to 14 mm in diameter, in the reported maximal sizes of normal mediastinal lymph nodes (6,17,46,49). Some of this variation relates to different levels in the mediastinum. Normal nodes rarely exceed 6 mm in diameter around the left brachiocephalic vein, in the supradiaphragmatic region, and in the retrocrural area. The largest size encountered is in the right tracheobronchial region, in the aortopulmonary window, and in the subcarinal space, where approximately 90% of normal nodes measure 11 mm in diameter or less. Upper paratracheal lymph nodes usually are smaller than lower paratracheal or tracheobronchial

nodes, and right-side tracheobronchial nodes are larger than those on the left side. Use of the short axis of a mediastinal node in the transverse plane has been advocated as a more predictable criterion of nodal enlargement (volume); 1.0 cm is considered the upper limit of normal (117). Such measurements were more accurate with right-side than with left-side lymph nodes. Besides the given limitation that CT cannot detect microscopic architectural alterations (e.g., metastatic neoplasm) in normal-size lymph nodes, it is obvious that no size criterion will allow both high sensitivity and high specificity for predicting abnormal nodal enlargement. For simplistic and pragmatic reasons, generally to enhance sensitivity at the expense of specificity, any lymph node exceeding 1 cm in diameter, in any dimension, is deemed abnormal and worthy of consideration for tissue sampling. In certain areas, such as the supradiaphragmatic region, a smaller size criterion (6 mm) can be used (6,17). A mildly enlarged lymph node, containing a center of low, near-fat density, can be considered a normal variant in the older population (Fig. 59). On occasion, with MRI, because of its inferior spatial resolution compared with CT, a closely clustered group of normal-size lymph nodes will appear as one conglomerate enlarged mass.

Pulmonary Hila

The anatomic pulmonary hilum, the pedicle joining the mediastinum to the lung, is composed of the main bronchi, pulmonary arteries, superior and inferior pulmonary veins, bronchopulmonary (hilar) lymph nodes and lymphatic vessels, nerve plexi, and areolar tissue, all enclosed within a connective-tissue envelope. However, the hila visible on plain chest radiographs are composed primarily of the pulmonary arteries, with the superior pulmonary veins contributing somewhat to their upper contour (69). The inferior pulmonary veins are too caudal to contribute to the hilar opacity, and the normal bronchial walls and lymph nodes are too small to add any substantial density.

Computed tomography can be very useful in hilar evaluation. There are fairly constant relationships among the various anatomic structures that generally allow their correct identification (102,153). Knowledge of the normal anatomy helps in identifying bronchial abnormalities, locating pulmonary lesions by segments, and recognizing hilar lymph node enlargement. The wide window levels obtained for the lung usually permit analysis of the bronchial tree and the interface between the pulmonary parenchyma and the soft-tissue structures of the hila. The narrower window levels primarily used to assess the mediastinum and chest wall are optimal for evaluating the pulmonary hilar vessels. Window settings optimized for the lung tend to underestimate the diameter of the bron-

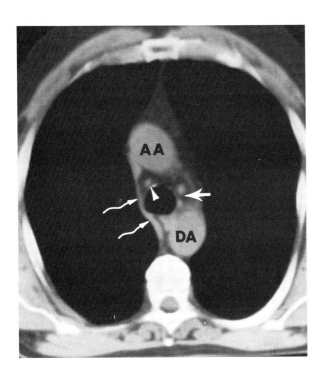

FIG. 56. Normal mediastinal lymph nodes. A small lymph node (*arrowhead*), a so-called azygos node that may range up to three in number, is seen in the pretracheal area just medial to the azygos vein arch (*curved arrows*). Two additional nodes (*arrow*), less than 1 cm in diameter, are seen in the aortopulmonary window; (AA) ascending aorta; (DA) descending aorta.

TABLE 1. *Modified American Thoracic Society classification of regional nodal stations*

Nodal stations	Definitions
X	Supraclavicular nodes.
2R	Right upper paratracheal nodes. Nodes to right of the midline of the trachea, between the intersection of the caudal margin of the brachiocephalic artery with the trachea and the apex of the lung or above the level of the aortic arch.
2L	Left upper paratracheal nodes. Nodes to the left of the midline of the trachea, between the top of the aortic arch and the apex of the lung.
4R	Right lower paratracheal nodes. Nodes to the right of the midline of the trachea, between the cephalic border of the azygos vein and the intersection of the caudal margin of the brachiocephalic artery with the right side of the trachea or the top of the aortic arch.
4L	Left lower paratracheal nodes. Nodes to the left of the midline of the trachea, between the top of the aortic arch and the level of the carina, medial to the ligamentum arteriosum.
5	Aortopulmonary nodes. Subaortic and paraaortic nodes, lateral to the ligamentum arteriosum or the aorta or left pulmonary artery, proximal to the first branch of the left pulmonary artery.
6	Anterior mediastinal nodes. Nodes anterior to the ascending aorta or the innominate artery.
7	Subcarinal nodes. Nodes arising caudal to the carina of the trachea, but not associated with the lower-lobe bronchi or arteries within the lung.
8	Paraesophageal nodes. Nodes dorsal to the posterior wall of the trachea and to the right or the left of the midline of the esophagus below the level of the subcarinal region (nodes around the descending aorta should also be included).
9	Right or left pulmonary ligament nodes. Nodes within the right or left pulmonary ligament.
10R	Right tracheobronchial nodes. Nodes to the right of the midline of the trachea, from the level of the cephalic border of the azygos vein to the origin of the right-upper-lobe bronchus.
10L	Left peribronchial nodes. Nodes to the left of the midline of the trachea, between the carina and the left-upper-lobe bronchus, medial to the ligamentum arteriosum.
11	Intrapulmonary nodes. Nodes removed in the right or left lung specimen, plus those distal to the main-stem bronchi or secondary carina (includes interlobar, lobar, and segmental nodes).
14	Superior diaphragmatic nodes. Nodes adjacent to the pericardium within 2 cm of the diaphragm.

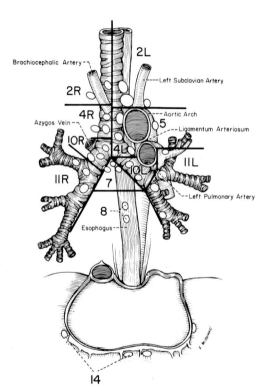

FIG. 57. Lymph node mapping scheme, modified from American Thoracic Society classification. Nodal stations 6 and 9 are not illustrated, because they superimpose other stations on the frontal view. (From ref. 51.)

chial lumen. If precise measurements are desired, a window mean of −150 HU is the most accurate (Fig. 60A); wall thickness is best determined using a mean window setting of −450 HU (Fig. 60B and C) (152). Depending on the clinical circumstances and the appearance of the hila on the routine non-contrast-enhanced scans (obtained at 8–10 mm collimation at 10-mm intervals), additional images may be acquired after intravenous administration of contrast material, with incremental dynamic techniques most optimal (Figs. 9 and 13). CT is more accurate than conventional radiographic techniques, including 55°

Table 2. *Lymph node sampling*

Method of sampling	Nodal stations
Mediastinoscopy	2R, 4R, 4L, 10R; 2L nodes adjacent to trachea; 7 nodes in anterior subcarinal area
Transbronchial needle aspiration	Same nodal groups as mediastinoscopy, but 7 nodes more easily accessible; 10L and 11 nodes can also be reached
Anterior parasternal thoracotomy	5, 6, and 2L nodes anterior to great vessels
Percutaneous needle biopsy	Under CT guidance, potentially can reach all nodal groups

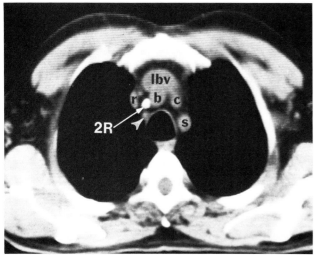

A

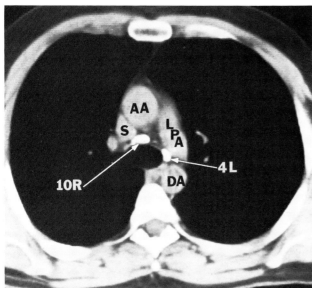

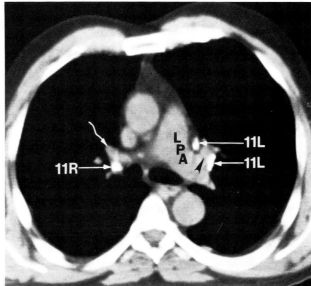

B,C

FIG. 58. Nodal stations of calcified mediastinal lymph nodes (see Fig. 57 for classification). **A:** Level of crossing left brachiocephalic vein (lbv); (r) right brachiocephalic vein; (b) brachiocephalic artery; (c) left carotid artery; (s) left subclavian artery; (*arrowhead*) normal pretracheal lymph node. **B:** Level of aortopulmonary window and top of left pulmonary artery (LPA); (AA) ascending aorta; (DA) descending aorta; (S) superior vena cava. **C:** Level of left pulmonary artery (LPA); (*curved arrow*) truncus anterior; (*arrowhead*) left-upper-lobe pulmonary artery. **D:** Level of right interlobar pulmonary artery (I); (aer) azygoesophageal recess. **E:** Level of cardiac ventricles; (IVC) inferior vena cava; (e) esophagus; (DA) descending aorta; (*curved arrow*) pericardium.

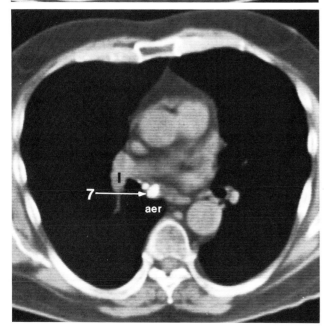

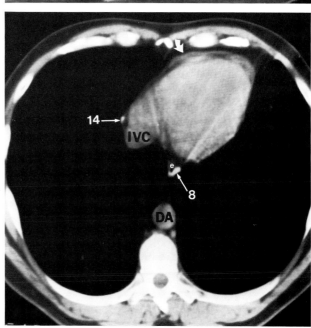

D,E

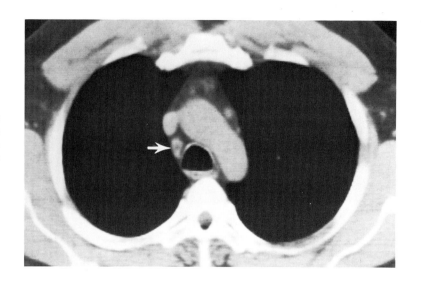

FIG. 59. Benign fibrolipomatous changes in a mildly enlarged paratracheal lymph node (*arrow*). Note that the central portion of the lymph node has an attenuation value similar to that for mediastinal and subcutaneous fat.

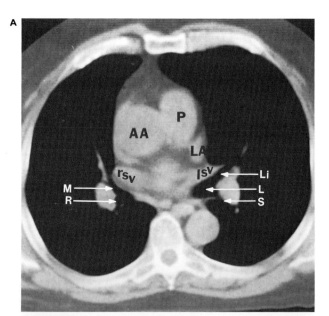

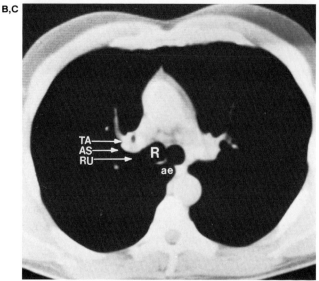

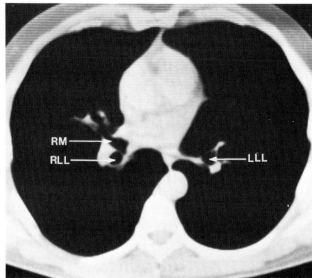

FIG. 60. Window-level settings for bronchi. **A:** Setting of −150 HU for measurement of diameter of bronchial lumen; (M) middle-lobe bronchus (with lateral and medial segmental orifices seen distally); (R) right-lower-lobe bronchus; (Li) lingular bronchus; (L) left-lower-lobe bronchus; (S) superior segmental bronchus of left lower lobe; (LA) left atrial appendage; (P) main pulmonary artery; (AA) ascending aorta; (rsv) right superior pulmonary vein; (lsv) left superior pulmonary vein. **B,C:** Setting of −450 HU for determination of wall thickness; (R) right main-stem bronchus; (ae) azygoesophageal recess (note thin posterior wall of right main bronchus, which should always be less than 0.5 cm in thickness); (RU) right-upper-lobe bronchus; (AS) anterior segment of right upper lobe; (TA) truncus anterior branch of right pulmonary artery; (RM) middle-lobe bronchus; (RLL) right-lower-lobe bronchus; (LLL) left-lower-lobe bronchus.

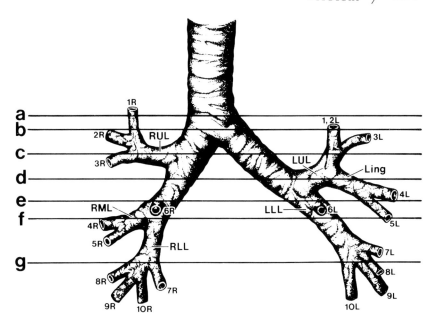

FIG. 61. Schematic depiction of segmental bronchi. Levels a–g represent key levels and correspond to the levels illustrated in Fig. 62; (RUL) right upper lobe with its segments; (1R) apical; (2R) posterior; (3R) anterior; (RML) right middle lobe with its segments; (4R) lateral; (5R) medial; (RLL) right lower lobe with its segments; (6R) superior; (7R) medial basal; (8R) anterior basal; (9R) lateral basal; (10R) posterior basal; (LUL) left upper lobe with its segments of the superior division 1; (2L) apical posterior; (3L) anterior; (Ling) lingular division with its segments; (4L) superior; (5L) inferior; (LLL) left lower lobe with its segments; (6L) superior; (7,8L) anteromedial basal; (9L) lateral basal; (10L) posterior basal.

posterior oblique tomography, for analyzing the myriad components of the true hila and for determining whether they are normal or pathologic (48,101). Although early reports assessing CT did not support this contention, they are of little more than historical interest. Such studies were conducted using CT scanners that did not always allow one to perform examinations during suspended respiration. More important, normal cross-sectional hilar anatomy was not fully appreciated, and dynamic scanning techniques to work out problem cases were not available.

The key to proper interpretation of cross-sectional images of the pulmonary hila is detailed knowledge of the bronchial anatomy (105). The bronchi are the most constant anatomic landmarks and can serve as easily identifiable reference points because the air within their lumina is a perfect natural contrast agent (Fig. 61). The bronchi form a lattice on which the pulmonary arteries and veins are draped in a characteristic fashion, and it can be used as a road map into the pulmonary parenchyma.

Because the bronchi are arranged perpendicular, obliquely, or parallel to the plane of the CT slice, the ability to demonstrate a particular bronchus depends not only on its size but also on its orientation. Simply imaging the thorax with 8- to 10-mm sections at 10-mm intervals will result in depicting only about 70% of the segmental bronchi. As previously emphasized, it is advocated that the radiologist monitor the CT examination while it is in progress. If a particular area or segment is of major clinical interest, a few extra sections through this region using 4- to 5-mm sequential scans usually will suffice for evaluation and will, at most, add only a few minutes to the study time. With such an approach, virtually all of the segmental bronchi can be demonstrated. Thin serial sections also may be beneficial in preventing overinterpretation of

bronchial narrowing resulting from the partial-volume averaging effect.

The origin and proximal portions of the horizontally coursing bronchi are routinely imaged on transaxial CT sections (Fig. 62). These include the right-upper-lobe bronchus (as well as its anterior and posterior segmental branches), the left-upper-lobe bronchus (and its anterior segment), the middle-lobe bronchus (and generally some portions of both the medial and lateral segmental branches), and the superior segments of both lower lobes. Bronchi having a vertical course are seen in cross section. These include the apical segmental bronchus of the right upper lobe, the apical posterior segmental bronchus of the left upper lobe, the bronchus intermedius, and the proximal portions of both lower-lobe bronchi (after the branching of the superior segments). The most difficult bronchi to recognize are those that run obliquely. These are the lingular bronchus (including the superior and inferior segments) and the basilar segmental bronchi. Sometimes the medial and lateral segments of the middle lobe course with a shallow obliquity. Although minor variations in bronchial anatomy are common, true anomalies are rare.

The most cephalad recognizable bronchus is that of the apical segment of the right upper lobe (Fig. 62A). Characteristic of upper-lobe relationships, this bronchus lies immediately lateral to the corresponding branch of the right-upper-lobe pulmonary artery and just medial to a branch of the right superior pulmonary vein.

The right-upper-lobe bronchus is seen just below the carina (Fig. 62C) and originates more cephalad than the left-upper-lobe bronchus. The posterior wall of the right-upper-lobe bronchus is in direct contact with the aerated posterior segment of the right upper lobe. The stripe of

A,B

C,D

E,F

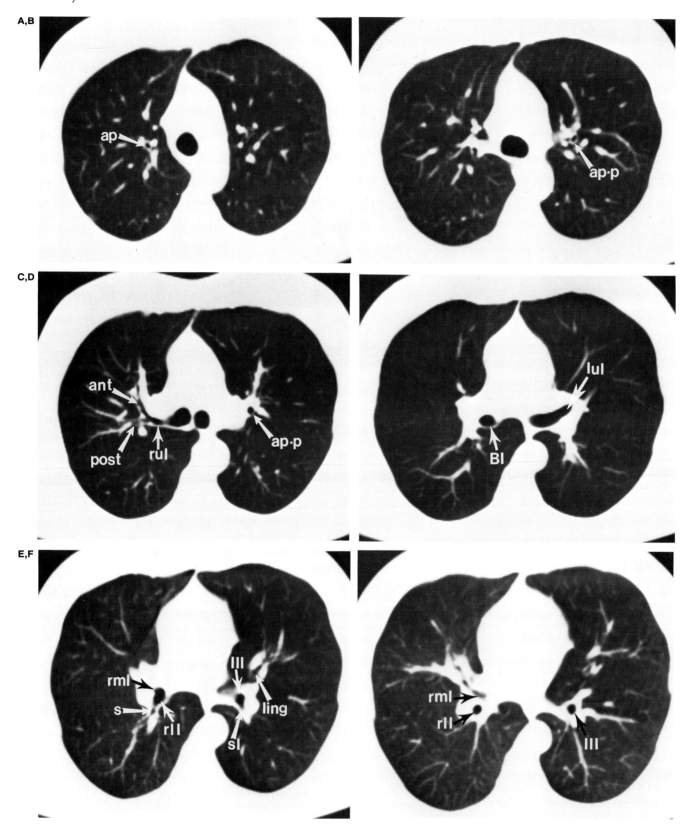

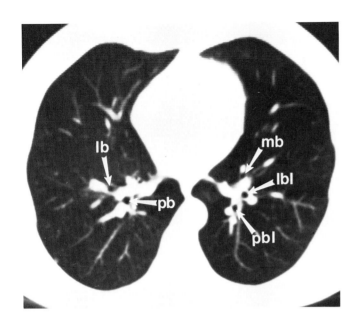

FIG. 62. Segmental bronchi. **A–F:** Facing page. **A:** Aortic arch (and distal trachea) level. The apical segmental bronchus (ap) of the right upper lobe is seen. **B:** Aortopulmonary window (and carinal) level. The apical posterior segmental bronchus (ap-p) of the left upper lobe is demonstrated. **C:** Left pulmonary artery level. The right-upper-lobe bronchus (rul) is seen arising from the right mainstem bronchus and bifurcating distally into the anterior segmental (ant) and posterior segmental (post) branches. The apical posterior segmental bronchus (ap-p) is again seen. **D:** Right pulmonary artery level. The bronchus intermedius (BI) is seen, with its thin posterior wall, along with the orifice for the left-upper-lobe bronchus (lul). **E:** Right interlobar pulmonary artery level. The superior segmental bronchus (s) is seen arising from the right-lower-lobe bronchus (rll); the origin of the right-middle-lobe bronchus (rml) is barely perceptible. The superior segmental bronchus (sl) is seen arising from the left-lower-lobe bronchus (lll); the lingular bronchus (ling) is seen coursing anteriorly. **F:** Left atrial level. The right-middle-lobe bronchus (rml) is seen anterior to the right-lower-lobe bronchus (rll). The left lower lobe bronchus (lll) is again demonstrated. **G:** Ventricular level. Only the posterior basal bronchus (pb) and lateral basal bronchus (lb) are identified on the right side. On the left, the medial basal (mb), lateral basal (lbl), and the posterior basal (pbl) bronchi are seen.

this wall generally is quite uniform in caliber and almost always less than 5 mm in thickness. A small focal bulge may be produced by a prominent azygos vein. The anterior and posterior segmental bronchi usually are visible as they bifurcate and course horizontally in the transaxial plane.

The bronchus intermedius, which is about 3 cm long, lies directly posterior to the right pulmonary artery and at a slightly more caudal level is just medial to the right interlobar pulmonary artery (Fig. 62D). The entire thin posterior wall of this bronchus is in contact with the aerated superior segment of the right lower lobe. Typically, pulmonary parenchyma also extends posteromedial to the bronchus intermedius into the azygoesophageal recess. As previously emphasized, except for patients with a narrow anteroposterior diameter of the thorax, this recess is normally concave (convex medially).

The middle-lobe bronchus courses caudally as well as anteriorly. In most patients the origin of the middle-lobe bronchus is demonstrated along with the proximal portion of the right-lower-lobe bronchus (Figs. 60A and C and 62E and F). The medial and lateral segmental bronchi usually are located in a slightly more caudal plane.

Although the superior segmental bronchus of the right lower lobe may arise at the same level as the orifice of the middle-lobe bronchus, it can also arise at a slightly more caudal or cephalad level (Fig. 62E).

There is considerable variability in the cross-sectional appearance of the right-lower-lobe basilar segmental bronchi (Fig. 62G). The medial basal segmental bronchus usually lies just anterior to the right inferior pulmonary

vein. The anterior, lateral, and posterior basal bronchi may be identifiable because of their positions relative to one another. Characteristic of lower-lobe relationships, the basal bronchi lie medial and anterior to the corresponding vertically coursing lower-lobe pulmonary arteries and peripherally are slightly lateral to the inferior pulmonary veins.

The left apical posterior segmental bronchus is seen in cross section at the level of the carina and right-upper-lobe orifice (Figs. 62B and C).

The left-upper-lobe bronchus (Fig. 62D) originates at a level more caudal than that of the right-upper-lobe bronchus; it forms a "sling" over which the left pulmonary artery passes. The orifice of the left-upper-lobe bronchus is large, and two serial CT sections may include it. The left-upper-lobe pulmonary artery, as it descends posteriorly, often produces a slight concavity to the posterior wall of the cephalad portion of the bronchus. The aerated superior segment of the left lower lobe abuts the posteromedial wall of the left-upper-lobe bronchus. The anterior segmental bronchus usually can be identified as the only bronchus arising from the left-upper-lobe bronchus that courses anteriorly in a horizontal plane.

A section through the caudal portion of the left-upper-lobe bronchus also often includes the origin of the left-lower-lobe bronchus (Fig. 60A). The lingular bronchus arises from the undersurface of the distal left-upper-lobe bronchus and has an oblique anterior and caudal course (Fig. 62E). Serial sections below the orifice of the lingular bronchus show progressively wider separation between the lingular bronchus anteriorly and the left-lower-lobe bronchus posteriorly (Fig. 62F). The superior and especially the inferior lingular segmental bronchi are rarely recognized on CT.

The left superior segmental bronchus may originate at a slightly more cephalad level than its opposite mate (Fig. 62E). The left-lower-lobe basal segmental bronchi generally have an anatomic distribution similar to that on the right side (Fig. 62G). The anterior and medial basal segmental bronchi on the left typically arise as a single structure.

At least the approximate positions of most of the bronchopulmonary segments can be recognized by identifying the distribution of the majority of the segmental bronchi (Fig. 63) (74,110). About 75% of the segments can be predicted with confidence, and the relative positions of the rest can be estimated.

The hilar vessels are more variable in position than the bronchi. The truncus anterior (right-upper-lobe pulmonary artery), the first main branch of the right pulmonary artery, arises within the pericardium and is commonly seen just anterior to the right-upper-lobe bronchus (Figs. 42C, 44B, and 58C). The posterior branch of the right superior pulmonary vein usually lies within the angle

formed by the bifurcation of the right-upper-lobe bronchus into the anterior and posterior segments; the anterior branch generally is located medial to the branches of the truncus anterior (Fig. 44B).

The right pulmonary artery initially crosses in front of the bronchus intermedius (Fig. 45) and then, at a more caudal level, lies alongside its lateral aspect as it becomes the right interlobar pulmonary artery (Fig. 46A), often causing a slightly nodular contour to the hilum at this level. More caudally, the right interlobar pulmonary artery assumes a vertical orientation and is positioned just lateral to the bifurcation of the middle- and lower-lobe bronchial orifices (Figs. 9B, 13B, and 46A). The right superior pulmonary vein now lies anteromedial to the middle-lobe bronchus as it enters the upper portion of the left atrium. Just caudal, the middle-lobe pulmonary artery lies between the medial and lateral segmental bronchi of the right middle lobe.

The right inferior pulmonary vein is oriented horizontally as it enters the lower portion of the left atrium (Fig. 46B).

The left-upper-lobe pulmonary artery and the left superior pulmonary vein have much less constant anatomic

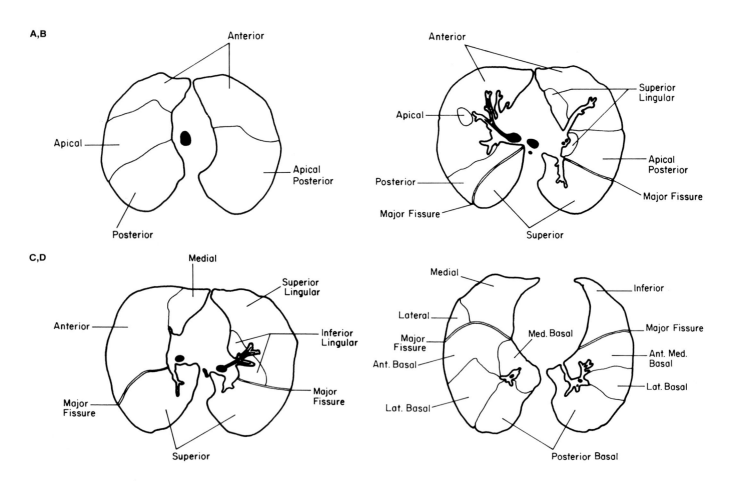

FIG. 63. Schematic drawings of segmental lung anatomy at representative levels. **A:** Aortic arch. **B:** Left pulmonary artery. **C:** Right pulmonary artery. **D:** Cardiac ventricles.

relationships to the left-upper-lobe bronchus than their counterparts on the right side. The apical posterior bronchus may lie medial or lateral to the branch of the left-upper-lobe pulmonary artery. The left pulmonary artery itself, first seen cephalad between the left main bronchus and the apical posterior bronchus, generally lies postero-lateral to the left superior pulmonary vein (Figs. 42C and 44). The posterior wall of the left-upper-lobe bronchus usually is concave where it is indented superiorly and posteriorly by the left pulmonary artery coursing over and around it (Fig. 45). The left superior pulmonary vein invariably lies in front of the left-upper-lobe bronchus as it courses to the left atrium; it frequently has a horizontal course at a slightly caudal level.

The left pulmonary artery extends caudally posterior to the left-upper-lobe bronchus to become the left inter-lobar pulmonary artery. Pulmonary parenchyma usually can be seen extending into a sulcus between the left interlobar pulmonary artery and the descending thoracic aorta (Figs. 44B, 45, and 60A and B). Obliteration of this space just behind the left-upper-lobe bronchus (or thickening of the left retrobronchial stripe), similar to the region behind the upper-lobe and intermediate bronchus on the right, is pathologic (147).

Just caudal to the left-upper-lobe bronchus, frequently at the level where the bronchus to the superior segment of the left lower lobe originates, the left interlobar pulmonary artery lies in the bifurcation behind the lingular bronchus and anterolateral to the lower-lobe bronchus.

The segmental lower-lobe pulmonary arteries generally lie more toward the periphery of the lung than their corresponding bronchi, and the segmental veins are positioned just central to the bronchi. Sometimes the segmental lower-lobe pulmonary arteries may be duplicated or even triplicated; such normal variations may simulate enlarged intersegmental lymph nodes.

Several normal areas of notable lobularity in the hila are caused by some of these described vascular relationships. The most marked regions of lobularity in the right hilum occur where the truncus anterior produces a convexity anterior to the right-upper-lobe bronchus (Figs. 42C and 44B), where the right superior pulmonary vein crosses anterolateral to the descending right interlobar pulmonary artery (Figs. 9 and 47), and just caudal to the right-middle-lobe bronchus where the basilar branches of the right-lower-lobe pulmonary artery divide. In the left hilum, the most prominent lobulation occurs where the descending left pulmonary artery branches posterior and caudal to the origin of the left-upper-lobe bronchus. If these lobulations cause any interpretive problem after viewing serial contiguous scans, contrast-enhanced dynamic scanning should allow confident recognition of vascular structures and eliminate confusion with a pathologic mass (Figs. 9 and 64).

The bronchopulmonary (hilar) lymph nodes, normally not appreciated as discrete structures on non-contrast-enhanced CT scans, are located adjacent to the bronchi in close relationship to the pulmonary vessels (Figs. 58C and D and 65A). Cephalad in the hila, the lymph nodes usually are medial to the segmental bronchi and lateral to the pulmonary arteries. Caudad in the hila, the nodes are situated lateral to the lower-lobe bronchi and medial to the pulmonary artery branches. Normal hilar lymph nodes and/or collections of fat frequently are visible on MRI (Figs. 65B and 66). Collections of tissue, representing both fat and normal-size lymph nodes, large enough to be confused with abnormally enlarged hilar lymph nodes, may be visible in three specific locations on MRI: on the right at the level of the bifurcation of the right pulmonary artery, at the origin of the middle-lobe bronchus, and on the left at the level of the upper-lobe bronchus (151). Generally, lymph nodes and fat are easily distinguished by virtue of their different signal intensities on T1-weighted images.

Trachea

The trachea is a cartilaginous and membranous tube that extends from the larynx (about the level of the C-6 vertebral body) to the carina (about the level of the T-5 vertebral body); the extrathoracic length is approximately 2 to 4 cm, and the intrathoracic length about 6 to 9 cm. As it becomes intrathoracic, it lies in the midline or slightly to the right; progressively caudal sections demonstrate a very gradual posterior course. At all levels, the trachea lies anterior or slightly to the right of the esophagus. Within the thorax, the right wall of the trachea is in contact with the mediastinal pleural reflections of the right upper lobe (Figs. 33, 37, and 39), creating the right paratracheal stripe seen on posteroanterior chest radiographs. Additionally, a potential space exists between the posterior right half of the trachea and the posteriorly positioned right lateral wall of the esophagus. This space, called the retro-tracheal recess, frequently is occupied by lung, creating the posterior tracheal band seen on lateral chest radiographs (77). A fair amount of normal variability in this space can create interfaces that simulate abnormalities on conventional roentgenography (23).

The normal tracheal wall is relatively thin and is defined internally by the central air column. The ring cartilages may be irregularly calcified in the elderly, especially in women. There is marked variability in the cross-sectional appearance of the trachea (42). It is generally circular in shape just below the cricoid cartilage and tends to be transversely ovoid near the carina. In between, it may be horseshoe-shaped; the anterior wall is convex, and the posterior wall, lacking cartilage, is flat. The trachea tends to be more uniformly round in children (62). In adults, the mean cross-sectional area of the normal trachea is 272 mm^2 (SD 33) in men and 194 mm^2 (SD 35) in women; values less than 190 mm^2 in men or 120 mm^2 in women

A,B

C,D

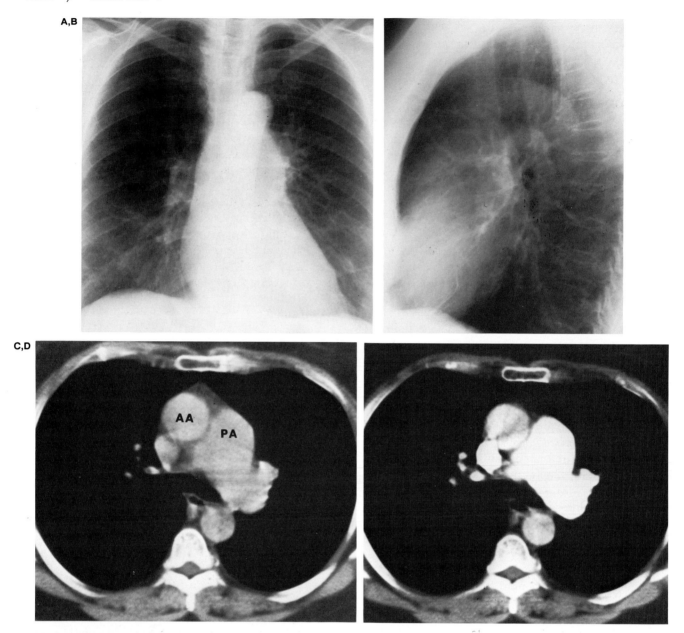

FIG. 64. A,B: Routine posteroanterior and lateral chest radiographs in a 64-year-old woman with a breast mass. The left hilum was interpreted as being too large and dense. **C:** Non-contrast-enhanced CT scan demonstrates marked enlargement of the main pulmonary artery (PA), compared with the ascending aorta (AA), consistent with clinically unsuspected pulmonary arterial hypertension. The left hilum is also enlarged and lobular. Is it all vascular? **D:** Contrast-enhanced scan demonstrates that all of enlarged left hilum is vascular; no lymphadenopathy is present.

should suggest abnormality (146). Abnormal variations in the configuration of the trachea are easily defined on CT. The most common is the saber-sheath trachea, typically associated with advanced chronic obstructive pulmonary disease (61). In this condition, there is marked narrowing of the width of the intrathoracic trachea, to about half to two-thirds of its widened anteroposterior diameter, often down to the level of the carina (Fig. 67). The ring cartilages frequently are densely calcified.

Esophagus

When sufficient posterior mediastinal fat is present, the esophagus can be adequately delineated with CT (Fig. 68). A collapsed esophagus may be confused with a lymph node mass on MRI (Fig. 69). The anterior wall of the esophagus generally contacts the posterior aspect of the trachea, the left main-stem bronchus, and the left atrium in its caudal descent. Distally it is bordered by the de-

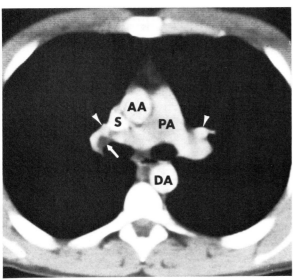
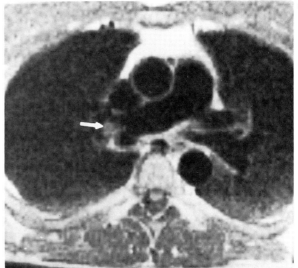

A,B

FIG. 65. Normal hilar lymph nodes. **A:** Contrast-enhanced CT scan demonstrates a normal-size lymph node (*arrow*) in the right hilum; (AA) ascending aorta; (DA) descending aorta; (PA) pulmonary artery; (S) superior vena cava; (*arrowheads*) superior pulmonary veins. **B:** T1-weighted SE MRI in same patient at slightly caudal level also shows the normal right hilar node (*arrow*) as an intermediate signal intensity structure.

scending aorta on its left and by the azygos vein on its right. Intraluminal air is a common finding, present in about 70% of normal patients. The lumen may appear to be divided into two or three sections by strands of mucus bridging the anterior and posterior walls (Fig. 70) (115). The apparent thickness of the wall is variable and dependent on the degree of distension. As a general guideline, a thickness of 3 mm or more should be considered abnormal (66).

Thymus

The morphology of the thymus changes drastically with age, and there are wide variations in its normal size,

weight, and consistency. Knowledge of these various appearances is essential for proper CT interpretation (33).

The thymus is a bilobed organ; each lobe has a separate fibrous capsule that is connected cephalically to the inferior lobes of the thyroid gland. The bulk of the organ is positioned anterior to the great vessels. The thymus is relatively largest (with respect to total body weight) in the

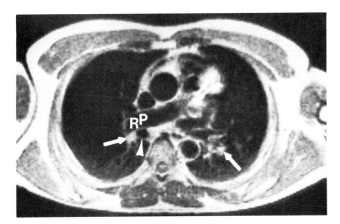

FIG. 66. Normal collections of fat (*arrows*) seen on T1-weighted MRI as relatively high-signal intensity structures; (RP) right pulmonary artery; (*arrowhead*) bronchus intermedius.

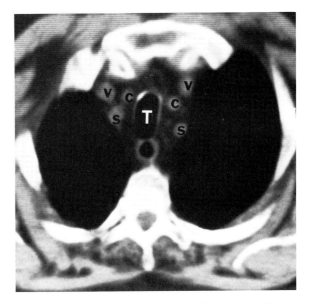

FIG. 67. Saber-sheath configuration of the trachea (T), characterized by an enlarged anteroposterior diameter and a narrow width, usually seen in patients with chronic obstructive pulmonary disease. Associated calcification of the ring cartilages is common; (v) brachiocephalic veins; (s) subclavian arteries; (c) carotid arteries.

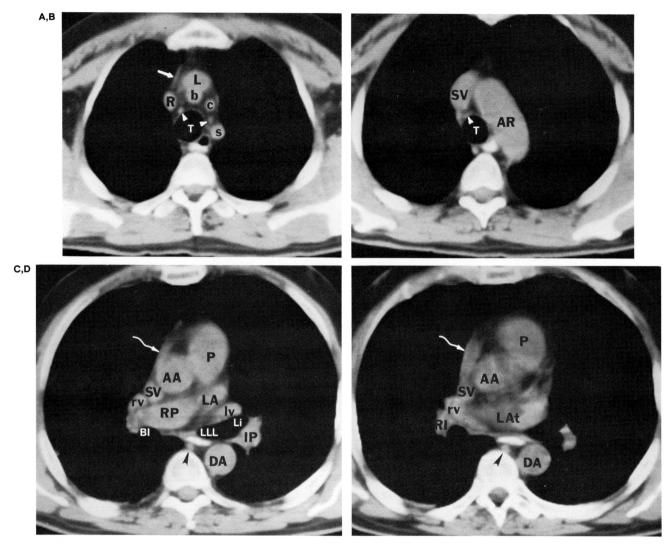

FIG. 68. Anatomic relationships of esophagus, filled with oral contrast material, at following levels: **A:** Crossing left brachiocephalic vein (L). **B:** Aortic arch (AR). **C:** Right pulmonary artery (RP). **D:** Left atrium (LAt); (R) right brachiocephalic vein; (T) trachea; (b) brachiocephalic artery; (c) left carotid artery; (s) left subclavian artery; (*straight arrow*) right internal mammary vein; (*white arrowheads*) normal mediastinal lymph nodes; (SV) superior vena cava; (AA) ascending aorta; (P) main pulmonary artery; (LA) left atrial appendage; (rv) right superior pulmonary vein; (lv) left superior pulmonary vein; (LLL) left-lower-lobe bronchus; (Li) lingular bronchus; (BI) bronchus intermedius; (IP) left interlobar pulmonary artery; (*black arrowhead*) azygos vein; (DA) descending aorta; (*curved arrow*) right atrial appendage; (RI) right interlobar pulmonary artery.

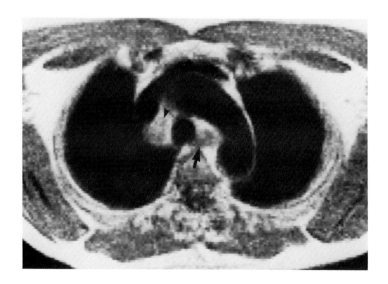

FIG. 69. Esophagus mimicking lymph node on MRI. On T1-weighted image, the esophagus (*arrow*) is similar in signal intensity to an enlarged right paratracheal lymph node (*arrowhead*) and could be confused with lymphadenopathy. They were also similar in signal intensity on the T2-weighted image. Review of sequential images permitted correct identification of structure as the esophagus.

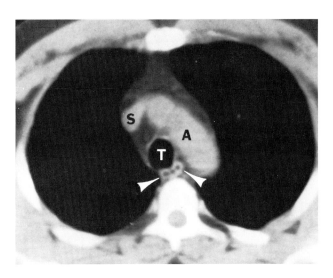

FIG. 70. Normal esophagus, filled with air (*arrowheads*), appears to contain multiple lumina due to apposition of anterior and posterior walls, perhaps by strands of mucus; (T) trachea; (S) superior vena cava; (A) aortic arch.

neonate and young infant (average weight 20 g), but increases slightly in size to reach a maximal weight at puberty (average 30 g). During this period, the thymus consists chiefly of parenchyma, composed mainly of a dense population of lymphocytes, separated by thin fibrous septa. Beginning at puberty, a phase of involution takes place, usually over a period of 5 to 15 years. There is a gradual reduction in the lymphocyte population, with progressive replacement of the atrophied thymic follicles by fat. After age 40, adipose tissue becomes the dominant constituent of the organ; the parenchymal elements and connective-tissue septa become increasingly sparse. By the age of 60, fat usually is the only thymic remnant present.

The appearance of the thymus on CT (and MRI) is directly related to these changes (10,37,100). From birth to puberty, the thymus is seen in the anterior mediastinum, demarcated cephalad by the horizontal portion of the left brachiocephalic vein and caudally by the horizontal portion of the right pulmonary artery (Fig. 71). Its largest portion is found in the 3- to 4-cm interval between the aortic arch and the main pulmonary artery. The thymus has a CT density comparable to that of the chest-wall musculature in this age group. Its outer contours may be convex laterally (Fig. 72). Although the lobes may appear to merge and assume a triangular (or arrowhead) configuration, they are not completely fused. The thymus often is rotated slightly to the left at the level of the aortic arch, and the junction between the two lobes may be about 2 cm to the left of midline. The left lobe usually is slightly larger and is the main caudal extension of the organ.

From puberty to 30 years of age, the appearance of the thymus begins to reflect the fatty infiltration that is occurring. Its overall density has diminished and is always less than that of skeletal muscle (Fig. 73). The thymus

may be seen as a discrete triangular or bilobed structure; its outer borders are now straight or concave laterally. As emphasized, there is broad variation in this involution. Some organs contain considerable fat in patients under age 20, whereas others have little fat even at age 30.

Over the age of 30, small islands of soft-tissue density are seen within a background of more abundant fat (Fig. 74). The residual thymic parenchyma may assume a linear, oval, or small round configuration. Never, however, is a focal alteration in the outer contour of the thymus normally seen in adults. Ultimately, in the older patient, only a thin fibrous skeleton remains of the thymus, and the anterior mediastinum is almost totally composed of fat within its remnant (Fig. 75). This fat may have a slightly higher density than that of the subcutaneous fat.

Although generally not necessary for accurate recognition of abnormality, the most reliable and meaningful measurements of the thymus relate to its thickness (largest distance across the long axis of each lobe) (Fig. 76). With the exception of some neonates, before the age of 20 when the thymus is most prominent, 1.8 cm is the normal maximal thickness. Thereafter, 1.3 cm should not be exceeded.

The thymus is also visible in all adults on MRI (Fig. 77) (28). Contrast between higher-intensity mediastinal fat and the lower-intensity thymus is optimal on T1-weighted images because of the long T1 of the thymus. The progressive decrease in T1 with advancing age likely reflects the fatty infiltration. The T2 relaxation times for the thymus do not change with age and overlap with those for fat. The thymus may appear slightly thicker on MRI than on CT in patients over the age of 20.

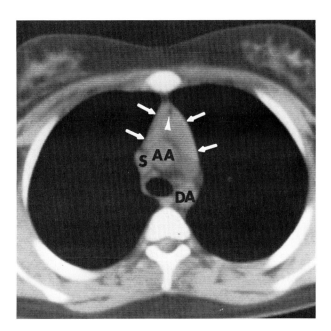

FIG. 71. Normal thymus, 14-year-old girl. At the level of the aortopulmonary window, the two lobes of the thymus (*arrows*) are separated by a thin cleft of fat (*arrowhead*); (S) superior vena cava; (AA) ascending aorta; (DA) descending aorta.

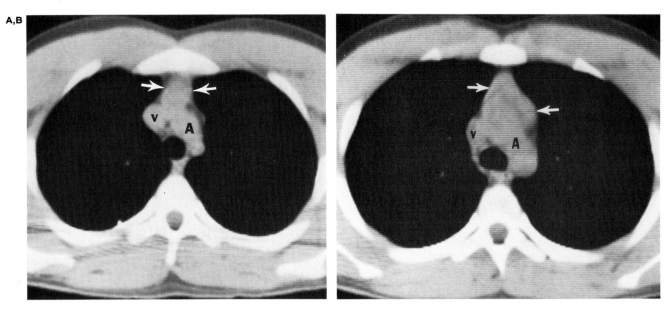

FIG. 72. Normal thymus, 15-year-old boy. **A:** At the level of the top of the aortic arch (A) and superior vena cava (V), both lobes of the thymus (*arrows*) are together. **B:** Caudad 1 cm, the two lobes (*arrows*) are relatively distinct; the left lobe has a bulbous, convex lateral margin. (From ref. 50.)

Azygos Venous System

The azygos and hemiazygos veins represent continuations into the thorax of the right and left ascending lumbar veins, respectively. The azygos vein traverses the diaphragm through a small opening, usually accompanied by branches of the sympathetic neural chain (Figs. 52 and 53). It ascends in the right prevertebral area, usually just posterolateral to the esophagus; laterally it is in contact with the pleural reflections of the right lower lobe, where it defines the medial border of the azygoesophageal recess (Figs. 4D, 42C, 44B, and 45). At the level of the T-5 or T-6 vertebra, the azygos vein arches toward the right and then anterior over the right main-stem bronchus to drain into the posterior aspect of the superior vena cava (Figs. 41 and 42A and B). Sometimes the azygos vein may be interposed between the posterior wall of the right main-stem or upper-lobe bronchus and lung in the azygoeso-

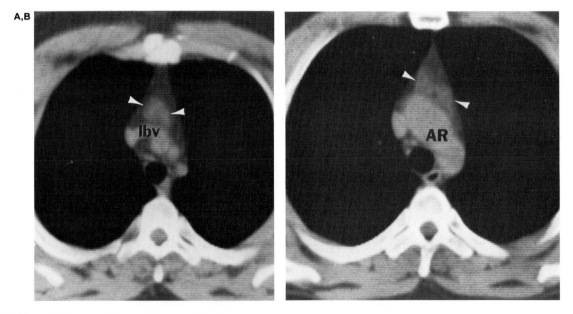

FIG. 73. Normal thymus, 28-year-old man. **A,B:** Sequential scans at level of the crossing left brachiocephalic vein (lbv) and the aortic arch (AR), respectively, show substantial fatty infiltration of the thymus (*arrowheads*), which is lower in density than the blood in the surrounding great vessels or the chest-wall musculature.

A,B

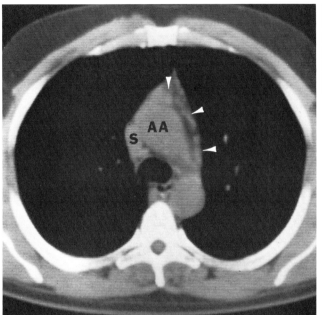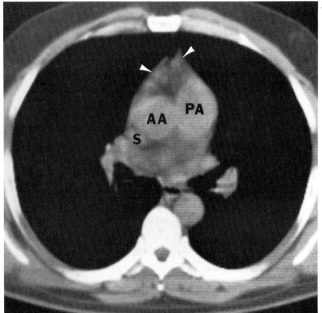

FIG. 74. Normal thymus, 35-year-old man. **A,B:** Scans at level of aortopulmonary window and top of left atrium demonstrate nodular remnants of normal thymus tissue (*arrowheads*) within surrounding fat; (AA) ascending aorta; (PA) main pulmonary artery; (S) superior vena cava.

phageal recess, simulating a mass or an enlarged lymph node (84). Tracing the course of the azygos vein on contiguous sections generally allows confident identification of this normal venous structure. On rare occasion, tortuosity of the azygos vein arch may simulate a pretracheal mass (123). Intravenous contrast enhancement can be used to ensure correct interpretation in perplexing cases (Fig. 78).

The right superior intercostal vein, which receives the effluent from the right second through fourth intercostal

veins, descends along the right anterolateral vertebral margin, where it may bulge slightly into the contour of the right upper lobe (Fig. 79) (85,89). It drains into the azygos vein posteriorly just prior to the formation of the azygos venous arch.

The hemiazygos vein on the left side, usually not seen on CT, parallels the posterior aspect of the descending aorta (Fig. 10) after penetrating the diaphragm through the aortic hiatus. The hemiazygos vein generally crosses the midline prevertebrally, passing posterior to the aorta at about the T-8 level, to drain into the azygos vein. The accessory hemiazygos vein, whose caudal course is also

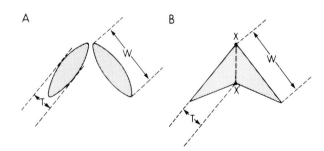

FIG. 76. Determining thymic size. **A:** In a bilobed organ, the short axis or thickness (T) is measured perpendicular to the long axis or width (W). **B:** When the two lobes are confluent, the thymus is arbitrarily divided in half by a line (x–x′) through the apex of the organ. The thickness (T) can then be measured. (From ref. 10.)

FIG. 75. Normal thymus, 75-year-old man. The thymic remnant (*arrows*) is composed of fat.

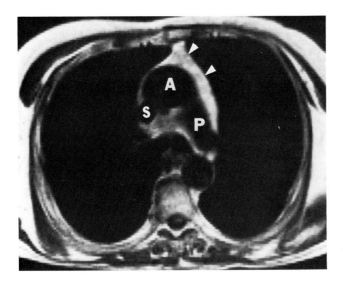

FIG. 77. MRI, normal thymus. On T1-weighted image, nodular remnants of normal thymus (*arrowheads*) are seen within the higher-intensity mediastinal fat; (A) aorta; (S) superior vena cava; (P) left pulmonary artery.

posterior to the descending aorta, usually joins the hemiazygos vein just before it crosses the midline.

The left superior intercostal vein, infrequently seen on CT, may communicate with the accessory hemiazygos vein at or just above the level of the aortic arch. The left superior intercostal vein then forms a horizontal arch that courses anteriorly along the superolateral border of the aortic arch (Fig. 80) or just cephalad (Fig. 81) to join the posterior aspect of the left brachiocephalic vein (8,38). On frontal plain chest roentgenograms, the left superior intercostal vein may be seen "on end," just lateral to or above the aortic knob, and has been termed the "aortic nipple" (94).

Mediastinal Vascular Anomalies

Anomalies of the intrathoracic vessels, including the superior vena cava and its tributaries, the aorta and its branches, and the pulmonary arteries and veins, can alter the radiographic appearance of the mediastinum. In some patients, such an anomaly is detected incidentally on CT scans performed for another reason, and its importance lies in not confusing it with pathologic alteration, such as an enlarged lymph node or a neoplastic mass (50,75,81,115,149). In other individuals, these vascular anomalies may have simulated a mediastinal mass on plain chest radiographs, thus prompting the CT study. In these circumstances, CT can serve as a relatively noninvasive procedure and often replace angiography, with the latter reserved for specific cases requiring further clarification (9,95). Identification of these vascular anomalies or variants, with the exclusion of significant pathologic conditions, has been one of the greatest benefits derived from thoracic CT (11).

An azygos lobe is the most frequent anomaly affecting the mediastinal veins, occurring in about 0.5% of the population. This variation is created during fetal development by anomalous lateral migration of precursors of the azygos vein through the right upper lobe (Fig. 82). The vein draws two layers each of the parietal and visceral pleura with it, forming a pleural mesentery. The lung trapped medial to this fissure is called the "azygos lobe" and consists of parts of the apical or posterior segments of the right upper lobe. In this anomaly, the azygos vein arch typically is located more cephalad than normal, generally about 2 cm above the carina; it may extend as high as the level of the right brachiocephalic vein (Fig. 83) (138). The superior vena cava tends to be rather elliptical in shape and has a much

A,B

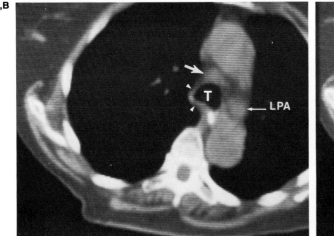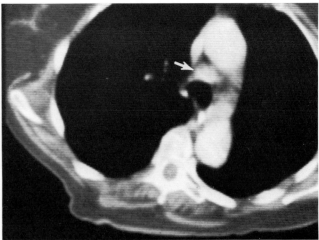

FIG. 78. Tortuous azygos vein. **A:** At the level of the aortopulmonary window, a soft-tissue density (*arrow*) is seen anterior to the trachea, simulating an enlarged lymph node; (*arrowheads*) azygos vein arch; (LPA) top of left pulmonary artery. **B:** After intravenous administration of contrast material, enhancement of the pretracheal density is demonstrated (*arrow*), which on serial scans was shown to be part of a tortuous azygos vein. (From ref. 50.)

A,B

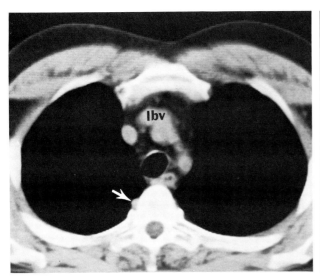 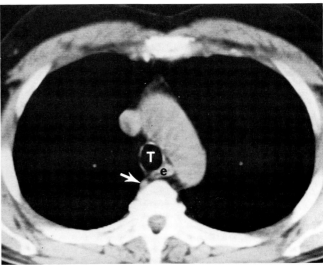

FIG. 79. Right superior intercostal vein. **A:** At level of the crossing left brachiocephalic vein (lbv), the right superior intercostal vein (*arrow*) is seen just lateral to the thoracic spine, slightly indenting the posterior segment of the right upper lobe. **B:** Caudad 1 cm, the right superior intercostal vein (*arrow*) has moved slightly anterior just behind the trachea (T) and lateral to the esophagus (e).

more coronal than sagittal axis. The superior vena cava is concomitantly displaced anteriorly with respect to the trachea, while the esophagus is rotated toward the left. This allows lung to intrude deep into the pretracheal and retrotracheal portions of the mediastinum. On a single scan, the laterally positioned prevertebral portion of the anomalous azygos vein arch can simulate a pulmonary

nodule; observing contiguous levels will clarify the true tubular nature of this structure.

A persistent left superior vena cava occurs in about 0.3% of the normal population (Fig. 84); there is a substantially higher incidence in patients with congenital heart disease (18). This anomaly, which drains at least the left jugular and left subclavian veins, results from em-

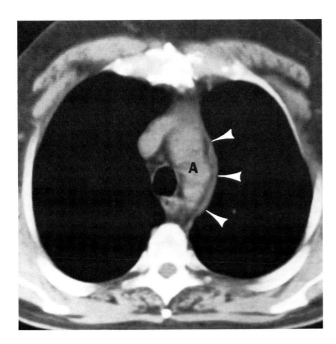 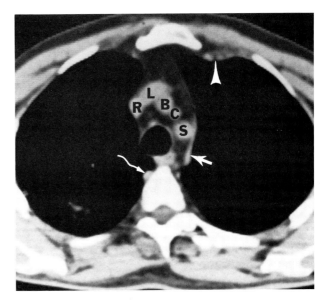

FIG. 80. The left superior intercostal vein (*arrowheads*) is seen coursing just lateral to the aortic arch (A). The mediastinal fat between the arch and the vein, seen only at this single level, should not be confused with an intimal flap in aortic dissection.

FIG. 81. Posterior portion of left superior intercostal vein (*straight arrow*) seen at level above aortic arch. The right superior intercostal vein (*curved arrow*) and the left internal mammary vessels (*arrowhead*) are also visible; (B) brachiocephalic artery; (C) left carotid artery; (S) left subclavian artery; (R) right brachiocephalic vein; (L) left brachiocephalic vein.

A,B

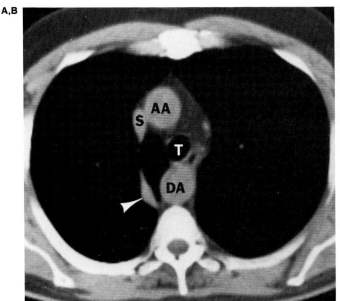
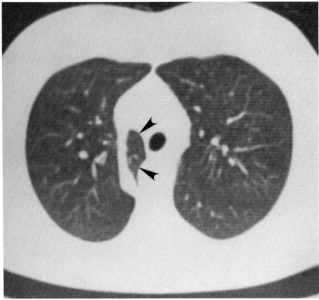

FIG. 82. Azygos fissure. **A:** The azygos vein arch (*arrowhead*) is separated from the mediastinum and trachea (T) as it enters the posterior aspect of the superior vena cava (S); (AA) ascending aorta; (DA) descending aorta. **B:** Lung window setting at same level demonstrates the azygos "lobe" (*arrowheads*) medial to the azygos arch.

bryologic failure of regression of parts of the left common and anterior cardinal veins. In most patients, a right superior vena cava is also present (Figs. 15 and 85), and the left brachiocephalic vein is small or absent. In about 20% of patients with a persistent left superior vena cava, it is joined by the left superior intercostal vein, which communicates with the hemiazygos vein to form an accessory azygos arch (Fig. 86), similar to the one on the right side. On CT, the left superior vena cava is positioned initially lateral to the left common carotid artery and anterior to

the left subclavian artery (71). The anomalous vessel descends lateral to the aortic arch, in approximately the same coronal plane as the normal right superior vena cava. It passes lateral to the main pulmonary artery and anterior to the left hilum and typically drains into a dilated coronary sinus posterior to the left ventricle. If necessary, contrast material injected into a left medial antecubital vein can corroborate that the structure in question is a vein.

Occasionally, anomalies of isolated partial pulmonary

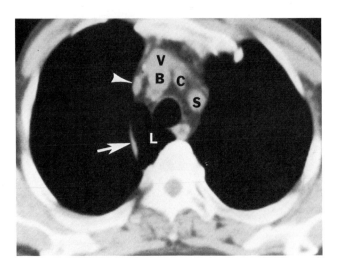

FIG. 83. Azygos fissure: cephalad-positioned azygos vein arch (*arrow*) entering the right brachiocephalic vein (*arrowhead*); the azygos "lobe" (L) is subtended medially; (V) left brachiocephalic vein; (B) brachiocephalic artery; (C) left carotid artery; (S) left subclavian artery.

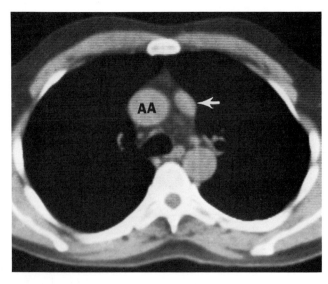

FIG. 84. Persistent left superior vena cava (*arrow*) to the left of the ascending aorta (AA). The right superior vena cava is absent.

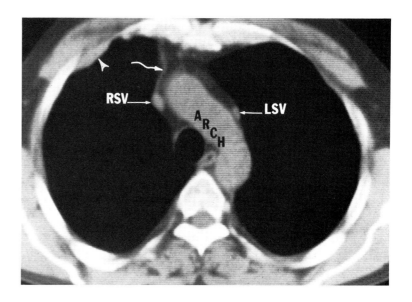

FIG. 85. Both a right superior vena cava (RSV) and a left superior vena cava (LSV) are seen surrounding the aortic arch (ARCH). A prominent right internal mammary vein (*curved arrow*) enters the anterior aspect of the right superior vena cava; a pleural plaque (*arrowhead*) is present. (From ref. 50.)

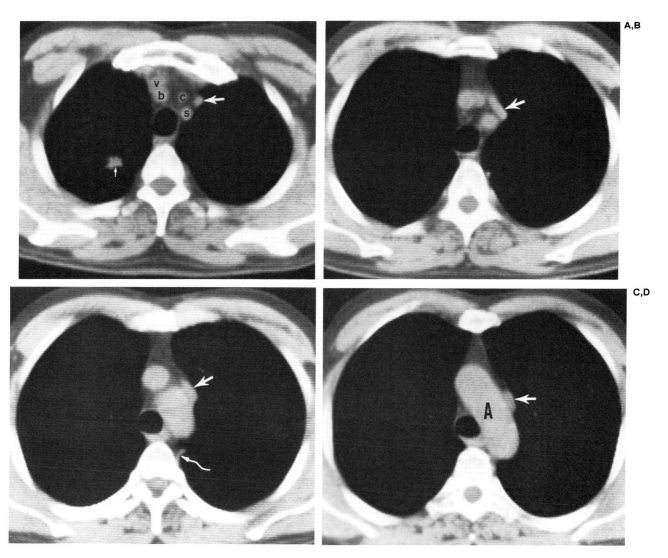

FIG. 86. Persistent left superior vena cava. **A:** The left brachiocephalic vein (*large arrow*) is seen descending along the upper left side of the mediastinum in a patient with a bronchogenic carcinoma of the right upper lobe (*small arrow*); (v) right brachiocephalic vein; (b) brachiocephalic artery; (c) left carotid artery; (s) left subclavian artery. **B:** Caudad 1 cm, the two brachiocephalic veins join to form a persistent left superior vena cava (*arrow*). **C:** Caudad 1 cm, an anterior-directed arch is being formed by the accessory hemiazygos vein (*curved arrow*) to join the persistent left superior vena cava (*straight arrow*). **D:** Caudad 1 cm, at the level of the aortic arch (A), the left superior vena cava (*arrow*) is seen laterally; the right superior vena cava is absent. (From ref. 50.)

venous drainage are detected on CT. When the left superior pulmonary vein empties into the left brachiocephalic vein, a vertical vein is seen coursing lateral to the aortic arch and aortopulmonary window, which looks identical in appearance with a persistent left superior vena cava. The correct diagnosis is possible when no left superior pulmonary vein is identified in its expected position in the left hilum (114). Other anomalies of pulmonary venous drainage that may be recognized include that from the right inferior pulmonary vein cephalad into the azygos vein (126) or caudad into an anomalous scimitar vein draining into the subdiaphragmatic inferior vena cava (108).

Idiopathic dilatation of virtually all of the major intrathoracic veins has been reported, including the superior vena cava (Fig. 87), the left innominate vein (Fig. 31), and the inferior vena cava (99).

Anomalies of the inferior vena cava can be associated with dilatation of the azygos and/or hemiazygos veins (21). When there has been embryologic failure of development of the infrahepatic segment of the inferior vena cava above the renal veins, blood from the lower half of the body returns to the heart via the persistent subcardinal veins, i.e., the azygos and hemiazygos veins. Azygos (and hemiazygos) continuation of the inferior vena cava, which can be present in asymptomatic individuals as well as those

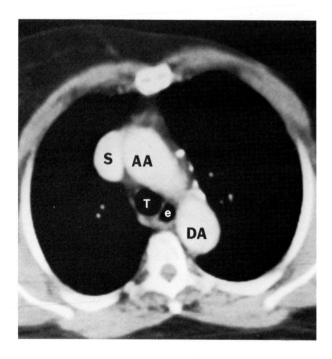

FIG. 87. Idiopathic dilatation of superior vena cava in a 67-year-old woman following left mastectomy referred because outside chest radiography demonstrated mediastinal widening. Contrast-enhanced scan demonstrates that widening results from dilatation of superior vena cava (S) and some tortuous vessels. No lymph node metastases present; (AA) ascending aorta; (DA) descending aorta; (T) trachea; (e) esophagus.

with congenital heart disease, may be mistaken on conventional radiography (or even CT) for a mass or enlarged lymph nodes in the right paratracheal, posterior mediastinal, or retrocrural areas. Careful examination of serial CT scans should readily facilitate the correct diagnosis from the characteristic constellation of findings (Fig. 88) (14,22). In this anomaly, there is dilatation of the azygos arch, the azygos vein, and the superior vena cava caudal to the azygos junction because of the increased blood flow. Similar enlargements of the paraspinal and retrocrural portions of the azygos and hemiazygos veins are present, and the suprarenal portion of the inferior vena cava is lacking on scans of the upper abdomen. Because the most cephalad portion of the inferior vena cava develops embryologically from the hepatic sinusoids, this segment draining the hepatic veins may be visible on both CT and plain chest radiographs in patients with congenital interruption of the inferior vena cava. Typically, the hemiazygos vein crosses over behind the aorta to join the azygos vein, although variations exist. The hemiazygos vein may serve as the major source of venous drainage and may empty into a persistent left superior vena cava and subsequently into the coronary sinus (2,25).

Anomalies of the aortic arch and great vessels can be categorized into three groups: left aortic arch, right aortic arch, and double aortic arch (132). CT can be a valuable technique for recognizing, and sometimes classifying, the various aortic arch anomalies (150). Although generally not of major clinical utility, other aortic anomalies, including coarctation, pseudocoarctation, transposition of the great vessels, and truncus arteriosus, also can be diagnosed.

The most common congenital anomaly of the aorta, occurring in close to 1% of the population, is an aberrant right subclavian artery originating from an otherwise normal left aortic arch (Fig. 89) (78). It rarely results in either symptoms or a detectable abnormality on plain chest roentgenograms; uncommonly, a posterior impression on the trachea is seen. The anomalous right subclavian artery is seen on CT arising as the last branch from the distal portion of the aortic arch. The vessel crosses the mediastinum obliquely from left to right behind the esophagus and trachea on its cephalad course. It is commonly dilated at its origin, and the adjacent esophagus may be compressed or displaced to the right. The aortic arch itself may be at a slightly higher level, and its orientation frequently is more directly anteroposterior. In its cephalad portion, the aberrant right subclavian artery often is positioned more dorsal than the normal vessel with respect to the right common carotid artery.

Although at least five potential right aortic arch anomalies can occur, depending on the exact point at which the normal arch is interrupted (133), only two are relatively common. The most frequent is the right aortic arch with an aberrant left subclavian artery (Fig. 90). In this anomaly, which is rarely associated with congenital heart disease, the origin of the left subclavian artery, the last branch from the aortic arch, frequently is dilated (diverticulum of Kommerrell). It crosses the mediastinum posterior to the esophagus. A right aortic arch with mirror-image branching has a high incidence of associated congenital heart disease, especially with tetralogy of Fallot. In this situation, because interruption of the normal left aortic arch occurred distal to the ductus arteriosus, there is no structure posterior to the trachea or esophagus.

The double aortic arch is characterized by two arches arising from a single ascending aorta, each generally giving rise to a subclavian and carotid artery, and then rejoining to form a single descending aorta. These arches surround the trachea and esophagus, and symptoms related to compression of these structures may arise. Typically, the right arch is larger and situated slightly more cephalad than the left arch. Portions of the left arch may be atretic, and it becomes difficult or impossible to distinguish this from right aortic arch anomalies.

Although CT can demonstrate aortic deformity at the site of a coarctation (54), MRI with oblique sagittal sections (Fig. 21) is the preferred noninvasive technique to demonstrate the size and extent of the narrowing in patients with abnormal physical and/or plain chest radiographic findings.

Pseudocoarctation, or kinking of the aortic arch in the region of the ligamentum arteriosum, is a rare anomaly that may be mistaken for a true coarctation or a mediastinal mass on conventional chest radiography (45). Typically, the ascending aorta is normal in position and caliber. However, the aortic arch is abnormally high, and as it descends it curves anteriorly, kinks, and then courses posteriorly to its normal position. Because the proximal descending aorta is located anteriorly, on CT, lung can be seen interposed between the descending aorta and the spine. The left subclavian artery may arise more distally than usual and sometimes can be seen posterior to the upper portion of the descending aorta.

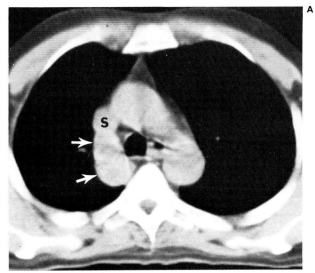

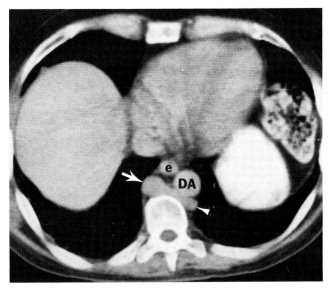

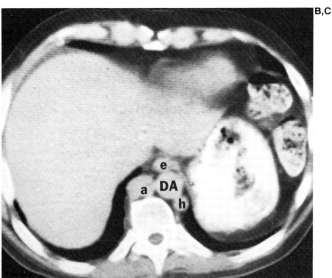

FIG. 88. Azygos continuation of inferior vena cava. **A:** At the level of the aortopulmonary window, a markedly dilated azygos vein arch (*arrows*) drains into the superior vena cava (S). **B:** At the ventricular level, a dilated hemiazygos vein (*arrowhead*) is seen crossing dorsal to the descending aorta (DA) to join a dilated azygos vein (*arrow*), which bulges into the azygoesophageal recess; (e) esophagus. **C:** At the top of the retrocrural space, dilated azygos (a) and hemiazygos (h) veins produced paraspinal line widening noted on a plain chest radiograph; (DA) descending aorta; (e) esophagus.

A

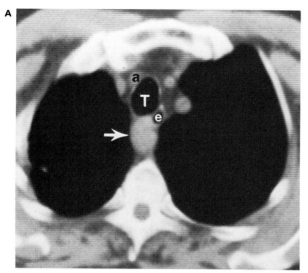

FIG. 89. Aberrant right subclavian artery. A,B: Sequential scans through superior mediastinum in patient with right-upper-lobe bronchogenic carcinoma (CA). A rounded, soft-tissue density (*arrow*) is seen posterior to the trachea (T) and adjacent to both the esophagus (e) and the posterior part of the top of the aortic arch (A). The apparent right brachiocephalic artery (a) is diminutive. C: After intravenous administration of contrast material, an aberrant right subclavian artery is demonstrated (*arrow*) arising from the aortic arch (A). The esophagus (*arrowhead*) is displaced slightly to the right; (r) right carotid (not the brachiocephalic) artery; (c) left carotid artery; (s) left subclavian artery; (v) brachiocephalic veins. (From ref. 50.)

B,C

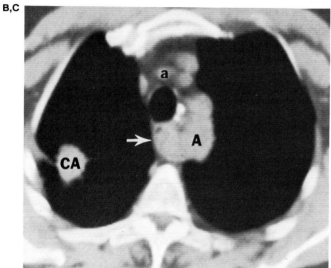
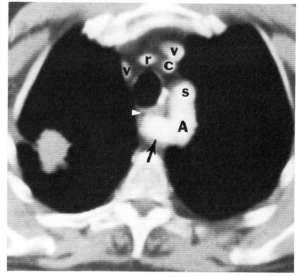

FIG. 90. Right aortic arch (ARCH) with aberrant left subclavian artery (*arrowhead*) adjacent to posterior aspect of arch; (V) superior vena cava; (T) trachea.

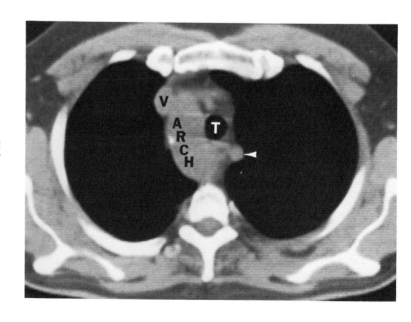

A,B

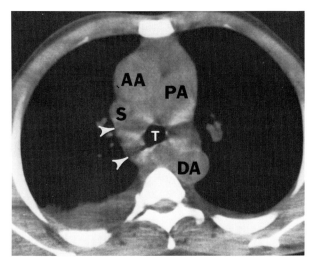

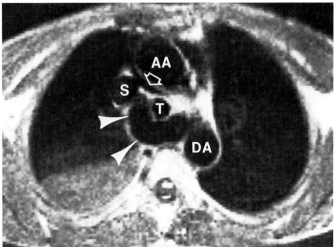

FIG. 91. Anomalous left pulmonary artery in a 45-year-old man with chronic renal failure on hemodialysis who developed renal cell carcinoma. Candidate for resection and renal transplantation. **A:** CT done to assess for possible thoracic metastasis demonstrates right paratracheal widening (*arrowheads*) and a probable retrotracheal mass. Is this due to lymphadenopathy? Clinician requested that intravenous contrast material not be administered. Bilateral pleural effusions present; (T) trachea; (S) superior vena cava; (AA) ascending aorta; (DA) descending aorta; (PA) pulmonary artery. **B:** T1-weighted SE MRI demonstrates that an anomalous left pulmonary artery (*arrowheads*) accounts for the right paratracheal and retrotracheal mass. A small pericardial effusion extending into the retroaortic recess (*open arrow*) is seen.

Transposition of the great vessels can be diagnosed on CT (or MRI) when the ascending aorta is seen arising from the anterior or right ventricle (9). The *l*-corrected form of transposition, the type generally encountered in adults, can be distinguished from the more clinically significant *d*-transposition by observing the side-to-side relationship of the aorta and pulmonary artery in the former. Also, the aorta descends to the left of the pulmonary artery in the *l*-corrected transposition.

Truncus arteriosus with absence of the right pulmonary artery may be diagnosed when CT shows a large central truncal artery giving rise to a right aortic arch and a left pulmonary artery (150).

Rarely in adults, an asymptomatic anomalous left pulmonary artery (pulmonary artery sling) may be encountered incidentally (Fig. 91) (142). In this condition, the main and right pulmonary arteries appear normal on CT. The anomalous left pulmonary artery arises from the posterior portion of the right pulmonary artery, passes above the right main bronchus lateral to the trachea, and then crosses the mediastinum interposed between the trachea and the esophagus to reach the left hilum.

Pulmonary Parenchyma

The appearance of the lung will vary somewhat depending on the slice thickness and the phase of respiration. Thoracic CT scanning usually is performed at full lung capacity (end-inspiratory volume), which has the effect of reducing crowding of the pulmonary vessels and potentially improving recognition of small pathologic pulmonary abnormalities. However, it may be more difficult to reproduce scans reliably at end inspiration than at breath holding at resting lung volume, and the latter may be used whenever anatomic reproducibility is critical, such as when sequential thin sections through a pulmonary nodule are required. At such resting lung volumes, there is considerable crowding of pulmonary vessels in the dependent portion of the lung. A similar phenomenon occurs in the posterior lung bases when CT is being used primarily for evaluation of the abdomen; such scans are obtained in expiration. Even with scans done in full inspiration in the supine position, there may be crowding of the vessels in the lung bases, making evaluation of abnormalities difficult. By scanning patients in the prone position, the normal distribution of the pulmonary vascularity can be altered; this may be effective for more confidently diagnosing or excluding small nodules in the posterior lung bases.

The normal range of pulmonary density generally is between −350 and −450 HU, with the differences less on inspiration than on expiration. Mean attenuation values in the posterior third of the lungs may be as much as 100 HU greater than in the anterior third; the gradient is reduced, but not abolished, on scans obtained in deep inspiration.

When the smaller peripheral pulmonary vessels course horizontally, it is generally possible to trace their origin to the major segmental vessels and verify their nature. If, however, a small vessel courses obliquely or in a cephalocaudal direction, demonstration of the origin (and thus the cause) of the ovoid or round density usually requires examination of sequential scans to verify that the structure is vascular. Similarly, a pulmonary arteriovenous malformation might be tracked and analyzed in such a fash-

A,B

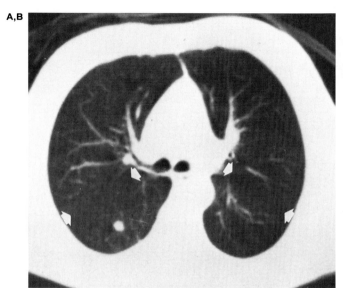 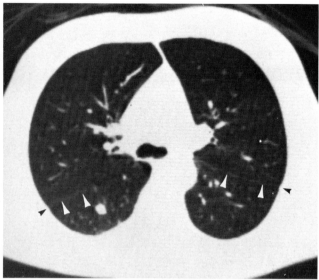

FIG. 92. Major interlobar fissures. **A:** On a standard 8-mm collimated section, the major (oblique) fissures are shown as vague areas of hypovascularity between the upper and lower lobes (*arrows*). **B:** On a 2-mm collimated scan, the major fissures (*white arrowheads*) can be recognized with confidence as lines. Very small pleural notches (*black arrowheads*) are seen peripherally. The right-lung nodule is posterior to the major fissure and thus definitely within the superior segment of the right lower lobe.

ion, and definitive diagnosis may not require intravenous contrast enhancement.

Pleura

A double serous membrane, the thicker parietal pleura, lines the thoracic cavity; it is separated from the musculature of the chest wall by a layer of loose areolar tissue. The visceral pleura, which intimately envelopes the lung, also extends between its lobes to line the major and minor fissures.

Delineation of the fissures on CT may become important, because they serve as major landmarks, allowing for accurate localization of disease within the pulmonary parenchyma (Fig. 63). Similarly, correct identification of loculated fluid within the fissures presupposes knowledge of their normal location and appearance.

The appearance of the major fissures, which are oriented relatively vertical (cephalocaudad), is variable, depending on the level and their exact axis with the cross-sectional plane (91). Most often, the major fissures can be identified as somewhat indistinct broad lucent bands within the pulmonary parenchyma (Fig. 92). They appear to be "avascular" because of the diminutive tapering of the pulmonary vessels in the most peripheral portions of the lungs. This is similar in appearance to the normal subpleural radiolucent zone, 3 to 5 mm in width, that usually is present in the nondependent portions of the lung where the peripheral blood vessels are too small to be seen. Less frequently, the major fissures may be seen as discrete lines; this occurs if the vertical axis of the fissure is exactly per-

pendicular to the plane of the CT section. Such a situation can almost always be achieved with narrow collimation (2–4 mm), and the major fissures can be recognized with certainty using this technical variation (Fig. 92B). A small collection of supradiaphragmatic fat occasionally is seen invaginating into the caudal aspect of one or both major interlobar fissures (Fig. 93) (41). This fat probably is a lateral extension of the pericardial fat pads. Similarly, fat from the anterior mediastinum may extend into the anterior junction line between the visceral pleura of the two lungs (Fig. 94).

The minor fissure, which is relatively parallel to the transaxial CT image, appears as a broad hypovascular area in the anterior portion of the right lung just lateral to the right interlobar pulmonary artery at the level of the bronchus intermedius (Fig. 95) (59). The orientation of the fissure at the level sectioned determines the pattern of the lucent zone, formed by the most peripheral portions of the adjacent right upper and middle lobes; most often it is triangular, but it may be round or ovoid. The latter two configurations are caused by slight cephalad doming of the fissure, with the right upper lobe completely surrounding the relatively avascular region. With narrow collimation, a portion of the domed minor fissure may be oriented vertical or slightly oblique to the cross-sectional CT plane and may appear as a discrete line or a hazy band on the section.

In addition to the normal major and minor fissures, accessory fissures may be recognized on CT. Most commonly seen is the previously described azygos fissure (Fig. 82B), which appears as a laterally convex curved line extending from the right brachiocephalic vein or superior

A,B

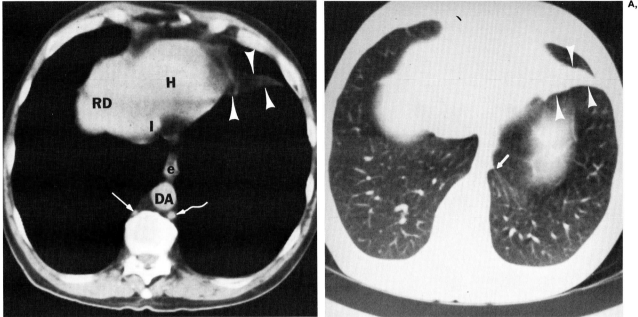

FIG. 93. A: At level of caudal portion of the heart (H), fat (*arrowheads*) is seen extending into the lower portion of the left major fissure; (RD) right hemidiaphragm; (I) inferior vena cava; (e) esophagus; (DA) descending aorta; (*straight arrow*) azygos vein; (*curved arrow*) hemiazygos vein. **B:** Same level, with lung window setting, shows apparent thickening of the left major fissure due to the extension of fat (*arrowheads*); (*arrow*) left inferior pulmonary ligament.

vena cava anteriorly to a posterior position alongside the lateral aspect of the T-4 or T-5 vertebra.

Additional accessory fissures may be formed at the boundaries of bronchopulmonary segments, but they are seldom visible or recognized on CT scans (55). An inferior accessory fissure (Fig. 96) may circumscribe the medial or anteromedial basal segments of the lower lobes. Also, a left minor fissure demarcating the lingula may create a

hypovascular area similar in appearance to the right minor fissure.

The inferior pulmonary ligaments constitute another normal, frequently recognizable, region of the pleura. These ligaments, a double-layered reflection of the parietal pleura, may envelope some bronchial veins and lymph nodes. They anchor the lower lobes to the mediastinum and extend from an apex just below the margins of the

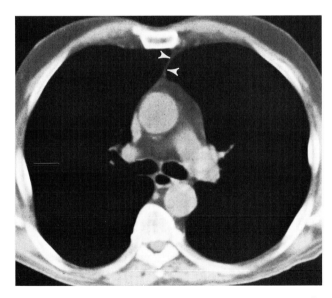

FIG. 94. Fat extending from the mediastinum into the anterior junction line (*arrowheads*) between the visceral pleura separating the two lungs.

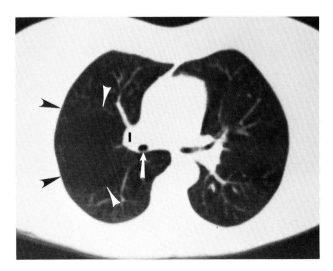

FIG. 95. Minor fissure. Lucent area in right midlung (*arrowheads*) represents the zone of the minor fissure that lies parallel to the transaxial CT section. Typically, the right interlobar pulmonary artery (I) and the bronchus intermedius (*arrow*) lie in the same plane.

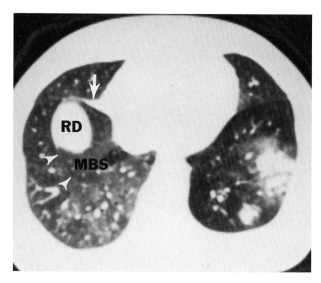

FIG. 96. An inferior accessory fissure (*arrowheads*) is seen circumscribing the medial basal segment (MBS) of the right lower lobe in a patient with a left-lower-lobe infiltrate. Fat is extending into the caudal portion (*arrow*) of the right major fissure; (RD) right hemidiaphragm.

inferior pulmonary veins in a caudal and posterior direction. On CT, the inferior pulmonary ligaments produce linear shadows arising from the mediastinum and extending laterally into the lung bases (26,56,125). They may be prominent in patients with emphysema and can be quite thick in those with pleural thickening, such as secondary to asbestos exposure. On the right side, the inferior pulmonary ligament lies adjacent to the inferior vena cava; on the left side, it lies alongside the distal esophagus (Figs. 93B and 97). Their caudal extensions are

variable; they may assume a triangular configuration as they reflect onto the diaphragm or more rarely end in a free falciform edge. The presence of these ligaments explains some of the unusual distributions of fluid or air within the caudal pleural space, as well as the configuration of lower-lobe atelectasis.

Pericardium

The pericardium is a double-layered, fibroserous sac that envelopes and anchors the heart. The thin, shiny visceral layer (or epicardium) is closely adherent to the heart, covering the subepicardial fat and myocardium. The thicker outer fibrous parietal layer forms a flask-like sac. Its narrowed upper segment is attached to the proximal portions of the great vessels; small pockets may be formed by these vascular reflections, including the transverse sinus between the superior vena cava and the ascending aorta. The wide caudal portion of the parietal pericardium is anchored to the central tendon of the diaphragm. Ventral insertions onto the sternum via the superior and inferior sternopericardial ligaments are generally present, and there may be attachments to the thoracic spine. The two layers of the pericardium have opposing serosal linings, the surface of which is lubricated by about 20 to 25 ml of fluid contained within the pericardial sac.

Although motion interferes with a well-defined image of the cardiac chambers to some degree on CT, at least a

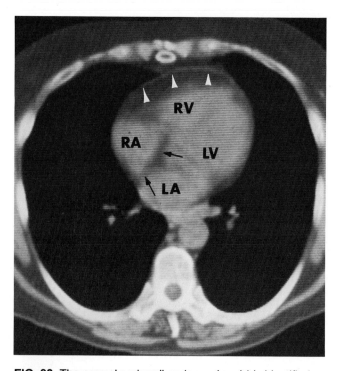

FIG. 98. The normal pericardium (*arrowheads*) is identified as a thin line of soft-tissue density between the pericardial (mediastinal) fat anteriorly and the underlying epicardial fat posteriorly; (RA) right atrium; (LA) left atrium; (*arrows*) interatrial groove; (RV) right ventricle; (LV) left ventricle.

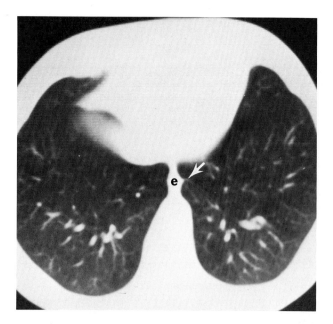

FIG. 97. The left pulmonary ligament (*arrow*) is seen extending from the esophagus (e) into the left lower lobe.

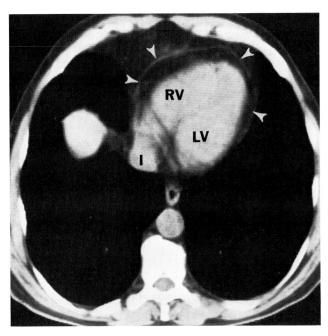

FIG. 99. The normal pericardium (*arrowheads*) is seen surrounding virtually the entire caudal portion of the heart because of the abundant internal epicardial fat present; (RV) right ventricle; (LV) left ventricle; (I) inferior vena cava.

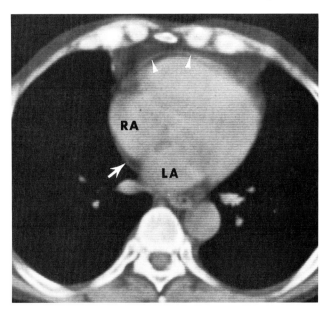

FIG. 100. The normal pericardium is seen not only overlying the anterolateral surface of the heart (*arrowheads*) but also posterolateral over the right atrium (*arrow*), where some underlying epicardial fat is present; (RA) right atrium; (LA) left atrium.

portion of the pericardium can be demonstrated in almost all cooperative adults (70,98,135). The part that is most commonly seen is over the anterior and caudal surfaces of the heart, where the pericardium is surrounded externally by mediastinal fat and internally by epicardial fat (Fig. 98). The fibrous parietal pericardium appears as a thin, curvilinear, soft-tissue-density line, generally 1 to 2 mm in thickness. The visceral pericardium, only a thin cellular membrane, casts no shadow in the normal individual. Its surface is identified at the edge of the epicardial fat. At the level of the left ventricle, the dorsal aspect of

the pericardium is visible in only a small minority of patients (Fig. 99), because of both a lack of underlying epicardial fat here and more vigorous pulsations along the free wall that produce blurring. In patients with abundant mediastinal and epicardial fat, the pericardium may be visible in some additional unusual locations, such as around the great vessels and near the interatrial septum (Fig. 100). Large lipomatous collections may form in the latter region; they are almost always incidental findings without clinical significance (Fig. 101). Also, abundant epicardial fat may be responsible for an echo-free space

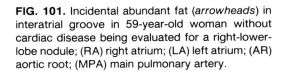

FIG. 101. Incidental abundant fat (*arrowheads*) in interatrial groove in 59-year-old woman without cardiac disease being evaluated for a right-lower-lobe nodule; (RA) right atrium; (LA) left atrium; (AR) aortic root; (MPA) main pulmonary artery.

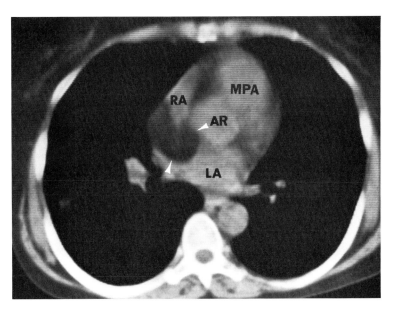

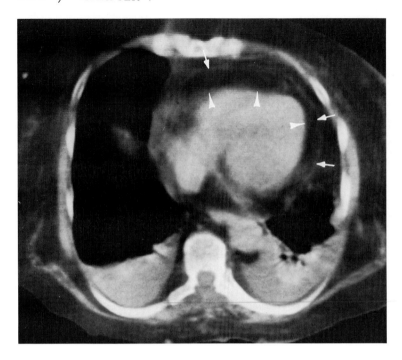

FIG. 102. A 78-year-old woman with congestive heart failure in whom both M-mode and 2-D echocardiograms demonstrated a sonolucent thick band surrounding the anterior and left lateral aspect of the heart, interpreted as secondary to a pericardial effusion. CT shows that the sonolucent band was simply abundant epicardial fat (*arrowheads*). The pericardium (*arrows*) itself is thin and normal; no pericardial effusion is present. Bilateral pleural effusions and atelectasis of the left lower lobe are seen.

on ultrasound that may be misinterpreted as a loculated anterior pericardial effusion (Fig. 102) (73). With gated MRI, the normal pericardium also may be superbly depicted (Fig. 103) (129).

The normal pericardial space and its contained fluid are not generally visible, with a few exceptions. Small physiologic amounts of fluid may collect in the recesses around the great vessels (88) and near the cardiac apex. The near-water-density transverse (or superior) sinus posterior to the ascending aorta (Fig. 104) may be seen in close to 50% of the normal population (7). The preaortic (pulmonary) recess in front of the main pulmonary artery (Fig. 105) and a sinus posterior to the left pulmonary artery are infrequently demonstrated. A pericardial recess anterior to the ascending aorta surrounding a relatively cephalad-positioned right atrial appendage may simulate

an anterior mediastinal mass (Fig. 106). Tracing its caudal contiguity with the right atrium on sequential images should facilitate its distinction as a normal anatomic structure. Around the caudal portion of the heart, the parietal pericardium has an oblique course as it inserts onto the central tendon of the diaphragm, and normal fluid up to 3 to 4 mm in thickness may be imaged on the transaxial sections here (Fig. 107), which can simulate pericardial thickening or an abnormal effusion. The normal fluid should be seen on only one or two scan levels near the diaphragm.

Occasionally, the normal phrenic nerve may be identified as a 1 to 3-mm rounded structure adjacent to the posterolateral surface of the pericardium, especially on the left side, that should not be mistaken for a small pulmonary nodule (metastasis) (143).

FIG. 103. On EKG-gated MRI, the normal pericardium (*black arrowhead*) is seen as a thin curvilinear area with absence of signal intensity over the anterior surface of the heart; (RA) right atrium; (LA) left atrium; (A) aortic root; (P) main pulmonary artery; (*white arrowhead*) left anterior descending coronary artery; (*arrow*) left circumflex coronary artery.

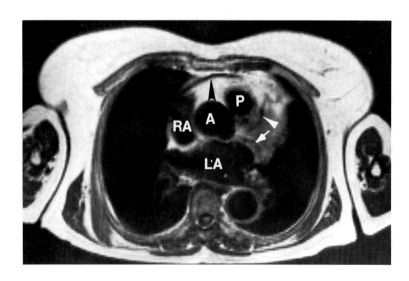

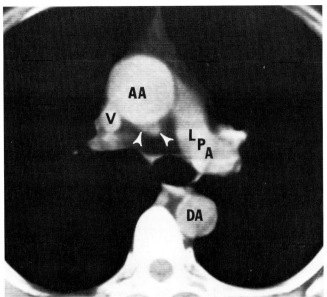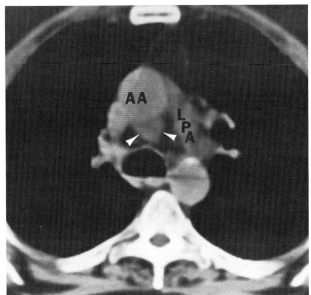

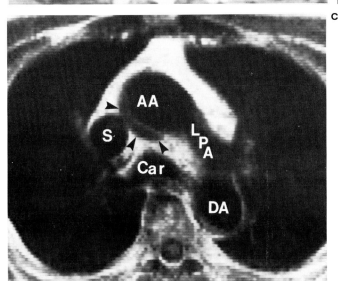

FIG. 104. Retroaortic pericardial recess. **A:** The transverse (or superior) sinus of the pericardium (*arrowheads*) appears as a semilunar near-water-density structure posterior to the ascending aorta (AA); (DA) descending aorta; (V) superior vena cava; (LPA) left pulmonary artery. (From ref. 50.) **B:** A large, 2.2-cm-diameter, near-water-density recess (*arrowheads*) in another patient; this could be confused with an enlarged lymph node; (AA) ascending aorta; (LPA) left pulmonary artery. (From ref. 4.) **C:** Recess (*arrowheads*) seen on MRI as an elliptical structure of very low signal intensity lateral and posterior to the ascending aorta (AA); (S) superior vena cava; (LPA) left pulmonary artery; (DA) descending aorta; (Car) carina. (From ref. 50.)

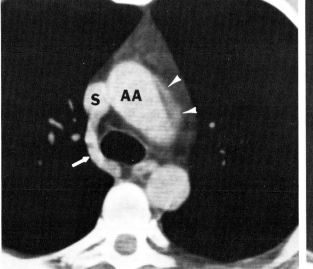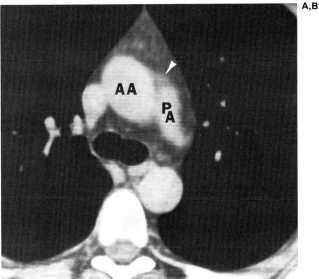

FIG. 105. Preaortic (aortopulmonary) pericardial recess. **A:** Near-water-density structure (*arrowheads*) lateral to ascending aorta (AA) near undersurface of aortic arch; (S) superior vena cava; (*arrow*) azygos vein arch. **B:** Caudad 1 cm, the pericardial recess (*arrowhead*) is seen insinuating between the ascending aorta (AA) and the top of the pulmonary artery (PA). (From ref. 50.)

A,B

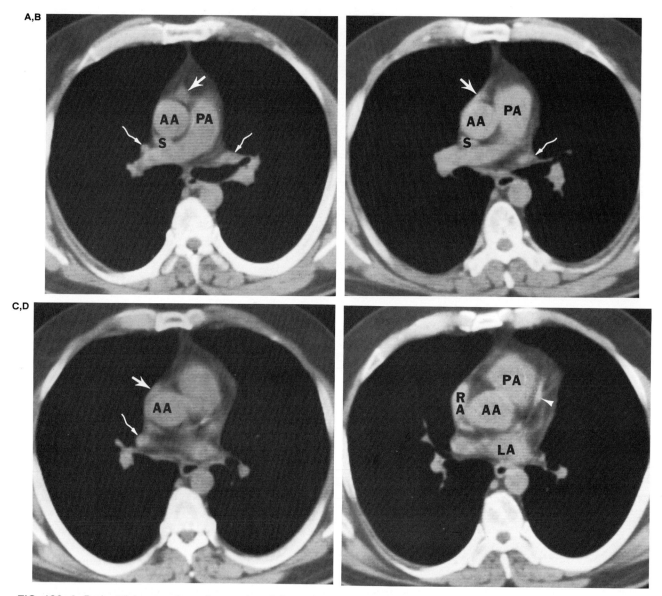

C,D

FIG. 106. **A:** Pericardial recess (*arrow*) around cephalad extension of right atrial appendage, anterior to ascending aorta (AA) and superior vena cava (S), at level of main and right pulmonary arteries (PA). This recess and appendage could simulate an enlarged lymph node or a thymic mass. **B–D:** Serial scans 1, 2, and 3 cm caudad show that recess and appendage (*straight arrow*) are contiguous with the right atrium (RA); (AA) ascending aorta; (PA) main pulmonary artery; (S) superior vena cava; (LA) left atrium; (*arrowhead*) anterior descending branch of left coronary artery; (*curved arrows*) superior pulmonary veins.

Diaphragm

A dome-shaped musculotendinous partition that separates the thorax from the abdomen, the diaphragm also is the chief muscle of respiration. It is composed of a central tendon and peripheral leaf-like muscle extensions bilaterally (Fig. 108). The anterior portion of the diaphragm is attached to the posterior surfaces of the six lowermost costal cartilages and the sternum. The posterior or lumbar portion, including the two crura that are attached to the anterolateral surface of the upper lumbar vertebral bodies, also is adherent to the medial and lateral arcuate ligaments, which are fascial thickenings over the anterior surfaces of the psoas and quadratus lumborum muscles. The pericardium is attached to the upper surface of the central tendon of the diaphragm. The superior diaphragmatic (cardiophrenic-angle) lymph nodes are located extrapleurally around this pericardial-diaphragmatic junction and can be divided into anterior, middle, and lateral groups (6). There are three major passageways through the diaphragm: one each for the inferior vena cava, esophagus and vagus nerves, and the aorta and thoracic duct.

The large domed portion of the diaphragm usually is not visible as a discrete structure on CT (104). This results from partial-volume averaging of the normally thin

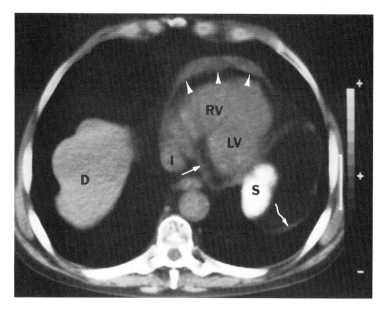

FIG. 107. Just before its caudal insertion into the central tendon of the diaphragm, there may be apparent anterior thickening of the pericardium (*arrowheads*), where small physiologic amounts of fluid accumulate and where transaxial CT scans image the pericardial sac tangentially; (I) inferior vena cava; (D) right hemidiaphragm and underlying liver; (RV) right ventricle; (LV) left ventricle; (S) stomach; (*straight arrow*) coronary sinus; (*curved arrow*) left hemidiaphragm.

diaphragm with adjacent structures that are of similar soft-tissue density (e.g., the liver and spleen). In addition, cardiac motion interferes with distinct imaging of the horizontal portion of the diaphragm. However, the positions of the hemidiaphragms can be inferred from knowledge of characteristic anatomic relationships (103). At all levels, the lungs and pleura lie adjacent and peripheral to the diaphragm, whereas the abdominal viscera and surrounding fat lie central to the hemidiaphragms. The peripheral, more vertically oriented portions of the hemidiaphragms may be distinctly defined on non-contrast-enhanced CT images when their inner aspects are marginated by abundant amounts of intraabdominal fat (Fig. 109). On contrast-enhanced scans, the densities of the liver and spleen usually are elevated to a much greater degree than that of diaphragmatic muscle, and the latter often may be seen as a discrete structure. A similar phenomenon occurs with fatty infiltration of the liver (Fig.

110). With deep inspiration, the individual muscle bundles for the costal insertions may be quite prominent because they are markedly foreshortened (Fig. 111). These fibers should not be confused with neoplastic peritoneal implants or small mural nodules even if they indent the stomach, colon, or liver. These pseudotumors are contiguous peripherally with the diaphragm and usually can be distinguished from the hollow viscera because of some subdiaphragmatic fat; their disappearance on scans performed in expiration permits conclusive diagnosis (Fig. 112) (124).

The most anterior portion of the diaphragm has a variable appearance on CT, depending on the cephalocaudal relationship of the xiphoid process to the central tendon of the diaphragm (39). The anterior diaphragm most often appears as a relatively smooth, slightly undulating soft-tissue arc, concave posteriorly and continuous across the midline. Sometimes there may be anterior divergence of

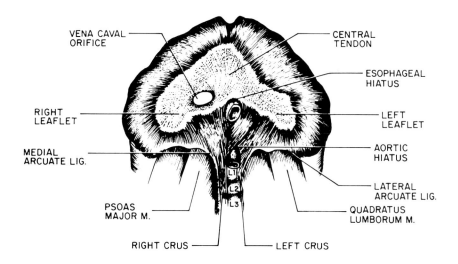

FIG. 108. Schematic drawing of diaphragm as viewed from below.

A,B

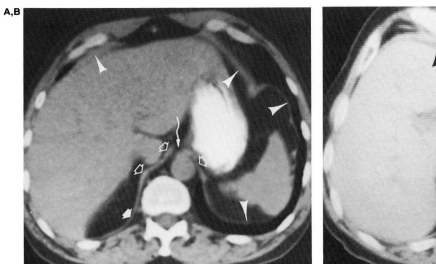
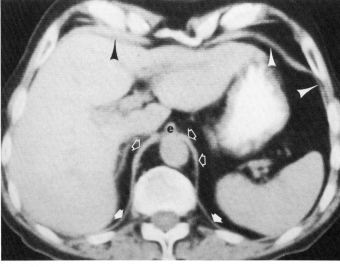

FIG. 109. A,B: Diaphragms in two different patients. Abundant intraabdominal fat marginates the peripheral muscular portions of the diaphragm (*arrowheads*), as well as the crura (*open arrows*) and the arcuate ligaments (*closed arrows*). A small gap (*curved arrow*) for passage of the esophagus (e) separates the medial ends of the crura.

A

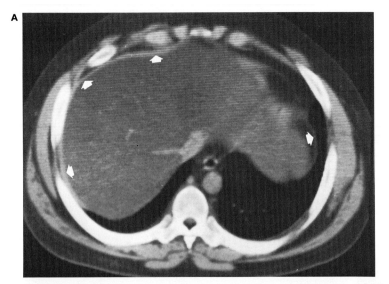

FIG. 110. A–C: Sequential caudal scans showing the peripheral diaphragmatic musculature (*closed arrows*) and crural insertions (*open arrows*) in a patient with fatty infiltration of the liver.

B,C

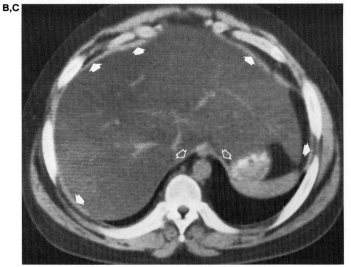
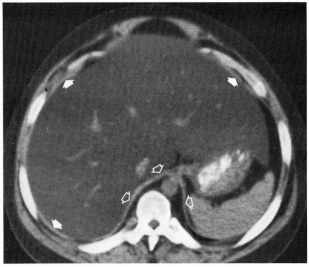

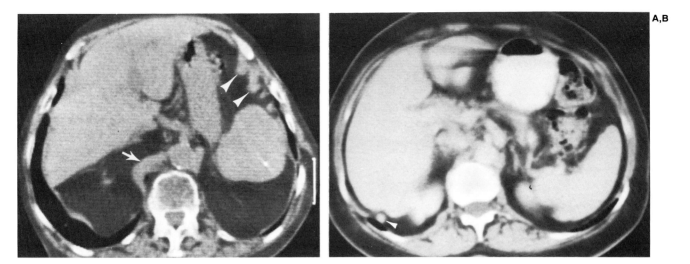

FIG. 111. Costal insertions of diaphragm. **A:** On scan in deep inspiration, the muscle bundles of the costal insertions (*arrowheads*) are quite prominent and could simulate peritoneal implants. The right diaphragmatic crus (*arrow*) is also thickened. **B:** In another patient, a costal insertion (*arrowhead*) could simulate a metastatic peritoneal implant posterior to the liver.

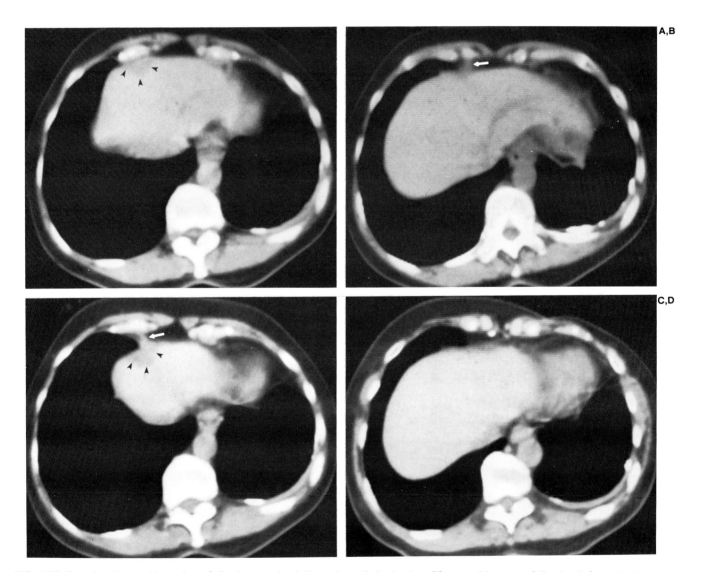

FIG. 112. Prominent costal insertion of diaphragm simulating a hepatic lesion in a 56-year-old woman following left mastectomy; she had a prior history of left tuberculous empyema. **A:** Non-contrast-enhanced scan performed in inspiration for study of the thorax suggests metastasis (*arrowheads*) in the dome of the liver. **B:** No lesion on non-contrast-enhanced scan performed in expiration to evaluate the liver. Prior low-density lesion was in region of a costal insertion of the diaphragm (*arrow*). **C:** Contrast-enhanced scan in inspiration shows pseudolesion (*arrowheads*) intimately associated with costal insertion (*arrow*). **D:** Pseudolesion disappears on contrast-enhanced scan performed in expiration.

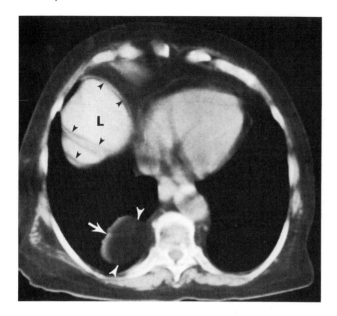

FIG. 113. Extension of retroperitoneal fat into an eventration (*white arrowheads*) medial to an irregular right hemidiaphragm (*arrow*). On lung window settings, this can simulate an intraparenchymal mass. Note also the prominent costal insertions of the diaphragm (*black arrowheads*) over the dome of the liver (L).

the diaphragmatic muscle fibers and apparent discontinuity as they insert onto the costal cartilages. Occasionally the anterior fibers lie in almost a single plane and are imaged as a broad angular band with poorly defined margins. The anterior diaphragmatic muscular attachments may not be identified at all on CT, either because the fibers are indistinguishable from adjacent structures (because of lack of surrounding fat) or because they are extremely short or even absent.

The posterior and caudal portions of the diaphragm, especially the crural part, which is oriented more vertically than the dome, generally are well defined on CT (16). The most cephalad section in which the crura can be identified usually is at the level of the esophageal hiatus (Figs. 52 and 53). The thicker right diaphragmatic crus arises from the first three lumbar vertebrae; the left crus is smaller and originates from the first two lumbar vertebrae. The medial aspects of the crura are demarcated by cephalad extensions of fat from the posterior pararenal space. The contained retrocrural space, bounded posteriorly by the spine, also encloses the aorta, azygos and hemiazygos veins, thoracic duct, and lymph nodes, which should not exceed 6 mm in diameter. In about 90% of patients, the transition from the crura to the medial arcuate ligament appears quite smooth and virtually imperceptible (Fig.

A,B

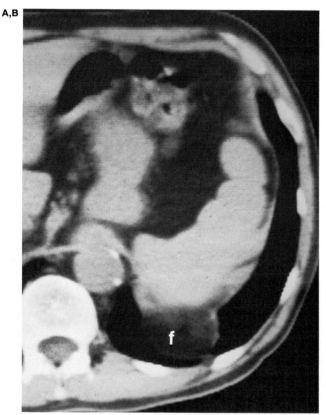
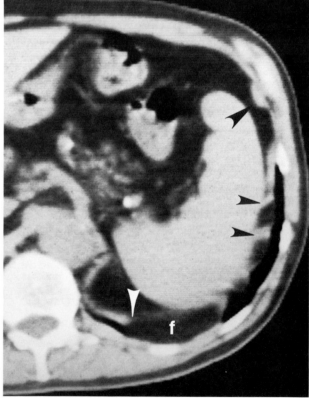

FIG. 114. A,B: Sequential caudal scans in inspiration demonstrate herniation of retroperitoneal fat (f) through a defect (*white arrowhead*) in the left hemidiaphragm into the thorax. Prominent costal insertions (*black arrowheads*) are noted lateral to the spleen.

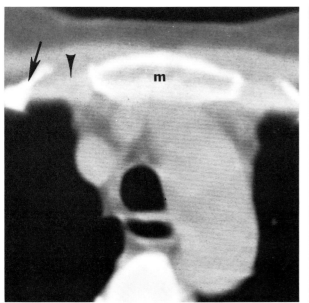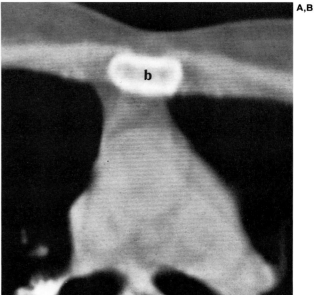

A,B

FIG. 115. A: The wide manubrium (m) of the sternum usually has an indistinct posterior margin as compared with the sharply defined anterior cortical boundary; (*arrow*) first rib; (*arrowhead*) first costal cartilage. **B:** The narrower body (b) of the sternum usually has sharp, cortical margins in its entire periphery.

109), but it may be abrupt. With an abrupt transition, most common in young patients with thick muscles, the crura, especially on the right, may appear quite lobulated or nodular (Fig. 53). This appearance tends to be maximal on deep inspiration (Fig. 111A) and should not be confused with enlarged lymph nodes (3).

Eventrations or small Bochdalek hernias, which result when a portion of the muscle of a hemidiaphragm becomes exceedingly thin or is absent, are relatively common congenital anomalies, occurring in about 5% of the population (40). They are more common on the left side and may be bilateral. Protrusions of abdominal fat through the weakened areas or defects may occur, which on CT images viewed at lung window settings through the lower thorax may simulate an intrapulmonary mass (Fig. 113). Recognition that this is simply a normal variation is contingent on identifying the fat density within the suspected mass (29). Tracing the "abnormality" in sequential sections to and through the level of the involved hemidiaphragm, often accompanied by a small defect or discontinuity in the hemidiaphragm, permits the correct interpretation (Fig. 114).

Chest Wall

Bilateral symmetry is relatively characteristic and facilitates radiographic analysis of the chest wall. Congenital absence (most usually incomplete) of the pectoralis major or minor muscles may rarely be encountered (30); this may be associated with other thoracic or hand anomalies. The shoulder girdle is quite mobile, and its appearance on CT varies with the position of the upper extremities.

Most cross-sectional illustrations in anatomy textbooks are based on adduction of the arms alongside the body. Whereas such positioning is used for MRI, it creates streak artifacts on CT, and most patients are optimally imaged with the arms abducted in external rotation and elevated alongside the head. This results in a different anatomic appearance of the normal shoulder girdle on CT scans. The scapulohumeral joint, the spine of the scapula, and the coracoid process are seen at about the level of the T-2 or T-3 vertebral body. The sternoclavicular joints usually are seen at about the T-4 level.

The sternum can be difficult to image with conventional radiography, and because the sternoclavicular joints are angled obliquely, their demonstration may be particularly difficult to accomplish. The three sections of sternum, its articulations with the clavicles (Figs. 28 and 29), and the contiguous soft tissues generally can be clearly depicted on transaxial CT sections (31,60,67,140). The manubrium is the widest part of the sternum (Fig. 115A) and forms the anterior boundary of the superior mediastinum. Part of its posterior cortical margin normally is unsharp and irregular, and the anterior margin may be indistinct. This appearance could simulate a destructive lesion. If desired, the gantry can be angulated so that it is perpendicular to the manubrium in an effort to improve cortical definition. The superior border of the manubrium has a rounded defect, the jugular (sternal) notch (Fig. 116). Just cephalad, the proximal portions of the clavicles have a steep obliquity and appear in cross section as enlongated or oval structures. Caudal to the jugular notch, there is an indentation (clavicular notch) on the posterolateral aspects of the manubrium for articulation with the clavicular heads.

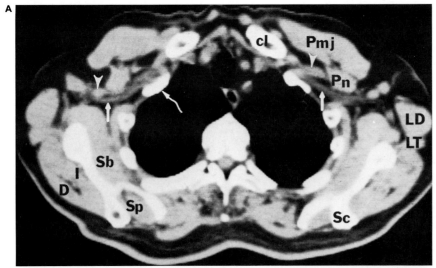

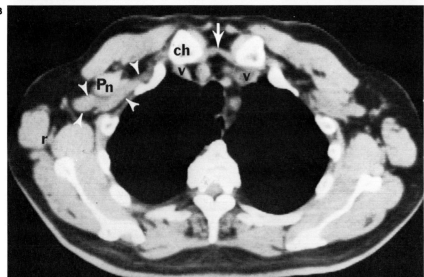

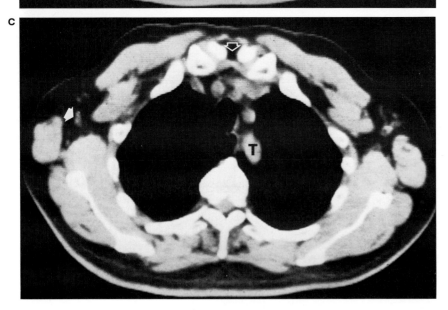

FIG. 116. Upper chest wall; sequential caudal scans at 1-cm intervals. **A:** At the level of the proximal heads of the clavicles (cl), the axillary arteries (*arrows*) can be seen just posterior to the axillary veins (*arrowheads*), external to the first rib (*curved arrow*); (LD) latissimus dorsi and teres major muscles; (LT) long head of triceps muscle; (Pmj) pectoralis major muscle; (Pn) pectoralis minor muscle; (D) deltoid muscle; (I) infraspinatus muscle; (Sb) subscapularis muscle; (Sp) supraspinatus muscle; (Sc) scapula. **B:** The axillary sheath (*arrowheads*) containing the axillary artery, veins, and nerves of the brachial plexus is seen posterior to the pectoralis minor muscle (Pn) at the level of the clavicular heads (ch); (*arrow*) sternothyroid muscle; (v) brachiocephalic veins. **C:** The sternal (jugular) notch (*open arrow*) along the cephalad portion of the manubrium is seen. Small axillary lymph nodes (*closed arrow*), one of which on the left side is calcified, are noted; (T) top of the aortic arch.

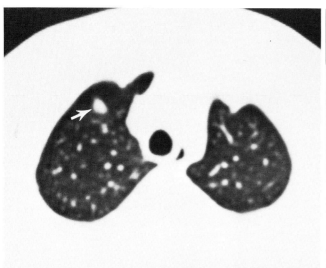 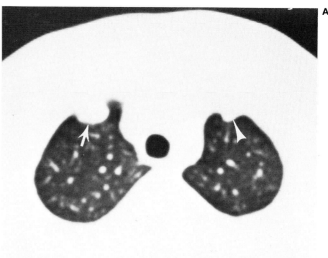

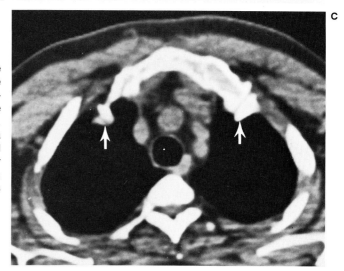

FIG. 117. First costochondral junction pitfall. **A:** Partial-volume averaging through the caudal portion of the junction of the first rib and its costal cartilage may simulate an intraparenchymal nodule (*arrow*) on lung window settings. No nodule was visible on same scan with mediastinal soft-tissue settings. **B:** Scan 1 cm cephalad shows that it is contiguous with a larger nodule shadow (*arrow*), in exactly the same vertical alignment, that abuts the anterior chest wall. A smaller anterior nodular projection (*arrowhead*) is seen on the left side. **C:** Same scan at mediastinal window settings shows that nodules are due to costochondral junctions (*arrows*).

The costal cartilages of the first ribs articulate with the manubrium anterolaterally. A very prominent first costochondral junction, a well-recognized pitfall on conventional chest radiography, can cause a rounded density on a lung-window-setting CT scan that may mimic a pulmonary nodule (Fig. 117) (111) or occasionally simulate a poorly defined area of parenchymal consolidation. Typically, this confusion arises on a CT section 1 cm below the junction of the first rib with its prominent costal cartilage, because the caudal edge of the junction is partial-volume-averaged with the surrounding lung. The "lesion" appears intraparenchymal rather than part of the anterior chest wall because of the rapid oblique caudal and anterior sloping of the latter. Correct, confident interpretation that the "nodule" or "infiltrate" is an artifact can be achieved by recognizing its precise vertical alignment with the costochondral junction on the prior cephalad scan.

The more caudal body of the sternum is ovoid or round in shape and usually has sharp cortical margins (Fig. 115B). Its lateral surfaces may be irregular at the various costochondral junctions; soft-tissue prominences also may surround these articulations. Similarly, sections through the transition between the manubrium and body of the sternum, and between the body and xiphoid process, typically demonstrate indistinct or sclerotic margins. Fusion anomalies may involve the lower half of the body of the sternum in 4% of the population. Clefts (slits) (Fig. 118) or wide gaps (foramen) may be seen on CT (139). In pectus excavatum deformities, the sternum not only is posteriorly displaced but also usually is rotated somewhat obliquely (Fig. 119).

The internal mammary vessels, located about 12 mm lateral to the sternal border, are only rarely seen on CT with standard soft-tissue settings (Figs. 33B and 41). On lung window settings, these vessels may cause tiny projections into the pulmonary parenchyma (115). The nor-

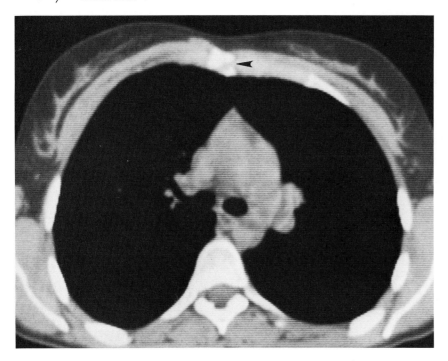

FIG. 118. At a single level, a congenital cleft (slit) (*arrowhead*) was incidentally noted in the upper body of the sternum.

mal adjacent parasternal (internal mammary) lymph nodes are too small to be seen on CT.

Comparable to the situation with mammography, and hardly a revelation, there is a wide range in the CT appearance of the normal female breast. The parenchyma may be dense and even somewhat mass-like, especially in young women, or quite sparse, with mainly fatty tissue seen in older adults.

The axillae typically are quite symmetric (Fig. 116), and the axillary artery and vein, accompanied by branches of the brachial plexus in a neurovascular sheath, often can be defined on CT as distinct structures (35). The axillary vein begins at the lower border of the teres major muscle and courses cephalad. With the arms positioned over the head, the axillary vein is completely anterior to the artery throughout its course, becoming the subclavian vein at the lateral border of the first rib. Contiguous scans at narrow collimation may be of value when trying to depict a possible small lesion in the course of the brachial plexus.

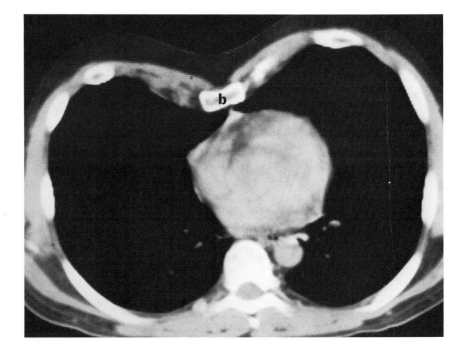

FIG. 119. Pectus excavatum deformity. The body of the sternum (b) not only is displaced posteriorly but also is rotated.

REFERENCES

1. Adler O, Rosenberger A. Computed tomography in guiding of fine needle aspiration biopsy of the lung and mediastinum. *Fortschr Röntgenstr* 1980;133:135–137.
2. Allen HA, Haney PJ. Left-sided inferior vena cava with hemiazygos continuation. *J Comput Assist Tomogr* 1981;5:917–920.
3. Anda S, Roysland P, Fougner R, Stovring J. CT appearance of the diaphragm varying with respiratory phase and muscular tension. *J Comput Assist Tomogr* 1986;10:744–745.
4. Aronberg DJ, Glazer HS, Sagel SS. MR and CT of the mediastinum: comparisons, controversies and pitfalls. *Radiol Clin North Am* 1985;23:439–448.
5. Aronberg DJ, Glazer HS, Madsen K, Sagel SS. Normal thoracic aortic diameters by computed tomography. *J Comput Assist Tomogr* 1984;8:247–250.
6. Aronberg DJ, Peterson RR, Glazer HS, Sagel SS. Superior diaphragmatic lymph nodes: CT assessment. *J Comput Assist Tomogr* 1986;10:937–941.
7. Aronberg DJ, Peterson RR, Glazer HS, Sagel SS. The superior sinus of the pericardium: CT appearance. *Radiology* 1984;153:489–492.
8. Ball JB Jr, Proto AV. The variable appearance of the left superior intercostal vein. *Radiology* 1982;144:445–452.
9. Baron RL, Gutierrez FR, Sagel SS, Levitt RG, McKnight RC. CT of anomalies of mediastinal vessels. *AJR* 1981;137:571–576.
10. Baron RL, Lee JKT, Sagel SS, Peterson RR. Computed tomography of the normal thymus. *Radiology* 1982;142:121–125.
11. Baron RL, Levitt RG, Sagel SS, Stanley RJ. Computed tomography in the evaluation of mediastinal widening. *Radiology* 1981;138:107–113.
12. Barrett HH, Gordon SK, Hershel RS. Statistical limitations in transaxial tomography. *Comput Biol Med* 1976;6:307–323.
13. Baxter BS, Sorenson JA. Factors affecting measurements of size and CT number in computed tomography. *Invest Radiol* 1981;16:337–341.
14. Breckenridge JW, Kinlaw WB. Azygos continuation of the inferior vena cava: CT appearance. *J Comput Assist Tomogr* 1980;4:392–397.
15. Brooks RA, Di Chiro G. Theory of image reconstruction in computed tomography. *Radiology* 1975;117:561–572.
16. Callen PW, Filly RA, Korobkin M. Computed tomographic evaluation of the diaphragmatic crura. *Radiology* 1978;126:413–416.
17. Callen PW, Korobkin M, Isherwood I. Computed tomographic evaluation of the retrocrural prevertebral space. *AJR* 1977;129:907–910.
18. Cha EM, Khoury GH. Persistent left superior vena cava: radiologic and clinical significance. *Radiology* 1972;103:375–381.
19. Chasen MH, McCarthy MJ, Gilliland JD, Floyd JL. Concepts in computed tomography of the thorax. *Radiographics* 1986;6:793–832.
20. Chew E, Weiss GH, Brooks RA, Di Chiro G. Effect of CT noise on detectability of test objects. *AJR* 1978;131:681–685.
21. Chuang VP, Mena CE, Hoskins PA. Congenital anomalies of the inferior vena cava: review of embryogenesis and presentation of a simplified classification. *Br J Radiol* 1974;47:206–213.
22. Churchill RJ, Wesby G III, Marsan RE, Moncada R, Reynes CJ, Love L. Computed tomographic demonstration of anomalous inferior vena cava with azygos continuation. *J Comput Assist Tomogr* 1980;4:398–402.
23. Cimmino CV. The esophageal-pleural stripe: an update. *Radiology* 1981;140:607–613.
24. Cohan RH, Newman GE, Braun SD, Dunnick NR. CT assistance for fluoroscopically guided transthoracic needle aspiration biopsy. *J Comput Assist Tomogr* 1984;8:1093–1098.
25. Cohen MI, Gore RM, Vogelzang RL, Rochester D, Neiman HL, Crampton AR. Accessory hemiazygos continuation of left inferior vena cava: CT demonstration. *J Comput Assist Tomogr* 1984;8:777–779.
26. Cooper C, Moss AA, Buy JN, Stark DD. CT appearance of the normal inferior pulmonary ligament. *AJR* 1983;141:237–240.
27. Crowe JK, Brown LR, Muhm JR. Computed tomography of the mediastinum. *Radiology* 1978;128:75–87.
28. de Geer G, Webb WR, Gamsu G. Normal thymus: assessment with MR and CT. *Radiology* 1986;158:313–317.
29. Demartini WJ, House AJS. Partial Bochdalek's herniation: computerized tomographic evaluation. *Chest* 1980;77:702–704.
30. Demos TC, Johnson C, Love L, Posniak H. Computed tomography of partial unilateral agenesis of the pectoralis muscles. *J Comput Assist Tomogr* 1985;9:558–559.
31. Destouet JM, Gilula LA, Murphy WA, Sagel SS. Computed tomography of the sternoclavicular joint and sternum. *Radiology* 1981;138:123–128.
32. Dickey JE, Haaga JR. Benign iatrogenic cause of mediastinal gas seen on computed tomography. *J Comput Assist Tomogr* 1984;8:330–331.
33. Dixon AK, Hilton CJ, Williams GT. Computed tomography and histological correlation of the thymic remnant. *Clin Radiol* 1981;32:255–257.
34. Federle MP, Moss AA, Boyd DP, Royal SA. Coronal and sagittal reconstruction using a 4.8 second CT body scanner: developments and applications. *AJR* 1979;133:625–632.
35. Fishman EK, Zinreich ES, Jacobs CG, Rostock RA, Siegelman SS. CT of the axilla: normal anatomy and pathology. *Radiographics* 1986;6:475–502.
36. Fink I, Gamsu G, Harter LP. CT-guided aspiration biopsy of the thorax. *J Comput Assist Tomogr* 1982;6:958–962.
37. Francis IR, Glazer GM, Brookstein FL, Gross BH. The thymus: reexamination of age-related changes in size and shape. *AJR* 1985;145:249–254.
38. Friedman AC, Chambers E, Sprayregen S. The normal and abnormal left superior intercostal vein. *AJR* 1978;131:599–602.
39. Gale ME. Anterior diaphragm: variations in the CT appearance. *Radiology* 1986;161:635–639.
40. Gale ME. Bochdalek hernia: prevalence and CT characteristics. *Radiology* 1985;156:449–452.
41. Gale ME, Greif WL. Intrafissural fat: CT correlation with chest radiography. *Radiology* 1986;160:333–336.
42. Gamsu G, Webb WR. Computed tomography of the trachea: normal and abnormal. *AJR* 1982;139:321–326.
43. Gamsu G, Webb WR, Sheldon P, et al. Nuclear magnetic resonance imaging of the thorax. *Radiology* 1983;147:473–480.
44. Gatenby RA, Mulhern CB Jr, Boroder GJ, Muldofsky PJ. Computed-tomographic-guided biopsy of small apical and peripheral upper-lobe lung masses. *Radiology* 1984;150:591–592.
45. Gaupp RJ, Fagan CJ, Davis M, Epstein NE. Pseudocoarctation of the aorta. *J Comput Assist Tomogr* 1981;5:571–573.
46. Genereux GP, Howie JL. Normal mediastinal lymph node size and number: CT and anatomic study. *AJR* 1984;142:1095–1100.
47. Glazer GM, Francis IR, Gebarski K, Samuels BI, Sorensen KW. Dynamic incremental computed tomography in evaluation of the pulmonary hila. *J Comput Assist Tomogr* 1983;7:59–64.
48. Glazer GM, Francis IR, Shirazi KK, Bookstein FL, Gross BH, Orringer MB. Evaluation of the pulmonary hilum: comparison of conventional radiography, 55° posterior oblique tomography, and dynamic computed tomography. *J Comput Assist Tomogr* 1983;7:983–989.
49. Glazer GM, Gross BH, Quint LE, Francis IR, Bookstein FL, Orringer MB. Normal mediastinal lymph nodes: number and size according to American Thoracic Society mapping. *AJR* 1985;144:261–265.
50. Glazer HS, Aronberg DJ, Sagel SS. Pitfalls in CT recognition of mediastinal lymphadenopathy. *AJR* 1985;144:267–274.
51. Glazer HS, Aronberg DJ, Sagel SS, Friedman PJ. CT demonstration of calcified mediastinal lymph nodes: a guide to the new ATS classification. *AJR* 1986;147:17–20.
52. Glazer HS, Gutierrez FR, Levitt RG, Lee JKT, Murphy WA. The thoracic aorta studied by MR imaging. *Radiology* 1985;157:149–155.
53. Gobien RP, Skucas J, Paris BS. CT-assisted fluoroscopically guided aspiration biopsy of central hilar and mediastinal masses. *Radiology* 1981;141:443–447.
54. Godwin JD, Herfkens RJ, Brundage BH, Lipton MJ. Evaluation of coarctation of the aorta by computed tomography. *J Comput Assist Tomogr* 1981;5:153–156.
55. Godwin JD, Tarver RD. Accessory fissures of the lung. *AJR* 1985;144:39–47.

56. Godwin JD, Vock P, Osborne DR. CT of the pulmonary ligament. *AJR* 1983;141:231–236.

57. Godwin JD, Webb WR. Contrast-related flow phenomena mimicking pathology on thoracic computed tomography. *J Comput Assist Tomogr* 1982;6:460–464.

58. Godwin JD, Webb WR. Dynamic computed tomography in the evaluation of vascular lung lesions. *Radiology* 1981;138:629–635.

59. Goodman LR, Golkow RS, Steiner RM, et al. The right mid-lung window. A potential source of error in computed tomography of the lung. *Radiology* 1982;143:135–138.

60. Goodman LR, Teplick SK, Kay H. Computed tomography of the normal sternum. *AJR* 1983;141:219–223.

61. Greene R. "Saber-sheath" trachea: relation to chronic obstructive pulmonary disease. *AJR* 1978;130:441–445.

62. Griscom NT. Cross-sectional shape of the child's trachea by computed tomography. *AJR* 1983;140:1103–1106.

63. Guthaner DF, Wexler L, Harell G. CT demonstration of cardiac structures. *AJR* 1979;133:75–81.

64. Haacke EM, Patrick JL. Reducing motion artifacts in two dimensional Fourier transform imaging. *Magn Reson Imaging* 1986;4:359–376.

65. Haaga JR, Reich NE, Havrilla TR, Alfidi RJ. Interventional CT scanning. *Radiol Clin North Am* 1977;15:449–456.

66. Halber MD, Daffner RH, Thompson WM. CT of the esophagus: normal appearance. *AJR* 1979;133:1047–1050.

67. Hatfield MK, Gross BH, Glazer GM, Martel W. Computed tomography of the sternum and its articulations. *Skeletal Radiol* 1984;11:197–203.

68. Heitzman ER. *The mediastinum: radiologic correlations with anatomy and pathology.* St. Louis: CV Mosby, 1977.

69. Herrnheiser G. Anatomic-roentgenological analysis of the normal hilar shadow. *AJR* 1962;45:595–612.

70. Houang MIW, Arozena X, Shaw DG. Demonstration of the pericardium and pericardial effusion by computed tomography. *J Comput Assist Tomogr* 1979;3:601–603.

71. Huggins TJ, Lesar ML, Friedman AC, Pyatt RS, Thane TT. CT appearance of persistent left superior vena cava. *J Comput Assist Tomogr* 1982;6:294–297.

72. Hyson EA, Ravin CE. Radiographic features of mediastinal anatomy. *Chest* 1979;75:609–613.

73. Isner JM, Carter BL, Roberts WC, Bankoff MS. Subepicardial adipose tissue producing echocardiographic appearance of pericardial effusion. *Am J Cardiol* 1983;51:565–569.

74. Jardin M, Remy J. Segmental bronchovascular anatomy of the lower lobes: CT analysis. *AJR* 1986;147:457–458.

75. Jasinski RW, Yang CF, Rubin JM. Vena cava anomalies simulating adenopathy on computed tomography. *J Comput Assist Tomogr* 1981;5:921–924.

76. Jost RG, Sagel SS, Stanley RJ, Levitt RG. Computed tomography of the thorax. *Radiology* 1978;126:125–136.

77. Kittredge RD. The right posterolateral trachea band. *J Comput Assist Tomogr* 1979;3:348–354.

78. Klinkhamer AC. Aberrant right subclavian artery: clinical and roentgenologic aspects. *AJR* 1966;97:438–446.

79. Koehler RP, Anderson RE. Computed angiotomography. *Radiology* 1980;137:843–845.

80. Koehler RP, Anderson RE, Baxter B. The effect of computed tomography viewer controls on anatomical measurements. *Radiology* 1979;130:189–194.

81. Kolbenstvedt A, Kolmannskog F, Aakhus T. Venous structures of the chest and abdomen at computer tomography. *Acta Radiol [Diagn] (Stockh)* 1979;20:513–522.

82. Krudy AG, Doppman JL, Herdt JR. Failure to detect a 1.5 centimeter lung nodule by chest computed tomography. *J Comput Assist Tomogr* 1982;6:1178–1180.

83. Kurujama K, Gamsu G, Stern RG, Cann CE, Herfkens RJ, Brundage BH. CT-determined pulmonary artery diameters in predicting pulmonary hypertension. *Invest Radiol* 1984;19:16–22.

84. Landay M. Azygos vein abutting the posterior wall of the right main and upper lobe bronchi: a normal CT variant. *AJR* 1983;140:461–462.

85. Lane EJ, Heitzman ER, Dinn WM. The radiology of the superior intercostal veins. *Radiology* 1976;120:263–267.

86. Levi C, Gray JE, McCullough EC, Hattery RR. The unreliability of CT numbers as absolute values. *AJR* 1982;139:443–447.

87. Levitt RG, Glazer HS, Roper CL, Lee JKT, Murphy WA. Magnetic resonance imaging of mediastinal and hilar masses: comparison with CT. *AJR* 1985;145:9–14.

88. Levy-Ravetch M, Auh YH, Rubenstein WA, Whalen JP, Kazam E. CT of the pericardial recesses. *AJR* 1985;144:707–714.

89. Lund G. The CT appearance of the superior intercostal veins. *Eur J Radiol* 1982;2:122–124.

90. Lund G, Lien HH. Computed tomography of the azygo-esophageal recess. Normal appearances. *Acta Radiol [Diagn] (Stockh)* 1982;23:225–230.

91. Marks BW, Kuhns LR. Identification of the pleural fissures with computed tomography. *Radiology* 1982;143:139–141.

92. Maue-Dickinson M, Trefler M, Dickson DR. Comparison of dosimetry and image quality in computed and conventional tomography. *Radiology* 1979;131:509–514.

93. McCullough EC, Morin RL. CT-number variability in thoracic geometry. *AJR* 1983;141:135–140.

94. McDonald CJ, Castellino RA, Blank N. The aortic "nipple." The left superior intercostal vein. *Radiology* 1970;96:533–536.

95. McLoughlin MJ, Weisbrod G, Wise DJ, Yeung HPH. Computed tomography in congenital anomalies of the aortic arch and great vessels. *Radiology* 1981;138:399–403.

96. Mencini RA, Proto AV. The high left and main pulmonary arteries: a CT pitfall. *J Comput Assist Tomogr* 1982;6:452–459.

97. Micklos TJ, Proto AV. CT demonstration of the coronary sinus. *J Comput Assist Tomogr* 1985;9:60–64.

98. Moncada R, Baker M, Salinas M, et al. Diagnostic role of computed tomography in pericardial heart disease. *Am Heart J* 1982;100:263–282.

99. Moncada R, Demos TC, Marsan R, Churchill RJ, Reynes C, Love L. CT diagnosis of idiopathic aneurysms of the thoracic systemic veins. *J Comput Assist Tomogr* 1985;9:305–309.

100. Moore AV, Korobkin M, Olanow W, et al. Age-related changes in the thymus gland: CT-pathologic correlation. *AJR* 1983;141:241–246.

101. Muller NL, Webb WR. Radiographic imaging of the pulmonary hila. *Invest Radiol* 1985;20:661–671.

102. Naidich DP, Khouri NF, Scott WW, Wang K, Siegelman SS. Computed tomography of the pulmonary hila: 1. Normal anatomy. *J Comput Assist Tomogr* 1981;5:459–467.

103. Naidich DP, Megibow AJ, Hilton S, Hulnick DH, Siegelman SS. Computed tomography of the diaphragm: peridiaphragmatic fluid localization. *J Comput Assist Tomogr* 1983;7:641–649.

104. Naidich DP, Megibow AJ, Ross CR, Beranbaum ER, Siegelman SS. Computed tomography of the diaphragm: normal anatomy and variants. *J Comput Assist Tomogr* 1983;7:633–640.

105. Naidich DP, Terry PB, Stitik FP, Siegelman SS. Computed tomography of the bronchi: 1. Normal anatomy. *J Comput Assist Tomogr* 1980;4:746–753.

106. Naidich DP, Zerhovni EA, Siegelman SS. Computed tomography of the thorax. New York: Raven Press, 1984.

107. O'Callaghan JP, Heitzman ER, Somogyi JW, Spirt BA. CT evaluation of pulmonary artery size. *J Comput Assist Tomogr* 1982;6:101–104.

108. Olson MA, Becker GJ. The scimitar syndrome: CT findings in partial anomalous pulmonary venous return. *Radiology* 1986;159:25–26.

109. Onitsuka H, Kuhns LR. Dextroconvexity of the mediastinum in the azygos-esophageal recess: a normal variant in young adults. *Radiology* 1980;135:126–128.

110. Osborne D, Vock P, Godwin JD, Silverman PM. CT identification of bronchopulmonary segments. *AJR* 1984;142:47–52.

111. Paling MR, Dwyer A. The first rib as the cause of a "pulmonary nodule" on chest computed tomography. *J Comput Assist Tomogr* 1980;4:847–848.

112. Parvey LS, Grizzard M, Coburn TP. Use of infusion pump for intravenous enhanced computed tomography. *J Comput Assist Tomogr* 1983;7:175–176.

113. Passariello R, Salvolino U, Rossi P, Simonetti G, Pasquini U. Automatic contrast media injector for computed tomography. *J Comput Assist Tomogr* 1980;4:278–279.

114. Pennes DR, Ellis JH. Anomalous pulmonary venous drainage of the left upper lobe shown by CT scans. *Radiology* 1986;159:23–24.

115. Proto AV, Rost RC. CT of the thorax: pitfalls in interpretation. *Radiographics* 1985;5:699–812.
116. Pugatch RD, Faling LJ, Robbins AH, Spira R. CT diagnosis of benign mediastinal abnormalities. *AJR* 1980;134:685–694.
117. Quint LE, Glazer GM, Orringer MB, Francis IR, Bookstein FL. Mediastinal lymph node detection and sizing at CT and autopsy. *AJR* 1986;147:469–472.
118. Rankin S, Faling LJ, Pugatch RD. CT diagnosis of pulmonary arteriovenous malformations. *J Comput Assist Tomogr* 1982;6:746–749.
119. Rao PS, Alfidi RJ. The environmental density artifact: a beam-hardening effect in computed tomography. *Radiology* 1981;141:223–227.
120. Reese DF, McCullough EC, Baker HL. Dynamic sequential scanning with table incrementation. *Radiology* 1981;140:719–722.
121. Robbins AH, Pugatch RD, Gerzof SG, et al. Further observations on the medical efficacy of computed tomography of the chest and abdomen. *Radiology* 1980;137:719–725.
122. Robinson PJ, Kreel L. Pulmonary tissue attenuation with computed tomography: comparison of inspiration and expiration scans. *J Comput Assist Tomogr* 1979;3:740–748.
123. Rockoff SD, Druy EM. Tortuous azygos arch simulating a pulmonary lesion. *AJR* 1982;138:577–579.
124. Rosen A, Auh YH, Rubenstein WA, Engel IA, Whalen JP, Kazam E. CT appearance of diaphragmatic pseudotumors. *J Comput Assist Tomogr* 1983;7:995–999.
125. Rost RC Jr, Proto AV. Inferior pulmonary ligament: computed tomographic appearance. *Radiology* 1983;148:479–483.
126. Schatz SL, Ryvicker MJ, Deutsch AM, Cohen HR. Partial anomalous pulmonary venous drainage of the right lower lobe shown by CT scans. *Radiology* 1986;159:21–22.
127. Schneider HF, Felson B. Buckling of the innominate artery simulating aneurysm and tumor. *AJR* 1961;85:1106–1110.
128. Schnyder PA, Gamsu G. CT of the pretracheal retrocaval space. *AJR* 1981;136:303–308.
129. Sechtem U, Tscholakoff D, Higgins CB. MRI of the normal pericardium. *AJR* 1986;147:239–244.
130. Shepard JO, Dedrick CG, Spizarny DL, McLoud TC. Dynamic incremental computed tomography of the pulmonary hila using a flow rate injector. *J Comput Assist Tomogr* 1986;10:369–371.
131. Shin MS, Berland LL. Computed tomography of retrocrural spaces: normal, anatomic variants, and pathologic conditions. *AJR* 1985;145:81–86.
132. Shuford WH, Sybers RG, Edwards FK. The three types of right aortic arch. *AJR* 1970;109:67–74.
133. Shuford WH, Sybers RG, Gordon IJ, Baron MG, Carson GC. Circumflex retroesophageal right aortic arch simulating a mediastinal tumor or dissecting aneurysm. *AJR* 1986;146:491–496.
134. Silverman PM, Godwin JD, Korobkin M. Computed tomographic detection of retrocrural air. *AJR* 1982;138:825–827.
135. Silverman PM, Harell GS. Computed tomography of the normal pericardium. *Invest Radiol* 1983;18:141–144.
136. Smathers RL, Buschi AJ, Pope TL Jr, Brenbridge AN, Williamson BR. The azygos arch: normal and pathologic CT appearance. *AJR* 1982;139:477–483.
137. Sones PJ, Torres WE, Colvin RS, Meier WL, Sprawls P, Rogers JV Jr. Effectiveness of CT in evaluating intrathoracic masses. *AJR* 1982;139:469–475.
138. Speckman JM, Gamsu G, Webb WR. Alterations in CT mediastinal anatomy produced by an azygos lobe. *AJR* 1981;137:47–50.
139. Stark P. Midline sternal foramen: CT demonstration. *J Comput Assist Tomogr* 1985;9:489–490.
140. Stark P, Jaramillo D. CT of the sternum. *AJR* 1986;147:72–77.
141. Steiner RM, Flicker S, Eldredge WJ, et al. The functional and anatomic evaluation of the cardiovascular system with rapid-acquisition computed tomography (cine CT). *Radiol Clin North Am* 1986;24:503–520.
142. Stone DN, Bein ME, Garris JB. Anomalous left pulmonary artery: two new adult cases. *AJR* 1980;135:1259–1263.
143. Taylor GA, Fishman EK, Kramer SS, Siegelman SS. CT demonstration of the phrenic nerve. *J Comput Assist Tomogr* 1983;7:411–414.
144. Trefler M, Haughton VM. Patient dose and image quality in computed tomography. *AJR* 1981;137:25–27.
145. Vock P, Owens A. Computed tomography of the normal and pathological thoracic inlet. *Eur J Radiol* 1982;2:187–193.
146. Vock P, Speigel T, Fram EK, Effmann EL. CT assessment of the adult intrathoracic cross section of the trachea. *J Comput Assist Tomogr* 1984;8:1076–1082.
147. Webb WR, Gamsu G. Computed tomography of the left retrobronchial stripe. *J Comput Assist Tomogr* 1983;7:65–69.
148. Webb WR, Gamsu G, Crooks LE. Multisection sagittal and coronal magnetic resonance imaging of the mediastinum and hila. *Radiology* 1984;150:475–478.
149. Webb WR, Gamsu G, Speckman JM, Kaiser JA, Federle MP, Lipton MJ. Computed tomographic demonstration of mediastinal venous anomalies. *AJR* 1982;139:157–161.
150. Webb WR, Gamsu G, Speckman JM, Kaiser JA, Federle MP, Lipton MJ. CT demonstration of mediastinal aortic arch anomalies. *J Comput Assist Tomogr* 1982;6:445–451.
151. Webb WR, Gamsu G, Stark DD, Moore EH. Magnetic resonance imaging of the normal and abnormal pulmonary hila. *Radiology* 1984;152:89–94.
152. Webb WR, Gamsu G, Wall SD, Cann CE, Proctor E. CT of a bronchial phantom: factors affecting appearance and size measurements. *Invest Radiol* 1984;19:394–398.
153. Webb WR, Glazer G, Gamsu G. Computed tomography of the normal pulmonary hilum. *J Comput Assist Tomogr* 1981;5:476–484.
154. Webb WR, Moore EH. Differentiation of volume averaging and mass on magnetic resonance images of the mediastinum. *Radiology* 1985;155:413–416.
155. Williams RA, Haaga JR, Karagiannis E. CT guided paravertebral biopsy of the mediastinum. *J Comput Assist Tomogr* 1984;8:575–578.
156. Zerhouni EA, Spivey JF, Morgan RH, Leo FP, Stitik FP, Siegelman SS. Factors influencing quantitative CT measurements of solitary pulmonary nodules. *J Comput Assist Tomogr* 1982;6:1075–1087.
157. Zylak CJ, Pallie W, Pirani M, Wandtke JC, Kothari K. Anatomy and computed tomography: a correlative module on the cervicothoracic junction. *Radiographics* 1983;3:478–530.

CHAPTER 8

Mediastinum

Stuart S. Sagel and Harvey S. Glazer

The greatest impact of thoracic computed tomography (CT) has been in the evaluation of the mediastinum. The cross-sectional CT images display the fine anatomic detail of this area with great precision and often yield unique and useful diagnostic information directly affecting the management or prognosis of a patient (5,115,125).

Compared with conventional radiographic techniques, transaxial CT sections provide an unparalleled view of the superimposed structures of the mediastinum. For recognition of a mediastinal lesion by standard X-ray films or tomography, sufficient expansion to deform the mediastinal contour and displace the pleuroparenchymal interface laterally is required. Using CT, detection of enlargement of an individual mediastinal component or mass is possible at an earlier stage. In addition, the superior contrast sensitivity of CT allows estimation of the density for most mediastinal structures. Even without intravenous administration of contrast material, in most adults the vessels, lymph nodes, airways, thymus, and esophagus can be distinguished. The size, homogeneity, site of origin, extent, and relation to normal mediastinal components of any abnormal mass usually can be defined. Distinction between benign lipomatous, calcific, and serous fluid collections from lymphadenopathy, soft-tissue masses, and vascular lesions and anomalies often is possible. It should be emphasized that CT is basically a morphologic technique, not a histologic technique, and reliable distinction between benign and malignant soft-tissue masses and enlarged lymph nodes generally is not feasible. When necessary, proper administration of intravenous contrast material can help distinguish between vascular and nonvascular abnormalities or allow determination of the effect of a pathologic process on a major vessel.

Because CT can simultaneously allow evaluation of the mediastinum along with the lung, pleura, and chest wall, it has revolutionized radiologic imaging of the thorax. Conventional tomography, barium studies, and angiography have been largely replaced for evaluation of me-

diastinal abnormalities seen or suspected on plain chest radiographs or when clinical findings suggest disease in this region. Studies such as the barium esophagogram are now reserved primarily for patients with dysphagia or those in whom an esophageal abnormality is strongly suggested as the cause of an abnormality seen on plain radiographic film. It is much less sensitive than CT for detecting mediastinal lymph node enlargement or other masses.

CT has emerged as the most thorough and most reliable radiologic technique for morphologic analysis of the mediastinum and surrounding tissues. For practical purposes, the anatomic information provided by magnetic resonance imaging (MRI) in the mediastinum is comparable in almost all cases to that from CT (2). It is rare that the coronal, sagittal, or other nontransaxial imaging plane will give vital, clinically relevant data. Almost never is MRI more specific in affording histologic distinction (e.g., separation of malignant neoplastic disease from benign inflammatory disease) of an enlarged lymph node or mediastinal mass. The inability of MRI to reveal calcification (or high iodine content) within a mediastinal mass, sometimes the hallmark of a benign lesion, can be a considerable limitation. Because of its superior spatial resolution, CT occasionally is better for distinguishing between adjacent disease (such as lung collapse or a focal pleural abnormality) and mediastinal abnormalities. The sole current major advantage of MRI is obviation of an intravenous contrast agent in allowing confident distinction between normal and abnormal blood vessels or vessels with disturbed flow (135). But because CT examination is substantially less expensive, can be accomplished in a notably shorter time, and is generally more widely available, and because intravenous administration of contrast material is required in the minority of cases, it is the preferred radiologic technique to further evaluate the mediastinum following conventional roentgenography in most patients. Certainly in critically ill individuals re-

A

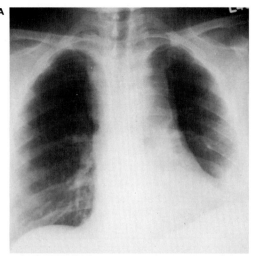

FIG. 1. Mediastinal lipomatosis. **A:** Chest radiograph demonstrates lobulated widening of the mediastinum in a 39-year-old man on corticosteroid therapy for 3 years. **B:** CT image at the level of the aortic arch demonstrates abundant amounts of normal-appearing fat throughout the mediastinum, with lateral bulging of the pleuromediastinal interface, accounting for the widening. Some extrapleural fat posterolaterally in both hemithoraces and exuberant subcutaneous fat also are present. **C:** T1-weighted MR image at comparable level shows identical findings. The mediastinal fat maintained the same signal intensity as the subcutaneous fat on the T2-weighted image.

B,C

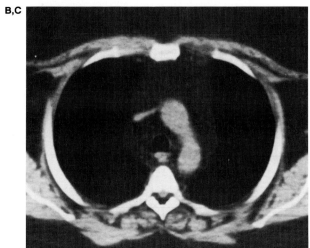 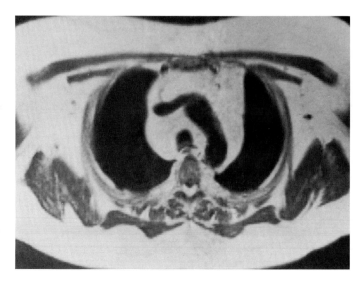

quiring close monitoring or life-support equipment, or in a patient with an implanted pacemaker or infusion pump, CT is the only option.

ABNORMALITIES OF MEDIASTINAL FAT

True fatty tumors of the mediastinum are not as common as diffuse lipomatosis or herniations of abdominal fat through the diaphragm (25,91,117). A lesion revealing a pure fat density, with well-defined margins, is almost invariably benign. In such cases, the CT diagnosis usually is conclusive, and no further diagnostic evaluation is warranted.

Mediastinal Lipomatosis

This is a benign condition in which large amounts of histologically normal, unencapsulated fat accumulate in the mediastinum. It is most commonly associated with obesity (79) or exogenous corticosteroid administration (73); it is less frequently seen with primary Cushing syndrome. As many as 25% of cases may have no predisposing factors.

The excess fat deposition is prominent mainly in the upper mediastinum. Smooth widening of the mediastinum is the most characteristic presentation on chest radiography. On CT, there may be gentle convex bulging of the pleuromediastinal contours (Fig. 1). Tracheal compression or displacement is uniformly absent. Less commonly, fat will accumulate preferentially in the paraspinal areas (Fig. 2) or near the cardiophrenic angles (pericardial fat pads). The fat in mediastinal lipomatosis should appear as a uniform low density of −80 to −120 Hounsfield units (HU) (9,65). If inhomogeneity is noted, an alternative diagnosis, such as liposarcoma (120), or superimposed processes, such as neoplastic infiltration, mediastinitis, or hemorrhage, must be considered. Small foci of residual thymic tissue in the anterior mediastinum should not be mistaken for infiltrated fat.

Focal Fatty Masses

These are most frequently seen in the peridiaphragmatic areas and usually represent herniations of abdominal fat (see Fig. 113 in Chapter 7). Omental fat can herniate through the foramen of Morgagni, almost always located

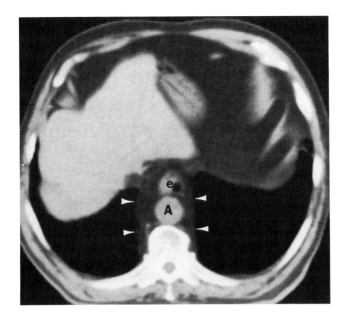

FIG. 2. Abundant fat is present in the paraspinal regions bilaterally (*arrowheads*), accounting for widening of the paraspinal lines noted on a chest radiograph; (A) descending aorta; (e) esophagus.

on the right side, to create the appearance of a cardiophrenic angle mass. Fine linear densities can sometimes be seen within the herniated fat that undoubtedly represent small omental vessels, and their presence can help distinguish herniated fat through the foramen of Morgagni from a pericardial fat pad.

Fat herniation through the foramen of Bochdalek is much more common on the left side (see Fig. 114 in Chapter 7), because the liver inhibits occurrence on the right.

Herniation of perigastric fat through the esophageal hiatus in the diaphragm may occur (Fig. 3). Extension alongside the aorta can create widening of the paraspinal line(s) or simulate a retrocardiac mass on conventional radiography.

True mediastinal lipomas are rare. These pliable neoplasms, which may be encapsulated, almost never produce compression of a mediastinal structure unless they are exceedingly large. Their boundaries are smooth and sharply defined. If the lesion is inhomogeneous or poorly demarcated, a benign lipoma cannot be diagnosed, and a liposarcoma, lipoblastoma, or a superimposed process must be suspected. The malignant fatty tumors, even the well-differentiated liposarcomas (Fig. 4), tend to show some soft-tissue-density elements besides the areas of fat density. Some liposarcomas have a predominantly soft-tissue attenuation value rather than a fat density. An inhomogeneous fatty mass in the anterior mediastinum most likely represents a teratoma or a thymolipoma; the former may also contain some areas of calcification.

LYMPHADENOPATHY

CT has emerged as the most sensitive and valuable radiologic technique for evaluating the mediastinal lymph

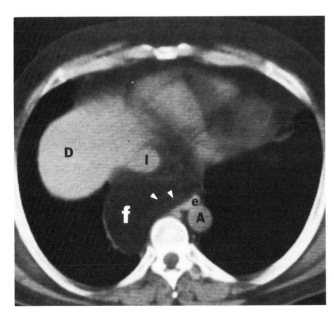

FIG. 3. Herniation of lesser omental fat (f) through the esophageal hiatus in the diaphragm is responsible for a right paraspinal mass noted on a plain chest radiograph. The contained linear soft-tissue densities (*arrowheads*) represent vessels; (D) diaphragm; (I) inferior vena cava; (e) esophagus; (A) descending thoracic aorta.

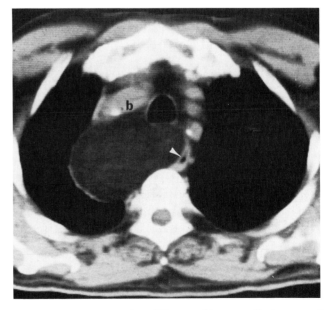

FIG. 4. Liposarcoma. In a 73-year-old man with true vocal cord paralysis on the right, an inhomogeneous mass composed largely of fat, but also containing some higher-density elements, is seen in the superior mediastinum displacing the brachiocephalic artery (b) anteriorly and the esophagus (*arrowhead*) laterally.

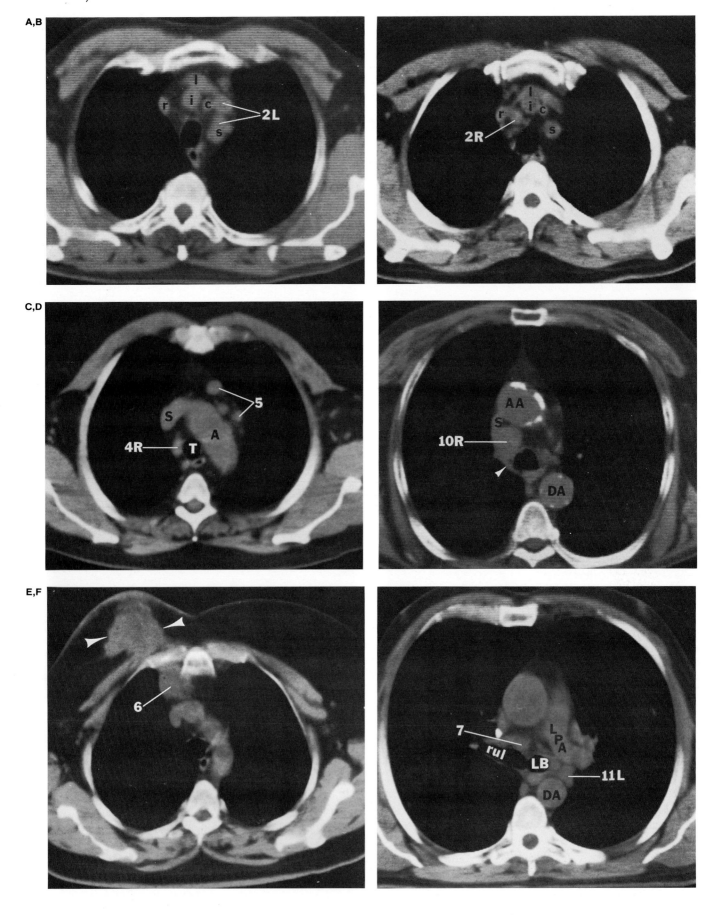

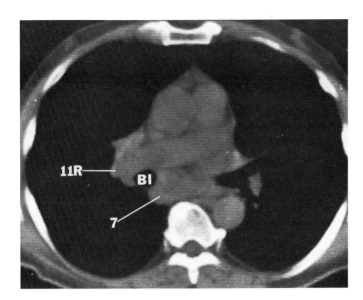

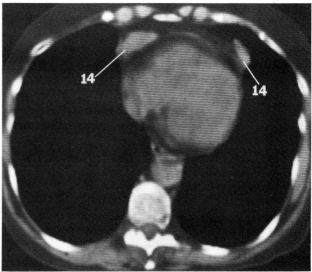

FIG. 5. Lymph node enlargement in various mediastinal regions. **A–F:** *Facing page.* **A:** Left brachiocephalic lymphadenopathy (2L) (see Fig. 57 in Chapter 7 for classification) due to non-Hodgkin lymphoma; these nodes cannot be sampled by transcervical mediastinoscopy, but can be reached via an anterior parasternal mediastinotomy; (r) right brachiocephalic vein; (l) left brachiocephalic vein; (i) innominate artery; (c) left carotid artery; (s) left subclavian artery. **B:** Mildly enlarged right brachiocephalic lymph nodes (2R) due to tuberculosis in the plane of mediastinoscopy. **C:** Lateral aortic (5) and right paratracheal (4R) lymphadenopathy secondary to metastatic renal cell carcinoma; (S) superior vena cava; (A) aortic arch; (T) trachea. **D:** Pretracheal lymphadenopathy (10R) due to metastatic bronchogenic carcinoma; (AA) ascending aorta; (DA) descending aorta; (S) superior vena cava; (*arrowhead*) azygos vein arch. **E:** Right internal mammary lymphadenopathy (6) secondary to metastatic breast carcinoma (*arrowheads*). **F:** Left posterior hilar (11L) and anterior subcarinal (7) lymphadenopathy due to Hodgkin disease; (LPA), left pulmonary artery; (DA) descending aorta; (LB) left main-stem bronchus; (rul) right upper lobe bronchus originating from right main-stem bronchus. **G:** Right hilar (11R) and posterior subcarinal (7) lymphadenopathy producing a convex bulge in the azygoesophageal recess, due to metastatic renal cell carcinoma; (BI) brochus intermedius. **H:** Superior diaphragmatic (pericardial) lymphadenopathy (14) due to non-Hodgkin lymphoma.

nodes. With this method, all lymph-node-bearing areas can be assessed (Fig. 5).

As previously emphasized, normal lymph nodes are demonstrable on CT in most adult patients with even a modest amount of mediastinal fat. The manifestations of lymphadenopathy (disease of lymph nodes) on both CT and MRI (Figs. 6 and 7; see Fig. 17 in Chapter 7), consisting mainly of enlargement, are relatively straightforward, but generally nonspecific as to etiology. When a lymph node exceeds 1.0 cm in diameter or in cross section, recognized by direct measurement, as described in the preceding chapter, it is considered pathologic. Also, a localized cluster of lymph nodes of borderline enlarged size should be regarded as highly suspect of disease. But the likelihood that a mediastinal lymph node is pathologically enlarged is a function not only of its size but also of its location. For example, a lymph node 8 mm in diameter in the paratracheal region is most likely normal, whereas such a node in the supradiaphragmatic or internal mammary chain probably is not (24,94,101,134). However, whether such enlargement is caused by metastatic neoplasm, lymphoma, or inflammation usually cannot be as-

certained by CT (or MRI) alone (Fig. 8). Even the patterns of lymph node enlargement in the mediastinum (and hilum) are not specific enough in a given individual to permit confident diagnosis as to etiology. Confirmation of abnormality and specific diagnosis may require histologic examination of material from the lymph nodes noted to be enlarged. Based on the precise location of the involved lymph nodes, when clinically necessary, the most appropriate method of tissue sampling (e.g., transcervical mediastinoscopy, parasternal mediastinotomy, percutaneous or transbronchoscopic needle aspiration biopsy) can be selected.

A well-recognized limitation for both CT and MRI is their inability in almost all cases to permit analysis of the internal architecture of a lymph node. If no enlargement is discerned, pathologic abnormality cannot be suspected or, obviously, excluded with certainty. Despite this restraint, CT allows detection of lymphadenopathy at an earlier stage than is possible with any other radiologic method. CT can be especially valuable in depicting mild to moderate mediastinal lymph node enlargement in areas where it is difficult or impossible to appreciate an abnor-

A,B

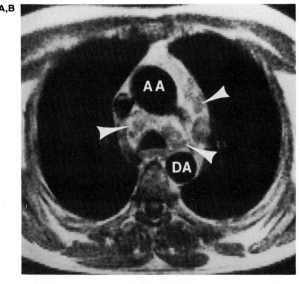

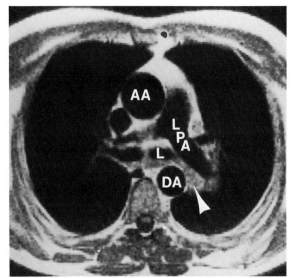

C

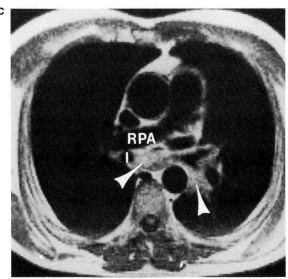

FIG. 6. Lymph node enlargement; MR demonstration. Multiple enlarged mediastinal and hilar lymph nodes (*arrowheads*) secondary to Hodgkin disease are seen on T1-weighted MR images; (AA) ascending aorta; (DA) descending aorta; (LPA) left pulmonary artery; (RPA) right pulmonary artery; (L) left bronchus; (I) bronchus intermedius.

mality on plain chest radiographs. This occurs when the abnormal lymph nodes lie within the mediastinum but are not sufficiently large to produce a distortion in the contour of the mediastinal pleural reflection. Paratracheal lymph node enlargement, anterolateral to the trachea and immediately posterior to the superior vena cava, frequently is not visible on conventional radiographs. Similar difficulties can be encountered in the aortopulmonary window, cardiophrenic angle (supradiaphragmatic), and subcarinal regions. Intravenous administration of contrast material may be beneficial to document the presence of an enlarged lymph node (Fig. 9).

Calcification within a lymph node generally connotes old granulomatous disease (Fig. 10A). However, there are some rare exceptions due to metastatic neoplasm (e.g., mucinous ovarian carcinoma, bronchioloalveolar cell carcinomas) (Fig. 10B) (85); the clinical history and associated findings most often permit distinction.

Necrosis within enlarged lymph nodes, resulting in low-density (near-water-density) central areas, usually with a preserved thick soft-tissue-density rim, can be seen with aggressive neoplastic involvement (Fig. 11), but occasionally is encountered with granulomatous infection. Also, low attenuation values within mediastinal lymph nodes, not due to necrosis, may occur secondary to involvement by metastatic testicular cancers (145).

Substantial enhancement of a lymph node after intravenous administration of contrast material may be noted, most typically with highly vascular metastatic neoplasms (e.g., renal cell or thyroid carcinoma). However, it also may be seen with benign conditions (e.g., angiofollicular lymph node hyperplasia) (43,107). Also, non-lymph-node masses in the mediastinum may exhibit marked contrast enhancement, such as intrathoracic goiter (see Chapter 6), paraganglioma, and hemangioma (48).

As disease advances in pathologically involved lymph

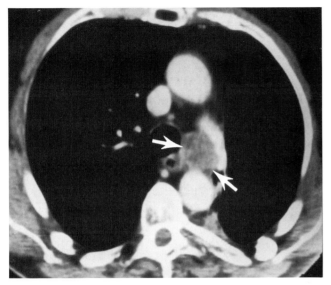

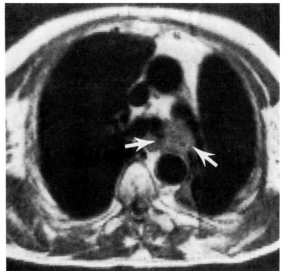

A,B

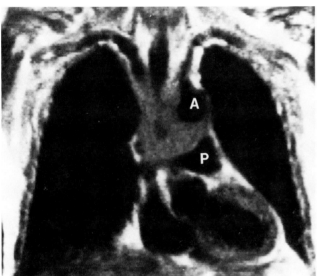

C

FIG. 7. Aortopulmonary window lymphadenopathy. **A:** Postcontrast CT image demonstrates aortopulmonary window lymphadenopathy (*arrows*) due to recurrent bronchogenic carcinoma, just medial to the left pulmonary artery. **B:** Similar findings are seen on a T1-weighted MR image; (*arrows*) lymphadenopathy. **C:** Mediastinal lymphadenopathy, with involvement of the aortopulmonary window, is seen on T1-weighted coronal MR image in a different patient; (A) aortic knob; (P) pulmonary artery.

nodes, the enlarged margins may lose their sharp definition, and the surrounding mediastinal fat may increase in density. Such changes are due to extension of the disease process through the nodal capsule and an associated fibrotic or inflammatory reaction. When the disease process extends through the capsule of several adjacent nodes, a single, larger coalescent mass may form. The resulting conglomerate mass may be difficult to ascribe confidently to lymphadenopathy, which, however, is the most common cause of a soft-tissue-density mass in the middle mediastinum. Sometimes, diffuse disease that has spread from the nodes into the surrounding mediastinal fat and connective tissue may be seen without any focal mass being recognizable. The only manifestations most typically occurring with metastatic adenocarcinoma may be apparent thickening of the walls of a vessel or airway and obliteration of the normal fat planes surrounding these structures.

Granulomatous Disease

Infections

Mediastinal lymph nodes may be involved in the primary phase of infection with tuberculosis or histoplasmosis (Fig. 5B). One or more groups of enlarged regional lymph nodes, most commonly the right paratracheal (azygos chain), may be seen, with or without a concomitant focal pulmonary parenchymal infiltrate. The involved nodal mass frequently has poorly defined margins and may be intimately adherent to surrounding mediastinal structures. Coalescence into a single soft-tissue-density mass may occur. However, as emphasized previously, such an appearance is not diagnostic; indistinguishable features may be seen with neoplastic lymphadenopathy. In the majority of cases, spontaneous regression occurs, often with resultant calcification of the affected lymph nodes (Fig. 10A). Healing, with extensive fibrosis, may

A,B

C,D

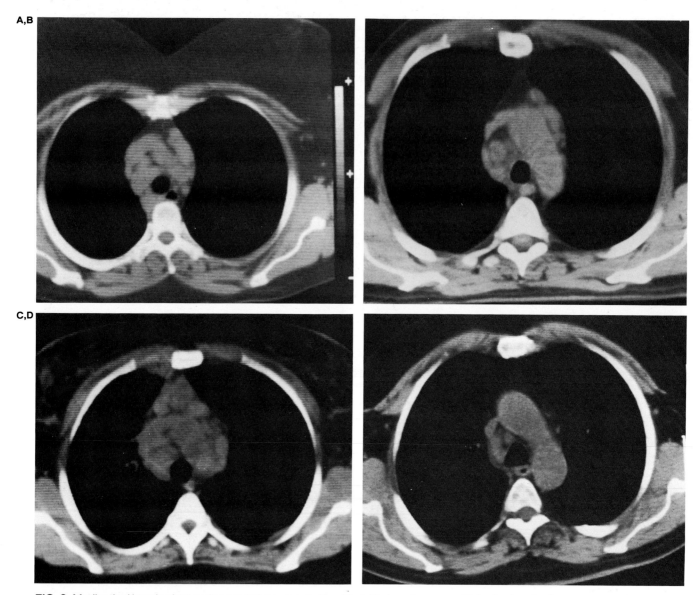

FIG. 8. Mediastinal lymphadenopathy, myriad causes. **A:** Non-Hodgkin lymphoma; multiple clustered enlarged superior mediastinal nodes. **B:** Hodgkin disease; enlarged pretracheal and lateral aortic nodes. **C:** Sarcoidosis: enlarged pretracheal, lateral aortic, right internal mammary, and anterior mediastinal nodes. **D:** Metastatic bronchogenic carcinoma; enlarged azygos-chain paratracheal nodes.

lead to such complications as superior vena caval (Fig. 12) or airway obstruction (56). Whereas CT and MRI are equivalent in depicting the mediastinal lymphadenopathy, CT is superior for demonstrating the contained calcifications, the recognition of which is critical in suggesting the correct diagnosis for the symptoms (114). MRI may supply complementary information in assessing vascular occlusion (or patency) if intravenous contrast material cannot be administered (39).

Sarcoidosis

CT has a very limited role in the diagnosis and management of this multisystem disease, which is most often detected on plain chest radiography. Hilar and paratracheal lymph node enlargement is the most typical presentation (10). Fiberoptic bronchoscopic biopsy of the bronchial walls and lung parenchyma usually suffices for histologic diagnosis. When this approach fails to secure adequate tissue for a definitive diagnosis, mediastinoscopy may be used. On rare occasion, CT may be beneficial to provide a map of the affected nodes prior to the procedure. Moderate enlargement of the involved lymph nodes, with typically well-defined margins, is most commonly seen on CT. Multiple regional groups of lymph nodes usually are enlarged, often in a relatively symmetrical fashion (Fig. 8C). Anterior mediastinal lymphadenopathy is commonly identified on CT, despite the classic conventional radiographic dogma that this is unusual.

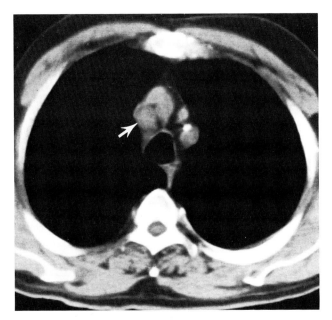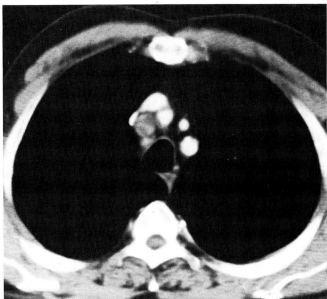

FIG. 9. Lymphadenopathy; value of intravenous contrast material. **A:** Non-contrast-enhanced CT image strongly suggests enlarged right pretracheal lymph node (*arrow*). **B:** Postcontrast image demonstrates definite adenopathy separate from the markedly enhancing surrounding great vessels.

Miscellaneous Inflammatory Conditions

Mild to moderate mediastinal lymph node enlargement may rarely be seen secondary to a variety of inflammatory conditions, such as infectious mononucleosis or Rocky Mountain spotted fever. Additionally, inhalational diseases, such as silicosis (which almost always is associated with characteristic pulmonary parenchymal changes), may cause lymphadenopathy, which frequently contains foci of calcification. When these abnormally enlarged nodes are not clearly related to a generalized disease process by clinical history and laboratory data, biopsy may be necessary for proper diagnosis.

Lymphoma

Malignant lymphoma frequently involves the thorax; mediastinal lymphadenopathy is its most common intrathoracic manifestation. At clinical presentation, approximately 65% of patients with Hodgkin lymphoma have intrathoracic disease; 90% of these have mediastinal disease, and in 40% it is the sole site of involvement (41,105). In patients with non-Hodgkin lymphoma, about 40% initially have intrathoracic disease, but in less than 10% is it purely mediastinal (82). Lymphomatous masses are most commonly found in the anterior mediastinum in Hodgkin disease; in the majority of cases this does not

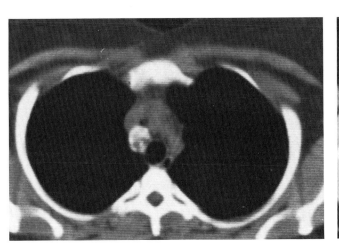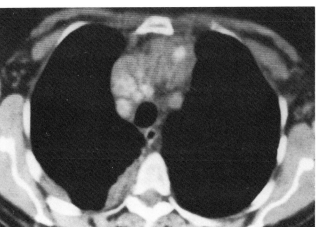

FIG. 10. Calcified mediastinal lymph nodes. **A:** Old healed histoplasmosis is responsible for the calcified right paratracheal nodal mass. **B:** Metastatic mucinous adenocarcinoma of the ovary is the cause of the multiple enlarged calcified mediastinal lymph nodes. Right pleural metastases also are present.

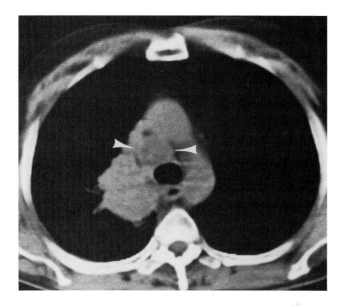

FIG. 11. Necrotic lymph node. An enlarged nodal mass (*arrowheads*), with soft-tissue-density rim and a lower-density, slightly inhomogeneous central portion, due to metastasis from a right-upper-lobe bronchogenic carcinoma, is seen in the pretracheal region. The high-density periphery, inhomogeneous center, and round shape allow confident distinction of this necrotic node from a prominent retroaortic pericardial recess (see Fig. 104 in Chapter 7).

reflect lymphadenopathy, but rather involvement of the lymphoid elements of the thymus (Fig. 13; see Fig. 18 in Chapter 7) (129). Concomitant lymph node disease elsewhere in the mediastinum (e.g., paratracheal, internal mammary, supradiaphragmatic) (Figs. 5F, 8B, and 14) (93) is frequent. Non-Hodgkin lymphoma predominantly presents as enlargement of the middle mediastinal lymph nodes (Figs. 5A, 8A, and 15) (19), but neither the localization pattern nor the appearance on CT of the abnormal nodes is distinct enough to play a vital role in differential diagnosis. The sizes and appearances of involved lymph nodes in lymphoma span the entire spectrum, from well-defined mildly enlarged lymph nodes in one region to large conglomerate soft-tissue-density masses in multiple areas. Typically, these nodal masses demonstrate little enhancement following intravenous administration of contrast material; in fact, their central areas may become relatively quite hypodense.

CT plays major roles in the detection and staging of disease in the thorax, the planning of therapy, and follow-up evaluation for many patients with lymphoma (45,71,118). This radiologic technique is useful in defining the sites and extent of involvement, as well as in detecting disease in regions difficult to assess on conventional radiographs. These areas include not only the mediastinal lymph nodes but also the chest wall (Fig. 16), pleura (Figs. 13 and 17), and pulmonary parenchyma (Fig. 18). Also, CT may enable diagnosis of a benign cause for a plain chest radiographic abnormality, such as mediastinal li-

A,B

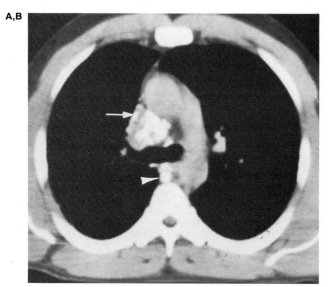

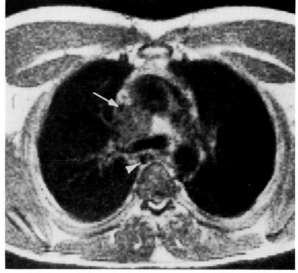

FIG. 12. Fibrosing mediastinitis. **A:** Postcontrast CT image demonstrates densely calcified precarinal lymph nodes, with secondary narrowing of the superior vena cava (*arrow*) and collateral enlargement of the azygos vein (*arrowhead*). **B:** On a T1-weighted MR image, severe compression of the superior vena cava (*arrow*) and enlargement of the azygos vein (*arrowhead*) are again seen. Calcifications shown by CT in the precarinal nodal mass are not appreciated as discrete areas of signal void. (From ref. 114.)

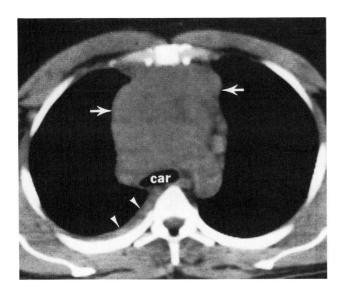

FIG. 13. Thymic Hodgkin disease; mixed-cellularity type. Large anterior mediastinal mass (*arrows*), shown by surgery to represent massive infiltration of the thymus, displacing the carina (car) posteriorly in a 39-year-old man with the superior vena caval syndrome. Concomitant enlargement of pretracheal and lateral thoracic lymph nodes is present. The neoplastic disease also is seen extending along the right posterior pleural surface (*arrowheads*).

pomatosis or hemorrhage, that can simulate lymphoma (5,14). Such information can be critical when radiation therapy is being considered as a treatment option, and it is sometimes helpful in selecting a site for biopsy or possible resection. Patients with Hodgkin disease who present clinically with stage I or II disease are most apt to benefit from CT (22). It is generally immaterial whether the plain chest radiographic findings are normal or abnormal if radiation therapy is contemplated (92). Intrathoracic involvement, especially mediastinal lymph node enlargement, may be detected in approximately 25% of patients with a normal chest radiographic examination. In as many as 40% of patients with "suspicious" conventional chest roentgenographic findings, CT documents the presence of disease. And even when chest radiographic findings are abnormal, additional sites or more extensive disease may be discovered. Overall staging is altered in about 15%, with radiation portals changed in nearly 40% of patients receiving primary or adjuvant radiation therapy for their disease. Partial-transmission lung blocks may be used when hilar, subcarinal, cardiophrenic angle, and/or paravertebral lymph node enlargement is detected. Localized boost therapy may be given when chest-wall invasion is discovered. Chemotherapy may be added to or substituted for radiotherapy in some cases, depending on the CT findings.

Leukemia, especially the chronic lymphocytic form, also may involve the mediastinal lymph nodes. Delineation of the extent of lymphadenopathy is almost never

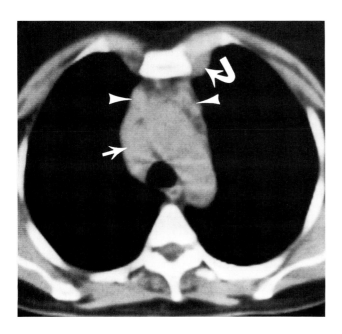

FIG. 14. Thymic Hodgkin disease; nodular sclerosing type. In addition to nodular enlargement of the thymus (*arrowheads*), there is right paratracheal (*straight arrow*) and left internal mammary (*curved arrow*) lymphadenopathy.

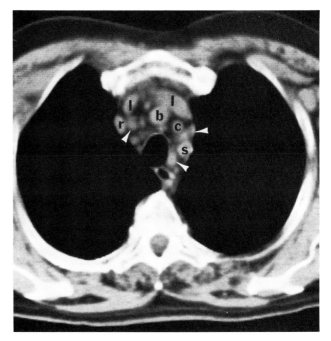

FIG. 15. Lymphadenopathy: non-Hodgkin lymphoma. Multiple mildly and borderline enlarged lymph nodes (*arrowheads*) are seen around the superior mediastinal vessels; (r) right brachiocephalic vein; (l) left brachiocephalic vein; (b) brachiocephalic artery; (c) left carotid artery; (s) left subclavian artery.

A,B

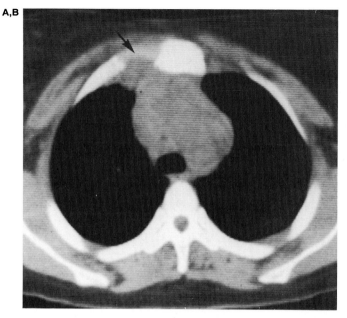

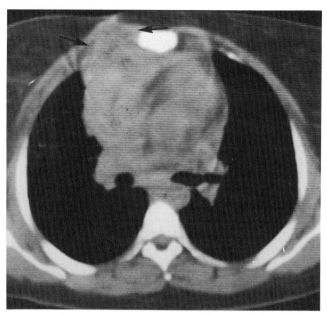

C

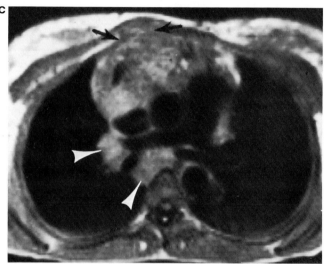

FIG. 16. Thymic Hodgkin disease; nodular sclerosing type. **A,B:** CT images showing direct extension of disease from a diffusely infiltrated and enlarged thymus into the right anterior chest wall (*arrows*). Right hilar and subcarinal lymphadenopathy also is present. **C:** In another patient, virtually identical findings are seen on T1-weighted MR image. A large mass infiltrates the thymus and extends into the chest wall (*arrows*). Right hilar and subcarinal lymphadenopathy (*arrowheads*) also is present.

crucial in treating the disease, because therapy is systemic rather than local.

CT also is helpful as a follow-up method in assessing treatment responses. It may aid in the readjustment of therapy (e.g., reduction in radiation-portal size as bulk tumor regresses). Relapse in the mediastinum may be detected when the plain chest radiographic findings are normal. CT is especially valuable in differentiating between recurrent mediastinal disease and paramediastinal radiation fibrosis, an especially difficult task with conventional roentgenography. Complete return to normal after successful treatment of mediastinal lymphadenopathy does not always occur. Follow-up CT examination may reveal some persistent, mildly enlarged lymph nodes, even though they contain no viable neoplasm. These "sterilized" nodes can pose a diagnostic and therapeutic dilemma (81). Although percutaneous needle aspiration with cytologic evaluation has been used, the cellular material obtained can be difficult to interpret after radiation

or chemotherapy. Serial CT examinations in patients otherwise doing well clinically after therapy usually suffice to determine the adequacy of treatment. Recurrence or failure of the initial therapy should be diagnosed only if an increase in the size of the lymph node subsequently occurs. In selected cases, MRI may be able to differentiate between posttherapeutic fibrosis (low signal intensity on both T1- and T2-weighted images) and lymphomatous involvement (Fig. 19) (50).

Metastatic Neoplasm

The overwhelming majority of mediastinal lymph node metastases originate from primary neoplasms within the thorax. Bronchogenic carcinoma is by far the most common etiology (Figs. 5D and 8D), with esophageal carcinoma a much less frequent cause. As will be emphasized in Chapter 9 in the section on bronchogenic carcinoma,

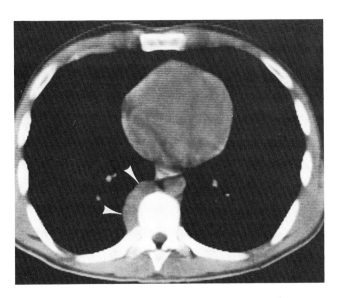

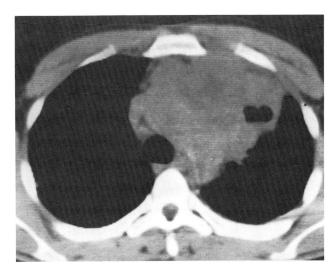

FIG. 17. Recurrent intrathoracic Hodgkin disease, manifesting as a pleural-based paravertebral mass (*arrowheads*), corroborated by percutaneous needle biopsy. Treated with local radiotherapy, it is uncertain whether the disease involved posterior mediastinal nodes, the pleura, or the lung, or various combinations.

FIG. 18. Thymic Hodgkin disease extending directly into adjacent left upper lobe, with resultant necrosis and cavitation.

CT is the best radiologic technique to demonstrate whether or not mediastinal lymph nodes are involved, as well as for delineating the extent of the primary pulmonary neoplasm. As previously described, lymph nodes 10 mm or larger in diameter are considered abnormal, emphasizing that the role of CT is in detection, not histologic diagnosis. Such a size criterion has been chosen to maximize sensitivity in identifying metastatic lymphadenopathy. This does result in a relatively low specificity (or substantial numbers of false positives) if pure statistical analysis is applied. Tissue sampling for corroboration of

metastatic neoplasm can be accomplished by a variety of semi–invasive methods (mediastinoscopy, percutaneous transthoracic or transbronchial needle aspiration), best chosen depending on the site of nodal enlargement.

Mediastinal lymph node metastases may also occur secondary to extrathoracic malignant neoplasms (88). The most likely primary sites are tumors of the head and neck, breast, and kidney and malignant melanoma (Fig. 5C, E, and G). If mediastinal lymph node enlargement is associated with atelectasis of a lobe or segment, bronchogenic carcinoma is the most likely cause.

A,B

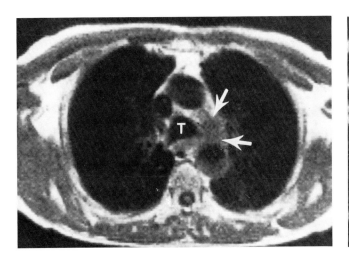

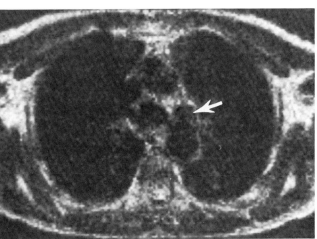

FIG. 19. Fibrosis in a nodal mass after radiation therapy. **A:** An intermediate-signal-intensity mass (*arrows*) is seen in the aorto-pulmonary window on a T1-weighted MR image; (T) trachea. **B:** On a T2-weighted image, the mass (*arrow*) is very low in signal intensity, similar to muscle.

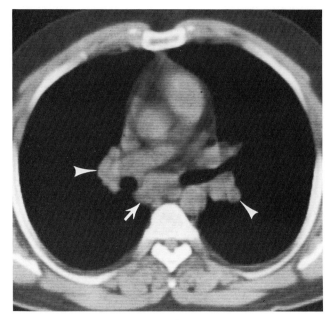

FIG. 20. Hilar lymphadenopathy. Small lobulated masses (*arrowheads*) are seen surrounding the interlobar pulmonary arteries bilaterally. Enlarged posterior subcarinal nodes (*arrow*) are also present in a patient with sarcoidosis.

Hilar Lymphadenopathy

Further assessment of an enlarged or questionably abnormal pulmonary hilum noted on plain chest radiography is a common radiologic problem. Usually the major decision to be made is whether the prominence is due to

a normal variation, enlargement of a pulmonary artery, enlargement of a lymph node, or a neoplastic mass. Although CT is capable of allowing these distinctions (see Fig. 64 in Chapter 7), in circumstances in which the hilum appears only questionably abnormal on standard radiographs and there is no compelling clinical reason to suspect hilar abnormality, conventional tomography (often in the 55° posterior oblique projection), which is less expensive and more readily available, generally suffices to resolve the dilemma. Standard tomography also may be used initially to document presumptive calcification within enlarged lymph nodes seen on plain chest radiographs (usually in a young individual). However, if the hilum is definitely abnormal, and it is uncertain whether this is due to enlarged lymph nodes, a mass, or vessels, CT is the preferred technique for differentiation. Similarly, CT would be used when the entire mediastinum (all lymph-node-bearing areas) needs to be assessed (e.g., patient with bronchogenic carcinoma or lymphoma).

The criteria for diagnosis of hilar lymph node enlargement on non-contrast-enhanced CT scans are similar to those used for conventional radiography: The hilum is too big and its contour is too nodular (Fig. 20) (102,124,137). In addition, there may be obliteration of some normal anatomic interfaces, such as convex bulging into the azygoesophageal recess or the space between the left-lower-lobe pulmonary artery and the descending aorta (Fig. 5F). Also, thickening of the posterior wall of the right-upper-lobe bronchus or the bronchus intermedius or of the left retrobronchial stripe may be present. With advanced hilar nodal enlargement, the central bronchi

A,B

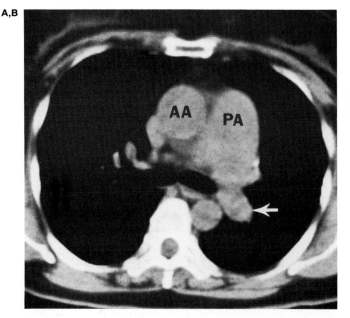
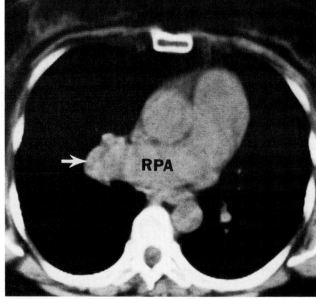

FIG. 21. Pulmonary arterial hypertension. **A:** The diameter of the main pulmonary artery (PA) is markedly dilated in comparison with the ascending aorta (AA). The left interlobar pulmonary artery (*arrow*) also is enlarged. **B:** More caudal, the horizontal intrapericardial portion of the right pulmonary artery (RPA) is substantially expanded, as is the right interlobar pulmonary artery (*arrow*) in the hilum.

A,B

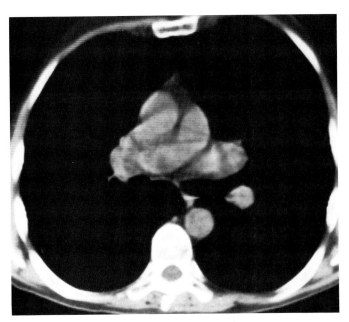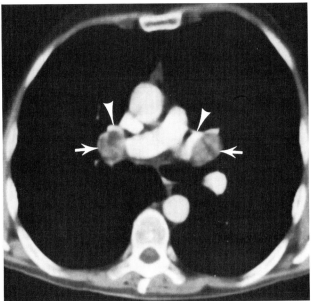

FIG. 22. Hilar lymphadenopathy; value of intravenous contrast material. **A:** Non-contrast-enhanced CT image shows enlargement of both hila. **B:** Postcontrast scan shows lymph node masses (*arrows*) to be the cause. Note that the superior pulmonary veins (*arrowheads*) are compressed by the enlarged nodes.

may be distorted and compressed. If the intrapericardial portion of the main pulmonary artery and its two major branches are enlarged, it is reasonable to assume that the extrapericardial portion of the vessel in the hilum is increased in size (Fig. 21). If doubt remains whether hilar enlargement is due to a lymph node mass or a vessel, it can almost always be dispelled by scanning following a bolus intravenous injection of contrast material (Figs. 22 and 23). Contrast enhancement also may be helpful in patients with adjacent pulmonary consolidation or atel-

ectasis to distinguish between any hilar nodal enlargement and central vessels. MRI is considered a supplementary technique if the CT examination is equivocal; it may assume a more primary role if there is a known contraindication to or inability to use intravenous contrast material. When contrast enhancement is used with CT (see Fig. 13 in Chapter 7), there is no difference in accuracy between the two techniques, and CT is superior for assessing the adjacent bronchial tree, which may be very important in evaluation of the hilum.

A,B

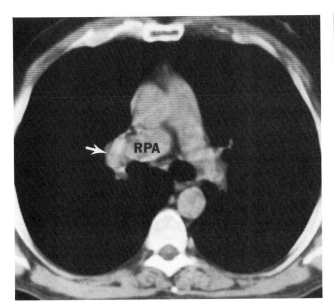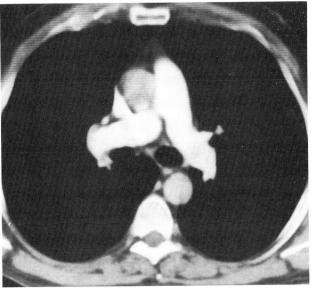

FIG. 23. Enlarged hilar pulmonary artery; value of intravenous contrast material. **A:** Non-contrast-enhanced CT image shows a big right hilum (*arrow*). This appears contiguous with the enlarged intrapericardial portion of the right pulmonary artery (RPA). **B:** Postcontrast CT image corroborates that a large right pulmonary artery accounts for the expanded hilum.

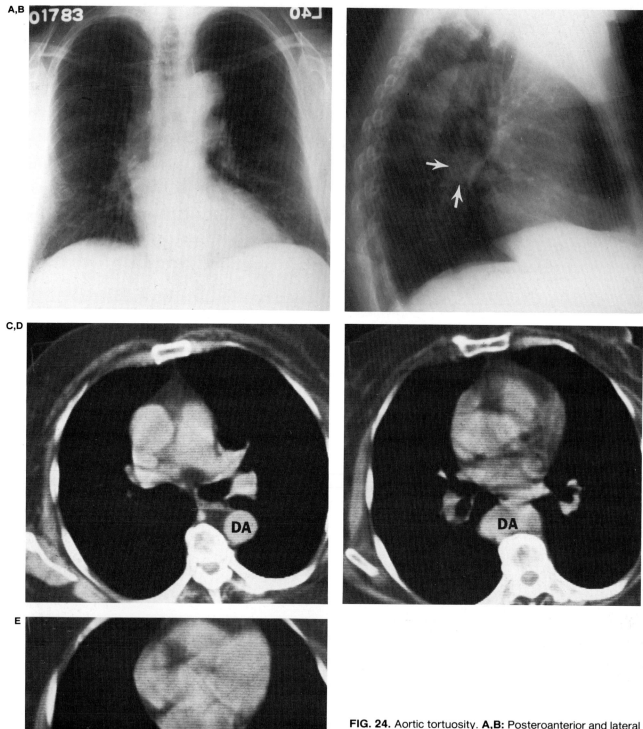

FIG. 24. Aortic tortuosity. **A,B:** Posteroanterior and lateral chest roentgenograms. A possible prevertebral mass (*arrows*) is suggested on the lateral view. **C–E:** Serial caudal CT images demonstrate that a tortuous descending aorta (DA), crossing in front of the thoracic spine and then descending on the right side, accounts for the suspected mass.

VASCULAR ABNORMALITIES

Tortuous Vessels

Excessively tortuous arteries (Fig. 24), relatively common in patients with hypertension and atherosclerosis, and vascular anomalies (see Figs. 87 to 91 in Chapter 7) may produce abnormalities in the mediastinal contours on plain chest radiographs that may be indistinguishable from a mass or aneurysm. Buckling of the brachiocephalic (innominate) artery, which produces a convex right superior interface, is the most frequently encountered example of this problem. CT can readily demonstrate the innocuous nature of this finding (see Fig. 32 in Chapter 7).

Aortic Aneurysm

Atherosclerosis

The majority of aneurysms involving the thoracic aorta are caused by atherosclerosis (112). A loss in strength of the media allows dilatation of all components of the aortic wall (true aneurysm) to occur. These aneurysms typically develop in the arch or descending aorta, where atherosclerosis predominates. Aneurysms of the ascending aorta are much less frequent, and their presence should suggest cystic medial necrosis, aortic dissection, or luetic aortitis as alternative causes. Because atherosclerosis affects long segments of the aorta circumferentially, these aneurysms tend to be fusiform rather than saccular.

Most atherosclerotic thoracic aortic aneurysms develop insidiously. The majority of patients are asymptomatic, and their aneurysms are detected incidentally on plain chest radiographs. Symptoms can be produced if the aneurysm is rapidly enlarging (or ruptures). Complaints arise due to pressure on adjacent structures—cough or dyspnea from compression of the airways, dysphagia from compression on the esophagus, hoarseness from pressure on the recurrent laryngeal nerve, and pain from erosion of bone. Survival is much better in patients without symptoms. In the evaluation of aneurysms, size is an important prognostic feature in any presurgical assessment. Based on data from conventional chest radiography, an aneurysm is diagnosed when the aorta exceeds 4 cm in diameter, or if the aorta enlarges distally. The risk of rupture increases with greater size of the aneurysm (112). It is approximately 10% for aneurysms between 5 and 10 cm in diameter, and about 50% for aneurysms greater than 10 cm. Surgical excision, when feasible, generally is advocated for aneurysms measuring more than 7 cm in diameter.

Although conventional radiographs usually raise the suspicion of an aortic aneurysm, they are often insufficient by themselves to confirm the diagnosis or to guide therapy.

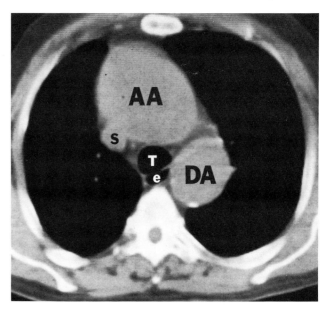

FIG. 25. Atherosclerotic aortic aneurysm. Fusiform dilatation of both the ascending (AA) and descending (DA) portions of the thoracic aorta is seen; (S) superior vena cava ; (T) trachea; (e) esophagus.

Direct imaging of the aortic lesion is required. Traditionally this has been accomplished by aortography, with its inherent risks and limitations in defining extraluminal abnormalities. In recent years, CT (and MRI) has provided sufficient diagnostic confirmation to obviate aortography and institute treatment in most cases. Ultrasound, another noninvasive procedure, usually is limited to the assessment of aortic abnormalities near the base of the heart in adults (30,66). In other regions, air-filled lung frequently scatters and deflects the sonic beam, making the technique unreliable.

Both CT and MRI, with their tomographic imaging formats, allow separation of the various portions of the aortic circumference from superimposed mediastinal structures. The lumen of the aorta, its wall, and the periaortic soft tissues are all well demonstrated. Both methods are effective in diagnosing an aortic aneurysm, distinguishing it from a soft-tissue-density lesion when the plain chest radiograph detects a mediastinal mass, and characterizing it further, including its measurement, location, and longitudinal extent (Figs. 25 and 26) (28,32,49,109,111).

CT can depict all of the gross pathologic features of an aortic aneurysm: dilatation, intraluminal thrombus (84), displacement or erosion of adjacent structures, and perianeurysmal hemorrhage (74). The aortic caliber can be precisely measured with CT. On non-contrast-enhanced images, intimal calcification, a common feature of atherosclerosis, frequently is seen at the periphery of the aneurysm (Fig. 26A). The location of these curvilinear calcifications not only assists in identifying the mediastinal abnormality as vascular but also serves to distinguish an

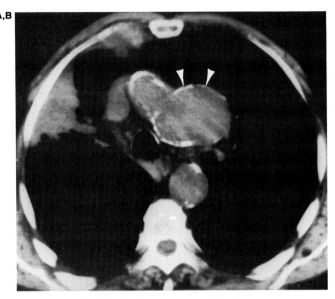
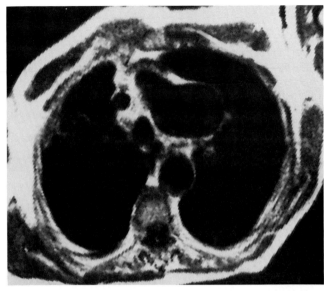

FIG. 26. Atherosclerotic aortic aneurysm. Chest radiograph in a 63-year-old man with chronic renal disease demonstrated consolidation and volume loss in the right upper lobe (subsequently proved secondary to a centrally obstructing epidermoid carcinoma) and a mediastinal mass. **A:** Non-contrast-enhanced CT image shows peripheral atherosclerotic calcification extending from the aortic arch around the mass (*arrowheads*), consistent with the diagnosis of an aneurysm. **B:** MR image corroborates an aneurysm by demonstrating its signal void contiguous with the aortic arch.

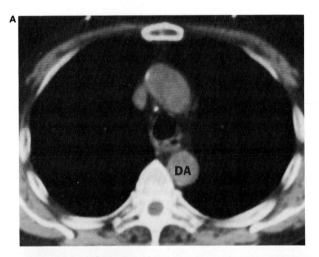

FIG. 27. Atherosclerotic aneurysm. **A:** Non-contrast-enhanced CT image at the level of the aortopulmonary window shows a normal proximal descending thoracic aorta (DA). **B:** Seven centimeters caudal, marked dilatation of the descending aorta is present. Peripheral atherosclerotic calcifications (*arrowhead*) can be noted. **C:** Image following intravenous administration of contrast material demonstrates a large thrombus (th) partially filling the aneurysm, with irregular dilatation of the remaining lumen.

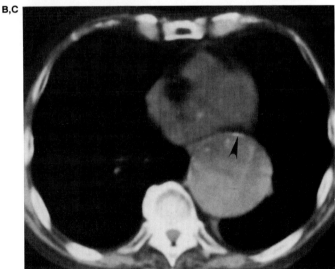
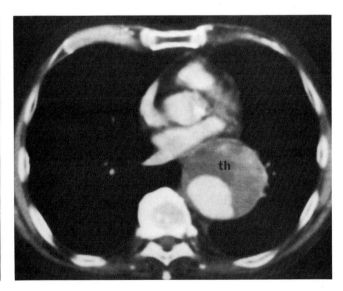

atherosclerotic aneurysm (Fig. 27) from aortic dissection. Intravenous administration of contrast material is used to corroborate the vascular nature of the mass (Fig. 28), to define portions that may be obscured by the mediastinum in an emaciated individual, and to assess its luminal contents.

In the past, using older CT equipment and slow-drip-

infusion techniques of administering contrast material, highly vascular lesions (e.g., intrathoracic goiter, leiomyosarcoma, angiofollicular lymph node hyperplasia) were described that were enhanced sufficiently to cause confusion with a vascular structure. Theoretically, a saccular aneurysm entirely filled with thrombus also could cause a major interpretive problem and simulate a soft-

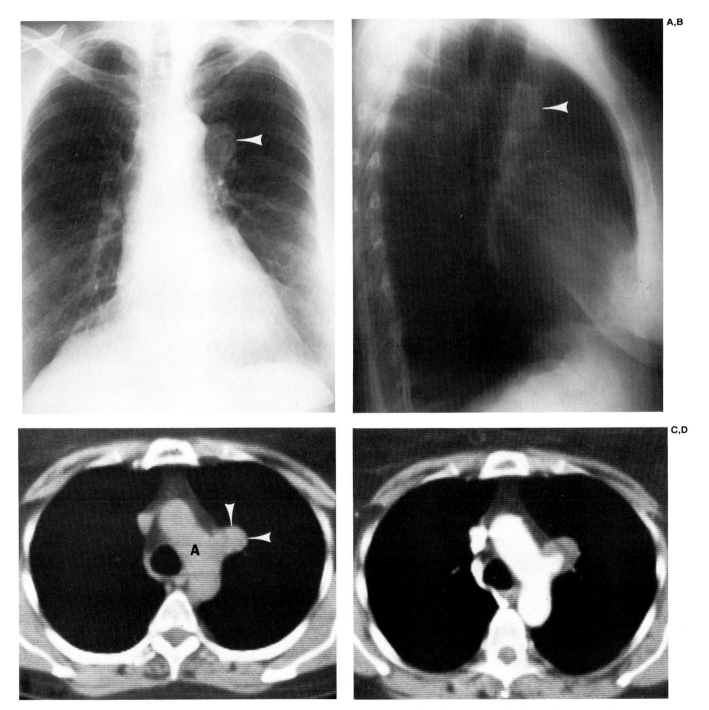

FIG. 28. Aortic aneurysm. **A,B:** Posteroanterior and lateral chest roentgenograms show a nodular lesion (*arrowheads*), perhaps in the left upper lobe, adjacent to the aortic arch. **C:** Non-contrast-enhanced CT image shows the mass (*arrowheads*), contiguous with the aortic arch (A). **D:** CT image after bolus intravenous injection of contrast material confirms a localized saccular aortic aneurysm, largely filled with thrombus, as its cause.

tissue neoplasm, similar to a well-described pitfall with angiography (123). However, if proper technique is used and serial CT levels are closely scrutinized (looking for changing aortic caliber and peripheral calcifications), CT after bolus contrast injection should almost always enable one to distinguish between an aneurysm and a soft-tissue-density mass (54,96). Problems may arise with poor vascular enhancement due to lack of adequate venous access, but this should be obvious at the time of the study.

In most cases, CT provides all of the information required for possible surgical intervention, and additional studies, such as aortography, are unnecessary. Because the upper and lower surfaces of the aortic arch cross the plane of the CT slice, dilatation in these areas may be difficult to diagnose. Similarly, the exact relationships of major branch vessels of the aorta to the aneurysm itself, especially one arising from the arch, may be difficult to ascertain. Supplemental MRI or angiography should be used when this information is critical to surgical planning.

CT can be used for serial follow-up examination to assess for possible interval growth of an aneurysm when it is decided that immediate operative intervention is not warranted.

There are several interpretive pitfalls with CT evaluation of suspected aortic aneurysm. When the aorta is tortuous and crosses the transaxial CT plane obliquely, its true caliber may be difficult to measure. The cross-sectional scan may incorporate both portions of a kink in the aorta, imaging them as a single structure that appears much larger than the actual diameter of either limb of the tortuous aorta. Similarly, the usual 10-mm-thick CT section can superimpose wider and narrower portions of an aneurysm of the ascending or descending aorta. This can lead to the false appearance of inwardly displaced intimal calcification and the erroneous suggestion of an

aortic dissection. On rare occasion, calcification may develop on the luminal surface of a thrombus within an atherosclerotic aneurysm, leading to a mistaken impression of displaced intima. Virtually all of these problems can be overcome by simply correlating the CT findings with the plain chest roentgenogram or preliminary computed radiograph; images obtained with thin collimation may occasionally help.

A major advantage of MRI is that there is no necessity for intravenous contrast material (142). Also, with MRI, the sagittal and coronal views may provide vital information regarding the relationship of an aneurysm to the branch arch vessels (Fig. 29) (106,136,138). In such congenital abnormalities as Marfan syndrome, MRI is effective for evaluating and monitoring aortic dimensions and can help screen kindred for the malady. Parasagittal sections may permit demonstration of the entire arch and descending thoracic aorta (see Fig. 19B in Chapter 7). However, with atherosclerosis, the aorta is frequently tortuous, preventing imaging of all of this portion on a single section. Slow-flowing blood within an aortic aneurysm may generate a signal and be difficult to distinguish from a thrombus. Distinction may be made by comparing the relative signal intensities between the first- and second-echo images (15), or with the phase-offset technique (34). Partial-volume averaging can also cause an interpretive pitfall with MRI (139).

Postoperative Complications

Complications involving the thoracic aorta may occur following cardiac surgery. These contained ruptures (false aneurysms), which most frequently involve the ascending portion, usually result from breakdown of an aortotomy

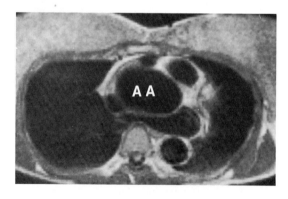

FIG. 29. Cystic medial necrosis. Transaxial and coronal MR images demonstrate generalized dilatation of the ascending aorta (AA) in a 28-year-old woman with Marfan syndrome. (From ref. 50.)

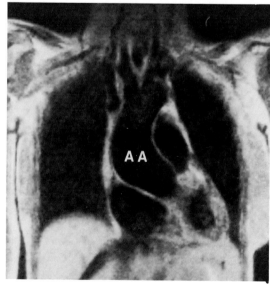

suture line (e.g., following aortic valve replacement) or at the site of prior cannulation for cardiopulmonary bypass. CT is a superb method for distinguishing between aortic abnormalities (Fig. 30) and other causes (Fig. 31) of mediastinal widening noted on conventional radiography following cardiac surgery (29,68,99,130,146). Fluid–fluid levels (due to separation of serum and formed blood elements in a subacute or chronic hematoma) secondary to rupture of a contained false aneurysm may be seen in the anterior mediastinum on non-contrast-enhanced images

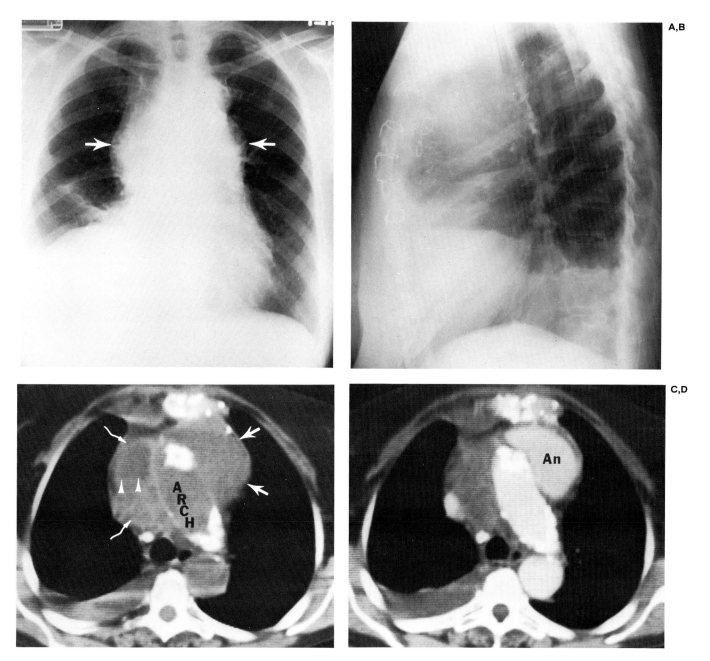

FIG. 30. False aneurysm of the aorta in a 72-year-old woman, asymptomatic 6 weeks after a coronary artery bypass procedure. **A,B:** Posteroanterior and lateral chest roentgenograms demonstrated a new mass (*arrows*) in the anterior mediastinum. The right pleural effusion was unchanged in size from that seen on a chest radiograph obtained on hospital discharge 4 weeks previously. **C:** Non-contrast-enhanced CT image shows a 7-cm soft-tissue-density mass (*straight arrows*) to the left of the top of the aortic arch (ARCH). Another mass (*curved arrows*), composed of near-water density anteriorly and soft-tissue density posteriorly, separated by a fluid level (*arrowheads*), characteristic of a subacute hematoma, is seen to the right of the aortic arch. **D:** Postcontrast image demonstrates a false (pseudo) aneurysm (An) to the left of the aortic arch. At surgery, performed under hypothermia because of the proximity of the pseudoaneurysm to the sternum, a small tear in the aorta next to a bypass graft was found responsible for the aneurysm and hematoma.

A,B

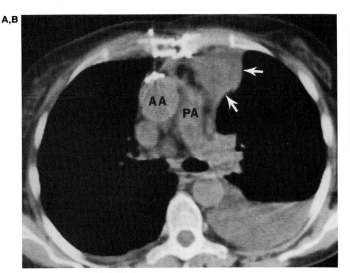
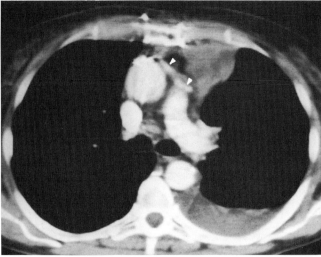

FIG. 31. Mediastinal hematoma in a 68-year-old woman 3 weeks after coronary artery bypass procedure, noted to have left anterior mediastinal mass on chest radiographs. **A:** Non-contrast-enhanced CT image shows a soft-tissue-density mass (*arrows*), consistent with a hematoma, in the mediastinum to the left of the ascending aorta (AA) and pulmonary artery (PA), and a high-density left pleural effusion. **B:** Image after bolus injection of contrast material shows opacification of a saphenous vein graft (*arrowheads*), but no aneurysm nor enhancement of the hematoma or effusion. Bleeding was presumed to be from a small artery or vein, and the patient was managed conservatively; the changes resolved spontaneously (compare with Fig. 30).

(Figs. 30C and 32). Images following a bolus injection of contrast material almost always demonstrate enhancement of the lumen of the false aneurysmal sac; such opacification may not be visible on aortography.

Trauma

Acute

Rupture of the thoracic aorta may result from a severe deacceleration injury, most typically an automobile accident. Although the thoracic aorta may be torn anywhere along its length (60), the most frequent site of the contained rupture, in those surviving the initial trauma, is the distal aortic arch at the insertion of the ligamentum arteriosum just after the origin of the left subclavian artery. A circumferential tear, constituting a complete transection, usually occurs. Expedient diagnosis and immediate surgical repair generally are essential to prevent progressive hemorrhage at the site of the aortic tear. Plain chest radiographs in these patients may demonstrate mediastinal widening. However, such widening may result from supine positioning or from shallow inspiration by the patient, or because of the use of the anteroposterior projection and a short X-ray-tube/film distance. In other patients, a real mediastinal hematoma may be present, but the source of rupture may be small arteries or veins that do not require surgical repair.

Aortography (oftentimes using digital technique), not CT (or MRI), remains the procedure of choice to evaluate possible aortic injury from blunt chest trauma (42). There

are several reasons for this recommendation. The major reason is that CT is not consistently or fully diagnostic. Patients who sustain major trauma may not be able to fully cooperate, and the images may be degraded by motion artifacts. Subtle changes in aortic caliber at the site

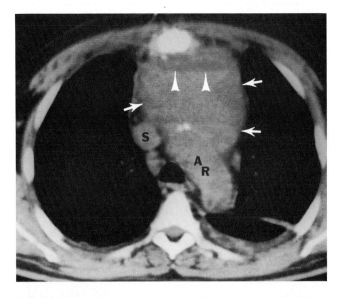

FIG. 32. Mediastinal hematoma in a 63-year-old man 9 months after an aortic valve replacement demonstrated marked interval mediastinal widening on a chest radiograph. CT image shows a huge anterior mediastinal mass (*arrows*) containing a fluid–fluid level (*arrowheads*), plus a small left pleural effusion. At surgery, a tear in the ascending aorta above the valve was found responsible for the hematoma; (S) superior vena cava; (AR) aortic arch.

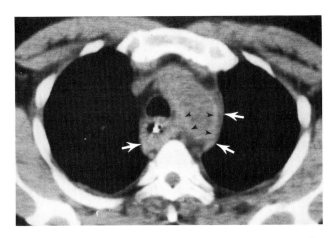

FIG. 33. Acute aortic rupture in a 47-year-old man involved in severe automobile accident. CT was requested primarily to evaluate suspected head and abdominal trauma; it was decided also to image the thorax because a portable supine chest radiograph showed some mild mediastinal widening. Mediastinal hemorrhage (*arrows*) is seen lateral to the aortic arch and posterior to the esophagus with its contained nasogastric tube. The distal aortic arch (*arrowheads*) appears dilated. Subsequent aortography corroborated a false aneurysm and aortic tear just distal to the left subclavian artery.

evaluation of intracranial or abdominal trauma), CT may be of value to look for a small traumatic aneurysm or a periaortic hematoma (Fig. 33). The presence of a normal aortic contour and the absence of a mediastinal hematoma usually are sufficient to obviate aortography. If a false aneurysm is recognized, or if a linear lucency caused by the torn edge of the aortic wall is seen, surgery will be indicated (62). Less specific findings, such as marginal irregularity of the aortic wall or a periaortic hematoma, will warrant angiography. In rare instances the mediastinal hemorrhage may extend across the posterior mediastinum into the extrapleural or pleural space of the right hemithorax.

Chronic

If the aorta is only partially transected following blunt trauma, and if such an injury is not suspected clinically and the patient survives, a localized false (pseudo) aneurysm may subsequently develop over a period of months to years. These lesions, which generally do not cause symptoms, again are most common near the aortic isthmus. They continue to communicate with the aortic lumen through the tear and tend to expand with time. Because rupture is unpredictable, in most clinical circumstances surgical excision is advised because of its low mortality (11,63). Contrary to the situation with suspected acute traumatic injury to the aorta, either CT or MRI usually is adequate for diagnostic confirmation of a chronic traumatic pseudoaneurysm suspected on plain chest radiography, and aortography is rarely required. The saccular or fusiform dilatation of the aortic isthmus can be detected and characterized by CT or MRI; peripheral calcification of the wall of the pseudoaneurysm usually is seen on CT (Fig. 34) (23). Because an MRI parasagittal

of a transection consequently can be missed. Traumatic disruption of an aortic arch vessel, which also usually requires surgical repair, may be virtually impossible to detect with CT. Although a mediastinal hematoma generally can be consistently demonstrated with CT, the source may not be the aorta or a major branch, but rather a small vein or artery.

In circumstances where the clinical suspicion of major mediastinal vascular trauma is low, or the injured patient requires a CT examination for another indication (e.g.,

A,B

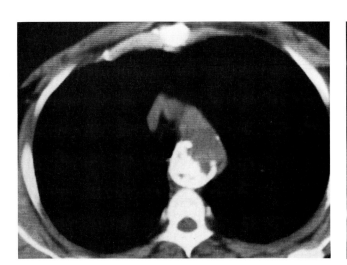 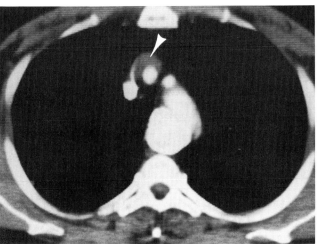

FIG. 34. Traumatic aortic aneurysm. **A:** Non-contrast-enhanced CT image demonstrates dense calcification within the dilated distal aortic arch in a 33-year-old man who had been in an automobile accident 8 years previously. **B:** Postcontrast image demonstrates enhancement of the dilated aortic knob. No opacification of the left brachiocephalic vein (*arrowhead*) has yet occurred because the bolus injection was into a right medial antecubital vein.

view of the aorta often can define the exact relationship of such an aneurysm to the left subclavian artery and determine the size of the communication with the aortic lumen, it is generally the preferred diagnostic technique in these stable individuals (see Fig. 20 in Chapter 7) (100).

Aortic Dissection

The most common acute catastrophe involving the aorta, dissection of the thoracic aorta, is approximately twice as frequent as a ruptured abdominal aortic aneurysm (116). An insidious onset also may occur. The peak incidence of the disease is seen in the sixth and seventh decades of life, and men are more commonly afflicted. Hypertension is the most common predisposing condition. In patients under the age of 40, aortic dissection usually is associated with cystic medial necrosis. Other factors such as aortic coarctation, congenital aortic valve disease, and pregnancy may play a role. Iatrogenic injury from catheterization or cardiac surgery may be causal. The exact etiology of aortic dissection is controversial. In most cases it probably begins as a tear in the intima of the aorta. Blood then enters the aortic wall through the tear, separating the layers of the media and creating a false channel. The intimal tear most commonly starts either in the proximal ascending aorta within several centimeters of the aortic valve or in the proximal descending aorta just beyond the origin of the left subclavian artery at the site of the ligamentum arteriosum. These two relatively fixed areas of the aorta are thought to bear the maximum force of each systolic pulse. The increased mechanical stress at these points, sometimes combined with an underlying abnormality of the media (e.g., cystic medial necrosis), is considered the dominant factor in its pathogenesis. However, because aortic dissection can occur in the absence of a documented intimal tear, an alternative postulated precipitating mechanism is that disease of the media leads to rupture of the vasa vasorum within the aortic wall that may subsequently propagate into the aortic lumen through an intimal tear. No matter what the primary event, a pulsating hematoma splits the media and may extend proximally or distally in the aortic wall. Distally created intimal tears can provide reentry points into the true lumen for the blood in the aortic wall.

The anatomic site of the aortic dissection influences both treatment and prognosis. The current classification of dissection reflects in a simple fashion the type of treatment usually selected. A type A dissection involves the ascending aorta, even if the initial intimal tear occurred in the descending aorta, with only proximal propagation of the medial hematoma affecting the ascending aorta. These patients usually are submitted to immediate surgery because of the high risks of the dissecting hematoma extending proximally into the pericardial sac, with development of cardiac tamponade, disruption of the aortic valve, with subsequent insufficiency, and occlusion of the coronary or brachiocephalic arteries. A type B dissection is limited to the descending aorta and usually is managed by medical therapy by reducing the peak systolic pressure to allow healing, unless there is persistent pain, ischemia to major organs, or rupture. These are allowed to enter a chronic phase, if no complication develops. Eventually, some type B dissections may require surgical repair, usually grafting for subsequent progressive aneurysmal dilatation. However, such surgery is associated with a much lower operative mortality if it can be delayed until fibrosis has developed and the aortic tissues are less friable.

The original surgical therapy for aortic dissection involved the excision of intimal tears, obliteration of the false lumen, reconstitution of the aorta, often with the interposition of a graft, and restoration of aortic valve competence by either reconstruction of the aortic annulus or replacement with an aortic valve prosthesis. Aortography was required then to provide preoperative information regarding the extent of the dissection, sites of intimal tears, patterns of flow in the true and false lumina, the source of perfusion of the major aortic branches, and the presence and degree of aortic insufficiency. With recent advances and changes in the surgical management of aortic dissection, such precise preoperative information generally is not required. Current surgical therapy is largely directed only at preventing proximal extension of the dissection (97,132). The proximal portion of the false channel is obliterated by resecting a segment of the ascending aorta and inserting a graft. Adequate perfusion of the coronary arteries is assured, sometimes by reimplantation. The aortic valve mechanism is made competent; aortic annuloplasty and valve reconstruction are performed routinely as part of the grafting of the ascending aorta. Neither operative mortality nor late mortality is influenced by surgical resection (or nonresection) of all the intimal tears. Residual patency of the distal false lumen is not associated with a worsened late functional status. The only information really required by the clinician is that necessary to rapidly and unequivocally diagnose an aortic dissection and to determine whether or not it involves the ascending aorta. Documentation of a type A dissection usually warrants immediate surgical repair.

Plain chest radiographs commonly demonstrate widening of the aorta, which, if acute in comparison with prior studies, is diagnostic. Inward displacement of calcification more than 6 mm from the outer aortic wall is a helpful sign, but must be applied with caution in the arch portion unless the finding is new because of foreshortening. However, findings on conventional chest roentgenograms may be normal. CT is a minimally invasive, reliable radiologic technique that generally can be used to definitively diagnose and classify the type of aortic dissection; it is at least as accurate as aortography and can obviate this more invasive method in most cases (38,52,78,131,133).

A,B

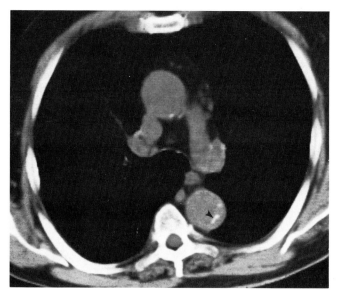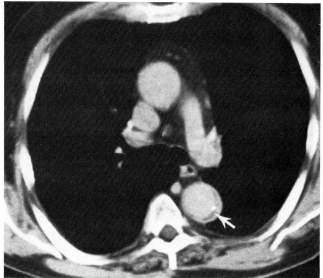

FIG. 35. Aortic dissection, type B. **A:** Non-contrast-enhanced CT image demonstrates internal displacement of intimal calcification (*arrowhead*). **B:** Postcontrast image demonstrates enhancement of the blood in the true lumen, with a false lumen (*arrow*) external to the calcification located posterolaterally in the proximal descending thoracic aorta. The ascending aorta is normal.

It may be worthwhile to obtain precontrast CT images of the thorax; they can be acquired at 2-cm intervals and occasionally will obviate subsequent contrast administration. Dynamic scanning is performed at a single level through the middle of the ascending aorta, following a bolus intravenous injection of 35 to 50 ml of contrast material. If these images show no dissection, an additional dynamic series more cephalad at the level of the aortic arch or more caudal may be of value, especially if the non-contrast-enhanced images demonstrate suspicious findings. If the dynamic sequence is positive for a dissection, especially a type B, a survey of the entire aorta is made during a subsequent rapid infusion of contrast material, from just above the aortic arch to at least the diaphragm. If the dissection is still present at the latter level, scanning is continued caudal into the abdomen until the aorta becomes normal or down to the iliac bifurcation.

The CT findings in aortic dissection may include the following:

A. Precontrast images
1. Internal displacement of calcified intimal atherosclerotic plaques (Fig. 35)
2. Higher density of the false lumen if it is acutely thrombosed, compared with the flowing blood in the true lumen (Fig. 36) (the reverse can occur with a chronic dissection)
3. Enlargement of a long segment of the aorta
4. Pericardial or mediastinal hemorrhage (Figs. 37 and 38)
B. Postcontrast images
1. Splitting of the aorta into two contrast-filled channels, with an intervening linear filling defect, the intimal flap (Figs. 39 and 40), which may be best

demonstrated with narrow window settings (the intimal flap may be seen on non-contrast-enhanced images in anemic patients) (Fig. 38) (31)
2. Delayed opacification of the false lumen on dynamic scanning
3. Opacification of only the true lumen, which is often compressed (Fig. 37C)

In the latter circumstance, in which the false lumen is thrombosed, distinction between a dissection and a fusiform atherosclerotic aneurysm may be a problem. Inward displacement of atheromatous calcification indicates a dissection, whereas peripheral aortic wall calcification is typical of an atherosclerotic aneurysm (61). In addition, narrowing or deformity of the residual opacified lumen strongly suggests a dissection; an atherosclerotic aneurysm has a larger, round or oval lumen. If an aneurysm involves the descending aorta, and the region of the aortic isthmus is spared, an atherosclerotic cause is favored (Fig. 41). There are several other problems and pitfalls (52) with CT diagnosis of aortic dissection:

1. Insufficient contrast enhancement may lead to failure to detect the intimal flap. Optimal aortic opacification cannot always be achieved, especially in patients with poor venous access or low cardiac output. This difficulty should be easily recognized at the time of the examination and can be circumvented with MRI.
2. Streak artifacts across the aorta induced by the moving heart may mimic an intimal flap (44). Artifacts usually are straight, and their orientation may change markedly from one CT image to another; they frequently extend beyond the confines of the aorta. In contradistinction, intimal flaps are persistent and generally show a mild curvature.

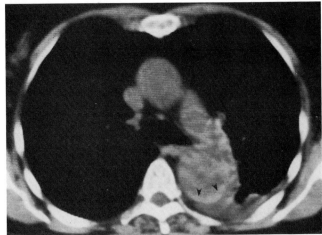

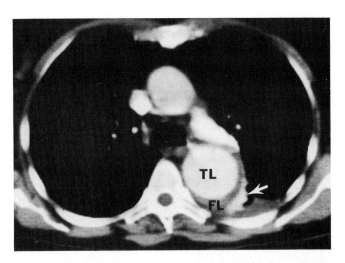

FIG. 36. Aortic dissection, type B. **A:** Non-contrast-enhanced CT image demonstrates a high-density peripheral rim (*arrowheads*) in the posterolateral portion of a dilated proximal descending thoracic aorta. There is a small associated left pleural effusion. **B:** Postcontrast image shows enhancement of the blood in a dilated true lumen (TL), presumably secondary to a preexisting atherosclerotic aneurysm; the thrombosed false lumen (FL) is now much less dense than the true lumen. The ascending aorta is normal. The enhancing crescentic density (*arrow*) external to the aorta represents atelectatic lung (undoubtedly secondary to some acute aortic dilatation) and should not be mistaken for extravasated contrast material.

A,B

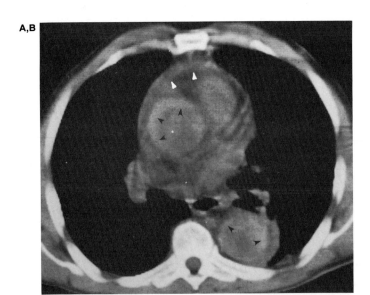

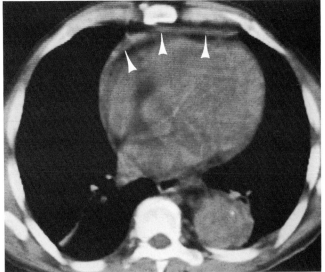

C

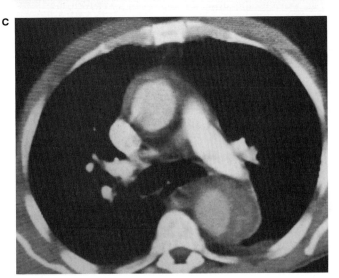

FIG. 37. Aortic dissection, type A. **A:** Non-contrast-enhanced CT image demonstrates a peripheral rim of high density (*black arrowheads*) in both the ascending and descending aortae. Some high-density thickening (*white arrowheads*) is also seen in the cephalad extension of the pericardial sac. **B:** On a more caudal scan at the ventricular level, a hemopericardium (*white arrowheads*) is demonstrated. An inwardly displaced intimal calcification is also seen in the distal descending aorta. **C:** Postcontrast CT image corroborates a type A dissection, with enhancement of blood in only the true lumen in both the ascending and descending aortae. In retrospect, there was no necessity to administer intravenous contrast material in this circumstance.

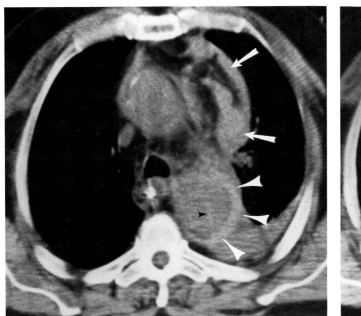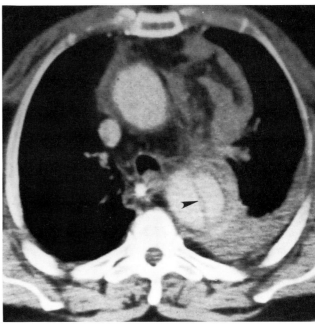

FIG. 38. Type B aortic dissection with rupture. **A:** Non-contrast-enhanced CT image demonstrates a mildly dilated descending aorta containing a faintly visible opaque line (*black arrowhead*), surrounded by a high-density thrombus (*white arrowheads*) as well as an acute hematoma in the mediastinum (*arrows*). In addition, there is a high-density left pleural effusion. **B:** Postcontrast image convincingly demonstrates an intimal flap (*arrowhead*) due to an acute dissection in the descending aorta that was the source of the leaking blood.

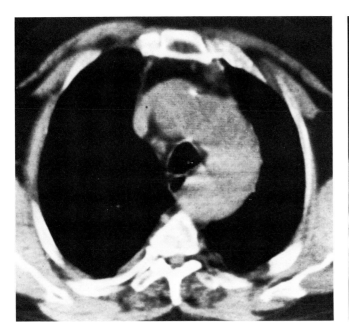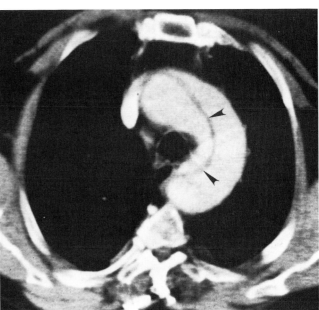

FIG. 39. Aortic dissection, type A. **A:** Non-contrast-enhanced CT image shows no definite abnormality of the aortic arch except mild dilatation. **B:** Postcontrast image demonstrates a linear lucency representing the intimal flap (*arrowheads*) separating the true and false lumina.

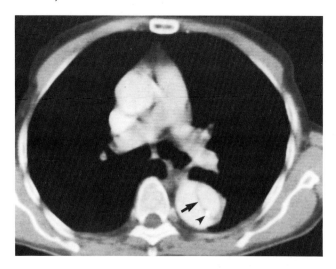

FIG. 40. Aortic dissection, type B. Postcontrast CT image demonstrates equal enhancement of both the true and false lumina within a dilated proximal descending thoracic aorta, compared with the ascending aorta; the lumina are separated by an intimal flap (*arrow*) with a contained atherosclerotic calcification (*arrowhead*).

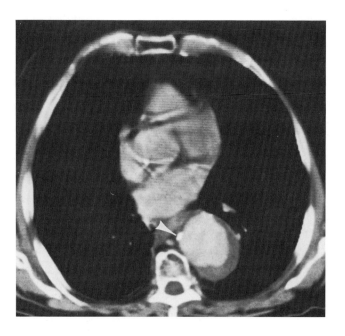

FIG. 41. Atherosclerotic aneurysm. Following intravenous contrast material, CT image shows a lobulated aneurysm of the descending thoracic aorta, with a contained eccentric peripheral thrombus. Peripheral atherosclerotic calcification (*arrowhead*) is present, but only around the opacified lumen. A normal-appearing, more proximal descending aorta, in conjunction with serial chest roentgenograms demonstrating gradual dilatation of the distal descending aorta, enables distinction from a dissecting aneurysm.

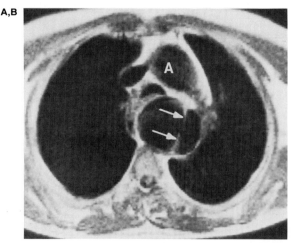
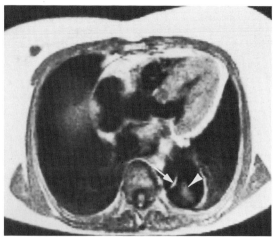

FIG. 42. Type B aortic dissection; MR images. **A:** The intimal flap (*arrows*) in the dilated descending aorta is seen separating the true and false lumina. The ascending aorta (A) is normal. The carina is displaced anteriorly. **B:** Similar findings are seen in another patient. A small amount of signal within the false lumen (*arrowhead*) is presumably secondary to slow flow; (*arrow*) intimal flap.

3. The left innominate vein anterior to the aortic arch (see Fig. 34 in Chapter 7), or the left superior intercostal vein lateral to it (see Fig. 80 in Chapter 7), may simulate a false lumen. The courses of these normal veins on contiguous images and their pattern of enhancement relative to the aorta should eliminate this pitfall.

4. A prominent preaortic or retroaortic pericardial recess (see Figs. 104 and 105 in Chapter 7) may be mistaken for a false channel; this is a more common problem with MRI than with CT.

5. Pseudodisplacement of intimal calcifications due to partial-volume averaging where the aorta is tortuous and crosses the CT plane obliquely, or at the junction where it is focally dilated, and the rare calcification on the luminal surface of a thrombus have already been detailed.

6. Thickened pleura adjacent to the aorta might simulate a surrounding chronic false lumen.

7. Atelectatic lung is common surrounding an acute aortic dissection with dilatation. These areas may be enhanced markedly on postcontrast images. Similarly, a small serous left pleural effusion commonly occurs. Neither finding should be construed as an ominous sign of rupture (Fig. 36B).

Similar to CT, transaxial MRI has a high sensitivity for detection of an intimal flap, the hallmark of a dissection (Fig. 42) (1,33,47). Accurate classification into types and depiction of the levels of involvement are possible. Coronal or sagittal images may be helpful in assessing the relationship of the dissection to the major arch vessels. When blood flow in both the true and false lumina exceeds a certain velocity, the intimal flap is displayed as a linear structure of medium signal intensity that is delineated by the flow voids in both lumina. An interpretive problem may arise when the false lumen is completely thrombosed. The commonly displaced atheromatous calcifications within the intimal flap, which frequently permit a definitive diagnosis of dissection and distinction from a thrombosed atherosclerotic aneurysm on CT, cannot be recognized with MRI. When flow is slow in the false lumen, the intimal flap is outlined on one side by the signal void from the normally flowing blood in the true lumen, and on the other side by the high anomalous intraluminal signal from the slowly flowing blood in the false lumen. Phase-shift techniques can be used to display differential flow rates in the true and false lumina.

Controversy still exists as to what is the most appropriate radiologic technique for the diagnosis of an aortic dissection. The sensitivity and specificity of CT (and probably MRI) are quite similar to those for aortography, with both exceeding 95%. Cases properly diagnosed by CT that were missed on angiography, and vice versa, have been reported. The obvious advantages of CT over aortography are that it can be performed much faster and the risks of arterial puncture and catheterization are avoided. In our hospital, surgical and/or medical management is almost exclusively predicated on the CT findings. CT generally is preferred to MRI because it is much more readily available, can be completed in a much shorter time, and usually is easier to perform in many of these patients who are hemodynamically unstable and require close monitoring. Although CT does not depict the site of an intimal tear, nor does it allow assessment of the aortic valve (incompetency usually can be determined with a stethoscope) or coronary arteries, this information either is not vital for surgical planning or can be ascertained intraoperatively. In a poor-operative-risk patient, aortography may be performed as a supplement to document clinically suspected occlusion of a major aortic branch, which might be a determinant in prompting surgical therapy. In a patient suspected of aortic dissection who has clinically detectable severe aortic regurgitation or is markedly hypotensive, in whom optimal aortic opacification might be difficult or impossible to achieve with CT, and who is too ill to be analyzed with MRI, aortography would be the preferred technique. A good-quality CT examination that shows no dissection generally is sufficient for exclusion of the diagnosis (Fig. 43). If strong clinical suspicion remains, or if CT demonstrates only nonspecific findings (e.g., hemopericardium) (95), angiography will be warranted.

CT also is extremely useful for follow-up evaluation of patients with aortic dissection treated either surgically or medically (53,87,143). These individuals are at risk from complications of the surgical procedure plus progression of the underlying disease. They are prone to redissection, extension of the dissection, and development of pseudoaneurysms due to suture dehiscence or progressive enlargement of the false lumen. These subsequent difficulties can be detected by CT (or MRI) in both symptomatic and asymptomatic patients.

Following surgical repair of aortic dissection, the prosthetic graft in the ascending aorta usually is visible on CT; it is only faintly more opaque than soft tissue when composed of Dacron, but quite dense if Teflon is used. Postoperatively, persistent patency of the false lumen is seen in the majority of patients. This supports the contention that surgical treatment of type A dissections is successful not because of obliteration of the false lumen or closure of the primary intimal tear but rather because proximal extension of the dissection is prevented by grafting or suturing, and a weakened portion of the aorta prone to rupture is removed or buttressed. The false lumen remains patent, presumably because of perfusion from a persisting intimal tear, with runoff back into the true lumen from a distal reentry site (59). In those patients treated medically, the false lumen shrinks, disappears, or totally thromboses in approximately 60%. These findings correlate with a favorable prognosis. In about 10% of patients, the false lumen progressively enlarges, with formation of a saccular aneurysm, which usually requires surgery to prevent future rupture.

Pulmonary Artery

CT is an accurate method of determining the size of the main pulmonary artery. Enlargement beyond a diameter of 29 mm is predictive of the presence of pulmonary arterial hypertension (77); it is usually accompanied by similar expansion of the major intrapericardial branches (Fig. 21). Idiopathic dilatation of the pulmonary artery or a localized aneurysm similarly can be recognized (27).

Obstruction of the central pulmonary arteries, most commonly partial, can be detected with CT. Encasement of these vessels is best demonstrated on postcontrast images. Neoplasm, specifically bronchogenic carcinoma, is the most frequent cause, but a variety of benign and malignant conditions may be responsible. The right pulmonary artery may be compressed by an aneurysm of the ascending aorta (26); clinically, pulmonary embolism may be simulated because of the unilateral diminished perfusion.

Superior Vena Cava

Contrast-enhanced CT is a rapid, informative, and cost-effective technique to demonstrate clinically suspected abnormality involving the superior vena cava (Fig. 44) (147). External compression, encasement, or intraluminal thrombus (see Fig. 8 in Chapter 7) can be depicted. Collateral circulation, especially through the internal mammary, azygos, or thoracic-wall veins, is commonly seen. Not only can superior vena caval obstruction be corroborated, but the extent and probable cause of the disease responsible may be depicted; neither venography nor scintiangiography can ascertain the cause of caval obstruction. The information acquired from CT may help in selecting the safest method for establishing a histologic diagnosis, which in some circumstances may be CT-guided percutaneous needle-aspiration biopsy. Superior vena caval obstruction may not have become clinically evident when it is demonstrable on CT (8), and palliative measures may be instituted to prevent its development.

MRI is similarly effective in demonstrating the site and extent of major venous obstruction; ancillary findings also may suggest the specific cause of the occlusion (89,141). Thrombus within a vessel typically has a decreased signal intensity on the second echo image, whereas slow flow, which may be encountered proximal to a stenosis, usually has a higher signal intensity on the second echo image.

MEDIASTINAL CYSTS

Most cysts of the mediastinum are congenital in origin; they include aerodigestive tract duplications (bronchogenic, foregut), neurenteric, lymphogenous, and pleuro-

A,B

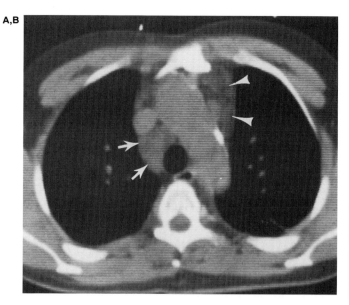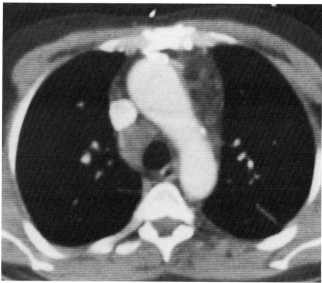

FIG. 43. Lymphoma, with no aortic dissection. A 64-year-old man, 9 months after coronary artery bypass, presented with chest pain. EKG findings were unchanged, and cardiac enzymes normal; chest roentgenography demonstrated new mediastinal widening. Aortic dissection was suspected clinically. **A:** Non-contrast-enhanced CT image demonstrates a normal-appearing aorta; right paratracheal lymphadenopathy (*arrows*) and some infiltration of the thymus (*arrowheads*) are noted. **B:** Postcontrast CT image confirms absence of dissection. Subsequent mediastinoscopic biopsy of the abnormal paratracheal nodes disclosed non-Hodgkin lymphoma.

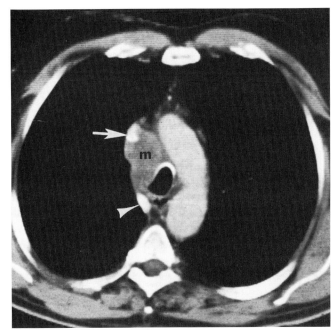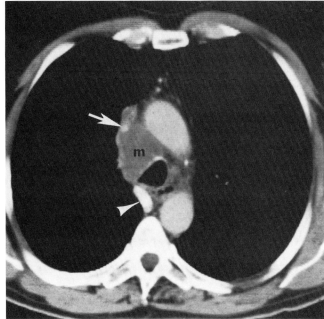

FIG. 44. Superior vena caval syndrome. **A,B:** Sequential caudal postcontrast CT images demonstrate marked narrowing and compression of the superior vena cava (*arrow*) by a large mediastinal nodal mass (m) due to oat cell carcinoma. Enhancement of collateral circulation through the azygos vein (*arrowhead*) and the anterior chest wall is noted.

pericardial. In adults, the majority are discovered as incidental findings on a plain chest radiograph, and only rarely do they produce clinical findings. On CT they are typically sharply marginated and have a near-water density; they are not enhanced after intravenous administration of contrast material (Fig. 45A). Generally, their appearance and attenuation values are so characteristic that in an asymptomatic patient surgery often may be avoided, and the patient can be managed conservatively, with only roentgenographic follow-up necessary to confirm their stability. Operation can be reserved for those unusually large cysts causing or potentially capable of causing compression of a major mediastinal structure, or when CT diagnosis is not definitive. Most mediastinal cysts are low in signal intensity on T1-weighted MR images and very high in signal intensity on T2-weighted images (Fig. 45B, C), reflecting the long T1 and T2 of fluid. However, hemorrhagic or proteinaceous cysts may have a higher signal intensity than that of simple cysts on T1-weighted images.

Bronchogenic Cysts

These result from abnormal budding of the tracheobronchial tree; approximately 90% are located within the middle mediastinum, near the carina or along the right paratracheal wall. Bronchogenic cysts are lined by columnar respiratory epithelium, which may secrete a variety of fluids. Their contents can range from clear serous ma-

terial to a milky white to brown mucoid material, with variable viscosities. Consequently, different CT densities may be observed with bronchogenic cysts, depending on their fluid composition (103). About half are of homogeneous, near-water density, reflecting their serous nature. This is the type of lesion, if relatively small, that can simply be followed radiologically. In the other half of cases, the density of a bronchogenic cyst can vary from the low soft-tissue range to substantially higher than muscle, usually because of viscid mucous contents (Fig. 46) (86,104). Cysts in this density range generally are indistinguishable from solid soft-tissue neoplasms, although their total lack of contrast enhancement may be a clue to the proper cause. In such circumstances, surgery or needle aspiration percutaneously or transbronchoscopically usually is required for definitive evaluation. Some cysts have very high attenuation values because the fluid contains calcium carbonate or calcium oxalate (144). Occasionally, calcification may develop in their walls. Rarely, when bronchogenic cysts become quite large, they may compress or obstruct the tracheobronchial tree or superior vena cava (Fig. 47) (3), requiring extirpation.

Foregut Cysts

These duplication cysts are lined by gastrointestinal-tract mucosa; if gastric epithelium is present, the produced secretions often result in symptoms. They are usually located in the posterior mediastinum near the spine and frequently are connected to the wall of the esophagus (75).

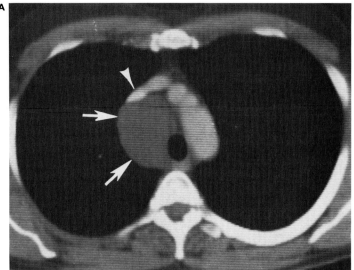

FIG. 45. Duplication cyst. **A:** Postcontrast CT image demonstrates a 6-cm nonenhancing, homogeneous, water-density paratracheal mass (*arrows*) in a 56-year-old man. The right brachiocephalic vein (*arrowhead*) is displaced anteriorly. The lesion did not change in size on subsequent chest radiographs during a 4-year follow-up period. **B:** On a T1-weighted coronal MR image in a different patient a sharply defined low signal intensity mass (*arrows*) is seen adjacent to the right side of the trachea (T). **C:** On a T2-weighted image the mass (*arrows*) increases in relative signal intensity and is much brighter than all surrounding tissues.

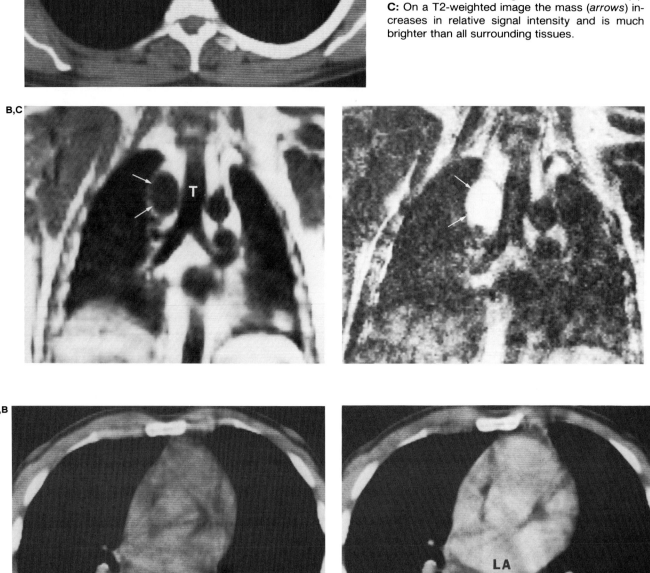

FIG. 46. Bronchogenic cyst. **A:** Non-contrast-enhanced CT image in a 47-year-old man demonstrates a soft-tissue density mass (*arrows*) filling the azygoesophageal recess. **B:** No enhancement of the mass, which is posterior to the left atrium (LA), is seen on a scan after intravenous administration of contrast material. Surgical removal disclosed a duplication cyst lined by respiratory epithelium filled with a viscid mucoid fluid.

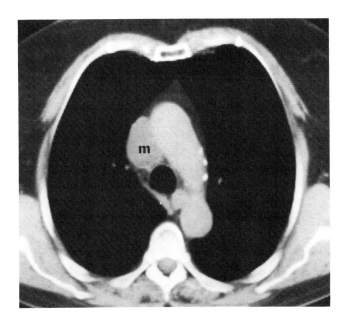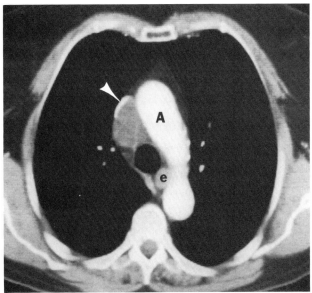

FIG. 47. Duplication cyst. **A:** Non-contrast-enhanced CT image demonstrates a well-circumscribed, homogeneous, near-water-density paratracheal mass (m) in a 67-year-old woman. **B:** Postcontrast CT image shows no enhancement of the mass. The superior vena cava (*arrowhead*) is compressed by the mass. Nonsurgical management was chosen because of associated cardiac disease and documentation on serial chest radiographs of slow interval growth during prior 3 years; (A) aorta; (e) esophagus.

Neurenteric Cysts

These rare cysts are connected to the meninges through a midline defect in one or more vertebral bodies. In contradistinction, an anterior meningocele, usually associated with neurofibromatosis, communicates with the subarachnoid space through an intervertebral foramen; MRI or CT with intrathecal contrast material (140) permits definitive diagnosis. Like the foregut cysts, neurenteric cysts also tend to occur in the posterior mediastinum. They may be distinguished by their usual association with spinal anomalies, such as dysraphism, butterfly vertebra or hemivertebra, and scoliosis; these defects may occur at different levels than the cyst.

Cystic Hygroma

These lymphogenous cysts typically occur in the superior mediastinum. On CT, they appear as round, occasionally multiloculated, smooth masses, with a homogeneous attenuation value sometimes lower than that for water (110,122). They commonly compress surrounding tissues.

Pleuropericardial Cysts

These cysts are secondary to defects in embryogenesis of the celomic cavities. They are most frequently located in the cardiophrenic angles. Typically, they have an attenuation value near that for water, with rare exception

(18). Although sharply marginated, they are commonly not round, but rather somewhat triangular, conforming to the space afforded by the lower portion of the major fissure.

MEDIASTINAL ABSCESS

CT can be valuable, especially in a febrile patient following median sternotomy, in detecting the presence and determining the extent of an abnormal mediastinal fluid collection (55). Reliable distinction between a diffuse mediastinitis and a drainable abscess usually is possible (21). Sometimes pockets of air are seen within the mass, even though they cannot be recognized on plain radiographs, supporting the diagnosis of an abscess. Percutaneous needle aspiration, under CT guidance, may be required to distinguish an abscess (in which the attenuation values may vary from 10 to 40 HU) from an uninfected seroma or hematoma. CT also is helpful in identifying other complications, such as an empyema. If communication is demonstrable between the mediastinal abscess and the empyema, thoracostomy-tube drainage of the latter collection alone usually suffices for treatment.

THYMIC MASS

CT should be the imaging procedure of choice following standard chest radiography when thymic abnormality is suspected (4). Scanning at 5-mm intervals using 5-mm collimation, sometimes after intravenous administration

A,B

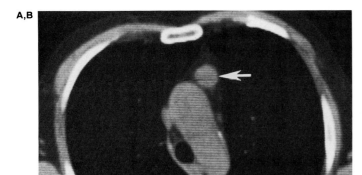 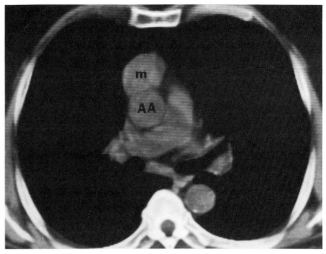

FIG. 48. Thymomas, myasthenia gravis. A: Homogeneous, sharply demarcated 2-cm round mass (*arrow*) in area of left lobe of thymus in a 33-year-old man; plain chest radiograph showed normal findings. Symptoms abated after surgical removal. B: Mass (m) of 4-cm in vicinity of right lobe of thymus anterior to ascending aorta (AA) in a 53-year-old man; plain chest radiograph showed questionable increased density in the retrosternal clear space. No clinical improvement was seen after removal of tumor.

of contrast material, may be valuable in selected cases when a small mass is suspected. No clinically important information is gained by adding or substituting MRI for CT; the latter technique provides better spatial resolution and can be accomplished quicker.

Thymoma

Thymomas are composed of both epithelial cells and lymphocytes, the proportions varying, sometimes with a mosaic of compositions within the same neoplasm (12,58).

This tumor is exceedingly rare before the age of 20; it occurs in association with myasthenia gravis or other less common conditions (red cell aplasia, hypogammaglobulinemia) or sporadically.

Thymomas are present in 10 to 15% of patients with myasthenia gravis. Plain chest radiographs are relatively insensitive, because most of the neoplasms associated with this condition are relatively small and are hidden by the surrounding mediastinal vessels. CT is a sensitive procedure for detection of these tumors; lesions as small as 1 cm in diameter can be reliably depicted (7,17,98). A thymoma typically appears on CT as a soft-tissue-density

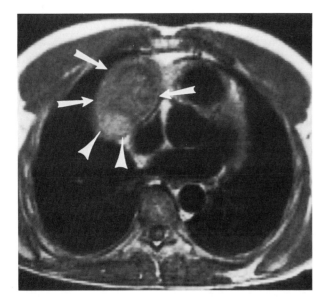

FIG. 49. Cystic thymoma. MR image shows a large, well-defined mass (*arrows*) adjacent to the right side of the heart. The more solid component of the mass (*arrowheads*) is higher in signal intensity than the cystic component (TR = 750 msec; TE = 30 msec).

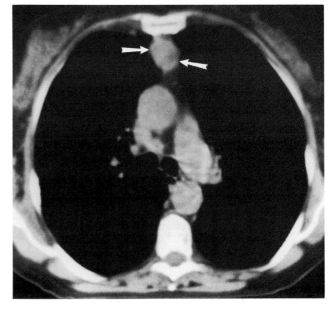

FIG. 50. Epidermoid carcinoma (*arrows*) of the medial portion of the right upper lobe simulating a thymoma.

mass that is oval, round, or lobulated and usually sharply demarcated (Fig. 48). Most often the neoplasm grows asymmetrically to one side of the mediastinum (Fig. 49). In a young adult, a distinct focal soft-tissue-density bulge may be seen along the normally smooth outer margin of the thymus. Over the age of 40, the mass is readily recognized, replacing a portion of a largely fat-filled organ. Focal areas of calcification may occur in about 25% of these tumors, which also usually are enhanced mildly and homogeneously after intravenous administration of contrast material. Occasionally, a pulmonary lesion adjacent to the anterior mediastinum may simulate a thymic mass (Fig. 50).

Approximately 10 to 15% of thymomas are classified as "malignant." Because the histologic appearance of a thymoma does not permit reliable distinction between the benign and malignant forms, the term "invasive" thymoma generally is preferred. The presence of neoplastic growth through the capsule determines whether or not the tumor is "invasive" ("malignant"). These neoplasms tend to be bulky and generally can be recognized on standard radiography. An invasive thymoma should be suspected on CT when, in addition to an anterior mediastinal mass in the vicinity of the thymus, infiltration into the surrounding mediastinal fat and fascia is seen (148). Caution should be used not to overdiagnose local invasion; mere contiguity of the mass with an adjacent mediastinal structure and the absence of a cleavage plane between it and an adjacent mediastinal structure are not reliable criteria to predict invasion. Invasive thymomas rarely metastasize hematogenously or via the lymphatics. Rather, this tumor typically extends locally into the adjacent mediastinum and further spreads by implanting along the

nearby pleural and pericardial surfaces, most commonly on only one side of the thoracic cavity (Fig. 51). Only rarely does it grow directly into the chest wall or through the visceral pleura into the lung. Following growth along the pleura, an invasive thymoma may extend caudally and involve the diaphragm. The tumor can extend through a hiatus or gap and invade the abdomen (e.g., the posterior pararenal space, perigastric tissues, liver surface). CT excels at demonstrating these additional sites of disease, which often are hidden on conventional radiography (119). This information can provide valuable guidance for the radiotherapist or chemotherapist in their treatment planning and monitoring for disease recurrence after as much as possible of the primary thymic tumor is resected. Therefore, a full examination of the thorax and upper abdomen is indicated when a thymic mass is detected.

About 65% of patients with myasthenia gravis and no thymoma have lymphoid hyperplasia of the organ. This is purely a histologic diagnosis, characterized by numerous lymphoid follicles with active germinal centers in the medulla surrounded by a plasma cell and lymphocytic infiltration, because the total thymic weight is not altered and the thymus usually is not enlarged. In some cases, with CT, the hyperplastic thymus appears larger than for appropriate age-matched controls; this may result from delayed fatty involution, which increases the volume of fat-free thymic tissue and causes it to seem larger. In most cases, lymphoid hyperplasia of the thymus is indistinguishable from a normal organ.

Controversy exists regarding the role of thymectomy in patients with myasthenia gravis and the necessity to search for an occult thymoma with CT. Cures and re-

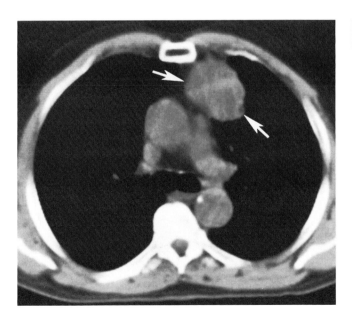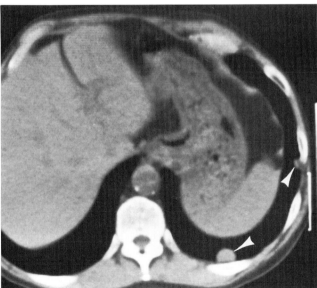

A,B

FIG. 51. Invasive ("malignant") thymoma. **A:** Irregularly marginated, 5-cm anterior mediastinal mass (*arrows*). **B:** More caudal scan demonstrates two pleural-based metastatic implants (*arrowheads*).

A,B

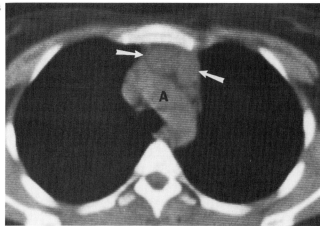 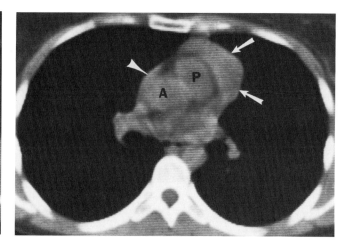

FIG. 52. Thymic Hodgkin disease, nodular sclerosing type. **A:** Enlargement of both lobes of the thymus (*arrows*) anterior to the aortic arch (A). **B:** Three centimeters caudad, the infiltrated left thymic lobe (*arrows*) drapes around the pulmonary outflow tract (P); (A) ascending aorta; (*arrowhead*) right atrial appendage.

missions can be induced in this disease following thymic removal, with or without a thymoma being present. Not all patients improve clinically after resection of a thymoma. Few convincing data exist to suggest that systematic removal of the thymus, whether normal, hyperplastic, or containing a thymoma, improves the clinical outcome in patients who are medically well controlled. It is for this reason that a positive CT diagnosis of hyperplasia or thymoma is not considered relevant to clinical decision making by some physicians. However, most still believe that radiologic detection of a thymoma is important, especially in the young adult with recent onset of the disease. Resection of the mass generally is recommended, along with

removal of adjacent tissue, not only because of the hope of inducing a remission but also to evaluate whether or not the thymoma is "invasive." There is no rationale for performing CT in a patient with a normal plain chest radiograph who will be undergoing thymectomy because of inadequate medical control of the myasthenia.

Lymphoma

The malignant lymphomas, particularly the nodular sclerosing form of Hodgkin disease, commonly infiltrate and enlarge the thymus, creating an anterior mediastinal

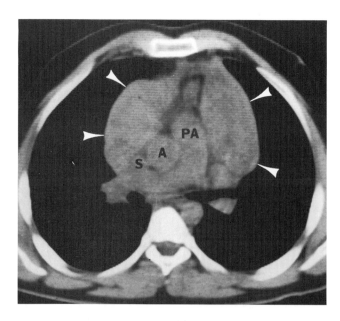

FIG. 53. Thymic non-Hodgkin lymphoma. Massive infiltration of both lobes of the thymus (*arrowheads*); (S) superior vena cava; (A) ascending aorta; (PA) main pulmonary artery.

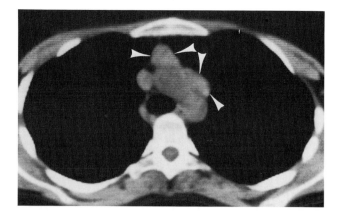

FIG. 54. Rebound thymic hyperplasia. A 29-year-old woman treated 6 months previously with chemotherapy for Hodgkin disease involving pelvic lymph nodes (the mediastinum was normal on a prior CT examination), now clinically well, has interval symmetric enlargement of both lobes of the thymus (*arrowheads*). The CT findings in this clinical context were believed most likely to represent rebound hyperplasia, and no biopsy was performed nor additional therapy given. A follow-up CT study 2 months later showed some spontaneous reduction in the size of the thymus.

mass (Figs. 52 and 53). Difficulty may arise in distinguishing *de novo* involvement from an invasive thymoma; even histologic distinction may be a problem, as a thymoma may contain abundant lymphocytes. On CT, the presence of lymph node enlargement elsewhere in the thorax (Figs. 13 and 14) (or abdomen) strongly favors a diagnosis of lymphoma, as does direct invasion of the anterior chest wall (Fig. 16). Multiple pleural implants at separate locations would suggest a thymoma. Calcification within the thymic mass also is more compatible with a thymoma; it is rare in untreated lymphoma.

Hyperplasia

A true hyperplasia involving both the cortex and medulla of the thymus, in which its weight and size are increased, can occur with hyperthyroidism secondary to Graves disease. On CT, diffuse enlargement of the organ is recognizable, especially in its thickness, with preservation of the normal shape. Similar enlargement may rarely be seen in patients with acromegaly or Addison disease.

Rebound hyperplasia of the thymus is well recognized in children and young adults recovering from severe illness. Analogous thymic enlargement may be observed after chemotherapy (most frequently when steroids have been part of the treatment regimen) (20) and following successful treatment of Cushing disease (35). The mechanism in most of these cases probably is initial lymphocyte depletion from the thymus, due in large part to high serum glucocorticoid concentrations, followed by substantial regrowth of the thymus. This immunological rebound phenomenon can occur as early as 3 to 4 weeks after the elevated cortisol levels drop. The overgrowth is transient and usually disappears after several months. This diffuse thymic enlargement, whether detected on plain chest radiographs or CT, may simulate a primary neoplasm or recurrent disease. It is a special problem in patients recovering from the cytotoxic effects of chemotherapy used for disease known to involve the thymus (e.g., lymphoma) (Fig. 54). If the patient is doing well clinically, and no recurrent or residual disease is evident in another location, our protocol is simply to follow the size of the thymus with repeat scanning, rather than to aggressively biopsy the organ. A gradual reduction in size corroborates the benign cause of this enlargement.

Germ Cell Tumors

Derived from one to three of the primitive embryonic germ cell layers, most of these lesions in the thorax arise within the thymus. Most cases occur during the second

to fourth decades of life. A variety of histologic types are encountered.

Dermoid cysts (containing elements of only the ectodermal layer of cells) and benign teratomas (containing elements of more than one of the three germinal layers) account for the majority of these tumors. On CT, both types are well demarcated, with a thick encapsulating wall; this rim may be enhanced after intravenous administration of contrast material (128). The internal contents of a benign teratoma typically are inhomogeneous, with a variable admixture of components exhibiting CT numbers in the range of fat, water, and soft-tissue densities (Fig. 55). They sometimes contain amorphous calcification or malformed teeth or bone. A specific diagnosis may be made with CT when these pleomorphic tissue densities are recognized within an anterior mediastinal mass. Layering of fat and fluid within such a mass also is presumptive evidence for this tumor (121). If only soft-tissue density and fat are present within the mass, a thymolipoma is an alternative possibility.

Local invasion is the only criterion that indicates a malignant neoplasm is present. For example, a malignant teratoma may be suggested on CT by irregular borders of the mass, with infiltration of the mediastinal fat (Fig. 56); compression or invasion of the mediastinal vessels and airways may also be present. The other rare malignant germ cell tumors (seminoma, embryonal cell carcinoma, choriocarcinoma, endodermal sinus) usually appear as irregular soft-tissue masses, often with central areas of cyst

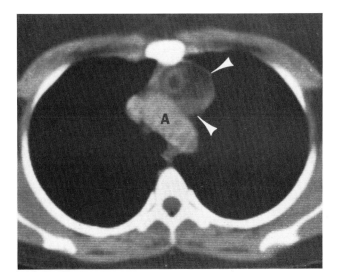

FIG. 55. Benign cystic teratoma. An encapsulated inhomogeneous mass (*arrowheads*), anterolateral to the aortic arch (A), arising from the left lobe of the thymus in a 22-year-old woman, is composed mainly of fat. A fat–fluid level separates a near-water-density posterior compartment. Wispy soft-tissue densities (due to matted hair) are scattered throughout the fatty portion.

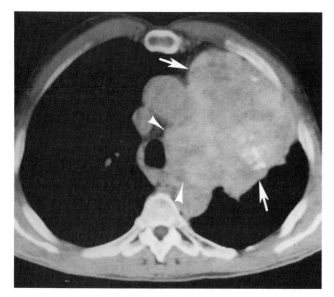

FIG. 56. Malignant teratoma in a 56-year-old man with left vocal cord paralysis. A huge inhomogeneous mass (*arrows*) containing focal areas of calcification is seen extending into the aortopulmonary window (*arrowheads*) where the left recurrent laryngeal nerve courses.

formation or necrosis (Fig. 57) (80). They may be indistinguishable in appearance from lymphoma or an invasive thymoma. The demonstration of their extent by CT can be valuable in monitoring response to treatment.

Thymolipoma

This entity is a rare, benign intrathymic neoplasm that typically causes no symptoms. It can grow exceedingly

large and may extend caudally to the cardiophrenic angles. On CT, the thymic mass may appear entirely of near-fat density, or it may contain some inhomogeneous areas of soft tissue. It does not compress or invade surrounding structures.

Carcinoid

A corticotropin-producing (ectopic ACTH) carcinoid tumor may arise within the thymus, resulting in Cushing syndrome. The lesions are often small and not detectable on plain chest radiographs (16). On CT, such a lesion appears identical with a small thymoma; distinction is based on the clinical findings.

Histiocytosis X

In children, this proliferative disease can involve the thymus and produce an anterior mediastinal mass. Massive cavitation may occur following chemotherapy when the necrotic tumor develops communications with the airways (37).

Cyst

This is a rare lesion that has features similar to a duplication or lymphogenous cyst, except it is located within the thymus (Fig. 58A) (57). Spontaneous hemorrhage into a thymic cyst may occur (Fig. 58B and C); pleuritic chest pain can result.

Thymic cysts also may occur in association with Hodg-

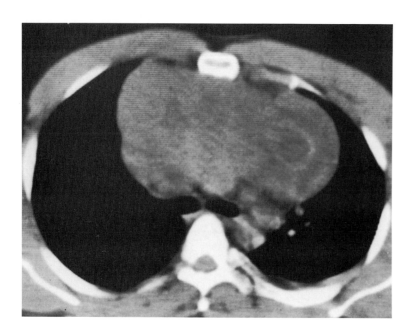

FIG. 57. Primary thymic seminoma in an 18-year-old man with large anterior mediastinal mass, containing some low-density foci of necrosis.

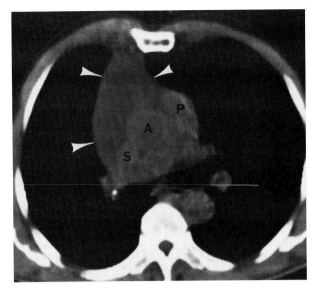 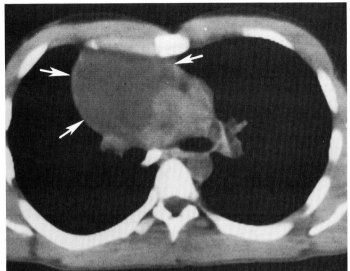

A,B

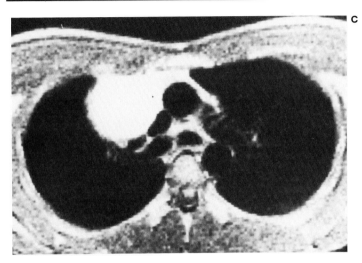

C

FIG. 58. Thymic cysts. **A:** A 77-year-old man with no intrathoracic symptoms. CT image shows a large near-water-density mass (*arrowheads*) corresponding to the configuration of the thymus (not proven); (S) superior vena cava; (A) ascending aorta; (P) main pulmonary artery. **B:** In another patient, a 23-year-old man who developed right anterior pleuritic chest pain while weight-lifting, a CT image demonstrates a well-circumscribed anterior mediastinal mass (*arrows*) with attenuation value of 30 HU. **C:** On a T1-weighted MR image, performed 3 weeks later because the patient was reluctant initially to have an operation, the mass is very high in signal intensity, reflecting T1 shortening secondary to the paramagnetic effect of methemoglobin. At surgery, a thymic cyst containing old hemorrhage was found.

kin disease; they probably are related to initial involvement of the organ with the disease, rather than being a consequence of radiotherapy or chemotherapy. Such cysts can persist or enlarge following successful treatment, while the lymphoma regresses, and they may simulate persistent or recurrent disease (6,72,83). Their CT appearance, sometimes combined with percutaneous needle-aspiration biopsy for corroboration, usually provides sufficient diagnostic information to obviate thoracotomy.

TRACHEA

Conventional tomography remains the appropriate radiologic technique for further evaluating the trachea in most conditions. Although tracheal stenosis can be corroborated on CT, with narrowly collimated images precisely defining its degree and length, generally such information can be more easily and equivalently achieved with conventional tomography and fluoroscopy. In tracheomalacia, fluoroscopy with videotape recording is the most practical method to delineate the severity and extent of involvement. In selected instances, CT may be valuable in documenting primary cartilaginous disease of the trachea, such as relapsing polychondritis (90), and assessing the degree of airway compromise.

CT may be beneficial in a patient with a primary tracheal neoplasm for demonstrating extension into the surrounding mediastinal structures (Fig. 59). This information, generally not available from conventional roentgenographic studies, may be important in planning possible surgery (46,126).

The trachea is a relatively flexible structure, allowing for substantial deviation before compression and symptoms are produced by an adjacent mass. Secondary neoplastic invasion can be diagnosed reliably only when there is marked irregularity of the tracheal wall and/or its lumen. Following radiation therapy for a bulky carcinoma of the esophagus, or rarely a bronchogenic carcinoma, a tracheoesophageal fistula may develop that may be demonstrable on CT (13).

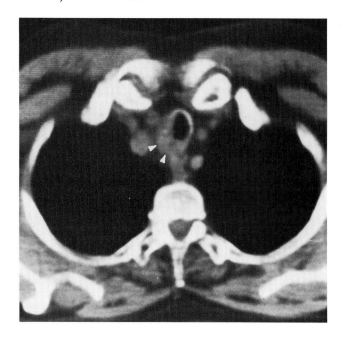

FIG. 59. Epidermoid carcinoma of the trachea. Arising along its right posterolateral wall, the neoplasm is seen extending directly into the adjacent mediastinal fat (*arrowheads*); it was managed successfully with radiation therapy alone.

POSTERIOR MEDIASTINAL MASSES

Esophageal Hiatal Hernia

A common abnormality incidentally encountered on CT, esophageal hiatal hernia appears as an air- and/or fluid-containing mass contiguous with the esophagus and gastric fundus. If the diagnosis is not clear on a CT ex-amination performed for evaluation of the thorax, oral administration of contrast material permits the correct interpretation. Obviously, a barium esophagogram, not CT, is the radiologic procedure of choice for corroboration of the diagnosis if a question arises on a plain chest radiograph.

Neurogenic Tumors

These account for about 80% of posterior mediastinal neoplasms, the majority of which are discovered incidentally on plain chest radiographs. These tumors can originate from the nerve roots (schwannomas, neurilemmomas, or neurofibromas) or from the sympathetic ganglia (neuroblastomas, ganglioneuromas, or ganglioneuroblastomas).

Nerve root tumors usually are spherical and tend to occur near the junction of the vertebral body with the adjacent rib (Fig. 60). Enlargement of an intervertebral foramen or pressure erosion of a rib is common. These neoplasms typically are sharply marginated and of homogeneous soft-tissue density on CT. Occasionally they may be lower in attenuation value because of high amounts of lipids within the neural tissue (76). Malignant neurogenic tumors tend to have poorly defined borders. Either MRI or CT (following opacification of the subarachnoid space with a nonionic contrast agent) is crucial in determining if an intraspinal component of the tumor is present.

Tumors arising from the sympathetic trunk tend to lie slightly anterior to the vertebral bodies and neural foramina. They usually are fusiform in shape in a cephalo-

A,B

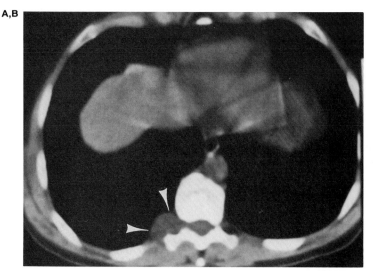 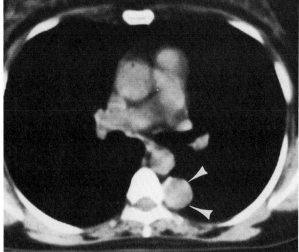

FIG. 60. Neurogenic tumors of the posterior mediastinum. **A:** Neurilemmoma (*arrowheads*). The mass is slightly lower in attenuation value than the paraspinal musculature and widens the right intervertebral foramen slightly. **B:** Neurofibroma (*arrowheads*).

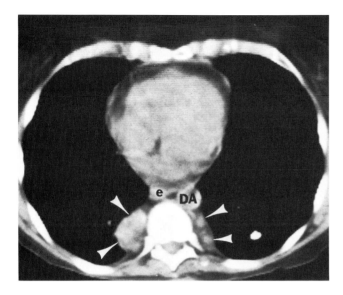

FIG. 61. Extramedullary hematopoiesis. Bilateral soft-tissue-density paraspinal masses (*arrowheads*) are identified in a 46-year-old woman with hemolytic anemia who had a splenectomy 5 years previously. An incidental calcified left-lower-lobe granuloma is present; (DA) descending aorta; (e) esophagus.

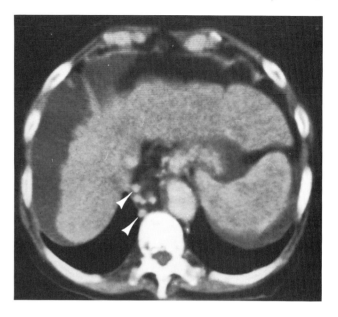

FIG. 62. Esophageal varices. A chest radiograph in a 55-year-old woman 3 years following a mastectomy showed right paraspinal widening; results of liver function tests were abnormal, and metastases were considered the likely explanation for these findings. A postcontrast CT image demonstrates enhancing esophageal varices (*arrowheads*) due to cryptic cirrhosis with ascites.

caudal direction. On CT, they typically appear as well-circumscribed soft-tissue-density masses. Calcification occasionally occurs within them, especially the ganglioneuroblastoma.

Extramedullary Hematopoiesis

This condition, usually secondary to severe hemolytic anemia (e.g., thalassemia major), may result in a paravertebral soft-tissue-density mass that typically is bilateral along the thoracic spine (Fig. 61). Associated expansion of the transverse processes of the vertebral bodies or of the ribs may be present.

Esophageal Varices

These may occasionally enlarge sufficiently to produce a paraspinal mass near the distal esophagus on conventional radiography (67). They can even simulate a parenchymal lung lesion if they extend markedly into the inferior pulmonary ligament. CT images after intravenous administration of contrast material generally permit definitive diagnosis (Fig. 62) (64); associated findings of cirrhosis and portal hypertension usually are present on other images through the upper abdomen. Varices treated with sclerotherapy also can mimic a neoplastic paraesophageal mass and do not demonstrate contrast enhancement; correlation with the clinical history obviously is critical for proper interpretation.

Pancreatic Pseudocyst

An extrapancreatic fluid collection may spread into the posterior mediastinum from the retroperitoneum via either the aortic or esophageal hiatus in the diaphragm. Typically, they are near-water-density masses, but their attenuation values may be higher if hemorrhage or infection is superimposed (108). Usually, contiguity can be demonstrated on serial images between the mediastinal fluid collection and peripancreatic inflammatory disease.

Miscellaneous

As described earlier, lymphoma may cause a paraspinal mass (Fig. 17). Infectious involvement of the thoracic spine, most typically tuberculosis, may secondarily cause a paraspinal abscess.

INDICATIONS

The relatively inexpensive and universally available standard chest roentgenogram continues to serve well as the initial radiologic examination in patients suspected of having mediastinal disease. CT is used as a supplementary or "problem-solving" technique when the cause of a demonstrated definite or questionable abnormality cannot be determined by simple radiologic methods (e.g., fluoroscopy) or clinical correlation, or when the plain chest radiographs are negative and strong clinical suspicion of

A,B

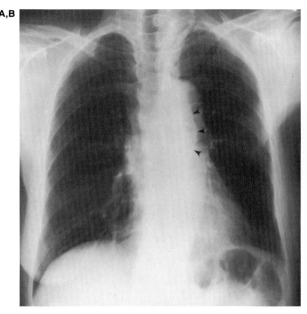
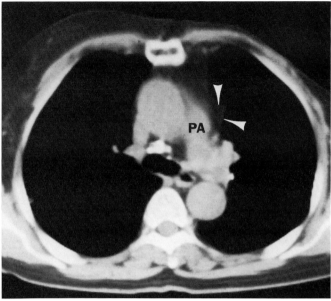

FIG. 63. Mediastinal ''mass'' (focal fat). **A:** Chest radiograph in a 54-year-old woman 4 years after a left mastectomy suggested a new mediastinal mass (*arrowheads*). **B:** CT image demonstrates that a focal collection of normal fat (*arrowheads*) anterolateral to the main and left pulmonary artery (PA) is responsible for the suspicious plain radiographic opacity. Retrospective questioning disclosed that the patient had recently gained weight.

disease remains. In patients with clinical problems known to affect the mediastinum, abnormalities may be detected with CT that are occult on conventional radiographs. Examples would include the demonstration of a small thymoma in a patient with myasthenia gravis or a mass responsible for recurrent laryngeal nerve paralysis when no cause in the neck is discovered (70). Similarly, CT would be indicated to assess the mediastinum for possible involvement by certain neoplastic diseases (e.g., bronchogenic carcinoma, lymphoma) to assist staging and treatment planning.

The significance of a mediastinal-contour abnormality identified on a plain chest radiograph is a common dilemma. The clinical circumstances may dictate whether or not a borderline abnormality requires further assessment. For example, a slight bulge in the right cardiophrenic angle in an obese individual generally would be attributed to a prominent pericardial fat pad, but in a patient with lymphoma it may need to be pursued because it could be secondary to lymphadenopathy.

In the great majority of cases in which the mediastinum is seen to be abnormal on conventional radiographs, CT is the next radiologic technique employed when further evaluation is required (115,125). The few exceptions would include suspected acute traumatic lesions of the aorta or great vessels, in which aortography is primarily

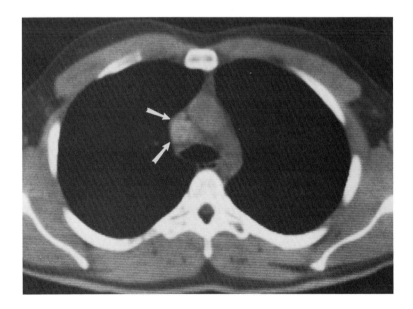

FIG. 64. Mediastinal mass, conglomerate calcified lymph nodes. A chest radiograph in a 29-year-old man with no intrathoracic symptoms showed a right paratracheal mass; conventional tomograms contributed no additional diagnostic information. A CT image demonstrates faint calcification throughout the mass (*arrows*), consistent with old healed granulomatous disease. The mass was unchanged in size on subsequent roentgenograms during the following year.

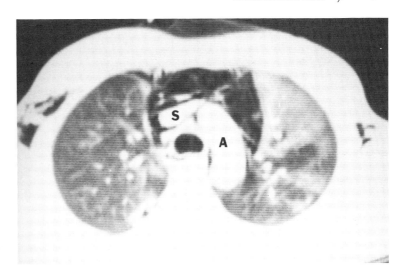

FIG. 65. Pneumomediastinum (posttraumatic). An extensive collection of air is seen in the anterior mediastinum, within and surrounding the thymus and small adjacent vessels, which also dissects around the superior vena cava (S) and aortic arch (A). Air in the axillae and pulmonary contusions also are present.

used, or probable esophageal abnormality, which should be studied first with barium esophagography.

Determination of the relative attenuation value of a mediastinal mass by CT may permit a definitive noninvasive diagnosis. The superior contrast sensitivity of CT is of paramount importance in the mediastinum, permitting confident differentiation among fat (Fig. 63), a serous cyst (Fig. 45), or a soft-tissue-density mass, and any contained calcification (Fig. 64) or air (Fig. 65). And with intravenous administration of relatively small amounts of contrast material, vascular abnormalities (Fig. 66) and anomalies may be distinguished. Focal lesions that present with values characteristic of benign fatty tissue (−80 to −120 HU), including a pericardial fat pad and omental herniations through the foramen of Morgagni or Bochdalek (see Fig. 114 in Chapter 7), usually can be conclusively diagnosed on CT, and no further diagnostic evaluation is indicated. Most benign cysts (pericardial, bronchogenic) have a near-water-equivalent density, with an imperceptible wall. Whereas malignant soft-tissue-density neoplasms, such as Hodgkin disease, can undergo necrosis and contain areas of near-water density (40), these lesions typically are either thick-walled or inhomogeneous, allowing distinction from benign cysts. Although CT may be valuable in determining the extent or origin of a soft-tissue-density mass, along with its relationship to other mediastinal structures (bronchi, vessels), precise histologic diagnosis is not possible. Demonstration of invasion into adjacent pleura, pericardium, or lung, with or without constriction of nearby vessels and bronchi, however, does strongly suggest malignant neoplasm as the cause. CT often can expedite the diagnostic process by supplanting multiple previously used imaging studies (conventional tomography, barium esophagography, radionuclide scans, and angiographic procedures such as cavography, pulmonary arteriography, and aortography), which in some cases even together accomplished only localization of the mass. It can also direct needed further investigation, including biopsy or resection.

When mediastinal widening is detected on a plain chest radiograph, the cause may be benign (Fig. 67), including such entities as abundant fat deposition (Fig. 1) or an unusual thoracic configuration (69,113). In addition, lymphadenopathy (Fig. 68), a soft-tissue neoplasm (Fig. 69), vascular dilatation (Fig. 30), or a hematoma (Figs. 32 and 70) may be responsible. CT is ideally suited for analysis and differentiation of these entities, and the necessity for invasive diagnostic procedures sometimes can be avoided (5). CT can demonstrate whether or not enlarged lymph nodes are present in the paratracheal area, accessible to biopsy via transcervical mediastinoscopy; such lymphadenopathy may not be recognizable by conventional roentgenographic studies. Vascular dilatation responsible for mediastinal widening should be diagnosable by CT in almost all cases, thus obviating angiography.

Similarly, when paraspinal-line widening is seen on a conventional roentgenogram, and its cause cannot be resolved by simple radiologic techniques (e.g., barium esophagogram, detailed spine views), CT is an excellent tool to clarify the cause. Such abnormalities as lymphadenopathy (Figs. 71 and 72), descending thoracic aortic aneurysms (Fig. 41), dilated veins (see Fig. 88 in Chapter 7), hernias (Fig. 3), thoracic spine lesions, or anatomic variations within the retrocrural space can be responsible for lateral displacement of the paraspinal lines noted on a plain radiograph (36,127).

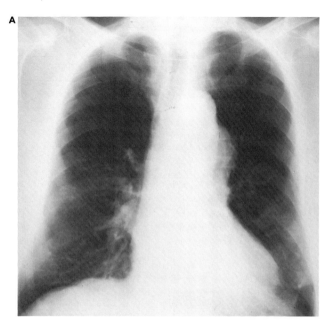

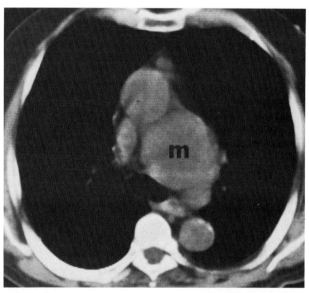

FIG. 66. Mediastinal mass, aortic aneurysm. **A:** Chest radiograph in a 69-year-old man with left vocal cord paralysis demonstrates a mass in the aortopulmonary window area; a bronchogenic carcinoma was considered the most likely explanation. **B,C:** Serial caudad non-contrast-enhanced CT images show that the mass (m) is contiguous with the undersurface of the aortic arch, and a portion of its periphery appears to contain an atherosclerotic calcification (*arrowhead*). **D,E:** Serial postcontrast CT images document an aortic aneurysm, containing a large thrombus, extending into the aortopulmonary window (the filling defect in the superior vena cava in **D** is a flow artifact).

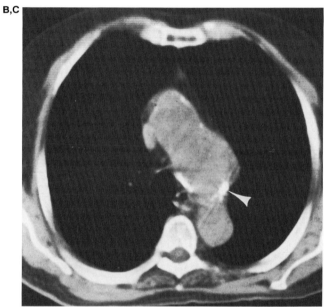

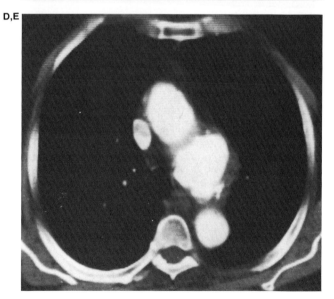

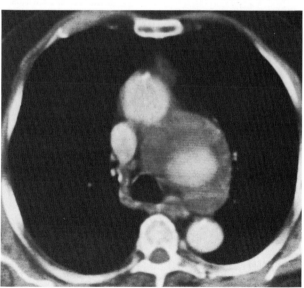

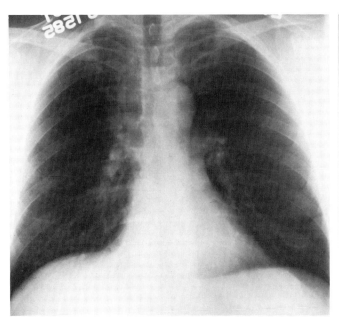 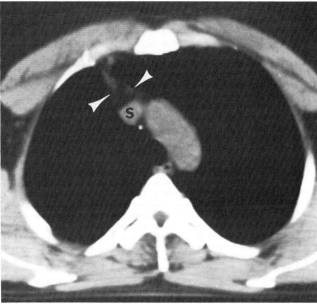

A,B

FIG. 67. Mediastinal widening, right-upper-lobe volume loss. **A:** Posteroanterior chest radiograph in a 38-year-old man demonstrates widening of the right mediastinal contour. **B:** CT image demonstrates marked deviation of the anterior junction line and contained thymic fat (*arrowheads*), accounting for the apparent mediastinal widening, with associated right-upper-lobe volume loss. Concomitant lung window settings showed fibrosis in the right upper lobe, presumably secondary to old granulomatous disease. A small calcified lymph node is seen posterior to the superior vena cava (S).

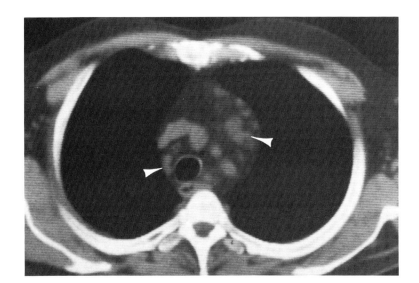

FIG. 68. Mediastinal widening, fat and lymphadenopathy. Multiple enlarged lymph nodes (*arrowheads*), subsequently proved due to non-Hodgkin lymphoma, are seen in addition to abundant fat to account for mediastinal widening noted on chest radiography.

A,B

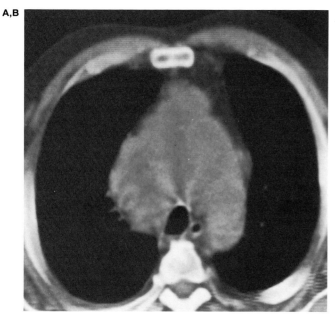

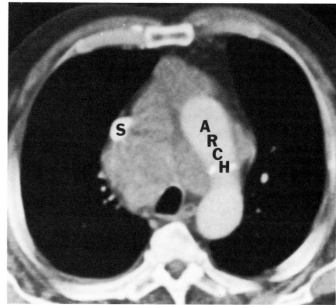

C

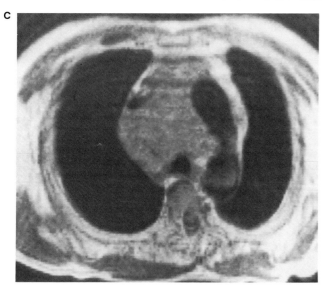

FIG. 69. Mediastinal widening, neoplasm (sarcoma). A: Non-contrast-enhanced CT image shows a soft-tissue-density mass widening and infiltrating the mediastinum. The trachea is displaced posteriorly. B: Postcontrast CT image demonstrates relationship of the primary mediastinal sarcoma to the major vessels at this level, the superior vena cava (S) and aortic arch (ARCH). C: T1-weighted MR image provides similar information.

FIG. 70. Mediastinal widening, hemorrhage. A 62-year-old woman on anticoagulant therapy developed chest pain; a chest radiograph demonstrated acute mediastinal widening. CT image shows a large hematoma in the anterior mediastinum infiltrating the thymus. The hemorrhage resolved spontaneously after readjustment of her therapy.

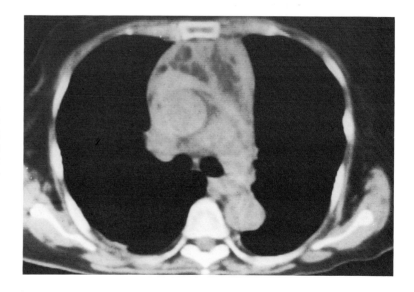

A,B

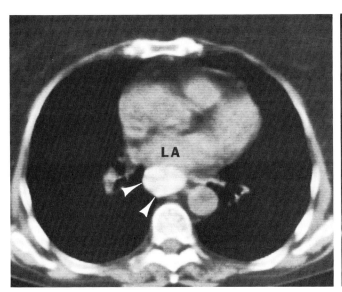 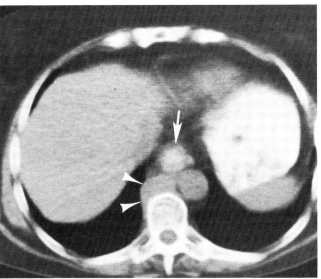

FIG. 71. Paraspinal-line widening, hiatus hernia and lymphadenopathy. A 61-year-old woman with right paraspinal-line widening noted on an excretory urogram. A barium swallow demonstrated a small hiatal hernia, but it did not appear to account for all of the abnormal density. **A:** CT at the level of the left atrium (LA) shows only a moderate-size esophageal hiatal hernia (*arrowheads*). **B:** However, 3 cm caudad, in addition to the hiatal hernia (*arrow*), there is a soft-tissue-density mass (*arrowheads*) in the right retrocrural area, subsequently proved to be caused by non-Hodgkin lymphoma.

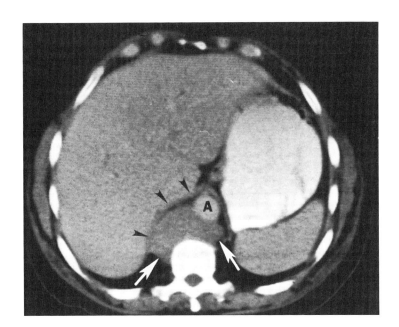

FIG. 72. Paraspinal-line widening, lymphadenopathy. Right paraspinal-line widening detected on a posteroanterior chest radiograph is due to a conglomerate lymph node mass (*arrows*) caused by metastatic breast carcinoma, which has displaced the fat in the retrocrural space. The right diaphragmatic crus (*arrowheads*) is pushed laterally and anteriorly; (A) aorta.

REFERENCES

1. Amparo EG, Higgins CB, Hricak H, Sollitto R. Aortic dissection: magnetic resonance imaging. *Radiology* 1985;155:399–406.
2. Aronberg DJ, Glazer HS, Sagel SS. MR and CT of the mediastinum: comparisons, controversies and pitfalls. *Radiol Clin North Am* 1985;23:439–448.
3. Bankoff MS, Daly BDT, Johnson HA, Carter BL. Bronchogenic cyst causing superior vena cava obstruction: CT appearance. *J Comput Assist Tomogr* 1985;9:951–952.
4. Baron RL, Lee JKT, Sagel SS, Levitt RG. Computed tomography of the abnormal thymus. *Radiology* 1982;142:127–134.
5. Baron RL, Levitt RG, Sagel SS, Stanley RJ. Computed tomography in the evaluation of mediastinal widening. *Radiology* 1981;138:107–113.
6. Baron RL, Sagel SS, Baglan RJ. Thymic cysts following radiation therapy for Hodgkin disease. *Radiology* 1981;141:593–597.
7. Batra P, Hermann C Jr, Mulder D. Mediastinal imaging in myasthenia gravis: correlation of chest radiography, CT, MR, and surgical findings. *AJR* 1987;148:515–519.
8. Bechtold RE, Wolfman NT, Karstaedt N, Choplin RH. Superior vena caval obstruction: detection using CT. *Radiology* 1985;157:485–487.
9. Bein ME, Mancuso AA, Mink JH, Hansen GC. Computed tomography in the evaluation of mediastinal lipomatosis. *J Comput Assist Tomogr* 1978;2:379–383.
10. Bein ME, Putman CE, McLoud TC, Mink JH. A reevaluation of intrathoracic lymphadenopathy in sarcoidosis. *AJR* 1978;131:409–415.
11. Bennett DE, Cherry JK: The natural history of traumatic aneurysms of the aorta. *Surgery* 1967;61:516–523.
12. Bergh N, Gatzinsky P, Larson S, Ludin P, Ridell B. Tumors of the thymus and thymic region: 1. Clinicopathological studies on thymomas. *Ann Thorac Surg* 1978;25:91–98.
13. Berkman YM, Auh YH. CT diagnosis of acquired tracheoesophageal fistula in adults. *J Comput Assist Tomogr* 1985;9:302–304.
14. Bethancourt B, Pond GD, Jones SE, Grogan T, Wasserman P. Mediastinal hematoma simulating recurrent Hodgkin disease during systemic chemotherapy. *AJR* 1984;142:1119–1120.
15. Bradley WG Jr, Waluch V. Blood flow: magnetic resonance imaging. *Radiology* 1985;154:443–450.
16. Brown LR, Augenbaugh GL, Wick MR, Baker BA, Salassa RM. Roentgenologic diagnosis of primary corticotropin-producing carcinoid tumors of the mediastinum. *Radiology* 1982;142:143–148.
17. Brown LR, Muhm JR, Sheedy PF II, Unni KK, Bernatz PE, Hermann RC. The value of computed tomography in myasthenia gravis. *AJR* 1983;140:31–35.
18. Brunner DR, Whitley NO. A pericardial cyst with high CT numbers. *AJR* 1984;142:279–280.
19. Burgener FA, Hamlin D. Intrathoracic histiocytic lymphoma. *AJR* 1981;136:499–504.
20. Carmosina L, Di Benedetta A, Feffer S. Thymic hyperplasia following successful chemotherapy: a report of 2 cases and review of the literature. *Cancer* 1985;56:1526–1528.
21. Carrol CL, Jeffrey RB Jr, Federle MP, Vernacchia FS. CT evaluation of mediastinal infections. *J Comput Assist Tomogr* 1987;11:449–454.
22. Castellino RA, Blank N, Hoppe RT, Cho C. Hodgkin disease: contributions of chest CT in the initial staging evaluation. *Radiology* 1986;160:603–605.
23. Chew FS, Panicek DM, Heitzman ER. Late discovery of a posttraumatic right aortic arch aneurysm. *AJR* 1985;145:1001–1002.
24. Cho CS, Blank N, Castellino RA. CT evaluation of cardiophrenic angle lymph nodes in patients with malignant lymphoma. *AJR* 1984;143:719–721.
25. Cohen WN, Seidelmann FE, Bryan PJ. Computed tomography of localized adipose deposits presenting as tumor masses. *AJR* 1977;128:1007–1011.
26. Cramer M, Foley WD, Palmer TE, et al. Compression of the right pulmonary artery by aortic aneurysms: CT demonstration. *J Comput Assist Tomogr* 1985;9:310–314.
27. Crivello MS, Hayes C, Thurer RL, Kim D, Cahalane M. Traumatic pulmonary artery aneurysm: CT evaluation. *J Comput Assist Tomogr* 1986;10:503–505.
28. Danza FM, Fusco A, Breda M, Bock E, Lemmo G, Colavita N. Ductus arteriosus aneurysm in an adult. *AJR* 1984;143:131–133.
29. Danza FM, Valentini AL, Colosimo C Jr, Vincenzoni M. Evolution of a mural thrombus in false aneurysm: CT demonstration. *J Comput Assist Tomogr* 1986;10:126–129.
30. DeMaria AN, Bommer W, Neuman A, Weinert L, Bogren H, Mason DT. Identification and localization of aneurysms of the ascending aorta by cross-sectional echocardiography. *Circulation* 1979;59:755–761.
31. Demos TC, Posniak HV, Churchill RJ. Detection of the intimal flap of aortic dissection on unenhanced CT images. *AJR* 1986;146:601–603.
32. Dinsmore RE, Liberthson RR, Wismer GL, et al. Magnetic resonance imaging of thoracic aortic aneurysms: comparison with other imaging methods. *AJR* 1986;146:309–314.
33. Dinsmore RE, Wedeen VJ, Miller SW, et al. MRI of dissection of the aorta: recognition of the intimal tear and differential flow velocities. *AJR* 1986;147:1286–1288.
34. Dinsmore RE, Wedeen V, Rosen B, Wismer GL, Miller SW, Brady TJ. Phase-offset technique to distinguish slow blood flow and thrombus on MR images. *AJR* 1987;148:634–636.
35. Doppman JL, Oldfield EH, Chrousos GP, et al. Rebound thymic hyperplasia after treatment of Cushing's syndrome. *AJR* 1986;147:1145–1147.
36. Efremidis SC, Dan SJ, Cohen BA, Mitty HA, Rabinowitz JG. Displaced paraspinal line: role of CT and lymphography. *AJR* 1981;136:505–509.
37. Eftekhari F, Shirkhoda A, Cangir A. Cavitation of a mediastinal mass following chemotherapy for histiocytosis X: CT demonstration. *J Comput Assist Tomogr* 1986;10:130–132.
38. Egan TJ, Neiman HL, Herman RJ, Malave SR, Sanders JH. Computed tomography in the diagnosis of aortic aneurysm dissection or traumatic injury. *Radiology* 1980;136:141–146.
39. Farmer DW, Moore E, Amparo E, Webb WR, Gamsu G, Higgins CB. Calcific fibrosing mediastinitis: demonstration of pulmonary vascular obstruction by magnetic resonance imaging. *AJR* 1984;143:1189–1191.
40. Federle MP, Callen PW. Cystic Hodgkin's lymphoma of the thymus: computed tomography appearance. *J Comput Assist Tomogr* 1979;3:542–544.
41. Filly R, Blank N, Castellino RA. Radiographic distribution of intrathoracic disease in previously untreated patients with Hodgkin's disease and non-Hodgkin's lymphoma. *Radiology* 1976;120:277–281.
42. Fisher RG, Hadlock F, Ben-Menachem Y. Laceration of the thoracic aorta and brachiocephalic arteries by blunt trauma. *Radiol Clin North Am* 1981;19:91–110.
43. Fiore D, Biondetti PR, Calabro F, Rea F. CT demonstration of bilateral Castleman tumors in the mediastinum. *J Comput Assist Tomogr* 1983;7:719–720.
44. Gallagher S, Dixon AK. Streak artefacts of the thoracic aorta: pseudodissection. *J Comput Assist Tomogr* 1984;8:688–693.
45. Gallagher GJ, White FE, Tucker AK, Fry JS, Malpas SS, Lister TA. The role of computed tomography in the detection of intrathoracic lymphoma. *Br J Cancer* 1984;49:621–629.
46. Gamsu G, Webb WR. Computed tomography of the trachea: normal and abnormal. *AJR* 1982;139:321–326.
47. Geisinger MA, Risius B, O'Donnell JA, et al. Thoracic aortic dissections: magnetic resonance imaging. *Radiology* 1985;155:407–412.
48. Glazer HS, Aronberg DJ, Sagel SS. Pitfalls in CT recognition of mediastinal lymphadenopathy. *AJR* 1985;144:267–274.
49. Glazer HS, Gutierrez FR, Levitt RG, Lee JKT, Murphy WA. The thoracic aorta studied by MR imaging. *Radiology* 1985;157:149–155.
50. Glazer HS, Lee JKT, Levitt RG, et al. Radiation fibrosis: differentiation from recurrent tumor by MR imaging. *Radiology* 1985;156:721–726.
51. Godwin JD, Breiman RS, Speckman JM. Problems and pitfalls in the evaluation of thoracic aortic dissection by computed tomography. *J Comput Assist Tomogr* 1982;6:750–756.
52. Godwin JD, Herfkens RJ, Skiödebrand CG, Federle MP, Lipton MJ. Evaluation of dissections and aneurysms of the thoracic aorta

by conventional and dynamic CT scanning. *Radiology* 1980;136: 125–133.

53. Godwin JD, Turley K, Herfkens RJ, Lipton MJ. Computed tomography for follow-up of chronic aortic dissections. *Radiology* 1981;139:655–660.

54. Godwin JD, Webb WR. Contrast-related phenomena mimicking pathology on thoracic computed tomography. *J Comput Assist Tomogr* 1982;6:460–464.

55. Goodman LG, Kay HR, Teplick SK, Mundth ED. Complications of median sternotomy: computed tomographic evaluation. *AJR* 1983;141:225–230.

56. Goodwin RA, Nickell JA, Des Pres RM. Mediastinal fibrosis complicating healed primary histoplasmosis and tuberculosis. *Medicine (Baltimore)* 1972;51:227–246.

57. Gouliamos A, Striggaris K, Lolas C, Deligeorgi-Politi H, Vlahos L, Pontifex G. Thymic cyst. *J Comput Assist Tomogr* 1982;6:172–174.

58. Gray GF, Gutowski WT III. Thymoma. A clinicopathologic study of 54 cases. *Am J Surg Pathol* 1979;3:235–249.

59. Guthaner DF, Miller DC, Silverman JF, Stinson EB, Wexler L. Fate of the false lumen following surgical repair of aortic dissections: an angiographic study. *Radiology* 1979;133:1–8.

60. Harrington DP, Barth KH, White RI Jr, Brawley RK. Traumatic pseudoaneurysm of the thoracic aorta in close proximity to the anterior spinal artery: a therapeutic dilemma. *Surgery* 1980;87: 153–156.

61. Heiberg E, Wolverson MK, Sundaram M, Shields JB. CT characteristics of aortic atherosclerotic aneurysm versus aortic dissection. *J Comput Assist Tomogr* 1985;9:78–83.

62. Heiberg E, Wolverson MK, Sundaram M, Shields JB. CT in aortic trauma. *AJR* 1983;140:1119–1124.

63. Heystraten FM, Rosenbusch G, Kingma LM, Lacquet LK. Chronic posttraumatic aneurysm of the thoracic aorta: surgically correctable occult threat. *AJR* 1986;146:303–308.

64. Hirose H, Takashima T, Suzuki M, Matsui O. "Downhill" esophageal varices demonstrated by dynamic computed tomography. *J Comput Assist Tomogr* 1984;8:1007–1009.

65. Homer MJ, Wechsler RJ, Carter BL. Mediastinal lipomatosis: CT confirmation of a normal variant. *Radiology* 1978;128:657–661.

66. Imaizumi T, Orita Y, Koiwaya Y, Hirata T, Nakamura M. Utility of two-dimensional echocardiography in the differential diagnosis of the etiology of aortic regurgitation. *Am Heart J* 1982;103:887–896.

67. Ishikawa T, Saeki M, Tsukune Y, et al. Detection of paraesophageal varices by plain films. *AJR* 1985;144:701–704.

68. Jacobs NM, Godwin JD, Wolfe WG, Moore AV Jr, Breiman RS, Korobkin M. Evaluation of the grafted ascending aorta with computed tomography: complications caused by suture dehiscence. *Radiology* 1982;145:749–753.

69. Jardin M, Lemaitre L, Remy J. Narrow superior mediastinum and pseudomasses: CT features. *J Comput Assist Tomogr* 1986;10:603–606.

70. Jolles PR, Shin MS, Jones WP. Aortopulmonary window lesions: detection with chest radiography. *Radiology* 1986;159:647–651.

71. Khoury MB, Godwin JD, Halvorsen R, Hanun Y, Putman CE. Role of chest CT in non-Hodgkin lymphoma. *Radiology* 1986;158:659–662.

72. Kim HC, Nosher J, Haas A, Sweeney W, Lewis R. Cystic degeneration of thymic Hodgkin's disease following radiation therapy. *Cancer* 1985;55:354–356.

73. Koerner HF, Sun DIC. Mediastinal lipomatosis secondary to steroid therapy. *AJR* 1966;98:461–464.

74. Kucich VA, Vogelzang RL, Hartz RS, LoCicero J III, Dalton D. Ruptured thoracic aneurysm: unusual manifestation and early diagnosis using CT. *Radiology* 1986;160:87–89.

75. Kuhlman JE, Fishman EK, Wang KP, Siegelman SS. Esophageal duplication cyst: CT and transesophageal needle aspiration. *AJR* 1985;145:531–532.

76. Kumar AJ, Kuhajda FP, Martinez CR, Fishman EK, Jezic DV, Siegelman SS. CT of extracranial nerve sheath tumors. *J Comput Assist Tomogr* 1983;7:857–865.

77. Kurujama K, Gamsu G, Stern RG, Cann CE, Herfkens RJ, Brundage BH. CT-determined pulmonary artery diameters in predicting pulmonary hypertension. *Invest Radiol* 1984;19:16–22.

78. Larde D, Belloir C, Vasile N, Frija J, Ferrane J. Computed tomography of aortic dissection. *Radiology* 1980;136:147–151.

79. Lee WJ, Fattal G. Mediastinal lipomatosis in simple obesity. *Chest* 1976;70:308–309.

80. Levitt RG, Husband JE, Glazer HS. CT of primary germ-cell tumors of the mediastinum. *AJR* 1984;142:73–78.

81. Libshitz HJ, Jing BS, Wallace S, Logothetis CJ. Sterilized metastases: a diagnostic and therapeutic dilemma. *AJR* 1983;140:15–19.

82. Lichtenstein AK, Levine A, Taylor CR, et al. Primary mediastinal lymphoma in adults. *Am J Med* 1980;68:509–513.

83. Lindfors KK, Meyer JE, Dedrick CG, Hassell LA, Harris NL. Thymic cysts in mediastinal Hodgkin disease. *Radiology* 1985;156: 37–41.

84. Machida K, Tasaka A. CT patterns of mural thrombus in aortic aneurysm. *J Comput Assist Tomogr* 1980;4:840–842.

85. Mallens WMC, Nijhuis-Heddes JMA, Bakker W. Calcified lymph node metastases in bronchioloalveolar carcinoma. *Radiology* 1986;161:103–104.

86. Marvasti MA, Mitchell GE, Burke WA, Meyer JA. Misleading density of mediastinal cysts on computerized tomography. *Ann Thorac Surg* 1981;31:167–170.

87. Mathieu D, Keita K, Loisance D, Cachera JP, Rousseau M, Vasile N. Postoperative CT follow-up of aortic dissection. *J Comput Assist Tomogr* 1986;10:216–218.

88. McLoud TC, Kalisher L, Stark P, Greene R. Intrathoracic lymph node metastases from extrathoracic neoplasms. *AJR* 1978;131:403–407.

89. McMurdo KK, deGeer G, Webb WR, Gamsu G. Normal and occluded mediastinal veins: MR imaging. *Radiology* 1986;159:33–38.

90. Mendelson DS, Som PM, Crane R, Cohen BA, Spura H. Relapsing polychondritis studied by computed tomography. *Radiology* 1985;157:489–490.

91. Mendez G, Isikoff MB, Isikoff SK, Sinner WN. Fatty tumors of the thorax demonstrated by CT. *AJR* 1979;133:207–212.

92. Meyer JE, Linggood RM, Lindfors KK, McLoud TC, Stomper PC. Impact of thoracic computed tomography on radiation therapy planning in Hodgkin disease. *J Comput Assist Tomogr* 1984;8: 892–894.

93. Meyer JE, McLoud TC, Lindfors KK. CT demonstration of cardiophrenic angle lymphadenopathy in Hodgkin disease. *J Comput Assist Tomogr* 1985;9:485–488.

94. Meyer JE, Munzenreider JE. Computed tomographic demonstration of internal mammary lymph node metastasis in patients with locally recurrent breast carcinoma. *Radiology* 1981;139:661–663.

95. Meziane MA, Fishman EK, Siegelman SS. CT diagnosis of hemopericardium in acute dissecting aneurysm of the thoracic aorta. *J Comput Assist Tomogr* 1984;8:10–14.

96. Miller GA Jr, Heaston DK, Moore AV Jr, Korobkin M, Braun SD, Dunnick NR. CT differentiation of thoracic aortic aneurysms from pulmonary masses adjacent to the mediastinum. *J Comput Assist Tomogr* 1984;8:437–442.

97. Miller DC, Stinson EB, Oyer PE, et al. Operative treatment of aortic dissections: experience with 125 patients over a sixteen-year period. *J Thorac Cardiovasc Surg* 1979;78:365–382.

98. Moore AV, Korobkin M, Powers B, et al. Thymoma detection by mediastinal CT: patients with myasthenia gravis. *AJR* 1982;138: 217–222.

99. Moore EH, Farmer DW, Geller SC, Golden JA, Gamsu G. Computed tomography in the diagnosis of iatrogenic false aneurysms of the ascending aorta. *AJR* 1984;142:1117–1118.

100. Moore EH, Webb WR, Verrier ED, et al. MRI of chronic posttraumatic false aneurysms of the thoracic aorta. *AJR* 1984;143: 1195–1196.

101. Müller NL, Webb WR, Gamsu G. Paratracheal lymphadenopathy: radiographic findings and correlation with CT. *Radiology* 1985;156: 761–765.

102. Naidich DP, Khouri NF, Stitik FP, McCauley DI, Siegelman SS. Computed tomography of the pulmonary hila: 2. Abnormal anatomy. *J Comput Assist Tomogr* 1981;5:468–475.

103. Nakata H, Nakayama C, Kimoto T, et al. Computed tomography of mediastinal bronchogenic cysts. *J Comput Assist Tomogr* 1982;6: 733–738.

104. Nakata H, Sato Y, Nakayama T, Yoshimatsu H, Kobayashi T.

Bronchogenic cyst with high CT numbers: analysis of contents. *J Comput Assist Tomogr* 1986;10:360–362.

105. North LB, Fuller LM, Hagemeister FB, Rodgers RW, Butler JJ, Shullenberger CC. Importance of initial mediastinal adenopathy in Hodgkin disease. *AJR* 1982;138:229–235.

106. O'Donovan PB, Ross JS, Sivak ED, O'Donnell JK, Meaney TF. Magnetic resonance imaging of the thorax: the advantages of coronal and sagittal planes. *AJR* 1984;143:1183–1188.

107. Onik G, Goodman PH. CT of Castleman disease. *AJR* 1983;140:691–692.

108. Owens GR, Arger PH, Mulhern CB Jr, Coleman BG, Gohel V. CT evaluation of mediastinal pseudocyst. *J Comput Assist Tomogr* 1980;4:256–259.

109. Peterson IH, Guthaner DF. Aortic pseudoaneurysm complicating Takayasu disease: CT appearance. *J Comput Assist Tomogr* 1986;10:676–678.

110. Pilla TJ, Wolverson MK, Sundaram M, Heiberg E, Shields JB. CT evaluation of cystic lymphangiomas of the mediastinum. *Radiology* 1982;144:841–842.

111. Pond GD, Hillman B. Evaluation of aneurysms by computed tomography. *Surgery* 1981;89:216–223.

112. Pressler V, McNamara JJ. Thoracic aortic aneurysm. *J Thorac Cardiovasc Surg* 1980;79:489–498.

113. Pugatch RD, Faling LJ, Robbins AH, Spira R. CT diagnosis of benign mediastinal abnormalities. *AJR* 1980;134:685–694.

114. Rholl KS, Levitt RG, Glazer HS. Magnetic resonance imaging of fibrosing mediastinitis. *AJR* 1985;145:255–259.

115. Robbins AH, Pugatch RD, Gerzof SG, et al. Further observations on the medical efficacy of computed tomography of the chest and abdomen. *Radiology* 1980;137:719–725.

116. Robert WC. Aortic dissection: anatomy, consequences, and causes. *Am Heart J* 1981;101:195–214.

117. Rohlfing BM, Korobkin M, Hall AD. Computed tomography of intrathoracic omental herniation and other mediastinal fatty masses. *J Comput Assist Tomogr* 1977;1:181–183.

118. Rostock RA, Siegelman SS, Lenhard RE, Wharam MD, Order SE. Thoracic CT enhancement for mediastinal Hodgkin disease: results and therapeutic implications. *Int J Radiat Oncol Biol Phys* 1983;9:1451–1457.

119. Scatarige JC, Fishman EK, Zerhouni EA, Siegelman SS. Transdiaphragmatic extension of invasive thymoma. *AJR* 1985;144:31–35.

120. Schweitzer DL, Aguam AS. Primary liposarcoma of the mediastinum. *J Thorac Cardiovasc Surg* 1977;741:83–97.

121. Seltzer SE, Herman PG, Sagel SS. Differential diagnosis of mediastinal fluid levels visualized on computed tomography. *J Comput Assist Tomogr* 1984;8:244–246.

122. Shin MS, Berland LL, Ho KJ. Mediastinal cystic hygromas: CT characteristics and pathogenetic considerations. *J Comput Assist Tomogr* 1985;9:297–301.

123. Smith TR, Khoury PT. Aneurysm of the proximal thoracic aorta simulating neoplasm: the role of CT and angiography. *AJR* 1985;144:909–910.

124. Sone S, Higashihara T, Morimoto S, et al. CT anatomy of hilar lymphadenopathy. *AJR* 1983;140:887–892.

125. Sones PJ, Torres WE, Colvin RS, Meier WL, Sprawls P, Rogers JR Jr. Effectiveness of CT in evaluating intrathoracic masses. *AJR* 1982;139:469–475.

126. Spizarny DL, Shepard JO, McLoud T, Grillo H, Dedrick CG. CT of adenoid cystic carcinoma of the trachea. *AJR* 1986;146:1129–1132.

127. Streiter ML, Schneider HJ, Proto AV. Steroid-induced thoracic lipomatosis: paraspinal involvement. *AJR* 1982;139:679–681.

128. Suzuki M, Takashima T, Itoh H, Choutoh S, Kawamura I, Watanabe Y. Computed tomography of mediastinal teratomas. *J Comput Assist Tomogr* 1983;7:74–76.

129. Tartas NE, Korin J, Dengra CS, Barazzutti LM, Blasetti A, Sanchez Avalos JC. Diffuse thymic enlargement in Hodgkin's disease. *JAMA* 1985;254:406.

130. Thorsen MK, Goodman LR, Sagel SS, Olinger GN, Youker JE. Ascending aorta complications of cardiac surgery: CT evaluation. *J Comput Assist Tomogr* 1986;10:219–225.

131. Thorsen MK, San Dretto MA, Lawson TL, Foley WD, Smith DF, Berland LL. Dissecting aortic aneurysms: accuracy of computed tomographic diagnosis. *Radiology* 1983;148:773–777.

132. Turley K, Ullyot DJ, Godwin JD, et al. Repair of dissection of the thoracic aorta. *J Thorac Cardiovasc Surg* 1981;81:61–68.

133. Vasile N, Mathieu D, Keita K, Lellouche D, Bloch G, Cachera JP. Computed tomography of thoracic aortic dissection: accuracy and pitfalls. *J Comput Assist Tomogr* 1986;10:211–215.

134. Vock P, Hodler J. Cardiophrenic angle adenopathy: update of causes and significance. *Radiology* 1986;159:395–399.

135. von Schulthess GK, McMurdo K, Tschalakoff D, deGeer G, Gamsu G, Higgins CB. Mediastinal masses: MR imaging. *Radiology* 1986;158:289–296.

136. Webb WR, Gamsu G, Crooks LE. Multisection sagittal and coronal magnetic resonance imaging of the mediastinum and hila. *Radiology* 1984;150:475–478.

137. Webb WR, Gamsu G, Glazer G. Computed tomography of the abnormal pulmonary hilum. *J Comput Assist Tomogr* 1981;5:485–490.

138. Webb WR, Jensen BG, Gamsu G, Sollitto R, Moore EH. Coronal magnetic resonance imaging of the chest: normal and abnormal. *Radiology* 1984;153:729–735.

139. Webb WR, Moore EH. Differentiation of volume averaging and mass on magnetic resonance images of the mediastinum. *Radiology* 1985;155:413–416.

140. Weinreb JC, Arger PH, Grossman R, Samuel L. CT metrizamide myelography in multiple bilateral intrathoracic meningoceles. *J Comput Assist Tomogr* 1984;8:324–326.

141. Weinreb JC, Mootz A, Cohen JM. MRI evaluation of mediastinal and thoracic inlet venous obstruction. *AJR* 1986;146:679–684.

142. White RD, Dooms GC, Higgins CB. Advances in imaging thoracic aortic disease. *Invest Radiol* 1986;21:761–778.

143. Yamaguchi T, Naito H, Ohta M, et al. False lumens in type III aortic dissections: progress CT study. *Radiology* 1985;156:757–760.

144. Yernault JC, Kuhn G, Dumortier P, Rocmans P, Ketelbant P, De Vuyst P. "Solid" mediastinal bronchogenic cyst: mineralogic analysis. *AJR* 1986;146:73–74.

145. Yousem DM, Scatarige JC, Fishman EK, Siegelman SS. Low-attenuation thoracic metastases in testicular malignancy. *AJR* 1986;146:291–293.

146. Yousem D, Scott WW Jr, Fishman EK, Watson AJ, Traill T, Gimenez L. Saphenous vein graft aneurysms demonstrated by computed tomography. *J Comput Assist Tomogr* 1986;10:526–528.

147. Zerhouni EA, Barth KW, Siegelman SS. Detection of venous thrombosis by computed tomography. *AJR* 1980;134:753–758.

148. Zerhouni EA, Scott WW Jr, Baker RR, Wharam MD, Siegelman SS. Invasive thymomas: diagnosis and evaluation by computed tomography. *J Comput Assist Tomogr* 1982;6:92–100.

CHAPTER 9

Lung, Pleura, Chest Wall

Stuart S. Sagel and Harvey S. Glazer

BRONCHI

The bronchi are the primary pathways connecting the mediastinum and hila with the pulmonary parenchyma. Computed tomography (CT) is a relatively sensitive technique for depicting anatomic distortions in the major bronchi (156,157). Approximately 85% to 90% of endobronchial lesions—which may produce associated changes in the distal pulmonary parenchyma, such as collapse, consolidation, and, rarely, focal overdistension—that are identified by fiberoptic bronchoscopy can be detected by CT, including virtually all primary neoplasms (93,149) (Fig. 1). Because of its better spatial resolution, CT is superior to magnetic resonance imaging (MRI) for demonstrating both normal bronchi and endobronchial masses (126). Occasionally, CT may be helpful in the selection of patients for bronchoscopy or an alternative diagnostic test. It can be used when the clinical suspicion of endobronchial disease is low to improve the potential diagnostic yield of bronchoscopy; that technique may be obviated if CT shows no bronchial abnormality (Fig. 2). Sometimes, a benign cause for a suspected lesion, such as broncholithiasis (105) (Fig. 3), is demonstrated. In a patient with congenital bronchial atresia, CT may depict concomitant regional lung hypodensity beyond a dilated mucus-filled bronchus more convincingly than conventional chest roentgenography (Fig. 4), perhaps allowing surgery to be avoided. Rarely, an occult abnormality, such as a neoplasm (55) or a foreign body (12), may be discovered. Predicting whether an abnormality seen on CT is endobronchial, submucosal, or extrinsic (peribronchial) is fraught with error, and CT is not as accurate as bronchoscopy in detecting submucosal spread of neoplasm. When transbronchial needle-aspiration biopsy is contemplated, CT is of major assistance because it allows detailed assessment of any possible associated mediastinal lymph node mass and its relationship to the adjacent major airways and vessels.

Bronchial Adenoma

Comprising a group of neoplasms that generally arise within the proximal bronchi or the trachea, the term bronchial "adenoma" is an acknowledged misnomer. All of the various histologic types—including carcinoid, cylindroma, adenocystic, and mucoepidermoid—should be considered low-grade carcinomas (220). These malignant neoplasms usually grow slowly, but may metastasize to the mediastinal lymph nodes or extrathoracic sites. The primary lesion may grow predominantly intraluminally or, alternatively, may have a small intraluminal component while extending deep into the adjacent peribronchial or paratracheal soft tissues. If the lesion is mainly intraluminal, the bronchus may become occluded. Although distal air trapping may occur, most commonly atelectasis or obstructive pneumonitis in the subtended lung results, which may be lobar or segmental, depending on the location and size of the lesion. Extrabronchial extension correlates with the tendency of these lesions to recur after local excision.

CT can be very helpful in the preoperative definition of the total extent of one of these infiltrating neoplasms, especially the extraluminal component (6,153). When no extension outside the bronchial wall is seen, local resection of the tumor, with plastic repair of the bronchus, may be feasible. Similarly, CT can be valuable in the follow-up of excised tumors, assessing for possible local recurrence or mediastinal lymph node metastases. The carcinoid variety of this tumor is highly vascular and may demonstrate substantial enhancement following intravenous administration of contrast material. It may also arise more pe-

A,B

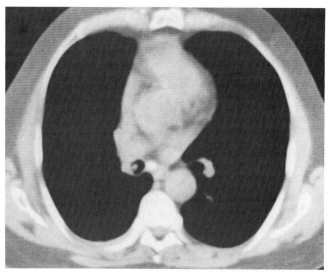

FIG. 1. Endobronchial mass. A: CT image at standard lung window setting (level of −600 HU, width of 800 HU) in a man with right-lower-lobe infiltrate and volume loss noted on plain chest radiographs demonstrates a smaller right lung, with infiltrate and some collapse in the right lower lobe. A mass (*arrowhead*) is seen in the bronchus intermedius. **B:** Same scan at window level of −150 HU and window width of 400 HU shows the true size of the epidermoid carcinoma partially occluding the right-lower-lobe bronchus.

ripherally in the lung, almost always in close proximity to a bronchus, and it usually appears as a sharply marginated nodule, frequently containing some stippled calcification.

Bronchogenic Carcinoma

Bronchogenic carcinoma currently is the leading cause of cancer death (27%) among both men and women over the age of 35 in the industrialized world. CT can sub-

stantially facilitate diagnostic evaluation and therapeutic planning for many patients suspected of having or known to have bronchogenic carcinoma.

In some patients, complex anatomic presentations on plain chest roentgenography often are resolved with CT. A benign condition (e.g., granuloma, aortic aneurysm, broncholithiasis) may be confidently distinguished from a suspected primary malignant neoplasm, and further work-up can be obviated or different investigation and management can be directed (Figs. 5 and 6). Because CT provides a detailed depiction of the segmental and sub-

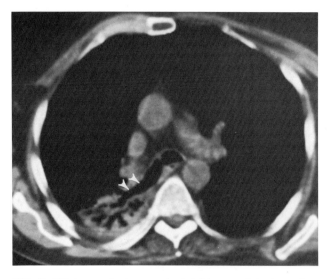

FIG. 2. CT demonstrates a patent right-upper-lobe bronchus (*arrowheads*), along with peripheral air bronchograms in the collapsed and consolidated apical and posterior segments of the right upper lobe. Minimal left pleural thickening is seen posterior to the descending aorta.

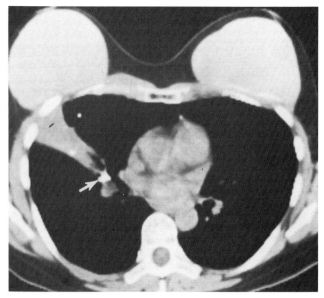

FIG. 3. CT demonstrates a broncholith (*arrow*) responsible for atelectasis of the lateral segment of the middle lobe; mammary implants are noted.

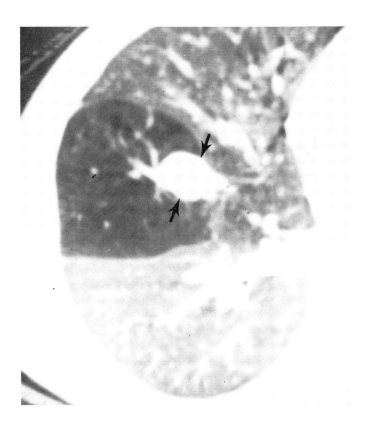

FIG. 4. CT demonstrates a branching, mucus-filled congenital bronchocele (*arrows*) as the cause of a pulmonary "nodule" noted on plain chest radiography. Hyperinflation of the lateral segment of the middle lobe, due to collateral air drift, is seen, but was not visible on conventional roentgenograms.

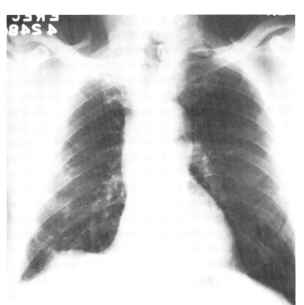

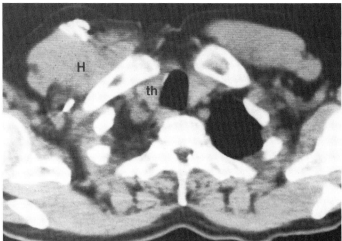

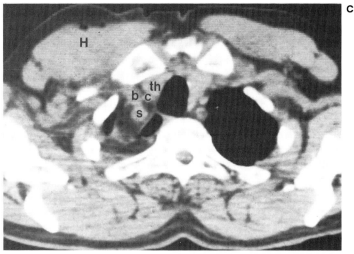

FIG. 5. Fibrosis mimicking a superior sulcus carcinoma. **A:** Posteroanterior chest radiograph from a man presenting with heart block demonstrates asymmetric opacification of the right-lung apex. **B,C:** Sequential caudal CT images obtained for clarification following the insertion of a pacemaker demonstrate predominantly fat, with several linear strands of fibrosis in the right superior sulcus, undoubtedly the result of old granulomatous disease. No soft-tissue mass or bone destruction is seen; (H) postoperative hematoma in right pectoralis major muscle; (th) right lobe of thyroid; (b) right brachiocephalic vein; (c) right carotid artery; (s) right subclavian artery.

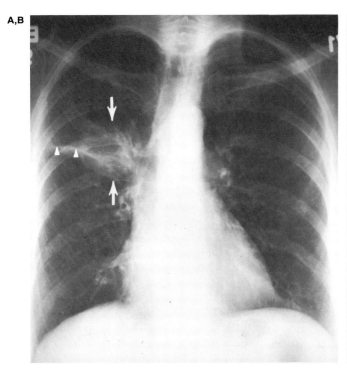
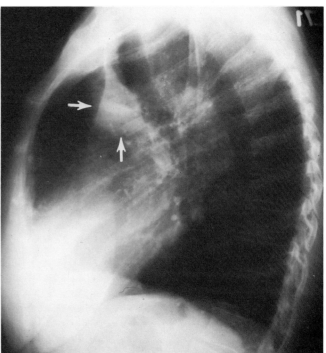

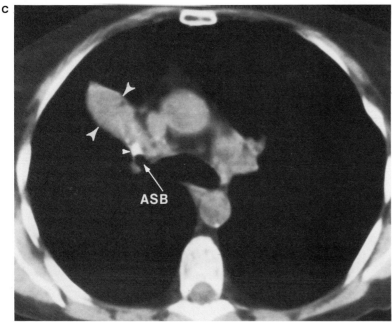

FIG. 6. Benign segmental collapse. **A,B:** Chest radiographs were initially interpreted as showing a mass (*arrows*), probably a bronchogenic carcinoma, in the anterior segment of the right upper lobe. In retrospect, there is slight elevation of the minor fissure (*arrowheads*), and the right lung is smaller than the left. **C:** CT demonstrates the "mass" to be a collapsed anterior segment of the right upper lobe (*large arrowheads*) caused by an occluding broncholith (*small arrowhead*) in the anterior segmental bronchus (ASB). (From ref. 65.)

segmental bronchi, in cases in which the suspected neoplasm is relatively peripheral, determination of the location of an endobronchial mass may be a helpful adjunct in directing the bronchoscopist to the appropriate biopsy site. When sputum analysis and fiberoptic bronchoscopy both yield negative results in a patient with a pulmonary mass, the findings on the CT examination can be valuable in directing further diagnostic evaluation. The next appropriate test may be suggested, be it transcervical mediastinoscopy (Fig. 7), anterior parasternal mediastinotomy (Fig. 8), percutaneous needle biopsy, or conventional

thoracotomy. Also, CT can be helpful in planning the best approach for percutaneous needle biopsy (see Fig. 25 in Chapter 7). For example, small subpleural blebs may be seen on CT that were not apparent on plain chest radiographs, prompting a revision in the direction of the biopsy needle, in order to reduce the risk of producing a pneumothorax.

There are at least a dozen different types of lung cancer. Over 95% arise from the bronchial or bronchiolar epithelium or from bronchial mucus glands; these carcinomas may be of the squamous-cell, adeno, large- or small-cell

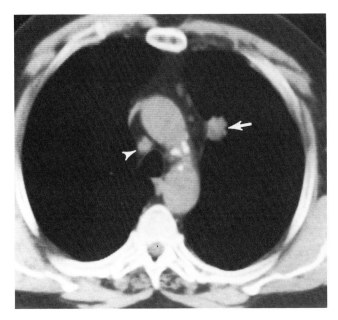

FIG. 7. Contralateral right paratracheal lymph node metastases (*arrowhead*) in patient with left-upper-lobe carcinoma (*arrow*).

undifferentiated type. Despite significant advances in chemotherapy and radiation therapy, cure of non-small-cell bronchogenic carcinoma basically is achievable only by surgical resection, and then only in certain categories of limited disease. Small-cell carcinomas are rarely amenable to surgical treatment because of their aggressive behavior and their usual widespread involvement at the time of presentation. Accurate preoperative staging is extremely desirable to select those patients with localized disease for curative surgery and those patients with more widespread neoplasm for palliative therapy. Ultimately, only about

40% of patients with newly diagnosed bronchogenic carcinoma are amenable to surgical resection with curative intent. Surgery should be restricted for complete tumor resection; incomplete "palliative" resection in patients with advanced disease should be avoided.

The purpose of any staging system is to provide consistency in communication about the cancer patient, to help determine prognosis, and to serve as a basis for evaluating various forms of treatment. Staging allows for predictability of cure in large populations. The TNM system, revised in 1986 (Table 1) (139), is that most commonly used for bronchogenic carcinoma, where T describes the extent of the tumor, N the regional lymph node involvement, and M the status of distant extrathoracic metastases. This classification is helpful in describing the anatomic extent of disease in an individual patient and can be used at any point in the disease process, not only at clinical presentation. The survival of patients with non-small-cell carcinoma correlates relatively well with the anatomic extent or stage (Table 2) of the disease, whereas survival in small-cell undifferentiated carcinoma generally does not (25,205,233). Thus, small-cell carcinoma is usually described as limited (confined to the ipsilateral hemithorax and the contained lymph nodes, without pleural effusion) or extensive (spread beyond these areas). When the TNM classification is used for non-small-cell carcinoma, overall 5-year survival in stage I, II, and III disease approximates 70%, 30%, and 10%, respectively. Lymph node status (N) is a better predictor of long-term results than is the size of the primary tumor (T). Modifications in the N category more precisely identify anatomic regions of mediastinal nodal involvement; nodal stations have been defined for each CT level for improved classification (see Fig. 57 in Chapter 7). There are several drawbacks to the TNM system: No histologic differentiation is inherent, and no dis-

A,B

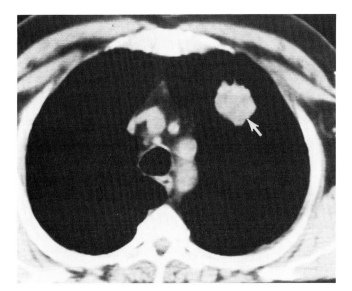
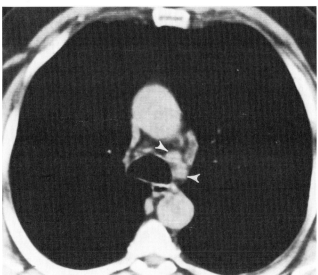

FIG. 8. **A:** Left-upper-lobe carcinoma (*arrow*). **B:** Aortopulmonary-window lymph node metastases (*arrowheads*) proved by parasternal mediastinotomy are seen at a more caudal level.

TABLE 1. *TNM categories for lung cancer*

Primary tumor (T):

T_1 3.0 cm or less in greatest diameter, surrounded by lung or visceral pleura, without invasion proximal to a lobar bronchus.

T_2 More than 3.0 cm in greatest diameter, or a tumor of any size that either invades the visceral pleura or has associated lobar atelectasis or obstructive pneumonitis. The proximal extent of demonstrable tumor must be within a lobar bronchus or at least 2.0 cm distal to the carina.

T_3 Tumor of any size, with direct extension into chest wall, diaphragm, mediastinal pleura, or pericardium; a tumor that involves a main bronchus within 2.0 cm of the carina (except for a superficial lesion).

T_4 Tumor of any size, with invasion of great vessels, trachea or carina, esophagus, heart, or vertebral body or presence of a malignant pleural effusion (positive cytology).

Nodal involvement (N):

N_0 No involvement of regional lymph nodes.
N_1 Metastasis to lymph nodes in the peribronchial or the ipsilateral hilar region.
N_2 Metastasis to ipsilateral mediastinal or subcarinal lymph nodes.
N_3 Metastasis to contralateral mediastinal or supraclavicular lymph nodes.

Distant metastasis (M):

M_0 No distant metastasis.
M_1 Distant metastasis present.

tinction is made between intracapsular nodal metastases and extracapsular matted nodes.

The location of the primary carcinoma determines the usual lymphatic pathways of tumor spread to the regional lymph nodes. Cancers originating in the right lung tend to metastasize initially to the ipsilateral tracheobronchial (hilar) nodes (10R) and subsequently to the right paratracheal nodes (4R, 2R). Such neoplasms rarely metastasize to contralateral lymph nodes, whereas cancers of the left lung commonly spread to the right paratracheal nodes subsequent to ipsilateral involvement. Carcinomas of the left upper lobe usually metastasize initially to nodes in the aortopulmonary window (5, 4L), and both left-upper-lobe and left-lower-lobe lesions may spread first to the left tracheobronchial region (10L). Cancers of the middle lobe and both lower lobes often affect the subcarinal nodes (7) early in their dissemination, and lower-lobe lesions also may extend to the paraesophageal (8), pulmonary

TABLE 2. *Stage grouping*

Stage I:
$T_{1,2}$, N_0, M_0
Stage II:
$T_{1,2}$, N_1, M_0
Stage IIIa (poor prognosis, technically resectable thoracic spread):
T_3, $N_{0,1}$, M_0
T_{1-3}, N_2, M_0
Stage IIIb (nonresectable thoracic spread):
T_{1-3}, N_3, M_0
T_4, N_{0-2}, M_0
Stage IV (extrathoracic spread):
Any T, any N, M_1

ligament (9), and supradiaphragmatic nodes (14). Knowledge of the expected drainage pattern can be valuable in selected cases. It would be extremely unlikely for a right-lung carcinoma to spread only to aortopulmonary lymph nodes, and isolated enlargement of nodes in this region noted on CT in such a patient generally can be presumed to be due to another cause, such as old granulomatous disease.

Surgical nodal sampling procedures, including transcervical mediastinoscopy and parasternal mediastinotomy, have been developed for staging purposes and have proved useful in selected groups of patients, reducing the percentage of "unnecessary" thoracotomies from 40% to 10% or less. Nevertheless, these procedures have definite limitations and are only 80% accurate in mediastinal nodal evaluation. The mediastinoscope cannot be used to evaluate all of the mediastinal compartments. Generally, only the middle mediastinum, anterior and lateral to the trachea and posterior to the major vessels (brachiocephalic arteries and veins, superior vena cava, and ascending aorta), is accessible to biopsy. A notable percentage of patients with bronchogenic carcinoma and negative findings on mediastinoscopy have mediastinal lymph node metastases at surgery. Such involved lymph nodes usually are in the anterior mediastinum (prevascular space), aortopulmonary window, and posterior subcarinal region, but sometimes metastases are detected in lymph nodes that are accessible to mediastinoscopy. In addition, these surgical procedures are unable to detect extramediastinal spread of bronchogenic carcinoma. The accuracy of these tissue sampling techniques, plus others such as percutaneous transthoracic needle biopsy and transbronchial needle aspiration (226), can be increased when directed by CT to areas of morphologic abnormality, including clinically unsuspected metastases in the adrenal and liver (228). Whereas the bronchoscopic recognition of widening and fixation of the carina may strongly suggest mediastinal involvement with tumor, CT or MRI demonstration of enlarged lymph nodes in the subcarinal area (Figs. 9 and 10) facilitates earlier appropriate selection of patients for transbronchial needle aspiration.

CT has assumed a major role in the staging of bronchogenic carcinoma, because it is the best method for its radiographic TNM classification. Although early reports were skeptical about the ability of CT to provide clinically meaningful data, investigations with improved equipment, more precise technique, and refined interpretive criteria have consistently demonstrated the clinical efficacy of this technique (23,24,48,57,62,102,185). CT staging of the thorax and upper abdomen is very helpful in predicting the likelihood of curative surgical resection and is indicated in the vast majority of patients in whom surgery is contemplated (61). But its role is not, by itself, to determine operability or establish prognosis. CT is an anatomic modality with definite limitations; in many cases, high specificity is impossible. Generally, it is used to direct the most appropriate invasive staging procedure for patients with positive findings and to obviate invasive staging for patients with negative findings. The detection of an enlarged mediastinal lymph node, or an enlarged adrenal gland or focal liver lesion, by CT alone should not constitute sufficient evidence for inoperability. Histologic corroboration of metastatic neoplasm within the enlarged node or abnormal organ is strongly recommended in patients otherwise considered operative candidates. Because an enlarged mediastinal lymph node or a mass in an adrenal or the liver may not be due to metastatic neoplasm, a decision against thoracotomy generally should not be based on CT findings alone. CT should be used not to replace invasive techniques of staging, such as transcer-

vical mediastinoscopy, anterior parasternal mediastinotomy, percutaneous needle biopsy, or transbronchoscopic needle-aspiration biopsy, but to optimize the selective use of these techniques. Based on CT localization of suspected disease, the appropriate biopsy procedure and access route can be determined.

Staging by CT is clearly superior to conventional radiologic techniques for the demonstration of direct extension of the primary neoplasm into the mediastinum or chest wall and the detection of enlarged mediastinal lymph nodes. Conventional radiography and tomography have proved inadequate for this task, with a sensitivity approximating only 50%. Enlarged lymph nodes in the pretracheal, aortopulmonary, and subcarinal areas can be more easily recognized than with standard roentgenography. Whether or not a staging CT examination needs to be performed in all patients with bronchogenic carcinoma is controversial; that it is appropriate for T_2 lesions is generally accepted. Some investigators believe that the relatively young, cigarette-smoking patient with a newly discovered small, irregular peripheral pulmonary nodule and a normal-appearing mediastinum on plain chest radiographs (presumed $T_1N_0M_0$) is unlikely to benefit from a CT examination (169). In this circumstance, mediastinal metastases are uncommon, and proceeding directly to needle biopsy or thoracotomy generally is justified providing there are no clinical contraindications. Others claim that CT staging of the mediastinum is cost-effective even in patients with T_1 lesions (Fig. 11), with a notable percentage having otherwise occult mediastinal lymph node or adrenal metastases, or a contralateral lung lesion (89). Those patients with clinically evident metastatic disease or unequivocal mediastinal lymphadenopathy on plain chest radiography precluding resection usually do not re-

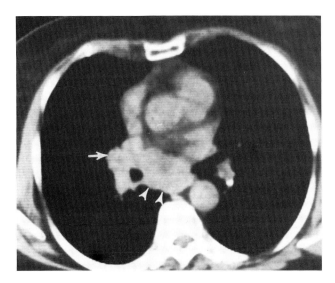

FIG. 9. Woman with right-lower-lobe carcinoma (not shown) with right hilar (*arrow*) and posterior subcarinal (*arrowheads*) lymph node metastases; the latter were documented by CT-guided percutaneous needle-aspiration biopsy.

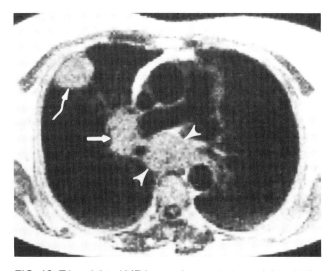

FIG. 10. T1-weighted MR image demonstrates a right-middle-lobe carcinoma (*curved arrow*), with right hilar (*straight arrow*) and posterior subcarinal (*arrowheads*) lymph node metastases; the latter were documented by transbronchial needle-aspiration biopsy caudally through the carina.

A,B

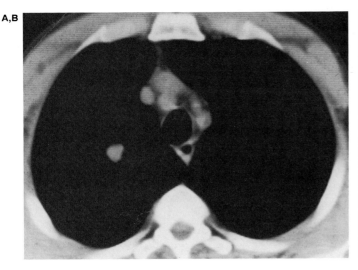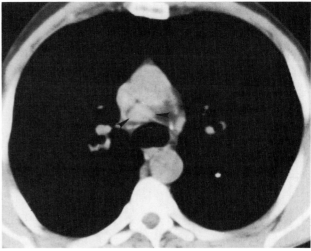

FIG. 11. A: A 1.5-cm right-upper-lobe carcinoma (T₁ lesion). B: At a more caudal level, pretracheal mediastinal lymph node metastases (*arrowheads*) are seen. The mediastinum appeared normal on conventional radiography.

quire a CT study for staging purposes. Nevertheless, such an examination may subsequently be valuable to pinpoint the exact location if necessary for biopsy planning or for radiation therapy planning. The anatomic information derived from CT images regarding the extent of the neoplastic disease and its relationship to surrounding structures, as well as measurements of tissue thickness, results in altering the design of the planned dose distribution in approximately one-third of patients to either a greater or lesser volume in order to maximize tumor coverage and minimize irradiation to uninvolved areas (46,174).

Contiguous extension of a primary bronchogenic carcinoma into the mediastinum generally precludes curative surgical resection. With conventional tomography, it is frequently difficult to determine whether a centrally situated pulmonary mass invades the mediastinum or merely lies in close proximity to it. CT can establish that the mediastinum is involved by direct extension of tumor when invasion of the mediastinal fat or invasion around the mediastinal vessels or airways is demonstrated (Figs. 12 and 13). It should be emphasized that a neoplastic mass simply contacting the mediastinal pleura, with no well-defined fat plane between the lesion and the mediastinum, does not indicate mediastinal invasion (Fig. 14). The tumor mass must infiltrate into (interdigitate with) the mediastinal fat or extend around the great vessels or major bronchi before extension can be confidently diagnosed. Imaging after a bolus intravenous injection of contrast material often is beneficial in confirming or excluding mediastinal vascular involvement (Figs. 15–17). Relatively central primary neoplasms, especially adenocarcinomas, frequently extend proximally in the sub-

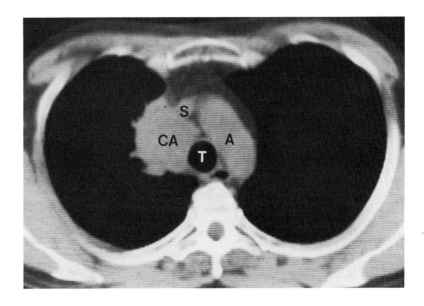

FIG. 12. Right-upper-lobe carcinoma (CA) directly invading the mediastinal fat deep to the superior vena cava (S) and in front of the trachea (T); (A) aortic arch.

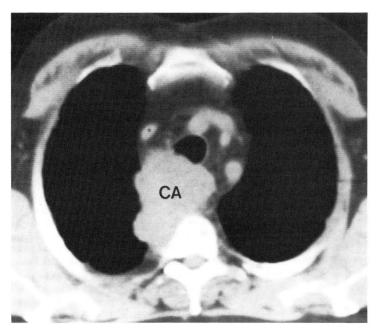

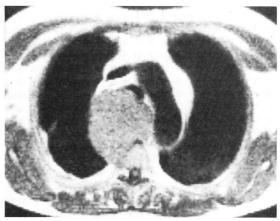

A,B

FIG. 13. A: CT demonstrates extensive infiltration of the mediastinal fat and the right posterolateral tracheal wall by a carcinoma (CA). **B:** T1-weighted MR image at a slightly lower level shows comparable findings.

mucosa of the bronchus for a considerable length. Peribronchial soft-tissue thickening may be depicted on CT (Fig. 18), sometimes with extension into the mediastinal fat. Such a finding should prompt a deep biopsy at bronchoscopy for corroboration. The ability of CT to depict the extrabronchial extent of carcinoma involving the distal trachea or proximal bronchi and its relation to adjacent major vascular structures (Fig. 19) can be very valuable if laser photoresection therapy is planned. The presence of substantial peribronchial tumor extrinsic to a bronchial obstruction, which cannot be evaluated by fiberoptic

bronchoscopy, is a predictor of poor response to laser photoresection therapy (170).

As in the case of the mediastinum, care should be taken not to overdiagnose invasion of the pleura and chest wall. Peripheral bronchogenic carcinoma may directly invade the adjacent pleura, sometimes by extending along the perivascular lymphatic sheaths. Involvement of the parietal pleura and chest wall may be present in the absence of a pleural effusion (Fig. 20). Assessment of such invasion by CT can be extremely difficult (66,171,197). When neoplasm simply abuts the pleura, even if it has obtuse mar-

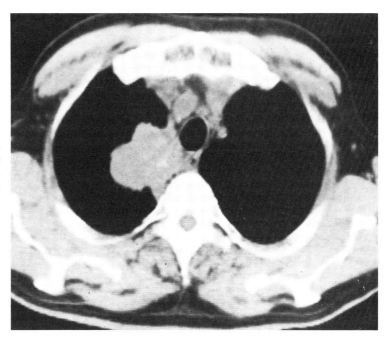

FIG. 14. Right-upper-lobe carcinoma abutting the mediastinum; no definite extension (interdigitation) into the mediastinal fat or deep to the major vessels is seen. At surgery, the lesion did not invade the mediastinum and was resectable.

A,B

C,D

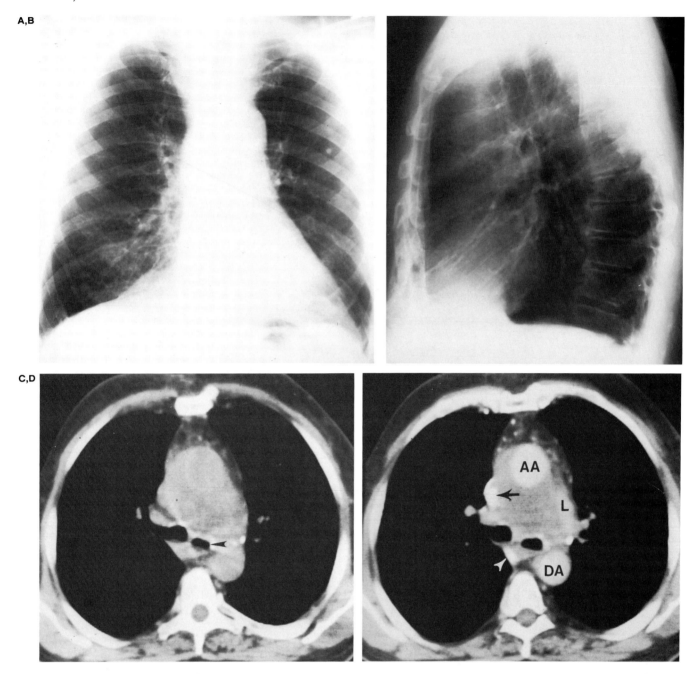

FIG. 15. A,B: Posteroanterior and lateral chest radiographs demonstrate some mild mediastinal widening and some increased pretracheal density. **C:** CT demonstrates extensive soft-tissue infiltration of the mediastinum, with posterior displacement and narrowing of the left main-stem bronchus (*arrowhead*). **D:** Contrast-enhanced CT image documents the extensive mediastinal mass (oat-cell carcinoma) causing partial obstruction of the superior vena cava (*arrow*), with collateral flow into several vessels, including the azygos vein (*arrowhead*); (AA) ascending aorta; (DA) descending aorta; (L) left pulmonary artery.

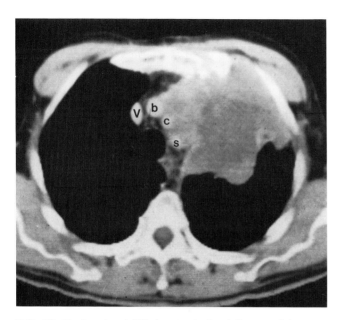

FIG. 16. Postcontrast CT demonstrates left-upper-lobe carcinoma invading the mediastinal fat surrounding the great vessels, and also extending into the left anterior chest wall; (V) superior vena cava; (b) brachiocephalic artery; (c) left carotid artery; (s) left subclavian artery.

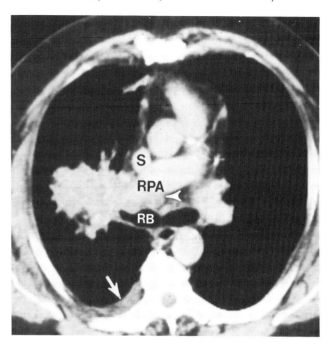

FIG. 17. Postcontrast CT demonstrating right-upper-lobe carcinoma directly invading the mediastinum (*arrowhead*) posterior to the right pulmonary artery (RPA) and anterior to the narrowed right upper lobe and right main-stem (RB) bronchus; (S) superior vena cava; (*arrow*) right pleural effusion.

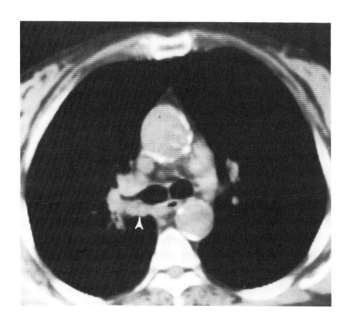

FIG. 18. Right-upper-lobe adenocarcinoma narrowing the lobar bronchus and extending proximally in the submucosa, producing thickening of the posterior wall of the right main-stem bronchus (*arrowhead*).

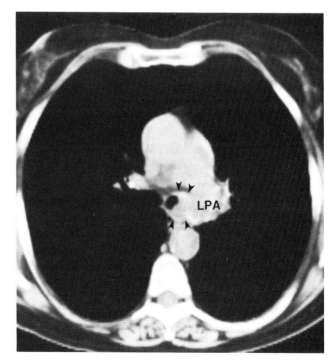

FIG. 19. Relatively bulky carcinoma (*arrowheads*) involving the left main-stem bronchus, extending adjacent to the left pulmonary artery (LPA).

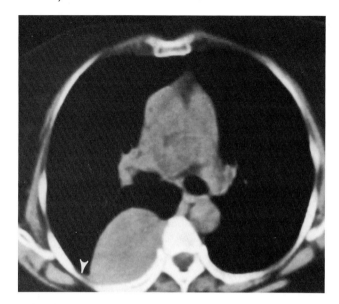

FIG. 20. Carcinoma of superior segment of right lower lobe abutting a vertebral body and rib in a patient with focal chest pain; no bone destruction identified. Minimal adjacent pleural reaction (*arrowhead*) is present. At surgery, the parietal pleura and rib were invaded by the neoplasm.

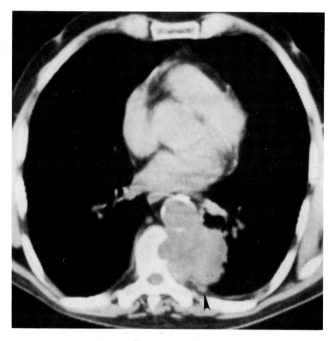

FIG. 21. Carcinoma of the left lower lobe invading and destroying the adjacent vertebral body. Neoplasm also extends externally (*arrowhead*) to left pleural thickening.

gins and is associated with local pleural thickening or a pleural effusion, true invasion of the parietal pleura may not be present. Associated inflammatory changes can result in these findings. A definite diagnosis of chest-wall invasion requires the demonstration of bone (rib or vertebral body) destruction (Fig. 21) or the depiction of a discrete extrapleural mass (Fig. 22). Slight asymmetry of the chest wall may be caused by improper patient positioning. If the CT findings are equivocal, MRI is occasionally helpful in definitively diagnosing chest-wall invasion (83). T2-weighted images best demonstrate the chest-wall thickening, which commonly contains a high-signal focus. The clinical presence of focal chest pain is probably a better indicator of chest-wall invasion than any CT or MRI finding. Even the demonstration of direct invasion of the chest wall by a peripheral bronchogenic carcinoma (stage IIIa spread), although a very poor prognostic sign, may not connote that the lesion is unresectable for cure (194). Resection of the involved chest wall, along with the primary tumor, can result in a reasonable survival rate in selected patients if the mediastinal lymph nodes are free of disease.

The presence of mediastinal lymph node metastases secondary to bronchogenic carcinoma presages a very poor prognosis and usually indicates incurable disease. In most medical centers it is a contraindication to thoracotomy, regardless of cell type or location. An exception may be the infrequently encountered patient with squamous-cell carcinoma with only intranodal growth within a node(s) in the ipsilateral superior tracheobronchial area (stage IIIa). CT can be very valuable in detecting me-

diastinal lymph node enlargement and can serve as a useful guide for selection of the optimal staging procedure for tissue sampling (e.g., mediastinoscopy, mediastinotomy, transtracheal or percutaneous needle biopsy) to corroborate lymph node metastases, before attempting cu-

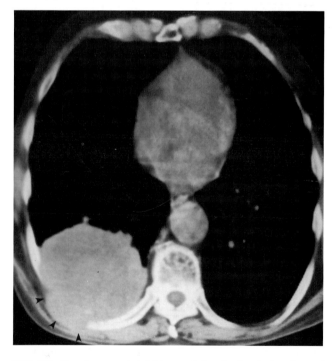

FIG. 22. Carcinoma of right lower lobe destroying a rib and invading the chest wall (*arrowheads*).

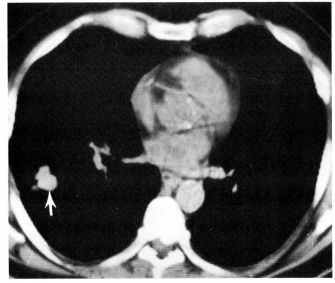
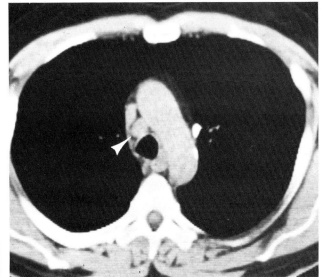
A,B

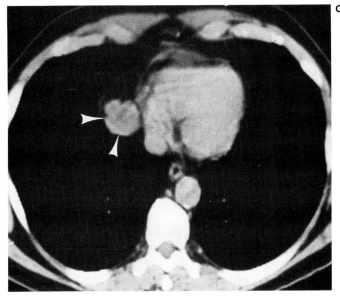

C

FIG. 23. Bronchogenic carcinoma with mediastinal lymph node metastases. **A:** A 3-cm irregularly lobulated mass (*arrow*) is seen in the right lower lobe. **B:** A 1.8-cm-diameter enlarged pretracheal lymph node (*arrowhead*) is present. Subsequent mediastinoscopy disclosed metastatic, poorly differentiated squamous-cell carcinoma. **C:** Concomitant enlarged right supradiaphragmatic lymph node (*arrowheads*), which was thought to represent a prominent pericardial fat pad on conventional chest radiography.

rative resection of a bronchogenic carcinoma (Figs. 23 and 24). Size criteria alone will never be totally reliable in staging the mediastinal lymph nodes (115,116). The demonstration of enlarged mediastinal lymph nodes in the patient with bronchogenic carcinoma does not automatically imply metastatic disease. CT cannot distinguish lymph node enlargement due to inflammatory disease from that due to neoplasm. Also, CT will fail to detect microscopic metastatic disease in normal-size lymph nodes. A receiver-operating-characteristic (ROC) curve, which relates the true-positive ratio (sensitivity) to the false-positive ratio, can be prepared for the CT assessment of mediastinal nodal involvement. If a diameter of 10 mm or greater is considered abnormal, then the sensitivity based on myriad studies will be between 90% and 95%, but the false-positive ratio will be about 40%. If a diameter greater than 6 mm is chosen, the specificity will be markedly worsened without any substantial improvement in

sensitivity. Using 15 mm as an indication of nodal abnormality, sensitivity will fall to about 60%, although specificity becomes greater than 90%. Recognizing these limitations, our diagnostic criterion on CT images, largely chosen to maximize sensitivity, is that any mediastinal lymph node 1 cm or larger in diameter is considered potentially involved with metastasis. Thus, nodes less than 1 cm in diameter are considered unlikely to harbor metastatic disease, whereas nodes 1 to 2 cm in diameter (or larger than 100 mm^2 in cross-sectional area) are considered suspicious; such mild enlargement can be caused by either neoplasm or granulomatous disease. Using this nodal measurement, CT is the most sensitive radiologic technique for the detection of metastatic mediastinal lymph node involvement (90–95%). This substantially exceeds the sensitivity of gallium scintigraphy (about 80%) and conventional chest radiography (about 50%) and is similar to that reported with MRI (by which basically the

A,B

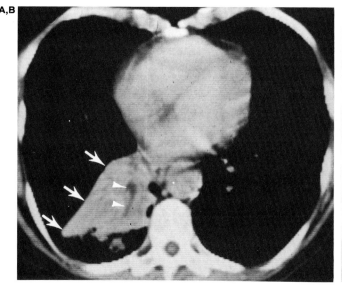
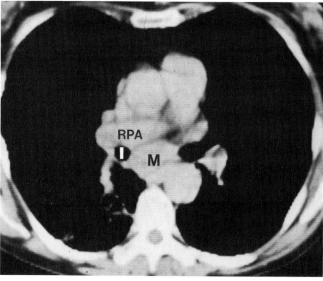

FIG. 24. Bronchogenic carcinoma with mediastinal lymph node metastases. **A:** Collapsed right lower lobe (*arrows*), distal to an obstructing lesion, containing some dilated mucus-filled bronchi (*arrowheads*). **B:** A large subcarinal lymph node mass (M) 4 cm cephalad is seen medial to the bronchus intermedius (I) and posterior to the right pulmonary artery (RPA). Fiberoptic bronchoscopy disclosed a carcinoma of the right-lobe bronchus; aspirates obtained from a caudally directed transcarinal needle biopsy of the nodal mass showed metastatic carcinoma.

same anatomic features are assessed). But as emphasized, CT is not highly specific for metastases using this criterion, approximating only 60%. Although mediastinal lymph nodes more than 2 cm in diameter in a patient with a known primary bronchogenic carcinoma almost always are due to neoplastic involvement, histologic corroboration is still strongly suggested in most instances.

Although some previous reports claimed that conventional tomography, especially in the 55° posterior oblique projection, was superior to CT in the analysis of the hilar lymph nodes, all of those studies were conducted with older equipment, more limited knowledge of the anatomy seen with CT, and often less than optimal technique (intravenous contrast material was not used routinely or even in problem cases). Currently, there is no doubt that contrast-enhanced CT (or MRI) gives a more sensitive depiction of hilar lymph node enlargement (Fig. 25), being able to detect lymph nodes 10 mm or larger in diameter,

A,B

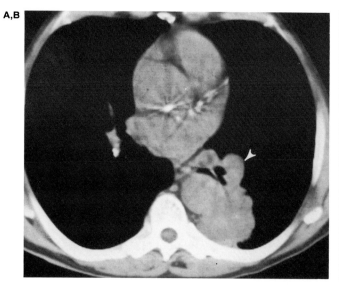
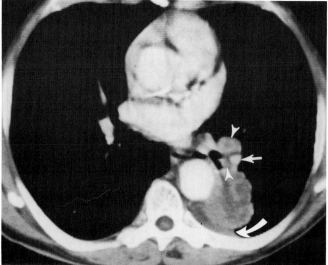

FIG. 25. Hilar lymph node metastases. **A:** Non-contrast-enhanced CT in patient with carcinoma of the left lower lobe demonstrates lobular enlargement (*arrowhead*) of the left hilum. **B:** Postcontrast image demonstrates nonenhancing enlarged lymph nodes (*arrowheads*) anteromedial to the left-lower-lobe pulmonary artery (*straight arrow*). Pleural reaction is noted posterior to the primary tumor (*curved arrow*).

A,B

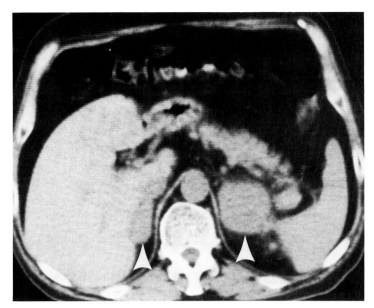
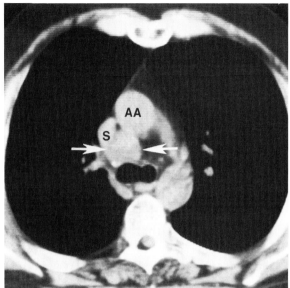

FIG. 26. Adrenal metastases. **A:** Image through upper abdomen demonstrates bilateral soft-tissue-density adrenal masses (*arrowheads*). **B:** Image through upper thorax shows concomitant precarinal mediastinal lymph node metastases (*arrows*) from right-upper-lobe bronchogenic carcinoma (not shown); (S) superior vena cava; (AA) ascending aorta.

whereas nodes must be approximately 20 mm in diameter to be routinely detected on oblique hilar tomography (60). Albeit far less sensitive, the larger critical size accounts for the better specificity of the conventional technique. Nevertheless, hilar lymph node assessment has little relevance in most patients with bronchogenic carcinoma. It is the presence of mediastinal metastatic disease (in the form of direct extension of the primary neoplasm or lymph node metastases) that contraindicates surgery. Although the presence of ipsilateral hilar lymph node involvement alters the stage classification and notably diminishes the prognosis for the patient, it neither makes the patient unresectable nor accurately predicts the presence of mediastinal lymph node involvement. Metastatic carcinoma may occur in mediastinal lymph nodes in 25% of patients with negative hilar nodes. Therefore, in the overall staging of bronchogenic carcinoma, hilar evaluation is of minor importance, and rigorous efforts at hilar staging usually are not warranted, unless the patient is clearly not a candidate for a pneumonectomy, which may be required if the nodal metastases are found to encase the central pulmonary artery at surgery.

CT is sufficiently sensitive to screen out patients who would not benefit from routine transcervical mediastinoscopy or left anterior parasternal mediastinotomy. In a patient with negative findings on CT examination of the mediastinum and upper abdomen, generally the surgeon can proceed directly to thoracotomy (80). Although there will always be a small percentage of false-negative findings on CT images because of microscopic metastases within normal-size lymph nodes, this may have little clinical significance. A relatively favorable prognosis still may

be achieved in patients with limited intranodal disease detected by routine biopsy of normal-appearing mediastinal lymph nodes draining the tumor, and thus resection still will be appropriate. Although the extent of the primary tumor and its cell type also influence prognosis, there is probably a salutary effect when high-dose postoperative mediastinal irradiation is administered in such individuals.

Some patients thought to be resectable for cure have metastatic disease present outside the thorax (10). Autopsies performed within 30 days of attempted "curative" resections have shown that the frequency of such occult metastases in non-small-cell bronchogenic carcinoma is approximately 20%. The adrenal is the most frequent site, followed by the liver. The staging examination for bronchogenic carcinoma should be extended into the upper abdomen to assess these sites. CT is very sensitive in detecting adrenal masses; the majority of patients with adrenal metastases do not have clinical signs of adrenal insufficiency. Although most patients with metastatic enlargement of the adrenals have CT evidence of mediastinal lymph node enlargement (Fig. 26), occasionally the adrenal is the only site of metastases to contraindicate surgery. An adrenal mass is not synonymous with metastasis; many represent incidental nonhyperfunctioning adenomas (164,190). A small adrenal mass with a homogeneous, relatively low attenuation value (0–20 Hounsfield units, HU) almost certainly represents an adenoma; this may be corroborated with other imaging techniques such as MRI (relatively low signal intensity on both T1- and T2-weighted images) (28,63) or adrenal scintigraphy (uptake with NP-59). Most lesions exceeding

A,B

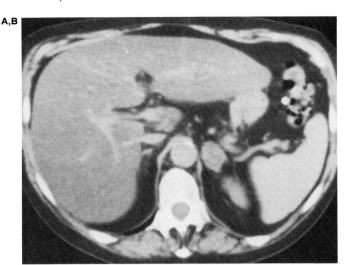 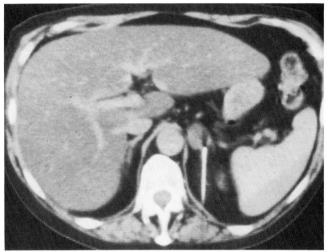

FIG. 27. Incidental nonhyperfunctioning adrenal adenoma in a patient with bronchogenic carcinoma. **A:** CT image (done prone) demonstrates 2-cm left adrenal mass; mild diffuse fatty infiltration of the liver is present. **B:** Image corroborating proper placement of tip of percutaneously inserted needle within adrenal mass. Cytologic samples disclosed "normal adrenal cells." Follow-up CT examination 9 months later, after resection of primary carcinoma, showed no change in the size of the adrenal mass.

3 cm in diameter, especially those that are inhomogeneous and have a thick wall, represent metastases. Percutaneous needle biopsy under CT-directed guidance may be required to document dissemination, because the histology of the lesion generally cannot be accurately determined from the morphologic appearance alone (Fig. 27). The liver is rarely the only demonstrable site of metastases (Fig. 28).

Studies thus far have failed to demonstrate any superiority for MRI in the detection of direct mediastinal extension or recognition of lymph node metastasis (91,114,123,146,231). MRI in most instances simply recapitulates the findings of CT. Calculation of relaxation times has not proved useful in distinguishing enlarged lymph nodes due to benign disease from those involved with metastatic neoplasm. As long as nodal size remains the sole criterion for the detection of metastatic lymphadenopathy, there will be no advantage for MRI compared with CT, as both techniques can accurately depict enlargement, and neither provides histologic specificity. Therefore, MRI should be reserved for patients in whom the CT findings are inconclusive (e.g., questionable chest-wall invasion) or in whom intravenous contrast material is contraindicated.

CT may provide unique information in specific clinical situations related to bronchogenic carcinoma. An occult primary tumor may be detected in a patient with a positive sputum cytologic examination or with a paraneoplastic syndrome and no lesion apparent on chest radiography or fiberoptic bronchoscopy. These carcinomas are frequently situated in areas poorly assessed by standard roentgenography, such as the lung apices, the paramediastinal areas (Fig. 29), or the juxtadiaphragmatic regions. CT may be valuable in distinguishing between the solitary

form of bronchioloalveolar-cell carcinoma and the diffuse variety, therefore changing the categorization and therapeutic approach (131). When planning radiation therapy, dynamic imaging after bolus intravenous administration of contrast material (or MRI) can be helpful in distinguishing between a central, partially endobronchial mass and more distal collapsed or consolidated lung (Fig. 30). With superior sulcus tumors, the extrapulmonary extent of the neoplasm and its relationship to surrounding struc-

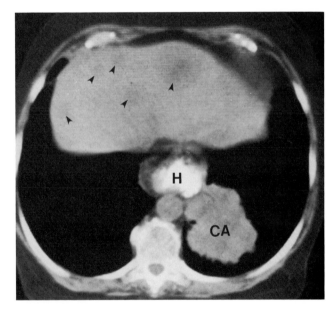

FIG. 28. Multiple liver metastases (*arrowheads*) are seen (later proved by percutaneous needle biopsy) in a patient with a left-lower-lobe carcinoma (CA); an esophageal hiatal hernia (H) is present. No mediastinal lymph node or adrenal enlargement was noted on CT.

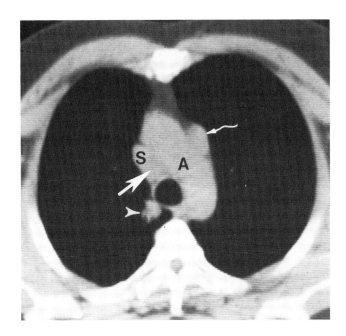

FIG. 29. Roentgenographically occult right-upper-lobe carcinoma in patient with inappropriate ADH secretion. CT demonstrates an irregular 1-cm mass (*arrowhead*) posterolateral to the trachea; mediastinal lymph node enlargement is also seen in the pretracheal (*straight arrow*) and lateral aortic (*curved arrow*) areas; (S) superior vena cava; (A) aortic arch.

tures, such as the subclavian vessels and the vertebral bodies, are much better assessed with CT than with conventional radiographs (162,214,230); invasion usually contraindicates surgery (Fig. 31). In some of these patients, coronal or sagittal MRI can facilitate the depiction of extrathoracic extension into the lower neck. CT may influence treatment and be of some prognostic value in patients with undifferentiated small-cell (oat-cell) carcinoma (78,136,223,236). Determination of disease extent may help in the decision whether or not to use adjuvant radiation therapy and to tailor portals. Initial pericardial or abdominal (liver, adrenals, lymph nodes) involvement is an especially poor prognostic indicator.

Bronchiectasis

Bronchiectasis, which represents irreversible dilatation of the bronchial tree that may require surgical therapy, has been classified pathologically into three forms, depending on the severity of the bronchial dilatation:

1. Cylindrical (tubular): uniform mild dilatation, with loss of normal tapering and abrupt termination
2. Varicose: greater dilatation, with irregular caliber due to areas of expansion and narrowing
3. Cystic (saccular): marked dilatation, with peripheral ballooning

The plain chest radiographic findings in bronchiectasis often are nonspecific, unless the disease is very advanced (81). Surrounding fibrosis, which may be causative (234) as well as a sequela, can obscure recognition of dilated,

A,B

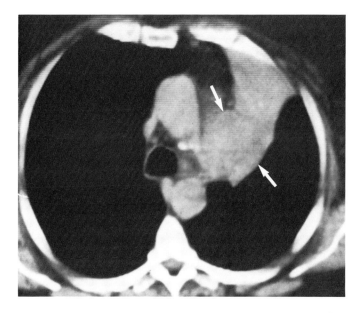 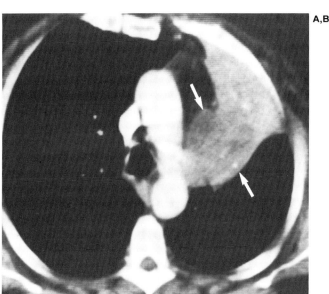

FIG. 30. Epidermoid carcinoma with distal atelectasis. **A:** Precontrast CT image at the level of the aortopulmonary window demonstrates left-upper-lobe collapse. The lobe widens proximally (*arrows*), suggestive of a central obstructing mass. **B:** On a postcontrast image, the proximal mass (*arrows*) is lower in attenuation value and well demarcated from the distal enhancing atelectatic lung.

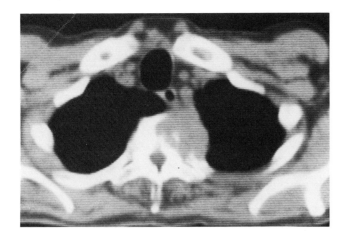

FIG. 31. Superior-sulcus tumor invading adjacent vertebral body.

thick-walled bronchi. In the past, bronchography usually was required for confirmation (or exclusion). However, this procedure not only is uncomfortable for the patient but also is associated with notable morbidity. In recent years, CT, which is clearly safer and easier to perform and causes no patient discomfort, has been used to establish the presence and extent of bronchiectasis (142,152,203) (Figs. 32 and 33).

Although the pathologic types of bronchiectasis have characteristic appearances on CT, differentiation between the various forms is much less important than simple identification of the disease process itself. Recognition of the anatomic changes produced by bronchiectasis and

distinction from the normal pulmonary parenchyma can be improved by obtaining the CT images with narrow collimation (77) (Fig. 34). When the diagnosis is suspected prospectively, this can be accomplished using 2-mm collimation, usually obtained at 10-mm intervals, or, alternatively, 4- to 5-mm collimation at 4- to 5-mm intervals to avoid skipping any area of lung (99).

Using standard collimation (8–10 mm), the normal bronchi usually are seen only in the central and middle portions of the lungs. Cylindrical bronchiectasis can be recognized on CT by the presence of dilated, thick-walled bronchi extending toward the lung periphery. When the changes are confined to the more central zones, allergic bronchopulmonary aspergillosis often is the cause. Such dilated bronchi coursing in a vertical direction appear as small, thick-walled circular lucencies. Branches of the pulmonary artery frequently are adjacent, sometimes producing a "signet-ring" configuration. A small emphysematous bleb usually can be differentiated from focal bronchiectasis because the former has a minimally thick wall and no accompanying vessel. With more advanced varicose bronchiectasis, the walls of the bronchi assume a beaded configuration, which is easier to identify if the involved bronchus has a horizontal course within the imaging plane. With cystic bronchiectasis, small, round, air–fluid collections commonly are seen because of retained secretions in the dependent portions of the dilated bronchi. If the bronchus involved is oriented horizontally, a linear array or cluster of thick-walled cysts may be seen. Branching nodular densities may be noted if the dilated

A,B

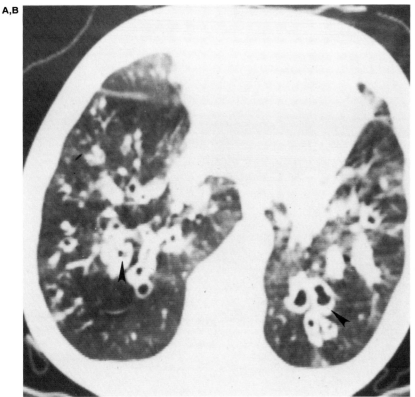

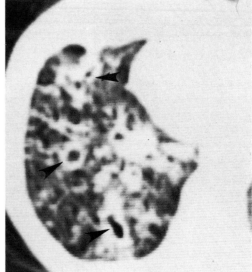

FIG. 32. Cystic bronchiectasis. **A:** Thick-walled, dilated bronchi are seen in both lower lobes, a few containing air–fluid levels (*arrowheads*). **B:** In another patient, thick-walled, dilated bronchi (*arrowheads*) are seen in both the right middle and lower lobes.

A,B

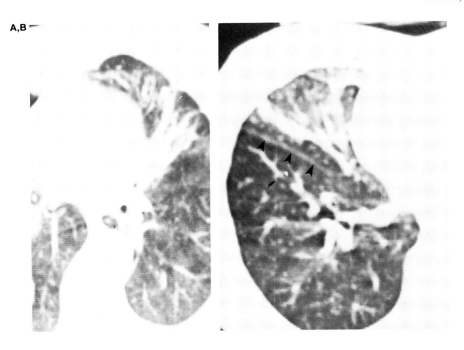

FIG. 33. Tubular bronchiectasis. **A:** An 8-mm collimated CT image demonstrates thick-walled, mildly dilated bronchi, some filled entirely with mucus and secretions, in the lingula. **B:** A 4-mm collimated CT image in another patient demonstrates mildly dilated, mucus-filled bronchi in the middle lobe, just anterior to the major fissure (*arrowheads*).

bronchi are entirely filled with fluid. More than one of these patterns may be present, sometimes on a single section.

Cylindrical bronchiectasis may be quite focal, and the changes produced may be exceedingly subtle or unrecognizable on CT. In addition, the concomitant presence of diseases that may distort or obscure the lung, such as pulmonary fibrosis, consolidation, or emphysema, may mask subtle bronchiectasis and result in false-negative CT findings (98). Although thin collimation, as previously described, improves definition, CT still is not as accurate as bronchography in the detection (or exclusion) of bronchiectasis nor as precise in determining its exact segmental distribution. Especially for the latter reason, bronchog-

raphy may still be required in a patient being considered for surgery. In most patients, however, CT is sufficiently sensitive and specific (both well over 90%) (99) to serve as both a screening procedure and often the definitive diagnostic procedure (especially if the disease is extensive). Another caveat, well recognized with bronchography, is that mildly dilated, somewhat thick-walled bronchi can be identified in patients with acute pneumonia. Yet, unlike true bronchiectasis, which by definition is irreversible, these bronchi may return to normal size when the pulmonary consolidation clears. Therefore, care should be taken in diagnosing bronchiectasis in the presence of acute infection. In questionable cases, a repeat examination can be obtained at a suitable interval following treatment.

A,B

FIG. 34. Tubular bronchiectasis; value of narrow collimation. **A:** Nonspecific patchy infiltrates are seen in the middle lobe and in the superior segment of the right lower lobe on a routine 8-mm collimated CT image. **B:** A 2-mm collimated image at the same level depicts dilated peripheral bronchi in an atelectatic middle lobe.

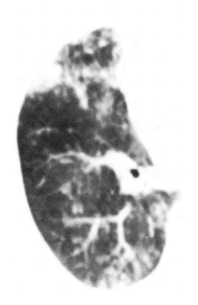
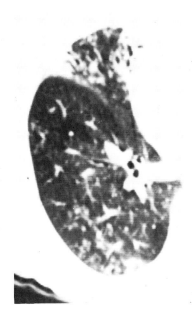

A,B

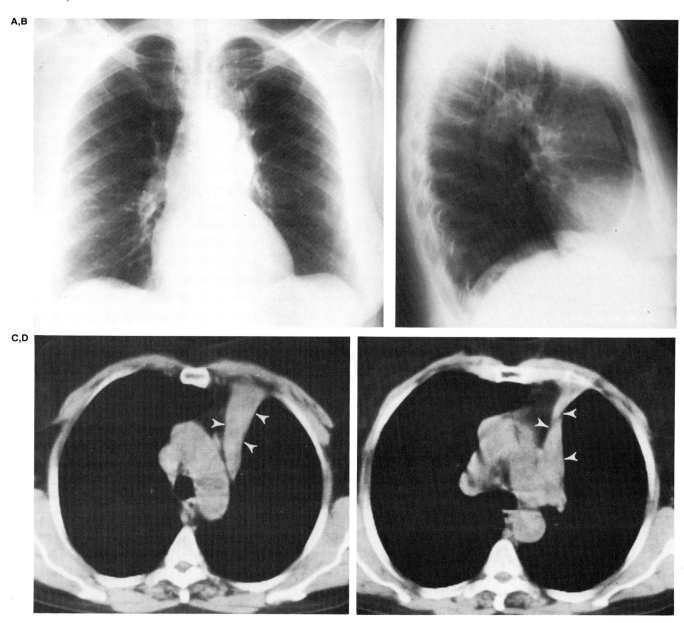

C,D

FIG. 35. Left-upper-lobe collapse. **A,B:** Posteroanterior and lateral roentgenograms show what was initially interpreted as a mass in the region of the pulmonary outflow tract. In retrospect, volume loss can be seen in the left hemithorax. **C,D:** Sequential caudal CT images demonstrate that the ''mass'' was simulated by atelectasis of the apical posterior and anterior segments of the left upper lobe (*arrowheads*). Note the smaller size of the left hemithorax.

Pulmonary Collapse

The patterns of pulmonary collapse seen on the plain chest radiograph have been well described. However, the appearance may be confusing, especially if scarring or adhesions exist between the lung and adjacent pleura. CT often is helpful in clarifying that the findings on plain radiographic film are secondary to collapse (65, 103,148,150,151,159,181) (Fig. 35), and it may also suggest the underlying cause and help determine the presence and extent of an obstructing process. Intravenous contrast material may be helpful in delineating a proximal obstructing tumor and distinguishing it from distal atelectatic lung as well as from adjacent mediastinal structures (Fig. 30). Collapsed lung usually is enhanced to a greater degree than neoplasm. Because this differential enhancement may be apparent only during certain phases of the injection of contrast material, it is important to obtain rapid serial images after bolus injection of contrast material. However, in some cases, distinction may not be possible, despite optimal technique. If the collapsed lung contains a large amount of water (e.g., drowned lung distal to tu-

A,B

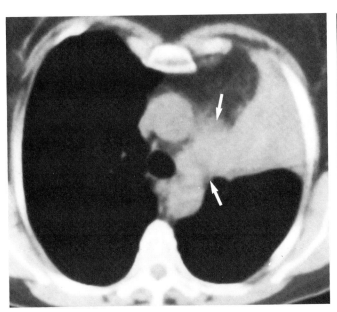 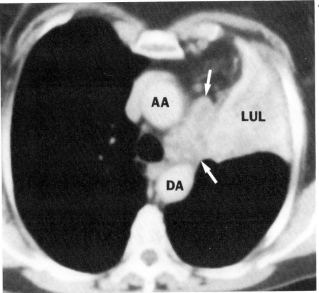

FIG. 36. Left-upper-lobe collapse. **A:** On a precontrast CT image it was uncertain whether the "mass" (*arrows*) in the aortopulmonary window proximal to the collapsed lobe was due to lymphadenopathy or a displaced left pulmonary artery. **B:** Postcontrast image demonstrates lymphadenopathy (*arrows*) separate from the higher-attenuation-value atelectatic lobe (LUL). More caudal images demonstrated a mass obstructing the lobar bronchus; (AA) ascending aorta; (DA) descending aorta.

mor), it may not be enhanced more than the tumor. Also, if the blood supply to the collapsed lobe is obstructed, or if the tumor is vascular, there may not be sufficient differences in enhancement patterns to allow distinction. In addition, with CT, the underlying mediastinum is not obscured by the collapsed lung and can be easily evaluated for coexistent lymphadenopathy (Figs. 24 and 36) or direct invasion by a bronchial neoplasm. Bronchoscopy, however, still plays a vital role in the evaluation of pulmonary collapse, especially in determining the histologic nature of an obstructing lesion.

General Observations

Both the direct (fissural displacement, hypoaeration, vascular/bronchial crowding) and indirect (mediastinal shift, hilar displacement, compensatory hyperaeration, decreased size of hemithorax, elevation of hemidiaphragm) signs of collapse seen on plain chest radiographs (177) can be applied to CT (65). This becomes important so as not to confuse the CT findings with a "mass." The lobes lose volume, while generally maintaining contact with the chest wall peripherally and the hilum centrally, resulting in a wedge shape on CT, which is not always apparent on conventional roentgenography. Although most observations can be made on a standard CT examination (8–10-mm-thick sections), several additional thin sections (4–5 mm) may be helpful in evaluating specific lobar or segmental bronchi for an obstructing mass.

Left-upper-lobe collapse

The left upper lobe (LUL) collapses predominantly in an anterosuperior direction against the anterior chest wall. Superior migration of the lung is limited somewhat by the left pulmonary artery passing over the LUL bronchus. As a result, the superior segment of the left lower lobe (LLL) frequently hyperexpands toward the left-lung apex. On CT, the atelectatic LUL appears as a triangular or V-shaped soft-tissue-density structure that abuts the chest wall anterolaterally, with the apex of the V merging with the pulmonary hilum (Figs. 30, 35, and 36). As the collapse increases, there is less contact of the LUL with the lateral chest wall. The collapsed lobe is bordered medially by the mediastinum and posteriorly by the major fissure, which is displaced anteriorly. Although the lobe usually is of homogeneous soft-tissue density, some crowded air-filled bronchi may be seen. Secondary signs of collapse that are visible include elevation of the left hilum, with foreshortening of the aortopulmonary window, along with mediastinal displacement, usually accompanied by herniation of the right lung anteriorly. With elevation of the left hilum, the LUL bronchus, which is normally lower than the right-upper-lobe bronchus, may be seen at approximately the same level. Moreover, the LLL bronchus may move anterolaterally. If the elevated left pulmonary artery is imaged lateral to the aortic arch, it may simulate lymphadenopathy (Fig. 37). The hyperexpanded superior segment of the LLL frequently extends between the collapsed LUL and aortic arch, accounting for the "periaortic

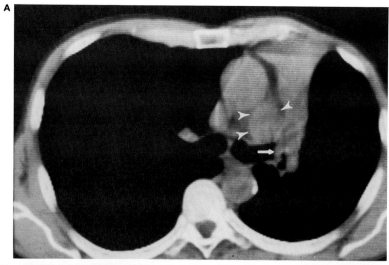

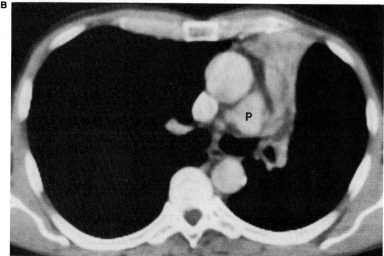

FIG. 37. Left-upper-lobe collapse; no mediastinal lymphadenopathy. **A:** A small, medially convex epidermoid carcinoma (*arrow*) is seen occluding the lobar bronchus. What is the ovoid structure (*arrowheads*) medial to the collapsed lobe? **B:** Postcontrast CT image shows the questionable mass to represent an elevated main pulmonary artery (P).

lucency" seen on the plain chest radiograph. Decreased size of the left hemithorax is also apparent and often is much more striking on CT than on the chest radiograph.

Several findings strongly suggest a proximal obstructing lesion, including bronchial narrowing or an intraluminal mass. It may be necessary to obtain several thin CT sections through the suspected level of obstruction to confidently identify subtle abnormalities. Careful attention to the contour of the collapsed lobe also may be helpful in confirming the presence of a proximal mass. In the absence of a large proximal obstructing lesion, the collapsed lobe should taper smoothly toward the hilum. If the obstructing mass (e.g., bronchogenic carcinoma, lymphadenopathy) is large enough, a contour bulge may be seen. The wedge of lung will be seen to widen focally, rather than taper, as it extends to the hilum (Fig. 30). This is the CT equivalent of the S sign of Golden and may be more apparent than on plain chest radiographs. Although the distinction between benign and malignant neoplasms only can be made histologically, in some cases CT can permit confident identification of a benign cause of obstruction (e.g., broncholithiasis) (Figs. 3 and 6).

Right-upper-lobe collapse

The pattern of right-upper-lobe (RUL) collapse is different than that of LUL collapse because of several anatomic differences between the two lobes. The RUL is smaller than the LUL (which incorporates the lingular division) and has two fissural borders (minor and major fissures). Furthermore, the right main-stem bronchus is more apt to shift as a result of lobar collapse, because it is not fixed at the hilum by the right pulmonary artery. These differences result in the RUL collapsing superiorly and medially, rather than predominantly anteriorly as in LUL collapse. On CT, the collapsed RUL is seen as a sharply defined triangular density bordered by the minor fissure laterally and the major fissure posteriorly (Fig. 38). The minor fissure, which is displaced more than the major fissure, has a straight border, whereas the major fissure may have a straight, concave, or convex border. With RUL collapse, there is elevation of the right hilum. As a result, the right pulmonary artery may be seen at a higher level than normal. In addition, the right main-stem bronchus may rotate anteriorly. Hyperexpansion of the right

A,B

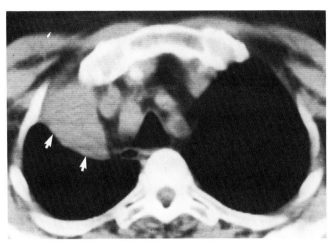 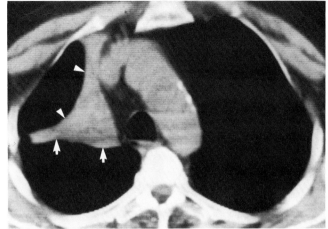

FIG. 38. Right-upper-lobe collapse. **A:** The collapsed lobe appears as a homogeneous triangular soft-tissue density, sharply marginated posteriorly by the right major fissure (*arrows*). **B:** On a more caudal image, both the minor (*arrowheads*) and major (*arrows*) fissures are seen.

middle lobe and RLL also occurs. The superior segment of the RLL may extend between the mediastinum and medial border of the collapsed RUL, but this is a less frequent finding than with collapse of the LUL. Moreover, anterior lung herniation is less common, probably because of the smaller size of the RUL.

Right-middle-lobe collapse

With collapse of the right middle lobe (RML), the minor fissure and lower half of the major fissure move close together. On CT images, the collapsed lobe is triangular or

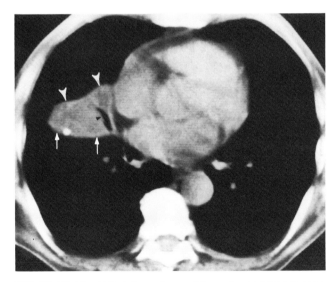

FIG. 39. Right-middle-lobe collapse. The collapsed lobe is seen as a relatively homogeneous wedge-shaped structure adjacent to the right heart border, bordered by the minor (*large arrowheads*) and major (*arrows*) fissures; air is seen in the medial segmental bronchus (*small arrowhead*). (From ref. 65.)

trapezoidal and is demarcated by the minor fissure anteriorly and major fissure posteriorly (Fig. 39). The interface between the RML and RUL frequently is less distinct than that between the RML and RLL, because the minor fissure is more nearly parallel to the imaging plane: The collapsed RML decreases its contact with the lateral chest wall, but maintains its contact with the anterior chest wall on more caudal images. Because of the small volume of the RML, usually there is no significant mediastinal shift, compensatory hyperinflation, or decreased volume of the hemithorax. Segmental middle-lobe collapse, which may be confusing on plain chest radiographs, is easily detected on CT by following the course of the middle-lobe bronchus as it bifurcates into medial and lateral segmental bronchi. The medial segment abuts the heart and anterior chest wall, whereas the lateral segment extends posterior to the hilum and does not contact the heart.

Lower-lobe collapse

The pattern of collapse is similar for the RLL and the LLL. Both collapse caudally, posteriorly, and medially toward the spine. On CT, the collapsed lower lobe appears as a wedged-shaped soft-tissue-density structure adjacent to the spine (Figs. 24 and 40). The major fissure, which forms the lateral border of the lobe, is displaced posteriorly. The upper border of the collapsed lobe usually is concave (in the absence of a large central mass), whereas the lower border may be straight, concave, or convex. The varying configurations relate to the extent of collapse, the presence or absence of a central mass, the degree of distal pneumonia, and the anatomy of the inferior pulmonary ligament. If the attachment of the pulmonary ligament to the hemidiaphragm is incomplete, the lower lobe may collapse more completely adjacent to the spine and have a rounded appearance. Secondary signs of col-

A,B

C,D

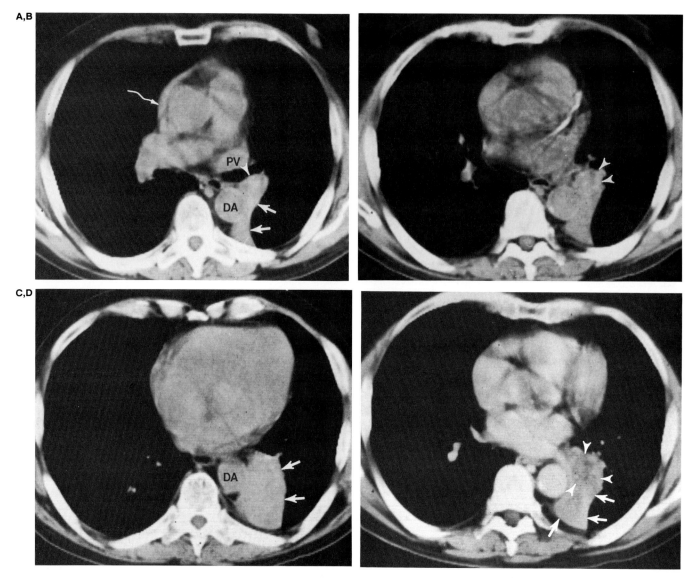

FIG. 40. Left-lower-lobe collapse. **A:** The upper concave lateral border of the atelectatic lobe is formed by the major fissure (*arrows*). A small convex mass (*arrowhead*) is seen occluding the left-lower-lobe bronchus; (*curved arrow*) right atrial appendage; (PV) left superior pulmonary vein; (DA) descending aorta. **B:** Image 2 cm caudal suggests a more extensive proximal obstructing mass because of a laterally convex central-contour bulge (*arrowheads*). **C:** Image 3 cm more caudal demonstrates the bulk of the collapsed left lower lobe (*arrows*); note the decreased size of the left lung; (DA) descending aorta. **D:** CT image, after intravenous administration of contrast material, at a level just caudal to (**B**), separates the enhanced collapsed lobe (*arrows*) from a proximal lower-attenuation-value epidermoid carcinoma (*arrowheads*).

lapse include inferior and medial displacement of the hilum, posteromedial displacement of the lower-lobe bronchus, ipsilateral mediastinal shift and hemidiaphragm elevation, compensatory hyperinflation, and decreased size of the hemithorax.

Role of MRI in Pulmonary Collapse

In most patients, MRI provides information comparable to that from CT with respect to identifying lobar collapse and evaluating the underlying mediastinum (216). Distinction between tumor and distal collapsed lung often is possible using a T2-weighted pulse sequence (Fig. 41). On T2-weighted images, the collapsed lung usually is higher in signal intensity than the more proximal tumor, most likely reflecting the higher water content of the collapsed lung. Because the water contents of tumors and collapsed lobes vary, distinction is not always possible. MRI is inferior to CT in delineating bronchial anatomy, and bronchial narrowing may be overestimated because of respiratory motion and poorer spatial resolution.

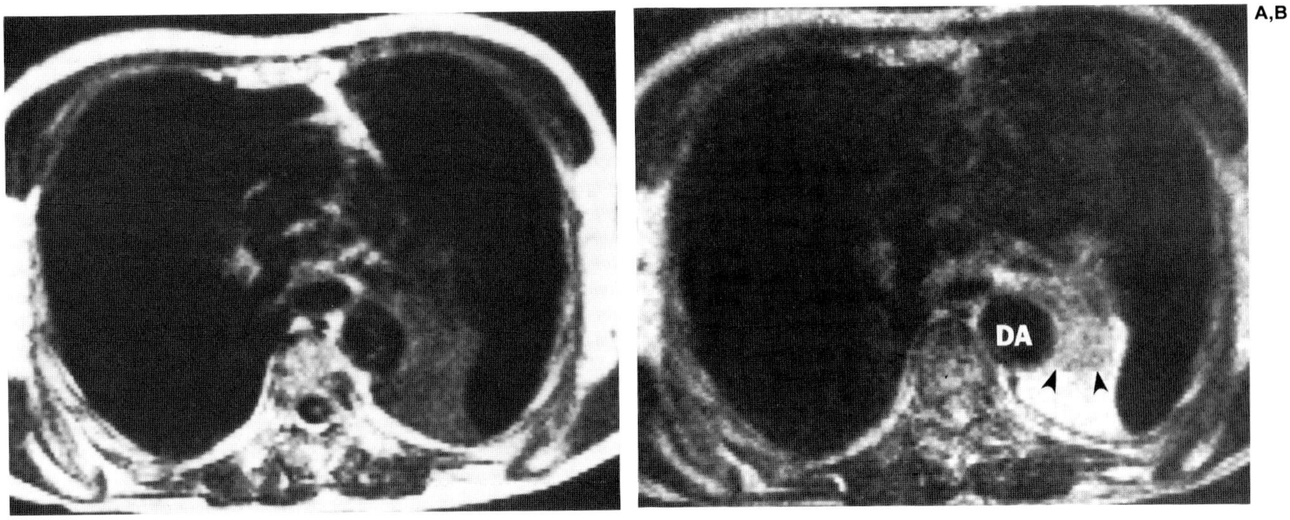

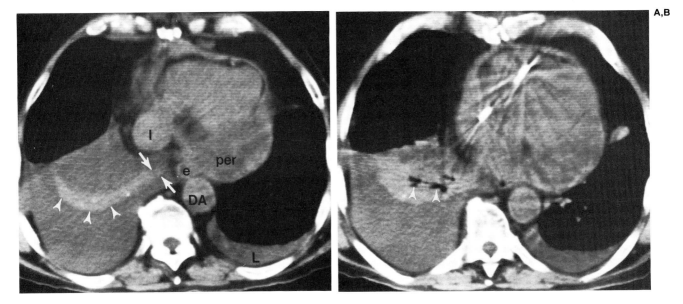

FIG. 41. Left-lower-lobe collapse. **A:** On T1-weighted MR image, the proximal obstructing mass and peripheral collapsed lung are both of medium signal intensity and indistinguishable. **B:** On T2-weighted MR image, the lower-intensity proximal bronchogenic carcinoma (*arrowheads*) is easily distinguished from the higher-intensity collapsed lung; (DA) descending aorta. (From ref. 216.)

Compressive Atelectasis

Compressive (or passive) atelectasis most frequently occurs secondary to fluid within the pleural space. Whereas a large pleural effusion can obscure parenchymal disease on the plain chest radiograph, CT can demonstrate atelectatic lung underlying the pleural effusion (166) (Fig. 42). If the bronchus is patent and air bronchograms are seen throughout the lobe, proximal obstruction is unlikely.

The distinction between the lower-density pleural fluid and relatively higher density collapsed lung can be appreciated on non-contrast-enhanced images, but the difference is accentuated by intravenous contrast material (Fig. 43). In patients with malignant pleural disease, the lung may be compressed by tumor masses as well as by pleural fluid. Neoplasm within the pleural space also is more easily seen following intravenous administration of contrast material.

FIG. 42. Pleural effusion with compressive atelectasis. **A:** A compressed right lower lobe (*arrowheads*) is surrounded by a moderate-size right pleural effusion; the medially extending inferior pulmonary ligament (*arrows*) divides the pleural space into anterior and posterior compartments. Pericardial thickening and a posteriorly loculated pericardial effusion (per) are also noted; (L) small left pleural effusion; (e) esophagus; (I) inferior vena cava; (DA) descending aorta. **B:** That the compressed right lower lobe is not a thickened diaphragm is convincingly demonstrated on an image 1 cm cephalad that shows contiguity with air bronchograms in the atelectatic lobe (*arrowheads*).

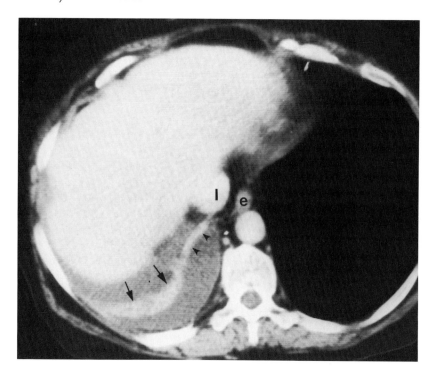

FIG. 43. Enhanced compressive atelectasis. On a postcontrast CT image, the enhanced atelectatic right lower lobe (*arrows*) is seen adjacent to the nonenhanced pleural effusion. The inferior pulmonary ligament (*arrowhead*) tethers the collapsed lobe to the mediastinum; (l) inferior vena cava; (e) esophagus.

The patterns of compressive atelectasis secondary to pleural effusion relate, in part, to the size of the pleural effusion. With small effusions, CT may demonstrate only segmental collapse of a lower lobe, seen anterior to the pleural effusion. The major fissure is visible farther anterior to the remainder of the aerated lower lobe. As the pleural effusion increases in size, most of the lower lobe is collapsed, and the major fissure is no longer visible as a discrete structure. With larger effusions, fluid can be seen extending into the major fissure anterior to the collapsed lobe. The inferior pulmonary ligament can be identified transfixing the medial border of the lower lobe to the mediastinum and dividing the medial pleural space into anterior and posterior compartments (56,188).

Cicatrization Atelectasis

Cicatrization atelectasis refers to volume loss secondary to scarring from previous inflammatory disease (151). Endobronchial obstruction is not present. The degree of volume loss usually is more marked than in cases of collapse secondary to endobronchial obstruction. Associated bronchiectatic changes and pleural thickening frequently are present. The pattern of collapse may be altered, probably secondary to pleural adhesions and parenchymal scarring. For example, the cicatrized RUL may collapse more posteriorly, with posterior rotation of the carina and RUL bronchus.

Rounded Atelectasis

Rounded atelectasis is a form of nonsegmental pulmonary collapse that may mimic a neoplasm. It is prob-

ably the residue of a previous pleural effusion, with entrapment of a peripheral portion of the underlying lung. This pulmonary pseudotumor is composed of a swirl of atelectatic parenchyma adjacent to thickened pleura. The subsequent mass may be 3 to 5 cm in diameter and most frequently is found in a basal and dorsal location. Although conventional radiography and tomography may demonstrate characteristic findings, especially a "tail" adjacent to the medial aspect of the mass, CT can be helpful in depicting the full extent of the disease process and confirming the diagnosis (44). The CT findings include (a) a rounded or oval mass that forms an acute angle with thickened pleura, with the pleura usually thickest at its contact with the mass, (b) vessels and bronchi converging in a curvilinear fashion into the lower border of the mass (CT equivalent of the "tail" or "comet" sign), (c) air bronchograms in the central portion of the mass (the periphery of the mass may be denser because it represents the area of most complete atelectasis), and (d) adjacent hyperinflated lung (Fig. 44). Rounded atelectasis often is associated with a history of asbestos exposure (132,221). In these patients, CT frequently demonstrates pleural plaques or parenchymal fibrosis in other areas of the thorax. Rounded atelectasis usually remains stable on serial radiographic studies; very slow growth may occur. In the majority of cases, the CT findings are so characteristic that further evaluation usually is not necessary. However, if the CT findings are equivocal, percutaneous needle biopsy of the "mass" can be very valuable for clarification; a specimen demonstrating fibrosis only solidifies the diagnosis.

A,B

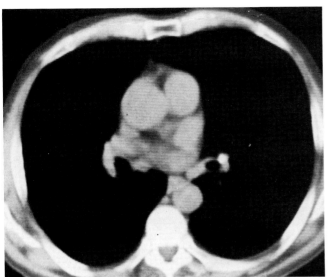

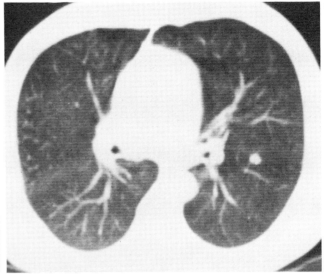

C

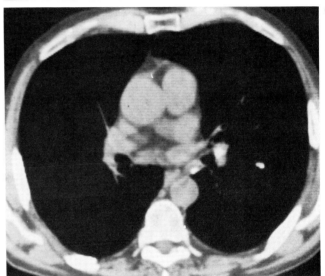

FIG. 47. Calcified pulmonary nodule. **A:** A left-lower-lobe pulmonary nodule is only faintly visible on the mediastinal window setting of a standard 8-mm-collimated CT image. A calcified left hilar lymph node is present. **B:** The nodule is easily seen on the lung window setting of the same image. **C:** A 2-mm collimated image through the nodule, overcoming the partial-volume-averaging effect, demonstrates that diffuse calcification is present within it, as well as in two hilar lymph nodes.

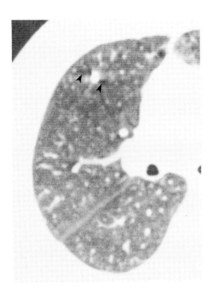

FIG. 48. Calcified pulmonary nodule. A 2-mm-collimated CT image demonstrates artifactual low-density streaking (*arrowheads*) adjacent to the nodule.

caudad to obtain sequential sections through the lesion; in cooperative patients, several images often can be obtained during a single breath-holding maneuver. The section in which the nodule is largest is chosen for analysis. If the nodule contains visible diffuse calcifications (which can be corroborated by cursor circle measurement), no further evaluation is necessary (Fig. 47). Linear, low-density artifactual streaking is sometimes seen adjacent to a calcified nodule (Fig. 48). Occasionally, other features are detected that permit confident diagnosis of a benign lesion, such as lucent areas of fat within the nodule consistent with a hamartoma (111,200). Similarly, an apparent solitary pulmonary nodule on conventional radiography may be shown on CT to represent part of a more extensive pulmonary parenchymal process (Fig. 49), pleural thickening, or a benign rib lesion, rather than a true intraparenchymal nodule. Conversely, in areas that are difficult to depict on standard radiographs, such as the lung bases or the paraspinal regions, CT may confirm the nodular nature of a questionable abnormality. Although there are

A

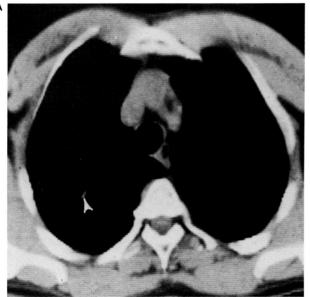

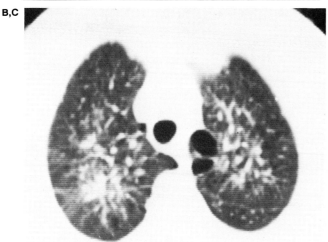

B,C

FIG. 49. Not solitary pulmonary nodules. **A:** CT image at a mediastinal window setting demonstrates an apparently solitary right-upper-lobe nodule (*arrowhead*), initially detected on a chest radiograph. **B:** Lung window setting at the same level discloses that the lesion is simply the largest of multiple bilateral upper-lobe nodules, surrounded by some emphysematous bullae. A history of prior silica exposure was subsequently obtained. **C:** In another patient thought to have an irregular pulmonary nodule in the right pulmonary apex on a conventional radiograph, CT shows only linear fibrotic changes in the area.

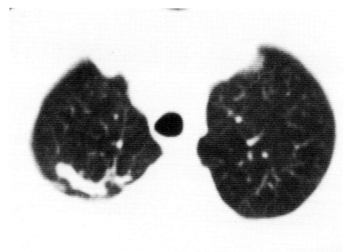

no pathognomonic radiologic features of a malignant pulmonary lesion, thin-section CT may strongly suggest that a small peripheral nodule represents a primary lung carcinoma (110). An outer margin that has a spiculated interface with lung (Fig. 50), is notched, or is hazy and less dense than centrally favors a malignant neoplasm. Convergence of a small peripheral pulmonary vessel and focal pleural retraction toward the lesion are additional signs of a malignant lesion. A heterogeneous internal composition, especially with small areas of necrosis, supports the diagnosis of a carcinoma.

If the nodular lesion in question is well circumscribed and not clearly benign, the attenuation values within it should be determined (Fig. 51). In the original investigation, a nodule containing representative CT numbers above 164 HU was considered calcified and benign (201). But using this criterion, others reported divergent results (68); explanations for these discrepancies are now well

established. A point that cannot be overemphasized is that CT numbers used for tissue characterization are not quantitatively absolute; they are relative values influenced by a variety of inherent technical and geometric factors (113,127,128,184,242). The numbers can vary substantially depending on the size and position of the object to be measured and the surrounding medium (beam-hardening effect), the reconstruction algorithm used, and the photon noise (scanning time, amperage). Attenuation values from a given lesion can be quite disparate when the images are generated by machines from different manufacturers with discordant hardware and software. Notable variations can occur with a given scanner from day to day because of voltage or detector drift. Therefore, it is impossible to establish a universal value that would document the presence of calcification within a pulmonary nodule.

The most practical method of overcoming these in-

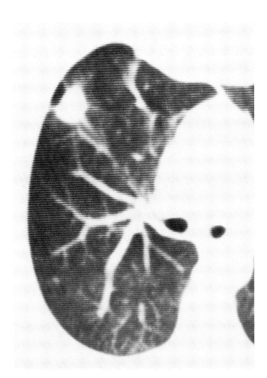

FIG. 50. Bronchogenic carcinoma. CT image with standard collimation demonstrates spiculated, irregular margins of the nodule, with infiltration into the surrounding pulmonary parenchyma.

trascanner and interscanner variations has been to develop an external standard, with the nodule measured (density assessed) relative to the standard. The anthropomorphic reference phantom devised by Zerhouni et al. (240) has proved helpful and reliable. Various attachments allow sufficient reproduction of patient anatomy at the level of the nodule to simulate the influence of surrounding structures. Small plastic rods of varying sizes, containing an amount of calcium adjusted to the 164-HU level derived from the original report, serve as the reference nodules. Because the CT density of a large lung nodule is always higher than that of a smaller nodule of identical composition, the simulated nodule chosen should never be smaller than the true nodule being measured.

Immediately after imaging the patient's nodule with thin collimation, the phantom and its attached parts are mounted on the scanning support in a configuration that is as similar as possible to the patient's anatomy at the level of the nodule. The phantom and an appropriate-size reference nodule are imaged using exactly the same technical factors used for the patient (Fig. 52). The images are then compared on a display monitor. By using a very narrow window width, it is easy to determine whether the patient's nodule is more or less dense than the reference nodule. A diagnosis of benign disease is rendered only when a substantial portion of the lesion exhibits attenuation values equivalent to or in excess of the reference standard. Such mean or threshold values must be located

centrally within the nodule, so as not to mistake a small calcified granuloma engulfed by a growing neoplasm for a benign lesion (Fig. 53). Also, the margins of the lesion must be relatively smooth (usually already established by conventional roentgenography) in order to permit confident diagnosis of a benign lesion, because a small percentage of primary bronchogenic carcinomas may contain foci of dystrophic calcification (73,213) (Fig. 54). This is most typically found in larger lesions, which almost always have markedly irregular margins. Relatively large and central carcinoid tumors also may contain foci of calcification; a clue to the proper cause is their location immediately adjacent to a secondary bronchus (Fig. 55). Motion artifacts may create spuriously high CT numbers. They typically are linear and usually are easily recognized on the image, extending through and outside the nodule. In such circumstances, most common with small lesions located near the heart border because of transmitted cardiac pulsations (Fig. 56), no conclusion should be reached regarding the attenuation value of the nodule. Similarly, falsely high numbers can occur with cavitary lesions, with streaking off the air interface; densitometry has no role in their characterization. As with conventional radiography, there are no pathognomonic features on CT to differentiate the various causes for cavitary lesions (Fig. 57).

Using this technique, a cooperative study from 10 institutions (243) demonstrated that approximately 17% (range 9–30%) of small solitary pulmonary nodules (8–30 mm in diameter) not seen to be definitely calcified on conventional radiographs can be diagnosed as benign when their attenuation values are equivalent to or higher than that of the reference nodule. Because thinly collimated images are "noisier" and subject to greater statistical variation, and it is known that malignant neoplasms may contain calcification, it is generally judicious to obtain a follow-up chest radiographic study in 3 to 6 months to

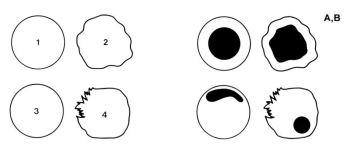

FIG. 51. Schematic drawing of representative pulmonary nodules. **A:** Edge analysis. Nodules 1 and 3 are sharp and smooth, whereas 2 is slightly lobulated. Nodule 4 has one edge that is spiculated; this type of lesion can never be diagnosed confidently as benign solely on the basis of CT. **B:** Patterns of calcification in the same nodules. Nodules 1 and 2 have extensive central calcification and are compatible with benign healed granulomas. Nodules 3 and 4 contain eccentric calcifications and do not meet the criteria for diagnosis of a benign lesion. (Adapted from ref. 199.)

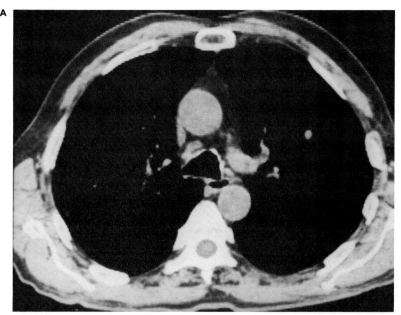

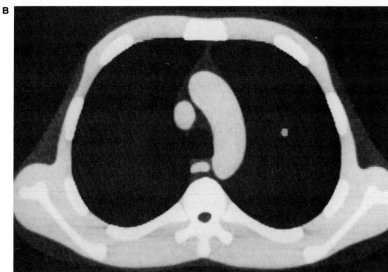

FIG. 52. Densitometry with anthropomorphic phantom. **A:** No calcification is visible within a well-circumscribed left-upper-lobe nodule on a 2-mm-collimated CT image reconstructed with a high-spatial-frequency algorithm. **B:** Simulated nodule imaged in phantom using the same technical factors. The attenuation values were slightly higher throughout the real nodule, enabling confident determination that it contained diffuse calcifications and was presumptively benign.

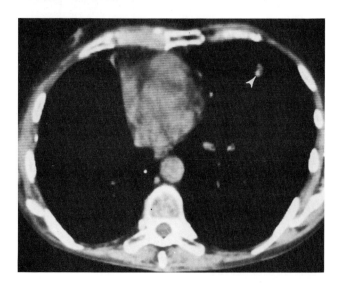

FIG. 53. Only eccentric calcification (*arrowhead*) was detected on a 2-mm-collimated CT image through a lobulated lingular nodule. Subsequent surgical resection disclosed a scar adenocarcinoma adjacent to a granuloma.

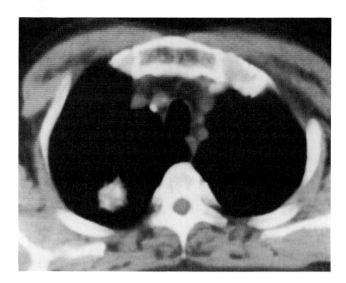

FIG. 54. Calcified epidermoid carcinoma. Diffuse punctate calcifications are seen throughout a right-upper-lobe nodule. However, the margins of the nodule are markedly irregular, precluding diagnosis of a benign lesion.

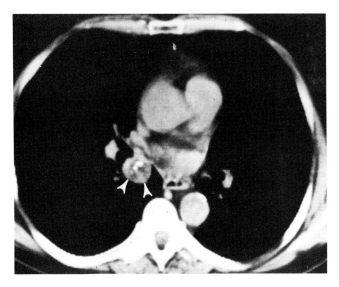

FIG. 55. Calcified carcinoid tumor. A well-circumscribed mass (*arrowheads*) containing punctate calcifications and arising from the superior segmental bronchus of the right lower lobe is noted to be located predominantly extrabronchially.

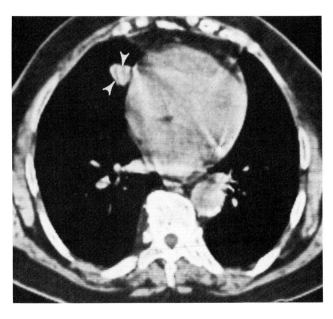

FIG. 56. Artifactual streaking due to transmitted cardiac pulsations is seen through a middle-lobe nodule (*arrowheads*) on a 2-mm-collimated CT image, preventing reliable determination of attenuation values.

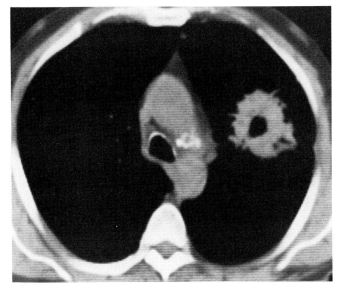

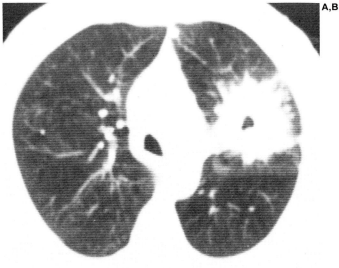

A,B

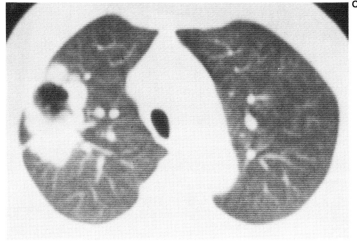

C

FIG. 57. Thick-walled cavitary masses. **A,B:** CT images at mediastinal and lung window settings, respectively, demonstrate a thick-walled left-upper-lobe cavity with irregular spiculated outer margins due to infection (torulosis). An additional small nodular infectious focus is seen just to the left of the anterior junction line. Calcification of the undersurface of the aortic arch is present. **C:** In another patient, a similar-appearing right upper cavity with lobulated outer margins is due to primary epidermoid carcinoma.

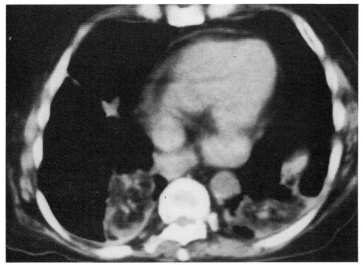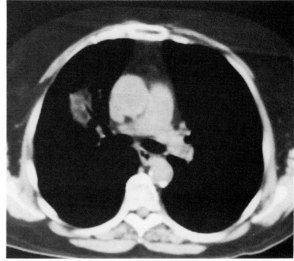

A,B

FIG. 58. Lipoid pneumonias. **A:** Fat-density areas are seen scattered throughout bilateral lower lobe "masses." **B:** Similar regions of fat density are seen in a solitary, irregular right-upper-lobe mass in another patient.

corroborate that the nodule has a stable growth pattern. The remaining nodules that are less dense than a comparable reference nodule are classified as indeterminate. Depending on the clinical situation, they may be surgically removed, biopsied via a percutaneous needle, or perhaps followed closely, with repeat chest radiographs and possible CT at 2- to 6-month intervals.

Alternative techniques may soon be available to determine precisely the amount of calcium present within a pulmonary nodule. Dual-energy CT imaging is one possible option (27). At low voltage levels, the CT numbers of a calcified nodule increase relative to the CT numbers obtained with higher voltage, whereas there would be no change with noncalcified nodules. However, maximal accuracy requires obtaining the data during the same suspended respiration and imaging cycle, and the X-ray-tube voltage cannot be switched so rapidly on most current scanners. Similar dual-energy techniques using digital radiography (or even digitized radiographs) may become quicker and less costly to perform. Whether or not these methods will be too sensitive to the detection of calcium (i.e., discovering very small amounts in neoplasms) is unknown.

A few other pulmonary masses besides healed granulomas may be diagnosed confidently with CT. As mentioned, small areas of fat density within a well-circumscribed nodule may be seen in a hamartoma. Large areas of fat within an irregular pulmonary mass or consolidated area strongly suggest exogenous lipoid pneumonia (235) (Fig. 58). Obtaining a history of chronic use of mineral oil or using percutaneous needle-aspiration biopsy can corroborate the diagnosis. Congenital bronchial atresia can be recognized by hyperinflated lung surrounding the mass-like, dilated, mucoid-filled bronchus (32,179) (Fig. 4). A variety of pulmonary lesions that either are com-

posed of abnormal vessels or have an aberrant blood supply can simulate a solitary lung nodule on chest radiography. Such abnormalities include a pulmonary arteriovenous malformation (see Fig. 10 in Chapter 7), pulmonary vein varix, and sequestration (Fig. 59). These entities sometimes can be definitively diagnosed with dynamic CT imaging following a bolus intravenous injection of contrast material, thus obviating angiography or directing further appropriate evaluation (4,71,168,183,227). Visual inspection of this rapid series of images almost always suffices to determine whether the vascular supply is primarily from the pulmonary artery or the aorta. If the lesion opacifies in phase with the pulmonary artery or vein, it is supplied by the pulmonary artery; if its peak opacification coincides with or immediately follows peak aortic enhancement, then its vascular supply is primarily systemic. Although some very vascular neoplasms, such as carcinoid tumor, can show an increase in CT number after contrast injection, the degree of opacification is less than that of the vascular lesions, and the enhancement persists for a longer period. MRI also may be used to define and characterize the size and course of anomalous arterial feeding vessels (82,155). Multiplanar imaging capabilities and nonreliance on contrast material to depict blood vessels may be valuable assets in their demonstration.

Occult Pulmonary Metastases

As cancer therapies have become increasingly successful and sophisticated, establishing the presence of pulmonary metastases often is important because it may dictate some modification of treatment or management. In the initial evaluation and follow-up of most patients with primary

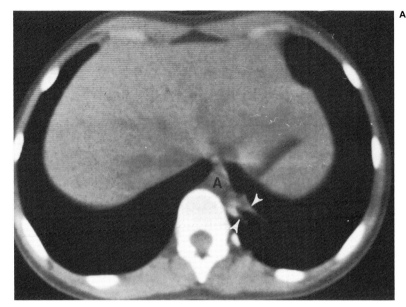

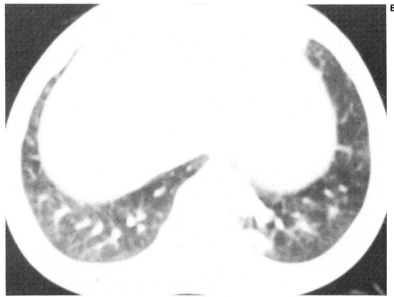

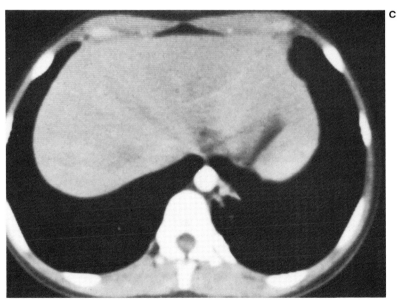

FIG. 59. Pulmonary sequestration. **A:** Branching structures (*arrowheads*) are demonstrated arising from the descending thoracic aorta (A) on a mediastinal window setting. **B:** On a lung window setting at the same level, a nodular infiltrate is seen in the adjacent left lower lobe, first detected on a chest radiograph in this 12-year-old boy. **C:** CT image following a bolus intravenous injection of contrast material demonstrates enhancement of vessels arising from the aorta.

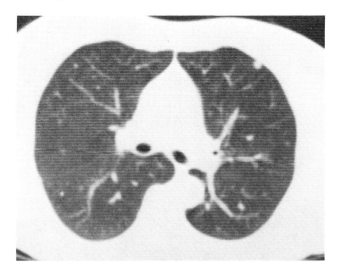

FIG. 60. Occult pulmonary metastasis. An 8-mm nodule is seen in the periphery of the left upper lobe that was not detected on prior conventional chest radiographs and tomograms.

neoplasms, standard chest radiography is the only radiological examination required. This diagnostic approach is dictated by its relatively low cost and good sensitivity, plus the difficulty of treating most lung metastases. CT is valuable in selected circumstances as a more sensitive method for identifying small metastases that are undetectable or poorly seen by standard chest radiography or tomography.

Noncalcified pulmonary nodules smaller than 6 mm in diameter generally will not be seen with conventional radiographic techniques, whereas those larger than 15 mm should be readily detectable (37). Not only is the size of the lesion important, but also the nature of the surrounding anatomic structures greatly affects detection. Certain unfavorable locations tend to mask lesions unless they are relatively large. Overlying bones, blood vessels, or the heart can obscure the outline of a nodule. Nodules about 6 mm in diameter usually are seen only when they are projected directly over rib interspaces. The vast majority of pulmonary metastases resulting from hematogenous dissemination occur in the peripheral third of the lung, frequently in a subpleural location (193). Such subpleural nodules may be difficult to detect even on conventional tomography, as the blurring produced by this technique frequently is insufficient to erase the obscuring densities of the overlying chest wall. The added yield of CT in detecting otherwise occult pulmonary nodules is in large part attributable to elimination of structural overlap. The transverse cross-sectional display of CT affords a more nearly ideal demonstration of these peripherally situated lung lesions, as well as improved detection of nodules in the retrocardiac, retrosternal, and perihilar areas, in the inferior recesses near the domes of the hemidiaphragms, and in the extreme lung apices (Figs. 60–62). In addition, the inherent superior contrast sensitivity of CT and the ability to make photographic adjustments also decrease

observer error. Pulmonary nodules frequently are overlooked on the "gray-on-gray format" of conventional chest radiographs or whole-lung tomograms in which the lesions lack a marked contrast difference from the surrounding parenchyma. The ability to display lung nodules on the CT format as white structures against the black background of the lung, rather than as light gray nodules against a darker gray background, enhances their density differences and consequently their detectability. Particularly with lesions 3 to 6 mm in diameter, CT frequently demonstrates one or more lung nodules when plain film tomography shows none, two or more nodules when tomography reveals only one, or bilateral nodules when tomography demonstrates only unilateral disease (133,140). Also, CT images the mediastinum and chest wall as well as the upper abdomen, with unsuspected metastases sometimes detected in these regions.

Identifying pulmonary nodules on CT generally is quite straightforward. Most lung metastases are round and well circumscribed, although some have irregular infiltrating margins; rarely, a predominantly interstitial ("lymphangitic") pattern occurs, which will be discussed later. If the nodular density is in the periphery of the lung and is separate from and larger than adjacent vascular structures located a similar distance from the chest wall, then the density represents a nodule. Because the lung is divided into lobes, a nodular metastasis may appear relatively central and yet actually be located subpleurally adjacent to a fissure. When pulmonary nodules are similar in size or smaller than vessels in the same area, interpretation is more difficult, and these lesions may be overlooked. Viewing sequential images is imperative; if the suspected lesion is continuous with a vascular structure on adjacent images, the density probably represents a vessel rather

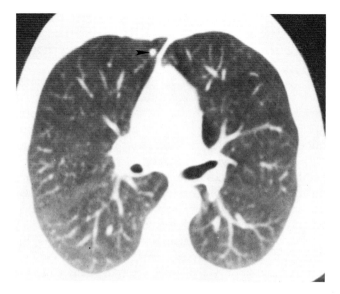

FIG. 61. An otherwise occult pulmonary metastasis (*arrowhead*) is detected just lateral to the anterior junction line.

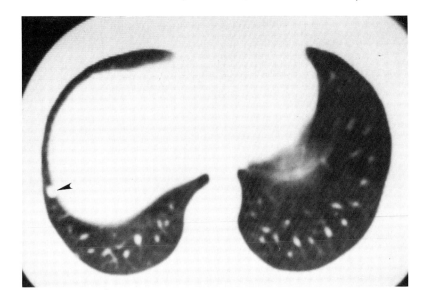

FIG. 62. An otherwise occult pulmonary metastasis (*arrowhead*) is seen just lateral to the right hemidiaphragm.

than a nodule. Repeating images of the area with the patient in a different position (prone, decubitus) sometimes is valuable in clarifying a suspicious nodular density (206); a vessel often changes in size and shape, whereas a true nodule is unaltered. Although 3 mm generally is accepted as the lower limit of detectability for peripheral lesions, more centrally located nodules must be 6 mm in size to be consistently distinguished from a vessel on the cross-sectional image. A pulmonary metastasis also may be missed on CT when a nodule goes undetected because it lies in a "skip area" produced by inconsistency in the depth of suspended respiration, which may vary up to 10 mm near the diaphragm even in cooperative patients (106). To diminish this problem, performing CT at end-tidal volume has been advocated if the primary objective of the study is to search for pulmonary metastases. Unnoticed patient movement in the scanner can result in similar exclusion of a portion of lung from the examination. Careful analysis of the CT images in a sequential fashion is mandatory to identify any missing anatomic levels.

Occasionally, the CT examination will detect a small linear density, sometimes irregular or angulated, in the periphery of the lung. Such a shape is not characteristic of a metastasis, which typically is round or lobulated, but rather is more consistent with a scar or focal atelectasis (79). A repeat image in approximately 2 months may be helpful if further clarification is required. Normal structures, such as the anterior portion of the first rib and costal cartilage (see Fig. 117 in Chapter 7), should not be mistakenly identified as a pulmonary nodule.

Although CT is more sensitive than conventional radiological studies in detecting small pulmonary nodules, a major limitation is that there are other causes besides metastases for such nodules (70,94,192). They can represent residue from previous infection or inflammation, an intrapulmonary lymph node, as well as a benign or primary malignant lung neoplasm. In areas where granulomatous disease (e.g., histoplasmosis) is endemic, approximately 30% of occult pulmonary nodules detected by CT are benign, even in patients with documented primary extrathoracic neoplasms. Nevertheless, most pulmonary nodules discovered, particularly in the pediatric age group (34) or in adults from areas in which granulomatous disease is rare, do represent metastases. And the more nodules detected, the greater is the presumption that metastases are present. Short of performing a limited thoracotomy for definitive histologic diagnosis (38), because fiberoptic bronchoscopy or percutaneous needle-aspiration biopsy would have exceedingly low yields with these small peripheral nodules, a repeat CT examination after waiting a period of approximately 6 weeks may be required before a definitive distinction between metastasis and granuloma is attempted. An increase in size or number of the nodules on the follow-up CT study may be assumed to represent *de facto* evidence of metastatic disease.

Not all patients with extrathoracic malignant neoplasms should undergo thoracic CT examination. Because of its relatively high cost, plus the problem of lack of tissue specificity, the clinical decision whether or not to proceed to a CT study when findings on chest roentgenography are negative should be based on answers to the following questions: (a) Would the demonstration of pulmonary metastases alter the clinical management of the patient's primary tumor? (b) What is the propensity of the specific type of tumor to metastasize to the lungs? (c) Is there effective therapy available for metastatic disease of this tumor type? If the overall incidence of lung metastases from the given tumor being evaluated is very low (e.g., stage I carcinoma of the cervix) (1,31), the extra effort to detect occult pulmonary nodules is not justified. However, with selected primary malignant neoplasms, an accurate assessment of the extent of metastatic disease may be crucial in reaching a therapeutic decision. CT will be indicated in some patients with primary tumors that have a high propensity for pulmonary metastases (e.g., osteosarcoma, melanoma of Clark level IV or V) (87,222), particularly when a major operation is being considered (e.g., amputation, extensive lymph node dissection) or when the likelihood of detecting additional lesions is high (e.g., presumed solitary lung metastasis or several closely grouped nodules in a lobe when surgical resection is being contemplated). CT may occasionally be used to provide a "road map" for surgical removal of metastases and may help to determine if a single procedure (i.e., a median sternotomy) or staging thoracotomies are required when bilateral lesions are present. Whole-lung CT can have a major clinical impact and is warranted in such patients when the detection of an otherwise occult nodule or nodules would alter treatment, including the institution of chemotherapy. In such circumstances, imaging evaluation beyond the standard chest radiograph is indicated, and CT should be the next examination performed because it is the most sensitive radiologic method for detection of pulmonary metastases, demonstrating more and smaller nodules than conventional tomography. Whereas MRI occasionally can demonstrate pulmonary nodules in close proximity to blood vessels that were undetected by CT (143), for the vast majority of patients either the techniques are equivalent or CT is superior because its greater spatial resolution permits better detection of nodules situated close to the pleura or diaphragm, as well as their relationship to a fissure. MRI should be reserved for a problem-solving role in very selected cases.

Other Occult Pulmonary Processes

Some lung lesions may be difficult to see or characterize on conventional radiographs because they are partially obscured or hidden by superimposed structures, such as tortuous mediastinal vessels, the heart, or the chest wall. Sometimes, technical factors, such as marked obesity or the inability of the patient to stand or sit, preclude optimal roentgenographic evaluation of a pulmonary process. CT commonly shows parenchymal pulmonary infiltrates, particularly in the lower lobes, due to aspiration or lung contusion in patients after nonpenetrating trauma for whom the chest radiograph (usually a supine portable) showed normal findings (135). A gas collection seen within the consolidated area immediately after trauma is indicative of a pulmonary laceration. In the immunosuppressed patient with a confluent bronchopneumonia noted on a portable chest radiograph, CT may be valuable in suggesting an earlier diagnosis of invasive pulmonary aspergillosis; a nonspecific pulmonary mass is seen surrounded by a zone of lower attenuation value (the "halo" sign) due to edema (108). On occasion, despite good-quality conventional chest radiographs, pathologic processes involving the lung parenchyma may be detectable on CT when findings on the former study are negative. These include small, otherwise occult cavitary lung lesions (22,107), emphysema, and interstitial disease due to a variety of causes. In addition, CT is more sensitive for detecting subtle (early) cavitation within a known nodule, and it can provide thorough assessment of the thickness and nodularity of the cavity wall. Early in the development of an aspergilloma, CT may demonstrate an irregular sponge-like network filling the cavity (186), before a mobile mass later becomes demonstrable (Fig. 63).

Diffuse Parenchymal Disease

Because of its low cost and excellent spatial resolution, plain chest radiography continues to be the primary imaging technique for evaluating diffuse parenchymal lung

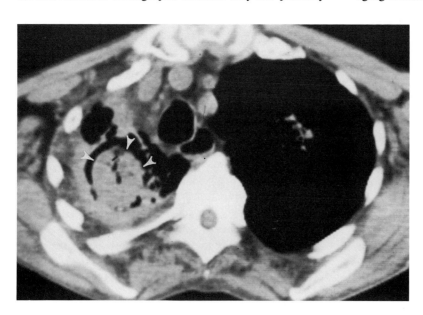

FIG. 63. Fungus ball (aspergilloma). In a patient previously treated for tuberculosis, a round mass (*arrowheads*) containing some aerated branching areas is seen in a right apical cavity. Marked surrounding pleural thickening is present, accompanied by notable volume loss in the right hemithorax. Parenchymal scarring also is present in the left upper lobe.

A, B

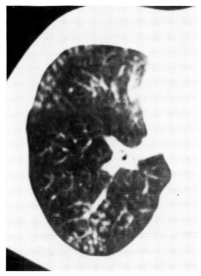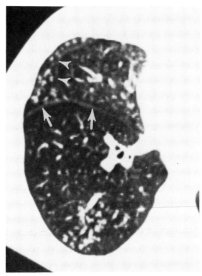

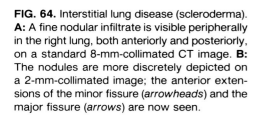

FIG. 64. Interstitial lung disease (scleroderma). **A:** A fine nodular infiltrate is visible peripherally in the right lung, both anteriorly and posteriorly, on a standard 8-mm-collimated CT image. **B:** The nodules are more discretely depicted on a 2-mm-collimated image; the anterior extensions of the minor fissure (*arrowheads*) and the major fissure (*arrows*) are now seen.

disease. However, the superior contrast sensitivity and the cross-sectional imaging plane of CT that diminishes superimposition may allow earlier detection and better characterization of diffuse pulmonary disease (16, 58,145,158,160,208,212,241), especially when the CT studies are performed using high-resolution 1.5- to 2-mm thin sections and edge-enhancement algorithms (125). With this technique, which results in much higher spatial resolution approaching that of conventional radiography, portions of the interlobular septa are commonly visible. It is unlikely that most diffuse parenchymal processes can be distinguished reliably with MRI on the basis of differences in signal intensity, although alveolar proteinosis may have notably short T1 values (137). However, MRI may be potentially useful in assessing disease activity (129).

Technique

Initially the thorax is studied with 8- to 10-mm-thick sections. Because all pathologic processes are higher in density than the normal lung, often they will be easily visible on these sections, which also allow easier orientation of blood vessels and bronchi. In patients known to have or suspected of having diffuse parenchymal disease, representative thin sections (1.5–2 mm) are obtained in the upper, middle, and lower lung or in the region of interest, as determined by thick-section CT or chest radiograph; reconstruction with a high-spatial-frequency algorithm for selected areas at several predetermined levels enhances spatial resolution. In many patients, especially those with thick chest walls, higher amperage settings may be valuable to decrease image noise. The role of high-resolution CT is to better define and characterize abnormalities already suspected from the conventional CT images (Fig. 64); it is exceedingly unlikely to be productive if findings on the original images are negative.

Lung Densitometry

Because CT numbers are linearly proportional to physical density and electron density, CT may have a role in the detection of diffuse pulmonary diseases that increase or decrease lung density. The diffuse interstitial lung diseases caused by inorganic dusts, drugs, or opportunistic infections increase lung density, whereas emphysema and possibly pulmonary embolism decrease it. Theoretically, such pathologic processes might be diagnosed before they can produce changes that are visible on conventional chest radiographs and possibly even before they are evident by pulmonary function testing.

In normal adults, the attenuation values of the lung vary from approximately −700 to −860 HU; lung densities are somewhat higher in children below the age of 10 years (90,187,232). Attenuation values may be up to 200 HU higher in the posterior dependent portions of the lung because of preferential blood flow received in the supine position, a phenomenon that is accentuated at full expiration. Full inspiration has the opposite effect, reducing the gradient as well as causing all attenuation values to become more negative.

Although various methods (e.g., computed automated regional-density calculations or frequency-distribution analysis of attenuation values) have been devised to measure lung density accurately, major limitations exist in their clinical application. The techniques used are tedious and time-consuming, and objective data collection is hampered by partial-volume averaging with a wide variety of intrathoracic tissue densities. For multiple technical reasons already detailed in discussing the solitary pulmonary nodule, besides the difficulty in obtaining precisely reproducible lung volumes, it is impossible to acquire absolute attenuation values for a given individual to be used for comparison between patients. Subjective (visual) inspection usually suffices to identify abnormal areas in diffuse lung disease, particularly when the process is focal or asymmetrically distributed. Some useful information may be provided by assessing the patient's anteroposterior gradient or by comparing the values obtained from a previous study on the same patient. Consequently, the use of CT to determine lung density is limited to physiologic investigations under controlled circumstances; it has no established clinical role.

Interstitial and Air-Space Patterns

Interstitial lung disease involves primarily the supporting structures that surround the air spaces. Several different CT signs of interstitial disease have been described (241). These are generally more apparent and better defined on thin-section images. The most common and earliest sign is obscuration of normal interfaces (Fig. 65), resulting in irregularity and thickening of the visceral pleura, including the major fissure, the pulmonary vessels, and the bronchial walls. The second most frequent sign is thickening of the interlobular septa. A reticular pattern develops that may range from a fine network of lines separated by 2 to 3 mm (sublobular) to a medium-size network measuring between 6 and 10 mm (the classic honeycomb pattern involving the primary lobules) to a large coarse polyhedral network with elements 15 to 25 mm in diameter centered around a central vessel (probably representing the secondary pulmonary lobule). Occasionally, a zonal alteration of lung density may occur. Patches of hazy increased density may surround nearby vessels, most typically at the lung periphery; in contradistinction to air-space consolidation, the vessels remain visible and are not "silhouetted." These patchy opacifications generally are seen in the earlier stages of interstitial disease and are due to alveolar septal inflammation and filling of some of the air spaces with mononuclear cells. Finally, nodules as small as 1 to 3 mm in diameter can be demonstrated, often in close contiguity to the vessels. CT may be valuable in patients suspected of having interstitial lung disease,

usually because of abnormal pulmonary function tests, who have normal or minimally abnormal plain chest radiographs: Interstitial disease may be confirmed, or the progress of the disease followed, or an appropriate biopsy site identified.

In its earliest stages, air-space ("alveolar") pulmonary disease usually starts as a collection of poorly defined 3- to 5-mm nodular densities; frequently the process is not recognizable on conventional radiography at this time (59,241). Typically, in a rapid fashion, these air-space nodules tend to fuse together and form a subsegmental region of opacification, often with air bronchograms being seen. Air-space processes tend to spare the most peripheral regions of the lung, whereas interstitial processes tend to be most prominent in the outer third ("cortex") of the lung parenchyma. The CT attenuation values do not allow distinction among exudative, transudative, and neoplastic processes. However, in some cases, density determination may allow a more specific diagnosis than is possible with conventional radiography. Areas of low attenuation secondary to fat can be seen in lipoid pneumonias (100) (Fig. 58). High-attenuation parenchymal infiltrates may occur with pulmonary calcification (e.g., secondary to chronic renal failure), with acute pulmonary hemorrhage, and in patients on amiodarone therapy, as a result of deposition of the iodine-containing drug and its metabolites (109) (Fig. 66).

Idiopathic pulmonary fibrosis

Also called fibrosing alveolitis, this condition is characterized pathologically by regions of fibrosis surrounding cystic spaces (honeycombing) accompanied by a mononuclear-cell interstitial infiltrate interspersed between areas of normal lung. CT usually demonstrates the aforementioned medium-thick reticular network of lines combined with cystic areas measuring 2 to 20 mm in diameter. Although the peripheral subpleural portion of the lung is characteristically involved, more severe cases may involve the entire lung (13,14,144) (Fig. 67). Small "honeycomb"

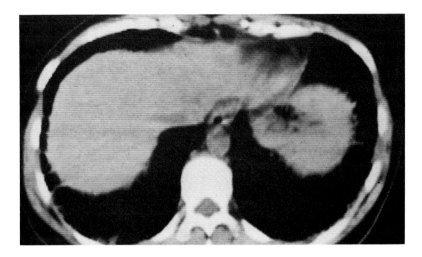

FIG. 65. Interstitial lung disease (rheumatoid arthritis). The normal sharp interfaces between the lung and the diaphragm (surrounding the liver and spleen) and with the pleura are obscured by the adjacent peripheral lung disease.

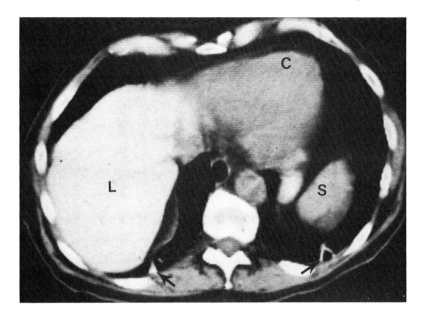

FIG. 66. High-density pleuroparenchymal lesions (*arrows*) are seen posteriorly in the lower lobes in a patient on amiodarone. Note also the high density of the liver (L) compared with the soft-tissue density of the cardiac musculature (C) and the spleen (S).

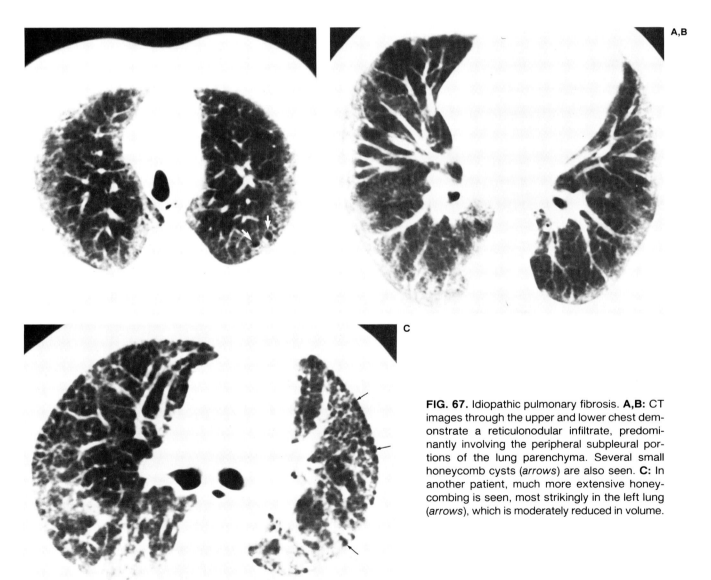

FIG. 67. Idiopathic pulmonary fibrosis. **A,B:** CT images through the upper and lower chest demonstrate a reticulonodular infiltrate, predominantly involving the peripheral subpleural portions of the lung parenchyma. Several small honeycomb cysts (*arrows*) are also seen. **C:** In another patient, much more extensive honeycombing is seen, most strikingly in the left lung (*arrows*), which is moderately reduced in volume.

A,B

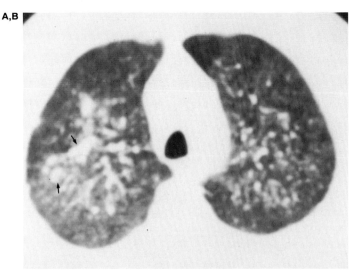
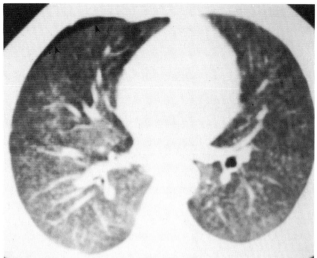

FIG. 68. Silicosis. **A:** Multiple small nodules are seen throughout both lungs, with areas of confluence (*arrows*) in the right upper lobe. **B:** On an image through the lower lung fields, the diffuse nodularity results in a ground-glass appearance. A small incidental right pneumothorax (*arrowheads*) is seen.

cysts are optimally seen on thin sections, and the intermingling of normal lung tissue with areas of fibrosis may be clearly appreciated only on thin-section images. The extent of disease can be better estimated with CT than with the plain chest radiograph, and CT findings correlate better with the clinical and functional severity of disease.

Pneumoconiosis

The CT characteristics of silicosis are similar to those described for the plain chest radiograph (9,16). Multiple nodules, most smaller than 1 cm, are seen predominantly in the upper lobes (Figs. 49B and 68). In most patients, more nodules are distributed posteriorly, a finding generally not apparent on the chest radiograph. Larger coalescent masses (progressive massive fibrosis) also may be more easily appreciated, usually in association with disruption of normal vascular markings and bullous formation (Fig. 69). Thickening of the interlobular septa (reticular densities) is not a prominent feature of silicosis. Emphysematous changes, which are not as easily detected on plain chest radiographs, may correlate well with pulmonary dysfunction. Poor correlation was found between pulmonary function tests and the extent of silicotic nod-

A,B

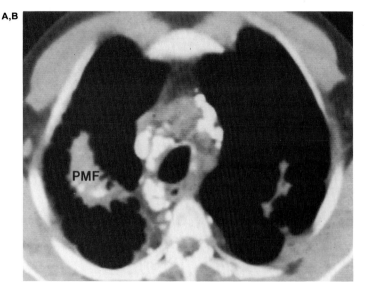

PMF

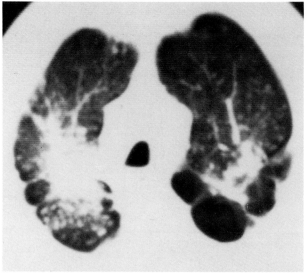

FIG. 69. Silicosis with progressive massive fibrosis (PMF). **A:** Areas of confluent nodulation (PMF) are seen, especially in the right upper lobe. Calcification is present within mediastinal lymph nodes, as well as in the areas of PMF. **B:** Lung window setting at the same level demonstrates surrounding areas of bullous emphysema and fine nodular infiltrates.

ules. No important role for CT has been defined in the evaluation of these patients, because pulmonary function tests suffice for determining the degree of pulmonary disability.

A potentially more widespread application of CT might be for evaluating the presence and extent of pulmonary parenchymal involvement caused by asbestos (101). Although CT clearly can detect the pleura-related changes caused by this dust earlier than conventional radiography, it is the presence of lung disease (asbestosis) rather than pleural plaques that is the main determinant of compensation (Fig. 70). In this analysis, CT also allows assessment that is more sensitive and less observer-dependent than that with the plain chest radiograph. Parenchymal abnormalities are seen most frequently in the dorsal aspect of the lung base. A subpleural curvilinear shadow, parallel to the inner chest wall, measuring 5 to 10 cm in length and usually in a lower lobe, may be seen in a high percentage of patients exposed to asbestos (239) (Fig. 71A). This may represent the initial phase of fibrosis that subsequently leads to honeycombing. However, the finding is not specific for asbestosis and may occur in other dis-

eases, such as idiopathic interstitial pneumonia or bleomycin lung toxicity (11) (Fig. 71B). Images obtained post lymphography suggest that these curvilinear shadows may result from thickening of the subpleural lymphatic network (173). In more advanced cases of asbestosis, reticular thickening and honeycombing may also be seen, initially in a subpleural location (like idiopathic pulmonary fibrosis) and later extending more centrally. These changes may be more easily seen on images obtained in the prone position, which also can demonstrate that they are fixed structural abnormalities and not simply subsegmental atelectasis and gravity-dependent blood flow secondary to less than full inspiration. Asbestos-related pleural disease is almost always present in patients who demonstrate parenchymal disease.

Lymphangitic Carcinoma

Pulmonary lymphangitic spread is most frequently seen secondary to adenocarcinomas of the breast, lung, stomach, colon, prostate, and pancreas. Pathologically there is

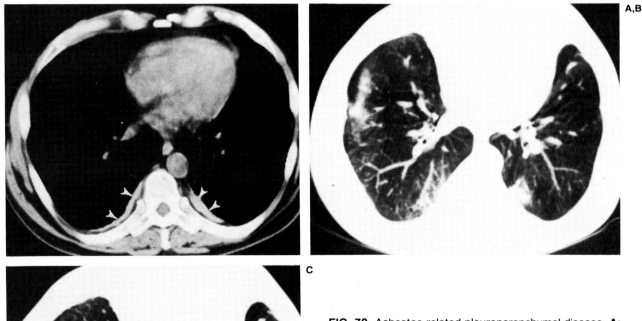

FIG. 70. Asbestos-related pleuroparenchymal disease. **A:** Bilateral pleural plaques are seen posteromedially (*arrowheads*). **B:** Lung window setting of the same CT image performed with standard collimation documents concomitant parenchymal infiltrates (asbestosis) in the middle and both lower lobes. **C:** A 2-mm-collimated image at the same level more sharply defines the parenchymal infiltrates and fibrosis. Some mild thickening of the right major fissure and the anterior extension of the minor fissure (*arrowheads*) is now visible.

A,B

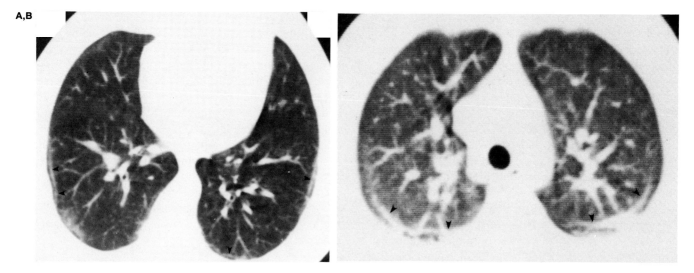

FIG. 71. A: Subpleural curvilinear shadows (*arrowheads*) are seen in the posterior and lateral subpleural lung in a patient with prior asbestos exposure. **B:** Similar subpleural curvilinear shadows (*arrowheads*) are seen in a patient on bleomycin.

thickening of the pulmonary interstitium by tumor cells, fibrous tissue, and edema. CT frequently shows irregularly thickened interlobular septa, generally centrally as well as in the lung periphery (14,211,241). As the disease worsens, a more nodular appearance may be seen superimposed on this reticular pattern, resulting in a characteristic appearance of small nodules connected to thickened lines. These findings generally are better appreciated on thin-section images and may be present when the findings on the chest radiograph are normal or equivocal. In addition to the parenchymal changes, hilar lymph node enlargement may be demonstrated.

Sarcoidosis

Interstitial lung disease secondary to sarcoidosis frequently is more apparent on CT than on plain chest radiographs. Small interstitial nodules may be seen throughout the lungs, as well as areas of confluent interstitial disease that may look similar to an alveolar process. Although CT generally is not used in patients suspected of having sarcoidosis, occasionally it may be helpful in demonstrating sites of mediastinal lymphadenopathy for possible biopsy (86). In most patients, however, a diagnosis can be made by transbronchial biopsy of the pulmonary parenchyma.

Emphysema

Emphysema is defined as an increase in air-space size distal to the terminal bronchioles, associated with destruction of the alveolar walls. Four different types of emphysema have been described pathologically: centrilobular, panlobular, paraseptal, and paracicatricial. Blebs and

bullae frequently are seen in association with emphysema, but they may be seen as localized processes in otherwise normal lungs. A bleb is an air collection within the layers of the visceral pleura, whereas a bulla is an intrapulmonary emphysematous space usually greater than 1 cm in diameter. The chest radiograph may demonstrate relatively advanced cases of emphysema, but it is much less sensitive in detecting mild or moderate disease. CT is more accurate in detecting and characterizing emphysema than is plain chest radiography, and CT findings often correlate better with the pathologic extent of disease than do pulmonary function tests (15).

Centrilobular Emphysema

Centrilobular emphysema is the most common type of emphysema and is characterized by nonuniform destruction of the secondary pulmonary lobule. The process tends to begin in the center of the lobule surrounding the respiratory bronchiole and more frequently involves the upper lobes. Corresponding to the emphysematous spaces seen pathologically, the CT findings range from small punctate holes within an otherwise normal lung to a moth-eaten pattern to more extensive areas of lung destruction (54) (Figs. 72–74). Pulmonary vascular pruning and distortion are also seen. Although the mean lung density is decreased in patients with emphysema, density measurements by themselves are not necessary; visual assessment alone is adequate.

Panlobular Emphysema

In panlobular emphysema there is uniform destruction of the secondary pulmonary lobule, predominantly in the

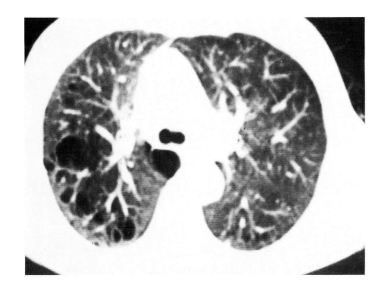

FIG. 72. Emphysema. Dilated distal air spaces and bullae, due to centrilobular emphysema, are seen in the right upper lobe and the superior segments of both lower lobes. Paraseptal bullae are noted just posterior to the carina.

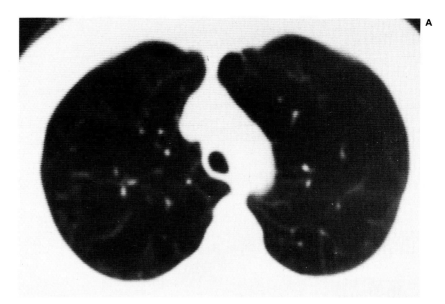

A

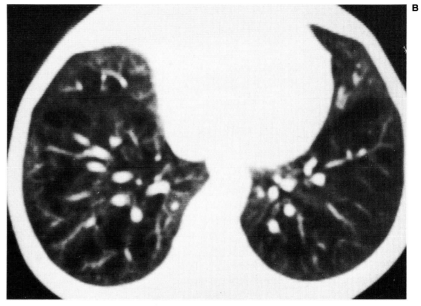

B

FIG. 73. Centrilobular emphysema. A: Severe emphysema, with multiple bullae, disrupts the normal bronchovascular anatomy in the upper lobes. B: Multiple smaller emphysematous spaces are seen scattered throughout areas of more-normal-appearing parenchyma at the lung bases.

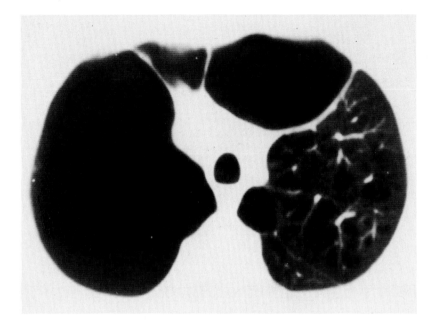

FIG. 74. Bullae. Enormous bullae replace the entire right lung and herniate into the left hemithorax. Moderately extensive centrilobular emphysematous changes are also seen in the smaller left lung.

lower lobes. On CT, the lung parenchyma is likely to appear diffusely abnormal, demonstrating widespread areas of low attenuation. The lower-lobe distribution may be more obvious on CT than on plain chest radiographs.

Paraseptal Emphysema

Paraseptal emphysema involves the distal portion of the lobule, and therefore it is characteristically seen adjacent to the pleura and interlobular septa. It may be seen in association with centrilobular or panlobular emphysema, or as an isolated phenomenon (180). On CT, multiple subpleural bullae (0.5–2 cm in diameter) are seen (Fig. 75), commonly in the azygoesophageal recess, adjacent to the anterior junction line, and next to the left ventricle.

Paracicatricial Emphysema

Paracicatricial emphysema is seen adjacent to scars and can result from a variety of diseases, including healed infectious granulomatous disease (e.g., tuberculosis) or progressive massive fibrosis (silicosis) (Fig. 69). The focal lung destruction may be obscured by the scarring on the plain chest radiograph.

Role of CT in Emphysema

CT is not recommended for routine evaluation of patients known to have or suspected of having emphysema. However, it may provide helpful additional information in patients who are being considered for bullectomy by

precisely defining the extent of the disease process (52,138). In rare circumstances, CT may be useful in patients in whom the clinical symptoms are more severe than suggested by plain chest radiographs and pulmonary function tests (17).

Radiation-Induced Pulmonary Injury

Patients who have undergone radiation therapy to the thorax usually are followed with plain chest radiographs. CT also can be helpful in the evaluation of these patients, particularly in the documentation of recurrent neoplastic

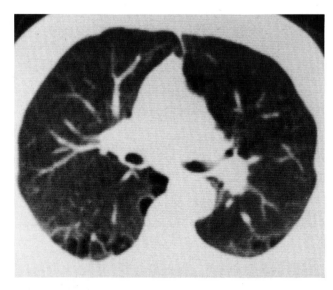

FIG. 75. Paraseptal emphysema. Multiple subpleural bullae are seen in the azygoesophageal recess and in the posterior subpleural lung.

to the X-ray beam; oblique views may help to bring a pleural mass into tangent for optimal demonstration. When conventional techniques fail in this differentiation, the superior contrast sensitivity and cross-sectional imaging format of CT can be very valuable for further analysis. Similarly, it may be difficult to assess the pulmonary parenchyma on plain radiographs when extensive pleural disease is present. CT is the best radiologic technique for detecting and distinguishing coexistent disease involving the lung, mediastinum, chest wall, or upper abdomen (178,238). The pleural, chest-wall, or pulmonary parenchymal contribution to a plain chest radiographic indication of abnormality can be assessed. A peripheral pulmonary nodule may be distinguished from localized pleural thickening, or a peripheral lung abscess from an empyema. Important information can be provided regarding the presence, location, and extent of any concomitant lung or mediastinal abnormality obscured by substantial pleural disease, be it thickening or a free or loculated effusion, especially when the fluid cannot be removed by thoracentesis. Although routine use of intravenous contrast material is unnecessary, its administration sometimes helps to distinguish pathologic pulmonary parenchyma (e.g., atelectasis, consolidation), which usually demonstrates marked enhancement, from a pleural tumor (e.g., metastasis), which is mildly enhanced, from a pleural fluid collection that is not enhanced (21). Contrast-enhanced images demonstrating pulmonary vessels within a lesion unequivocally identify it as parenchymal. Contrast material is helpful in defining both components when there is combined parenchymal and pleural involvement.

Peripheral lesions in the thorax generally are classified by location as extrapleural, pleural, or parenchymal. On conventional radiography, pleural lesions usually have a characteristic obtuse angle between the lesion and the chest wall. Similar changes usually are seen with extrapleural lesions, although associated features, such as rib destruction, may help to confirm the precise site of origin of the disease process. Pedunculated pleural lesions may invaginate into the pulmonary parenchyma, creating an acute angle with the lung and chest wall and simulating an intraparenchymal lesion. Similar difficulties may be encountered on the cross-sectional imaging techniques (CT and MRI), although distinction generally is easier. The CT features characteristic of pleural lesions include (a) a lenticular or crescentic shape, (b) an obtuse or tapering angle at the interface with the chest wall, and (c) well-defined margins with the adjacent lung (Fig. 83). But exceptions to these rules occur. Loculated pleural fluid collections may bulge into the lung, creating an acute angle between the pleural lesion and the chest wall. If a parenchymal lesion (e.g., bronchogenic carcinoma) infiltrates the pleura, an obtuse angle rather than an acute angle with the chest wall may be formed. Thus, overlap in the appearance of extrapleural, pleural, and peripheral parenchymal lesions can also exist on CT. Even if distinction

is not possible with CT, it still may provide more precise delineation of the extent of the pathologic process than can conventional radiography.

Pleural Effusion

The most common pleural abnormality, free pleural fluid initially collects in the most dependent portion of the pleural space, which is posteromedial and caudal to the lung base in the usual supine position used for CT imaging. Subpulmonic fluid in this pleural recess lies just posterior to the medial portion (crus) of the hemidiaphragm (which may be displaced anterolaterally), in close proximity to the posterior mediastinum (esophagus or descending aorta) anterolateral to the thoracic spine (Fig. 84). Occasionally, a very small pleural effusion may be depicted on CT that was not visible on standard chest radiography. If there is any difficulty in differentiating between such a small effusion and pleural thickening (fibrosis), images obtained with the patient prone or in a lateral decubitus position should clarify the problem. As an effusion increases in size, it conforms to the pleural

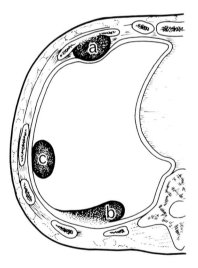

FIG. 83. Schematic drawing of the cross-sectional appearance of extrapleural (a), pleural (b), and peripheral pulmonary parenchymal (c) lesions. Extrapleural lesions displace the overlying parietal and visceral pleura, resulting in an obtuse angle between the lesion and the chest wall. Associated chest-wall abnormality (e.g., rib erosion) may further help define the lesion as extrapleural. Pleural lesions may remain confined between the two pleural layers and cause similar obtuse angles with the chest wall, or they may become pedunculated and protrude into the pulmonary parenchyma, resulting in an acute angle between the lesion and chest wall. Subpleural parenchymal lesions generally result in an acute angle with the chest wall. Infiltration of the pleura may cause obtuse angulation. Thus, there may be considerable overlap in the appearances of these lesions. (Adapted from ref. 159.)

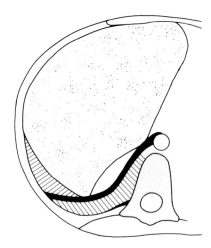

FIG. 84. Schematic drawing illustrating relationship of pleural effusion and ascites to the diaphragmatic crus. The thick black line represents the right hemidiaphragm and its medially extending crus. A pleural effusion lies posterior (external) to the diaphragm and extends medially adjacent to the spine. Large amounts of pleural fluid may displace the crus anteriorly and laterally. Ascites lies anterior (internal) to the diaphragm and does not extend medially (blocked by the coronary ligament on the right side). (Adapted from ref. 84.)

space and generally extends toward the lateral chest wall (Fig. 85). The lateral aspects of the major fissures may become filled with fluid pointing toward the hilum (Fig. 86). In the presence of a moderate-size pleural effusion, volume loss (compressive atelectasis) commonly develops in the adjacent lung, most typically the lower lobe or a portion thereof. Large effusions usually result in a major degree of lower-lobe collapse. The collapsed lobe tends to be displaced anterior by the fluid ("floating" on it) and compressed toward the hilum, with consequent stretching and tethering of the inferior pulmonary ligament. This subsegmental basilar atelectasis may create a curvilinear band density on some CT sections simulating the hemidiaphragm (202); the pleural fluid anterior to the atelectasis may mimic an intraabdominal collection. This atelectatic lung can be easily distinguished from the diaphragm because it is thicker and tapers laterally, and most important, it can be followed on contiguous cephalad images into the lung (which initially can be recognized by patchy aeration) (Fig. 42). When pleural fluid becomes sufficiently massive to cause inversion of a hemidiaphragm, again intraabdominal fluid may be simulated on some images. However, a real diagnostic dilemma rarely occurs, because it is almost always known that a large pleural effusion exists from a prior chest radiograph or the preliminary computed digital radiograph, or from more cephalad images. Once more, it should be emphasized that individual CT sections should never be analyzed in isolation; the configuration of fluid and the appearances

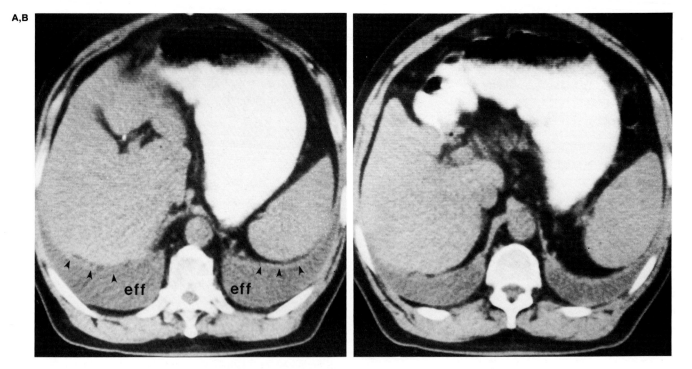

FIG. 85. Bilateral pleural effusions. **A:** Near-water-density collections are seen posteriorly in the caudal costophrenic sulci dorsal (external) to the hemidiaphragms (*arrowheads*). Note how the effusions (eff) extend medially behind the crura and adjacent to the spine. **B:** Caudally, the amount of pleural fluid diminishes; it still remains external to the hemidiaphragms.

A,B

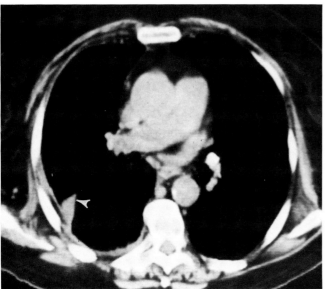 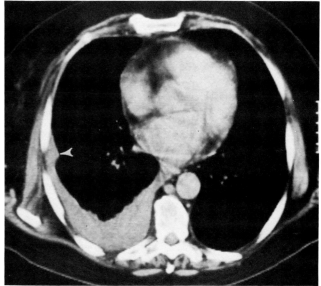

FIG. 86. Pleural effusion. **A:** A moderate-size right effusion is seen extending into the major fissure (*arrowhead*). **B:** At 6 cm caudad, the amount of pleural fluid is greater. It still extends into the major fissure (*arrowhead*) and also medially in front of the spine.

of adjacent structures over multiple contiguous levels enable precise localization in almost all cases.

Virtually all pleural effusions (transudative, exudative, and chylous) have a homogeneous, near-water attenuation value and are not distinguishable on CT. This is because the expected differences between them are small, and technical limitations prevent precise densitometry. Attenuation values slightly higher than those for soft tissue, oftentimes inhomogeneous, may be seen with an acute hemothorax. Loculation of fluid within a fissure due to prior adhesions, relatively common in patients with congestive heart failure, may simulate an intrapulmonary mass. Its margins may be poorly defined if the fissure is not perpendicular to the imaging plane. The near-water density of the collection should be a clue to the correct cause.

Distinguishing Pleural Fluid and Other Abnormalities

Pleural effusion in the caudal recesses near the diaphragm may be confused with subdiaphragmatic fluid. The key to accurate localization of the fluid is identification of the hemidiaphragm (154), which usually is directly visible as a thin, soft-tissue-density (Fig. 87) stripe, or whose position can be inferred by lung lateral and abdominal fat central to it. Once the position of the hemidiaphragm is clarified, differentiation between intrathoracic disease and intraabdominal disease, particularly fluid collections, is facilitated (Fig. 88). The pleura and lung lie peripheral to the hemidiaphragm and posterior to the crus and arcuate ligament, whereas the intraperitoneal spaces (and abdominal viscera and fat) lie central to the hemidiaphragm and anterior to the crus and arcuate lig-

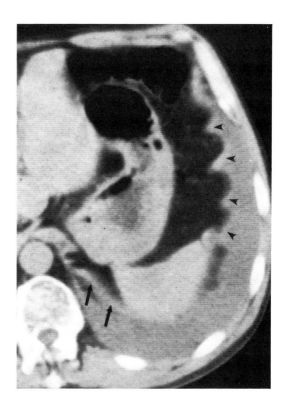

FIG. 87. Left pleural effusion. The near-water-density collection is seen lateral (external) to a contracted left hemidiaphragm (*arrowheads*) on an image obtained during deep inspiration. The fluid also is noted extending medially behind the left diaphragmatic crus (*arrows*).

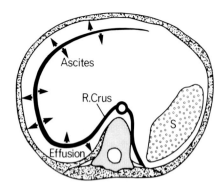

FIG. 88. Schematic drawing illustrating relationship of pleural effusion and ascites to the diaphragm. The solid black line represents the diaphragm. The position of the fluid relative to the diaphragm identifies where the fluid lies. Fluid inside the diaphragm is ascites; fluid outside (peripheral to) the diaphragm is pleural; (S) spleen. (Adapted from ref. 84.)

ament. Intraabdominal fluid may collect in the peritoneal spaces or in the retroperitoneum; differentiation between these locations generally is not difficult and will be discussed thoroughly in Chapters 11 and 16.

Certain generalizations help in distinguishing pleural fluid from abdominal fluid (50,84,85). Individually, any of these criteria (or signs) may be indeterminate or misleading, but distinction should be possible in almost all cases when their combined features are used. A pleural fluid collection usually diminishes in size gradually on more caudal images, and as emphasized earlier, its most caudal extent usually is located posteromedial to a diaphragmatic crus (Fig. 85). Anterolateral displacement of a crus by fluid is a pathognomonic sign that it is in the pleural space. In contradistinction, subdiaphragmatic fluid generally increases in amount on caudal images into the upper abdomen, usually extending progressively lateral to the liver and the spleen (Fig. 89). Ascitic fluid is re-

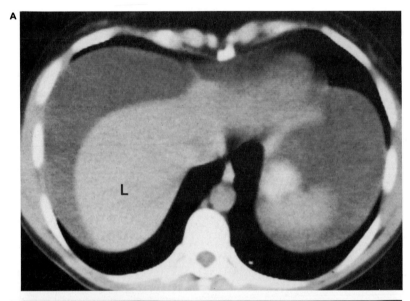

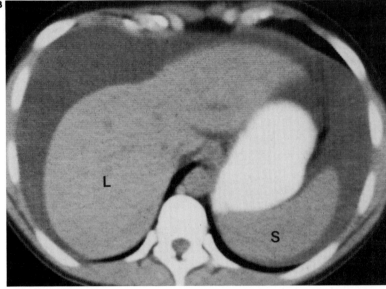

FIG. 89. Ascites. **A,B:** Sequential caudal CT images separated by a 2-cm interval demonstrate near-water-density fluid surrounding the liver (L) and spleen (S). Note that the ascites does not extend posteromedially behind these organs; the posterior caudal recesses of the lungs are seen dorsally.

stricted by the peritoneal reflections. On the right side, peritoneal fluid is restricted from moving posteromedially to the bare area of the liver (not covered by peritoneum) by the right coronary ligament. A corresponding, albeit smaller, 2- to 3-cm bare area of the spleen demarcated by the splenorenal ligament prevents posteromedial egress of peritoneal fluid on the left side (224). However, when ascites is massive, fluid may collect immediately beneath the domes of the hemidiaphragms and extend medially above the bare areas on both sides (Fig. 90). Aerated lung surrounded by fluid indicates that the fluid is intrathoracic, whereas fluid central or anterior to aerated lung is sub-diaphragmatic (Fig. 91). Rarely, ascitic fluid can extend into the posterior mediastinum through the esophageal hiatus; tracing such fluid on contiguous sections into the abdomen should permit proper diagnosis (69). A hazy interface between pleural fluid and the liver or spleen has been described, as opposed to a sharp demarcation between these organs and ascites (215). This is a relatively unimportant feature that may not even be seen with modern CT equipment and its short scanning times; other

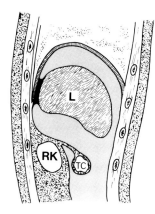

FIG. 90. Schematic drawing of sagittal section through the right upper quadrant of the abdomen; left side of diagram is posterior (dorsal). Ascitic fluid (*fine-dotted area*) cannot extend behind the liver (L) into the nonperitonealized bare area (*solid black*) demarcated by the superior and inferior coronary ligaments, whereas pleural fluid (*coarse-lined area*) can go behind the liver in the deep posterior sulcus. When ascites is massive, a small amount of fluid may extend posterior to the liver along its most cephalad and caudad margins outside the bare area; (RK) right kidney; (TC) transverse colon. (Adapted from ref. 84.)

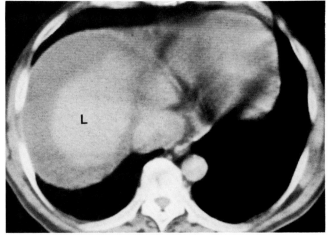

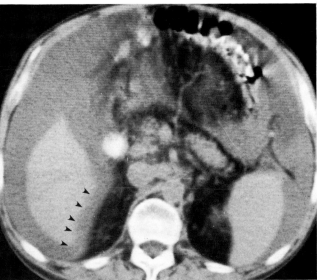

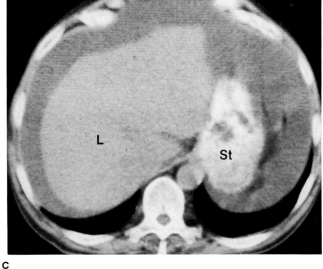

FIG. 91. Massive ascites. A,B: Sequential caudal images separated by a 2-cm interval demonstrate some ascitic fluid extending posteromedially just beneath the domes of the hemidiaphragms. On the more cephalad section, because of the oblique orientation of the dome of the liver (L), there is an indistinct interface with the ascites; (St) stomach. C: At 7 cm caudal, ascites also extends posterior to the liver into the hepatorenal fossa (*arrowheads*).

findings should convincingly demonstrate whether the fluid is pleural or ascitic.

Rarely, relatively low density consolidation within a lower lobe might be mistaken for pleural or perhaps intraabdominal fluid. As with pleural fluid collections, parenchymal lung disease lies peripheral to the hemidiaphragm, and the medial portions may extend in close proximity to the descending aorta and esophagus in the posterior mediastinum. However, consolidated lung never has a near-water density like a pleural effusion or ascites, and residual areas of parenchymal aeration (air bronchograms) usually are discernible to further aid proper identification. If needed, imaging with intravenous contrast material at the plane of major abnormality usually is diagnostic; parenchymal pulmonary processes and their contained vessels are enhanced, whereas pleural fluid is not.

Empyema

By definition, empyema means pus (white blood cells more than 500/mm^3) in the pleural space. Pleural infection most commonly follows a primary infection within the adjacent lung, such as acute bacterial pneumonia, lung abscess, or septic pulmonary infarction. Less frequently, infection spreads to the pleura from contiguous extrapulmonary sites, such as osteomyelitis of the spine or a subdiaphragmatic abscess. Iatrogenic pleural infection may result from prior thoracic surgery or percutaneous needle aspiration.

The incidence of parapneumonic pleural effusions is dependent to some degree on the infecting organism, ranging from about 10% for pneumonias caused by *Streptococcus pneumoniae* to over 50% for those caused by *Staphylococcus pyogenes.* Most parapneumonic effusions, which are composed of thin uninfected fluid resulting from inflammation of the visceral pleura and increased capillary permeability, resolve with appropriate antibiotic treatment. However, some do become infected and progress to true empyema, in which large numbers of polymorphonuclear leukocytes accumulate in the pleural space, with fibrin deposited over the visceral and parietal pleura. Thickening of the pleura may develop within several days, and as a consequence there is impairment of fluid resorption and a tendency toward loculation.

Generally, plain chest roentgenography, sometimes in conjunction with decubitus or oblique X-ray films, suffices to diagnose a pleural fluid collection and distinguish it from a peripheral pulmonary parenchymal process. Ultrasound also can be extremely helpful in corroborating pleural fluid, although it is of little value in confirming parenchymal disease. At times, however, distinction between a loculated pleural collection and a parenchymal process may not be possible with conventional radiologic techniques. This also can be true when a bronchopleural

fistula is present, producing air in the pleural space; this occurs in approximately 50% of empyemas when peripheral lung necrosis creates a communication between an airway (usually a bronchiole) and the pleural space. CT can be valuable in differentiating such a pyopneumothorax from a necrotizing parenchymal process, each of which may appear on plain radiographs as a "cavitary" lesion containing an air–fluid level adjacent to the chest wall. Accurate diagnosis is critical because of the disparate treatments for these serious suppurative lesions. Proper therapy for empyema requires closed tube drainage, whereas a lung abscess is appropriately managed with antibiotics and postural and perhaps bronchoscopic drainage. The cross-sectional CT images better delineate the three-dimensional shape of the lesion and its pleuroparenchymal interface, generally permitting accurate localization and distinction of the predominant process (Fig. 92). Several morphologic features are helpful for differentiation between a pleural and a parenchymal process; because none is infallible, they are best used in combination (7,210,237):

1. An empyema generally conforms to the shape of the chest wall and has a lenticular configuration, with gradually tapering obtuse margins toward the thoracic cage (Fig. 93). In contradistinction, a peripheral lung abscess usually has a spherical shape and forms an acute angle with the chest wall (Fig. 94A); concomitant pleural disease may cause the angle to become obtuse. Although generally not necessary, imaging the patient in a different position (e.g., lateral decubitus or prone) may provide some complementary information. Pleural-space contents may be somewhat mobile, and the shape of an empyema, as well as the length of any contained air–fluid level, may change

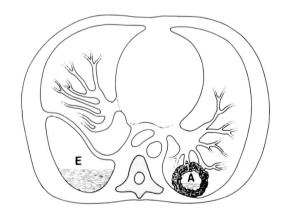

FIG. 92. Schematic drawing demonstrating cross-sectional features of empyema (E) and a lung abscess (A). The empyema is lenticular-shaped, with thin walls and smooth inner surfaces, forming an obtuse margin with the chest wall; the pulmonary vessels are compressed and displaced around the empyema. In contradistinction, the lung abscess is spherical, with thick irregular walls, and forms an acute angle with the chest wall; pulmonary vessels extend directly toward the lesion. (Adapted from ref. 237.)

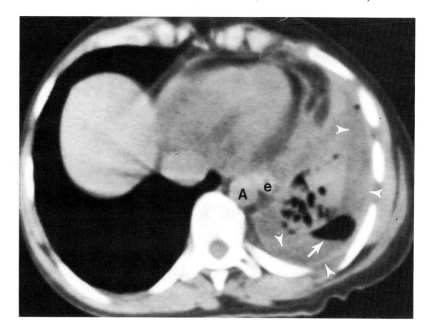

FIG. 93. Empyema. A smooth, thin-walled, largely elliptical, near-water-density collection (*arrowheads*), containing an air–fluid level (*arrow*) due to a bronchopleural fistula, is seen external and posterolateral to a collapsed consolidated left lower lobe demarcated by air bronchograms. Volume loss is noted in the left hemithorax; (A) aorta; (e) esophagus.

slightly, whereas a lung abscess tends to remain rigidly spherical, with an equidimensional air–fluid level.

2. An empyema generally has thin, smooth walls, especially along its inner margin (Fig. 95). Imaging at the plane of major abnormality following intravenous administration of contrast material may help define the separate visceral and parietal pleural layers (the "split-pleura" sign) around an empyema; hyperemia induced by inflammation causes their marked enhancement (Fig. 96). In comparison, a lung abscess usually has thick, irregular walls, especially internally (Fig. 97); multiple small side pockets may be present.

3. The adjacent lung frequently is compressed by an empyema, resulting in gradual displacement and bowing of peripheral pulmonary vessels and bronchi around its circumference; sharp separation from the pulmonary parenchyma often is apparent. The parenchyma surrounding a lung abscess often is also infected, and no distinct boundary may be visible; the pulmonary vessels and bronchi usually extend directly toward the periphery of a lung abscess (Fig. 94B).

Fluid may accumulate in a subpleural bulla, analogous to a parapneumonic pleural effusion (an inflammatory response of the wall to adjacent pneumonitis). In most

A,B

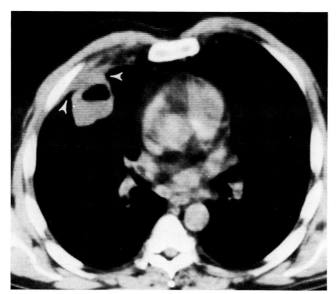

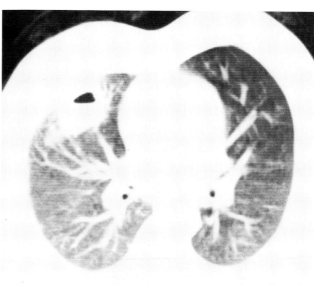

FIG. 94. Lung abscess. **A:** A cavitary pulmonary mass (cryptococcosis) abuts a thickened pleural surface, but maintains acute angles (*arrowheads*) with the chest wall. **B:** Lung window setting at the same level shows pulmonary vessels extending directly toward the mass.

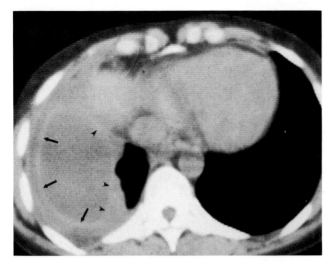

FIG. 95. Empyema; split pleura sign. Near-water-density fluid is seen between thickened parietal (*arrows*) and visceral (*arrowheads*) pleura on a nonenhanced CT image. Some fluid is also present external to the parietal pleura.

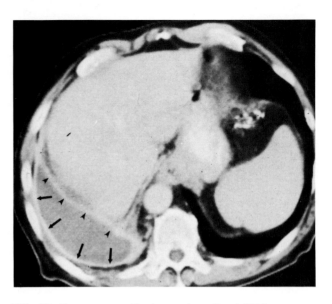

FIG. 96. Empyema; split pleura sign. On a CT image post intravenous administration of contrast material, fluid is seen between enhanced thickened parietal (*arrows*) and visceral (*arrowheads*) pleura. Volume loss in the right hemithorax is demonstrated.

A,B

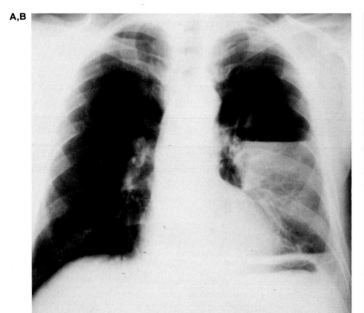

C

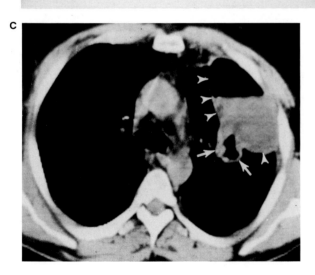

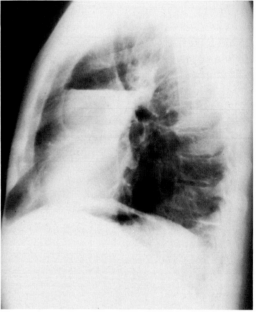

FIG. 97. Empyema and lung abscess. **A,B:** Posteroanterior and lateral chest radiographs demonstrate a loculated pleural collection containing air and fluid. A cavitary left-upper-lobe lesion was questioned. **C:** CT image documents an irregular thick-walled cavity (*arrows*) due to histoplasmosis adjacent to the loculated empyema (*arrowheads*).

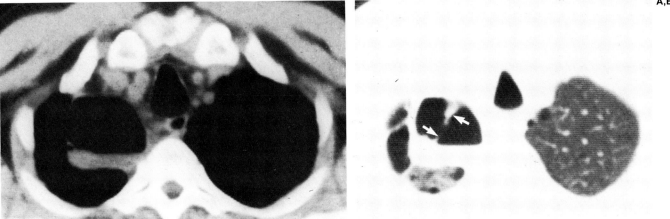

FIG. 98. Pneumonia and bulla containing fluid. **A,B:** Just anterior to a right-upper-lobe pneumonia, air and fluid are seen within a large bulla containing a septa (*arrows*) in the right-lung apex, simulating a lung abscess or empyema. Smaller bullae are seen in the adjacent lung.

circumstances, the bullae themselves are not truly "infected." Obstruction of adjacent bronchioles due to inflammation and mucus plugging may play a role in preventing or impairing adequate drainage. CT may be performed in such patients, and the findings may simulate a loculated hydropneumothorax or empyema (244) (Fig. 98). Accurate radiologic diagnosis usually requires comparison with earlier chest radiographs or a prior CT examination to document the presence of preexisting bullous lung disease. Suggestive, but less definitive, would be demonstration of contralateral or adjacent bullae. A pleural process may be more likely if coexistent pleural collections are seen at other sites. In some cases, distinction between fluid within a bulla and fluid within the pleural space may not be possible.

Infected pleural fluid may extend directly through the soft tissues of the thoracic wall and present as a subcutaneous mass. Such an empyema necessitatis is most commonly secondary to tuberculosis, but also may occur as a consequence of actinomycosis or blastomyocosis or even following thoracentesis of a pyogenic empyema. CT not only can demonstrate contiguity of the subcutaneous abscess with a pleural-space collection (Fig. 99) but also may show areas of lung destruction beneath the pleural disease that were obscured on conventional roentgenograms (19).

An additional important application of CT is for precise localization of empyema pockets to assist in proper thoracostomy tube placement and drainage (209). Clearer depiction of the exact site(s) and extent of the empyema

FIG. 99. Tuberculous empyema necessitatis. In a woman thought clinically to have a large left-breast mass, in whom a chest radiograph showed hazy opacification of the left upper hemithorax, CT demonstrates a loculated empyema (*arrows*) with a contiguous chest-wall abscess (*arrowheads*) extending into the retromammary area. Several small calcifications are noted within the empyema, as well as a large calcified paratracheal lymph node.

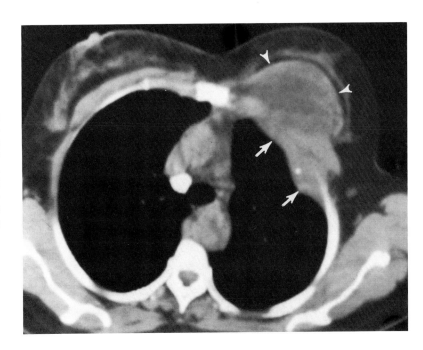

is more possible than with plain chest radiographs; otherwise occult loculations may be identified (Figs. 100 and 101). An unsuspected condition may be discovered (Fig. 102). Safe insertion of a thoracostomy tube into certain areas, such as the posterior costophrenic recess, may be better ensured. In patients not responding well clinically to the usual thoracostomy tube drainage, CT can demonstrate the position of the tube relative to the extent of any residual pleural collection (Figs. 103 and 104). Similarly, any undrained hemothorax following trauma, which might serve as a nidus for a subsequent empyema or restrict full lung reexpansion, can be identified (217). An improperly drained empyema is much more commonly a consequence of tube malposition rather than clogging with fibrin or debris. A persistent air leak may be documented to be caused by inadvertent lung puncture

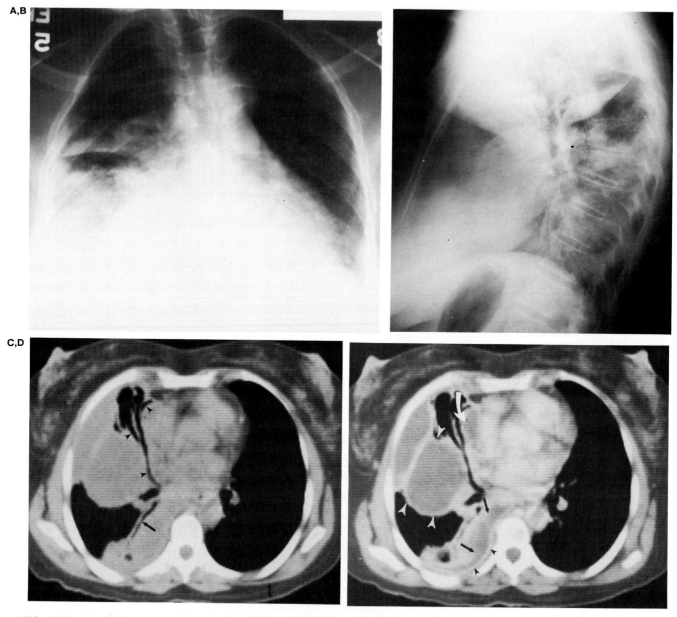

FIG. 100. Loculated empyemas secondary to staphylococcal pneumonia. **A,B:** Posteroanterior and lateral chest radiographs show right-middle-lobe and right-lower-lobe consolidation. The amount and site of concomitant pleural effusion were uncertain, although some fluid clearly was present in the posterior aspect of the right major fissure. Decubitus views showed no change in the appearance of the right hemithorax. **C:** Noncontrast CT image shows air bronchograms within the right middle lobe (*arrowheads*) and posterior basal segment of the right lower lobe (*arrow*). Opacification is noted lateral to the former and posterior to the latter. **D:** CT image post intravenous administration of contrast material clearly demarcates loculated nonenhanced fluid collections in the right major fissure (*white arrowheads*) and in the paraspinal area (*straight arrows*) internal to thickened parietal pleura (*black arrowheads*). Thoracostomy tube drainage of both of these regions resulted in dramatic clinical improvement. A smaller additional loculated fluid collection is noted medial to the middle lobe (*curved arrow*).

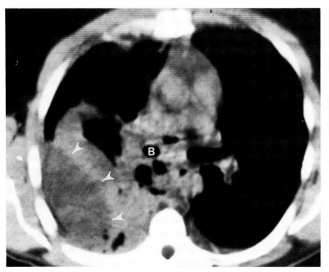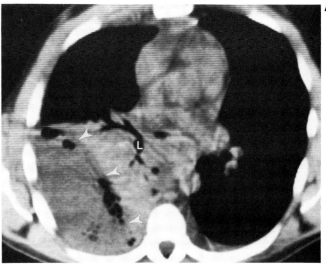

FIG. 101. Empyema. **A,B:** Sequential caudal noncontrast CT images demonstrate consolidation and volume loss within the right lower lobe and lateral segment of the middle lobe. An elliptical collection of slightly lower density (*arrowheads*) containing multiple air bubbles is seen posterolateral to the lower lobe. In addition, air and fluid collections are noted communicating posteromedially to the bronchus intermedius (B) and the right-lower-lobe bronchus (L) in the pleural space of the azygoesophageal recess and possibly within the mediastinum. A single thoracostomy tube inserted into the posterolateral empyema sufficed to drain all the collections.

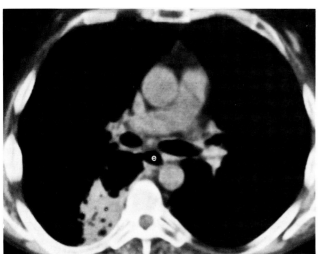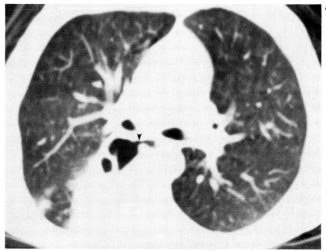

FIG. 102. Bronchoesophageal fistula. **A:** CT image at soft-tissue window setting in a patient with an unresponsive pneumonia demonstrates consolidation in the superior segment of the right lower lobe. No complicating empyema is identified, but the lateral wall of the esophagus (e) is not seen. **B:** Same image at lung window setting corroborates an apparent communication (*arrowhead*) between the esophagus and a cavity in the right lower lobe. **C:** Repeat image at the same level following oral barium administration documents a fistulous tract between the esophagus and lung.

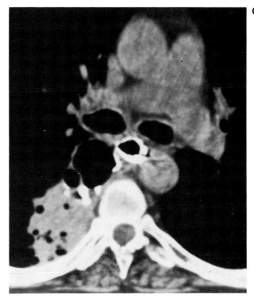

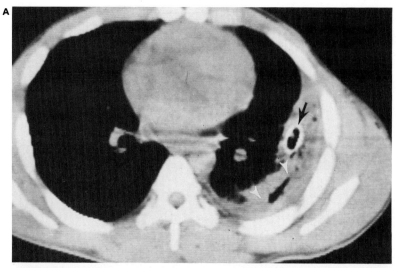

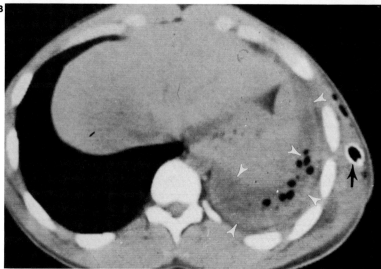

FIG. 103. Malpositioned thoracostomy tube for empyema drainage. **A,B:** CT images at the atrioventricular level and more caudally through the lung bases demonstrate that the thoracostomy tube (*arrow*) has been placed in the pleural space anterior and cephalad to the location of the empyema (*arrowheads*).

by the tip of the tube. Impending damage may be signaled by noting the tube tip directly against the mediastinum. The radiologist also can use CT to directly guide a relatively large (about 12 Fr) angiographic-type catheter into an empyema space for primary drainage (Fig. 105). The catheter, which is anchored and sealed with a "stomadhesive" disk or petroleum-jelly-impregnated gauze, generally can be removed after a few days when drainage ceases, the cavity closes, and the patient's fever subsides and white blood count returns to normal.

An undiagnosed or improperly treated empyema may progress to a chronic organized stage. Fibrosis may occur along the fibrin lining the visceral and parietal pleura surrounding the loculated pleural fluid, resulting in an inelastic membrane trapping the lung. Eventually the pleura may calcify, particularly if the cause of the empyema is tuberculous infection (96) (Fig. 106). The ipsilateral hemithorax usually becomes contracted, sometimes accompanied by an increase in the amount of extrapleural fat (Fig. 107). Although pleural calcification and fibrosis are the end results of long-standing pleural infection, nei-

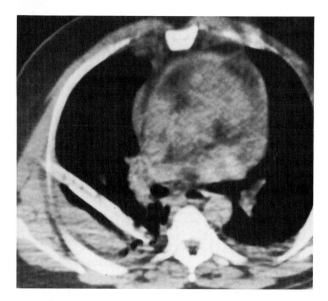

FIG. 104. Malpositioned thoracostomy tube. CT image documents that the tube has been placed in the major fissure anterior to a posteriorly loculated empyema (seen best on more caudal images).

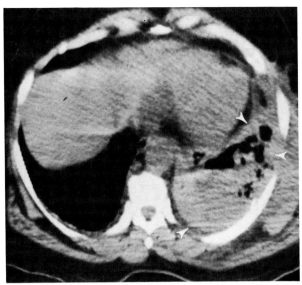
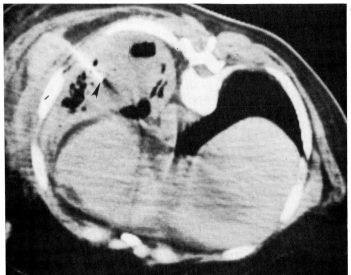

A,B

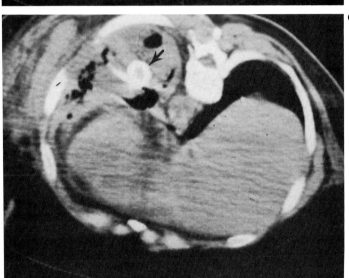

C

FIG. 105. CT-guided percutaneous drainage of empyema. **A:** CT demonstrates a large residual empyema (*arrowheads*) containing air and fluid caudally in the left pleural space in an obese man unsuccessfully drained by a poorly positioned, surgically placed thoracostomy tube. **B:** Prone CT image documents needle tip (*arrowhead*) within pleural-space collection; purulent material was aspirated. The subcutaneous hematoma resulted from the prior thoracostomy tube placement. **C:** Subsequent prone CT image shows a large pigtailed catheter (*arrow*) appropriately positioned within the empyema.

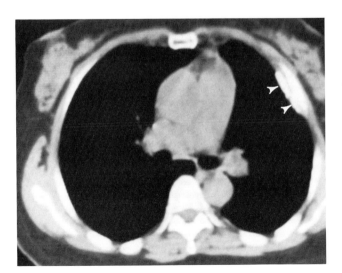

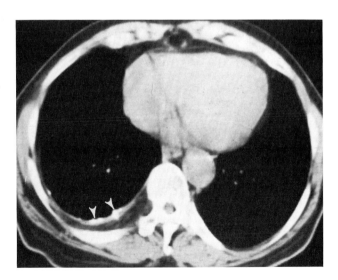

FIG. 106. Calcified thickened pleura (*arrowheads*) secondary to an old tuberculous empyema. Note the associated volume loss in the left hemithorax.

FIG. 107. Calcified thickened pleura (*arrowheads*) secondary to a prior tuberculous empyema. The abundant surrounding extrapleural fat is indicative of a chronic process.

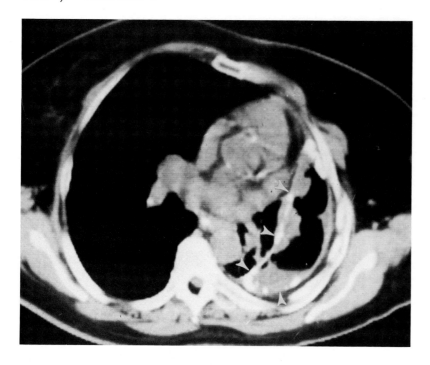

FIG. 108. Air and fluid are seen within a loculated pleural cavity with calcified walls (*arrowheads*) in a woman with a prior history of a tuberculous empyema. The left hemithorax and underlying lung are markedly contracted. Percutaneous aspiration of the pleural collection yielded only anaerobic streptococci; antibiotic therapy directed at this organism resulted in clinical improvement.

ther indicates quiescent disease. The presence of near-water-density fluid within the chronic pleural rind may be secondary to active, ongoing infection (Fig. 108). Once the pleura has fibrosed, effective therapy requires surgical intervention, including pleural decortication.

Asbestos-Related Pleural Disease

Persons exposed to asbestos dust have a notably increased incidence of various pleural disorders (plaque, thickening, and effusion), as well as pulmonary fibrosis and malignant neoplasms of the lung and pleura. Asbestos-related pleural disease should not be called "asbestosis," a term that should be restricted to the pulmonary parenchymal fibrosis caused by asbestos exposure. The diagnosis of asbestos-related pleural disease relies almost exclusively on radiologic changes.

Focal, smooth parietal pleural thickening, usually less than 1 cm thick, usually occurring bilaterally along the posterolateral thoracic wall, is the most common radiographic manifestation of asbestos exposure. Plaques may also occur within the pleura overlying the mediastinum, diaphragm, and pericardium; rarely they may be present in the visceral pleura of an interlobar fissure (229). On microscopic sectioning, these plaques are located beneath the mesothelial layer of cells and are actually extrapleural. Plaques do not undergo malignant degeneration, but are simply indicators of asbestos exposure. Because a history of such exposure may be difficult to obtain or may not be sought, conventional chest radiographs may provide the first indication of such exposure, with oblique views accentuating questionable pleural changes. The latent period between the time of first exposure and roentgeno-

graphic demonstration of the plaques is approximately 20 years. CT is more sensitive than conventional radiography in demonstrating pleural plaques, especially in depicting involvement of the mediastinal and paravertebral pleura. On CT, pleural plaques first appear as focal areas of soft-tissue thickening (Fig. 109), usually most prominent around the basilar paravertebral and posterior pleural surfaces. Initially, the disease process is discontinuous, with the plaques seen as "skip lesions" along the pleura, most notably on lung-window-setting images (Fig. 110). Calcification may be observed within the plaques, which may be punctate (Fig. 111), linear (Fig. 112), or "cake-

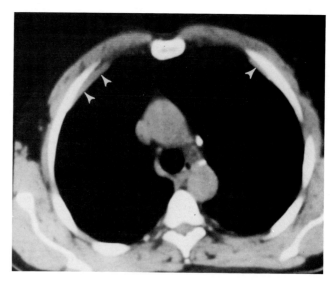

FIG. 109. Asbestos-related pleural plaques are seen as focal bilateral soft-tissue thickening (*arrowheads*) just internal to the ribs.

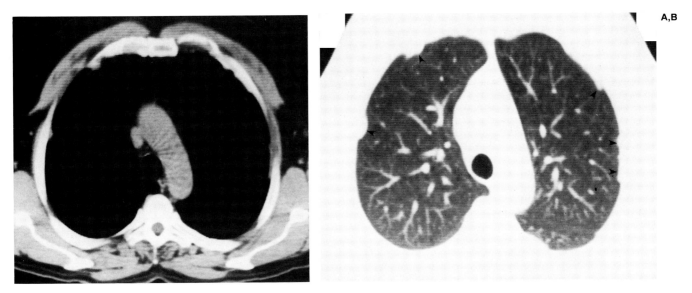

A,B

FIG. 110. Asbestos-related pleural plaques. **A:** CT image at soft-tissue window setting shows focal bilateral pleura-based nodulation. **B:** The presence and extent of the pleural plaques (*arrowheads*) are more easily demonstrated on a lung window setting at the same level.

like," the latter especially prevalent along the diaphragmatic surface (Fig. 113). Most times, the calcification predominates in the center of the plaque; calcified and noncalcified plaques frequently coexist (Fig. 114). On histologic examination, 85% of pleural plaques contain calcification. With CT, calcification is demonstrable in approximately 60% of pleural plaques; visible calcification on conventional radiography occurs in only 10%. Most plaques are noted in the absence of interstitial pulmonary

disease or fibrosis. Although CT may demonstrate more numerous or otherwise occult pleural plaques, routine use of this costly procedure is not justified, because demonstration of plaques indicates only exposure, not the presence of a financially compensable occupational disease nor malignant precursors. CT may be valuable when there is uncertainty on plain roentgenograms as to whether the observed pleural-based changes are due to plaques or extrapleural muscles or abundant fat (191) or whether in-

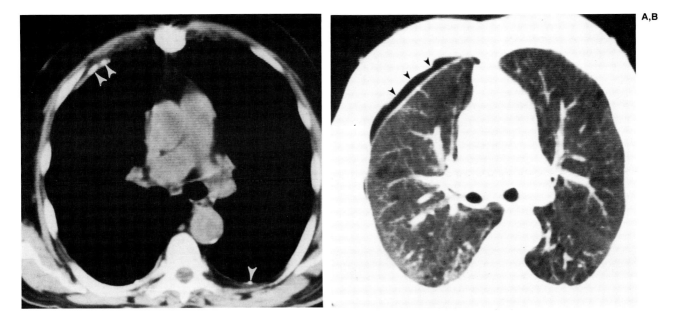

A,B

FIG. 111. Calcified pleural plaques. **A:** Punctate calcifications (*arrowheads*) are seen within areas of focal pleural thickening on a soft-tissue-window-setting CT image. **B:** Same image at lung window setting shows small concomitant right pneumothorax and demonstrates that maximal pleural thickening involves the parietal pleura (*arrowheads*). Scattered emphysematous changes are noted, as well as some interstitial disease in the superior segment of the right lower lobe.

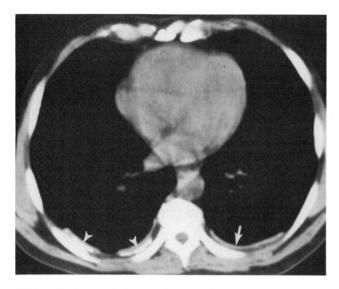

FIG. 112. Calcified pleural plaques. Linear calcifications (*arrowheads*) are seen within areas of focal pleural thickening in the right hemithorax. Soft-tissue-density pleural thickening (*arrow*) is present on the left side.

terstitial lung disease is present (Fig. 70). Also, CT can be beneficial in distinguishing focal plaques from intraparenchymal nodules (possibly carcinoma) or a complicating mesothelioma (Fig. 115), as well as in determining whether thoracic masses are pulmonary, mediastinal (Fig. 116), or pleural or indicate a combined benign pleuroparenchymal fibrotic condition (see previous section on rounded atelectasis).

Diffuse pleural thickening, with involvement from the apex to the base, also may be due to asbestos exposure (2,130). Unlike the case with pleural plaques, this radiologic appearance is nonspecific. The fibrosis usually involves both the parietal and visceral pleura, encasing the lung(s) in a dense rind (Fig. 117). When extensive, marked restrictive lung disease may be produced. Visceral pleural thickening may be recognized with certainty only when it is seen thickening the major interlobar fissure (Fig. 118). In other locations, it is indistinguishable from the adjacent parietal pleura. In a minority of patients, diffuse pleural thickening is associated with underlying pulmonary fibrosis.

A pleural effusion usually is a harbinger of a malignant pleural or pulmonary neoplasm in a patient with a substantial asbestos exposure, and this should be the initial presumption. However, a pleural effusion related to asbestos exposure may be benign in nature; it is typically an exudate and may be hemorrhagic (47).

Mesothelioma

Benign Fibrous Mesothelioma

A relatively rare, generally asymptomatic, slowly growing neoplasm arising from the fibrous elements of the mesothelium, this tumor usually originates from the visceral pleural layer and may occur within a fissure (207). On CT, a benign mesothelioma usually appears as a sharply defined soft-tissue-density mass, sometimes with

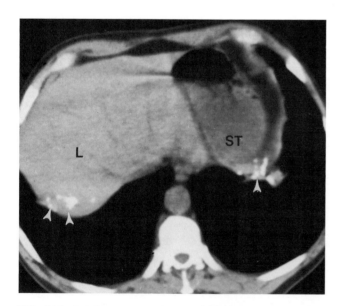

FIG. 113. Calcified pleural plaques. Irregular "cake-like" calcifications (*arrowheads*) are seen within focal pleural thickenings adjacent to the diaphragm on CT image in deep inspiration; (L) liver; (ST) stomach.

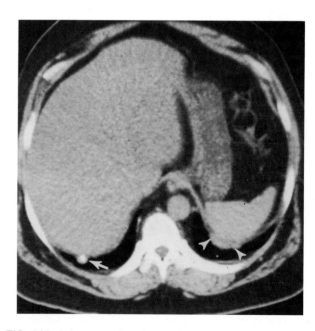

FIG. 114. Asbestos-related pleural plaques. Both calcified (*arrow*) and noncalcified (*arrowheads*) plaques along the diaphragmatic surface are seen.

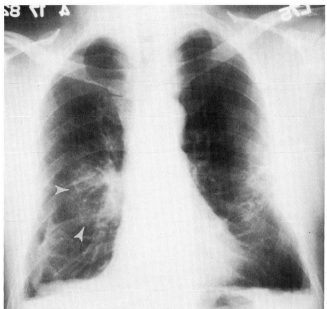
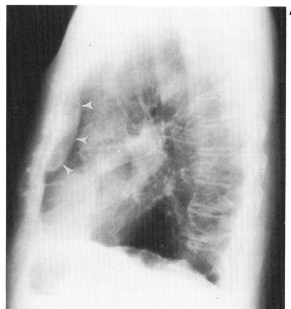

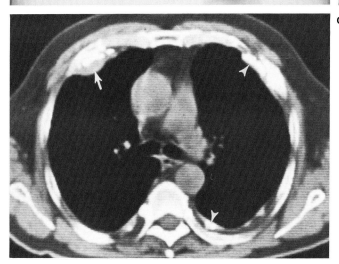
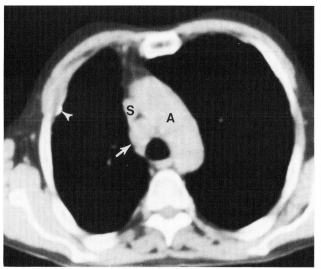

C

FIG. 115. Asbestos-related pleural plaques. **A,B:** Posteroanterior and lateral chest radiographs clearly demonstrate pleural plaques. However, it was questioned whether the mass (*arrowheads*) anteriorly in the right hemithorax could represent a complicating mesothelioma. **C:** CT shows that the mass (*arrow*) contains abundant calcification, compatible with a large benign plaque. Additional calcified plaques (*arrowheads*) are also noted.

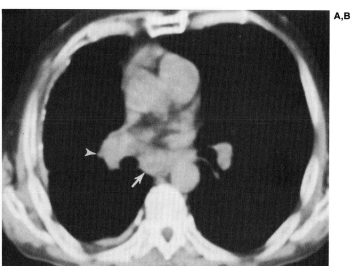

FIG. 116. Asbestos-related pleural plaques and bronchogenic carcinoma. **A:** CT image in a patient with right paratracheal widening noted on conventional chest radiography, in addition to pleural plaques and volume loss in the right hemithorax, demonstrates lymphadenopathy (*arrow*) as the cause of the widening, rather than medial pleural thickening or simple mediastinal shift; (S) superior vena cava; (A) aortic arch; (*arrowhead*) calcified pleural plaque. **B:** At 4 cm caudad, subcarinal (*arrow*) and right hilar (*arrowhead*) lymphadenopathy is also seen, in addition to the plaques. Subsequent mediastinoscopy disclosed undifferentiated small-cell carcinoma.

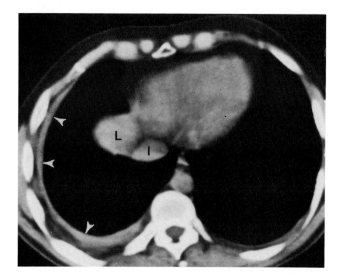

FIG. 117. Asbestos-related diffuse pleural thickening. Marked smooth, soft-tissue-density pleural thickening (*arrowheads*) is associated with notable volume loss in the right hemithorax. Abundant fat external to the thickened pleura is indicative of a chronic process; (I) inferior vena cava; (L) dome of liver and right hemidiaphragm.

lobulated margins, in close relationship to a pleural surface (40) (Fig. 119). The typical obtuse margins of a pleural mass may not be present; no invasion of the chest wall or lung is seen. Inhomogeneous enhancement after intravenous administration of contrast material may be observed.

Malignant Mesothelioma

The incidence of this highly aggressive, primary pleural neoplasm has increased in recent years, concomitant with other manifestations of asbestos exposure. Malignant mesothelioma is at least five times more frequent among asbestos workers than among the general population. The exposure to asbestos often has been only mild to moderate, and generally a 30-year latent period ensues between the initial exposure and development of this neoplasm. A malignant mesothelioma may arise from any mesothelial surface, but the vast majority originate in the pleura. Most are epithelial in type, but fibrous and mixed varieties also occur.

The most frequent plain chest radiographic manifestation is that of a pleural effusion that is often large and may obscure the pleural neoplasm. When the tumor itself is visible, it usually appears as a lobular mass or masses between the lung and chest wall. CT generally discloses that the neoplasm is much more extensive than appreciated on conventional radiographic studies (3,76). On CT, a malignant mesothelioma usually appears as a diffuse

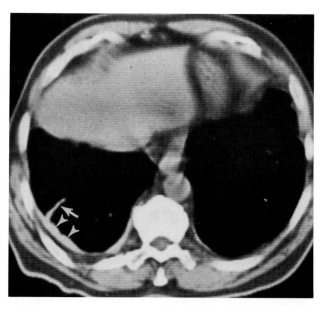

FIG. 118. Asbestos-related pleural thickening. Somewhat lobulated, diffuse, soft-tissue-density thickening (*arrowheads*) is seen extending into the right major fissure (*arrow*). Abundant extrapleural fat denotes a chronic process. Scattered plaques are also demonstrated in the left hemithorax.

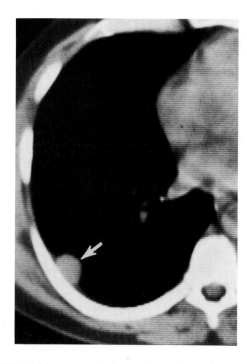

FIG. 119. Benign mesothelioma. A well-circumscribed soft-tissue-density mass (*arrow*) involving the pleura has obtuse margins with the chest wall.

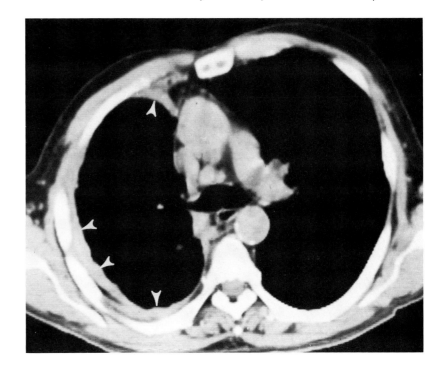

FIG. 120. Malignant mesothelioma. Circumferential, irregularly lobulated pleural thickening (*arrowheads*) is seen encasing and diminishing the volume of the right lung. Precarinal lymphadenopathy also is noted.

soft-tissue-density pleural thickening (Fig. 120) or mass (Fig. 121) encasing and having an irregular lobulated interface with a large portion of adjacent lung; rarely the lesion may be relatively localized (134) (Fig. 122). An associated pleural effusion, often loculated, usually is present (Fig. 123). The tumor commonly extends into the fissures and may cause volume loss in the ipsilateral lung. It can spread into the mediastinum, pericardium, lateral chest wall (Fig. 124), or contralateral hemithorax. Pene-

tration of the diaphragm, with involvement of the retroperitoneum or peritoneal cavity, may be detected. Such findings have obvious implications in treatment planning; the prognosis is poor, and neither surgery nor radiation therapy is universally accepted as a treatment option. Coexistent signs of asbestos exposure, including pleural thickening or plaques at remote sites and interstitial lung disease, are relatively common. Although CT may be valuable in suggesting this diagnosis in a patient with an

A,B

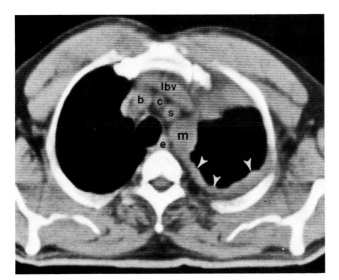
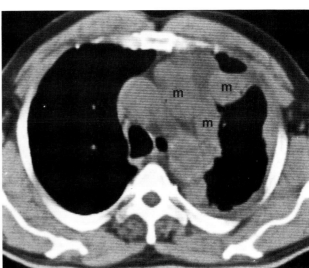

FIG. 121. Malignant mesothelioma. **A:** CT demonstrates irregular pleural thickening (*arrowheads*) surrounding the left lung, with a medial soft-tissue-density mass (m) invading the mediastinal fat; (lbv) left brachiocephalic vein; (r) right brachiocephalic vein; (s) left subclavian artery; (c) left carotid artery; (b) brachiocephalic artery; (e) esophagus. **B:** At 4 cm caudad, additional large lobulated masses (m) are seen involving the mediastinum, and there is diffuse circumferential pleural thickening.

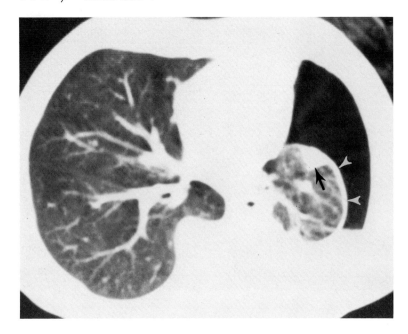

FIG. 122. Malignant mesothelioma. In a patient who presented with a spontaneous left hydro-pneumothorax on plain chest radiography, CT demonstrates a focal pleura-based mass (*arrow*) along with diffuse thickening of the visceral pleura (*arrowheads*).

unexplained persistent pleural effusion on plain chest radiography, occasionally it may be difficult to differentiate between a malignant mesothelioma and advanced benign pleural disease such as thickening (Fig. 125) or rounded atelectasis (Fig. 126) resulting from asbestos exposure (182). Irregular nodularity of the pleura is highly suspicious of a neoplastic process, but not specific.

Pleural Metastases

Abundant lymphatic channels and lymphoid aggregates are present in the subpleural region of the lung. Both met-astatic carcinoma and lymphoma can involve these areas just beneath the visceral pleura. In addition, pleural extension may occur from tumor emboli lodged in distal branches of the pulmonary arteries. Metastases constitute the overwhelming majority of malignant neoplasms involving the pleura. Besides bronchogenic carcinoma, primary neoplasms of the breast, gastrointestinal tract, ovary, and kidney are the most frequent sources. Generally, because of infiltration of the pleural surfaces, such metastases first become manifest as a pleural effusion. Substantially less commonly, pleural metastases may present as pleural-based nodules or masses, although even then they usually are accompanied by an effusion. CT has an advantage

A,B

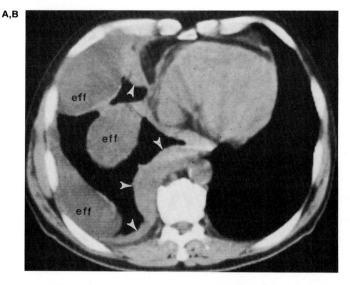
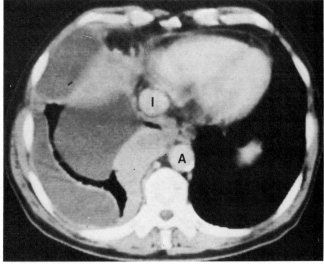

FIG. 123. Malignant mesothelioma. A: Noncontrast CT image shows only a subtle higher density of the pleural masses and thickening (*arrowheads*) compared with associated loculated exudative pleural effusions (eff). B: A contrast-enhanced image at approximately the same level demonstrates accentuation of the density differences between the enhanced pleural neoplasm and the nonenhanced fluid; (I) inferior vena cava; (A) aorta.

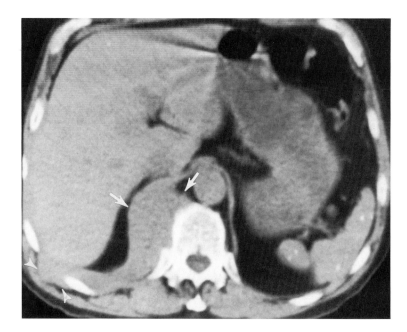

FIG. 124. Malignant mesothelioma. Extension through the chest wall (*arrowheads*), as well as caudally into the retrocrural space (*arrows*), is seen on an image of the upper abdomen.

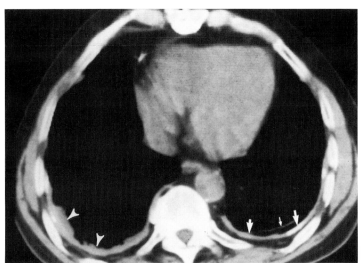

FIG. 125. Benign asbestos-related pleural thickening. Markedly irregular pleural thickening (*arrowheads*) is seen posteriorly in the right hemithorax, simulating a complicating mesothelioma. Pleuroscopic biopsies disclosed only fibrosis, and follow-up CT study demonstrated stability of the pleural abnormalities. Similar, but smoother, partially calcified pleural thickening (*large arrows*) is noted on the left side, as well as subpleural linear fibrosis (*small arrow*).

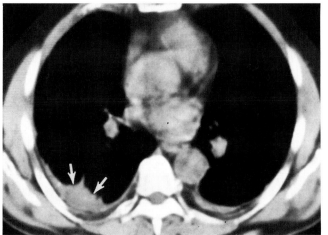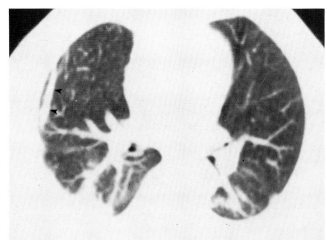

A,B

FIG. 126. Asbestos-related rounded atelectasis. **A:** An irregular mass (*arrows*) is seen adjacent to the pleura in the right hemithorax on a CT image at a soft-tissue window setting. Concomitant smooth pleural thickening is noted posteriorly on the left side. **B:** On the lung window setting of the same image, vessels are seen to approach, but not swirl around, the mass. Because of the absence of definitive findings of rounded atelectasis, percutaneous needle biopsy of the mass was performed. This disclosed only fibrosis, and follow-up CT examinations have shown no change. Some subpleural linear fibrosis (*arrowheads*) is noted in the middle lobe.

A,B

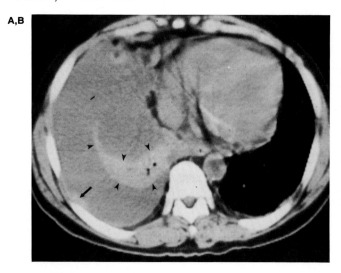 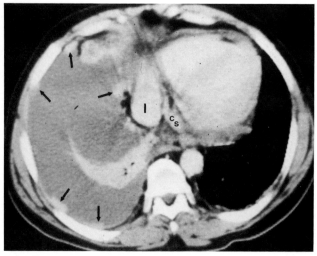

FIG. 127. Pleural metastases. **A:** On a noncontrast CT image in a patient with a large exudative pleural effusion, a single nodular pleural mass (*arrow*) is barely perceptible. Compressive atelectasis of the underlying right lower lobe (*arrowheads*) is present. **B:** On an image at the same level following intravenous administration of contrast material, multiple enhanced pleural metastases (*arrows*) are seen. A small pericardial effusion also is noted; (I) inferior vena cava; (cs) coronary sinus.

over plain chest roentgenography in demonstrating this malignant disease because of its capability to distinguish relatively subtle pleural nodularity from surrounding fluid. Images following intravenous administration of contrast material are particularly effective in this differentiation because the metastases frequently are enhanced (Fig. 127), although sometimes foci of tumor are difficult or impossible to identify within the effusion. Pleural metastases usually appear as relatively small lenticular masses having obtuse margins with the chest wall. Rarely, especially with metastatic adenocarcinoma, diffuse involvement of the pleura may occur (Fig. 128), mimicking a malignant mesothelioma; histologic distinction also can be a problem. Ancillary findings on CT, such as mediastinal lymph node enlargement, lung nodules, rib lesions, or a subcutaneous mass, would support a presumptive diagnosis of pleural metastases (Fig. 129). With inflammatory pleural disease (e.g., granulomatous infection or asbestos-related), although the pleural surfaces become thickened, they are rarely nodular and irregular, and associated notable volume loss in the ipsilateral hemithorax occurs when it is extensive and chronic pleural fibrosis ensues.

Involvement of the pleura by lymphoma is seldom the solitary initial manifestation of the disease (198). Usually it is due to recurrence (see Fig. 23 in Chapter 7) or is an additional intrathoracic site at presentation along with mediastinal (thymic and/or nodal) and sometimes pulmonary parenchymal disease. Pleural lymphoma characteristically presents as a localized, broad-based pleural mass that may be difficult to recognize on conventional

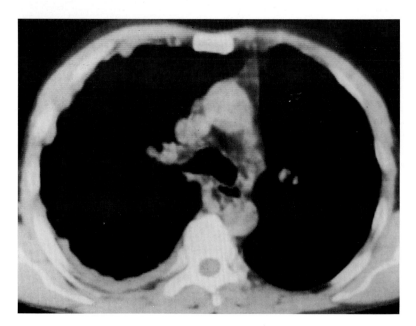

FIG. 128. Pleural metastases. Multiple lobulated soft-tissue-density right pleural masses due to metastatic renal-cell carcinoma are seen without an associated pleural effusion. The appearance simulates a malignant mesothelioma. Concomitant mediastinal lymph node metastases are present.

A,B

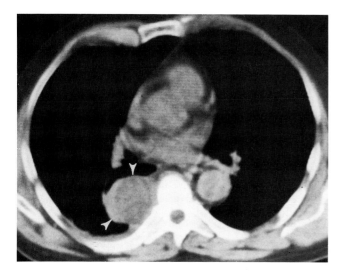
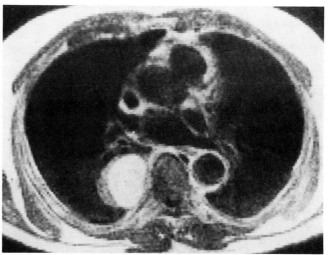

FIG. 129. Pleural metastasis. **A:** Noncontrast CT image in a patient with melanoma and right posterior chest pain demonstrates an inhomogeneous pleural-based mass (*arrowheads*). Most of the mass has an attenuation value (30 HU) slightly lower than that of soft tissue, except for the periphery, especially laterally. A small associated pleural effusion of relatively high attenuation value is present. **B:** On a T1-weighted MR image, most of the mass has a very high signal intensity, identical in distribution to the relatively low density portion noted on CT. The explanation for the high signal was a combination of the paramagnetic effect of melanin and a small amount of subacute internal hemorrhage.

radiography, especially if there is a coexistent pleural effusion (Fig. 130).

Pneumothorax

Following severe trauma, thoracic injury frequently coexists with damage to other areas (e.g., abdomen, head). Identification of a small pneumothorax or even a relatively large anteromedial air collection in the pleural space can be very difficult on a supine or semirecumbent chest radiograph, often performed with portable apparatus. Forthcoming mechanical ventilation or surgery under general anesthesia makes it imperative to detect such a pneumothorax and institute thoracostomy tube drainage. In traumatized patients undergoing abdominal CT examination, the most cephalad images should be examined with lung window settings to attempt to identify an otherwise occult pneumothorax (225). A limited thoracic study has even been advocated following serious trauma if the patient requires a CT examination for another indication, assessing for possible mediastinal hemorrhage, sternoclavicular dislocation, pericardial effusion, or a diaphragmatic tear, as well as an occult pneumothorax (218,219). CT also may be valuable in selected patients for characterizing confusing paramediastinal air collections, distinguishing a medial pneumothorax from a pneumomediastinum or a parenchymal pneumatocele. An unsuspected pneumothorax may be depicted in any critically ill patient with progressive pulmonary insufficiency, as may a substantial pleural fluid collection in a septic individual that was not visible on a portable chest radiograph (135). Additionally, CT can demonstrate a

coexistent pneumothorax in a patient with extensive subcutaneous air.

Postpneumonectomy Space

The space created following pneumonectomy, bordered by the residual subcostal and mediastinal parietal pleura, initially contains serosanguinous fluid, after absorption

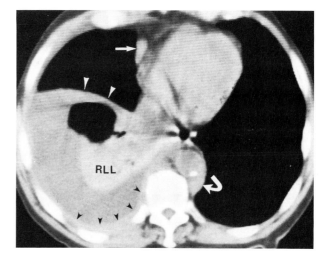

FIG. 130. Pleural lymphoma. In a patient presenting with weight loss noted to have a large right pleural effusion on chest radiography, CT demonstrates diffuse smooth thickening (*black arrowheads*) of the right-side pleura. Compressive atelectasis of the right lower lobe (RLL) is noted, and some fluid extends into the major fissure (*white arrowheads*). Otherwise occult concomitant, mildly enlarged right supradiaphragmatic (*straight arrow*) and left paraaortic (*curved arrow*) lymph nodes are seen. Pleuroscopic biopsy disclosed non-Hodgkin lymphoma.

A,B

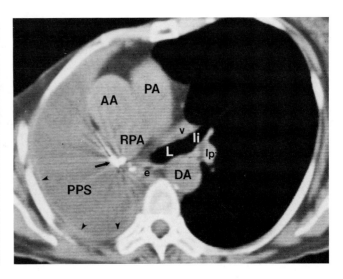

FIG. 131. Normal anatomy post right pneumonectomy. **A,B:** CT images at the level of the aortic arch (ARCH) and right pulmonary artery (RPA), respectively, demonstrate the postpneumonectomy space (PPS), which is low in attenuation value (25 HU) compared with the soft-tissue density of the chest-wall musculature and blood within the great vessels. The space, demarcated externally by the residual parietal pleura (*arrowheads*), is contained within a notably contracted right hemithorax. Slight motion in the metallic vascular or bronchial-stump surgical clips (*arrow*) can produce minor streak artifacts; (S) superior vena cava; (T) trachea; (e) esophagus; (AA) ascending aorta; (DA) descending aorta; (PA) main pulmonary artery; (L) left main-stem bronchus; (li) left upper lobe and lingular bronchus; (v) left superior pulmonary vein; (lp) left-lower-lobe pulmonary artery.

of the gas in the immediate postoperative period. Some of this fluid also is eventually resorbed, and the postpneumonectomy space is gradually reduced in size. However, in only about 20% of patients does it become completely obliterated and occupied by relocated mediastinal structures. In the remainder, a space persists for many years following surgery, varying from 1 to 5 cm in transverse diameter. A range of anatomic alterations may occur consequent to rotation and displacement of the mediastinal structures as well as hyperexpansion of the contralateral lung. Knowledge of these various appearances on CT is essential so as not to confuse distorted normal anatomy and a pathologic condition (20). The postpneumo-

nectomy space itself is relatively homogeneous and of lower density than soft tissue because of the contained residual fluid. Following a right pneumonectomy, the mediastinum tends to rotate, with a resultant transverse orientation of the aortic arch, and the contralateral lung herniates anteriorly (Fig. 131). In general, the smaller the postpneumonectomy space, the greater the lung herniation (Figs. 132 and 133). The mediastinal shift may be so extreme following a right pneumonectomy in childhood

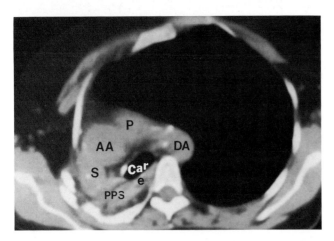

FIG. 132. Diminutive right postpneumonectomy space (PPS). Marked counterclockwise rotation of the mediastinum is seen, and the ascending aorta (AA) and descending aorta (DA) have assumed a coronal orientation; (P) main pulmonary artery; (Car) carina; (e) esophagus; (S) superior vena cava.

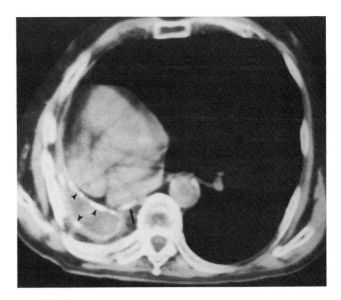

FIG. 133. Calcification is present in the parietal pleura (*arrowheads*) surrounding a small right postpneumonectomy space 12 years after surgery for bronchogenic carcinoma. The left lung has herniated anterior to the heart; (*arrow*) esophagus containing barium.

A,B

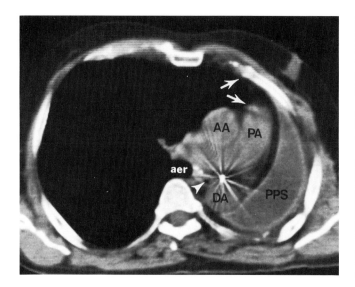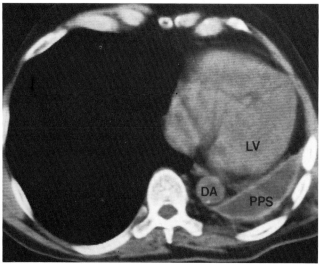

FIG. 134. Normal anatomy post left pneumonectomy. **A,B:** CT images at the level of the main pulmonary artery (PA) and left ventricle (LV), respectively, demonstrate the residual, relatively low density postpneumonectomy space (PPS). Note that the medial border of the space is either concave or straight in its interface with the mediastinum. Motion in a left-bronchial-stump clip creates some streak artifacts. The right lung has herniated (*arrows*) anterior to the ascending aorta (AA), as well as posterior to the bronchus intermedius into the azygoesophageal recess (aer); (DA) descending aorta; (*arrowhead*) esophagus.

or adolescence that the distal trachea and remaining left main-stem bronchus are partially compressed between the aorta and left pulmonary artery, resulting in dyspnea or recurrent left-lung infections (196). Following a left pneumonectomy, the mediastinum shifts so that the usual anteroposterior orientation of the aortic arch generally is maintained; the contralateral lung may herniate posteriorly as well as anteriorly (Figs. 134–136).

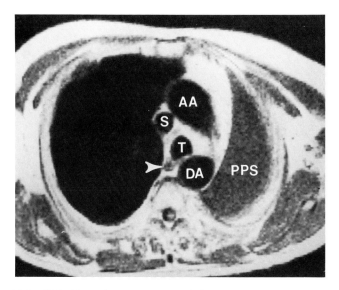

FIG. 135. Normal anatomy post left pneumonectomy. T1-weighted MR image demonstrates medium signal intensity in the postpneumonectomy space (PPS), which is clearly demarcated from the high-signal-intensity mediastinal fat; (AA) ascending aorta; (DA) descending aorta; (S) superior vena cava; (T) trachea; (*arrowhead*) esophagus.

As a result of a previous pneumonectomy, opacification of the hemithorax makes evaluation of the postpneumonectomy space and ipsilateral mediastinum extremely difficult with conventional radiography. Disease in this area can be detected only when it is so gross that mediastinal shift occurs. CT (or MRI) is a more sensitive and useful technique for detecting recurrent neoplasm or another complication at an earlier stage (64,172). Recurrence of bronchogenic carcinoma within the thorax most commonly occurs near the bronchial stump or in the mediastinal lymph nodes (Figs. 137 and 138). Sometimes it can be identified as a soft-tissue-density mass projecting into the lower-density postpneumonectomy space (Fig. 139). Palliative radiation therapy may be targeted to the recurrent tumor. CT also may be of value in confirming infection in the postpneumonectomy space (88) (Fig. 140). Convex expansion of the medial border may be a relatively early sign of a complicating empyema; it may be accompanied by air in the postpneumonectomy space. With advanced infection, the mediastinum may shift back toward the midline.

Miscellaneous

Pleural thickening, nodularity, and/or a large mass may occur as manifestations of intrapleural aspergillosis (36). Although this complication may be engrafted on prior granulomatous disease, it also can follow resection for bronchogenic carcinoma and needs to be distinguished from recurrent neoplasm.

Pleural calcification along the hemidiaphragm may be seen on CT as a consequence of previous pancreatitis (26),

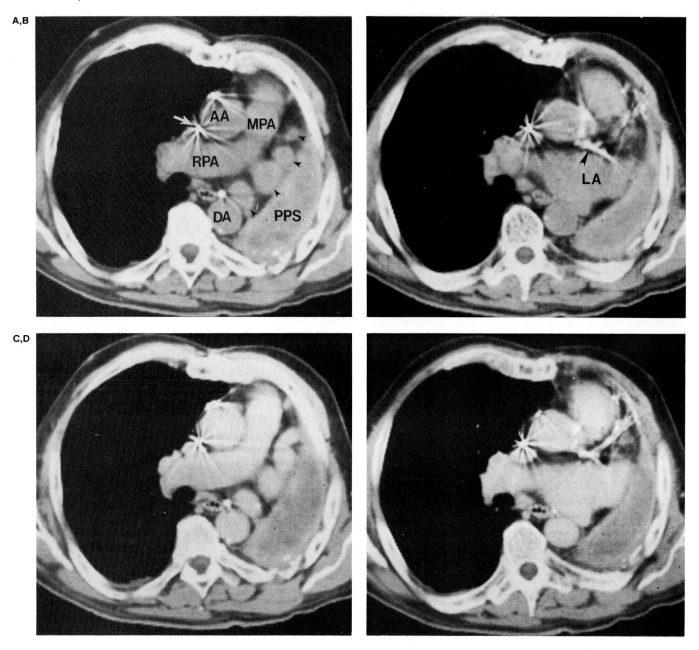

FIG. 136. Anatomic variation post left pneumonectomy; value of contrast enhancement. **A:** Noncontrast CT image at the level of the right pulmonary artery (RPA) demonstrates multiple round mediastinal "masses" (*arrowheads*), of questionable etiology, anteromedial to the postpneumonectomy space (PPS). Streak artifacts are produced by a transvenous pacemaker (*arrow*) in the superior vena cava and by clips anterior to the ascending aorta (AA) from a previous coronary artery bypass procedure; (DA) descending aorta; (MPA) main pulmonary artery. **B:** At 1 cm caudad, the questioned round opacities merge with the top of the left atrium (LA); (*arrowhead*) extensive calcification in left coronary artery. **C,D:** Sequential caudal CT images at same levels as (**A**) and (**B**) following intravenous administration of contrast material demonstrate enhancement of the tubular "masses" to the same degree as blood in the great vessels and the left atrium. The questioned masses therefore represent a dilated left atrial appendage.

A,B

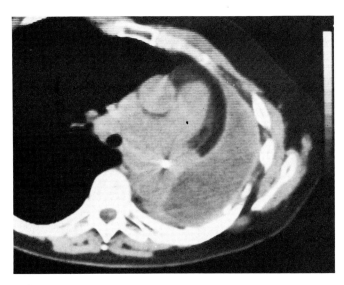
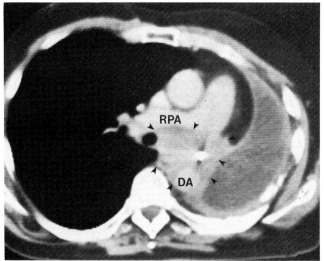

FIG. 137. Recurrent bronchogenic carcinoma post left pneumonectomy. **A:** Noncontrast CT image shows a poorly defined soft-tissue mass surrounding the surgical clip. **B:** On a contrast-enhanced image at the same level, the extensive mediastinal tumor recurrence around the bronchial stump is more clearly demarcated (*arrowheads*), compressing the right pulmonary artery (RPA) and extending medial and lateral to the descending aorta (DA).

FIG. 138. Recurrent bronchogenic carcinoma post left pneumonectomy. On a T1-weighted MR image, the neoplasm (*arrowheads*) is seen as an interme-diate-signal-intensity mass clearly demarcated from the signal void in the mediastinal vessels and right bronchi. The recurrent tumor has a slightly higher signal intensity than the fluid in the postpneumo-nectomy space (PPS).

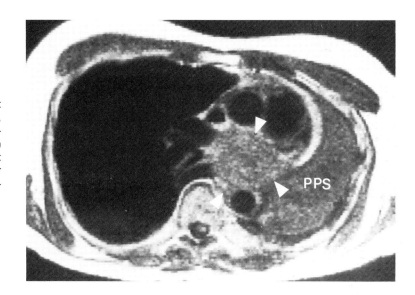

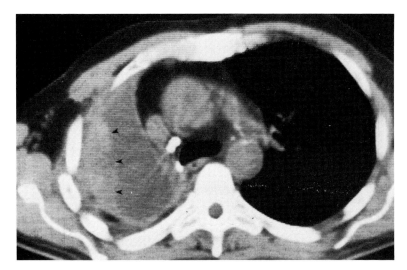

FIG. 139. Recurrent bronchogenic carcinoma in postpneumonectomy space. A soft-tissue-density mass (*arrowheads*) fills the lateral aspect of the space. Subsequent CT-guided needle-aspiration biopsy of the mass corroborated recurrent neo-plasm.

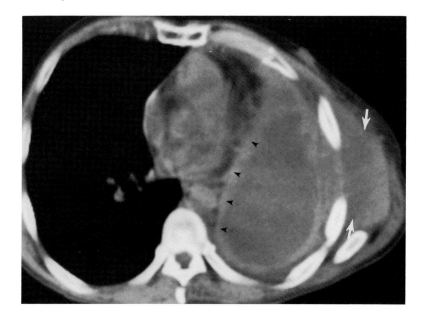

FIG. 140. Empyema in the postpneumonectomy space. Convex expansion of the medial border of the space (*arrowheads*) is seen, resulting in some contralateral displacement of the mediastinum. The mediastinal fat is poorly defined and infiltrated by irregular linear densities. Spread of infection also has occurred into the left lateral chest wall (*arrows*). Needle aspiration of the space yielded purulent material containing *Staphylococcus aureus*.

as well as asbestos exposure. Also, high-density (about 160 HU) pleuroparenchymal lesions may be noted near the lung bases in patients on amiodarone therapy (109); the concomitant increased liver density should suggest the proper diagnosis (Fig. 66).

DIAPHRAGM

A variety of abnormalities involving the diaphragm may arise from a disturbance in its barrier function, including a congenital defect, acquired hernia, or traumatic rupture.

Certainly, most esophageal hiatus hernias do not require CT for diagnosis. However, CT may uniquely demonstrate transhiatal herniation of fat (see Fig. 3 in Chapter 8), which may be mistaken for a mediastinal mass. Morgagni (anterior) (Fig. 141) and Bochdalek (posterior) (see Figs. 113 and 114 in Chapter 7) hernias are less likely to contain gastrointestinal loops and therefore usually are better evaluated by CT than by conventional barium studies if corroboration is necessary.

Rupture of the diaphragm following blunt trauma may be overlooked initially because of other, more salient injuries; obscuring parenchymal and pleural disease may

A,B

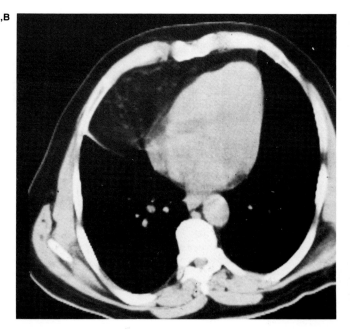
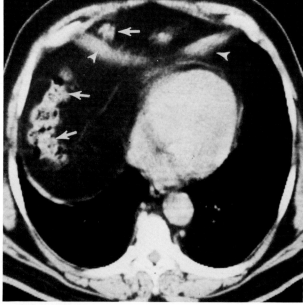

FIG. 141. Diaphragmatic herniation through the foramen of Morgagni. **A:** The hernia contains omental fat and associated mesenteric vessels; the latter feature allows differentiation from a large pericardial fat pad. **B:** In another patient, the hernia contains colon (*arrows*) in addition to omental fat and vessels; (*arrowheads*) anterior diaphragmatic muscle insertions.

prevent diagnosis (8). Of special note, herniation of abdominal contents may not develop until months or years after the injury. Left-sided herniation predominates, accounting for about 90% of cases; the liver probably reduces its development on the right side. Most tears originate in the peripheral portion of the diaphragm at the junction of its tendon and posterior leaves. Conventional radiography may disclose air-containing bowel within the thorax, which can be confirmed with barium studies. Diagnosis is much more difficult when the herniation does not include bowel. The condition may be misdiagnosed as an abnormally contoured, elevated hemidiaphragm or a pleural mass. Omental fat accompanying the herniated contents may simulate a pleural effusion on plain radiographs. CT can demonstrate the intrathoracic location of the abdominal organs, such as the liver, spleen, kidney, or omental fat, passing through a discontinuity in the diaphragm (92) (Fig. 142). Loops of bowel may be seen posterior or lateral to the diaphragm in the thorax.

A normal, intact diaphragm is not an impermeable barrier to either inflammatory or neoplastic disease. With a subphrenic abscess, the accompanying pleural effusion usually is reactive, but infective organisms can penetrate the diaphragm and cause a concomitant empyema. Similarly, fluid collections resulting from pancreatitis may extend through a hiatus into the mediastinum; their origin generally is readily documented on CT. Conversely, infection may spread from the thorax into the abdomen. With neoplastic disease, CT can be valuable in determining if a disease process is confined to the chest or abdomen or if it penetrates the diaphragm, a determination some-

times of critical staging importance (159). Irregular thickening of the diaphragm may be a sign of neoplastic infiltration, with extension beyond the diaphragm manifested by a soft-tissue-density mass protruding above or below it.

Primary and metastatic neoplasms involving the diaphragm are rare. Although intimately associated with the diaphragm, the source of origin frequently is impossible to determine definitively with CT.

CHEST WALL

The ability to use direct palpation to define precisely the extent of a chest-wall lesion and determine its origin is relatively limited, especially in obese patients. Except for some osseous abnormalities, the information provided by plain-film roentgenography regarding the thoracic wall is similarly restricted, and even the detail of the bones may be insufficient. Again, the ability of CT to distinguish among fat, soft-tissue, and bone densities and display the individual components of the chest wall in cross section can be valuable in providing important clinical information (75). CT is particularly beneficial in demonstrating the precise anatomic location and extent of a disease process, which may be critical for treatment planning. In some patients, the CT findings in the chest wall are incidental and unsuspected because the examination was directed primarily toward evaluation of the mediastinum or lungs. Rarely, a specific diagnosis of a chest-wall lesion (e.g., lipoma) may be provided. Furthermore, because of the

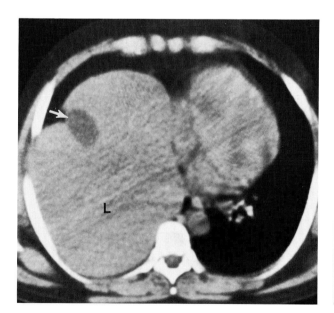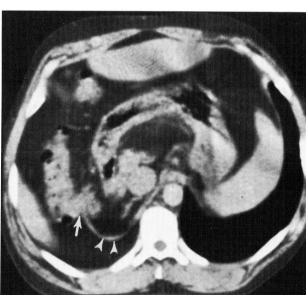

A,B

FIG. 142. Traumatic rupture of the diaphragm. **A:** In a patient noted on chest radiography to have apparent marked elevation of the right hemidiaphragm, CT shows the true cause to be herniation of the liver (L) into the lower right hemithorax. The liver has rotated on its horizontal axis during its ascent, with the gallbladder fossa (*arrow*) now directed anterolaterally. **B:** A more caudal image demonstrates the torn free end (*arrow*) of the right diaphragmatic crus (*arrowheads*), adjacent to the ascending colon. On questioning, the patient related involvement in an automobile accident 9 years previously.

complex anatomy of the thoracic skeleton, when conventional roentgenograms including special views are not conclusive, CT is preferred over plain-film tomography, especially if involvement of the contiguous soft tissues is questioned; both sides can be seen simultaneously, and there is better separation from superimposed structures. In selected cases, CT may be helpful in providing information about congenital thoracic-cage deformities such as pectus excavatum or absence of a pectoral muscle (41).

Trauma

Sternoclavicular Dislocation

The more common anterior dislocation of the clavicular head is easier to diagnose clinically because of the usually obvious anterior chest-wall deformity. A posterior dislocation, however, is difficult to diagnose both clinically and roentgenographically and is a much more serious disorder because of the proximity of the medial end of the clavicle to the great vessels in the mediastinum. Rarely, superior dislocation of the clavicular head may occur. The cross-sectional CT images enable easy demonstration of any of these types of dislocation (see Fig. 112 in Chapter 21) (42,112).

Rib Fracture

Clearly, these common fractures generally can be evaluated satisfactorily with conventional radiography. Rib fractures may be discovered incidentally on CT while evaluating the thorax following trauma; attention should be directed toward contiguous vital structures, including

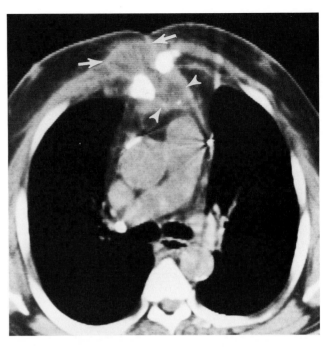

FIG. 144. Subcutaneous and mediastinal abscess. In a febrile patient 3 months after a coronary artery bypass procedure, sclerosis and nonunion of the body of the sternum are seen. A poorly circumscribed mass (*arrows*) is seen in the anterior chest wall, communicating through the sternum with an inhomogeneous collection with a low-density central area (*arrowheads*) within the anterior mediastinum.

the great vessels, tracheobronchial tree, pericardium, and the solid upper abdominal organs.

A diagnostic problem can occur in a patient with a history of carcinoma and an abnormal radionuclide bone scintigram when a corresponding abnormality cannot be seen on standard radiography; CT may be helpful in dem-

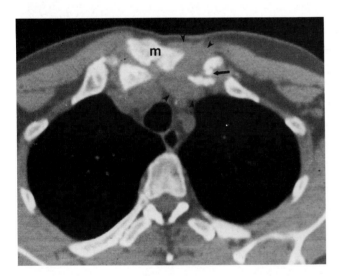

FIG. 143. Sternoclavicular osteomyelitis and septic arthritis. A soft-tissue mass (*arrowheads*) is seen surrounding the left sternoclavicular joint. The manubrium (m) is deformed and sclerotic, and the left clavicular head (*arrow*) is sclerotic and fragmented.

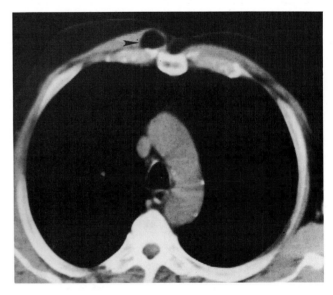

FIG. 145. Lipoma. A well-defined homogeneous fat collection (*arrowhead*) is seen within the right pectoralis major muscle, accounting for a palpable anterior-chest-wall mass.

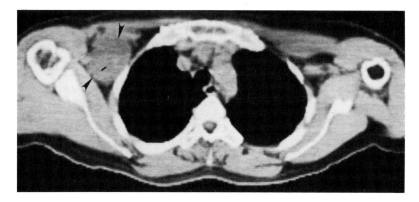

FIG. 146. Neurilemoma, right brachial plexus. CT image, performed with arms at patient's side, demonstrates a well-circumscribed 5-cm mass (*arrowheads*) in the right axilla, which is slightly lower in attenuation value than the surrounding chest-wall muscles.

onstrating a callus and rib deformity characteristic of a healing fracture. If the fracture is acute, CT may be beneficial to evaluate for an underlying destructive lesion.

Infection

Infection of the sternum and sternoclavicular joint is uncommon, and usually it occurs following thoracic surgery or radiation therapy. Drug addiction and infective endocarditis are other causes of osteomyelitis and septic arthritis (Fig. 143) in these sites. The radiographic findings can be subtle and difficult to detect because of the complex skeletal anatomy and any associated osteopenia; concomitant pulmonary infiltrates or pleural effusions also may obscure osseous detail. In postoperative patients, nuclear medicine imaging often is not beneficial because the radionuclide normally concentrates in surgical sites. CT can more effectively demonstrate small areas of bone destruction, periosteal reaction, and the presence of any associated soft-tissue abscess (Fig. 144).

Chest-wall infection may occur secondary to disease of the pleura or pulmonary parenchyma. Reactivation of pleural tuberculosis may result in a "cold" thoracic-wall abscess (Fig. 99). Actinomycosis may secondarily invade the chest wall from a focus of infection originating in the pulmonary parenchyma. The appearances of these conditions on CT may be indistinguishable from that of a neoplastic process; hypervascular walls may be seen on contrast-enhanced images.

Neoplasm

A variety of tumors can arise within the soft tissues of the chest wall, including lipoma, hemangioma, and those of fibrous or neurogenic origin. A lipoma can be specifically diagnosed on CT by its characteristic homogeneous low density (approximately −80 HU) (Fig. 145); when transmural extension is present, an apparent destructive bone lesion noted on a conventional radiograph may be shown to be due to pressure erosion (49). Distinction from a liposarcoma, which almost always has areas of higher

density, usually is possible. Neurogenic tumors often have a relatively low density (Fig. 146) approaching that of water, for a variety of reasons, including an abundant lipid content, myxoid matrix, hypocellularity, and/or regions of cystic degeneration (33,39). Malignant transformation may not be present even when inhomogeneous attenuation values are seen. CT cannot provide a specific diagnosis for lesions that have a soft-tissue density, and benign histology may be indistinguishable from a malignant lesion, because neither size nor the sharpness of the border is a reliable diagnostic criterion. For example, elastofibroma dorsi, a benign connective-tissue mass occurring in elderly patients that arises between the chest wall and the inferior angle of the scapula, usually appears on CT as an infiltrating, incompletely marginated, soft-tissue-density mass (18,121). Subcutaneous metastases may appear well circumscribed (Fig. 147).

CT rarely provides additional useful information with most benign bone lesions, other than reassurance that they

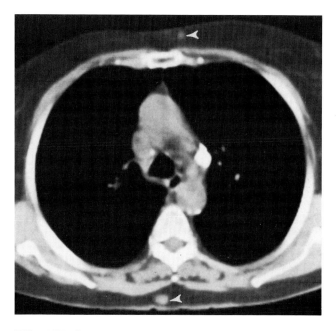

FIG. 147. Subcutaneous metastases (*arrowheads*) due to melanoma manifested as soft-tissue-density nodules within the predominantly fatty background.

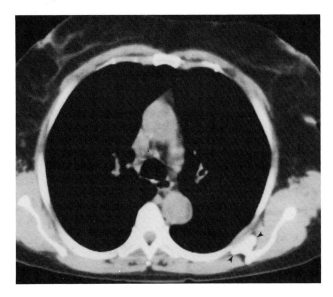

FIG. 148. Osteochondroma (*arrowheads*) of left scapula. No abnormally thickened soft-tissue-density cartilaginous cap is present to suggest malignant transformation.

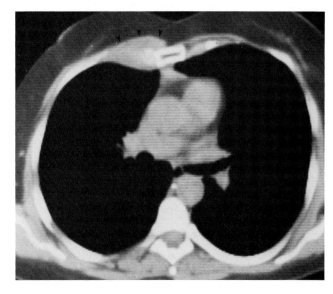

FIG. 150. A soft-tissue mass (*arrowheads*) involving a rib and costal cartilage was the sole manifestation of recurrent non-Hodgkin lymphoma.

are clearly benign (Fig. 148), such as a developmental anomaly or posttraumatic lesion (45). In Tietze syndrome, CT may demonstrate enlargement or ventral angulation of the costal cartilage at the site of the complaint and exclude the presence of a soft-tissue mass. With a hemangioma, the intact cortical margin surrounding an expansile lesion containing internal trabeculations may be shown (165).

The ribs and thoracic spine are frequent sites of neoplastic metastases. Although radionuclide bone scintigraphy is the preferred technique for detection, CT occasionally discloses a previously undiagnosed lesion. Skeletal metastases generally appear as areas of subtle or complete lytic destruction (Figs. 149–151) and may be first noted because they were obscured on conventional radiographs by the heart, diaphragm (Fig. 152), or an underlying lung

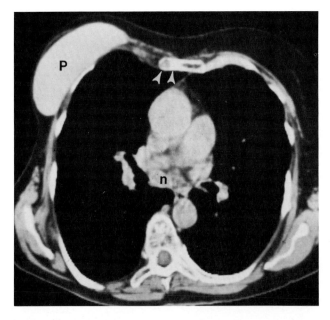

FIG. 149. Sternal metastasis. Metastatic breast carcinoma producing a mixed lytic and blastic lesion (*arrowheads*) involving the right side of the body of the sternum. A breast prosthesis (P) is noted, and concomitant subcarinal lymphadenopathy (n) is present.

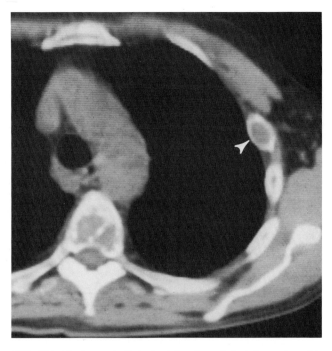

FIG. 151. Myeloma. Lytic lesions involve a left rib (*arrowheads*), which is also expanded, and a thoracic vertebral body.

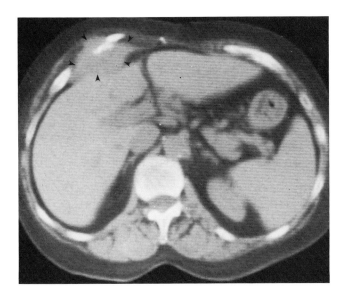

FIG. 152. Rib metastasis. In a patient who presented with a palpable "right-upper-quadrant" abdominal mass, CT shows the cause to be a destructive rib lesion, with a surrounding soft-tissue mass (*arrowheads*). More caudal images demonstrated a primary renal tumor.

mass or pleural effusion. Occasionally, CT may be helpful in characterizing a lesion that is poorly seen on conventional radiography (Fig. 153); features present may strongly suggest metastasis as the likely cause. In addition, with malignant bone lesions, CT can be useful in determining the presence and delineating the total extent of any associated soft-tissue infiltration (Fig. 154), an assessment that may affect the decision regarding radiation therapy, radical surgery, or some palliative measure, or where to conduct a percutaneous biopsy if histologic corroboration is required (Fig. 155). Certain primary tumors, such as myeloma, chondrosarcoma, and Ewing sarcoma, are accompanied by a soft-tissue mass, whereas this is a much less frequent finding with metastases.

When studying the thorax for other reasons, an incidental breast mass (e.g., carcinoma) (Fig. 156) may be detected (144). Dedicated CT units for depicting breast abnormalities have been abandoned because of limited specificity and the impractical requirement for intravenous administration of contrast material to detect carcinomas with a high sensitivity (29). Very rarely, CT may be useful for three-dimensional localization of a clinically occult lesion detected on a single mammographic projection (43,104). There may be some value in using CT if chest-wall invasion or regional lymph node involvement

A

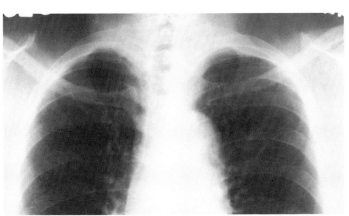

FIG. 153. Rib metastasis. **A,B:** Posteroanterior and lateral chest radiographs demonstrate an abnormal density (*arrowheads*) seen only on the lateral projection, questioned to represent an anterior mediastinal mass. **C:** CT image shows the cause to be a soft-tissue mass (*arrowheads*) arising from the anterior end of a left rib.

B,C

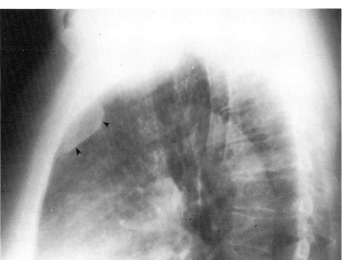

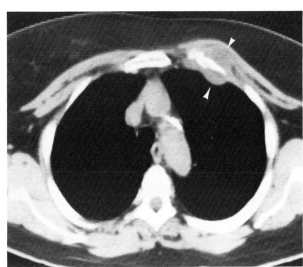

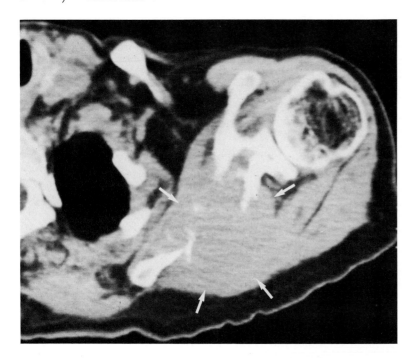

FIG. 154. Lymphoma of scapula. CT documents the extent of the soft-tissue mass (*arrows*) associated with the destructive bone lesion prior to radiation therapy.

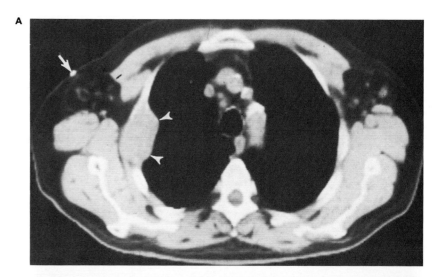

A

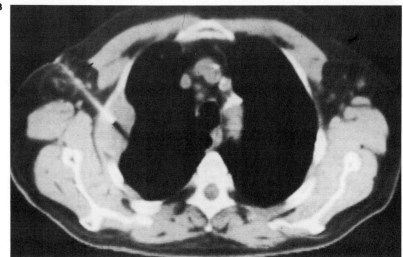

B

FIG. 155. Rib metastasis; CT-guided percutaneous needle biopsy. **A:** A soft-tissue mass (*arrowheads*) arising from a destroyed rib is well delineated. A small metallic marker (*arrow*) demarcates the planned skin entry site, allowing calculation of the appropriate angle and depth. Two small pretracheal lymph nodes are noted. **B:** Repeat image documents that the tip of the needle is within the center of the mass.

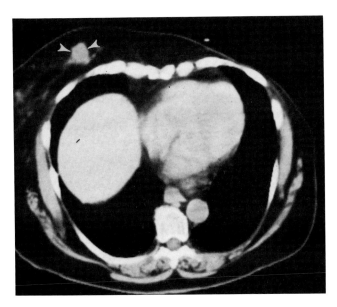

FIG. 156. Breast carcinoma. On a CT study performed to evaluate for possible liver metastases in a patient with a prior left mastectomy, a new mass (*arrowheads*) was discovered in the right breast.

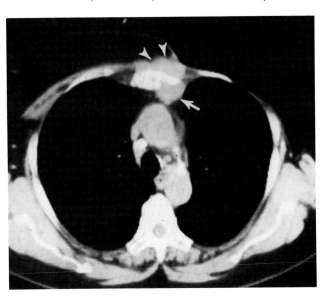

FIG. 157. Recurrent breast carcinoma. Subcutaneous metastases (*arrowheads*) communicating through the costal cartilage with a soft-tissue mass in the anterior mediastinum (*arrow*) are documented in a woman who had a previous left radical mastectomy.

(e.g., internal mammary, axillary) is strongly suspected; the findings may be helpful in radiation therapy planning (118). Mastectomy results in asymmetric absence of breast and fatty tissue and, depending on how radical the surgery was, the pectoral muscles. After resolution of the immediate postoperative changes, there should be no localized soft-tissue mass either outside or inside the ribs. Locally recurrent breast carcinoma, sometimes clinically unsuspected or difficult to document, usually can be demonstrated with CT when the lesion exceeds 1 cm in diameter (195) (Fig. 157): A soft-tissue-density mass will be seen in the subcutaneous tissues; this should be distinguished from the wispy linear soft-tissue densities within the fat seen in patients following radiation therapy that are confined to the portal used. Displacement or penetration of the intercostal muscles or the ribs themselves may be caused by recurrent carcinoma. CT-guided percutaneous needle biopsy may be helpful to corroborate (or exclude) recurrence.

The anterior chest wall frequently is invaded secondary to lymphoma originating in the thymus. CT can be helpful in detecting such invasion and depicting its extent, subsequently guiding radiation therapy and assessing the re-

sponse (30,175). Enlarged thoracic-wall lymph nodes, especially in the axilla, also may be discovered (Fig. 158).

Miscellaneous

Enlarged subcutaneous collateral veins may be noted, with occlusion of a major vein in the thorax (or abdomen). They appear on CT as round or tubular structures that are enhanced after intravenous administration of contrast material (see Fig. 8B in Chapter 7 and Fig. 44 in Chapter 8). Very transient enhancement of normal thoracic-wall veins, particularly around the scapula, may be seen because the hyperabduction of the arms required for thoracic CT can result in some compression of the subclavian veins.

CT can be valuable in demonstrating a mass involving the brachial nerve plexus (Figs. 146 and 159). Anatomic depiction of this area and the surrounding vessels and muscles is more exquisite with MRI, with coronal-plane images especially valuable, and this technique can be used primarily or for problem-solving if CT findings are negative or equivocal.

A,B

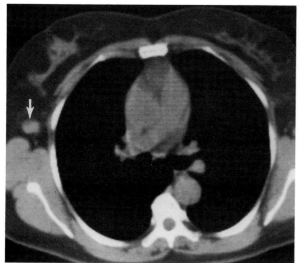 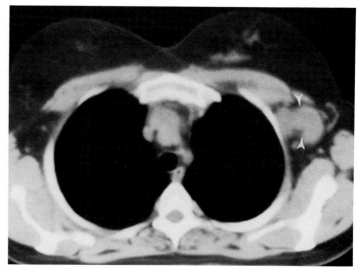

FIG. 158. Axillary lymphadenopathy due to non-Hodgkin lymphoma. **A:** An enlarged right axillary lymph node (*arrow*) is seen. **B:** In another patient, a left-side nodal mass (*arrowheads*) is noted.

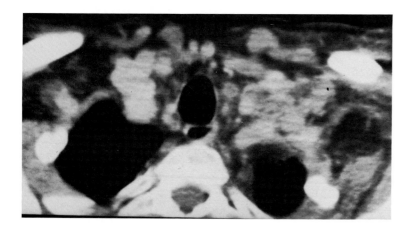

FIG. 159. Brachial plexus metastases. A poorly defined, infiltrating soft-tissue-density mass due to metastatic breast carcinoma is seen surrounding the vessels and nerves in the left thoracic inlet.

REFERENCES

1. Abrams HL, Spiro R, Goldstein N. Metastases in carcinoma. *Cancer* 1950;3:74–85.
2. Albelda SM, Epstein DM, Gefter WB, Miller WT. Pleural thickening: its significance and relationship to asbestos dust exposure. *Am Rev Respir Dis* 1982;126:621–624.
3. Alexander E, Clark RA, Colley DP, Mitchell SE. CT of malignant pleural mesothelioma. *AJR* 1981;137:287–291.
4. Ang JGP, Proto AV. CT demonstration of congenital pulmonary venolobar syndrome. *J Comput Assist Tomogr* 1984;8:753–757.
5. Aronberg DJ, Sagel SS. High CT attenuation values of a benign pulmonary nodule. *J Comput Assist Tomogr* 1981;5:563–564.
6. Aronchick JM, Wexler JA, Christen B, Miller W, Epstein D, Gefter WB. Computed tomography of bronchial carcinoid. *J Comput Assist Tomogr* 1986;10:71–74.
7. Baber CE, Hedlund LW, Oddson TA, Putman CE. Differentiating empyemas and peripheral pulmonary abscesses: the value of computed tomography. *Radiology* 1980;135:755–758.
8. Ball T, McCrory R, Sonik JO, Clements JL. Traumatic diaphragmatic hernia: errors in diagnosis. *AJR* 1982;138:633–637.
9. Begin R, Bergeron D, Samson L, Boctor M, Cantin A. CT assessment of silicosis in exposed workers. *AJR* 1987;148:509–514.
10. Bell JW. Abdominal exploration in one hundred lung carcinoma suspects prior to thoracotomy. *Ann Surg* 1968;167:199–203.
11. Bellamy EA, Husband JE, Blaquiere RM, Law MR. Bleomycin-related lung damage: CT evidence. *Radiology* 1985;156:155–158.
12. Berger PE, Kuhn JP, Kuhns LR. Computed tomography and the occult tracheobronchial foreign body. *Radiology* 1980;134:133–135.
13. Bergin CJ, Müller NL. CT in the diagnosis of interstitial lung disease. *AJR* 1985;145:505–510.
14. Bergin CJ, Müller NL. CT of interstitial lung disease: a diagnostic approach. *AJR* 1987;148:8–15.
15. Bergin CJ, Müller NL, Miller RR. CT in the qualitative assessment of emphysema. *J Thorac Imag* 1986;1:94–103.
16. Bergin CJ, Müller NL, Vedal S, Chan-Yeung M. CT in silicosis: correlation with plain films and pulmonary function tests. *AJR* 1986;146:477–483.
17. Bergin C, Müller N, Nichols DM, et al. The diagnosis of emphysema. A computed tomographic-pathologic correlation. *Am Rev Respir Dis* 1986;133:541–546.
18. Berthoty DP, Shulman HS, Miller HAB. Elastofibroma: chest wall pseudotumor. *Radiology* 1986;160:341–342.
19. Bhatt GM, Austin HM. CT demonstration of empyema necessitatis. *J Comput Assist Tomogr* 1985;9:1108–1109.
20. Biondetti PR, Fiore D, Sartori F, Colognato A, Ravasini R, Romani S. Evaluation of the post-pneumonectomy space by computed tomography. *J Comput Assist Tomogr* 1982;6:238–242.
21. Bressler EL, Francis IR, Glazer GM, Gross BH. Bolus contrast medium enhancement for distinguishing pleural from parenchymal

lung disease: CT features. *J Comput Assist Tomogr* 1987;11:436–440.

22. Breuer R, Baigelman W, Pugatch RD. Occult mycetoma. *J Comput Assist Tomogr* 1982;6:166–168.
23. Breyer RH, Karstaedt N, Mills SA, et al. Computed tomography for evaluation of mediastinal lymph nodes in lung cancer: correlation with surgical staging. *Ann Thorac Surg* 1984;38:215–220.
24. Brion JP, Depauw L, Kuhn G, et al. Role of computed tomography and mediastinoscopy in preoperative staging of lung carcinoma. *J Comput Assist Tomogr* 1985;9:480–484.
25. Buell PE. The importance of tumor size in prognosis for resected bronchogenic carcinoma. *J Surg Oncol* 1971;3:539–551.
26. Bydder GM, Kreel L. Pleural calcification in pancreatitis demonstrated by computed tomography. *J Comput Assist Tomogr* 1981;5:161–163.
27. Cann CE, Gamsu G, Birnberg FA, Webb WR. Quantification of calcium in solitary pulmonary nodules using single and dual energy CT. *Radiology* 1982;145:493–496.
28. Chang A, Glazer HS, Lee JKT, Ling D, Heiken JP. Adrenal gland: MR imaging. *Radiology* 1987;163:123–128.
29. Chang CHJ, Nesbit DE, Fisher DR, et al. Computed tomographic mammography using a conventional body scanner. *AJR* 1982;138:553–558.
30. Cho CS, Blank N, Castellino RA. Computerized tomography evaluation of chest wall involvement in lymphoma. *Cancer* 1985;55:1892–1894.
31. Chiles C, Ravin CE. Intrathoracic metastasis from an extrathoracic malignancy: a radiographic approach to patient evaluation. *Radiol Clin North Am* 1985;23:427–438.
32. Cohen AM, Solomon EH, Alfidi RJ. Computed tomography in bronchial atresia. *AJR* 1980;135:1097–1099.
33. Cohen LM, Schwartz AM, Rockoff SD. Benign schwannomas: pathologic basis for CT inhomogeneities. *AJR* 1986;147:141–143.
34. Cohen M, Grosfeld J, Baehner R, Weetman R. Lung CT for detection of metastases: solid tissue neoplasms in children. *AJR* 1982;139:895–898.
35. Coscina WF, Arger PH, Mintz MC, Coleman BG. CT demonstration of pulmonary effects of tangential beam radiation. *J Comput Assist Tomogr* 1986;10:600–602.
36. Costello P, Rose RM. CT findings in pleural aspergillosis. *J Comput Assist Tomogr* 1985;9:760–762.
37. Crow J, Salvin G, Kreel L. Pulmonary metastasis: a pathologic and radiologic study. *Cancer* 1981;47:2595–2602.
38. Daly BDT, Pugatch RD, Faling LJ, Jung-Legg Y, Gale ME, Snider GL. Computed-tomographic-guided minithoracotomy. A preliminary report of a new approach to open lung biopsy. *Radiology* 1983;146:543–544.
39. Daneman A, Mancer K, Sonley M. CT appearance of thickened nerves in neurofibromatosis. *AJR* 1983;141:899–900.
40. Dedrick CG, McLoud TC, Shepard JO, Shipley RT. Computed tomography of localized pleural mesothelioma. *AJR* 1985;144:275–280.
41. Demos TC, Johnson C, Love L, Posniak H. Computed tomography of partial unilateral agenesis of the pectoralis muscles. *J Comput Assist Tomogr* 1985;9:558–559.
42. Destouet JM, Gilula LA, Murphy WA, Sagel SS. Computed tomography of the sternoclavicular joint and sternum. *Radiology* 1981;138:123–128.
43. Dixon GD. Preoperative computed-tomographic localization of breast calcifications. *Radiology* 1983;146:836.
44. Doyle TC, Lawler GA. CT features of rounded atelectasis of the lung. *AJR* 1984;143:225–228.
45. Edelstein G, Levitt RG, Slaker DP, Murphy WA. CT observation of rib abnormalities: spectrum of findings. *J Comput Assist Tomogr* 1985;9:65–72.
46. Emami B, Melo A, Carter BL, Munzenreider JE, Piro AJ. Value of computed tomography in radiotherapy of lung cancer. *AJR* 1978;131:63–67.
47. Epler GR, McLoud TC, Gaensler EA. Prevalence and incidence of benign asbestos pleural effusion in a working population. *JAMA* 1982;247:617–622.
48. Faling LJ, Pugatch RD, Jung-Legg Y, et al. Computed tomographic scanning of the mediastinum in the staging of bronchogenic carcinoma. *Am Rev Respir Dis* 1981;124:690–695.

49. Faer MJ, Burnam RE, Beck CL. Transmural thoracic lipoma: demonstration by computed tomography. *AJR* 1978;130:161–163.
50. Federle MP, Mark AS, Guillaumin ES. CT of subpulmonic pleural effusions and atelectasis: criteria for differentiation from subphrenic fluid. *AJR* 1986;146:685–689.
51. Fennessy JJ. Irradiation damage to the lung. *J Thorac Imag* 1987;2:68–79.
52. Fiore D, Biondetti PR, Sartori F, Calabro F. The role of computed tomography in the evaluation of bullous lung disease. *J Comput Assist Tomogr* 1982;6:105–108.
53. Fisher MR, Higgins CB. Central thrombi in pulmonary arterial hypertension detected by MR imaging. *Radiology* 1986;158:223–226.
54. Foster WL Jr, Pratt PC, Roggli VL, Godwin JD, Halvorsen RA Jr, Putman CE. Centrilobular emphysema: CT–pathologic correlation. *Radiology* 1986;159:27–32.
55. Foster WL Jr, Roberts L Jr, McLendon RE, Hill RC. Localized peribronchial thickening: a CT sign of occult bronchogenic carcinoma. *AJR* 1985;144:906–908.
56. Friedman PJ. CT demonstration of tethering of the lung by the pulmonary ligament. *J Comput Assist Tomogr* 1985;9:947–948.
57. Friedman PJ, Feigin DS, Liston SE, et al. Sensitivity of chest radiography, computed tomography, and gallium scanning to metastasis of lung carcinoma. *Cancer* 1984;54:1300–1306.
58. Genereux GP. Computed tomography and the lung: review of anatomic and densitometric features with their clinical application. *J Can Assoc Radiol* 1985;36:88–102.
59. Genereux GP. CT of acute and chronic distal air space (alveolar) disease. *Semin Roentgenol* 1984;19:211–221.
60. Glazer GM, Gross BH, Aisen AH, Quint LE, Francis IR, Orringer MB. Imaging of the pulmonary hilum: a prospective comparative study in patients with lung cancer. *AJR* 1985;145:245–248.
61. Glazer GM, Gross BH, Quint LE, Francis IR, Orringer MB. Staging of non-small cell lung cancer. *Contemp Issues Comput Tomogr* 1986;7:101–121.
62. Glazer GM, Orringer MB, Gross BH, Quint LE. The mediastinum in non-small cell lung cancer: CT–surgical correlation. *AJR* 1984;142:1101–1105.
63. Glazer GM, Woolsey EJ, Borrello J, et al. Adrenal tissue characterization using MR imaging. *Radiology* 1986;158:73–79.
64. Glazer HS, Aronberg DJ, Sagel SS, Emami B. Utility of CT in detecting postpneumonectomy carcinoma recurrence. *AJR* 1984;142:487–494.
65. Glazer HS, Aronberg DJ, VanDyke JA, Sagel SS. CT manifestations of pulmonary collapse. *Contemp Issues Comput Tomogr* 1984;4:81–119.
66. Glazer HS, Duncan-Meyer J, Aronberg DJ, Moran JF, Levitt RG, Sagel SS. Pleural and chest wall invasion in bronchogenic carcinoma: CT evaluation. *Radiology* 1985;157:191–194.
67. Glazer HS, Lee JKT, Levitt RG, et al. Radiation fibrosis: differentiation from recurrent tumor by MR imaging. *Radiology* 1985;156:721–726.
68. Godwin JD, Fram EK, Cann CE, Gamsu GG. CT densitometry of pulmonary nodules: a phantom study. *J Comput Assist Tomogr* 1982;6:254–258.
69. Godwin JD, MacGregor JM. Extension of ascites into the chest with hiatal hernia: visualization on CT. *AJR* 1987;148:31–32.
70. Godwin JD, Speckman JM, Fram EK, et al. Distinguishing benign from malignant pulmonary nodules by computed tomography. *Radiology* 1982;144:349–351.
71. Godwin JD, Webb WR. Dynamic computed tomography in the evaluation of vascular lung lesions. *Radiology* 1981;138:629–635.
72. Godwin JD, Webb WR, Gamsu G, Ovenfors CO. Computed tomography of pulmonary embolism. *AJR* 1980;135:691–695.
73. Goldstein MS, Rush M, Johnson P, Sprung CL. A calcified adenocarcinoma of the lung with very high CT numbers. *Radiology* 1984;150:785–786.
74. Good CA. The solitary pulmonary nodule: a problem of management. *Radiol Clin North Am* 1963;1:429–437.
75. Gouliamos AD, Carter BL, Emami B. Computed tomography of the chest wall. *Radiology* 1980;134:433–436.
76. Grant DC, Seltzer SE, Antman KH, Finberg HJ, Koster K. Computed tomography of malignant pleural mesothelioma. *J Comput Assist Tomogr* 1983;7:626–632.

77. Grenier P, Maurice F, Musset D, Menu Y, Nahum H. Bronchiectasis: assessment of thin-section CT. *Radiology* 1986;161:95–99.
78. Griffin CA, Lu C, Fishman EK, et al. The role of computed tomography of the chest in the management of small-cell lung cancer. *J Clin Oncol* 1984;12:1359–1365.
79. Gross BH, Glazer GM, Bookstein FL. Multiple pulmonary nodules detected by computed tomography: diagnostic implications. *J Comput Assist Tomogr* 1985;9:880–885.
80. Gross BH, Glazer GM, Orringer MB, Spizarny DL, Flint A. Bronchogenic carcinoma metastatic to normal-sized lymph nodes: frequency and significance. *Radiology* 1988;166:71–74.
81. Gudbjerg CE. Roentgenologic diagnosis of bronchiectasis. An analysis of 112 cases. *Acta Radiol (Stockh)* 1955;43:209–226.
82. Gutierrez FR, Glazer HS, Levitt RG, Moran JF. NMR imaging of pulmonary arteriovenous fistulae. *J Comput Assist Tomogr* 1984;8:750–752.
83. Haggar AM, Pearlberg JP, Froelich JW, et al. Chest wall invasion by carcinoma of the lung: detection by MR imaging. *AJR* 1987;148:1075–1078.
84. Halvorsen RA, Fedyshin PJ, Korobkin M, Foster WL Jr, Thompson WM. Ascites or pleural effusion? CT differentiation: four useful criteria. *RadioGraphics* 1986;6:135–149.
85. Halvorsen RA, Fedyshin PJ, Korobkin M, Thompson WM. CT differentiation of pleural effusion from ascites. An evaluation of four signs using blinded analysis of 52 cases. *Invest Radiol* 1986;21:391–395.
86. Hamper UK, Fishman EK, Khouri NF, Johns CJ, Wang KP, Siegelman SS. Typical and atypical CT manifestations of pulmonary sarcoidosis. *J Comput Assist Tomogr* 1986;10:928–936.
87. Heaston DK, Putman CE, Rodan BA, et al. Solitary pulmonary metastasis in high-risk melanoma patients: a prospective comparison of conventional and computed tomography. *AJR* 1983;141:169–174.
88. Heater K, Revzani L, Rubin JM. CT evaluation of empyema in the post pneumonectomy space. *AJR* 1985;145:39–40.
89. Heavey LR, Glazer GM, Gross BH, Francis IR, Orringer MB. The role of CT in staging radiographic $T_1N_0M_0$ lung cancer. *AJR* 1986;146:285–290.
90. Hedlund LW, Vock P, Effmann EL. Computed tomography of the lung. Densitometric studies. *Radiol Clin North Am* 1983;21:775–788.
91. Heelan RT, Martini N, Westcott JW, et al. Carcinomatous involvement of the hilum and mediastinum: computed tomographic and magnetic resonance evaluation. *Radiology* 1985;156:111–115.
92. Heiberg E, Wolverson MK, Hurd RN, Jagannadharao B, Sundaram M. CT recognition of traumatic rupture of the diaphragm. *AJR* 1980;135:369–372.
93. Henschke CI, Davis SD, Auh Y, et al. Detection of bronchial abnormalities: comparison of CT and bronchoscopy. *J Comput Assist Tomogr* 1987;11:432–435.
94. Hidalgo H, Korobkin M, Finney TR, Falletta J, Heaston DH, Kirks DR. The problem of benign pulmonary nodules in children receiving cytotoxic chemotherapy. *AJR* 1983;140:21–24.
95. Higgins GA, Shields TW, Keehn RJ. The solitary pulmonary nodule. Ten year follow-up. Veterans Administration–Armed Forces cooperative study. *Arch Surg* 1975;110:570–575.
96. Hulnick DH, Naidich DP, McCauley DI. Pleural tuberculosis evaluated by computed tomography. *Radiology* 1983;149:759–765.
97. Huston J III, Muhm JR. Solitary pulmonary opacities: plain tomography. *Radiology* 1987;163:481–485.
98. Jacobsen LE, Houston CS, Habbick BF, Genereux GP, Howie JL. Cystic fibrosis: a comparison of computed tomography and plain chest radiographs. *J Can Assoc Radiol* 1986;37:17–21.
99. Joharjy IA, Bashi SA, Abdullah AK. Value of medium-thickness CT in the diagnosis of bronchiectasis. *AJR* 1987;149:1133–1137.
100. Joshi RR, Cholankeril JV. Computed tomography in lipoid pneumonia. *J Comput Assist Tomogr* 1985;9:211–213.
101. Katz D, Kreel L. Computed tomography in pulmonary asbestosis. *Clin Radiol* 1979;30:207–213.
102. Khan A, Gersten KC, Garvey J, Khan FA, Steinberg H. Oblique hilar tomography, computed tomography, and mediastinoscopy for prethoracotomy staging of bronchogenic carcinoma. *Radiology* 1985;156:295–298.
103. Khoury MB, Godwin JD, Halvorsen RA Jr, Putman CE. CT of obstructive lobar collapse. *Invest Radiol* 1985;20:708–716.
104. Kopans DB, Meyer JE. Computed tomography guided localization of clinically occult breast carcinoma—the "N" skin guide. *Radiology* 1982;145:211–212.
105. Kowal LE, Goodman LR, Zarro VJ, Haskin ME. CT diagnosis of broncholithiasis. *J Comput Assist Tomogr* 1983;7:321–323.
106. Krudy AG, Doppman JL, Herdt JR. Failure to detect a 1.5 centimeter lung nodule by chest computed tomography. *J Comput Assist Tomogr* 1982;6:1178–1180.
107. Kruglik GD, Wayne KS. Occult lung cavity causing hemoptysis: recognition by computed tomography. *J Comput Assist Tomogr* 1980;4:407–408.
108. Kuhlman JE, Fishman EK, Siegelman SS. Invasive pulmonary aspergillosis in acute leukemia: characteristic findings on CT, the CT halo sign, and the role of CT in early diagnosis. *Radiology* 1985;157:611–614.
109. Kuhlman JE, Scatarige KC, Fishman EK, Zerhouni EA, Siegelman SS. CT demonstration of high attenuation pleural-parenchymal lesions due to amiodarone therapy. *J Comput Assist Tomogr* 1987;11:160–162.
110. Kuriyama K, Tateishi R, Doi O, et al. CT–pathologic correlation in small peripheral lung cancers. *AJR* 1987;149:1139–1143.
111. Ledor K, Fish B, Chaisse L, Ledor S. CT diagnosis of pulmonary hamartomas. *CT* 1981;5:343–344.
112. Levinsohn EM, Bunnell WP, Yuan HA. Computed tomography in the diagnosis of dislocations of the sternoclavicular joint. *Clin Orthop* 1979;140:12–16.
113. Levi C, Gray JE, McCullough EC, Hattery RR. The unreliability of CT numbers as absolute values. *AJR* 1982;139:443–447.
114. Levitt RG, Glazer HS, Roper CL, Lee JKT, Murphy WA. Magnetic resonance imaging of mediastinal and hilar masses: comparison with CT. *AJR* 1985;145:9–14.
115. Libshitz HI, McKenna RJ Jr. Mediastinal lymph node size in lung cancer. *AJR* 1984;143:715–718.
116. Libshitz HI, McKenna RJ Jr, Haynie TP, McMurtrey MJ, Mountain CT. Mediastinal evaluation in lung cancer. *Radiology* 1984;151:295–299.
117. Libshitz HI, Shuman LS. Radiation-induced pulmonary change: CT findings. *J Comput Assist Tomogr* 1984;8:15–19.
118. Lindfors KK, Meyer JE, Busse PM, Kopans DB, Munzenrider JE, Sawicka JM. CT evaluation of local and regional breast cancer recurrence. *AJR* 1985;145:833–837.
119. Mah K, Poon PY, Van Dyk J, Keane T, Majesky IF, Rideout DF. Assessment of acute radiation-induced pulmonary changes using computed tomography. *J Comput Assist Tomogr* 1986;10:736–743.
120. Maltby JD, Gouverne ML. CT findings in pulmonary venoocclusive disease. *J Comput Assist Tomogr* 1984;8:758–761.
121. Marin ML, Austin JHM, Markowitz AM. Elastofibroma dorsi: CT demonstration. *J Comput Assist Tomogr* 1987;11:675–677.
122. Martin KW, Sagel SS, Siegel BA. Mosaic oligemia simulating pulmonary infiltrates on CT. *AJR* 1986;147:670–673.
123. Martini N, Heelan R, Westcott J, et al. Comparative merits of conventional, computed tomographic, and magnetic resonance imaging in assessing mediastinal involvement in surgically confirmed lung carcinoma. *J Thorac Cardiovasc Surg* 1985;90:639–648.
124. Matsumoto AH, Parker LA, Delany DJ. CT demonstration of central pulmonary venous and arterial occlusive diseases. *J Comput Assist Tomogr* 1987;11:640–644.
125. Mayo JR, Webb WR, Gould R, et al. High-resolution CT of the lungs: an optimal approach. *Radiology* 1987;163:507–510.
126. Mayr B, Heywang SH, Ingrisch H, Huber RM, Häussinger K, Lissner J. Comparison of CT with MR imaging of endobronchial tumors. *J Comput Assist Tomogr* 1987;11:43–48.
127. McCullough EC. Factors affecting the use of quantitative information from a CT scanner. *Radiology* 1977;124:99–107.
128. McCullough EC, Morin RL. CT-number variability in thoracic geometry. *AJR* 1983;141:135–140.
129. McFadden RG, Carr TJ, Wood TE. Proton magnetic resonance imaging to stage activity of interstitial lung disease. *Chest* 1987;92:31–39.
130. McLoud TC, Woods BO, Carrington CB, Epler GR, Gaensler EA. Diffuse pleural thickening in an asbestos-exposed population: prevalence and causes. *AJR* 1985;144:9–18.
131. Metzger RA, Mulhern CB Jr, Arger PH, Coleman BG, Epstein

DM, Gefter WB. CT differentiation of solitary from diffuse bronchioloalveolar carcinoma. *J Comput Assist Tomogr* 1981;5:830–833.

132. Mintzer RA, Gore RM, Vogelzang RL, Holz S. Rounded-atelectasis and its association with asbestos-induced pleural disease. *Radiology* 1981;139:567–570.

133. Mintzer RA, Malave SR, Neiman HL, Michaelis LL, Vanecko RM, Sanders JH. Computed vs. conventional tomography in the evaluation of primary and secondary pulmonary neoplasms. *Radiology* 1979;132:653–659.

134. Mirvis S, Dutcher JP, Haney PJ, Whitley NO, Aisner J. CT of malignant pleural mesothelioma. *AJR* 1983;140:665–670.

135. Mirvis SE, Tobin KD, Kostrubiak I, Belzberg H. Thoracic CT in detecting occult disease in critically ill patients. *AJR* 1987;148:685–689.

136. Mirvis SE, Whitley NO, Aisner J, Moody M, Whitacre M, Whitley JE. Abdominal CT in the staging of small-cell carcinoma of the lung: incidence of metastases and effect on prognosis. *AJR* 1987;148:845–847.

137. Moore EH, Webb WR, Müller N, Sollitto R. MRI of pulmonary airspace disease: experimental model and preliminary clinical results. *AJR* 1986;146:1123–1128.

138. Morgan MDL, Denison DM, Strickland B. Value of computed tomography for selecting patients with bullous lung disease for surgery. *Thorax* 1986;41:855–862.

139. Mountain C. A new international staging system for lung cancer. *Chest* 1986;89:225–233.

140. Muhm JR, Brown LR, Crowe JK, Sheedy PF II, Hattery RR, Stephens DH. Comparison of whole lung tomography and computed tomography for detecting pulmonary nodules. *AJR* 1978;131:981–984.

141. Muller JWT, van Waes PFGM, Koehler PR. Computed tomography of breast lesions: comparison with x-ray mammography. *J Comput Assist Tomogr* 1983;7:650–654.

142. Müller NL, Bergin CJ, Ostrow DN, Nichols DM. Role of computed tomography in the recognition of bronchiectasis. *AJR* 1984;143:971–976.

143. Müller NL, Gamsu G, Webb WR. Pulmonary nodules: detection using magnetic resonance and computed tomography. *Radiology* 1985;155:687–690.

144. Müller NL, Miller RR, Webb WR, Evans KG, Ostrow DN. Fibrosing alveolitis: CT–pathologic correlation. *Radiology* 1986;160:585–588.

145. Murata K, Itoh H, Todo G, et al. Centrilobular lesions of the lung: demonstration by high-resolution CT and pathologic correlation. *Radiology* 1986;161:641–645.

146. Musset D, Grenier P, Carette MF, et al. Primary lung cancer staging: prospective comparative study of MR imaging with CT. *Radiology* 1986;160:607–611.

147. Nabawi P, Mantravadi R, Breyer D, Capek V. Computed tomography of radiation-induced lung injuries. *J Comput Assist Tomogr* 1981;5:568–570.

148. Naidich DP, Ettinger N, Leitman BS, McCauley DI. CT of lobar collapse. *Semin Roentgenol* 1984;19:222–234.

149. Naidich DP, Lee JJ, Garay SM, McCauley DI, Aranda CP, Boyd AD. Comparison of CT and fiberoptic bronchoscopy in the evaluation of bronchial disease. *AJR* 1987;148:1–7.

150. Naidich DP, McCauley DI, Khouri NF, Leitman BS, Hulnick DH, Siegelman SS. Computed tomography of lobar collapse. 1. Endobronchial obstruction. *J Comput Assist Tomogr* 1983;7:745–757.

151. Naidich DP, McCauley DI, Khouri NF, Leitman BS, Hulnick DH, Siegelman SS. Computed tomography of lobar collapse. 2. Collapse in absence of endobronchial obstruction. *J Comput Assist Tomogr* 1983;7:758–767.

152. Naidich DP, McCauley DI, Khouri NF, Stitik FP, Siegelman SS. Computed tomography of bronchiectasis. *J Comput Assist Tomogr* 1982;6:437–444.

153. Naidich DP, McCauley DI, Siegelman SS. Computed tomography of bronchial adenoma. *J Comput Assist Tomogr* 1982;6:725–782.

154. Naidich DP, Megibow AJ, Hilton S, Hulnick DH, Siegelman SS. Computed tomography of the diaphragm: peridiaphragmatic fluid localization. *J Comput Assist Tomogr* 1983;7:641–649.

155. Naidich DP, Rumanick WM, Lefleur RS, Estioko MR, Brown SM. Intralobar pulmonary sequestration: MR evaluation. *J Comput Assist Tomogr* 1987;11:531–533.

156. Naidich DP, Stitik FP, Khouri NF, Terry PB, Siegelman SS. Computed tomography of the bronchi. 1. Normal anatomy. *J Comput Assist Tomogr* 1980;4:746–753.

157. Naidich DP, Stitik FP, Khouri NF, Terry PB, Siegelman SS. Computed tomography of the bronchi. 2. Pathology. *J Comput Assist Tomogr* 1980;4:754–762.

158. Naidich DP, Zerhouni EA, Hutchins GM, Genieser NB, McCauley DI, Siegelman SS. Computed tomography of the pulmonary parenchyma. Part 1: Distal air-space disease. *J Thorac Imag* 1985;1:39–53.

159. Naidich DP, Zerhouni EA, Siegelman SS. *Computed tomography of the thorax.* New York: Raven Press, 1984.

160. Nakata H, Kimoto T, Nakayama T, Kido M, Miyazaki N, Harada S. Diffuse peripheral lung disease: evaluation by high-resolution computed tomography. *Radiology* 1985;157:181–185.

161. Nathan MH, Collins VP, Adams RA. Differentiation of benign and malignant pulmonary nodules by growth rate. *Radiology* 1962;79:221–227.

162. O'Connell RS, McLoud TC, Wilkins EW. Superior sulcus tumor: radiographic diagnosis and workup. *AJR* 1983;140:25–30.

163. O'Keefe ME Jr, Good CA, McDonald JR. Calcification in solitary nodules in the lung. *AJR* 1957;77:1023–1033.

164. Oliver TW Jr, Bernardino ME, Miller JI, Mansour K, Greene D, Davis WA. Isolated adrenal masses in non-small-cell bronchogenic carcinoma. *Radiology* 1984;153:217–218.

165. Ortega W, Mahboubi S, Dalinka MK, Robinson T. Computed tomography of rib hemangiomas. *J Comput Assist Tomogr* 1986;10:945–947.

166. Paling MR, Griffin GK. Lower lobe collapse due to pleural effusion: a CT analysis. *J Comput Assist Tomogr* 1985;9:1079–1083.

167. Pagani JJ, Libshitz HI. CT manifestations of radiation-induced change in chest tissue. *J Comput Assist Tomogr* 1982;6:243–248.

168. Paul DJ, Mueller CF. Pulmonary sequestration. *J Comput Assist Tomogr* 1982;6:163–165.

169. Pearlberg JL, Sandler MA, Beute GH, Madrazo BL. $T_1N_0M_0$ bronchogenic carcinoma: assessment by CT. *Radiology* 1985;157:187–190.

170. Pearlberg JL, Sandler MA, Kvale P, Beute GH, Madrazo BL. Computed-tomographic and conventional linear-tomographic evaluation of tracheobronchial lesions for laser photoresection. *Radiology* 1985;154:759–762.

171. Pennes DR, Glazer GM, Wimbish KJ, Gross BH, Long RW, Orringer MB. Chest wall invasion by lung cancer: limitations of CT evaluation. *AJR* 1985;144:507–511.

172. Peters JC, Desai KK. CT demonstration of postpneumonectomy tumor recurrence. *AJR* 1983;141:259–262.

173. Pilate I, Marcelis S, Timmerman H, Beeckman P, Osteaux MJC. Pulmonary asbestosis: CT study of subpleural curvilinear shadow. *Radiology* 1987;164:584.

174. Prasad S, Pilepich MV, Perez CA. Contribution of CT to quantitative radiation therapy planning. *AJR* 1981;136:123–128.

175. Press GA, Glazer HS, Wasserman TH, Aronberg DJ, Lee JKT, Sagel SS. Thoracic wall involvement by Hodgkin disease and non-Hodgkin lymphoma: CT evaluation. *Radiology* 1985;157:195–198.

176. Proto AV, Thomas SR. Pulmonary nodules studied by computed tomography. *Radiology* 1985;156:149–153.

177. Proto AV, Tocino I. Radiologic manifestations of lobar collapse. *Semin Roentgenol* 1980;15:117–173.

178. Pugatch RD, Faling LJ, Robbins AH, Snider GL. Differentiation of pleural and pulmonary lesions using computed tomography. *J Comput Assist Tomogr* 1978;2:601–606.

179. Pugatch RD, Gale ME. Obscure pulmonary masses: bronchial impaction revealed by CT. *AJR* 1983;141:909–914.

180. Putman CE, Godwin JD, Silverman PM, Foster WL. CT of localized lucent lung lesions. *Semin Roentgenol* 1984;19:173–188.

181. Raasch BN, Heitzman ER, Carsky EW, Lane EJ, Berlow ME, Witwer G. A computed tomographic study of bronchopulmonary collapse. *RadioGraphics* 1984;4:195–232.

182. Rabinowitz JG, Efremidis SC, Cohen B, et al. A comparative study of mesothelioma and asbestosis using computed tomography and conventional chest radiography. *Radiology* 1982;144:453–460.

183. Rankin S, Faling LJ, Pugatch RD. CT diagnosis of pulmonary arteriovenous malformations. *J Comput Assist Tomogr* 1982;6:746–749.

184. Rao SP, Alfidi RJ. The environmental density artifact: a beam

hardening effect in computed tomography. *Radiology* 1981;141: 223–227.

185. Rea HH, Shevland JE, House AJS. Accuracy of computed tomographic scanning in assessment of the mediastinum in bronchial carcinoma. *J Thorac Cardiovasc Surg* 1981;81:825–829.

186. Roberts CM, Citron KM, Strickland B. Intrathoracic aspergilloma: role of CT in diagnosis and treatment. *Radiology* 1987;165:123–128.

187. Rosenblum LJ, Mauceri RA, Wellenstein DE, et al. Density patterns in the normal lung as determined by computed tomography. *Radiology* 1980;137:409–416.

188. Rost RC Jr, Proto AV. Inferior pulmonary ligament: computed tomographic appearance. *Radiology* 1983;148:479–483.

189. Sagel SS, Stanley RJ, Evens RG. Early clinical experience with motionless whole-body computed tomography. *Radiology* 1976;119:321–330.

190. Sandler MA, Pearlberg JL, Madrazo BL, Gitschlag KF, Gross SC. Computed tomographic evaluation of the adrenal gland in the preoperative assessment of bronchogenic carcinoma. *Radiology* 1982;145:733–736.

191. Sargent EN, Boswell WD Jr, Ralls PW, Markovitz A. Subpleural fat pads in patients exposed to asbestos: distinction from non-calcified pleural plaques. *Radiology* 1984;152:273–277.

192. Schaner EG, Chang AE, Doppman JL, Conkle DM, Flye MW, Rosenberg SA. Comparison of computed and conventional whole lung tomography in detecting pulmonary nodules: a prospective radiologic-pathologic study. *AJR* 1978;131:51–54.

193. Scholten ET, Kreel L. Distribution of lung metastases in the axial plane. A combined radiological-pathological study. *Radiol Clin (Basel)* 1977;46:248–265.

194. Scott IR, Müller NL, Miller RR, Evans KG, Nelems B. Resectable stage III lung cancer: CT, surgical and pathological correlation. *Radiology* 1988;166:75–79.

195. Shea WJ Jr, de Geer G, Webb WR. Chest wall after mastectomy. Part II. CT appearance of tumor recurrence. *Radiology* 1987;162:162–164.

196. Shepard JO, Grillo HC, McLoud TC, Dedrick CG, Spizarny DL. Right-pneumonectomy syndrome: radiologic findings and CT correlation. *Radiology* 1986;161:661–664.

197. Shin MS, Anderson SD, Myers J, Ho KJ. Pitfalls in CT evaluation of chest wall invasion by lung cancer. *J Comput Assist Tomogr* 1986;10:136–138.

198. Shuman LS, Libshitz HI. Solid pleural manifestations of lymphoma. *AJR* 1984;142:269–273.

199. Siegelman SS, Khouri N, Leo FP, Fishman EK, Braverman RM, Zerhouni EA. Solitary pulmonary nodules: CT assessment. *Radiology* 1986;160:307–312.

200. Siegelman SS, Khouri N, Scott WW Jr, et al. Pulmonary hamartoma: CT findings. *Radiology* 1986;160:313–317.

201. Siegelman SS, Zerhouni EA, Leo FP, Khouri NF, Stitik FP. CT of the solitary pulmonary nodule. *AJR* 1980;135:1–13.

202. Silverman PM, Baker ME, Mahony BS. Atelectasis and subpulmonic fluid: a CT pitfall in distinguishing pleural from peritoneal fluid. *J Comput Assist Tomogr* 1985;9:763–766.

203. Silverman PM, Godwin JD. CT/bronchographic correlations in bronchiectasis. *J Comput Assist Tomogr* 1987;11:52–56.

204. Sinner WN. Computed tomographic patterns of pulmonary thromboembolism and infarction. *J Comput Assist Tomogr* 1978;2:395–399.

205. Smith RA. Evaluation of the long-term results of surgery for bronchial carcinoma. *J Thorac Cardiovasc Surg* 1981;82:325–333.

206. Spirt BA. Value of the prone position in detecting pulmonary nodules by computed tomography. *J Comput Assist Tomogr* 1980;4:871–873.

207. Spizarny DL, Gross BH, Shepard JO. CT findings in localized fibrous mesothelioma of the pleural fissure. *J Comput Assist Tomogr* 1986;10:942–944.

208. Staples CA, Müller NL, Vedal S, Abboud R, Ostrow D, Miller RR. Usual interstitial pneumonia: correlation of CT with clinical, functional and radiologic findings. *Radiology* 1987;162:377–381.

209. Stark DD, Federle MP, Goodman PC. CT and radiographic assessment of tube thoracostomy. *AJR* 1983;141:253–258.

210. Stark DD, Federle MP, Goodman PC, Podrasky AE, Webb WR. Differentiating lung abscess and empyema: radiography and computed tomography. *AJR* 1983;141:163–167.

211. Stein MG, Mayo J, Müller N, Aberle DR, Webb WR, Gamsu G. Pulmonary lymphangitic spread of carcinoma: appearance on CT scans. *Radiology* 1987;162:371–375.

212. Steinberg DL, Webb WR. CT appearances of rheumatoid lung disease. *J Comput Assist Tomogr* 1984;8:881–884.

213. Stewart JG, MacMahon H, Vyborny CJ, Pollak ER. Dystrophic calcification in carcinoma of the lung: demonstration by CT. *AJR* 1987;148:29–30.

214. Takasugi JE, Godwin JD, Halvorsen RE, Williford ME, Silverman PM, Putman CE. Computed tomographic evaluation of lesions in the thoracic apex. *Invest Radiol* 1985;20:260–266.

215. Teplick JG, Teplick SK, Goodman L, Haskin ME. The interface sign: a computed tomographic sign for distinguishing pleural and intra-abdominal fluid. *Radiology* 1982;144:359–362.

216. Tobler J, Levitt RG, Glazer HS, Moran J, Crouch E, Evens RG. Differentiation of proximal bronchogenic carcinoma from postobstructive lobar collapse by magnetic resonance imaging. Comparison with computed tomography. *Invest Radiol* 1987;22:538–543.

217. Tocino TM, Miller MH. Computed tomography in blunt chest trauma. *J Thorac Imag* 1987;2:45–59.

218. Tocino TM, Miller MH, Frederick PR, Bahr AL, Thomas F. CT detection of occult pneumothorax in head trauma. *AJR* 1984;143:987–990.

219. Toombs BD, Sandler CM, Lester RG. Computed tomography of chest trauma. *Radiology* 1981;140:733–738.

220. Turnbull AD, Huvos AG, Goodner JT, Beattie EJ. The malignant potential of bronchial adenoma. *Ann Thorac Surg* 1972;14:453–464.

221. Tylen U, Nilsson U. Computed tomography in pulmonary pseudotumors and their relation to asbestos exposure. *J Comput Assist Tomogr* 1982;6:229–237.

222. Vanel D, Henry-Amar M, Lumbroso J, et al. Pulmonary evaluation of patients with osteosarcoma: roles of standard radiography, tomography, CT, scintigraphy, and tomoscintigraphy. *AJR* 1984;143:519–523.

223. Vas W, Zylak CJ, Mather D, Figueredo A. The value of abdominal computed tomography in the pre-treatment assessment of small cell carcinoma of the lung. *Radiology* 1981;138:417–418.

224. Vibhakar SD, Bellon EM. The bare area of the spleen: a constant CT feature of the ascitic abdomen. *AJR* 1984;141:953–955.

225. Wall SD, Federle MP, Jeffrey RB, Brett CM. CT diagnosis of unsuspected pneumothorax after blunt abdominal trauma. *AJR* 1983;141:919–921.

226. Wang KP, Terry P, Marsh B. Bronchoscopic needle aspiration biopsy of paratracheal tumors. *Am Rev Respir Dis* 1978;118:17–21.

227. Webb WR. CT of solitary pulmonary vascular lesions. *Semin Roentgenol* 1984;19:189–198.

228. Webb WR. Plain radiography and computed tomography in the staging of bronchogenic carcinoma: a practical approach. *J Thorac Imag* 1987;2:57–65.

229. Webb WR, Cooper C, Gamsu G. Interlobar pleural plaque mimicking a lung nodule in a patient with asbestos exposure. *J Comput Assist Tomogr* 1983;7:135–136.

230. Webb WR, Jeffrey RB, Godwin JD. Thoracic computed tomography in superior sulcus tumors. *J Comput Assist Tomogr* 1981;5:361–365.

231. Webb WR, Jensen BG, Sollitto R, et al. Bronchogenic carcinoma: staging with MR compared with staging with CT and surgery. *Radiology* 1985;156:117–124.

232. Wegener OH, Kaeppe P, Oeser H. Measurement of lung density by computed tomography. *J Comput Assist Tomogr* 1978;2:263–273.

233. Weiss W, Boucot KE, Cooper DA. Survival of men with peripheral lung cancer in relation to histologic characteristics and growth rate. *Am Rev Respir Dis* 1968;98:75–92.

234. Westcott JL, Cole SR. Traction bronchiectasis in end-stage pulmonary fibrosis. *Radiology* 1986;161:665–669.

235. Wheeler PS, Stitik FP, Hutchins GM, Klinefelter HF, Siegelman SS. Diagnosis of lipoid pneumonia by computed tomography. *JAMA* 1981;245:65–66.

236. Whitley NO, Fuks JZ, McCrea ES, et al. Computed tomography of the chest in small cell lung cancer: potential new prognostic signs. *AJR* 1984;142:885–892.

237. Williford ME, Godwin JD. Computed tomography of lung abscess and empyema. *Radiol Clin North Am* 1983;21:575-583.

238. Williford ME, Hidalgo H, Putman CE, Korobkin M, Ram PC. Computed tomography of pleural disease. *AJR* 1983;140:909-914.

239. Yoshimura H, Hatakeyama M, Otsuji H, et al. Pulmonary asbestosis: CT study of subpleural curvilinear shadow. *Radiology* 1986;158:653-658.

240. Zerhouni EA, Boukadoum MA, Siddiky MA, et al. A standard phantom for quantitative CT analysis of pulmonary nodules. *Radiology* 1983;149:767-772.

241. Zerhouni EA, Naidich DP, Stitik FP, Khouri NF, Siegelman SS. Computed tomography of the pulmonary parenchyma. Part 2: Interstitial disease. *J Thorac Imag* 1985;1:54-64.

242. Zerhouni EA, Spivey JF, Morgan RH, Leo FP, Stitik FP, Siegelman SS. Factors influencing quantitative CT measurements of solitary pulmonary nodules. *J Comput Assist Tomogr* 1982;6:1075-1087.

243. Zerhouni EA, Stitik FP, Siegelman SS, et al. CT of the pulmonary nodule: a cooperative study. *Radiology* 1986;160:319-327.

244. Zinn WL, Naidich DP, Whelan CA, Litt AW, McCauley DI, Ettenger NA. Fluid within preexisting pulmonary air spaces: a potential pitfall in CT differentiation of pleural from parenchymal disease. *J Comput Assist Tomogr* 1987;11:441-448.

CHAPTER 10

Heart and Pericardium

P. H. Nath, Robert G. Levitt, and Fernando Gutierrez

The anatomy of the heart and its great arteries and veins is seen on both unenhanced and contrast-enhanced computed tomographic (CT) images of the thorax. It is important for the radiologist to be familiar with the normal and pathologic anatomy of the heart and great vessels, because chest examinations now account for about 20% of body CT studies. Clinical use of magnetic resonance imaging (MRI) in cardiac diagnosis is based on its ability to depict detailed intracardiac anatomy (50). Cardiac magnetic resonance (MR) images result from signal-intensity differences between flowing blood and myocardium, pericardium, and epicardial fat; spatial resolution can be improved by synchronizing data acquisition to a fixed part of the cardiac cycle (48). Although cardiac anatomy generally is perceived in coronal and sagittal planes, as demonstrated on chest radiographs and angiocardiograms, cross-sectional anatomy has advantages, as it removes interference with overlapping structures and is easy to learn.

TECHNIQUE OF EXAMINATION

CT

The heart is a constantly moving, blood-filled organ with a complex contractile pattern. Its internal architecture produces no natural contrast, and its motion degrades the spatial resolution. Hence, the ideal technique requires contrast enhancement and some way to limit the effects of motion. The latter is more difficult and can be achieved either by prospective or retrospective electrocardiographic (EKG) gating or use of millisecond imaging times that are possible with the new instruments utilizing multiple X-ray tubes or scanning electron beams (9,66). Such instruments can provide measurements of left ventricular dimensions, wall thickness, and wall motion, but they are costly devices that are primarily dedicated to cardiac studies (65). However, when functional information is not crucial, adequate anatomic information usually can be obtained with non-EKG-gated CT images (43,60).

Contrast enhancement is essential in most instances. Some exceptions might be the detection of pericardial disease or follow-up of the size of an aortic aneurysm. When contrast material is used, it is important to use an adequate amount and to give a bolus injection into a large peripheral vein through a large-bore needle (such as 18.0 g). Approximately 100 ml of 60% contrast material injected as a rapid bolus usually is adequate to opacify and image the cardiovascular structures from the ascending aorta to the inferior vena cava if rapid scanning is used. The timing and sequence of imaging need to be tailored to the clinical situation. The area of interest should be imaged during the phase of maximum contrast enhancement. In a person with a normal circulation time, the right side of the heart and pulmonary artery are maximally opacified after 4 to 6 sec. The left-side heart chambers, ascending aorta, and its branches (including coronary artery grafts) are well opacified after 8 to 10 sec. For example, if left-side heart chambers are being evaluated for a source of systemic emboli, images should be obtained from the level of the aortic root to the base of the ventricles so that the entire left atrium and the left ventricle are imaged. The five or six images needed to cover the area should be obtained beginning 8 to 10 sec after a bolus of contrast material is given by hand injection or power injector. If EKG gating is employed, a sustained infusion is preferred to a simple bolus injection.

MRI

EKG gating of images is required to display internal cardiac anatomy in detail (47). Gating systems have been

387

developed that do not interfere with the imaging process and are not themselves affected by the switching of the magnetic field or radiofrequency pulses (12). With the gating technique, the gating signal is initiated by the R wave, and the pulse repetition rate (TR) is determined by the subject's heart rate (R-R interval in the QRS complex). TR varies from 1,000 msec to 600 msec when the heart rate is 60 to 100 beats per minute. The echo delay time (TE) is kept short (15–30 msec) for single-echo imaging. A multisection, double-echo imaging technique is commonly utilized in gated cardiac studies. The first slice is synchronous with the R wave (end-diastole). Additional slices are imaged within the R-R interval, with a delay of 100 msec for each subsequent slice. If double-echo imaging is used, e.g., TE = 15 msec, 30 msec, five slices can be obtained within the cardiac cycle (12). With this technique, each slice is out of phase by 100 msec with the previous slice and represents a different portion of the cardiac cycle. Gated images are degraded by the presence of artifacts (signal variation along the phase-encoding direction due to periodic heart motion), long echo delays (second-echo imaging), inconsistent triggering due to premature ventricular contractions and atrial fibrillation or poor R-wave amplitude, and imaging at the cardiac apex

(61). A rapid heart rate does not preclude satisfactory gating; the signal intensity may be increased by gating to every second or third heart beat. This results in a long TR (R-R interval × 2 or 3), which allows for greater recovery of magnetization between pulses (47), but increases the time required to produce the images.

The presence or absence of signal from blood within vessels and cardiac chambers depends on the velocity of blood flow. At high velocities there is no signal, but stationary blood shows strong signal, and slow flow produces spin-enhancing effects, i.e., increased signal on the second-echo image (93).

Signal is shown in the cardiac chambers and aorta during portions of the cardiac cycle when flow is slow. Healthy patients show signal in the left ventricle, aorta, and pulmonary arteries during end-diastole and isovolumic systole (R wave ± 50 msec when heart rate is 50–80/min), but may not show signal if the heart rate is greater than 80/min. Normally, no signal is seen in the left ventricle, aorta, or pulmonary arteries during systole (80–300 msec post R wave). In the left atrium, signal often is seen during ventricular systole. The right atrium and right ventricle show little signal throughout the cardiac cycle. When signal is seen in a cardiac chamber or the aorta due to slow

A,B

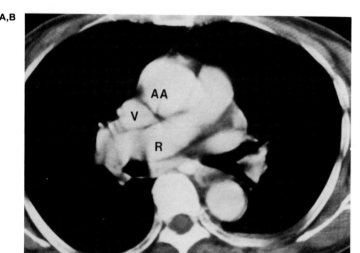

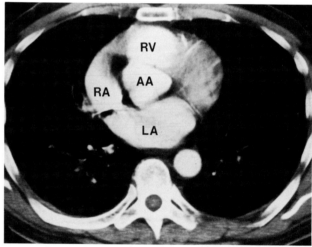

C

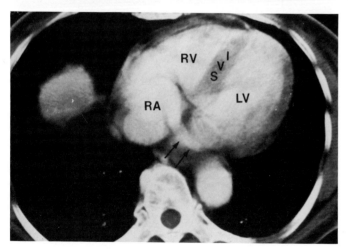

FIG. 1. Normal CT anatomy of the heart. **A:** Level of the right pulmonary artery. The horizontal portion of the right pulmonary artery (R) is well seen. The ascending aorta (AA) and the superior vena cava (V) are anterior to the right pulmonary artery. **B:** Level of the aortic root. The ascending aorta (AA) has a cloverleaf shape. The left atrium (LA) is behind it, and the right atrium (RA) is along its right lateral margin. A portion of the right ventricular outflow tract (RV) is seen anterior to the aorta. **C:** Ventricular level. The right ventricle (RV), interventricular septum (IVS), and left ventricle (LV) are clearly seen. The right atrium (RA) is seen posterolateral to the right ventricle, and the coronary sinus (arrows) is identified as a tubular structure entering the right atrium.

flow, the second-echo signal is stronger than the first-echo signal (93). Cine MRI, a new pulse sequence with low flip angles and gradient-refocused echoes, acquires images of the heart so rapidly that a cine display can assess cardiac function. On cine MRI of normal subjects, blood yields high signal intensity relative to myocardium.

NORMAL CARDIAC ANATOMY BY CT AND MRI

Transaxial imaging is the standard method for acquiring CT images. With MRI, sagittal, coronal, and oblique planes of the heart can be imaged directly, which increases the diagnostic yield. CT and MRI show similar cardiac anatomy on transverse images (Figs. 1 and 2). Moving in a cephalocaudal direction, different structures are seen at different levels (41).

Level of Right Pulmonary Artery

This level demonstrates the vascular structures at the base of the heart between the aortic arch above and the aortic root below. The structures regularly seen are the proximal right and main pulmonary arteries, the superior vena cava (SVC), and the ascending aorta (Figs. 1A and 2A). The pulmonary trunk and horizontal portion of the right pulmonary artery are seen as the latter courses from left to right anterior to the right main-stem bronchus. The size of the pulmonary arteries is related to the pulmonary blood flow and pulmonary artery pressure. They are enlarged when either or both are increased. The SVC is constantly seen as a circular structure slightly to the right of the midline, in front of the right pulmonary artery and posterolateral to the ascending aorta. The shape and size of the SVC are rarely influenced by respiratory cycle, in contrast to the situation for the inferior vena cava (IVC).

Aortic Root Level

The aortic root is visualized 4 to 5 cm caudal to the level of the carina (Figs. 1B and 2B). The aorta is seen as an ovoid, well-delineated structure anterior to the left atrium. The size of the ascending aorta at the level of the aortic root ranges from 32 to 38 mm and about 30 to 35 mm at the level of the right pulmonary artery (41). If the

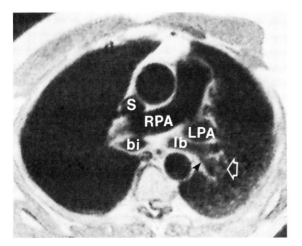

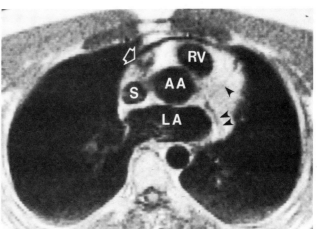

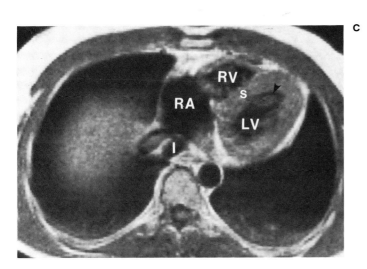

FIG. 2. Normal gated MRI anatomy of the heart (SE 500/30). **A:** Level of the right pulmonary artery. The right pulmonary artery (RPA) courses posterior to the superior vena cava (S) and anterior to the bronchus intermedius (bi); (LPA) left pulmonary artery; (lb) left main-stem bronchus; (*arrowhead*) left-lower-lobe bronchus; (*open arrow*) left-lower-lobe pulmonary artery. **B:** Level of aortic root. The left atrium (LA) is a quadrangular structure posterior to the ascending aorta (AA). The right ventricular outflow tract (RV) is anterolateral to the ascending aorta. A portion of the right atrial appendage (*open arrow*) is seen; (S) superior vena cava; (*single arrowhead*) left anterior descending coronary artery; (*double arrowheads*) circumflex coronary artery. **C:** Ventricular level. The interventricular septum (s) separates the thin-walled right ventricle (RV) from the thick-walled left ventricle (LV); (RA) right atrium; (I) inferior vena cava; (*arrowhead*) papillary muscle.

ratio of the ascending aorta to descending aorta at the level of aortic root exceeds 1.7, dilatation of the ascending aorta is present.

The right atrium and its appendage are seen along the right lateral aspect of the aortic root. The atrial appendage is seen as a curved triangular structure lateral to the aorta. The SVC is slightly posterior, projecting below the atrial appendage. The left atrium is a quadrangular structure seen posterior to the aorta directly in front of the vertebral body. This structure is easily recognized because of its shape and the pulmonary veins entering the left atrium posterolaterally. The right ventricular outflow tract is seen as an ovoid structure along the left anterolateral aspect of the aorta.

Ventricular Level

On contrast-enhanced images, both ventricles are well seen. The ventricular septum courses from right posterior to left anterior, separating the ventricular chambers (Figs. 1C and 2C). Septal structures and papillary muscles can sometimes be identified, even without EKG gating, if the patient is anemic. EKG gating and cine CT significantly increase the ability to clearly define these structures. On ungated CT, the thickness of the left ventricular wall is estimated to range from 7 to 18 mm; on gated studies, the thickness is about 10 mm during diastole and 14 mm during systole (60). The angle between the sagittal plane and ventricular septum is normally about 38°. It is possible to estimate left ventricular muscle mass, volumes, wall-thickness dynamics, and ejection fraction from EKG-gated scans. On the transaxial images, the curving posterior and inferior walls of the left ventricle are seen tangentially. Caudal to the ventricles, the IVC is seen as an ovoid structure entering the right atrium. The coronary sinus can be identified in the fat of the atrioventricular groove as a curvilinear density slightly above and medial to the IVC.

Additional anatomic information can be acquired from MRI that generally is not present on CT images. On MRI, the myocardium is of medium signal intensity; the endothelial surface is sharply outlined by the signal void of the blood within the cardiac chambers. The papillary muscles and chordae can be seen in most patients (Fig. 2C). Cusps of the mitral, tricuspid, and aortic valves also may be identified in some normal patients, but assessment of the valves is difficult using orthogonal planes because the images are not perpendicular to the valve leaflets and because of the thickness of the images relative to the thinness of valve leaflets (16). The atrial septum is well defined, but is very thin and has low intensity at the fossa ovalis. Both anterior (outlet) and posterior (inlet) portions of the ventricular septum are depicted on different transverse levels. Sagittal images show the normal connection of the pulmonary artery to the right ventricle and the origin of the aorta from the left ventricle (48). The proximal parts of the coronary arteries can be seen in some patients (Fig. 3) (47,63).

Pericardium

The normal pericardium is a fibroserous sac that surrounds and supports the heart and the great vessels. According to anatomic textbooks, the pericardium consists of an outer sac known as the fibrous pericardium and an inner double-layer sac known as the serous pericardium. The fibrous pericardium is composed of dense collagenous fibers and is anchored to the sternum anteriorly and to the central tendon of the diaphragm inferiorly, blending with the coats of the great vessels superiorly. The serous pericardium has two layers, an outer parietal layer that is associated with the fibrous pericardium and an inner visceral layer that is intimately related to the external surface of the heart. To most clinicians, the pericardium is regarded as two layers: the visceral and parietal pericardium, separated by a small amount of fluid. Under the visceral pericardium there is usually abundant fat in which lie the coronary arteries, veins, and coronary sinus. The parietal pericardium invaginates the heart like a bursa, reflecting off the great vessels leaving or entering the heart such as the aorta, pulmonary artery, venae cavae, and pulmonary veins. At these reflections are the preaortic and retroaortic pericardial recesses, which normally contain a small amount of lymph fluid (Fig. 3) (62). The thickness of normal pericardium has been determined to be 1 to 2 mm by anatomic studies.

The pericardium is identified on CT because of the presence of fat in the mediastinum and epicardial space. Pericardium is seen as a curvilinear density between these two fat planes (Fig. 4). It is most frequently identified anterior to the ventricles, and less frequently inferolaterally. Normal pericardium is identifiable in 95% of adult patients (84). It is less frequently seen in children. The normal thickness of pericardium on nongated CT images does not exceed 4 mm. However, many patients normally exhibit variable, short segments of apparent pericardial thickening particularly around the anterior sternopericardial ligaments where the pericardial sac is imaged tangentially.

EKG gating is necessary to clearly identify the normal pericardium during MRI. The pericardium is seen as a curvilinear line of low signal intensity separating higher-intensity myocardium or epicardial fat from mediastinal fat (86). Normal pericardium is best seen in systole along the anterior surface of the right ventricle posterior to the sternum because of the increased amount of epicardial and mediastinal fat in this region (Fig. 5) (81). Average pericardial thickness by MRI is 1.3 to 2.5 mm in systole when measured anterior to the right ventricle at the mid-ventricular level (81). Pericardial thickness is measured

A,B

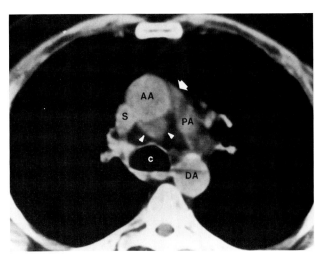 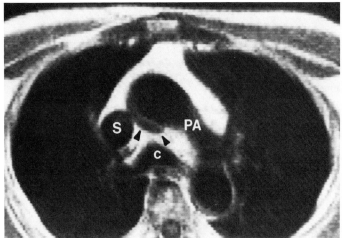

FIG. 3. Normal pericardial recesses. **A:** CT image shows the retroaortic recess (*arrowheads*) and the preaortic recess (*arrow*); (AA) ascending aorta; (DA) descending aorta; (S) superior vena cava; (PA) top of pulmonary artery; (c) carina. **B:** Transverse MR image (SE 500/30) in a different patient shows the retroaortic recess (*arrowheads*); (PA) top of pulmonary artery; (S) superior vena cava; (c) carina. (From ref. 31.)

on a first-echo image because the pericardial line may be blurred and appears thicker on second-echo images (81).

The thickness of the pericardial line on MRI is made up by the fibrous layer of the pericardium and the small amount of serous fluid normally present in the pericardial cavity. The low signal intensity of the pericardium is due to the low signal intensity of fibrous pericardium and low signal intensity of serous fluid in nonlaminar motion (81). The thickness of the pericardium is greater in systole than in diastole because of shifting of pericardial fluid. The pericardium is also thicker on more caudal sections of the heart in systole because pericardial fluid shifts from

the base of the heart in diastole to the apex of the heart in systole (81,86). The preaortic recess and the retroaortic recesses are particularly well seen because of the low signal intensity of the recesses compared with the high intensity of mediastinal fat (68).

MULTIPLANAR CARDIAC MRI

Using MRI, direct images can be obtained in sagittal, coronal, or oblique planes. Direct imaging avoids the loss of spatial resolution that occurs with reformatting. Coronal views are best for showing the inferior (diaphragmatic) wall of the left ventricle, and sagittal views show the entire length of the normal thoracic aorta.

Gated images of the heart in sagittal and coronal planes produce good detail of the heart and great vessels. How-

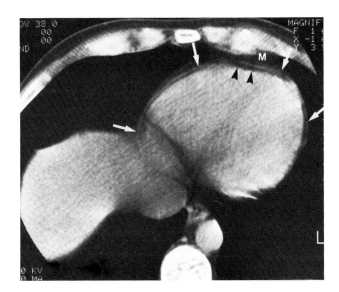

FIG. 4. CT image of normal pericardium. A transverse image at the midventricular level. Pericardium is seen as a thin line (*arrows*) around most of the circumference of the heart, separating the epicardial fat (*arrowheads*) from the outer mediastinal fat (M).

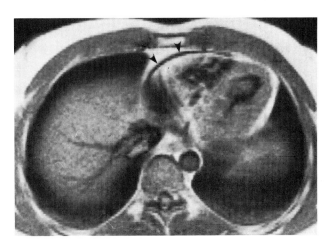

FIG. 5. Gated MRI of normal pericardium (TE = 30 msec) overlying right ventricle. The low-signal-intensity pericardium (*arrowheads*) is surrounded by high-signal-intensity mediastinal and epicardial fat.

ever, because the left ventricle and ventricular and atrial septa lie in oblique planes, accurate measurements of left ventricular wall thickness, ventricular volume, and ejection fraction and clear delineation of ventricular and atrial septa (and defects therein) are possible only on oblique images.

An image plane through the long axis of the left ventricle parallel to the interventricular septum is comparable to an angiographic right anterior oblique view. In this projection, the aortic valve, aortic root, and segments of the left ventricular wall are seen (Fig. 6). An image plane through the long axis of the left ventricle perpendicular to the interventricular septum is comparable to an angiographic left anterior oblique (LAO) view with cranial angulation (18). This plane demonstrates the septa, mitral valve, left atrium, and left ventricle. Interatrial and interventricular septal defects are well seen using this imaging plane (19). An imaging plane oriented to the short axis of the left ventricle shows the ventricular apex, septum, aorta, and pulmonary artery (Fig. 7). All of the foregoing oblique imaging planes are obtained by electronic rotation of the magnetic fields (19,25).

CONGENITAL HEART DISEASE

The primary imaging methods for diagnosis and management of congenital heart disease (CHD) are angiography and two-dimensional echocardiography. In a few conditions, such as atrial septal defect or ductus arteriosus, echocardiographic diagnosis is sufficient prior to surgical therapy. In the majority of congenital anomalies, cardiac catheterization and angiocardiography are needed to provide accurate anatomic and hemodynamic information.

CT

CT can demonstrate aortic arch anomalies, including coarctation and pseudocoarctation, and positional anomalies such as levoposition of the ascending aorta, e.g., corrected transposition (Fig. 8) (7,24,27). Whereas CT can demonstrate positional abnormalities, ventriculoarterial connections are not as easily demonstrable.

CT demonstration of coarctation and pseudocoarctation (nonobstructive coarctation) is valuable because it may obviate the need for angiography (36). In coarctation, the narrowed segment of the aorta can be identified. Collateral circulation is also seen, establishing the hemodynamic significance of the lesion (34,36). In pseudocoarctation, collateral vessels are not present. The aortic arch is unusually high, and the aortic isthmus lies anterior to its usual location adjacent to the spine (Fig. 9) (34). The left subclavian artery has a more caudal and posterior origin; however, this may also be seen in true coarctation. The clinical role of CT in coarctation is questionable, because the clinical diagnosis is readily made when typical chest roentgenographic findings are present; angiography is not always needed. Even when the diagnosis is in question, MRI or digital-subtraction angiography generally is preferred to CT examination. However, pseudocoarctation may occasionally be confused with a mediastinal mass or aortic aneurysm on conventional radiography, and CT is helpful in making a proper diagnosis.

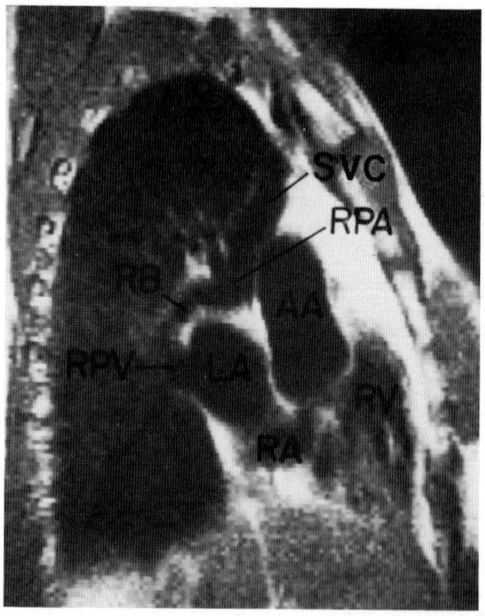

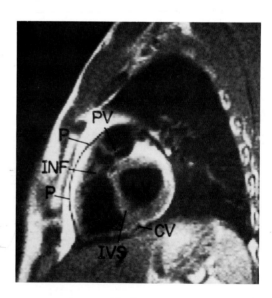

FIG. 6. Gated oblique MRI (TE = 30 msec) through the long axis of the left ventricle parallel to the interventricular septum (angiographic RAO) demonstrates the aortic root and ascending aorta (AA); (SVC) superior vena cava; (RB) right bronchus; (RPV) right pulmonary veins; (LA) left atrium; (RA) right atrium; (RV) right ventricle. (From ref. 78.)

FIG. 7. Gated oblique MRI (TE = 30 msec) oriented to the short axis of the left ventricle (angiographic LAO) demonstrates the pulmonary infundibulum (INF) and pulmonic valve (PV); (P) pericardium; (RV) right ventricle; (IVS) interventricular septum; (LV) left ventricle; (CV) coronary vein. (From ref. 78.)

A,B

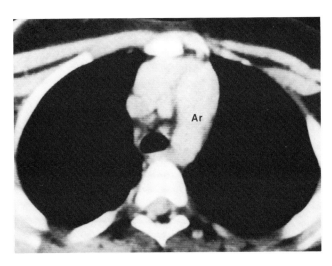 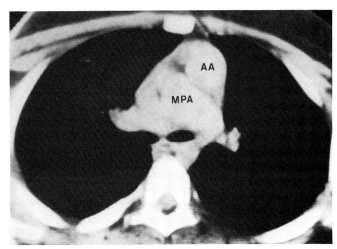

FIG. 8. An 11-year-old boy with corrected transposition of the great vessels. **A:** CT image at the aortic-arch level shows that the aortic arch (Ar) is directed anteroposteriorly. **B:** CT image at the level of the carina shows the ascending aorta (AA) to be anterior and to the left of the main pulmonary artery (MPA).

A,B

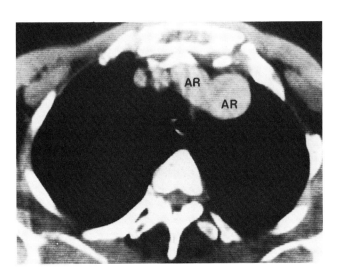 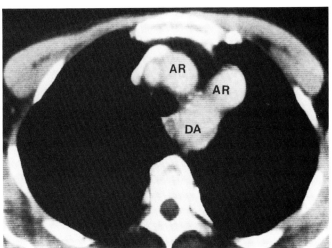

C

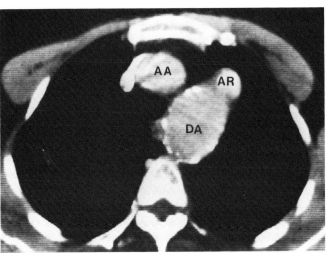

FIG. 9. Contrast-enhanced CT images of the thorax in a patient with cervical aortic arch, pseudocoarctation, and aneurysm of descending thoracic aorta. The images **A–D** are obtained in a cephalocaudal direction. **A:** The aortic arch (AR) is unusually high and extends from right to left instead of in an anteroposterior direction. **B:** The aortic arch (AR) appears to be discontinuous because of its tortuosity. Fusiform dilatation of proximal descending aorta (DA) is seen. **C:** The ascending aorta, distal aortic arch (AR), and dilated descending aorta (DA) are seen.

Some congenital abnormalities of the pulmonary arteries and veins and the systemic veins may appear as mediastinal masses on chest radiographs of children and adults (37,87). Examples include interruption of the IVC, partial anomalous pulmonary venous connection to the right or left SVC, and aberrant left pulmonary artery (pulmonary artery sling) (10,87). Using CT, the correct diagnosis may be established noninvasively (see Chapter 7).

Diagnosis of many intracardiac defects such as ventricular septal defect (6,24,27), atrial septal defect, tetralogy of Fallot, and visceroatrial anomalies is possible by CT. However, CT has not been widely used because slow scanning times degrade spatial resolution. Additional factors that limit the clinical utility of CT in evaluation of congenital heart disease include (a) limited field of view, (b) inability to visualize cardiac valves, (c) inability to see branch pulmonary arteries, (d) difficulties in reformatting imaging planes other than axial views, and (e) difficulties in imaging infants and young children. The recent development of cine CT with acquisition times of 33 to 50 msec/scan has overcome some of the foregoing limitations (6,66). Cine CT can also be triggered at a specific phase of the EKG, allowing physiologic data collection, such as cardiac output and shunts. But this technology is not yet widely available.

MRI

Great-Vessel Anomalies

Using transverse, coronal, and sagittal images, abnormalities of the positions of the great vessels are reliably identified (16). In patients with transposition of the great arteries, sagittal images show the aorta arising from the anatomic right ventricle, and the pulmonary artery from the anatomic left ventricle. The relationship of the great vessels to each other is easily appreciated on transverse images. In complete transposition, the aorta is anterior and to the right of the pulmonary artery (Fig. 10). In corrected transposition, the aorta is anterior, but to the left of the pulmonary artery (16). Sagittal images are also useful in persistent truncus arteriosus; a series of images will show the truncal vessel straddling the two ventricles (45).

The abnormalities of the pulmonary outflow tract, such as pulmonary stenosis in tetralogy of Fallot or atresia in pulmonary atresia and ventricular septal defect (Fig. 11), are identified on transverse and coronal images. The status of the central pulmonary arteries also can be defined, but stenoses in their branches are less clearly seen.

Coarctation of the aorta (Fig. 12) is best demonstrated on sagittal or long-axis (LAO) views of the aorta, as these projections depict the ascending aorta, aortic arch, and proximal descending aorta in children and young adults on a single image. Imaging in more than one plane is useful to avoid misinterpretations resulting from partial-volume effects. The presence of coarctation, its site and extent, and any involvement of the arch vessels are accurately defined by MRI (94).

Other congenital abnormalities of the aorta and pulmonary artery have been demonstrated by MRI, including left aortic arch with aberrant right subclavian artery, right aortic arch with aberrant left subclavian artery, Marfan's syndrome (Fig. 13), and Takayasu disease. Dilatation of the ascending aorta may be monitored by serial MRI examinations, and MRI may be used as an alternative to CT to diagnose complicated aortic dissection when contrast material is contraindicated or CT findings are equiv-

A,B

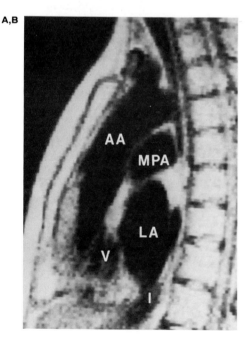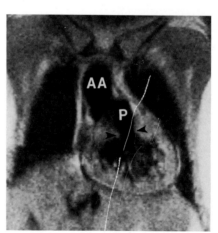

FIG. 10. A 24-year-old woman with double-inlet ventricle (left ventricular type) and transposition of the great vessels. **A:** Gated sagittal MRI (TE = 30 msec) shows the ascending aorta (AA) arising anterior to main pulmonary artery (MPA). The inferior vena cava (I) passes posterior to the left atrium (LA) as it courses rightward to join the right atrium; (V) single ventricle. **B:** Coronal MR image shows the ascending aorta (AA) to the right of the main pulmonary artery (P). Subvalvular pulmonary artery stenosis (*arrowheads*) is present.

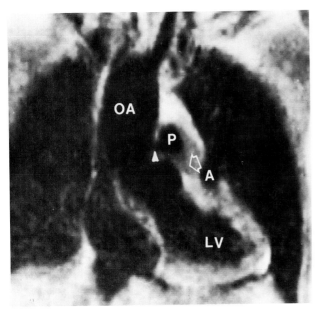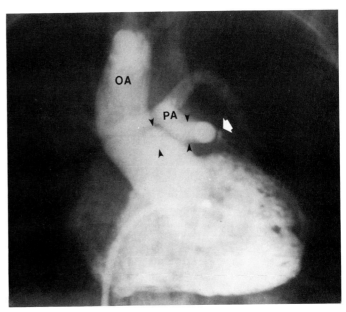

FIG. 11. A 24-year-old woman with pulmonary atresia and ventricular septal defect. **A:** Coronal MRI (SE 500/30) through left ventricle (LV) demonstrates a right ventricular infundibular stenosis (*open arrow*). The right ventricular chamber was seen on more anterior images. A fistula (*arrowhead*) from an overriding aorta (OA) supplies the pulmonary artery (P) distal to the stenosis. This fistula was appreciated on MRI only retrospectively, after an angiogram was performed; (A) left atrial appendage. **B:** Right ventriculogram in AP projection opacifies right ventricle and left ventricle via a ventricular septal defect. A hypertrophied left coronary artery (*arrowheads*) is identified as the fistula between an overriding aorta (OA) and pulmonary artery (PA). No pulmonary outflow tract is identified; (*arrow*) left anterior descending coronary artery.

ocal. In Takayasu disease, stenoses and occlusions of branch vessels of the aortic arch may be identified by MRI, but false-positive and false-negative errors are found when MRI is compared with angiography (32,72). A pulmonary sling may be demonstrated by MRI when an aberrant left pulmonary artery arises from the right pulmonary artery and passes between the trachea and esophagus (see Fig. 91 in Chapter 7).

Determination of Visceroatrial Situs and Ventricles

With transverse and coronal images extending through the heart and upper abdomen, visceroatrial situs can be determined. The tracheal bifurcation is identified, and the relations of the main-stem bronchi to the right and left pulmonary arteries are seen. The relationship of the stomach to the aortic arch and the position of the liver are identified (Fig. 14). Morphologic details of the anatomic right and left ventricles can be recognized (16). The anatomic right ventricle is triangular and has a coarse internal trabecular pattern and moderator band at its apex. The anatomic left ventricle has an elliptical shape and smooth internal trabecular pattern (16).

Ventricular Septal Defects/Ventricular Abnormalities

Perimembranous and muscular ventricular septal defects (VSD) are well defined using transverse images (Figs.

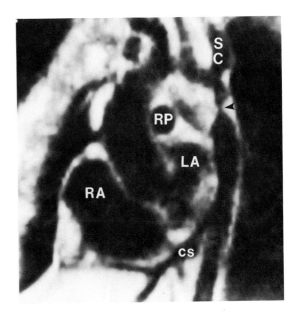

FIG. 12. A 10-year-old boy with coarctation of the aorta. Gated left anterior oblique MRI (TE = 30 msec) demonstrates a 6-mm-long coarctation (*arrowhead*) 12 mm distal to the origin of the left subclavian artery (SC). The aortic arch is hypoplastic; (RA) right atrium; (RP) right pulmonary artery; (LA) left atrium; (cs) coronary sinus.

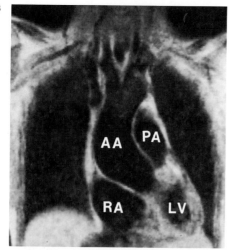
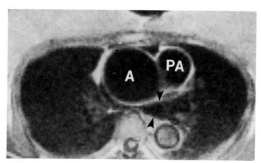
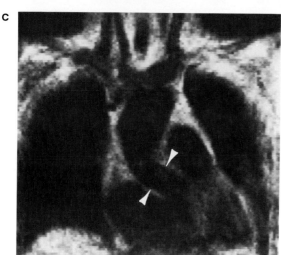

FIG. 13. A 26-year-old woman with Marfan's syndrome. **A:** Gated coronal MRI (TE = 30 msec) shows aneurysmal dilatation of ascending aorta (AA); (RA) right atrium; (PA) pulmonary artery; (LV) left ventricle. **B:** Transverse MR image just above sinuses of Valsalva demonstrates 5-cm aortic root (A). The left atrium (*arrowheads*) is compressed by the aortic root. High-intensity signal in the descending aorta results from diastolic pseudogating; (PA) pulmonary artery. **C:** Coronal MRI 2 months following insertion of composite aortic graft. The tubular graft (*arrowheads*) is seen in the aortic root.

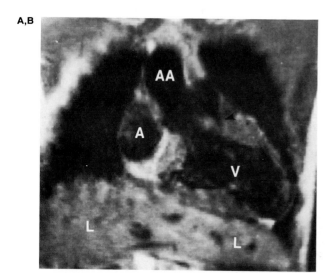
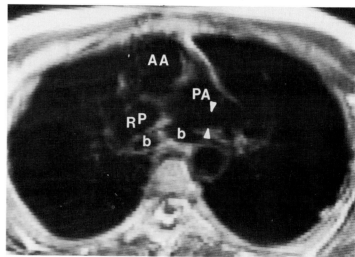

FIG. 14. A 16-year-old girl with asplenia. Associated congenital heart disease includes pulmonic stenosis, single atrium, single ventricle, and *d*-malposition of the great vessels. **A:** Gated coronal MRI (TE = 28 msec) demonstrates transverse liver (L) and infundibular pulmonic stenosis (*arrowhead*). The ascending aorta (AA) arises from a single ventricle (V); (A) single atrium. **B:** Transverse MR image just below the carina demonstrates both pulmonary arteries anterior to the main-stem bronchi (b). The great vessels are transposed; the ascending aorta (AA) is anterior and to the right of the pulmonary artery (PA); (RP) right pulmonary artery; (*arrowheads*) left pulmonary artery.

A,B

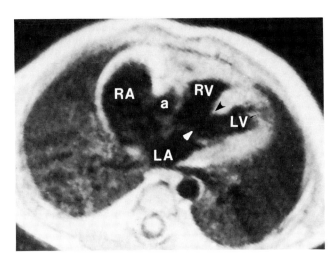 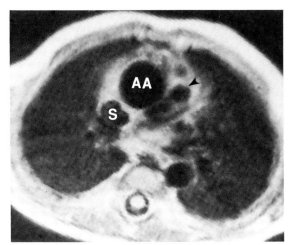

FIG. 15. A 6-year-old boy with subvalvular pulmonic stenosis and ventricular septal defect with right-to-left shunting. **A:** Gated transverse MRI (TE = 30 msec) depicts perimembranous ventricular defect (*arrowheads*). The right ventricular wall is hypertrophied secondary to pulmonary stenosis; (RA) right atrium; (RV) right ventricle; (LV) left ventricle; (LA) left atrium; (a) aortic valve. **B:** Transverse MRI 4 cm above **A** demonstrates a small pulmonary artery (*arrowhead*) due to subvalvular pulmonic stenosis; (AA) ascending aorta; (S) superior vena cava.

15 and 21B); the associated enlargements of the pulmonary artery and right ventricle are also seen. Small septal defects may be missed when transverse images alone are used, and imaging in a plane along the long axis of the left ventricle perpendicular to the septum is recommended (19). The atrioventricular (AV) septal defect is especially well demonstrated by MRI (53,55). On transverse images, these patients demonstrate absence of the primum atrial septum and inlet ventricular septum. In complete form, a "common" AV valve is also recognized.

Ebstein's anomaly consists of a downward displacement of implantation of the septal leaflet of the tricuspid valve into the right ventricle. The displaced valve divides the ventricle into a proximal "atrialized" portion and a small distal functional portion. Transverse and coronal images display the displaced leaflets as well as the dilated right atrium and the functionally small right ventricle (Fig. 16).

Dilatation and/or hypertrophy of the right ventricle are also seen on transverse images in patients with transposition of the great vessels, pulmonary stenosis or atresia, and Eisenmenger syndrome. In patients with elevated right ventricular pressure, the ventricular septum, which is normally convex to the right ventricle, is straightened or concave to the right ventricle (16). In patients with severe pulmonary artery hypertension (systolic pressure > 80 mm Hg) and severe pulmonary vascular resistance (>787 dynes-cm/sec), the normal pulmonary artery signal in diastole persists into systole (15).

Atrial Septal Defects/Systemic and Pulmonary Venous Abnormalities

Defects at the superior portion of the atrial septum near its junction with the superior vena cava (sinus venosus

defects) (Fig. 17), defects in the midportion of the septum (ostium secundum defects) (Fig. 18), and defects in the lower septum near the AV valves (ostium primum defects) are identified (16,17). When using transverse images, the normal thinning of the atrial septum at the fossa ovalis may produce signal dropout and mimic a secundum septal defect. This appearance typically appears on only a single slice of an imaging series, whereas true secundum defects usually are seen on more than one image. Also, the thickness of the septum at the edges of a true secundum defect increases and does not thin out (17). False-positive diagnoses in atrial septal defects can be avoided by using planes oriented to the cardiac axes, particularly a plane along the long axis of the left ventricle perpendicular to

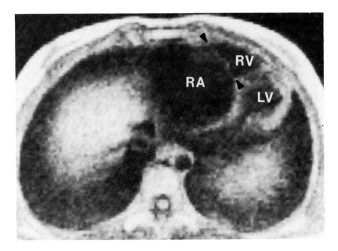

FIG. 16. A 30-year-old woman with Ebstein's anomaly. Gated transverse MRI (TE = 30 msec) shows the septal leaflet (*arrowheads*) of the tricuspid valve displaced downward, resulting in a dilated right atrium (RA) and small functional right ventricle (RV); (LV) left ventricle.

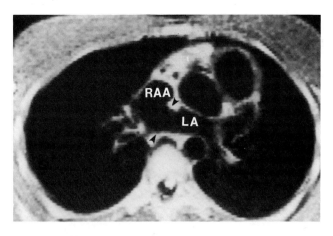

FIG. 17. A 30-year-old woman with sinus venosus atrial septal defect (*arrowheads*); (RAA) right atrial appendage; (LA) left atrium.

the atrial and ventricular septa (20). Cor triatriatum may be diagnosed using MRI (Fig. 19); the common pulmonary vein persists as an accessory chamber that communicates with the left atrium. The membrane between the true left atrium and accessory chamber produces hemodynamic changes similar to those of mitral stenosis.

A variety of venous anomalies can be defined by MRI. Anomalous pulmonary venous connections, dilated pulmonary veins in large left-to-right shunts, a persistent left SVC draining to a dilated coronary sinus, and azygos continuation of an interrupted IVC are all seen (26,80) (see Fig. 88 in Chapter 7).

Postoperative Evaluation of Palliative Procedures

The patency of palliative systemic–pulmonary-artery shunts can be accurately determined by MRI (54,58). Patency is determined by absence of signal from inside the lumen of the shunt. The optimal imaging plane depends on the type of shunt and the individual patient (54,58). Blalock-Taussig shunts (anastomosis of subclavian artery to pulmonary artery) are best demonstrated on coronal or axial images (Fig. 14B). Glenn shunts (anastomosis of SVC to right pulmonary artery) are seen optimally on coronal images. Pott's shunts (anastomosis of descending

A,B

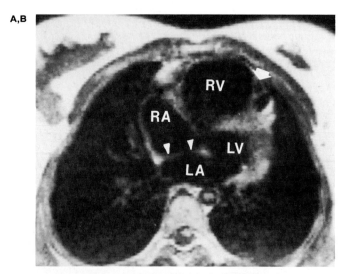

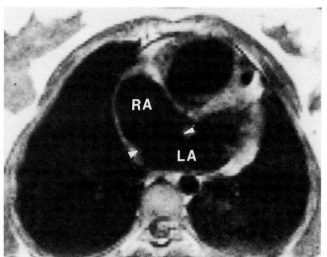

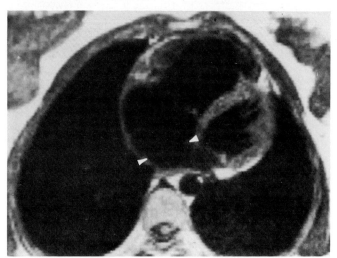

FIG. 18. A 20-year-old woman with ostium secundum atrial septal defect (ASD). **A:** Gated transverse MRI (TE = 35 msec) 1 cm above secundum ASD shows normal atrial septum (*arrowheads*) separating right atrium (RA) and left atrium (LA). A thickened trabeculation (*arrow*) is present in the right ventricle (RV) (the tricuspid valve was in normal position at cardiac catheterization); (LV) left ventricle. **B:** Transverse MR image 1 cm below **A** shows large secundum ASD (*arrowheads*); (RA) right atrium; (LA) left atrium. **C:** Transverse MR image 1 cm below **B** demonstrates that a true ASD (*arrowheads*) usually is seen on more than one image.

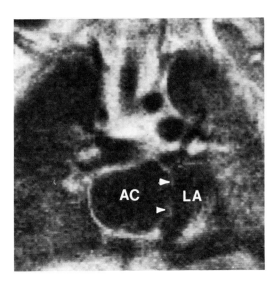

FIG. 19. A 5-year-old boy with cor triatriatum. Gated coronal MRI (TE = 30 msec) demonstrates a septum (*arrowheads*) between left atrium (LA) and accessory chamber (AC) formed by persistent common pulmonary vein.

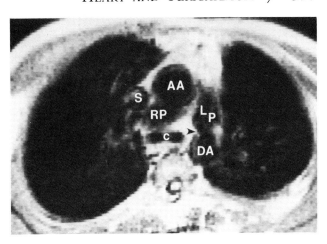

FIG. 20. A 13-year-old boy with pulmonary atresia. Gated transverse MRI (TE = 30 msec) shows a patent Potts anastomosis (*arrowhead*) between left pulmonary artery (LP) and descending aorta (DA); (AA) ascending aorta; (S) superior vena cava; (RP) right pulmonary artery; (c) carina.

aorta to left pulmonary artery) and Waterston shunts (anastomosis of ascending aorta to right pulmonary artery) are well identified on transaxial images (Fig. 20) (54,58). Using MRI, an entire palliative shunt may not be imaged on a single section. Blalock-Taussig shunts usually course posteriorly as they descend to the right or left pulmonary artery, and multiple coronal images are needed to image different portions of the shunt (54).

Determination of stenoses in these palliative shunts is less reliable than determination of patency using MRI. Tortuous shunts may not be entirely seen even after superimposing contiguous sections manually or electronically. Using current MRI technology, stenoses in grafts less than 10 mm in diameter may be missed (58). Improved resolution and use of thinner sections will be necessary for complete assessment of smaller vessels, especially in neonates and infants (58).

The postoperative aorta is best evaluated in the long-axis (LAO) imaging plane. This plane displays the entire aortic arch and the origins of the innominate, left common carotid, and left subclavian arteries. The problem of vessel tortuosity is minimized by superimposing contiguous images. Postoperative studies following repair of coarctation of the aorta (Fig. 21) can identify restenosis, postoperative aneurysm, and perianastomotic hematoma (58,94). Patients with mild (<25%) aortic narrowing on postoperative MRI exhibit no Doppler-measured blood-pressure drop between the right arm and legs. Increasing gradients correspond to increasing narrowing of the luminal diameter on MRI (58).

When a patch is used to repair a VSD, the patch is identified as a thin layer of low intensity surrounded by a thin layer of higher intensity. Intraatrial baffles in repairs of transposition of the great vessels are clearly seen (16).

Clinical Application of MRI

MRI can show many of the congenital defects depicted by echocardiography and Doppler studies and has several unique capabilities. MRI provides better delineation of central pulmonary arteries in pulmonary atresia or pulmonic stenosis (29); echocardiography does not demonstrate these arteries adequately. Antegrade cardiac catheterization of the pulmonary arteries may not be possible, and only partial opacification may be achieved by pulmonary venous-wedge angiograms or by contrast injection of collateral vessels or palliative shunts (29).

MRI is also an excellent noninvasive means of evaluating the aortic arch for coarctation beyond the isthmus in older children and adults. This portion of the arch is the least accessible for ultrasound in older subjects (29). MRI does not provide information on the pressure gradient across a coarctation that catheterization does; this pressure gradient is an indicator of the severity of the lesions and is critical information for patient management.

MRI can noninvasively demonstrate complex anomalies of the great vessels and ventricles. Recently, MRI has been shown to be very accurate (>90%) in achieving the correct anatomic diagnosis without knowledge of prior clinical, echocardiographic, or angiographic data. These cases were studied with a complete set of transverse images and one or more other imaging planes (16).

ISCHEMIC HEART DISEASE

CT

One of the earliest interests in cardiac applications of CT concerned detecting myocardial infarction (1,42). Demonstration of infarction and estimation of the size of

A,B

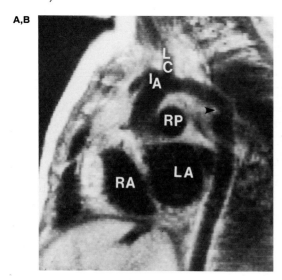 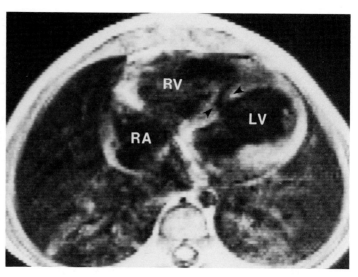

FIG. 21. A 2-year-old girl following Waldhausen repair of aortic coarctation. The left subclavian artery has been taken down to repair the coarctation. A muscular ventricular septal defect (VSD) was closed with a patch at the same operation. **A:** LAO gated MRI (TE = 30 msec) shows expected postoperative deformity at site of coarctation repair (*arrowhead*); (IA) innominate artery takeoff; (LC) left common carotid artery; (RA) right atrium; (RP) right pulmonary artery; (LA) left atrium. **B:** Transverse MR image shows residual VSD (*arrowheads*) in the trabecular septum; (RV) right ventricle; (LV) left ventricle; (RA) right atrium. (From ref. 58.)

infarction are valuable for two reasons: There are few reliable methods for *in vivo* demonstration of myocardial infarction in its early stages, and improving methods for altering the natural history of evolving myocardial infarction (use of streptokinase, tissue plasminogen activator, angioplasty, surgical revascularization, etc.) make detection, quantification, and follow-up of infarction clinical necessities rather than experimental investigations.

In experimental studies, normal myocardium and ischemic myocardium exhibit differences in X-ray attenuation with and without the use of intravenous contrast material. There is decreased attenuation of jeopardized myocardium compared with the normal (a reduction of 5–10 HU), secondary to intracellular edema (95). With administration of contrast material, there is increased accumulation of contrast material in infarcted myocardium, whereas ischemic but uninfarcted tissue does not show such a change. Using EKG-gated CT and cine CT, ischemic myocardium exhibits loss of normal systolic thickening (Fig. 22), with paradoxical thinning, whereas normal segments show compensatory increases in systolic thickening (71). There is good correlation between estimates of infarct volume from contrast-enhanced CT and pathology examination; this estimation is believed to be superior to that from radionuclide studies (30). These findings make CT a promising technique for studying acute myocardial infarction (44,60,64,67).

Myocardial infarction can lead to formation of ventricular aneurysm or, less commonly, pseudoaneurysm. These can be readily detected by CT (38,64). Contrast enhancement is necessary to detect localized dilatation of the myocardium, mural thrombus formation, and wall thinning. The infarcted myocardium not only is thin but also does not contract normally. On nongated CT images, the normal contraction of the healthy myocardium causes blurring, making the wall appear thicker than it actually is. An infarcted segment is more sharply defined because of its akinesis.

Pseudoaneurysm results from rupture of the free wall of the ventricle that is contained by the pericardium and surrounding mediastinal structures; pseudoaneurysms tend to be posterior or inferior in comparison with the anterior or apical location of the true aneurysms (Fig. 23). On CT images, true aneurysm and pseudoaneurysm can look alike; both can calcify and contain mural thrombus (Fig. 24). The narrow neck of the pseudoaneurysm, which distinguishes it from true aneurysm, can be recognized on contrast ventriculography and echocardiography, but seldom on CT images.

MRI

Acutely infarcted myocardium has a higher signal intensity than normal myocardium on T1- and T2-weighted images (28). Overlap exists between the T1 values of infarcted and normal myocardium, but not between the T2 values of infarcted and normal myocardium (69). Greater T2 weighting results in greater contrast between infarcted and normal myocardium (50). An intracavitary flow signal usually is identified adjacent to the infarcted myocardial wall, but this is a nonspecific finding, because a similar flow signal may be seen in normal individuals during diastole (69).

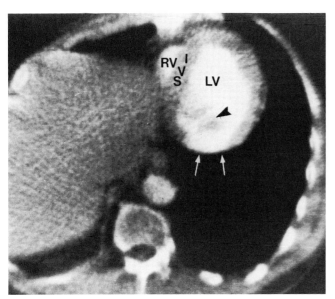 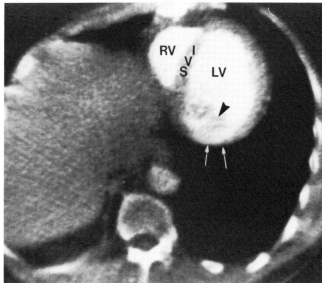

FIG. 22. Cine CT in a patient with posterior myocardial infarction and thinning of posterior wall (*arrows*). **A:** End-diastolic image; (RV) right ventricle; (IVS) interventricular septum; (LV) left ventricle. **B:** End-systolic image. Notice the akinesis and absence of posterior-wall thickening during systole. There are intraluminal filling defects representing left ventricular thrombus (*arrowhead*). (Courtesy of Dr. Martin J. Lipton, University of California, San Francisco.)

Myocardial wall thinning (50% of adjacent wall thickness) often can be demonstrated at the site of the prior infarction (Fig. 25). The transition between normal myocardium and wall thinning is well defined (46). The thinned wall often has a very low signal intensity because of a shortened T2 in that segment, consistent with replacement of myocardium by fibrous scar (70). When a prior myocardial infarction is complicated by left ventricular aneurysm (Fig. 26), the extreme wall thinning and bulging of the wall are well seen (46). If slow flow or stasis of blood is present within the aneurysm, the first-echo image usually will show a signal void within the aneurysm, but the second-echo image will show high signal intensity (46).

Cardiac thrombi complicating myocardial infarction usually occur in association with ventricular aneurysms. On MRI, cardiac thrombi are broadly attached to the wall of the cardiac chamber (or aneurysm) and may be homogeneous or heterogeneous in signal intensity (22). The signal intensity of a thrombus is greater than that of normal myocardium on the first-echo image and may increase or decrease on second-echo images (22). It is not always possible to differentiate an intracardiac thrombus from

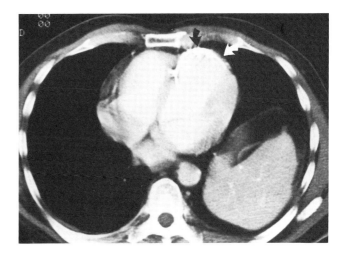

FIG. 23. Chronic apical left ventricular aneurysm. CT image shows a focal, abnormal dilatation of the apical portion of the left ventricle (LV). A mural thrombus (*arrows*) is seen as a crescentic lucency between the contrast-filled cavity and the thin apical wall.

FIG. 24. CT image shows calcification in chronic apical myocardial infarct (*arrows*).

A,B
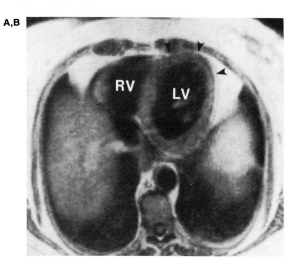
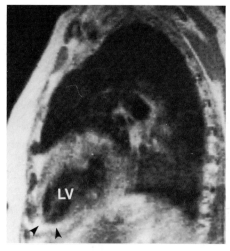

FIG. 25. A 64-year-old woman who had anterolateral myocardial infarction 1 year earlier. **A:** Gated transverse MRI (TE = 30 msec) at ventricular level during diastole shows thinning of anterolateral (*arrowheads*) wall of left ventricle (LV). Septal and posterior wall thicknesses are normal; (RV) right ventricle. **B:** Sagittal MRI through left ventricular apex during diastole shows extreme wall thinning (*arrowheads*) at the ventricular apex; (LV) left ventricle.

slow flow. Typically, slow flow shows little or no signal intensity on the first-echo image and high signal intensity on the second-echo image. But sometimes slow flow in a cardiac chamber shows medium to high signal intensity on the first-echo image that increases in relative intensity on the second-echo image, preventing differentiation from thrombus (4).

CARDIOMYOPATHY

CT

Cardiomyopathy is classified into (a) dilated or congestive, (b) hypertrophic, and (c) restrictive types. CT can demonstrate dilated chambers in the dilated form, and increased ventricular mass in the hypertrophic variety. In restrictive cardiomyopathy, the ventricular wall thickness, the ventricular chamber size, and the pericardium are normal; but the atrial chambers are dilated, and signs of systemic venous hypertension are present. Although abnormal findings may be seen on CT (67), this method is rarely used as the primary or even secondary investigative technique.

MRI

Accurate measurements of normal wall thickness, as well as accurate measurements of normal left ventricular cavity diameter and ejection fraction, are best obtained using imaging planes oriented along the long axis of the left ventricle perpendicular to the septum and oriented to the short axis of the left ventricle (59,88). In congestive cardiomyopathy, MRI usually demonstrates dilatation of the left ventricle; left atrial and right ventricular enlarge-

ments are seen less often (Fig. 27). Wall thickness is seen to be normal or mildly reduced. Disproportionate thinning of the ventricular septum is sometimes seen (46).

MRI accurately defines the presence, severity, and distribution of abnormal wall thickness in hypertrophic cardiomyopathies (Fig. 28). Although early angiographic reports suggested that hypertrophic cardiomyopathy was limited to the infundibular septum, two-dimensional echocardiography and MRI have shown a variable distribution of disease, including midventricle and apical forms (49). In amyloid heart disease, MRI has shown ab-

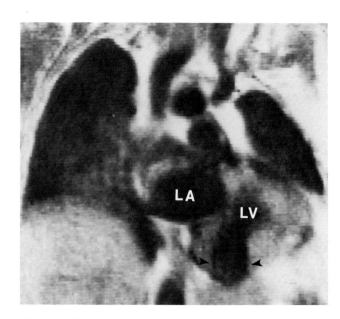

FIG. 26. A 65-year-old man 2 years after a posterior myocardial infarction. Right anterior oblique gated MRI (TE = 35 msec) of a left ventricular pseudoaneurysm (*arrowheads*); (LV) left ventricle; (LA) left atrium.

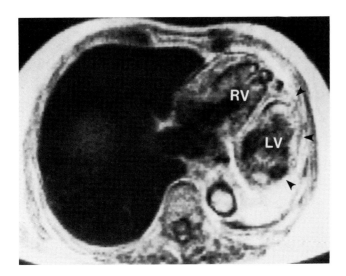

FIG. 27. A 75-year-old alcoholic man with congestive cardio-myopathy. Gated transverse MRI (TE = 30 msec) at low ventricular level demonstrates dilated right ventricular (RV) and left ventricular (LV) chambers. Signal in the ventricles and ventricular walls is inhomogeneous. The left ventricular wall is thinned (arrowheads). High signal intensity in the descending aorta is due to diastolic pseudogating.

normal wall thickness, with decreased regional wall thickening during systole; increased regional wall thickening is normally seen in left ventricular hypertrophy (50). No characteristic changes in T1 or T2 values have been identified in the myocardium in hypertrophic or congestive cardiomyopathies (50).

INTRACARDIAC AND PARACARDIAC MASSES

CT

Masses may be found in any cardiac chamber. The most common form of cardiac mass is thrombus, which is most frequent in the left ventricle. Thrombus may form in any situation associated with sluggish flow, such as myocardial infarction, dilated cardiomyopathy, mitral stenosis, and atrial fibrillation. Thrombi may be sessile or pedunculated. Most ventricular thrombi are detected by echocardiography, but sessile thrombi and thrombi on the diaphragmatic surface of the heart can be missed by echocardiography (14). Contrast-enhanced CT can detect thrombus as a focal mass with a different attenuation than blood and myocardium (Fig. 23). Small thrombi may be invisible on CT because of blurring caused by cardiac motion. In one small series, CT was more sensitive than echocardiography or angiography in detecting ventricular thrombi (90), but CT is not a practical method to routinely screen patients suspected of having cardiac thrombi. CT would be indicated in investigating a patient with systemic embolization in whom echocardiography fails to reveal a cardiac source (33).

Echocardiography has a limited role in detecting thrombi in the left atrium. Atrial thrombus occurs along its roof or in the appendage, both of which are difficult to image by echocardiography. Contrast-enhanced CT has been successfully used to demonstrate atrial thrombi in small numbers of patients (83,89,91). Atrial thrombi need to be distinguished from myxoma. The distinguishing

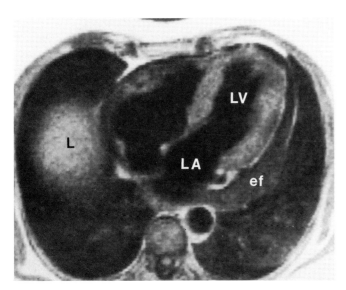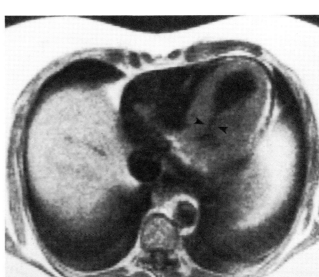

A,B

FIG. 28. A 52-year-old woman with hypercontractile ventricular septum. A: Gated transverse MRI (TE = 30 msec) at ventricular level during diastolic filling of left ventricle (LV) shows normal wall thickness of septum and free wall of left ventricle. A pericardial effusion (ef) is present; (LA) left atrium; (L) liver. B: Transverse MR image 2 cm below A shows narrowing of left ventricular chamber (arrowheads) during systole by hypercontractile ventricular septum.

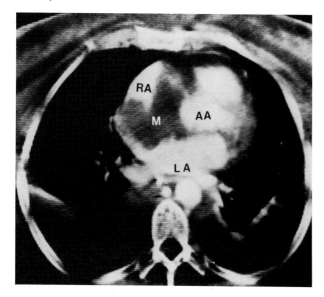

FIG. 29. Non-Hodgkin lymphoma presenting as a right atrial mass. CT shows a large irregular mass (M) filling the right atrium (RA). No mediastinal lymphadenopathy was seen; (AA) ascending aorta; (LA) left atrium.

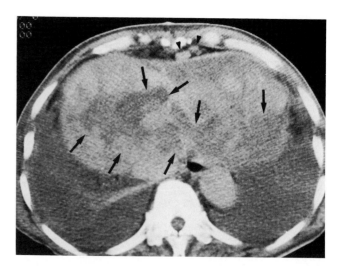

FIG. 30. Right atrial angiosarcoma invading the pericardium. Contrast-enhanced CT image of the thorax at the midventricular level shows extensive replacement of cardiac chambers by a complex mass (arrows) that produces an unrecognizable disorganization of the cardiac anatomy. Large bilateral pleural effusions and enlarged supradiaphragmatic lymph nodes (arrowheads) are present.

features are as follows: (a) myxoma characteristically arises near the atrial septum, whereas thrombi are along the posterior wall or in the atrial appendage; (b) myxomas are inhomogeneous and have lobulated margins (39,91). Although thrombi may be homogeneous or inhomogeneous, most have smooth or discrete, angulated margins (51,91).

Metastatic tumors of the heart, most frequently from carcinoma of the breast or lung or secondary to melanoma or lymphoma, are more common than primary neoplasms (Fig. 29) (2). Angiosarcoma and rhabdomyosarcoma are the common primary malignant neoplasms and appear as irregular, pedunculated masses (Fig. 30). In most suspected cases, echocardiography is the primary mode of diagnosis.

MRI

Location on the interatrial septum is an important criterion for differentiating atrial myxoma from thrombus. Demonstration of tumor attachment to the interatrial septum or tumor prolapse through the mitral valve may require imaging in the sagittal or coronal plane. Both myxoma and intracardiac thrombus produce medium to high signal intensities on first-echo images. Both may also show a relative increase on second-echo images, so that differentiation by signal intensity may not be possible (4,22).

Paracardiac masses and masses involving the septa (Fig. 31) may be identified as distinct from cardiac chambers because of the signal void in cardiac chambers. Signal intensities on T1- and T2-weighted images may identify

paracardiac or septal masses as pericardial cysts, pericardial fat pads, loculated pericardial effusions, enlarged or displaced cardiac chambers, or soft-tissue masses. Invasion of the pericardium and cardiac chambers by pulmonary or mediastinal malignancies can be demonstrated when a paracardiac mass projects into a cardiac chamber. When the mass simply deforms or displaces the cardiac chamber, invasion may or may not be present (4).

PATENCY OF CORONARY ARTERY BYPASS GRAFTS

CT has been proposed as a noninvasive method for evaluating patency of coronary artery bypass grafts (CABG), with accuracy ranging up to 97% (3,8,11, 40,57,79). Rapid-sequence dynamic CT demonstrates a patent graft as a densely opacified tubular structure at its anticipated location. But there are several limitations to this technique: (a) Enhancing structures such as native coronary arteries, atrial appendages, etc., can mimic a patent graft (35). (b) When multiple grafts are present, their origins may be so close together that distinction between grafts becomes impossible. (c) Rarely, a graft that is distally occluded may enhance over a short segment proximally (11,35,40,73). (d) Stenoses in grafts may not be identified or may mimic occlusions. Hence, except in limited numbers of patients in the immediate perioperative period, CT has no useful clinical role in evaluating CABG (13,35,92).

Using MRI, the right coronary artery and proximal left coronary artery branches can be identified, but spatial resolution is not sufficient to detect coronary artery ste-

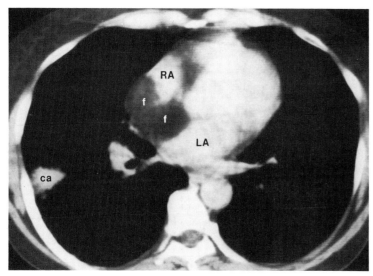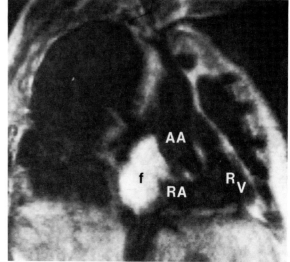

FIG. 31. A 61-year-old woman with right-lower-lobe bronchogenic carcinoma and lipomatous infiltration in the interatrial septum. **A:** CT demonstrates a large collection of fat (f) within the interatrial septum displacing the right atrium (RA) anteromedially; (LA) atrium; (ca) carcinoma. **B:** Right anterior oblique ungated MRI (SE 500/45) demonstrates abundant fat (f) in expected position of right atrium (RA), which is displaced medially; (AA) ascending aorta; (RV) right ventricle.

nosis or occlusions at this time. CABG can also be detected, but graft stenosis cannot be determined.

POSTOPERATIVE COMPLICATIONS

At a second cardiac operation involving sternotomy, catastrophic hemorrhage resulting from entering an adherent retrosternal cardiovascular structure is an uncommon but important risk. Such a complication is more serious in patients with external cardiac conduits and aortic aneurysms, with mortality ranging from 20 to 43% (21). Mortality can be reduced by anticipating such a complication and reducing the risk of hemorrhage by instituting partial cardiopulmonary bypass prior to sternotomy. Contrast-enhanced CT can be a useful technique to demonstrate the relationship of the sternum to the cardiovascular structures behind it (76). CT can demonstrate pressure effects on the sternum by the conduits (Fig. 32) and loss of fat plane between aortic aneurysms and the posterior cortex of the sternum when postoperative fibrosis makes these structures adherent to the sternum.

PERICARDIUM

CT

Because of its ability to consistently demonstrate the pericardium, CT is an excellent tool to noninvasively image the pericardium. Although echocardiography is the mainstay in the diagnosis in pericardial disease, CT may be complementary to it in several clinical settings. In ad-

dition, pericardial abnormalities frequently are visible on thoracic CT images obtained for other indications.

The pericardium is equally well seen on unenhanced and contrast-enhanced CT images, so that intravenous contrast material is not essential when the primary indication is imaging the pericardium. However, enhanced CT can give additional information about cardiac chambers, particularly in constrictive disease, and should be used in appropriate circumstances.

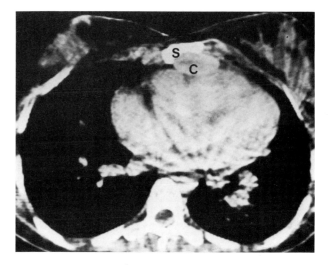

FIG. 32. CT image of the thorax in a patient 7 years following placement of an external conduit from right ventricle to pulmonary artery for ventricular septal defect and pulmonary atresia. The conduit (C) is eroding the posterior sternal cortex (S).

Congenital Anomalies of the Pericardium

Congenital diseases of the pericardium are rare. These are classified as (a) partial or total absence of pericardium and (b) cyst or diverticulum (23). Congenital absence of the pericardium is further divided into a partial defect (almost always occurring on the left), absence of the left hemipericardium, or total absence; among these, absence of the left hemipericardium is the most common. Absence of the left pericardium almost always is asymptomatic and is detected as an abnormality of mediastinal or cardiac contour on a chest radiograph. If confident diagnosis is not possible on plain films alone, CT, instead of angiocardiography or diagnostic pneumothorax, can be used

for corroboration (Fig. 33). The characteristic CT findings are (a) inability to identify the fibrous layer of parietal pericardium along the left cardiac border, (b) change in the axis of the main pulmonary artery, which bulges toward the left lung (this feature explains the prominence of the hilum and the left side of the mediastinum noted on plain radiographs of the chest), and (c) direct contact of lung and heart structures (5,74).

A pericardial diverticulum has an open communication with the pericardial cavity; a cyst results when the communication is closed or pinched off during development. Pericardial diverticula are very rare, whereas pericardial cysts are far more common. Pericardial cysts are mostly asymptomatic, are encountered during adult life, and most

A

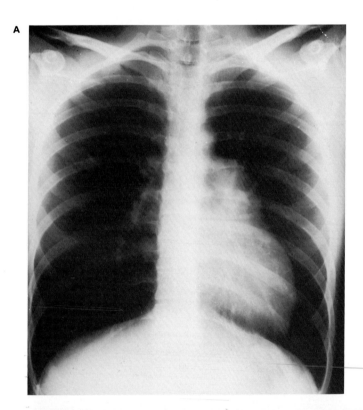

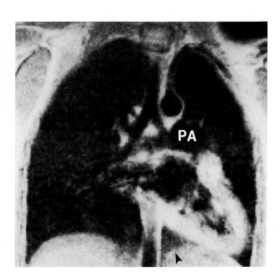

FIG. 33. An 18-year-old man with congenital absence of the left hemipericardium evident on chest radiograph. **A:** Chest radiograph shows the heart shifted to the left, but the trachea is in the midline. The pulmonary artery segment is prominent, and the left-heart border is more distinct than usual. **B:** CT image just below carina shows prominence of main pulmonary artery (PA) and left pulmonary artery (LP). Lung is insinuated between the main pulmonary artery and the ascending aorta (AA). **C:** Coronal MR image (SE 500/30) demonstrates pulmonary artery (PA) prominence. Air (*arrowhead*) is between the left hemidiaphragm and heart; this occurs in the absence of the left hemipericardium because of failure of fusion of the diaphragm and parietal pericardium.

B,C

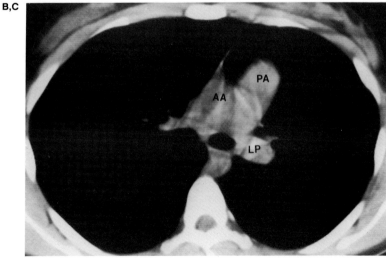

often appear as mediastinal masses on radiographs of the chest. When encountered in infants and newborn, these cysts can cause hemodynamic compromise and can be confused with pericardial teratomas.

Pericardial Effusion

Echocardiography is the method of choice for detecting pericardial effusions. Its advantages include ease of examination, portability, and high sensitivity, as well as its being totally noninvasive. However, interposition of lung between thoracic wall and heart and several interpretive pitfalls can result in errors of diagnosis.

CT can also detect pericardial effusion with a high degree of accuracy. Most effusions are recognized as near-water-density collections located between the mediastinal and epicardial fat. When the effusion is exudative or hemorrhagic, the collection may have soft-tissue density. Yet benign and malignant pericardial effusions cannot be reliably differentiated based on attenuation values (74,85). The CT appearance of the pericardial effusion will depend on its quantity. Small effusions collect behind the left ventricle and to the left of the left atrium as thin elliptical fluid collections (Fig. 34). With larger volumes, fluid also accumulates ventral and lateral to the right ventricle, forming an asymmetric halo around the heart (Fig. 35). With very large, chronic effusions, the heart appears to float within the pericardial fluid and is displaced somewhat cephalad (Fig. 36). Pericardial effusions may infrequently

be loculated because of adhesions. Although such loculation may occur anywhere in the pericardial space, posterior and right anterolateral loculations seem to be more common (74). Such loculations usually are results of previous surgery or pericarditis (56).

Small pericardial effusions may be distinguished by CT from symmetric pericardial thickening resulting from fibrosis or tumor. Pericardial effusions do not show contrast enhancement and generally change configuration with positional change; the reverse is true of pericardial thickening. Linear and nodular irregularities are common in pericardial thickening (Fig. 37). Also, thickening tends to predominate over the anterolateral cardiac surface, whereas small effusions most commonly occur posteriorly. If thickening and effusion coexist, they generally may be distinguished by their differing densities.

Constrictive Pericarditis

Constrictive pericarditis is an uncommon form of pericardial disease in which diseased pericardium impairs the distensibility of cardiac chambers, resulting in progressive diastolic dysfunction of both ventricles. This may result from infections such as tuberculosis or viral pericarditis, from inflammatory conditions such as uremia, rheumatoid arthritis, and primary or metastatic tumors, or from idiopathic causes.

Differentiation of constrictive pericarditis from restrictive cardiomyopathy is a major diagnostic problem. Findings at cardiac catheterization can be identical in both conditions. Echocardiography can help distinguish between the two conditions, but misdiagnosis is not uncommon. Endomyocardial biopsy is another useful investi-

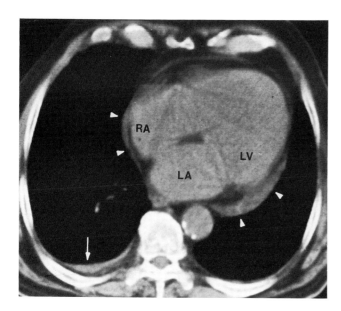

FIG. 34. A 70-year-old man with bronchogenic carcinoma. CT image at the midventricular level demonstrates a small pericardial effusion (*arrowheads*) dorsal to the left ventricle (LV) and lateral to the right atrium (RA). The density of the pericardial effusion is near that of soft tissue, consistent with an exudative effusion. A small right pleural effusion (*arrow*) is present; (LA) left atrium.

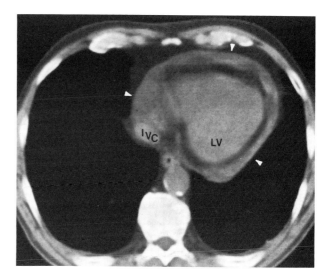

FIG. 35. A 65-year-old man with bronchogenic carcinoma. CT image at low ventricular level shows an asymmetric halo of pericardial fluid (*arrowheads*) surrounding the heart; (IVC) inferior vena cava; (LV) left ventricle.

A,B

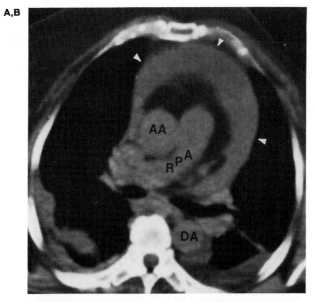
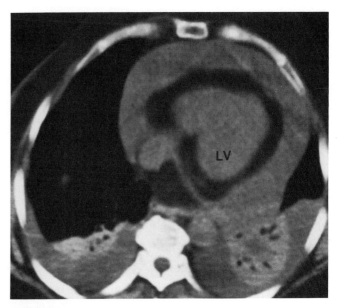

C

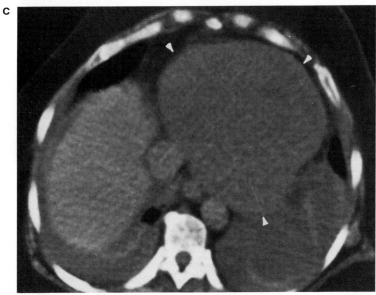

FIG. 36. A 65-year-old woman with lymphoma. **A:** CT image at level of right pulmonary artery (RPA) shows a halo of pericardial effusion (*arrowheads*) surrounding the great vessels; (AA) ascending aorta; (DA) descending aorta. Bilateral pleural effusions are present. **B:** CT image 7 cm caudad demonstrates a larger halo of pericardial effusion surrounding the left ventricle (LV). Bilateral lower-lobe consolidation, volume loss, and pleural effusions are present. **C:** CT image 3 cm below **B** shows a large collection of pericardial fluid (*arrowheads*) beneath the heart. Large pleural effusions are present.

gation to establish myocardial disease. In the past, thoracotomy was needed to diagnose the operable constrictive pericarditis from the untreatable restrictive cardiomyopathy.

CT is a useful technique to distinguish constrictive pericarditis from other forms of heart disease under appropriate clinical circumstances. The major CT feature of constrictive pericarditis is pericardial thickening (ranging from 0.5 to 2.0 cm), which is characteristically diffuse, but may not be uniform (Fig. 37) (52,74,77). Some of the areas of thickening may contain calcification. In addition, signs of systemic venous hypertension, e.g., dilated SVC and IVC, ascites, hepatomegaly, pleural effusions may be present. On postcontrast images, dilated right and left atria, with small, tubular ventricular chambers, may be seen, along with a straightened, hypertrophied ventricular septum.

Although CT is very sensitive in detecting abnormalities of the pericardium, it cannot provide hemodynamic information in most cases. Pericardial thickening may be found on CT images due to several causes, such as radiation, pericarditis, or trauma, without hemodynamic compromise. Hence, the presence of focal or diffuse pericardial thickening on CT should not be interpreted as evidence of constrictive pericarditis without clinical or CT signs of systemic venous hypertension.

Tumors

Primary pericardial tumors include mesothelioma, teratoma, and various sarcomas (Fig. 38) (75). All are likely to have varying amounts of pericardial effusion with nodular masses. Metastatic tumors are more common than primary neoplasms. Carcinoma of breast and lung and lymphoproliferative disorders account for more than 70%

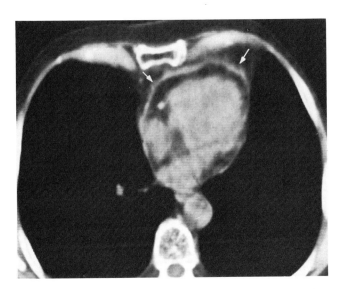

FIG. 37. A 77-year-old woman with clinical signs of constrictive pericarditis. The pericardium is irregularly thickened (*arrows*) over the anterolateral surface of the heart.

of pericardial metastases. As with primary tumors, the most common CT finding is pericardial effusion. Pericardial fluid often is not hemorrhagic in these cases, so that attenuation numbers may not be helpful (2). Metastases produce a locally or diffusely thickened pericardium (Fig. 39); large masses are infrequently seen (Fig. 40).

MRI

Pericardial effusions produce an increase in thickness of the pericardial line. Fluid collects mainly behind the left ventricle, but also behind the right atrium (82). Non-hemorrhagic effusions show low signal intensity; effusions with high protein or cell content may have focal areas of increased signal intensity corresponding to fibrinous material adherent to the pericardium (Fig. 41) (82). Hemopericardium shows medium and high signal intensities on MR images; the range of signal intensities reflects the thrombus and serum components of the hemopericardium (82).

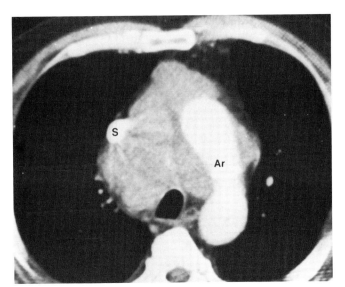

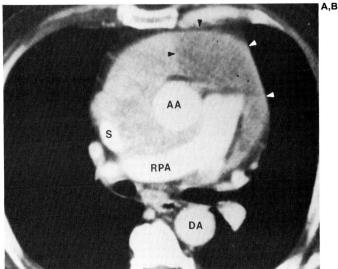

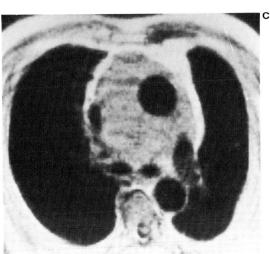

FIG. 38. A 67-year-old man with fibrosarcoma of the pericardium. **A:** CT image at level of the aortic arch (Ar) demonstrates soft-tissue mass infiltrating mediastinum and displacing superior vena cava laterally. **B:** CT image 4 cm caudad shows that mass is confined by pericardium and extends into the retroaortic recess. At this level, a loculated pericardial effusion (*arrowheads*) is also present; (AA) ascending aorta; (DA) descending aorta; (S) superior vena cava; (RPA) right pulmonary artery. **C:** Ungated transverse MRI (SE 500/30) at a level between **A** and **B** shows mediastinal vessels encased by pericardial tumor.

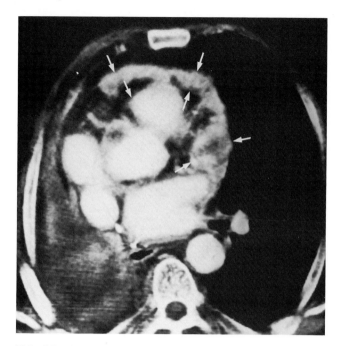

FIG. 39. Metastatic involvement of pericardium. Patient had prior right pneumonectomy for carcinoma of the lung. CT image at the level of the aortic root shows a nodular, thickened pericardium (*arrows*) surrounding the heart.

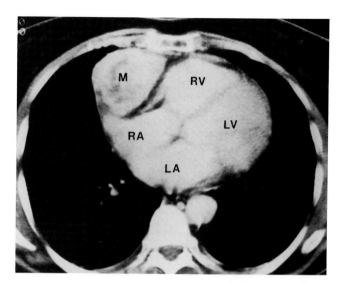

FIG. 40. A 30-year-old woman with metastatic fibrous histiocytoma. A preoperative chest radiograph showed an unsuspected mediastinal abnormality. CT image of the chest shows an intrapericardial mass (M) that is compressing the anterior wall of the right atrium (RA); (LA) left atrium; (RV) right ventricle; (LV) left ventricle.

Pericardial thickening can appear as low or medium signal intensities on MR images. Associated pericardial effusions (low signal intensity) can be distinguished from medium-intensity pericardial thickening. Differentiation of low-signal-intensity effusion from low-signal-intensity thickening or calcified pericardium relies on certain MRI findings: (a) an enlarged preaortic recess may be found in effusion, but not with thickening; (b) effusions typically collect dorsolateral to the left ventricle or right atrium; (c) only effusions change thickness during the cardiac cycle; (d) calcifications have irregular borders. MRI cannot distinguish between chronic pericardial thickening and calcification (Fig. 42) (82). As with CT, pericardial thickening alone does not indicate pericardial constriction.

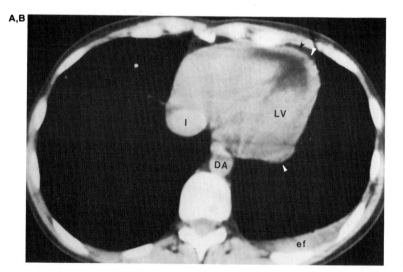
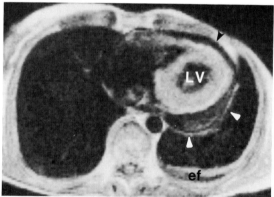

FIG. 41. A 60-year-old woman with malignant pericardial effusion and left pleural effusion from breast carcinoma. **A:** Non-contrast-enhanced CT image near cardiac apex shows pericardial effusion (*arrowheads*) loculated anterior and posterior to the left ventricle (LV). A left pleural effusion is present (ef); (I) inferior vena cava; (DA) descending aorta. **B:** Gated transverse MRI (TE = 30 msec) at same level as **A** shows low-intensity anterior and posterior pericardial effusion (*arrowheads*). The pericardial effusion posterior to the left ventricle (LV) has higher signal intensity, possibly due to gravitation of protein elements within the effusion. The pleural effusion (ef) is seen.

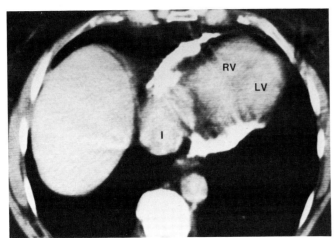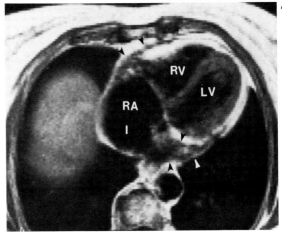

FIG. 42. A 64-year-old woman with calcific constrictive pericarditis. **A:** CT image at low ventricular level shows thick calcific pericardium anterior to the right ventricle (RV) and posterior to the left ventricle (LV). The inferior vena cava (I) is dilated. **B:** Gated transverse MRI (TE = 30 msec) at same level as **A** shows apparently "thickened" pericardium in locations corresponding to calcific pericardium on CT (*arrowheads*). The septum does not have its normal convex curve, but is straightened due to constrictive pericarditis. The inferior vena cava (I) is dilated; (RA) right atrium; (RV) right ventricle; (LV) left ventricle.

INDICATIONS FOR CARDIAC CT AND MRI

Both CT and MRI can provide anatomic and limited physiologic information in normal and diseased hearts. The superiority of CT and MRI in regard to spatial resolution has not yet overcome the ease of use, portability, and temporal resolution of two-dimensional echocardiography. Technical improvements in Cine CT and MRI are continually evolving. The recent introduction of Cine MR imaging, a technique that implies low flip angles and gradient refocused echoes, holds considerable promise in cardiac diagnosis. The current practical clinical applications of CT and MRI in heart disease include the following:

1. Loculated pericardial effusion (CT)
2. Differentiation between constrictive pericarditis and restrictive cardiomyopathy (CT)
3. Delineation of central pulmonary arteries in pulmonary atresia or pulmonic stenosis (MRI)
4. Evaluation of patency of palliative systemic–pulmonary-artery shunts (MRI)
5. Coarctation of aorta (MRI)
6. Hypertrophic cardiomyopathy (MRI)
7. Paracardiac masses (CT)
8. Intracardiac tumors (MRI)
9. Cardiac volumes and regurgitant fractions (MRI)

REFERENCES

1. Adams DF, Hessel SJ, Judy PF, Stein JA, Abrams HL. Computed tomography of the normal and infarcted myocardium. *Radiology* 1976;126:786–791.
2. Adenle AD, Edwards JE. Clinical and pathologic features of meta-static neoplasms of the pericardium. *Chest* 1982;81:166–169.
3. Albrechtsson U, Stahl E, Tylen U. Evaluation of coronary artery bypass graft patency with computed tomography. *J Comput Assist Tomogr* 1981;5:822–826.
4. Amparo EG, Higgins CB, Farmer D, Gamsu G, McNamara M. Gated MRI of cardiac and paracardiac masses: initial experience. *AJR* 1984;143:1151–1156.
5. Baim RS, MacDonald IL, Wise DJ, Lenkel SC. Computed tomography of absent left pericardium. *Radiology* 1980;135:127.
6. Bali C, Chomka EV, Fisher EA, Brundage BH. Ultra-fast computed tomography in congenital heart disease. *Circulation* 1985;72:28.
7. Baron RL, Gutierrez FR, Sagel SS, Levitt RG, McKnight RC. CT of anomalies of the mediastinal vessels. *AJR* 1981;137:571–576.
8. Bateman TM, Whiting JS, Forrester JS, et al. Noninvasive evaluation of aorto-coronary bypass grafts using cine CT. *JACC* 1986;7:154.
9. Behrenbeck T, Kinsey JH, Harris LD, Robb RA, Pitman EL. Three-dimensional spatial, density and temporal resolution of the dynamic spatial reconstructor. *J Comput Assist Tomogr* 1982;6:1138–1147.
10. Berdon WE, Baker DH, Wung JT, et al. Complete cartilage-ring tracheal stenosis associated with anomalous left pulmonary artery: the ring-sling complex. *Pediatr Radiol* 1984;152:57–63.
11. Brundage BH, Lipton MJ, Herfkens RJ, et al. Detection of patent coronary bypass grafts by computed tomography: a preliminary report. *Circulation* 1980;61:826–831.
12. Crooks LE, Barker B, Chang H, et al. Magnetic resonance imaging strategies for heart studies. *Radiology* 1984;153:459–465.
13. Daniel WG, Dohring W, Stender HS, Lichtlen PR. Value and limitations of computed tomography in assessing aortocoronary bypass graft patency. *Circulation* 1983;67:983–987.
14. DeMaria AN, Bommer W, Neumann A, et al. Left ventricular thrombi identified by cross-sectional echocardiography. *Ann Intern Med* 1979;90:14–18.
15. Didier D, Higgins CB. Estimation of pulmonary vascular resistance by MRI in patients with congenital cardiovascular shunt lesions. *AJR* 1986;146:919–924.
16. Didier D, Higgins CB, Fisher MR, Osaki L, Silverman NH, Cheitlin MD. Congenital heart disease: gated MR imaging in 72 patients. *Radiology* 1986;158:227–235.
17. Diethelm L, Dery R, Lipton MJ, Higgins CB. Atrial level shunts: sensitivity and specificity of MR in diagnosis. *Radiology* 1986;162:181–186.
18. Dinsmore RE, Wismer GL, Leurne RA, Ikada RD, Brady TJ. Magnetic resonance imaging of the heart: positioning and gradient angle selection for optimal imaging planes. *AJR* 1984;143:1135–1142.

19. Dinsmore RE, Wismer GL, Miller SW, et al. Magnetic resonance imaging of the heart using image planes oriented to cardiac axes: experience with 100 cases. *AJR* 1985;145:1177–1183.

20. Dinsmore RE, Wismer GL, Guyer D, et al. Magnetic resonance imaging of the interatrial septum and atrial septal defects. *AJR* 1985;145:697–703.

21. Dobell ARC, Jain AK. Catastrophic hemorrhage during redo sternotomy. *Ann Thorac Surg* 1984;37:273–278.

22. Dooms GC, Higgins CB. MR imaging of cardiac thrombi. *J Comput Assist Tomogr* 1986;10:415–420.

23. Edwards JE. Malformations of the pericardium. In: Gould SE, ed. *Pathology of the heart and great vessels,* 3rd ed. Springfield, Illinois: Charles C Thomas, 1968:376–378.

24. Farmer DW, Lipton MJ, Webb WR, Ringertz H, Higgins CB. Computed tomography in congenital heart disease. *J Comput Assist Tomogr* 1984;8:677–687.

25. Feiglin DH, George CR, MacIntyre WJ, et al. Gated cardiac magnetic resonance structural imaging: optimization by electronic axial rotation. *Radiology* 1985;154:129–132.

26. Fisher MR, Hricak H, Higgins CB. Magnetic resonance imaging of developmental venous anomalies. *AJR* 1985;145:705–709.

27. Fisher MR, Lipton MJ, Higgins CB. Magnetic resonance imaging and computed tomography in congenital heart disease. *Semin Roentgenol* 1985;20:272–282.

28. Fisher MR, McNamara MT, Higgins CB. Acute myocardial infarction: MR evaluation in 29 patients. *AJR* 1987;148:247–251.

29. Fletcher BD, Jacobstein MD. MRI of congenital abnormalities of the great arteries. *AJR* 1986;146:941–948.

30. Gerber KH, Higgins CB. Quantitation of size of myocardial infarctions by computerized transmission tomography: comparison with hot-spot and cold-spot radionuclide scans. *Invest Radiol* 1983;18:238–255.

31. Glazer HS, Aronberg DJ, Sagel SS. Pitfalls in CT recognition of mediastinal lymphadenopathy. *AJR* 1985;144:267–274.

32. Glazer HS, Gutierrez FR, Levitt RG, Lee JKT, Murphy WA. The thoracic aorta studied by MR imaging. *Radiology* 1985;157:149–155.

33. Godwin JD, ed. Intracardiac masses. In: *Computed tomography of the chest.* New York: JB Lippincott, 1984:316.

34. Godwin JD, ed. The thoracic aorta. In: *Computed tomography of the chest.* New York: JB Lippincott, 1984:332.

35. Godwin JD, Califf RM, Korobkin M, Moore AV, Vreiman RS, Kong Y. Clinical value of coronary bypass graft evaluation with CT. *AJR* 1983;140:649–655.

36. Godwin JD, Herfkins RJ, Brundage BH, Lipton MJ. Evaluation of coarctation of the aorta by computed tomography. *J Comput Assist Tomogr* 1981;5:153–156.

37. Godwin JD, Tarver RD. Scimitar syndrome: four new cases examined with CT. *Radiology* 1986;159:15–20.

38. Goldstein J, Lipton M, Schiller N, Ports T, Brundage B. Evaluation of left ventricular aneurysms with contrast enhanced computed tomography and two-dimensional echocardiography. *Clin Res* 1982;30:10A.

39. Greenwood WF. Profile of atrial myxoma. *Am J Cardiol* 1968;21:367–375.

40. Guthaner DF, Brody WR, Ricci M, Oyer PE, Wexler L. The use of computed tomography in the diagnosis of coronary artery bypass graft patency. *Cardiovasc Intervent Radiol* 1980;3:3–9.

41. Guthaner DF, Wexler L, Harell G. CT demonstration of cardiac structures. *AJR* 1979;133:75–81.

42. Hessel SJ, Adams DF, Judy PF, Fishbein MC, Abrams HL. Detection of myocardial ischemia in vitro by computed tomography. *Radiology* 1978;127:413–418.

43. Higgins CB. Computed tomography of the heart. *Radiology* 1981;140:525–526.

44. Moncada R, Baker M. Metastatic involvement of the pericardium. In: Higgins CB, ed. *CT of the heart and great vessels: experimental evaluation and clinical application.* New York: Futura Publishing, 1983:313.

45. Higgins CB, Byrd BF, Farmer DW, Osaki L, Silverman NH, Cheitlin MD. Magnetic resonance imaging in patients with congenital heart disease. *Circulation* 1984;70:851–860.

46. Higgins CB, Lanzer P, Stark D, et al. Imaging by nuclear magnetic resonance in patients with chronic ischemic heart disease. *Circulation* 1984;69:523–531.

47. Higgins CB, Stark D, McNamara M, Lanzer P, Crooks LE, Kaufman L. Multiplane magnetic resonance imaging of the heart and major vessels: studies in normal volunteers. *AJR* 1984;142:661–667.

48. Higgins CB, Byrd BF, McNamara MT, et al. Magnetic resonance imaging of the heart: a review of the experience in 172 subjects. *Radiology* 1985;155:671–679.

49. Higgins CB, Byrd BD, Stark D, et al. Magnetic resonance imaging in hypertrophic cardiomyopathy. *Am J Cardiol* 1985;55:1121–1125.

50. Higgins CB. Overview of the heart. *AJR* 1986;146:907–918.

51. Huggins TJ, Huggins MJ, Schnapf DJ, Brott WH, Sinnott RC, Shawl FA. Left atrial myxoma: computed tomography as a diagnostic modality. *J Comput Assist Tomogr* 1980;4:253–255.

52. Isner JM, Carter BL, Bankoff MS, et al. Differentiation of constrictive pericarditis from restrictive cardiomyopathy by computed tomographic imaging. *Am Heart J* 1983;105:1019–1025.

53. Jacobstein MD, Fletcher BD, Nelson AD, Goldstein S, Alfidi R, Riemenschneider TA. ECG-gated nuclear magnetic resonance imaging: appearance of the congenitally malformed heart. *Am Heart J* 1984;107:1014–1020.

54. Jacobstein MD, Fletcher DB, Nelson AD, Clampitt M, Alfidi RJ, Reimenschneider TA. Magnetic resonance imaging: evaluation of palliative systemic-pulmonary artery shunts. *Circulation* 1984;70:650–656.

55. Jacobstein MD, Fletcher BD, Goldstein S, Reimenschneider TA. Evaluation of atrioventricular septal defect by magnetic resonance imaging. *Am J Cardiol* 1985;55:1158–1161.

56. Johnson MA, Kirji MK, Hennig RC, Williams D. Pericardial abscess: diagnosis using two-dimensional echocardiography and CT. *Radiology* 1986;159:419–421.

57. Kahl FR, Wolfman NT, Watts LE. Evaluation of aortocoronary bypass graft status by computed tomography. *Am J Cardiol* 1981;48:304–310.

58. Katz ME, Glazer HS, Siegel MJ, Gutierrez F, Levitt RG, Lee JKT. Post-operative evaluation of mediastinal vessels by magnetic resonance imaging. *Radiology* 1986;161:647–651.

59. Kaul S, Wismer GL, Brady TJ, et al. Measurement of normal left ventricular heart dimensions using optimally oriented MR images. *AJR* 1986;146:75–79.

60. Lackner K, Thorn P. Computed tomography of the heart: ECG-gated and continuous scans. *Radiology* 1981;140:413–420.

61. Lanzer P, Barta C, Botvinick EH, Wiesendanger HUD, Modin G, Higgins CB. ECG-synchronized cardiac MR imaging: method and evaluation. *Radiology* 1985;155:681–686.

62. Levy-Ravetch M, Auh YH, Rubenstein WA, Whalen JP, Kazam E. CT of the pericardial recesses. *AJR* 1985;144:707–714.

63. Lieberman JM, Alfidi RJ, Nelson AD, et al. Gated magnetic resonance imaging of the normal and diseased heart. *Radiology* 1984;152:465–470.

64. Lipton MJ, Higgins CB. Evaluation of ischemic heart disease by computerized transmission tomography. *Radiol Clin North Am* 1980;18:557–576.

65. Lipton MJ, Farmer DW, Killebrew EJ, et al. Regional myocardial dysfunction: evaluation of patients with prior myocardial infarction with fast CT. *Radiology* 1985;157:735–740.

66. Lipton MJ, Higgins CB, Farmer D, Boyd DP. Cardiac imaging with a high-speed cine-CT scanner: preliminary results. *Radiology* 1984;152:579–582.

67. Lipton MJ, Higgins CB, Boyd DP. Computed tomography of the heart: evaluation of anatomy and function. *JACC* 1985;5:55S–69S.

68. McMurdo KK, Webb WR, von Schulthess GK, Gamsu G. MRI of the superior pericardial recesses. *AJR* 1985;145:985–988.

69. McNamara MT, Higgins CB, Schechtmann N, Botvinick E, Amparo EG, Chatterjee K. Detection and characterization of acute myocardial infarctions in man using gated magnetic resonance imaging. *Circulation* 1985;71:717–724.

70. McNamara MT, Higgins CB. Magnetic resonance imaging of chronic myocardial infarction in man. *AJR* 1986;146:315–320.

71. Mattrey RF, Slutsky RA, Long SA, Higgins CB. In vivo assessment of left ventricular wall and chamber dynamics during transient myocardial ischemia using prospectively ECG-gated computerized transmission tomography. *Circulation* 1983;67:1245–1251.

72. Miller DR, Reinig JW, Valkman DJ. Vascular imaging with MRI: inadequacy in Takayasu's arteritis compared with angiography. *AJR* 1986;146:949–954.

73. Moncada R, Salinas M, Churchill R, et al. Patency of saphenous

aortocoronary bypass grafts demonstrated by computed tomography. *N Engl J Med* 1980;303:503–505.

74. Moncada R, Baker M, Salinas M, et al. Diagnostic role of computed tomography in pericardial heart disease: congenital defects, thickening, neoplasms, and effusions. *Am Heart J* 1982;103:263–282.

75. Moncada R, Baliga K, Moguillansky SJ, et al. CT diagnosis of congenital intrapericardial masses. *J Comput Assist Tomogr* 1985;9:56–59.

76. Nath PH, Soto B. Computed tomography in assessing a high risk patient for "redo" sternotomy. *Circulation* 1985;72:182.

77. Reinmuller R, Doppman JL, Lissner J, Kemkes BM, Strauer BE. Constrictive pericardial disease: prognostic significance of a nonvisualized left ventricular wall. *Radiology* 1985;156:753–755.

78. Rholl KS, Levitt RG, Glazer HS, et al. Oblique magnetic resonance imaging of the cardiovascular system. *Radiographics* 1986;6:177–188.

79. Rumberger JA, Feiring AJ, Kiratzka LE, Reiter SJ, Stanford W, Marcus ML. Determination of changes in coronary bypass graft flow rate using cine-CT. *JACC* 1986;7:155.

80. Schultz CL, Morrison S, Bryan PJ. Azygos continuation of inferior vena cava: demonstration by NMR imaging. *J Comput Assist Tomogr* 1984;8:774–776.

81. Sechtem V, Tscholakoff D, Higgins CB. MRI of the normal pericardium. *AJR* 1986;147:239–244.

82. Sechtem V, Tscholakoff D, Higgins CB. MRI of the abnormal pericardium. *AJR* 1986;147:245–252.

83. Shimada E, Asano H, Kurasawa T, Matsumoto K, Yamane Y. Clinical study on left atrial thrombi: comparative study between echocardiography and CT scan (in Japanese). *J Cardiogr* 1981;11:933–944.

84. Silverman PM, Harell GS. Computed tomography of the normal pericardium. *Invest Radiol* 1983;18:141–144.

85. Silverman PM, Harell GS, Korobkin M. Computed tomography of the abnormal pericardium. *AJR* 1983;140:1125–1129.

86. Stark DD, Higgins CB, Lanzer P, et al. Magnetic resonance imaging of the pericardium: normal and pathologic findings. *Radiology* 1984;150:469–474.

87. Stone DN, Bein ME, Garris JB. Anomalous left pulmonary artery: two new adult cases. *AJR* 1980;135:1259–1263.

88. Stratemeier EJ, Thompson R, Brady TJ, et al. Ejection fraction determination by MR imaging: comparison with left ventricular angiography. *Radiology* 1986;158:775–777.

89. Tomoda H, Hoshiai M, Tagawa R, et al. Evaluation of left atrial thrombus with computed tomography. *Am Heart J* 1980;100:306–310.

90. Tomoda H, Hoshiai M, Furuya H, Shotsu A, Ootaki M, Matsuyama S. Evaluation of left ventricular thrombus with computed tomography. *Am J Cardiol* 1981;48:573–577.

91. Tsuchiya F, Kohno A, Saitoh R, Shigeta A. CT findings of atrial myxoma. *Radiology* 1984;151:139–144.

92. Ullyot DJ, Turley K, McKay CR, Brundage BH, Lipton MJ, Ebert PA. Assessment of saphenous vein graft patency by contrast-enhanced computed tomography. *J Thorac Cardiovasc Surg* 1982;83:512–518.

93. von Schulthess GK, Fisher M, Crooks LE, Higgins CB. Gated MR imaging of the heart: intracardiac signals in patients and healthy subjects. *Radiology* 1985;156:125–132.

94. von Schulthess GK, Higashino SM, Higgins SS, Didier D, Fisher MR, Higgins CB. Coarctation of the aorta: MR imaging. *Radiology* 1986;158:469–474.

95. Wittenberg J, Powell WJ, Dinsmore RE, Miller SW, Maturi RA. Computerized tomography in ischemic myocardium: quantitation of extent and severity of edema in an in vitro canine model. *Invest Radiol* 1977;12:215–223.

CHAPTER 11

Normal Abdominal and Pelvic Anatomy

Dennis M. Balfe, Roy R. Peterson, and Jerrold A. van Dyke

NORMAL ABDOMINAL ANATOMY

The basic science of anatomy has seen no major advances in the past century, but in the last decade our ability to image abdominal structures has been so radically improved that the radiologist has been forced to assimilate a wealth of detailed information related to transverse, sagittal, and coronal sectional images. Furthermore, in the last five years, we have witnessed the explosion of interventional techniques in the abdomen. As a result, anatomic details that were hitherto of little practical importance have become critical: The relationships of the celiac ganglia and the complex folding of the upper peritoneal spaces are but two examples.

Of primary importance is the ability to recognize a normal abdominal structure as normal; every radiologist has learned that the full range of normal variation must be completely grasped in order to confidently diagnose what is abnormal.

Most of the examples of normal anatomy will be displayed via transverse images, because, in most cases, transaxial sections provide the most easily understandable means to depict interorgan relationships. The internal structure of abdominal viscera will be briefly described; a more detailed discussion of the anatomy of each organ accompanies the chapter dealing with that specific system. Particular emphasis will be placed on those anatomic points that have practical applications to daily imaging procedures and to those regions in which pathologic processes are likely to occur. The experience recently acquired in magnetic resonance imaging (MRI) makes it clear that in specific areas, coronal or sagittal images are superior to transaxial sections in clarifying some anatomic details. Sagittal images are useful in tracing the course and configuration of the thoracic and abdominal aorta; coronal images may be useful in detecting masses in either renal pole. Moreover, sagittal and coronal planes add significant information regarding the relationships of the bladder and the genital structures in both males and females.

A brief and necessarily very general discussion of the comparative merits of computed tomography (CT) and MRI in displaying abdominal and pelvic anatomy may therefore be useful. CT images provide superb spatial resolution of anatomic structures. However, the separation between any two adjacent anatomic structures can be detected only if those structures differ appreciably in attenuation coefficient. Thus, contrast sensitivity is an important consideration when adjacent structures are to be resolved. Problems for CT occur when processes (such as tumors) with soft-tissue attenuation values abut normal structures that are also of soft-tissue density. MRI has appreciably better contrast sensitivity than CT, although its spatial resolution is generally somewhat worse (Fig. 1).

One factor greatly affecting the sharpness of an image is its acquisition time. CT images are acquired in a very short time interval, well within the breath-holding capabilities of most individuals. Many MRI sequences can also be obtained rapidly, but those sequences involving long repetition times may take several minutes to complete. Breathing, cardiac motion, and alimentary tract peristalsis produce motion unsharpness, with concomitant image degradation. These factors are most relevant to MRI of the upper abdomen and alimentary tract. The pelvis is relatively motionless, even over long time periods; accordingly, motion unsharpness is less a problem for pelvic imaging.

When two structures of similar attenuation values are separated from one another by a plane of different attenuation value, it is easy to distinguish the two structures as being separate. An obvious example is the separation of the bladder wall from the seminal vesicles by a plane of fat. Separation is optimized when the fat plane is perpendicular to the imaging plane. In the pelvis, however, fat planes often course obliquely or parallel to the transverse plane; in such cases, coronal or sagittal sections are advantageous. Unless special maneuvers are employed, CT images are always obtained in a transverse plane; MR images can be acquired in any plane desired, with no loss of resolution due to reformatting.

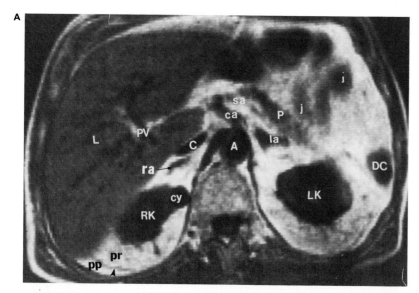

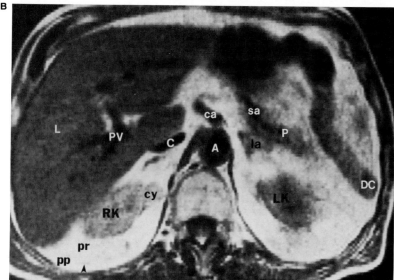

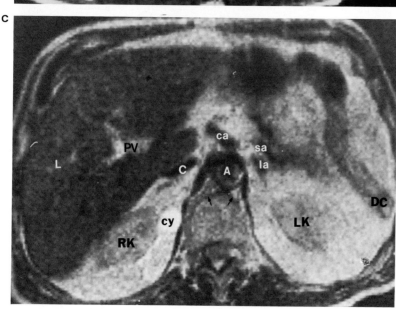

FIG. 1. MRI anatomy of the upper abdomen: effect of differing pulse sequences. **A:** Inversion-recovery sequence (TR = 1,500 msec, TE = 30 msec, TI = 400 msec). Generally, spatial resolution is poorer than that with CT. Respiratory and peristaltic motion each contribute to the image unsharpness. However, ready identification of the adrenals (la and ra) and separation of the left lateral limb of the adrenal from the adjacent pancreas (P) and splenic artery (sa) is possible. Previous renal obstruction has produced diminished intensity of the perirenal fat (pr) compared with the posterior pararenal fat (pp), allowing identification of the posterior renal fascia (*arrowhead*). Flowing blood in the aorta (A), inferior vena cava (C), and portal veins (PV) produces a signal void, allowing ready identification of these moderately large vascular structures. A small right renal cyst (cy) is also low in signal intensity on this sequence. **B:** Same anatomic section, spin-echo sequence (TR = 2,100 msec, TE = 35 msec). The image is predominantly a map of proton density, with a mixed T1 and T2 effect. Vascular structures, e.g., portal vein (PV), inferior vena cava (C), aorta (A), celiac axis (ca), and splenic artery (sa), are well seen, but the contrast differences between the perinephric (pr) and posterior pararenal fat (pp), between the renal cyst (cy) and renal parenchyma (RK), and between the left lateral adrenal (la) and adjacent pancreas (P) are visibly diminished. Note that the intensity of the renal cyst has increased relative to adjacent fat; (*arrowhead*) posterior renal fascia. **C:** Same anatomic section, spin-echo sequence (TR = 2,100 msec, TE = 90 msec). The image is strongly T2-weighted. Overall, the signal-to-noise ratio of this image is worse than that of **B**. The inferior vena cava (C) and celiac trunk (ca) have low signal intensities, but the aorta (A), retrocrural veins (*arrows*) and portal veins (PV) have increased signal intensities. The perirenal and posterior pararenal spaces cannot be distinguished at all, and the kidneys (RK and LK) are only slightly lower in intensity than the perinephric fat. The renal cyst (cy), however, has become hyperintense on this sequence; (sa) splenic artery; (DC) descending colon; (L) liver; (la) left adrenal.

The physical characteristic that produces the brightness of any CT pixel is the calculated linear attenuation coefficient for that volume of tissue. That coefficient varies only slightly with changes in beam energy within the range used for body imaging. The situation is quite different in MRI; the signal intensity that designates the brightness of any MRI pixel is a complex function heavily dependent on the sequence used to acquire it. Images obtained with short repetition and echo times contain predominantly T1 information: Fat is of high intensity; body fluids with high water content, such as urine, cerebrospinal fluid, and bile, are of low intensity; liver, spleen, and kidney parenchyma are intermediate. Images of the same structures obtained with very long repetition and echo times appear strikingly different and contain predominantly T2 information: Body fluids are of high intensity, muscle and liver of low intensity, and spleen, kidney, and fat of intermediate intensity. Therefore, the ability of any given image to resolve two structures may depend entirely on the sequence chosen.

Abdominal Contents

Body-Wall Muscles and Fascia

The body-wall musculature in the abdomen (Fig. 2) consists of the paired rectus abdominis muscles that occupy a paramedian position anteriorly. Three muscles make up the anterolateral surface: Listed from superficial to deep, they are the external oblique muscle, which arises from the external surface of the lower eight ribs, the internal oblique muscle, and the transverse abdominal muscle. The latter two muscles arise from the iliac crest and fascia to insert on the medial aspect of the lower three ribs. Posterolaterally, the latissimus dorsi muscle arises from the broad posterior surface of the iliac crest. Its lateral border forms an angle with the insertion of the external oblique, which the iliac crest converts into the lumbar triangle. Hernias may occur in this location (7). Most posteriorly lie the vertebral column, psoas muscles, and quadratus lumborum muscles.

The rectus sheath is formed chiefly by the aponeurosis of the internal oblique and transverse abdominal muscles. On sections obtained cephalic to a crescentic line (called the semicircular line), the transverse abdominal aponeurosis passes behind the rectus muscles; on sections caudal to the semicircular line, the aponeurosis passes in front. Therefore, a potential communication exists between the rectus sheath and the anterior extraperitoneal spaces of the lower abdomen and pelvis (5).

Diaphragm and Esophageal Hiatus

The diaphragm is a large, dome-shaped muscle that incompletely divides the thorax from the abdomen. Its fibers take origin from the sternum, from the medial surfaces of the lower ribs, and from the upper lumbar vertebral bodies. They insert on an aponeurosis, the central tendon, which is shaped like an inverted "V." The apex of the central tendon lies just anterior to the inferior vena cava; its limbs descend posterolaterally to enclose the vena cava on the right and pass anterior to the esophageal hiatus on the left. The appearance of the relatively short anterior fibers depends on body habitus. Normally, the central tendon lies 2 to 3 cm cephalic to the xiphoid process, so that cross-sectional images of the diaphragm show a thin soft-tissue stripe coursing roughly parallel to the anterior body wall (Fig. 5C). A more caudally positioned central tendon produces a confusing image (22). In this situation, anterior diaphragmatic fibers course anterior and lateral to their origin on costal cartilage and enclose abdominal fat, forming an arch anterior to the liver and heart (Fig. 3). This orientation produces fan-like soft-tissue stripes projecting from the base of the heart to the anterior body wall. If the central tendon and the xiphoid are at the same level, most of the anterior diaphragm will be imaged on a single slice and will appear as a very broad soft-tissue band (22).

In most patients, the lateral and posterior portions of the diaphragm are perpendicular to the plane of section and are thus seen as thin soft-tissue stripes separating lung from abdominal perivisceral fat. Suspended inspiration, particularly in a patient performing a Valsalva maneuver, allows the muscular slips of the diaphragm to relax and become folded near their rib insertions. They are then imaged as discrete, thick, sometimes nodular soft-tissue densities (Fig. 4).

The diaphragmatic crura, right and left, take origin from the anterolateral surface of the upper lumbar vertebral bodies. They unite anteriorly to form the median arcuate ligament surrounding the aorta immediately cephalic to the celiac trunk. The crura continue upward, the right crus dividing to enclose the esophagus within the esophageal hiatus.

The right crus is larger and originates lower than the left; it extends to the left of the midline, and it is the right crural fibers that divide to admit the esophagus. At the level of the esophageal hiatus, crural fibers extend almost directly anterior and the most anterior portion may have a bulbous or nodular configuration, simulating left gastric adenopathy (Fig. 6B). The smaller left crural fibers remain posterior at this level, in contact with the anterolateral surface of the descending aorta. The anterior portion of the right crus lies immediately posterior to the superior recess of the lesser sac and posterior aspects of the caudate

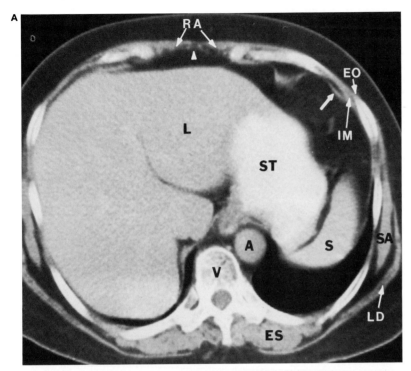

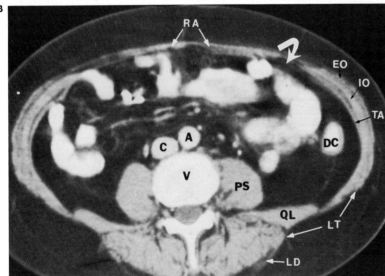

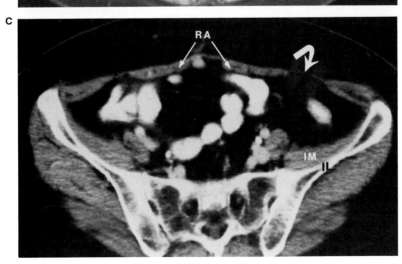

FIG. 2. Musculoskeletal structures forming the abdominal wall. **A:** Two centimeters below the xiphoid, the anterior surface of the body is composed of the rectus abdominis muscles (RA), joined at the linea alba (*arrowhead*). Laterally lie the external oblique (EO), ribs, and intercostal muscle (IM), deep to which is the diaphragm (*arrow*). Posterolaterally are the larger fibers of the serratus anterior (SA) and latissimus dorsi (LD) muscles. In a median location posteriorly is the vertebral body (V) and erector spinae muscles (ES). **B:** Seventeen centimeters caudal, in the middle abdomen, the rectus muscles (RA), atrophied in this patient, continue to occupy the midline. Anterolaterally, fat outlines the three major muscles of the anterior abdomen: external oblique (EO), internal oblique (IO), and transversus abdominis (TA). Posteriorly, there is separation of the thin aponeurotic fibers of the latissimus dorsi (LD) muscle from the posterior boundary of the external oblique. This gap is the lumbar triangle (LT); the quadratus lumborum muscles (QL) extend over a portion of this space, and hernias may occur through it. At this level, the most anterior fibers of the transverse abdominal muscle (*curved arrow*) pass posterior to the rectus muscle; (A) aorta; (C) inferior vena cava; (V) vertebral body; (PS) psoas muscle; (DC) descending colon. **C:** Eight centimeters caudal, the lower abdomen is supported by the broad iliac wings (IL) and iliacus muscles (IM). There is diastasis of the rectus muscles (RA). At this level (below the semilunar line) the thin aponeurotic fibers of the transverse abdominal muscle (*curved arrow*) pass anterior to the rectus muscle.

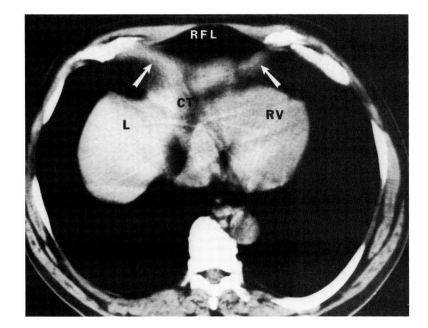

FIG. 3. Unusual appearance of the anterior diaphragm. In this patient, the xiphoid process lies cephalic to the central tendon of the diaphragm (CT). Accordingly, the anterior diaphragmatic fibers (*arrows*) course nearly parallel to the plane of axial section, producing thick soft-tissue stripes radiating outward toward the anterior ribs. They enclose abdominal fat lying in the root of the falciform ligament (RFL). This should not be confused with a herniation; (L) liver; (RV) right ventricle.

lobe. The posterior aspects of both crura lie against the pleural spaces.

The two crura enclose a retrocrural space (Fig. 5) anterior to the upper lumbar vertebral bodies (57). The major component of this space is the aorta, but the thoracic duct and azygos/hemiazygos veins also lie within it. This space connects the posterior mediastinum with the abdominal retroperitoneum; pathologic processes in this space are well contained on cephalic sections near the diaphragm, but below the median arcuate ligament may escape anteriorly into the space anterior to the great vessels. Caudal to the median arcuate ligament, the vertebral origins of the diaphragm are seen as fusiform soft-tissue densities lying on the lateral surface of the vertebral body anterior

to the psoas muscles. On more caudal sections, the right crus may be quite nodular in appearance, mimicking paraaortic adenopathy (Fig. 5F).

Gastroesophageal Junction

The distal esophagus is easily identified on CT sections as a round, soft-tissue-attenuation structure of 2 to 3 cm lying immediately anterior to the aorta. As it enters the abdomen, it curves anteriorly and to the left to enter the stomach (Fig. 6). Throughout its short abdominal course, it is fixed to the right crus by the phrenoesophageal ligament, a collagenous band of variable strength. The an-

FIG. 4. Nodular crura and diaphragmatic insertions. Image performed in inspiration shows nodularity of both crura (more marked on the left) (*arrows*) as well as "thickening" of an anterior diaphragmatic insertion (*arrowhead*) adjacent to the liver (L); (A) aorta; (S) spleen; (V) vertebral body.

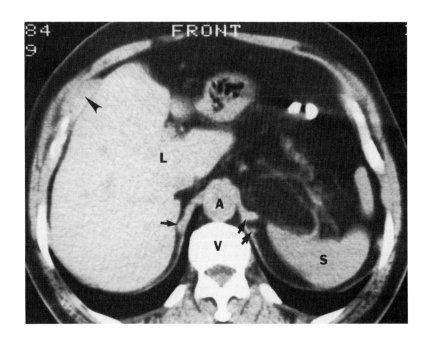

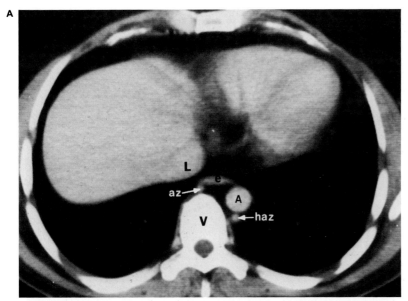

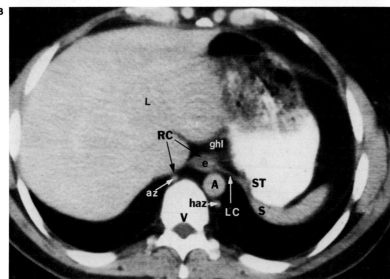

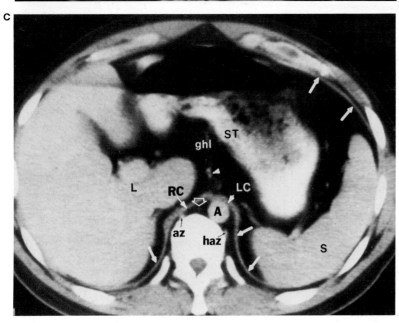

FIG. 5. Retrocrural space and crura. **A:** In the posterior mediastinum above the diaphragm are the aorta (A), azygos (az) and hemiazygos (haz) veins, and the esophagus (e). No crural fibers are present at this level. **B:** Three centimeters caudal, thin crural fibers are present (RC and LC), under which pass the aorta (A), and through which pass the esophagus (e). Immediately anterior and to the left of the right crus is the gastrohepatic ligament (ghl), which attaches the lesser curve of the stomach (ST) to the liver (L); (az) azygos vein; (haz) hemiazygos vein. **C:** Four centimeters caudal to the esophageal hiatus there is a well-defined retrocrural space, containing fat, the thoracic duct (*open arrow*), and the azygos (az) and hemiazygos (haz) veins. The anterior portion of the crura are closely applied to the aorta (A). Fat outlines many segments of the diaphragm (*arrows*) that course parallel to the body wall both anteriorly and posteriorly; (ghl) gastrohepatic ligament; (RC) right crus; (LC) left crus; (*arrowhead*) left gastric vessels; (S) spleen; (L) liver. Parts **D–F** on *facing page.*

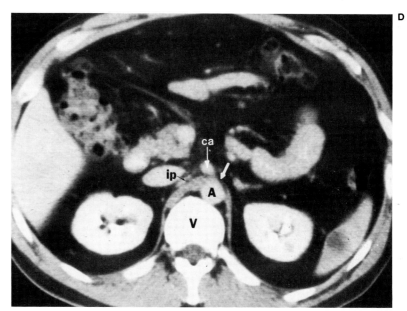

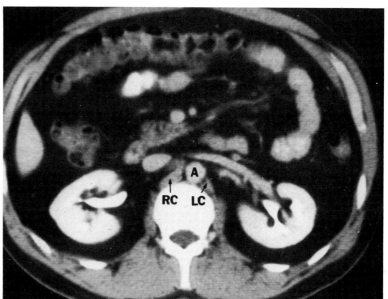

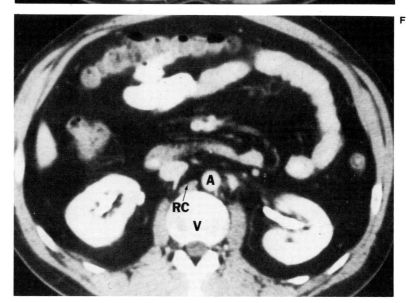

FIG. 5. (*Continued.*) Parts **A–C** on *facing page.* **D:** Four centimeters caudal, the crural fibers are separated by the celiac axis (ca), which emerges just caudal to the median arcuate ligament (*arrow*). The space enclosed by the crura becomes progressively smaller as sections proceed caudally; (A) aorta; (v) vertebral body; (ip) inferior phrenic artery arising from celiac axis. **E:** Three centimeters caudal, both right (RC) and left crura (LC) persist on either side of the aorta (A) as thick soft-tissue bands. **F:** One centimeter more caudal, only the right crural fibers (RC) are present on the anterolateral surface of the vertebral body (V). This should not be confused with an enlarged lymph node; (A) aorta.

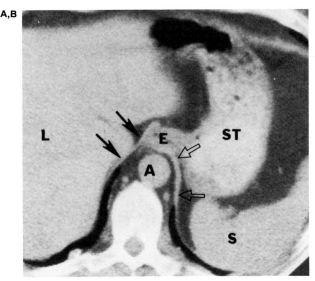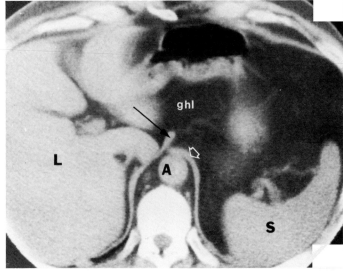

FIG. 6. The gastroesophageal junction. **A:** At the esophageal hiatus, the right crus (*arrows*) is anteriorly positioned, and the left crural fibers (*open arrows*) remain in apposition with the aorta (A). The abdominal portion of the esophagus (E) passes through the gap in the right crural fibers to join the stomach (ST). **B:** Two centimeters more caudal, most of the right crural fibers return to a position anterior to the aorta (A), but the anterior portion of the crus (*arrow*) is bulbous and remains relatively vertical in orientation. If its continuity with the rest of the right crus is not obvious, it may mimic a pathologic mass in the gastrohepatic ligament (ghl); (L) liver; (S) spleen; (*open arrow*) left crus.

terior and caudal margins of the abdominal esophagus are apposed to the lesser omentum and a portion of the superior recess of the lesser sac; perforations of the esophagus, particularly by longitudinally directed forces (as occur in endoscopy), can cause fluid collections within either space (1).

As the esophagus enters the stomach, both structures are relatively firmly tethered to the hepatic fissure for the ligamentum venosum by the gastrohepatic ligament. As a result of this fixation, a portion of the stomach wall runs in a transverse plane and therefore appears thicker than the rest of the stomach on transverse sections. This "pseudomass" has been noted in 25% to 30% of normal subjects (Fig. 7) (40,62). It is most apparent in patients with large left hepatic lobes.

The Alimentary Tract and Intramesenteric Viscera

The intraperitoneal contents of the abdomen derive from one of the following sources: the alimentary tube (foregut, midgut, and hindgut), its supporting mesentery, or the intramesenteric viscera that arise within the ventral or dorsal mesenteries, many of which are formed, at least in part, by diverticula from the foregut. A brief review of gastrointestinal embryogenesis serves as an introduction to the formation of adult anatomy. Although the peritoneal spaces molded by the complex rotation of abdominal viscera are not imaged on normal CT sections, they exert

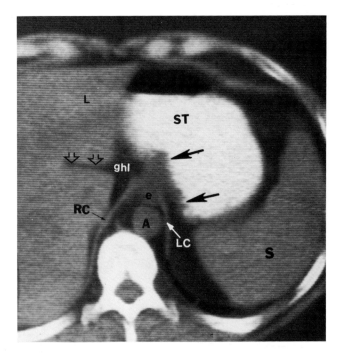

FIG. 7. Pseudomass in stomach. CT section through the stomach immediately caudal to the gastroesophageal junction shows an apparent mass (*arrows*) on the posterior gastric wall. At this level, the stomach (ST) is relatively well tethered to the liver (L) by the gastrohepatic ligament (ghl), which enters the fissure for the ligamentum venosum (*open arrows*); (A) aorta; (e) esophagus; (RC) right crus; (LC) left crus; (S) spleen.

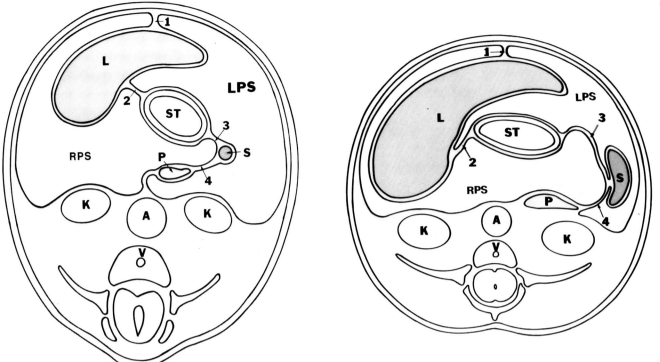

FIG. 8. Line drawings of the mesenteries attached to the stomach and the developing intramesenteric viscera. (Adapted from ref. 73.) **A:** Schematic drawing of a section obtained in an embryo, near the end of the fifth week of development. The stomach (ST) is supported by two major mesenteries, ventral and dorsal. Developing within the ventral mesentery, and distorting its surface, the liver (L) grows chiefly at the expense of the right peritoneal space (RPS). Maternal blood courses through the ventral part of the ventral mesentery, which thins to form the falciform ligament (1). The dorsal portion of the ventral mesentery (2) carries the left gastric artery and, more caudally, the hepatic artery, portal vein, and biliary duct within its leaves. It will become the lesser omentum. The primordial spleen (S) takes shape in the ventral part of the dorsal mesentery; the gastrosplenic ligament (3) formed thereby contains the short gastric vessels. While the head of the pancreas (P) arises in the dorsal mesoduodenum, its tail grows in a cephalic direction to occupy the dorsal mesogastrium within the splenorenal ligament (4); (A) aorta; (K) kidney; (V) vertebral body; (LPS) left peritoneal space. **B:** Approximately 1 week later, the rapid hepatic growth forces considerable rotation of the stomach (ST). Meanwhile, the pancreatic tail (P) has fused to the dorsal body wall, reducing the posteromedial extent of the left peritoneal cavity (LPS). This line of fusion generally continues along the splenorenal ligament to form a posteromedial splenic "bare" or nonperitonealized region. Occasionally, the peritoneal cavity can extend posterior to the pancreatic tail when fusion with the posterior abdominal wall is incomplete; (1) falciform ligament; (2) lesser omentum; (3) gastrosplenic ligament; (4) splenorenal ligament; (A) aorta; (K) kidney; (V) vertebral body; (L) liver; (S) spleen.

a profound effect on the distribution of pathologic fluid collections in the abdomen and will also be briefly described.

Embryology

Embryologically, the gut develops from the yolk sac; it is suspended from the anterior and posterior body walls by ventral and dorsal mesenteries, which separate to enclose the developing alimentary tube. Early in fetal life, important viscera develop within the mesentery of the caudal part of the foregut (79) (Fig. 8). The dorsal mesogastrium is the site for the developing spleen, whereas the liver expands within the ventral mesogastrium. The pancreas takes origin from foregut diverticula and grows

within the dorsal mesoduodenum. Major fetal arteries course anteriorly through the dorsal mesenteries from the aorta to supply the developing gut and intramesenteric structures. As the liver grows, the ventral mesogastrium thins greatly; the anterior part of it, which in the adult contains the obliterated umbilical vein (ligamentum teres), becomes the falciform ligament. On transaxial images performed in adults, the fat within this ligament has a triangular appearance and courses just deep to the rectus abdominis muscles from the umbilicus to the xiphoid (Fig. 16A). The fatty triangle is much smaller on cephalic than on caudal sections. Some of this fat accompanies the ligamentum teres as it enters the liver substance; this forms an incomplete separation between the lateral and medial segments of the left hepatic lobe (54).

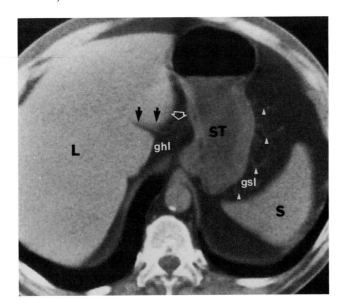

FIG. 9. Ligaments of the upper abdomen. Section through the gastroesophageal junction shows fat within the gastrohepatic ligament (ghl) extending between the fissure for the ligamentum venosum (*arrows*) and the lesser gastric curvature (ST). An accessory left hepatic artery (*open arrow*) is present. The gastrosplenic ligament (gsl) is marked by the short gastric vessels (*arrowheads*) and lies between the greater curvature of the stomach fundus and the visceral surface of the spleen (S); (L) liver.

The dorsal part of the ventral mesogastrium also thins appreciably to form the lesser omentum. In the adult, this structure, with its accompanying fat, stretches between the lesser gastric curvature and the slit-like fissure for the ligamentum venosum, forming a partial separation between the caudate lobe and the lateral segment of the left hepatic lobe. Within this gastrohepatic ligament are the left gastric artery and coronary vein and part of the celiac lymph node chain (8) (Fig. 9).

More caudally, the ventral mesoduodenum forms the remainder of the lesser omentum, the hepatoduodenal ligament (71). This structure encloses the portal vein, hepatic artery, common hepatic/common bile duct, and the hepatic group of celiac lymph nodes.

The spleen grows within the leaves of the dorsal mesogastrium, and there is similar thinning of its ventral and caudal portions. The ventral part of this mesentery, the gastrosplenic ligament, becomes greatly reduplicated by the growth of the lesser sac. On cephalic sections, the gastrosplenic ligament is short and relatively posterior; it transmits the short gastric vessels behind the inferior recess of the lesser sac. The elongated caudal portion of the gastrosplenic ligament fuses with the transverse colon to form the gastrocolic ligament and with the dorsal mesentery of the colon to become the definitive adult transverse mesocolon. The gastrocolic ligament (greater omentum) is easily recognized because of its abundant fat content. It lies on the anterolateral surface of the stomach and continues inferiorly anterior to the transverse colon. Within its leaves lie the gastroepiploic vessels (14).

The dorsal segment of the dorsal mesogastrium extends between the spleen and the posterior body wall; it encloses the tail of the pancreas, splenic artery, and the splenic vein within its leaves. In virtually all patients, this segment fuses with the posterior body wall to form the splenorenal ligament. Because of this fusion, the posteroinferior surface of the spleen (near the upper pole of the left kidney) is not peritonealized. This "bare area" limits the distribution of fluid in the perisplenic space (66) (Fig. 12).

Adult peritoneal spaces

Complex rotation and fusion of mesenteric structures alter the peritoneal anatomy; growth of intramesenteric viscera, particularly the liver, further distorts its appearance. A schematic overview of the distribution of peritoneal spaces in the adult is shown in Fig. 10.

The left peritoneal space in the adult can be divided into four compartments (all of which intercommunicate): two perihepatic spaces, anterior and posterior, and two subphrenic spaces, anterior and posterior. The anterior perihepatic space is limited on the right by the falciform ligament. The posterior perihepatic space (69) follows the undersurface of the lateral segment of the left hepatic lobe, extending deep within the fissure for the ligamentum venosum, where it reflects from the gastrohepatic ligament.

The left anterior subphrenic space is the continuation of the anterior perihepatic space (27). It courses over the gastric fundus just posterior to the diaphragm. Large collections can extend posterolaterally into the posterior subphrenic (or perisplenic) space (15,52). This space covers the superior and inferolateral surfaces of the spleen, but is limited medially by the gastrosplenic ligament, the fusion of which forms the splenic "bare area." Below the spleen, the phrenicocolic ligament separates the perisplenic space from the rest of the peritoneal cavity.

The right peritoneal space has two major divisions: the perihepatic space (51) and the lesser sac (omental bursa) (18,33,44). The right perihepatic space continues along the anterior and lateral surfaces of the right hepatic segments. It is limited on the left by the falciform ligament and reflects posteriorly near the diaphragm at the coronary ligament, which marks the lateral aspect of the large bare area of the liver (Figs. 11 and 12). On successively caudal images, the peritoneal recess extends more and more medially, then turns anterior to follow the visceral liver surface between the kidney and right posterior hepatic segment. This posterior recess is named "Morison's pouch." On images below the gallbladder fossa, the perihepatic space completely encircles the right hepatic segments.

The anatomy of the lesser sac attests to the complexity of embryologic rotation (18). It began, in the embryo, as a portion of the right peritoneal space just to the right of the lesser omentum (dorsal part of the ventral mesogas-

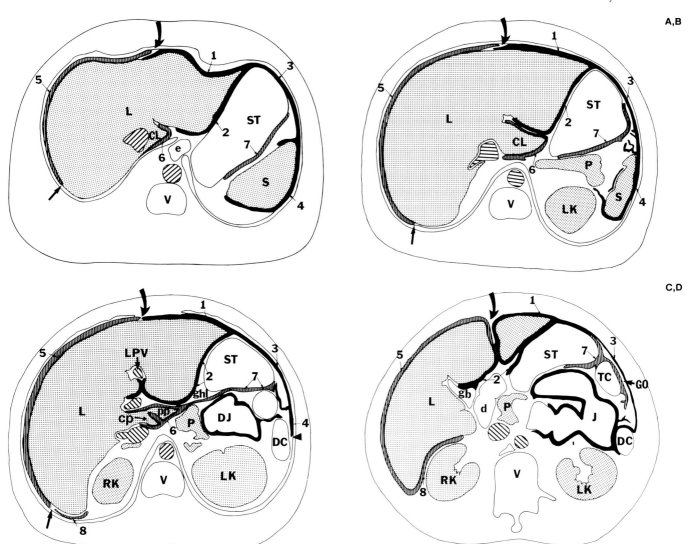

FIG. 10. Peritoneal spaces of the upper abdomen. On these schematic drawings, the left peritoneal spaces are drawn with heavy black lines, and the right peritoneal spaces have vertical hatching. **A:** Near the gastroesophageal junction, four divisions of the left peritoneal space are present. Anterior to the liver, medially limited by the falciform ligament (*curved arrow*), is the left anterior perihepatic space (1). Curving posterior to cover the visceral hepatic surface is the left posterior perihepatic space (2). The anterior subphrenic space (3) separates the gastric fundus (ST) from the diaphragm, while the posterior subphrenic (perisplenic) space (4) surrounds the spleen (S). The right peritoneal space consists of the perihepatic spaces and the lesser sac. The former has a diaphragmatic surface (5), limited on the left by the falciform ligament and posteromedially by the hepatic bare area (*arrow* marks the peritoneal reflection). The lesser sac has two components: The superior recess (6) surrounds the caudate lobe (CL) and is separated from the inferior recess (7) by the lesser omentum; (L) liver; (e) esophagus; (V) vertebral body. **B:** Two centimeters caudal, the superior recess of the lesser sac (6) surrounds the caudate lobe (CL) on three sides. The peritoneal reflection at the hepatic bare area (*arrow*) is more posterior and medial than on the previous section; (*curved arrow*) falciform ligament; (ST) stomach; (S) spleen; (P) pancreas; (LK) left kidney; (V) vertebral body; (L) liver. **C:** Two centimeters caudal, the posterior subphrenic (perisplenic) space (4) is limited inferiorly by the phrenicocolic ligament (*arrowhead*) formed at the proximal descending colon (DC). At this level, the posterior left perihepatic space (2) extends deep into the visceral surface of the liver, near the left portal vein (LPV). The superior recess of the lesser sac surrounds the papillary process (pp) and caudate process (cp). The cephalic portion of the visceral right perihepatic peritoneum (8) is limited laterally by the triangular ligament (*arrow*); (L) liver; (*curved arrow*) falciform ligament; (ST) stomach; (L) liver; (DJ) duodenojejunal flexure; (P) pancreas; (RK) right kidney; (LK) left kidney; (V) vertebral body. **D:** Four centimeters more caudal, the left posterior perihepatic space (2) contacts the anterior wall of the gallbladder (gb). The inferior recess of the lesser sac (7) extends into the leaves of the greater omentum (GO), which forms a drape over the distal transverse colon (TC); (L) liver; (*curved arrow*) falciform ligament; (RK) right kidney; (LK) left kidney; (V) vertebral body; (J) jejunum; (ST) stomach; (d) duodenum; (DC) descending colon.

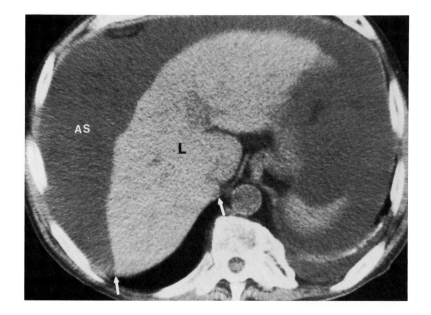

FIG. 11. The bare area of the liver. Embryologic fusion between the posterior liver surface (L) and the right hemidiaphragm produces a large non-peritonealized surface (*arrows*). Ascites (AS) cannot extend medial to the peritoneal reflection and thus outlines the bare area in this patient.

FIG. 12. Triangular ligament. In this patient with malignant ascites, the cephalic portion of the right perihepatic peritoneal space (5) is distended, as is the right subdiaphragmatic peritoneum (8). Outlined between these spaces is the triangular ligament (*open arrow*). Note also that the ascitic collection is limited medially on the left by the bare area of the spleen (*arrowheads*), a feature consistently observed on the posteromedial splenic boundary at the level of the anterior renal fascia; (*closed arrow*) falciform ligament; (1) left anterior perihepatic space; (3) left anterior subphrenic space; (4) perisplenic space; (7) inferior recess of lesser sac; (6) superior recess of lesser sac.

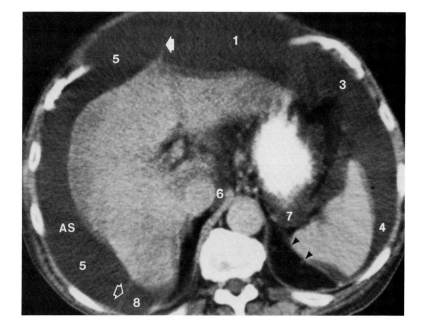

trium). As the liver grows and rotates into the right peritoneal space, the stomach also undergoes counterclockwise rotation, so that this bit of peritoneal cavity lies posterior to the lesser omentum and extends behind the stomach. As a result of this extension, the ventral part of the dorsal mesogastrium (gastrosplenic ligament) is stretched, and the right peritoneal space extends between its reduplicated folds. This space later fuses when the adult greater omentum is formed.

In the adult, two major recesses are present (Fig. 13C–E). The superior recess completely encloses the medial surface of the caudate lobe. At the porta hepatis, the superior recess lies just posterior to the portal vein; on more cephalic sections, it lies immediately behind the lesser

FIG. 13. Peritoneal spaces of the upper abdomen: MRI demonstration. Parts **A–C** on *facing page*. **A:** Transverse section through the upper abdomen shows low-intensity ascites (AS) filling the right perihepatic space (5), which continues along the falciform ligament (*curved arrow*) into the liver surface (L). The greater omentum (gastrocolic ligament) (gcl) floats in the ascites within the left anterior (1) and posterior (2) perihepatic space. There is a small quantity of fluid in the anterior (3) and posterior (4) subphrenic space as well as in the inferior recess of the lesser sac (7); (tm) transverse mesocolon; (TC) transverse colon; (S) spleen; (gsl) gastrosplenic ligament; (ghl) gastrohepatic ligament. **B:** Sagittal section obtained through the lateral margin of the right hepatic lobe shows the bare area (*arrows*) attached to the posterior boundary of the liver. The perihepatic space (5) encircles the liver and is continuous with the posterior hepatorenal recess (8) (Morison's pouch). **C:** Two centimeters to the left, fluid in the superior recess of the lesser sac (6) is separated from left perihepatic ascites (2) by the hepatoduodenal ligament (hdl) (*arrow*), which encompasses the portal vein (pv) and hepatic artery. Note that the caudate lobe (CL) is bathed in the superior portion of the lesser sac collection; (d) duodenum. Figures and legends for parts **D–E** on *facing page*.

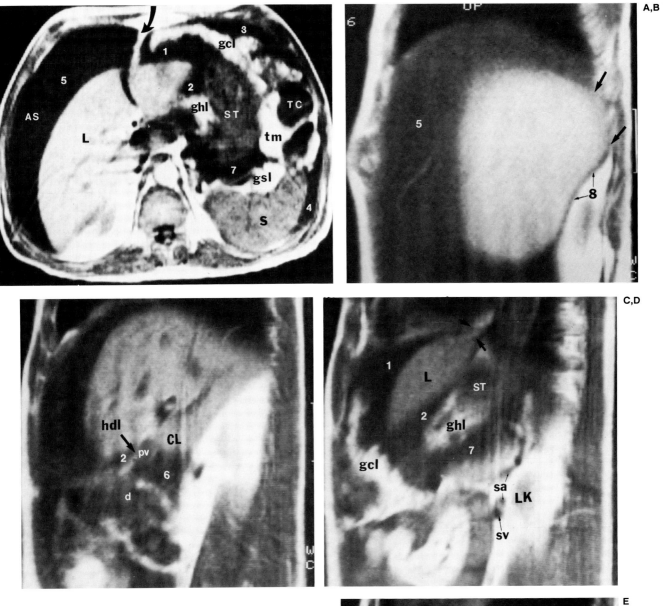

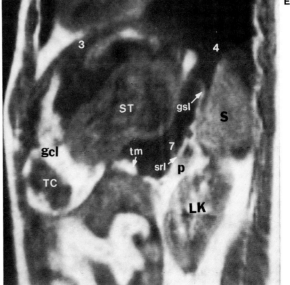

FIG. 13. Legend for Parts **A–C** on *facing page.* **D:** Six centimeters to the left, the left side of the liver's bare area (or left coronary ligament) (*arrows*) suspends the left lateral hepatic segment from above. Fluid in the posterior portion of the left perihepatic space (2) is separated from the inferior recess of the lesser sac (7) by the stomach (ST) and gastrohepatic ligament (ghl). The latter contains segments of the left gastric artery and vein; (1) left anterior perihepatic space; (gcl) gastrocolic ligament; (LK) left kidney; (sa) splenic artery; (sv) splenic vein. **E:** Four centimeters to the left, the boundaries of the lesser sac (7) are easily appreciated: superiorly and posterosuperiorly is the thin gastrosplenic ligament (gsl), superior to which lies the left posterior subphrenic space (4); posteriorly and posteroinferiorly the splenic vessels and pancreas (p) within the splenorenal ligament (srl); inferiorly, the root of the transverse mesocolon (tm); anteriorly, the posterior wall of the stomach (ST). There is potential communication of this part of the lesser sac anteriorly into the greater omentum (gcl), which floats in the anterior subphrenic space (3) in this patient; (S) spleen; (LK) left kidney; (TC) transverse colon.

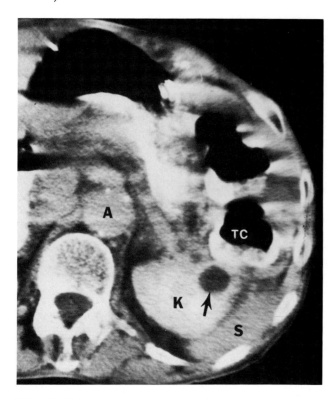

FIG. 14. Retrorenal spleen. The peritoneal space extends posteriorly in this individual, so that the intraperitoneal spleen (S) lies in a retrorenal location. Since the descending colon lies in the retroperitoneum immediately caudal to the splenic tip, it may also lie in a retrorenal site. This variation in normal anatomy presents an obvious hazard if percutaneous catheter manipulation is attempted; (K) kidney; (A) aorta; (TC) distal transverse colon. Incidentally noted is a renal cyst (*arrow*).

omentum deep within the fissure for the ligamentum venosum and follows the caudate lobe surface posteriorly and to the right, extending almost to the inferior vena cava. Near the diaphragm, the posterior part of this space lies adjacent to the right diaphragmatic crus. The inferior recess of the lesser sac lies between the stomach and the visceral surface of the spleen; on lower sections, it separates the stomach from the pancreas and the transverse mesocolon (24,45). Part of this space may potentially extend between the leaves of the greater omentum.

Posterior recesses of the peritoneum

The precise distribution of the most posterior recesses of the peritoneal spaces depends on the completeness of fusion between the dorsal mesenteries and the posterior abdominal retroperitoneum. When fusion is incomplete, peritoneum may extend posterior to the renal margin on either side (38). Because mobile structures in the peritoneal cavity can inhabit any portion of the peritoneal space, it is possible for the colon (29,56) or spleen (Fig. 14) to lie in a retrorenal position. Clearly, this variation may be a considerable hazard to patients undergoing percutaneous renal procedures.

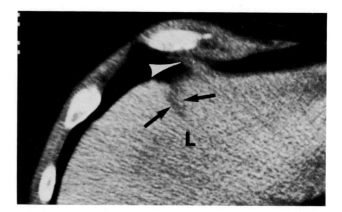

FIG. 15. Accessory hepatic fissure. Image through the dome of the liver shows a narrow fatty cleft (*arrows*) invaginating the anterior hepatic surface near a diaphragmatic insertion (*arrowhead*). This is a typical location for an accessory fissure; (L) liver.

Adult anatomy of the gut and intramesenteric viscera

Liver and Gallbladder.   The liver is the largest abdominal organ. It forms within the ventral mesogastrium and grows rapidly, so that its cephalic margin grows within the septum transversum. In the adult, that connection to the developing diaphragm is reflected by the presence of the bare area of the liver, a large posterior nonperitonealized surface over which the liver is inseparable from the diaphragm. The inferior vena cava (IVC) is recognized on sections near the dome of the liver, and it receives three major hepatic veins. These veins define the location of the planes dividing the major hepatic segments—the central vein runs in the course of the interlobar fissure (see Fig. 6 in Chapter 15) (9,21,46). The liver presents a large, smooth diaphragmatic surface; in some individuals, the smooth diaphragmatic surface may be indented by incomplete accessory fissures (6) (Fig. 15). The visceral surface of the liver is related to the lesser curve of the stomach on the left, to the pancreas and duodenum posteriorly near the midline, and to the right kidney and adrenal posteriorly on the right (Fig. 16). Immediately

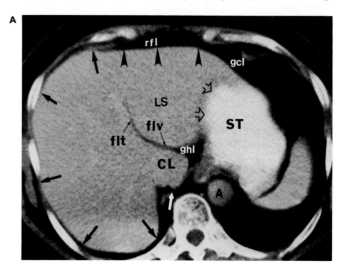

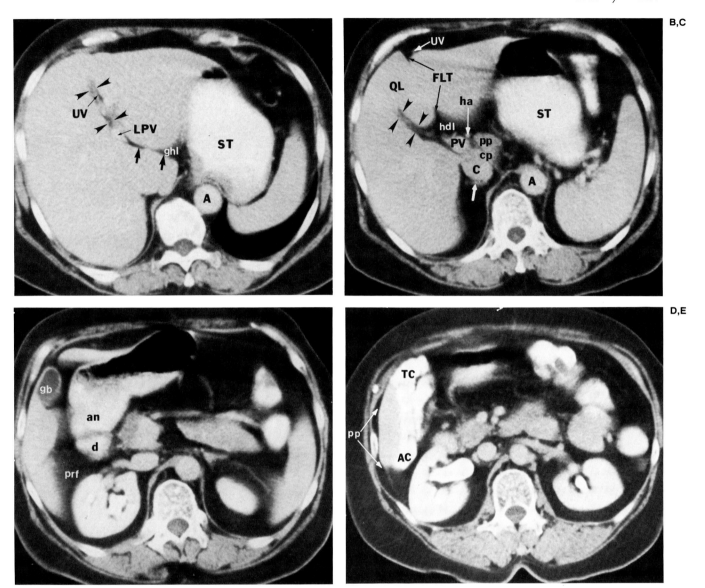

FIG. 16. Fissures and relationships of the liver. **A:** (Part **A** on *facing page.*) Image through the upper portion of the liver shows the smooth diaphragmatic surface (*arrows*) contacting the right hemidiaphragm over nearly a 180° arc. On the left anteriorly, the liver surface (*arrowheads*) is related to fat in the root of the falciform ligament (rfl) and in the greater omentum (gcl). The visceral surface of the liver (*open arrows*) is related to the stomach (ST) anteriorly; posteriorly, its contour is interrupted by the fissure for the ligamentum venosum (flv) dividing the caudate lobe (CL) from the left lateral segment (LS). On this section it intersects the deepest margin of the fissure for the ligamentum teres (flt). More posteriorly, the caudate lobe is related to the right diaphragmatic crus (*white arrow*); (A) aorta; (ghl) gastrohepatic ligament. **B:** One centimeter caudal, the deep portion of the fissure for the ligamentum teres (*arrowheads*), containing the fibrous umbilical vein remnant (UV), ends at the margin of the left main portal vein (LPV); (*arrows*) fissure for the ligamentum venosum; (ghl) gastrohepatic ligament; (ST) stomach; (A) aorta. **C:** Two centimeters caudal, the caudate lobe divides into an anterior papillary process (pp) and a posterior caudate process (cp); the latter lies between the inferior vena cava (C) posteriorly and the portal vein (PV) anteriorly. At this level, the separation between the caudate lobe and the lateral segment of the left lobe has widened to form the porta hepatis (hepatoduodenal ligament) (hdl), within which courses the hepatic artery (ha), portal vein (not visible), and common hepatic duct. Another fatty fissure has appeared to the right of the fissure for the ligamentum teres (FLT); it is the true interlobar fissure (*arrowheads*), and on sections obtained caudally, it opens inferiorly to enclose the gallbladder fossa. The quadrate lobe (QL) (medial segment of the left hepatic lobe) is the parenchyma between the interlobar fissure and the fissure for the ligamentum teres. Farthest posteriorly, the visceral surface of the liver contacts the perirenal fat and right adrenal gland (*white arrow*); (UV) fibrous umbilical vein; (ST) stomach; (A) aorta. **D:** Three centimeters caudal, the posterior visceral surface of the liver contacts the perirenal fat (prf) and the gastric antrum (an) immediately posterior to the gallbladder (gb); (d) duodenum. **E:** Three centimeters caudal, the right lobe's visceral surface is related to the ascending colon (AC) and proximal transverse colon (TC) at the hepatic flexure. The posterior pararenal space (pp) lies posterolateral to the liver at this level.

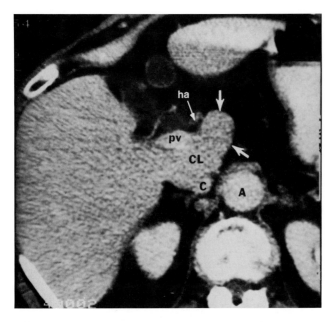

FIG. 17. Papillary process. An unusually large papillary process (*arrows*) extends anteromedially from the cuadate lobe (CL), mimicking a mass in the left gastric nodal distribution; (A) aorta; (C) inferior vena cava; (pv) portal vein; (ha) hepatic artery.

lateral to the duodenal bulb, aligned in the plane of the interlobar fissure, lies the fossa for the gallbladder. Sections caudal to this level show the gallbladder fundus progressively more to the right and anterior. Medial to the anterior part of the right hepatic lobe is the proximal transverse colon, which derives its name ("hepatic flexure") from this proximity. The posteroinferior part of the right lobe extends caudally just lateral to the ascending colon.

In some patients, a portion of the caudate lobe (the papillary process) may extend between the lesser gastric curve and the portal vein, in a position usually occupied by gastrohepatic lymph nodes. Serial images will document its attachment to the rest of the caudate lobe (3) (Fig. 17). Another inconstant portion of the caudate lobe, the caudate process, extends caudally between the IVC and portal vein.

Biliary Anatomy. Intrahepatic bile ducts follow a branching pattern virtually identical with that of the portal veins. On contrast-enhanced images, dilated bile ducts can be observed as water-attenuation structures usually lying immediately anterior to the opacified portal vein. Variations in biliary anatomy are common, and on any section a bile duct may normally lie posterior to its accompanying portal vein. As sections proceed caudally to

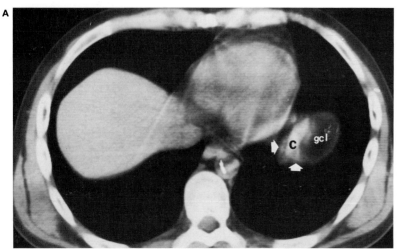

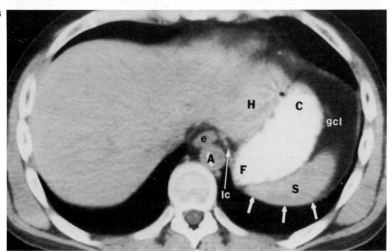

FIG. 18. Anatomic relationships of the normal stomach and spleen. **A:** The gastric cardia (C) is related to the medial portion of the left diaphragmatic dome (*arrows*). Laterally, it is abutted by fat in the greater omentum (gcl). **B:** One centimeter caudal, the fundus (F) is apposed to the crus (lc) of the left hemidiaphragm and heart (H) and spleen (S); the posterior margin of the spleen contacts the diaphragm over a wide arc (*arrows*). Omental fat (gcl) persists laterally and also inferiorly; (A) aorta; (e) esophagus; (C) gastric cardia. Parts **C–E** on *facing page*.

include the hepatoduodenal ligament, the intrahepatic segments join to form the common hepatic duct; this junction usually is just anterior to the confluence of the right portal vein with the main portal vein. Throughout the hepatoduodenal ligament, the bile duct occupies a position anterior and lateral to the portal vein. In many individuals, the cystic duct can be traced from the gallbladder neck to its point of insertion into the common duct. Usually, the cystic duct courses posterior to the common hepatic duct for a variable distance. On images obtained caudal to the hepatoduodenal ligament, the bile duct courses medially and posteriorly to a position on the posterolateral surface of the pancreatic head. At the ampulla of Vater, there may be slight dilatation of the normal common bile duct, just before it turns to the right to enter the duodenal papilla.

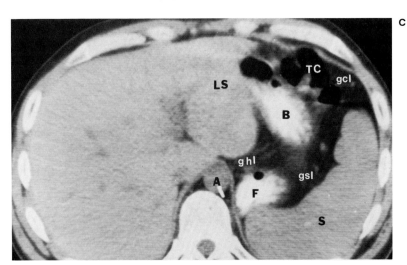

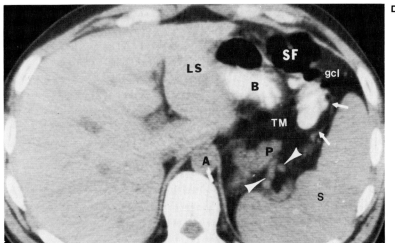

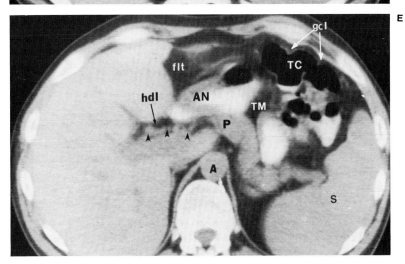

FIG. 18. (Continued.) Parts **A** and **B** on facing page. **C:** Three centimeters more caudal, at the incisura angularis, the gastric fundus (F) continues anteriorly lateral to the gastrohepatic ligament (ghl) to become the gastric body (B), which courses medial to the distal transverse colon (TC). The stomach and spleen (S) remain tethered by the gastrosplenic ligament (gsl), through which course the short gastric arteries and veins; (LS) left lateral hepatic segment; (gcl) gastrocolic ligament; (A) aorta. **D:** One centimeter caudal lie the pancreatic tail (P) and hilar splenic vessels (*arrowheads*), which are separated from the gastric body (B) by the root of the transverse mesocolon (TM) supporting the splenic flexure (SF). The left gastroepiploic vessels (*arrows*) arise from the splenic hilus and pass anteriorly to enter the greater omentum (gcl); (LS) left lateral hepatic segment; (A) aorta. **E:** Two centimeters more caudal, the gastric antrum (AN) courses anterior to the pancreas (P) and hepatic vessels (*arrowheads*) within the porta hepatis (hdl). The tail of the pancreas marks the course of the splenorenal ligament. The distal transverse colon (TC) posterior to its drape of omentum (gcl) courses toward its junction with the descending colon, which lies just caudal to the anterior tip of the spleen; (flt) fissure for the ligamentum teres; (TM) transverse mesocolon; (A) aorta.

A,B

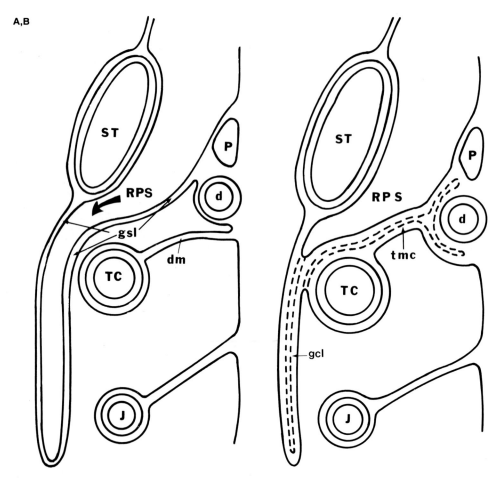

FIG. 19. Formation of the gastrocolic ligament. (Adapted from ref. 73.) **A:** Schematic drawing of a sagittal section through a developing embryo. Growth of the right peritoneal space (RPS) behind the stomach (ST) has greatly elongated the gastrosplenic ligament (GSL), so that it hangs like a drape over the transverse colon (TC) and its attached dorsal mesentery (dm); (p) pancreas; (d) duodenum; (J) jejunum. **B:** Fusion occurs between anterior and posterior surfaces of the gastrosplenic ligament, obliterating part of the right peritoneal space (RPS) and forming the gastrocolic ligament (gcl). The posterior surface of the fused ligament in turn fuses to the transverse colon (TC) and its dorsal mesentery to form the adult transverse mesocolon (tmc); (P) pancreas; (d) duodenum; (J) jejunum; (ST) stomach.

Stomach. The stomach (Fig. 18) has a diaphragmatic surface related to the dome and anterolateral portion of the left hemidiaphragm. Its lesser curvature is, in nearly all patients, related to the lateral segment of the left hepatic lobe. The greater omentum is attached to the posterolateral surface of the greater curvature; this structure becomes larger and more anterior in location as images proceed caudally. It can be identified by the presence of gastroepiploic vessels within its fat. Posteriorly, the greater curve of the stomach is separated from the spleen by the lesser sac; on more caudal images, the lesser sac separates it from the pancreas and transverse mesocolon. The junction of the antrum with the duodenum reliably occurs posterior to the left hepatic lobe; its position is marked by the increased thickness of the pyloric musculature as well as by the proximity of the gastroduodenal artery on the anterolateral surface of the pancreas.

Spleen. The spleen (Fig. 18) presents a diaphragmatic surface that lies against the lateral and posterolateral por-

tions of the left hemidiaphragm, separated from it by the perisplenic space. Its posterior surface may also lie against the diaphragm; in some individuals, the most cephalic portion of the left perirenal space is found between the spleen and the diaphragm. The anteromedial surface of the spleen faces the stomach, to which it is connected via the gastrosplenic ligament, containing the short gastric vessels. On more caudal images, the splenic artery and vein enter the hilus behind the pancreatic tail. At this level or slightly more caudal, the anterior tip of the spleen is related to the beginning of the descending colon.

Transverse Colon. The transverse mesocolon results from a complex fusion: Its anterior leaf is derived from the posterior portion of the redundant gastrosplenic ligament. Thus, the lesser sac is immediately anterior to the mesocolon (Fig. 19). The remainder of the mesocolon forms from the dorsal mesentery of the distal midgut. The artery to the transverse colon, the middle colic artery, arises as the first branch of the superior mesenteric artery.

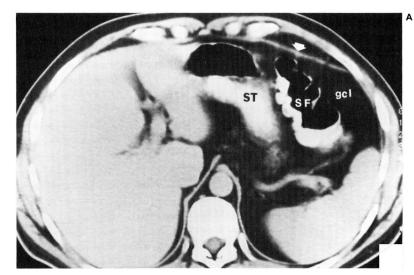

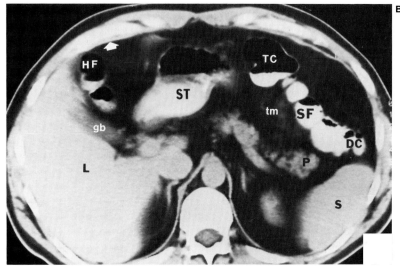

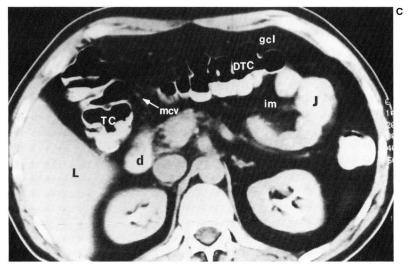

FIG. 20. Relationships of the transverse colon. **A:** The splenic flexure (SF) passes just lateral to the gastric body (ST) and immediately posterior to the anterior left hemidiaphragm (*arrow*). The abundant fat on its lateral surface is in the greater omentum (gcl). **B:** Two centimeters caudal, the distal part of the hepatic flexure (HF) passes anteromedial to the gallbladder (gb) and lies just posterior to the diaphragm (*arrow*). Here, the contrast-filled stomach (ST) lies just anterior to the root of the transverse mesocolon (tm), in which runs the vascular supply to the transverse colon (TC). On the left, the descending loop of the splenic flexure (SF) fuses to the retroperitoneum to form the origin of the descending colon (DC) anterior to the spleen (S) and just medial to the left diaphragm, to which it is attached by the phrenicocolic ligament. In its descent, it passes close to the tail of the pancreas (P); (L) liver. **C:** Three centimeters caudal, adjacent to the visceral surface of the liver (L), the proximal transverse colon (TC) at the hepatic flexure turns anterior, passing just lateral to the duodenum (d). Middle colic vessels (mcv) are evident medial to the hepatic flexure. A more distal portion of the transverse colon (DTC) is also present on this section; the fat anterior to it is in the greater omentum (gcl). On the left, the colon contacts a loop of jejunum (J) and lies anterior to fat in the small intestinal mesentery (im).

It enters the mesocolon immediately anterior to the gastroduodenal artery just caudal to the gastric antrum, then courses to the right and left to supply the entire transverse colon. The mesocolon can be recognized on CT by its position posterior to the transverse colon and by its middle colic vessels. There are important attachments of the transverse colon as it passes from right to left (Fig. 20): The right colic flexure begins as the ascending colon passes

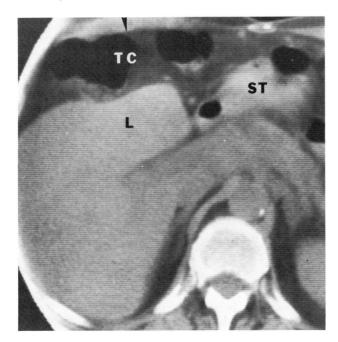

FIG. 21. Colonic interposition (Chiladiti's syndrome). The transverse colon (TC) occupies a position directly anterior to the liver (L) and posterior to the diaphragm (*arrowhead*); (ST) stomach.

anteriorly immediately lateral to the transverse duodenum. As it proceeds more anteriorly, it is attached to the medial part of the gallbladder by the hepatocolic ligament. Throughout its mesenteric course, the transverse colon is in contact with the greater omentum, which drapes over its anterior surface. In some individuals, the right side of the transverse colon lies interposed between the anterior surface of the liver and the right hemidiaphragm (Fig. 21). In fact, the mesenteric portion of the colon can occupy any portion of the upper abdominal peritoneal space (Fig. 22). On the left, the colon reenters the retroperitoneum, passing posteriorly and cephalad. In this part of its course, it passes behind the greater curvature of the stomach and caudal to the anterior splenic tip. As it passes into the retroperitoneum, it is fixed to the left hemidiaphragm by the phrenicocolic ligament.

Small Intestine. The small-bowel mesentery winds from the duodenojejunal flexure in the left upper abdomen to the ileocecal valve in the right lower abdomen. Into the root of this mesentery (Fig. 23) runs the superior mesenteric artery, which emerges from the periaortic fat at the same level as, or immediately caudal to, the pancreatic body and continues inferiorly, anterior to the duodenum, giving off leftward branches to jejunal segments. The artery then continues to the right and anteriorly as the ileocolic branch.

While the mesenteric root is relatively short, the coils of attached small bowel fill the majority of the middle abdomen and false pelvis. Normal mesentery contains fat, small lymph nodes, and segmental vessels that can be identified by CT. When adequately distended by oral contrast material, the normal jejunum has an almost imperceptible wall, but thin transverse stripes (representing plica circularis) are often seen. These stripes are almost never observed within the normal ileum (32) (Fig. 24).

A,B

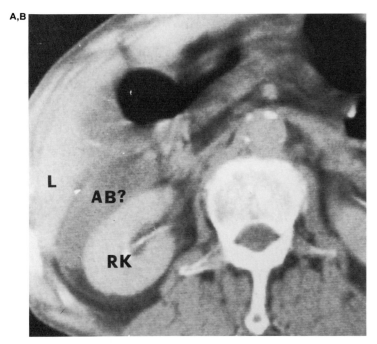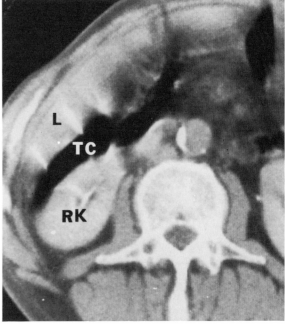

FIG. 22. Transverse colon in Morison's pouch. **A:** Section through hepatorenal fossa demonstrates a fluid collection that might represent an abscess (AB) anterolateral to the right kidney (RK); (L) liver. **B:** Section obtained in left lateral decubitus position demonstrates that the fluid was within the lumen of the transverse colon (TC), which is now gas-filled; (RK) right kidney; (L) liver.

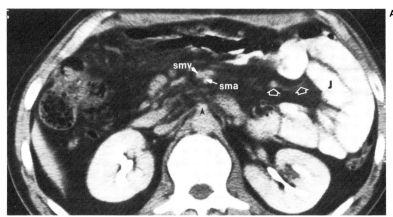

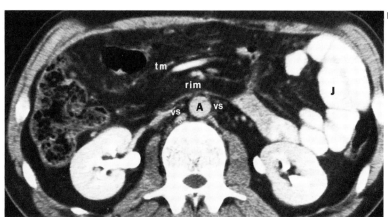

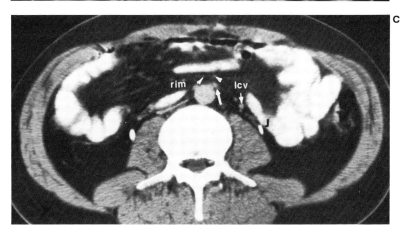

FIG. 23. Small-intestine mesentery. **A:** Section through the renal hila shows the superior mesenteric artery (sma) and vein (smv) coursing within the root of the small intestinal mesentery. From this origin, the leaves of the mesentery fan out—one leaf with its associated jejunum (J) and central vascular core (*open arrows*) is visible on this section; (*arrowhead*) origin of superior mesenteric artery from the aorta. **B:** Three centimeters caudal, the root of the mesentery (rim) is placed more to the right than on the previous section. Posterior to it lies the aorta (A) and vascular space (vs); anterior to it is the transverse mesocolon (tm). **C:** Five centimeters more caudal, the mesenteric root (rim), identified by its major vessels, lies farther to the right; its contained vessels have become somewhat attenuated (*arrowheads*). At this level, the inferior mesenteric artery (*arrow*) and its left colic vessels (lcv) pass posterior to a jejunal loop (J) and its mesenteric leaf.

Retroperitoneal Spaces

The retroperitoneum is a layered space including all of the abdominal contents between the transversalis fascia posteriorly and the parietal peritoneum anteriorly. It extends from the diaphragm to the pelvic brim. The retroperitoneum is a complex anatomic region. Many careful clinicoradiologic studies have shown that fascial boundaries established by anatomic studies do not always correlate with patterns of disease spread observed clinically. Accordingly, this discussion will be based on both clinical observations of the distribution of retroperitoneal processes and anatomically documented fascial boundaries. The retroperitoneum will be divided into five separate

components: (a) a poorly defined space surrounding the great vessels, (b) the psoas spaces, (c) the kidneys and perirenal spaces, (d) the posterior pararenal space (or properitoneal compartment), and (e) the complex anterior pararenal space produced by fusion of the dorsal mesenteries of the stomach, duodenum, and colon with the posterior body wall.

Great vessels

The aorta and its major visceral branches, as well as the IVC and its tributaries, course within an ill-defined space anterior to the vertebral bodies. This space is a caudal continuation of the posterior mediastinum, but no

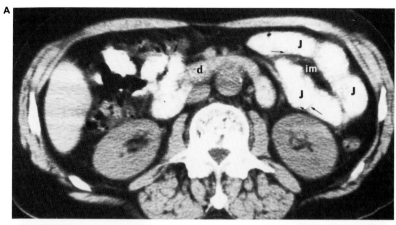

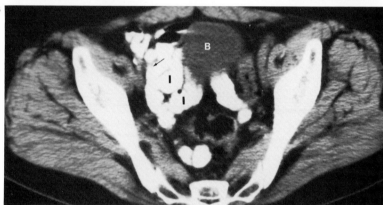

FIG. 24. Normal small intestine. A: Image through the level of the transverse duodenum (d) shows the normal jejunum (J) enclosing a fatty mesenteric leaf (im). Even when well distended, the jejunal plica circulares (*arrows*) can be identified in most patients. B: Image through the pelvis demonstrates that the ileum (I) is relatively featureless; only one fold (*arrow*) is visible; (B) bladder.

fascial planes confine it, and processes may extend from it to involve any other retroperitoneal space. Paraaortic and paracaval lymph nodes accompany the entire course of the abdominal aorta and vena cava (Fig. 25). The diaphragmatic crura enclose the upper part of the abdominal aorta, ending in a fibrous arch, the median arcuate ligament, immediately cephalic to the level of the celiac trunk. Lying 1 to 2 cm caudal is the origin of the superior mes-

enteric artery, whose course parallels the aorta over several centimeters. Approximately 1 to 2 cm more caudal, the renal arteries exit the aorta laterally or posterolaterally to enter the renal hila (Fig. 26). The right renal artery passes behind the IVC in its course. At 1 to 2 cm above the aortic bifurcation, the inferior mesenteric artery (Fig. 23C) exits the left anterolateral surface of the aorta and gives off left colic, sigmoid, and superior rectal branches.

The IVC passes through its hiatus within the central tendon of the diaphragm. Just caudal to this level, it re-

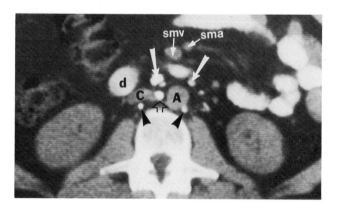

FIG. 25. Great vessels and accompanying lymph nodes. Image obtained in a patient after bipedal lymphangiogram. Section just below renal hila shows lymph nodes posterior to (*arrowheads*), anterior to (*arrows*), and between (*open arrow*) the aorta (A) and inferior vena cava (C). Note the proximity of the root of the small intestinal mesentery, marked by the superior mesenteric artery (sma) and vein (smv), and the distal duodenum (d) to the anterior group of nodes.

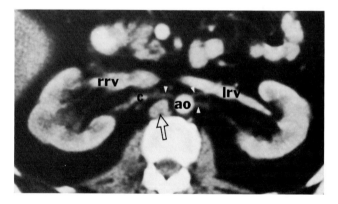

FIG. 26. Renal hilar vessels. Section through the hila of both kidneys shows the typical arrangement of renal vessels. A single, right renal artery and two left renal arteries (*arrowheads*) are imaged. Major portions of the left renal vein (lrv) and right renal vein (rrv) course anterior to the renal arteries to enter the inferior vena cava. Note thick right crus (*open arrow*).

ceives the three major hepatic veins, which serve to mark the boundaries of the four major liver segments. Inferiorly, it is situated on a groove on the posterior surface of the caudate lobe; fat is rarely seen interposed between the two. At its lower intrahepatic margin, the IVC is imme-

diately anterior to the right adrenal gland; a fat plane separates it from the right diaphragmatic crus. It is in this space that the right portion of the celiac ganglion ramifies. Just inferior to its hepatic course, the IVC is close to the portal vein; the fat between them has been termed the

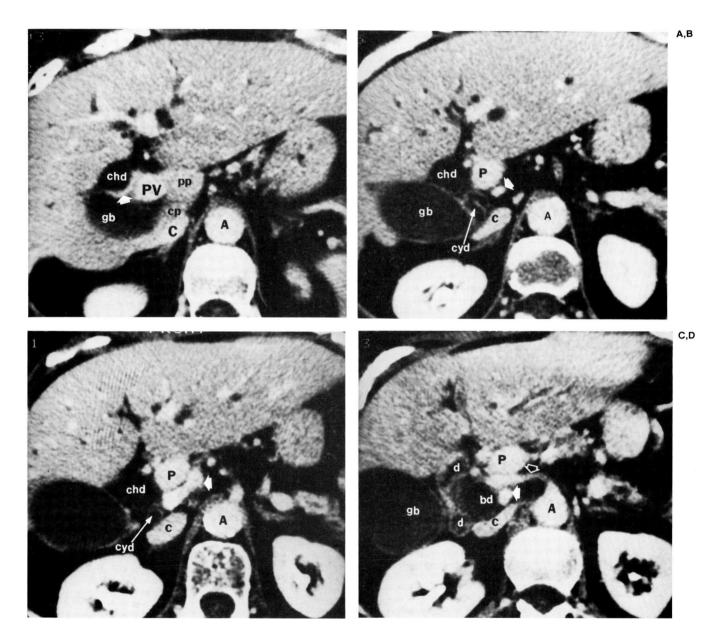

FIG. 27. The portacaval space. Structures lying between the inferior vena cava (C) and the portal vein (PV) occupy the so-called portacaval space, which is chiefly formed by the hepatoduodenal ligament and its extension into the perivascular retroperitoneum. Postcontrast images in a patient with ampullary carcinoma. **A:** Section through the unbranched portal vein (PV) shows the common hepatic duct (chd) and right hepatic artery (*arrow*) in the lateral portion of the hepatoduodenal ligament. Occupants of the portacaval space are the neck of the dilated gallbladder (gb) and the caudate process (cp) of the caudate lobe; (pp) papillary process of the caudate lobe; (C) inferior vena cava; (A) aorta. **B:** Eight millimeters caudal, the spiraling cystic duct (cyd) and a calcified lymph node (*arrow*) lie within the portacaval space; (gb) gallbladder; (chd) common hepatic duct; (P) portal vein; (A) aorta; (c) inferior vena cava. **C:** Eight millimeters more caudal, the common hepatic duct (chd) and cystic duct (cyd) course on the right of the portacaval space. More medially lies a lymph node (3 × 1 cm) (*arrow*), which was pathologically benign; (P) portal vein; (c) inferior vena cava; (A) aorta. **D:** Twelve millimeters caudal to **C,** the hepatoduodenal ligament contents have extended into the retroperitoneum medial to the duodenum (d). Another normal component of the portacaval space, an accessory right hepatic artery (*open arrow*), is visible in this patient; (gb) gallbladder; (P) portal vein; (c) inferior vena cava; (A) aorta; (*closed arrow*) lymph node.

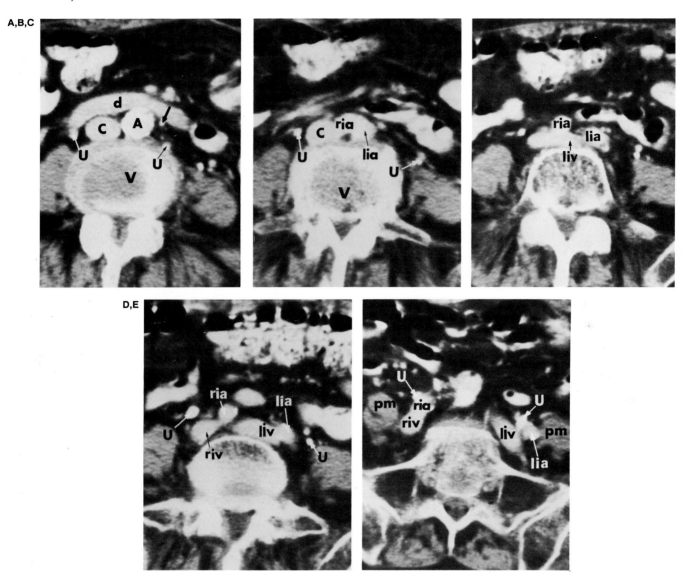

FIG. 28. Aortic bifurcation. **A:** Image through the transverse duodenum (d) shows the distal aorta (A) and inferior vena cava (C). The perivascular space at this level contains the left colic vessel (*arrow*) and both ureters (U); (V) vertebral body. **B:** One centimeter caudal, the proximal right common iliac artery (ria) courses anterior to the undivided inferior vena cava (C). The left common iliac artery (lia) maintains a position just anterior to the vertebral body. **C:** One centimeter more caudal, the left common iliac vein (liv) has a nearly transverse course as it passes posterior to the iliac arteries. **D:** One centimeter more caudal, the right common iliac vein on this and subsequent sections is positioned posterolateral to the right common iliac artery. The left common iliac vein on this section is posteromedial to its accompanying artery. **E:** Two centimeters caudal to **D,** the iliac vessels continue posterolaterally medial to the psoas muscles (pm) and lateral to the sacral vertebral body.

portacaval space (72) (Fig. 27). This space contains the hepatic group of lymph nodes, lying within the hepatoduodenal ligament. More caudally, the uncinate process of the pancreas is interposed between the superior mesenteric vein and the IVC.

Both the IVC and the aorta are crossed anteriorly by the transverse part of the duodenum. Caudal to this, the IVC is related predominantly to the root of the small intestinal mesentery. The IVC divides approximately 1 to 2 cm caudal to the aorta bifurcation. The left common iliac vein then passes posterior to the right common iliac

artery before arriving at a point posterior and slightly medial to the left common iliac artery (Figs. 28 and 29).

Psoas spaces

The fascia around the psoas muscles form a pyramidal space that potentially connects the mediastinum with the lower limb (65). The psoas muscle begins at the vertebral body and intervertebral space of T12–L1 and passes posterior to the crura of the diaphragm under the medial arcuate ligaments (Fig. 30). Its anterior and lateral borders

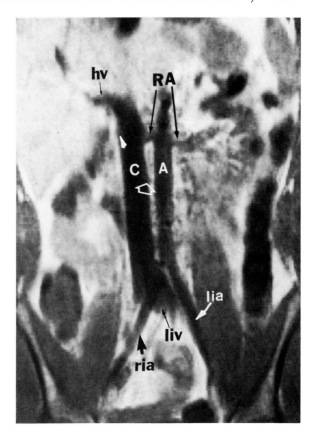

FIG. 29. Great-vessel anatomy: Coronal MR image (TR = 500 msec, TE = 15 msec) shows entry of a major hepatic vein (hv) into the inferior vena cava (C). Alterations in intensity mark the site of entry of the right renal vein (*arrowhead*) and a small left renal vein (*open arrow*). The broad left common iliac vein (liv) passes behind the right common iliac artery (ria). Both renal arteries (RA) are well defined.

are ensheathed with fascia, which effectively prevents communication with the perirenal space above the renal hilus. Below that level, the posterior renal fascia inserts directly onto the psoas fascia, and the two spaces may communicate.

On the medial surfaces of the psoas muscles there are tendinous arches coursing over the constricted middle portion of the vertebral bodies. Medial to these arches are the lumbar veins, lumbar arteries, and sympathetic trunks. Posterolaterally, the psoas muscles cover the intervertebral foramina, so that lumbar nerves course caudally within the substance of the muscle. These nerves then pass anterolaterally to form the following peripheral nerves (Fig. 31): The genitofemoral nerve lies on the anterior surface of the psoas muscle near the ureter; the lateral femoral cutaneous nerve lies on its posterolateral surface (within the posterior pararenal space); the femoral nerve passes behind the psoas muscle in a groove between it and the iliac muscle; the obturator nerve remains on the postero-medial surface of the psoas, posterolateral to the iliac arteries and veins. Thus, processes arising in the psoas space can produce symptoms in every lower limb distribution except the sciatic.

The medial portion of the psoas space also contains lymphatics, and it is this space that enlarges in patients with neoplastic or inflammatory lymph node disease, displacing the psoas fibers laterally and anteriorly (Fig. 32).

Kidneys and perirenal spaces

The kidney and its associated suprarenal gland are enclosed in an envelope of perirenal fat that in turn is sheathed within the renal fascia (Fig. 33). On CT sections, the posterior renal fascia is well defined and smoothly continuous with the lateroconal fascia, which extends anteriorly just lateral to the ascending or descending colon. The thinner, less well defined anterior renal fascia intersects the posterior renal fascia at an acute angle. The posterior renal fascia is laminar (50), and fluid collections can dissect between its leaves to extend posterior to the kidney (Fig. 34), simulating involvement of the posterior pararenal space.

The perirenal space contains the kidneys, adrenal glands, renal hilar vessels, renal pelvis and proximal ureter, and a substantial quantity of fat. They are enclosed between the renal fascial layers; medially, they communicate by way of the hilar vessels with the space surrounding the aorta and vena cava (61). The largest fat accumulation in the perinephric space is medial to the lower pole; abscesses, hematomas, and urinomas have a tendency to accumulate in this location. The fat within the perirenal space contains numerous septations that may produce loculations within perinephric fluid collections (35).

The adrenal glands lie superior and medial to each kidney; the right adrenal is related to the posterior surface of the IVC, and the lateral limb may be so closely apposed

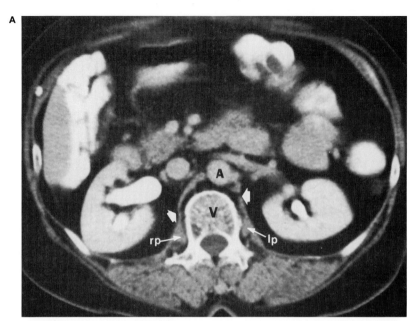

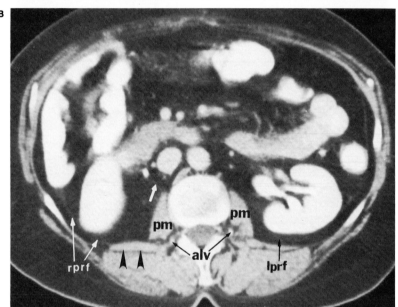

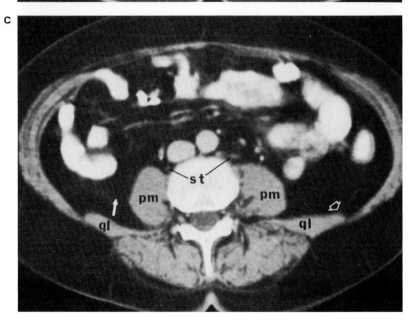

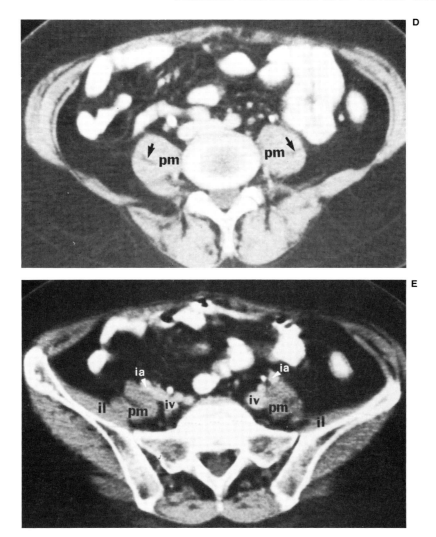

FIG. 30. Psoas muscle relationships. Parts **A–C** on *facing page.* **A:** The psoas muscles (rp and lp) begin as thin triangular stripes whose tendinous anterior borders (*arrows*) (the medial arcuate ligaments) give rise to the crural fibers of the diaphragm; (V) vertebral body; (A) aorta. **B:** Two centimeters caudal, the thin right anterior renal fascia (*arrow*) intersects the anterior margin of the psoas muscle (pm). Posteriorly the psoas muscles come into contact with the quadratus lumborum muscle (*arrowheads*). There is a fat cleft on the posteromedial surface of the psoas muscle adjacent to the neural foramen. It contains the lumbar nerves and ascending lumbar veins (alv); (rprf) right posterior renal fascia; (lprf) left posterior renal fascia. **C:** Six centimeters more caudal, the contour of the psoas muscles is nearly circular. The right posterior renal fascia (*arrow*) intersects the lateral margin of the psoas; the left posterior renal fascia fuses laterally (*open arrow*) with the edge of the quadratus lumborum (ql). The sympathetic trunk (st) can be seen on the anterior medial border of the psoas at this level. **D:** Four centimeters more caudal, a thin fat crescent (*arrow*) appears in the belly of the psoas (pm); the psoas tendon lies in this crescent, and the femoral nerve passes immediately behind it. **E:** Four centimeters more caudal, the psoas muscles (pm) pass laterally to accompany the iliacus (il). The common iliac artery (ia) and vein (iv) lie on the anteromedial surface of the psoas muscle.

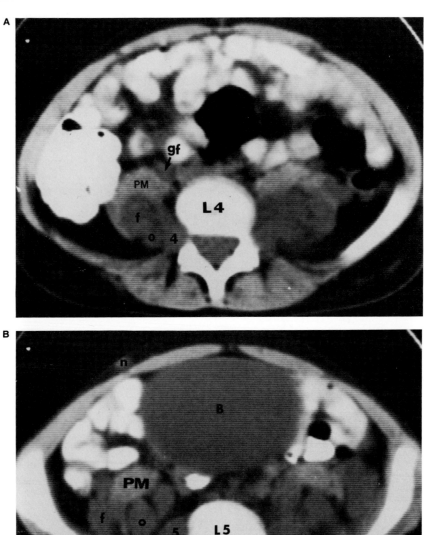

FIG. 31. Psoas space: neuroanatomy. Sections obtained through the lower abdomen in a patient with neurofibromatosis. **A:** Image through the fourth lumbar vertebra (L4) shows neurofibromata involving the fourth lumbar nerve (4), the obturator nerve (o) and the femoral nerve (f) on the posterior aspect of the psoas muscle (PM). Anteriorly lies the genitofemoral nerve (gf). **B:** Three centimeters more caudal, the imaging plane is near the origin of the fifth lumbar nerve (5). Fibromata of the obturator nerve (o) and femoral nerve (f) are again seen. Note multiple subcutaneous neurofibromata (n) and distended neurogenic bladder (B); (PM) psoas muscle; (L5) fifth lumbar vertebral body.

to the liver that it is invisible (Fig. 35). The medial limb lies close to the right diaphragmatic crus; between it and the crus lies the celiac ganglion. The left adrenal is closely related to the tail of the pancreas and its vessels, the splenic artery and vein. It also presents a medial surface close to the left diaphragmatic crus. Congenital gastric diverticula or dilated peripancreatic vessels occur in the region of the left adrenal and may mimic adrenal abnormality (43,53,58).

The ureter occupies the perirenal space caudal to the renal hilum (Fig. 36). At the level of the lower pole, it passes into the space surrounding the great vessels and accompanies the anterior border of the psoas muscle into the pelvis.

Posterior pararenal space

Lateral to the lateroconal fascia, posterior to the renal fascia, but within the transversalis fascia, lies the posterior pararenal space (Fig. 37), which is continuous with the

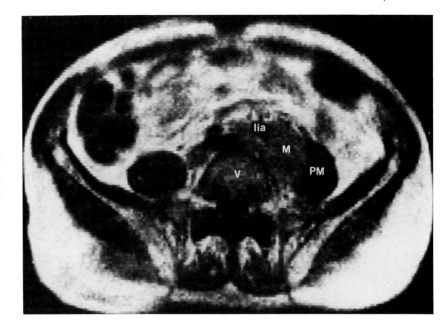

FIG. 32. MR image (TR = 900 msec, TE = 30 msec) from a patient with lymphoma. Marked enlargement of lymph nodes (M) that lie in the space medial to the psoas muscle (pm) has produced lateral displacement of the muscle and of the left common iliac artery (lia) anteriorly; (V) vertebral body.

properitoneal flank stripe. It contains no organs, but is closely related to the posterior surfaces of the ascending and descending colon; inflammatory processes originating in these colonic segments (e.g., diverticulitis, retrocecal appendicitis) easily extend into this space. Above the level of the renal hilum, the posterior pararenal space is quite small and posteriorly located. In perihilar sections, it extends anteriorly and becomes thicker. It may be medially limited by the lateral boundary of the quadratus lumborum muscle; in some individuals it extends farther medially to end at the psoas muscle. Caudal to the kidneys, the posterior pararenal fat continues anterior to the iliacus muscle and posterior to the ascending and descending colon.

Anterior pararenal space

The space between the anterior renal fascia and posterior peritoneum is a complex area formed by fusion of the dorsal mesenteries of the stomach (pancreatic tail and splenorenal ligament), duodenum (mesoduodenum and head of pancreas), and ascending and descending colon. It has been declared a single intercommunicating space by some authors (39) and a multilaminar area by others (17). It is certain that this space contains most of the duodenum, ascending colon, descending colon, and pancreas and that pathologic processes arising within any of these organs can and do spread to involve the others. In turn, the anterior pararenal space communicates readily with the other ligamentous structures fused with it: the root of the small intestinal mesentery, the root of the transverse mesocolon, the phrenicocolic, duodenocolic, and splenorenal ligaments, and the lesser omentum. In this way, subperitoneal spread of very aggressive processes can fill the retroperitoneal spaces of the upper abdomen.

Less fulminant processes, however, seem to be confined within predictable subcompartments within the anterior pararenal space. A frequent observation in patients with moderately severe pancreatitis is pancreatic fluid extending along the pancreatic tail, dividing the posterior renal fascia to extend behind the kidney, and proceeding anterolaterally along or within the lateroconal fascia (Fig. 46). The fat within what was originally the dorsal descending mesocolon is spared, as is the posterior pararenal space. This distribution does suggest a separation between the relatively anterior mesocolic space and the relatively posterior pancreaticoduodenal space (17) (Fig. 38).

Pancreas, Duodenum, and Mesenteric Roots. The pancreas arises from two sources: the larger dorsal pancreas, which originates within the dorsal mesoduodenum, and the ventral pancreas, which originally occupies the ventral mesoduodenum. The dorsal pancreas grows in a posterocephalic direction so that the tail comes to lie behind the developing spleen within the mesogastrium. This segment, within the splenorenal ligament, subsequently fuses with the posterior body wall on the left (Fig. 39). Meanwhile, the pancreatic head and apposed duodenum and dorsal mesoduodenum likewise fuse with the posterior body wall on the right. The ventral pancreas rotates 270° around the superior mesenteric vessels to lie posterior and medial to the superior mesenteric vein. This most caudal portion of the pancreas is called the uncinate process.

The pancreas is seldom imaged on a single transverse section (Fig. 40). As could be predicted from its embryology, images near the splenic hilum routinely demonstrate the pancreatic tail. Pancreatic tissue is characteristically somewhat lobular in outline, with retroperitoneal fat within its sulci. The splenic artery and vein lie posterior to the pancreatic surface. In younger individuals, both vessels are straight and parallel to the pancreatic contour,

Text continues on page 452.

A

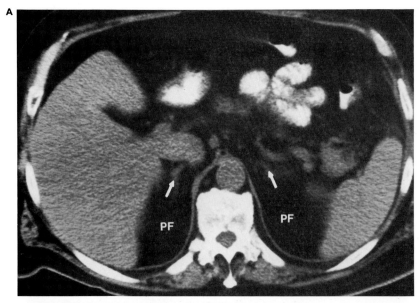

B

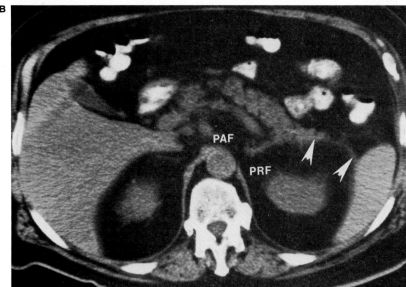

C

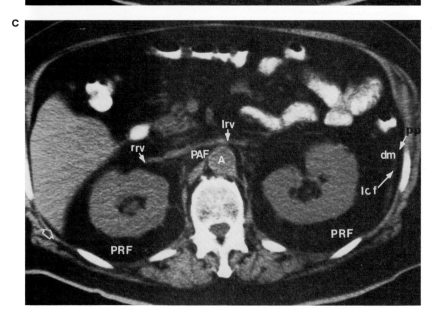

FIG. 33. Renal fascia and retroperitoneal spaces. Images obtained in a patient whose retroperitoneal fascial planes were thickened from a previous inflammatory process. **A:** (Parts **D** and **E** on *facing page.*) Section through the adrenal glands (*arrows*). At this level, the renal fascia are not well defined. The perirenal fat (PF) is elliptical, extending from the diaphragm posteriorly and medially to encompass the adrenals anteriorly. **B:** Three centimeters caudal, the left anterior renal fascia (*arrowheads*) is well seen. There is no clear-cut anteromedial boundary separating the perirenal fat (PRF) from the preaortic fat (PAF) in the root of the hepatoduodenal ligament. The shape of both perirenal spaces is more circular than in image **A. C:** Two centimeters more caudal, the renal hilar vessels, such as the veins (lrv and rrv), provide a potential communication between the preaortic space (PAF) and the perirenal spaces (PRF). At this level the lateroconal fascia (lcf), well seen at left, separates the fat in the fused dorsal colonic mesentery (dm) from the properitoneal fat in the posterior pararenal space (pp). On the right, a thin crescent of properitoneal fat extends posterior to the liver (*open arrow*), forming a potential communication with the bare hepatic area; (A) aorta. Parts **D** and **E** on *facing page.*

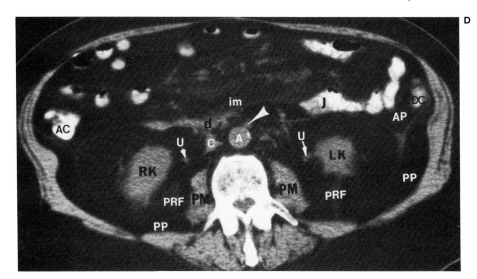

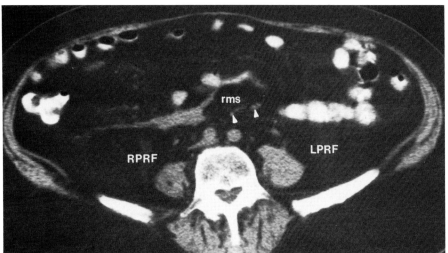

FIG. 33. (Continued.) Parts **A–C** on facing page. **D:** Seven centimeters more caudal, all of the retroperitoneal divisions are well outlined. Behind the mesentery (im) lies a portion of the transverse duodenum (d) and the fat surrounding the inferior mesenteric artery that extends leftward toward the descending colon (DC), behind a jejunal loop (J). These colonic segments lie in the anterior pararenal space (AP). A roughly circular space, whose lateral borders are poorly defined, surrounds the aorta (A), inferior vena cava (C), and the origin of the inferior mesenteric artery (*arrowhead*). The perirenal spaces (PRF), containing the lower renal poles (RK, LK) and ureters (U), are separated from the posterior pararenal space (PP) by the posterior renal fascia. Note that the posterior pararenal spaces extend medially behind the psoas muscles (PM) in this subject. **E:** Four centimeters more caudal, the perirenal spaces (LPRF, RPRF) no longer contain the kidneys, but maintain their well-defined boundaries, becoming more fusiform in shape. An inferior continuation of the anterior pararenal space is the fat in the root of the mesosigmoid (rms), surrounding inferior mesenteric branches (*arrowheads*).

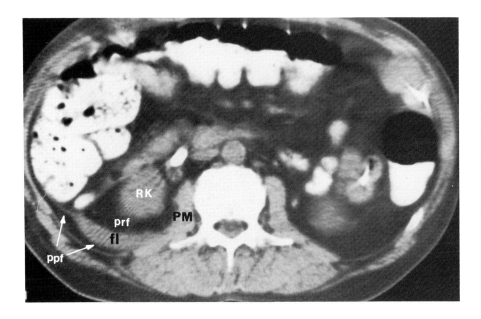

FIG. 34. Fluid collection within the posterior renal fascia. Image through the lower pole of the right kidney (RK) shows a pancreatitis-related fluid collection (fl) that spares both the posterior pararenal fat (ppf) and perirenal fat (prf). The fluid, therefore, lies within the laminae of the posterior renal fascia; (PM) psoas muscle.

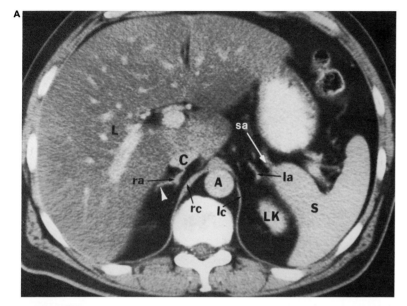

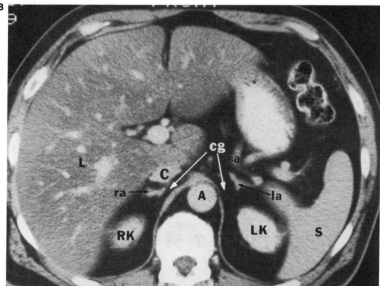

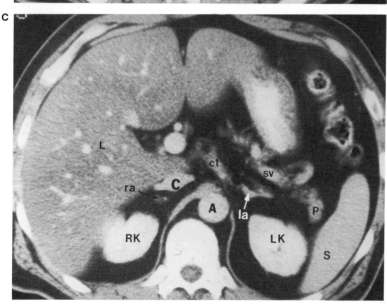

FIG. 35. Normal adrenal relationships. **A:** The right adrenal (ra) is an arrowhead-shaped structure whose lateral segment (*arrowhead*) lies close to the visceral surface of the liver (L). The medial limb is close to the right diaphragmatic crus (rc). The apex of the right adrenal lies just posterior to the inferior vena cava (C). The left adrenal (la) has a similar shape. Its lateral limb lies adjacent to the spleen (S), its medial limb parallels the left crus (lc), and its posterior surface lies anterior to the upper pole of the left kidney (LK). The apex of the adrenal is very close to the splenic artery (sa) in this patient; (A) aorta. **B:** One centimeter caudal, the contour for both adrenal glands (ra, la) is somewhat flattened. The fat between the medial adrenal limbs and the diaphragm contains branches of the celiac nerve plexus (cg); (L) liver; (A) aorta; (RK) right kidney; (LK) left kidney; (S) spleen; (sa) splenic artery. **C:** One centimeter more caudal, the caudal portion of the right adrenal (ra) lies just anterior to the right upper renal pole (RK); (L) liver; (C) inferior vena cava; (A) aorta; (ct) celiac trunk; (la) left adrenal; (LK) left kidney; (sv) splenic vein; (P) pancreas; (S) spleen.

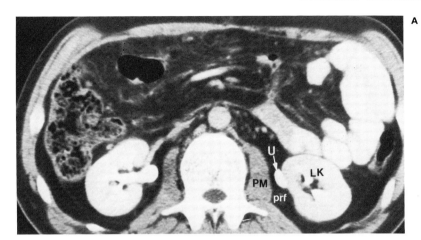

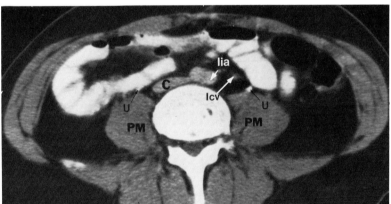

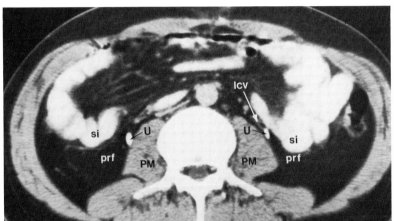

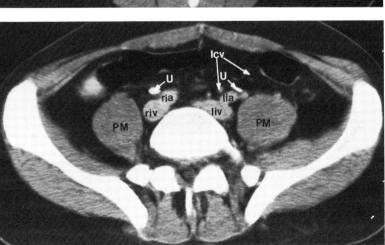

FIG. 36. Abdominal course of the ureters. **A:** The ureters (U) begin within the perinephric space (prf) as an extension of the renal pelvis; (PM) psoas muscle; (LK) left kidney. **B:** Five centimeters caudal, as the ureters (U) exit the perinephric space (prf), they lie on the anterolateral surface of the psoas muscles (PM); (si) small intestine; (lcv) left colic vessels. **C:** Four centimeters more caudal, the ureters (U) lie at the lateral margins of the fat surrounding the great vessels. On the left, this space is more voluminous because it contains the inferior mesenteric and left colic vessels (lcv) as well as the proximal left common iliac artery (lia); (PM) psoas muscles. **D:** Four centimeters more caudal, the ureter (U) occupies the anterolateral margin of the space surrounding the common iliac vessels (ria, riv, lia, liv); (PM) psoas muscles; (lcv) left colic vessels.

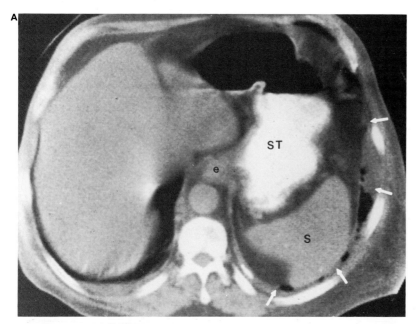

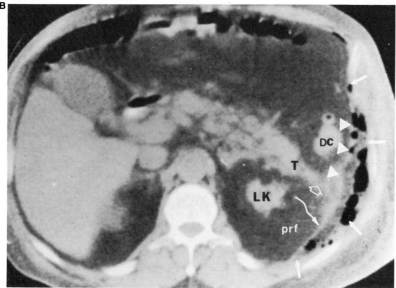

FIG. 37. The posterior pararenal space. In this patient, an extensive diverticular abscess occupies the posterior pararenal space, exemplifying its cephalocaudal extent. **A:** (Part **D** on *facing* page.) Image near the gastroesophageal junction shows the superior portion of the posterior pararenal space (*arrows*) between the spleen (S) and the diaphragm; (e) esophagus; (ST) stomach. **B:** Six centimeters caudal, near the pancreatic tail (T), the process (*arrows*) thickens the posterior renal (*curved arrow*) and lateroconal (*arrowheads*) fascia as well as the anterior renal fascia (*open arrow*). The descending colon (DC) lies in the notch formed by the anterior renal and lateroconal fascia. **C:** Eight centimeters more caudal, there is perirenal fat (PRF) present well below the atrophic left kidney. The posterior pararenal space (*arrows*) extends medially as far as the quadratus lumborum muscle (QLM); (DC) descending colon; (PM) psoas muscle. Part **D** on *facing page.*

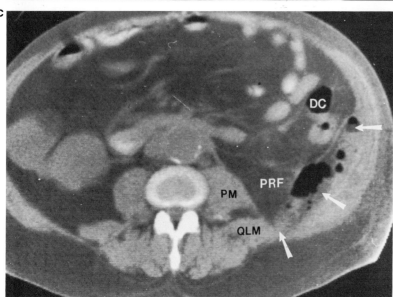

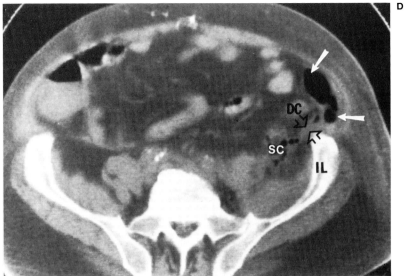

FIG. 37. (Continued.) Parts **A–C** on *facing page.*
D: Six centimeters more caudal, the inferior extent of the posterior pararenal space (*arrows*) is anterior to the iliac wing (IL) and remains just lateral to the descending colon (DC). Note the fistula (*open arrows*) arising from a diverticular abscess that produced the extensive inflammation within the posterior pararenal space; (SC) sigmoid colon.

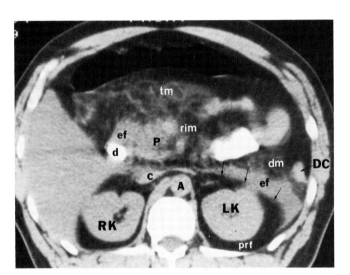

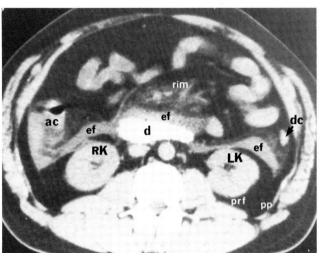

FIG. 38. The pancreaticoduodenal space. Images obtained in a patient with moderately severe acute pancreatitis. **A:** Section through the uncinate process of the pancreas (P) shows effusion (ef) surrounding pancreatic tissue, extending to the medial wall of the duodenum (d). The effusion also extends leftward anterior to the left anterior renal fascia (*arrows*). There is relative sparing of the transverse mesocolon (tm) and the fat around the descending colon. This fat represents the fused dorsal mesentery (dm) of the colon and is part of the anterior pararenal space; (rim) root of the small intestinal mesentery; (c) inferior vena cava; (A) aorta; (RK) right kidney; (LK) left kidney; (prf) perirenal fat. **B:** Section 4 cm caudal shows effusion (ef) chiefly involving the transverse duodenum (d), with relative sparing of the fat surrounding the ascending and descending colon (dc); (rim) root of small intestinal mesentery; (RK) right kidney; (LK) left kidney; (prf) perirenal fat; (pp) posterior pararenal space.

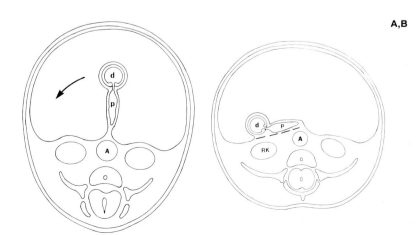

FIG. 39. Rotation and fusion of the pancreas and duodenum. **A:** Schematic diagram of a transverse section through a developing embryo. The ventral mesentery of the duodenum (d) and all other distal intestinal segments have been resorbed. The pancreas (p) and duodenum (*arrow*) rotate in a counterclockwise direction to meet with the posterior abdominal wall; (A) aorta. **B:** Fusion eventually takes place, limiting the posteromedial extent of the right peritoneal space. There is potential for extension of the peritoneum posterior to the duodenum and pancreas (*dashed line*); (d) duodenum; (P) pancreas; (RK) right kidney; (A) aorta.

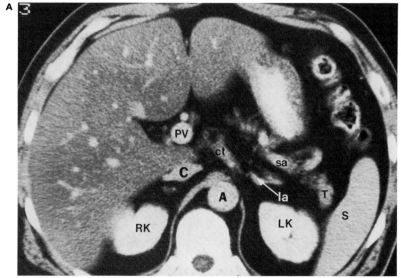

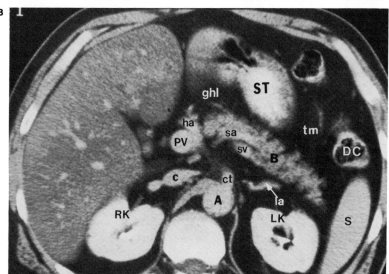

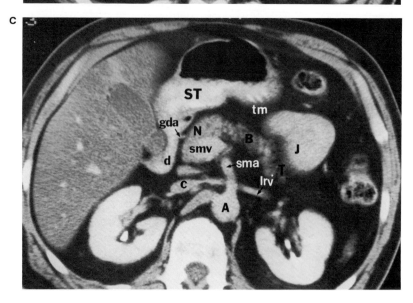

FIG. 40. Pancreas: normal relationships. **A:** Image through the celiac trunk (ct) shows the pancreatic tail (T), which is the most cephalic portion in this patient. Note that the distal tip of the tail dips posterior to the splenic artery (sa); (PV) portal vein; (C) inferior vena cava; (A) aorta; (RK) right kidney; (LK) left kidney; (la) left adrenal; (S) spleen. **B:** One centimeter caudal, the pancreatic body (B) is displayed; the normal lobular parenchymal pattern is well seen. On the left, the pancreas lies anterior to the left adrenal (la) and kidney (LK), medial to the spleen (S), and posteromedial to the descending colon (DC). The stomach (ST) lies just anterior to the more proximal pancreas. On this section, the splenic artery (sa) lies anterior to the splenic vein (sv); both are posterior to the pancreatic body. The hepatic artery (ha) passes to the right of the pancreas; (ghl) gastrohepatic ligament; (tm) transverse mesocolon. **C:** Two centimeters more caudal, the neck of the pancreas (N) is adjacent to the confluence of the splenic vein with the superior mesenteric vein (smv); no fat plane separates these structures. The inferior part of the pancreatic tail (T) is adjacent to the proximal jejunum (J). On the right, the duodenum (d) is separated from the pancreatic neck by a fat plane containing the gastroduodenal artery (gda); (ST) stomach; (tm) transverse mesocolon; (sma) superior mesenteric artery; (C) inferior vena cava; (lrv) left renal vein; (A) aorta. Parts **D–F** on *facing page*.

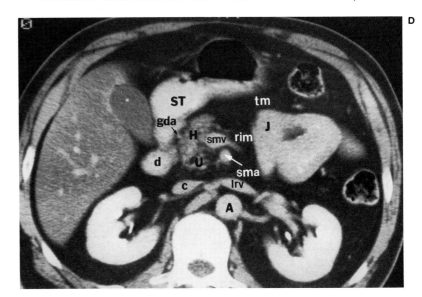

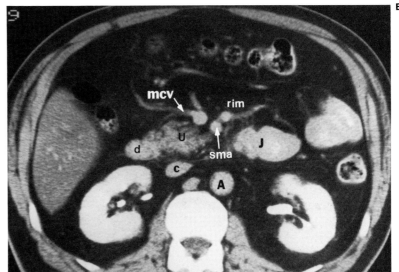

FIG. 40. (*Continued*.) Parts **A–C** on facing page. **D:** One centimeter more caudal, arising from the posterior surface of the pancreatic head (H), the uncinate process (U) curves posterior to the superior mesenteric artery (sma) and vein (smv). It lies just anterior to the inferior vena cava (c) at the same level as the left renal vein (lrv); (d) duodenum; (ST) stomach; (gda) gastroduodenal artery; (rim) root of small intestinal mesentery; (A) aorta; (tm) transverse mesocolon. **E:** Two centimeters more caudal, the uncinate process (U) is the only pancreatic tissue present. On sections near the ampulla of Vater, the fat plane separating the duodenum (d) from the pancreas disappears; (mcv) middle colic vein; (rim) root of small intestinal mesentery; (c) inferior vena cava; (A) aorta; (J) jejunum. **F:** One centimeter more caudal, the transverse duodenum (d) lies in close apposition to the posterior surface of the uncinate. The medial boundary of the uncinate has a biconcave appearance, but the posterolateral aspect is convex. Convexity of the entire surface of the uncinate is suspicious for pancreatic neoplasm; (A) aorta; (c) inferior vena cava; (rim) root of small intestinal mesentery; (J) jejunum.

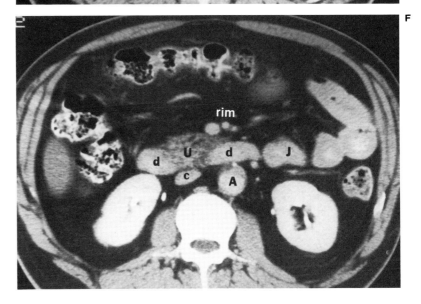

A,B

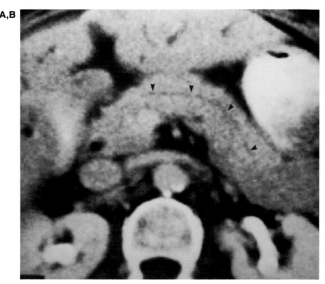
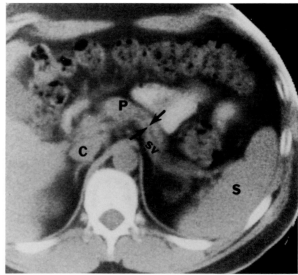

FIG. 41. Pancreatic duct and pseudopancreatic duct. **A:** Contrast-enhanced image through the neck of the pancreas shows a thin, water-density line coursing through the center of the pancreas: the normal pancreatic duct (*arrowheads*). **B:** In another patient, the fat plane (*arrows*) between the pancreas (P) and the splenic vein (SV) mimics a pancreatic duct; (S) spleen; (C) inferior vena cava.

separated from it by a thin plane of fat. The splenic artery generally lies cephalic and slightly anterior to the splenic vein. With age, the splenic artery becomes tortuous and may loop in any direction on its way to the splenic hilum; the course of the splenic vein is not altered. In a few individuals, the tip of the pancreatic tail may curl posteriorly to lie behind the splenic vessels. Anomalies of the peripancreatic abdominal vessels are not uncommon.

The rotation and fusion of the dorsal mesoduodenum and mesogastrium causes the posterior surface of the pancreatic body to lie anterior to the original posterior body wall. A dome-shaped collection of fat is thus enclosed; this fat is contained in the root of the dorsal mesentery of the midgut. This space is bounded by the aorta and diaphragmatic crura posteriorly and the pancreas and splenic vessels anteriorly and laterally. The origin of the superior mesenteric artery is contained within it. Pancreatic inflammation tends to involve adjacent leaves of mesoduodenum or mesogastrium, sparing the fat around the superior mesenteric artery; carcinoma, however, can infiltrate this fat space to encase the artery.

While the superior mesenteric artery is isolated from the pancreas by an envelope of periaortic fat, the superior mesenteric vein lies in the notch formed by the junction of the head and neck of the pancreas; only rarely is there fat separating them. On sections caudal to this junction, the uncinate process abuts the posterolateral and posterior surface of the superior mesenteric vein. The most posterior portion of the uncinate process lies immediately anterior to the IVC; a fat plane usually is present between them, but its absence is not necessarily pathologic. Most com-

monly, on the same section, the left renal vein can be seen crossing anterior to the aorta and posterior to the superior mesenteric artery to drain into the IVC (34).

High-resolution CT sections, particularly with intravenous contrast enhancement, will sometimes depict a normal pancreatic duct as a thin, water-attenuation stripe parallel to the pancreatic surface (Fig. 41).

The duodenum originates immediately distal to the pylorus (Fig. 42); the first portion (or "bulb") generally courses posterior and lateral with respect to the gastric antrum. This segment often lies close to the body or neck of the gallbladder or the quadrate lobe of the liver. The duodenum turns farther posterior to enter the retroperitoneum, passing just lateral to the common duct as the duct exits the hepatoduodenal ligament. At this level, the gastroduodenal artery separates the head of the pancreas from the duodenum. The duodenum then passes directly caudal, passing lateral to the pancreas and medial to the hepatic flexure. Often there is no fat plane between the medial duodenal wall and the pancreas in this segment, which includes the ampulla of Vater. This segment frequently passes anterior to the right renal pelvis. Immediately caudal to the uncinate process, the duodenum turns to the left, passing anterior to the IVC and aorta, posterior to the superior mesenteric vein and artery. Finally, the duodenum turns anteriorly and leftward to exit the retroperitoneum at the ligament of Treitz.

Ascending and Descending Colon. The ascending colon has variable fixation; in most subjects, it is related to the anterior surface of the iliacus muscle. On its medial wall is the ileocecal valve, attached to the ileal mesentery.

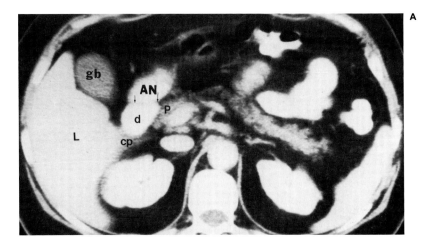

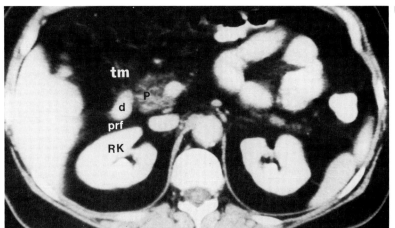

FIG. 42. Normal relationships of the duodenum. **A:** The duodenum (d) originates immediately distal to the gastric antrum (AN); a ridge of muscle representing the pylorus (*arrows*) is occasionally evident. Normal relationships of the first portion of the duodenum include the gallbladder (gb), the caudate process (cp) of the liver (L), and the lateral margin of the pancreas (P). **B:** One centimeter caudal, the lateral surface of the duodenum (d) is closely related to the transverse mesocolon (tm); its posterior surface lies against the right anterior renal fascia and subjacent perirenal fat (prf). Often, no fat plane separates the uncinate process of the pancreas (P) from the medial duodenal wall; (RK) right kidney. **C:** Two centimeters more caudal, the posterior margin of the duodenum (d) abuts the right renal margin (RK). The distal duodenum (dd) exits the retroperitoneum on this section that shows the most proximal jejunal loop (J); (tm) transverse mesocolon; (HF) hepatic flexure; (P) pancreas; (c) inferior vena cava. **D:** Three centimeters more caudal, the duodenum (d) passes from right to left, coursing posterior to the superior mesenteric vein (smv) and artery (sma) and anterior to the inferior vena cava (c) and aorta (A); (tmc) transverse mesocolon; (prf) perirenal space.

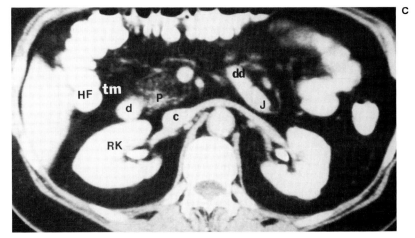

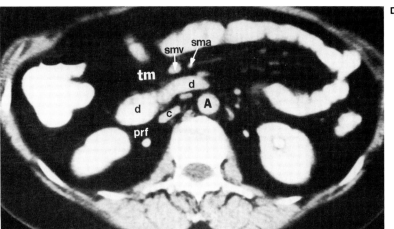

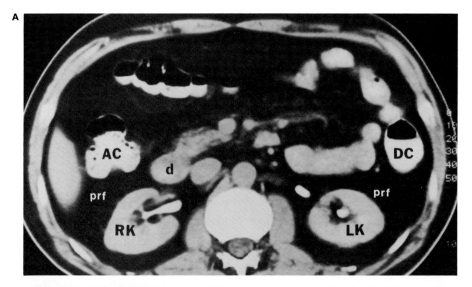

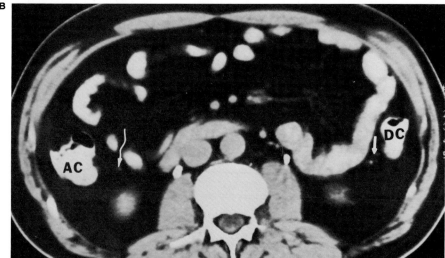

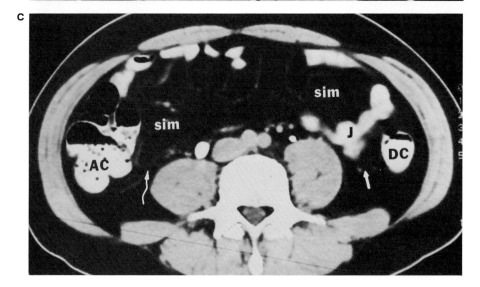

FIG. 43. Normal relationships of the ascending and descending colon. **A:** Both the distal ascending colon (AC) and proximal descending colon (DC) lie within the anterior pararenal space, formed (in part) by the fusion of their dorsal mesenteries to the posterior body wall. They lie anterior and lateral to the kidneys (RK, LK), separated from them by the renal fascia and the perirenal envelope of fat (prf); (d) duodenum. **B:** Three centimeters caudal, the space containing the ascending and descending colon is triangular and contains vessels arising from the superior mesenteric (*curved arrow*) (on the right) and inferior mesenteric (*straight arrow*) (on the left) arteries. **C:** Six centimeters more caudal, the perirenal envelope is no longer present. On the left, the descending colon (DC) and its vascular supply (*straight arrow*) lie posterolateral to the jejunum (J) and small intestinal mesentery (sim). Similarly, the ascending colon (AC) receives its vascular supply (*curved arrow*) posterior to the small-bowel mesentery. Parts **D** and **E** on *facing page.*

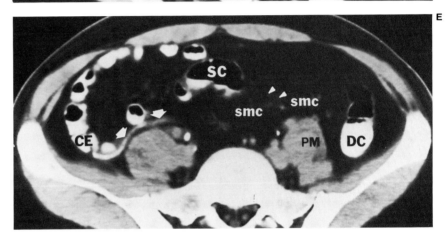

FIG. 43. (*Continued.*) Parts **A–C** on *facing page.* **D:** Four centimeters more caudal, the ascending colon (AC) and descending colon (DC) course between the iliacus (IM) and psoas (PM) muscles. The terminal ileum (ti) enters the medial portion of the colon at the ileocecal valve. Some of the blood supply to this region arises from the ileocolic vessels (icv). **E:** Two centimeters more caudal, the base of the cecum (CE) and its attached appendix (*arrows*) are visible. Just caudal to the plane of this section, the descending colon (DC) turns medially and anteriorly over the psoas muscle (PM) to become the sigmoid segment. Vessels (*arrowheads*) within the sigmoid mesentery (smc) and a cephalic loop of distal sigmoid colon (SC) are visible on this section.

On its posteromedial surface, the vermiform appendix may sometimes be imaged (Fig. 43). The ascending colon occupies the right abdomen just anterior to the caudal portion of the posterior pararenal space, then turns abruptly anterior, lateral to the transverse duodenum and inferior or medial to the gallbladder to become the transverse colon. In this segment, the gas-filled colon may pass medial to the right lobe of the liver or, less commonly, the right renal hilum (10,59). In the latter situation, the kidney may be displaced laterally. Infrequently, the posterior renal fascia of either kidney may fuse with the anterior renal fascia in a posterior location, so that the ascending or descending colon can come to lie in a retrorenal position.

The descending colon begins at the phrenicocolic ligament and is related to the anterior tip of the spleen and to the greater omentum. As it descends, it passes anterolateral to the pancreatic tail and anterior renal fascia, and lateral to jejunal segments. Farther caudal, the inferior mesenteric vascular branches can be traced medially; the veins drain into the inferior mesenteric vein, which courses anterior to the ureter and the psoas space (55) (Fig. 44). The latter vessel can in turn be traced cephalad toward its junction with the splenic vein. At the pelvic brim, the descending colon turns anteriorly to lie in a space anterior to the iliopsoas muscle. From there it curves posterior, medial to the external iliac vessels, to become the sigmoid colon.

THE PELVIS

Major Musculoskeletal Landmarks

The pelvic inlet is bounded posteriorly by the lower lumbar and upper sacral vertebral bodies. As sections continue caudally from the abdomen to the pelvis, the sacral vertebrae slope abruptly posterior to form the posterior wall of the true pelvis (Fig. 45A). Laterally, the pelvis is bounded by the large iliac bones, which are joined to the sacrum by the sacroiliac joints. Caudal to the sacroiliac joints there is discontinuity between the sacrum and the ilium; this space, the greater sciatic notch, allows communication between the pelvis and the lower limb. At the same level, a deep fossa for the femoral head (the acetabulum) is formed by the three portions of the hip bones. This surface is formed superiorly by the ilium, anteriorly by the superior pubic ramus, and posteroinferiorly by the

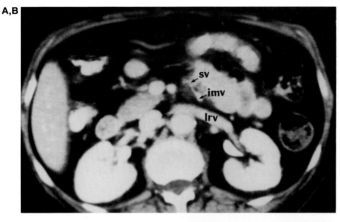
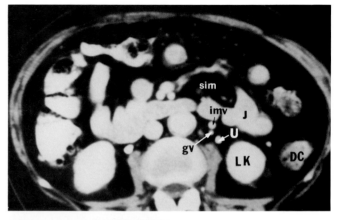
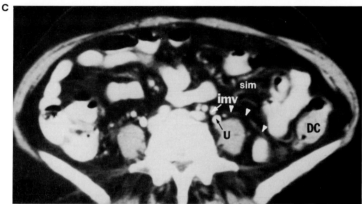

FIG. 44. The inferior mesenteric vein. **A:** The inferior mesenteric vein (imv) passes in front of the left renal vein (lrv) to join the splenic vein (sv). **B:** Four centimeters caudal, the inferior mesenteric vein (imv) courses through what was embryologically the dorsal mesentery of the descending colon (DC), passing anterior to the left kidney (LK), ureter (U), and gonadal vein (gv) and posterior to the jejunum (J) and its mesentery (sim). **C:** Four centimeters caudal, the descending colon (DC) near its junction with the sigmoid is drained by venous structures (*arrowheads*) that can be traced medially behind the small intestinal mesentery (sim) and in front of the left ureter (U) to the inferior mesenteric vein (imv).

body of the ischium. The ischium extends posteriorly and caudally, then circles anteromedially to connect to the inferior ramus of the pubis. The foramen thus formed between the pubis and the ischium is called the obturator foramen and is another communication between the pelvis and the lower limb (16,41,42). A long, strong sacrotuberous ligament extends between the ischial tuberosity to a broad attachment over the lateral and posterior surfaces of the sacrum, while a shorter sacrospinous ligament extends from a smaller portion of the anterior surface of the sacrum laterally, caudally, and slightly anteriorly to affix to the ischial spine. These two ligaments convert the sciatic notches into greater (cephalic) and lesser (caudal) sciatic foramina (Fig. 45B).

The anterior portion of the pelvis is defined chiefly by soft-tissue structures. Anteriorly, the paired rectus abdominis muscles course in a nearly sagittal plane. Lateral to them lie the three major muscles of the flank; from superficial to deep, they are the external oblique, the internal oblique, and the transverse abdominal muscles.

These muscles become thinner as sections proceed more caudally, and their tendons blend with the rectus sheath. Posterior to the rectus abdominis muscles near the umbilicus and separated from them by the rectus fascia are the median umbilical ligament (the fibrotic remnant of the urachus) and the paired medial umbilical ligaments (obliterated umbilical arteries). The former retains its anterior position as it passes toward the bladder dome, while the latter pass posteriorly on more caudal sections, to connect to the superior vesicle arteries within the medial umbilical folds of peritoneum (Fig. 46).

The muscular walls of the pelvis, anteriorly and anterolaterally, are the muscles listed earlier. Posterolaterally, the iliacus muscle covers the broad surface of the iliac bone. Below the sacroiliac joint, the iliacus fuses with the psoas, and the combined muscle lies on the anterior surface of the acetabulum as it courses toward the lesser trochanter of the femur. Medially, the obturator internus muscles cover the surface of the ischium and attach to the posterior surface of the pubic symphysis. The pos-

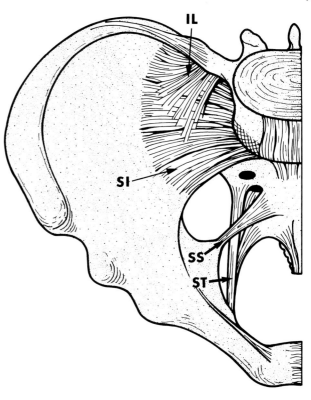

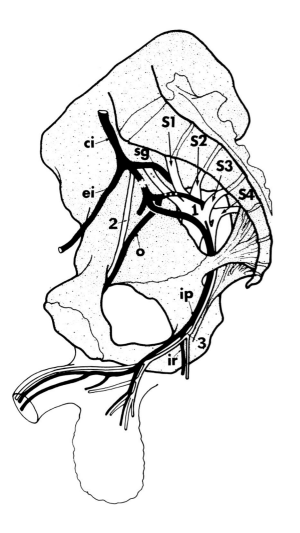

C

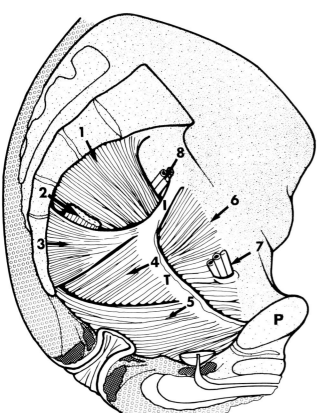

FIG. 45. Major pelvic landmarks. **A:** Neurovascular landmarks. (Adapted from ref. 74.) Schematic drawing showing major blood vessels and neural structures in the male pelvis. The left side of the pelvis has been removed, and the structures of the right are viewed from the side. The common iliac artery (ci) gives off external and internal (*) branches. The latter immediately gives off the major superior (sg) and inferior gluteal (· · ·) arteries. The obturator artery (o) emerges from the inferior gluteal and exits anteriorly through the obturator canal. The terminal branch of the internal iliac artery is the internal pudendal artery (ip), from which emerges the inferior rectal (ir) and penoscrotal vessels. The obturator nerve (2) formed by fibers from upper lumbar nerves leaves via the obturator canal. Fibers contributed by lower lumbar nerves give rise to the lumbosacral trunk (**), which then merges with the first four sacral nerves (S1–4) to form the sciatic plexus. The pudendal nerve arising from the plexus accompanies the internal pudendal vessels through its canal to supply the perineum. **B:** Ligamentous structures. (Adapted from ref. 75.) Schematic drawing of the right side of the pelvis viewed from the front. Support for the sacroiliac articulation is provided by the tough iliolumbar (IL) and ventral sacroiliac (SI) ligaments. The sacrospinous ligament (SS) and sacrotuberous ligament (ST) attach the sacrum to the ischium; the sacrospinous separates the greater (cephalic) and lesser (caudal) sciatic foramina. **C:** Muscular landmarks. (Adapted from ref. 75.) Schematic drawing of a male pelvis viewed from the left side. The sciatic nerve (2) forms on the pelvic surface of the pyriformis muscle. Anteriorly the wall of the pelvis is covered by the obturator internus muscle (6). The floor of the pelvis is covered by a bowl-shaped tripartite muscle, collectively known as the pelvic diaphragm; posterocephalically is the coccygeus (3), anterocaudally the pubococcygeus (5), and in between the iliococcygeus (4). The iliococcygeus muscle arises from a tendinous arch (T) that courses from the ischial spine to the body of the pubis (P); (7) obturator vessels and nerve; (8) superior gluteal neurovascular bundle; (1) pyriformis muscle.

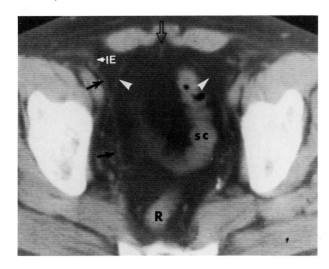

FIG. 46. Umbilical ligaments. The anterior segments of the superior vesical arteries (*arrowheads*) represent the fibrous remnant of the umbilical artery coursing within the medial umbilical ligament. They arc anteromedially toward the remnant of the urachus (*open arrow*), which lies within the median umbilical ligament. Crossing the umbilical artery is the vas deferens (*arrows*), which passes lateral to the inferior epigastric vessel (IE) after entering the abdomen through the deep inguinal ring; (sc) sigmoid colon; (R) rectum.

terolateral surface of the pelvic inlet is covered by the pyriformis muscles, which on more caudal sections exit through the greater sciatic notch to attach to the greater femoral trochanter. The smaller coccygeus muscles arise from the lateral surface of the coccyx to form the posterolateral wall of the pelvic outlet. As the pelvis curves forward toward the perineum, its floor (the pelvic diaphragm) is formed by the levator ani and coccygeus muscles.

External to the pelvic skeletal structure lie the bulky gluteal muscles; from superficial to deep, they are the gluteus maximus, medius, and minimus. Branches of the superior and inferior gluteal vessels occupy the planes between them (70).

Neuroanatomy

Major neural structures ramify over this musculoskeletal framework (Fig. 45C). The lumbosacral trunk can be routinely identified anterior to the sacroiliac junction at the pelvic inlet. This trunk, as well as large sacral nerves, gives rise to the sciatic nerve, which forms on the anterior surface of the pyriformis muscle and exits the pelvis through the greater sciatic foramen at the level of the acetabular roof (23,36,47). The much smaller pudendal nerve exits on the superior surface of the ischial spine, then curves anteromedially into the pudendal canal, on the lateral surface of the ischiorectal fossa. The femoral

and obturator nerves have abdominal roots, as discussed in a previous section.

Vascular Anatomy

There are two major tiers containing the arterial supply and venous drainage of the pelvis (Fig. 45). The common iliac artery enters the pelvis medial to the psoas muscle; the accompanying common iliac vein lies just posterior to it. At the level that the sacrum begins its posterior curve, the internal iliac artery arises and rapidly courses posteriorly to lie anterior to the sacroiliac joints and, more caudally, on the anteromedial aspect of the pyriformis muscle. Meanwhile, the external iliac artery and vein continue to course medial to the psoas muscle, passing behind the inguinal ligament to become the femoral vessels.

A small middle tier of vessels is present lateral to the ureter; it is the obturator artery and vein, which arises from the internal iliac vessels to course inferiorly, exiting the pelvis through the obturator foramen. The latter can be recognized on CT as a triangular space bounded by the pectineus muscle anteriorly, the pubic symphysis and obturator internus muscle medially, and the acetabulum laterally.

Pelvic Peritoneal Spaces

The urinary bladder subdivides the pelvic peritoneal spaces into left and right paravesical spaces. Indentations are formed into each paravesical space by the medial and lateral umbilical folds. The urachus, with its surrounding fat, occupies the midline and may indent large supravesical fluid collections (Fig. 47).

The supravesical space lies between and posterior to the obliterated umbilical arteries in the medial umbilical fold (4). Lateral to this fold, lying medial to the inferior epigastric vessels, is the inguinal fossa, which is continuous with the femoral canal. The lateral part of the inguinal fossa is continuous with the inguinal canal.

Posterior to the bladder, in females, the peritoneum is reflected from the anterior surface of the uterus to form a shallow vesicouterine space. Posterior to the uterus, the peritoneum reflects again from the anterior rectal surface to form the rectouterine pouch (of Douglas). This space is bounded anteriorly by the broad ligaments as well. This peritoneal space extends lateral to the rectum. The anterolateral portion of this extension is the ovarian fossa, which is separated by the rectouterine folds that reflect over the vesical and uterine vessels, from the space immediately lateral to the rectum.

In males, only the rectovesical pouch is present; the sacrogenital folds separate the pararectal space from the remainder of the rectovesical pouch.

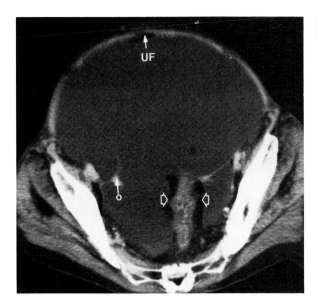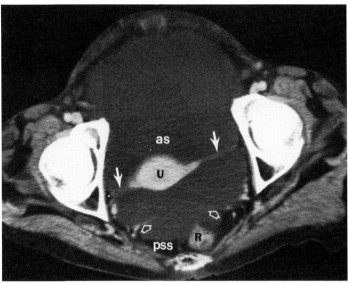

FIG. 47. Peritoneal spaces in the female pelvis. **A:** CT image from a patient with voluminous ascites (as). The upper margin of the broad ligament encloses the right ovary (o). The mesosigmoid fat (*open arrows*) divides the right posterior peritoneal space from the left. A small amount of periurachal fat (UF) indents the anterior peritoneal collection, which is otherwise featureless. **B:** Four centimeters caudal, the broad ligament (*arrows*) and uterus (U) effectively divide the peritoneum into anterior and posterior spaces. At this level, the posterior spaces are partially divided by the rectouterine folds (*open arrows*); (R) rectum; (pss) presacral space.

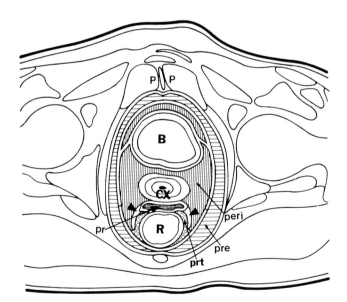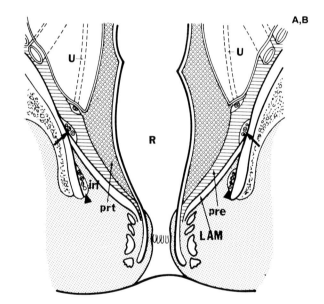

FIG. 48. Pelvic extraperitoneal spaces. (Adapted from ref. 25.) **A:** Schematic diagram of a transverse section through the female pelvis shows the concentric arrangement of the extraperitoneal spaces. The perivesical space (peri, *vertical hatching*) surrounds the urinary bladder (B). Its posterior component is larger; there, it encompasses the areolar tissue surrounding the cervix (CX)—in males, the prostate and seminal vesicles occupy this position. The most caudal peritoneum (*crosshatched*), the rectouterine pouch (pr), descends anterior to the rectum (R) and behind the uterus. Its line of fusion anterior to the perirectal fat forms the rectouterine folds (*arrowheads*). A second circular region, the perirectal space (prt, *small circles*), surrounds the rectum and contains fat and rectal vessels. It is continuous with the fat in the mesosigmoid. Surrounding both perivesical and perirectal spaces is the prevesical space (pre, *horizontal hatching*), which is continuous with the presacral space and the fat surrounding obturator and external iliac vessels. On cephalic sections it is continuous with the properitoneal fat and rectus sheath; (P) pubis. **B:** Schematic diagram of a coronal section through the midportion of the rectum (R) shows the perirectal fat envelope (prt, *small circles*) surrounded by the prevesical fat (pre) within which course the ureters (U) in the sacrogenital fold. Also, this space contains the obturator vessels (*arrow*) and, anterior to this section, the external iliac vessels. Note that the gluteal fat (*stippled*) in which runs the pudendal canal (*arrowhead*) is continuous with the ischiorectal fossa (irf), but is separated from the prevesical fat by the levator ani muscle (LAM).

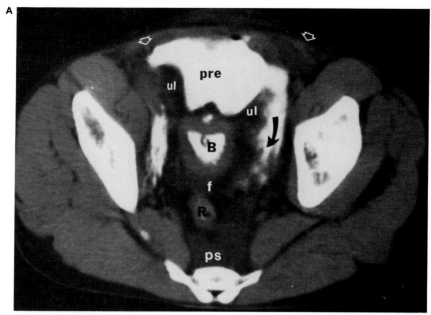

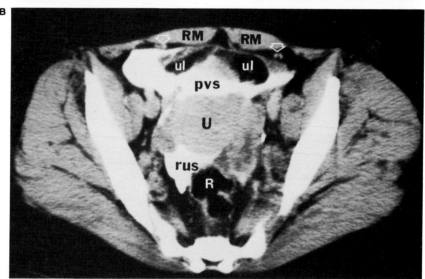

FIG. 49. Intraperitoneal and extraperitoneal spaces in the pelvis. **A:** In a patient with extraperitoneal bladder rupture, contrast extravasation into the prevesical space (pre) is seen. The configuration of this collection has been likened to a "molar tooth," which separates the preserved fat within the medial umbilical ligaments (ul). Note the continuity of the contrast collection (*curved arrow*) with the space medial to the psoas and obturator muscles. Unopacified urine in the same space has dissected posterior to the perirectal space into the presacral space (ps). The majority of the perivesical space (surrounding the bladder and in continuity with the medial umbilical ligaments) is spared, but a small amount of fluid (f) is present posterior to the bladder (B). Although there is preservation of the lateral umbilical ligaments and their contained inferior epigastric vessels (*open arrows*), the fat posterior to the rectus muscles is diffusely obscured by fluid. **B:** In a patient with intraperitoneal bladder rupture, unopacified fluid surrounds the medial umbilical ligaments (ul) and extends posterior to the uterus (U). Note that, in comparison with prevesical collections, the medial umbilical ligaments are close to the rectus muscles (RM), which are surrounded by an intact fat plane. No perivascular or presacral fluid is present; (*open arrows*) inferior epigastric vessels; (rus) rectouterine space; (R) rectum.

Images obtained cephalad to the rectum show division of the pararectal fossae by the sigmoid colon and its mesentery.

Extraperitoneal Spaces

The extraperitoneal spaces surrounding the urinary bladder are complex, exhibiting a laminar arrangement similar to the perirenal spaces (5,49) (Fig. 48).

On sagittal sections in the midline, just deep to the rectus abdominis muscles, lies the transversalis fascia. Between this fascial layer and the fascia covering the bladder and urachus (the umbilicovesical fascia) lies the prevesical fat. This space, while normally small, is greatly expansile; its immediate retropubic portion is known as the space of Retzius and has achieved a well-justified notoriety for the quantity of fluid it can conceal. Collections in this space may extend laterally to the external iliac vessels (Fig. 49). Here, the umbilicovesical fascia is continuous with the parietal pelvic fascia; so fluid collections may track posterior to the perirectal fascia in the presacral space.

Below the semilunar line, the prevesical space communicates with the rectus muscle and may progress into the rectus sheath. Similarly, large collections may extend along the round ligament or vas deferens into the inguinal canal, along the external iliac vessels into the femoral canal, and upward into the posterior pararenal space.

Between the umbilicovesical fascia and the peritoneum lies the perivesical space, in which is contained the bladder, umbilical arteries, and urachus. In females, the supravaginal portion of the cervix and anterior portion of the vagina are continuous with the perivesical space. In males, there is similar continuity of the perivesical space with the prostate and seminal vesicles.

Separate from (and, in fact, encircled by) the perivesical space is the perirectal space (13,25,26). The anterior portion of the fascia defining it lies immediately behind the posterior layer of prostatic fascia; together, these form an effective barrier (Denonvilliers' fascia) separating the two structures. On cephalic sections, the fat in the perirectal compartment is continuous with the mesosigmoid. The superior rectal (hemorrhoidal) vessels are contained within it.

Distinctive Features of the Male Pelvis

Prostate, Seminal Vesicles, and Vasa Deferentia

The prostate is situated in the midline posterior to the symphysis pubis, anterior to the rectum, and medial to the levator ani (pubococcygeus) muscles (Fig. 50). The fascia of the pelvic diaphragm ensheaths the prostate in a tough fibrous capsule that extends upward to surround the bladder base as well. Anteriorly, the prostate is fixed to the symphysis pubis by the puboprostatic ligament. This compartment is endowed with fat and contains the rich prostatic venous plexus. Posteriorly, an extension of the rectovesical peritoneum fuses to form the rectovesical septum. This thick fascia effectively prevents processes arising in the prostate from entering the perirectal space. Posterosuperiorly lie the paired seminal vesicles. On the medial aspect of the junction between the seminal vesicles, the vasa deferentia enter. On transaxial images, a portion of the ductus deferens (Fig. 51) can be traced as it passes anterolaterally just medial to the ureter to a position deep to the transversalis fascia on the lateral aspect of the rectus abdominis muscle. At the deep inguinal ring, it joins the testicular artery, the pampiniform plexus, and the processus vaginalis to become the spermatic cord. This structure passes caudally and medially through the superficial inguinal ring (see Fig. 72 in Chapter 20), then parallels the medial surface of the pectineus muscle on its way to the scrotum.

The prostate is well shown on MR images (Fig. 52), in part because its clinically important relationships to the seminal vesicles and bladder base are best evaluated by sagittal (Fig. 53) or coronal (Fig. 54) imaging techniques (11,12,31,37,48,60). On sagittal images, the prostate is a round 2- to 4-cm structure immediately posterior to the symphysis pubis. Midline images show the urethra passing through the anterior portion of the gland. Its median lobe indents the inferior aspect of the bladder base, from which it is virtually inseparable. On coronal images, the seminal vesicles are seen as oval structures projecting obliquely from the posteromedial surface of the prostate.

The penis and penile urethra are seen in cross section on coronal body images. Paired corpora cavernosa occupy the dorsal penile shaft, while the single spongiosum lies ventrally in the midline.

Text continues on page 465.

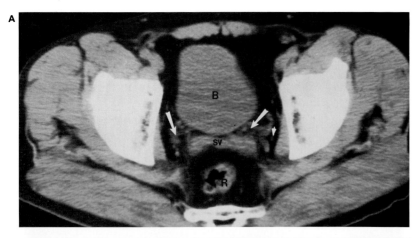

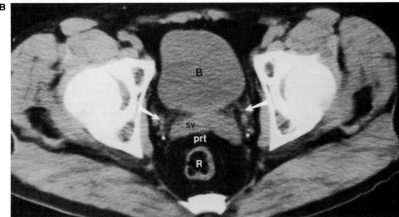

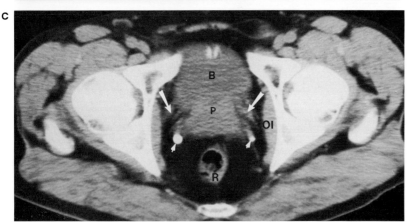

FIG. 50. Male pelvis: transaxial anatomy of the bladder, prostate, and seminal vesicles. **A:** On this image centered at the acetabular roof, there is complete separation of the medial portion of the seminal vesicles (sv) from the bladder (B) by a fat plane. Laterally, there are multiple branches of the prostatic venous plexus (*arrows*); farther lateral, adjacent to the obturator internus muscle, are the obturator vessels (*arrowhead*). **B:** One centimeter caudal, the lateral portions of the seminal vesicles (sv) drape obliquely over the perirectal fat (prt). A deep fat cleft is present between the bladder (B) and the seminal vesicles, containing tributaries of the prostatic venous plexus (*arrows*); (R) rectum. **C:** One centimeter caudal, the superior margin of the prostate (P) blends with the bladder base (B), with which it is structurally continuous. Lateral to their junction lies the rich prostatic venous plexus (*arrows*); (OI) obturator internus muscle; (R) rectum; (*arrowheads*) phleboliths in prostatic plexus. **D:** One centimeter caudal, the prostatic venous plexus is quite prominent on the anterior (*arrow*) and lateral (*arrowhead*) margin of the gland; (P) prostate; (R) rectum; (OI) obturator internus muscle; (pc) pudendal canal; (irf) ischiorectal fossa; (prt) perirectal space. Part **E** on *facing page.*

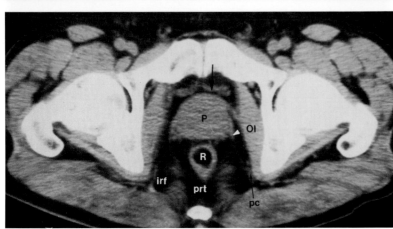

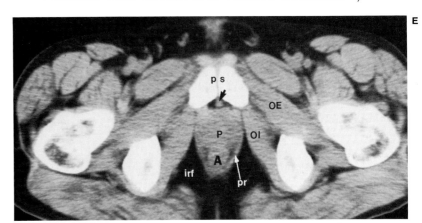

E

FIG. 50. (*Continued.*) Parts **A–D** on *facing page.* **E:** Two centimeters caudal, the puborectalis muscle (pr) encirles the prostate (P) and anorectal junction (A). A small triangular fat plane posterior to the public symphysis (ps) contains the dorsal vein of the penis (*arrow*); (irf) ischiorectal fossa; (OI) obturator internus muscle; (OE) obturator externus muscle.

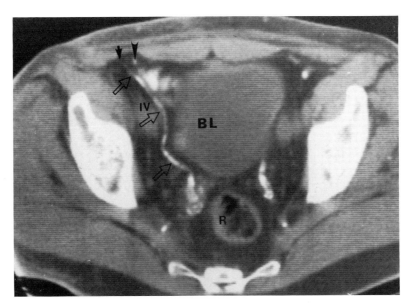

FIG. 51. The vas deferens. In this diabetic patient, the vasa deferentia are diffusely calcified. The characteristic course of the right vas deferens (*open arrows*) is illustrated on this single section. The vas enters the abdominal cavity just lateral to the inferior epigastric artery (*arrowhead*) at the deep inguinal ring (*arrow*). It then courses posteriorly medial to the external iliac vessels (IV), then turns medially posterior to the bladder (BL). It finally turns caudally, where it joins the excretory duct of the seminal vesicle to form the ejaculatory duct; (R) rectum.

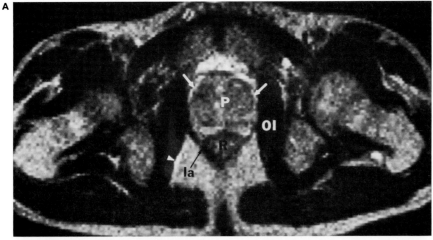

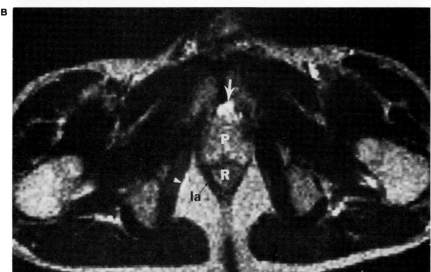

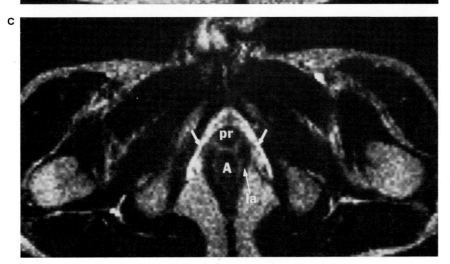

FIG. 52. Series of transverse MR images of a normal male pelvis (TR = 2,100 msec, TE = 90 msec). With this pulse sequence, slowly flowing blood emits a high-intensity signal. **A:** Image through the middle of the prostate (P) shows the rich prostatic venous plexus (*arrows*) immediately anterolateral to the prostate. Obscuration of these vessels suggests extracapsular extension of prostatic tumor; (la) levator ani; (R) rectum; (OI) obturator internus; (*arrowhead*) internal pudendal vessels. **B:** Thirteen millimeters caudal, the dorsal vein of the penis (*arrow*) lies anterior to the prostate (P); (R) rectum; (la) levator ani muscle; (*arrowhead*) internal pudendal vessels. **C:** Thirteen millimeters caudal, the corpora cavernosa of the penis (*arrows*) course in an anteromedial direction lateral to the levator ani (la); (A) anus; (pr) base of the prostate. Part **D** on *facing page.*

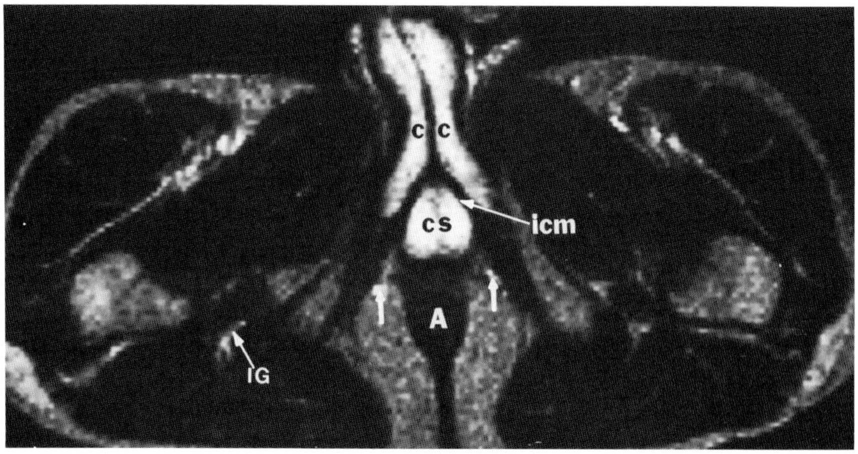

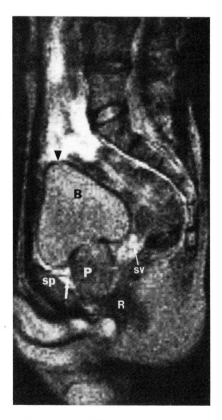

FIG. 52. (*Continued*.) Parts **A–C** on *facing page*. **D**: Thirteen millimeters caudal, an image through the perineum shows the corpora cavernosa (cc) extending along the penile shaft. The crus of the penis is outlined by the ischiocavernosus muscles (icm), which arch over the corpus spongiosum (cs); (*arrows*) internal pudendal vessels; (IG) inferior gluteal vessels; (A) anus.

Male Perineum

Transaxial images obtained caudal to the prostate demonstrate the male perineum (63) (Figs. 55 and 56). At this level, the ischial tuberosities lie posterolaterally inferior to the pubic symphysis. The ischiocavernosus muscle forms an arch over the vertically oriented corpus cavernosum. More medially, the bulbospongiosus muscle encloses the corpus spongiosum and within it the bulbous urethra. Immediately posterior to the bulbospongiosus muscles lie the transverse perineal muscles; lateral to them are the ischiorectal fossae (Fig. 57). Most posteriorly in the perineum are the internal anal sphincter and the levator ani muscles.

Distinctive Features of the Female Pelvis

Uterus and Cervix

The uterus is a pear-shaped organ that is relatively unfixed in its pelvic location (Figs. 58 and 59). The least movable portion, the supravaginal part of the cervix, is connected anteriorly to the bladder base by loose connective tissue. A number of ligamentous structures attach or enfold the uterus, but provide little mechanical support.

The broad ligament is formed at the lateral margin of the uterus and extends laterally to the pelvic wall. In so doing, it encloses the loose connective tissue called the parametrium (67,68) (Fig. 60), the uterine (Fallopian) tubes, the ovarian and round ligaments, and the uterine artery and vein. The cardinal ligaments extend posterolaterally from the cervix. These ligaments merge with the fascia of the pelvic diaphragm. The round ligaments follow

FIG. 53. Midline sagittal MR image of a male pelvis (TR = 2,100 msec, TE = 90 msec) shows a distended urinary bladder (B) with a low-signal thin muscular wall (*arrowhead*). An enlarged prostate (P) is immediately subjacent to the bladder base, and part of a seminal vesicle (sv) is displayed posterior to it. The rich plexus of veins (*arrow*) draining the bladder and prostate lies in the anterior space behind the pubic symphysis (sp); (R) rectum.

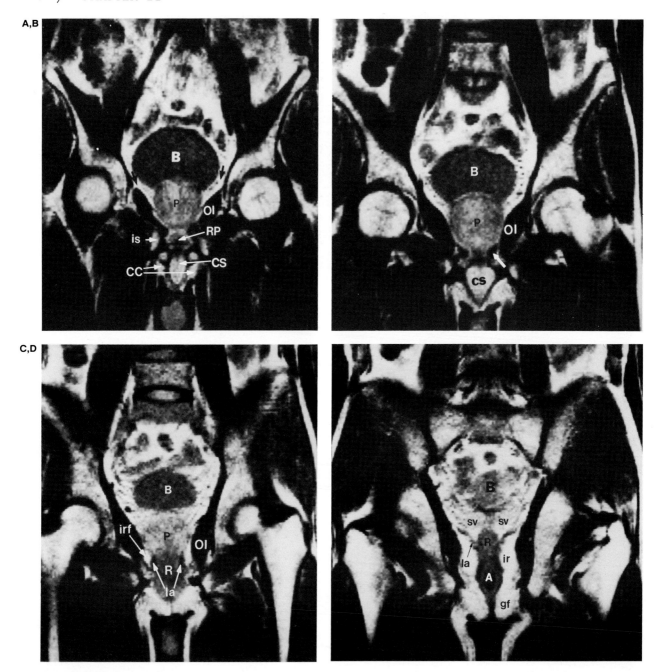

FIG. 54. Coronal MR images obtained in a patient with prostatic hypertrophy (TR = 2,100 msec, TE = 35 msec). **A:** Coronal section through the anterior femoral heads shows the urinary bladder (B) superior to the enlarged prostate (P). A portion of the prostatic plexus (*arrows*) is noted just lateral to the prostate and medial to the obturator internus muscle (OI); (cc) corpora cavernosa; (rp) root of penis; (is) ischium; (cs) corpus spongiosum. **B:** Thirteen millimeters posterior, the obturator internus muscles (OI) flank the prostate (P) on its lateral surface, while its base is encircled by the puborectalis muscle (*arrow*), a part of the levator ani; (cs) corpus spongiosum. **C:** Thirteen millimeters more posterior, the obturator internus muscle (OI) is separated from the prostate by the apex of the ischiorectal fossa (irf) just lateral to the puborectalis (la). A portion of the anterior rectal margin (R) is imaged on this section; (P) prostate; (B) bladder. **D:** Thirteen millimeters more posterior, the seminal vesicles (sv) are displayed immediately superior to the lateral fibers of the levator ani (la) contributed by the pubococcygeus muscle. The cephalic extent of the ischiorectal fossa (ir) is well displayed; (B) bladder; (sv) seminal vesicles; (R) rectum; (A) anus; (gf) gluteal fat.

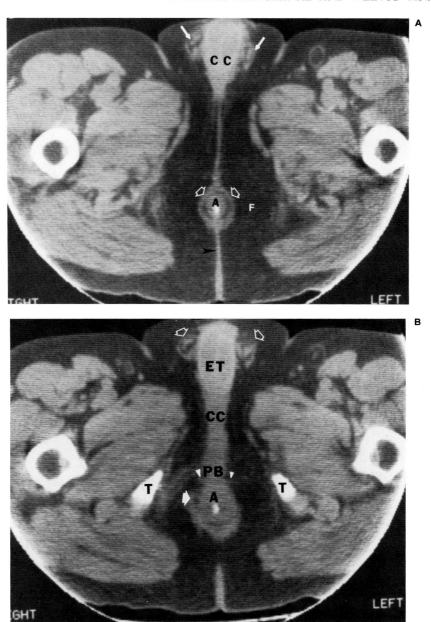

FIG. 55. Male perineum: central structures. **A:** In the perineum, the fat (F) within the ischiorectal fossa becomes continuous with the medial part of the thigh. The natal cleft (*arrowhead*) is traced to the anus (A) and surrounding anal sphincters (*open arrows*). Anteriorly, the erectile bodies of the penis (CC) are flanked by the spermatic cords (*arrows*). **B:** One centimeter cephalad, the ischial tuberosities (T) are identified. The contrast-containing anus (A) is supported by the levator ani muscle (*arrow*). The vertical structure anterior to the anus is made up of the three portions of the erectile tissues. The posterior portion is the bulb of the penis (PB). The narrower portions are the cavernous bodies (CC). The anterior part (ET) is compared of all three bodies. The superficial transverse perineal muscle (*small arrowheads*) is present just anterior to the anus; (*open arrows*) spermatic cords.

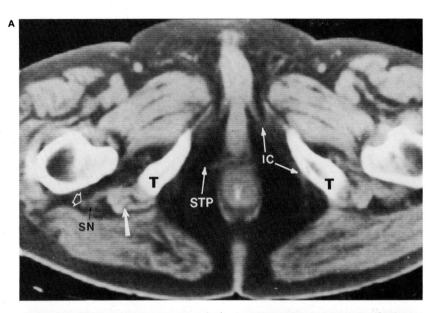

FIG. 56. Male perineum: musculoskeletal and neurovascular landmarks. **A:** The tendons of the semimembranous, semitendinous, and biceps femoris muscles (*arrow*) form a bulky attachment lateral to the ischial tuberosities (T). The sciatic nerve (SN) and inferior gluteal vessels (*open arrow*) are imaged lateral to this attachment. More anteriorly, the slender ischiocavernous muscles (IC) course anteriorly to ensheath the crus of the penis; (STP) superficial transverse perineal muscle. **B:** One centimeter caudal, the curved tendons of the gracilis muscles (*curved arrows*) identify the level of the perineum. The large fatty cleft between the gluteus maximus (GM) and the adductors (AD) medial to the femur (F) contains the sciatic nerve (*arrow*), the semitendinous muscle (ST), and the tendon of the semimembranous muscle (*open arrow*). Anteriorly, between the sartorius muscle (SM) and the adductors is another fat cleft. It contains the femoral artery (1), vein (2), and nerve (3). The great saphenous vein (*arrow*) lies immediately anterior to the adductor longus muscle (ALM); (n) superficial inguinal node.

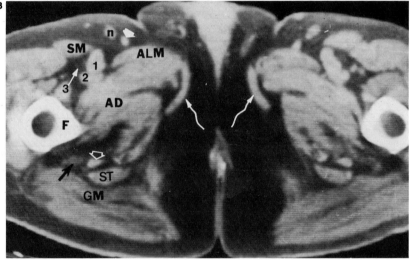

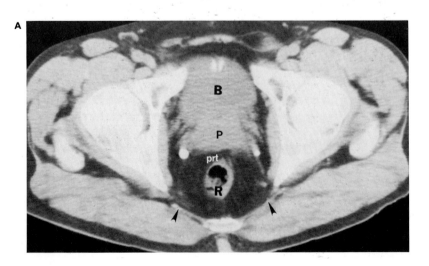

FIG. 57. Male pelvis: perirectal and ischiorectal spaces. **A:** The perirectal fat (prt) surrounds the rectum (R), separating it from the prostate (P), which lies in the perivesical space along with the bladder neck (B). Posteriorly lie the sacrospinous ligaments (*arrowheads*). This ligament separates the greater (cephalic) and lesser (caudal) foramina. Parts **B–E** on *facing page*.

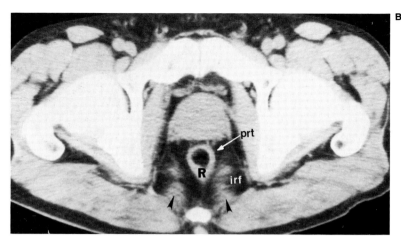

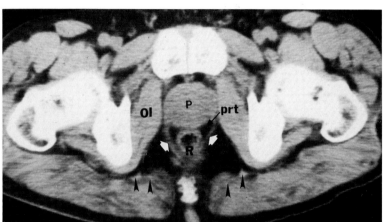

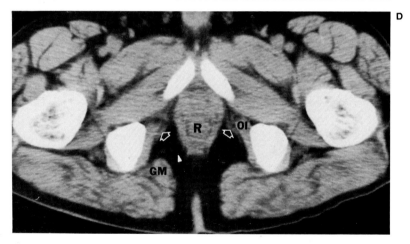

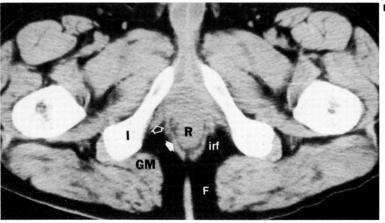

FIG. 57. (*Continued*.) Part **A** on *facing page*. **B:** One centimeter caudal, only the apex of the ischiorectal fossa (irf) is present just lateral to the fibers of the levator ani (*arrowheads*). The perirectal fat (prt) also increases in volume on cephalic sections; (R) rectum. **C:** One centimeter caudal, the area encompassed by the levator ani (*arrows*) widens as the more lateral fibers contributed by the pubococcygeus and iliococcygeus muscles are encountered. On the posterolateral border of the ischiorectal fossa lie the sacrotuberous ligaments (*arrowheads*), which attach on the ischial tuberosity; (P) prostate; (prt) perirectal space; (R) rectum; (OI) obturator internus muscle. **D:** One centimeter caudal, the internal pudendal vessels (*open arrows*) course within the pudendal canal superolaterally within the ischiorectal fossa. A small inferior rectal vessel (*small arrowhead*) traverses the fossa more posteriorly. The obturator internus muscle (OI) forms the lateral boundary of the fossa at this and all higher levels; (R) rectum. **E:** One centimeter caudal, an image through the ischium (I) shows the pyramidal ischiorectal fossa (irf) bounded by the pubrectalis muscle (*arrow*) medially, the ischiocavernosus muscle (*open arrow*) anteriorly, the ischial tuberosity (I) laterally, and the gluteus maximus (GM) muscle posterolaterally. Posteromedially it is continuous with the gluteal fat (F); (R) rectum.

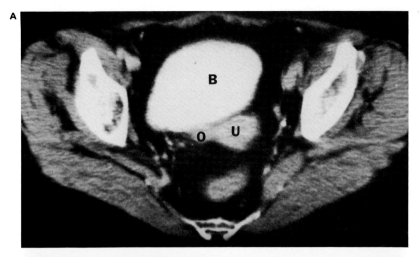

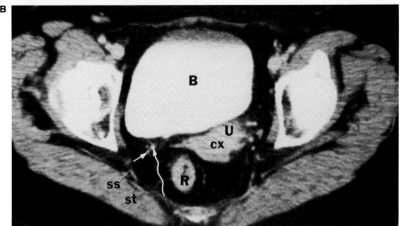

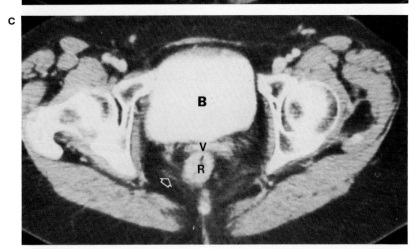

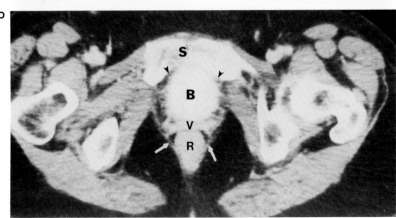

FIG. 58. Normal female pelvis. **A:** Two centimeters more cephalad is the uterine fundus (U). The right ovary (O) is imaged immediately behind the bladder (B). **B:** Two centimeters more caudal, the cervix (cx) and part of the uterine corpus (U) are imaged on the same section. A uterine vessel (*arrow*) lies just lateral to the distal ureter (*curved arrow*); (st) sacrotuberous ligament; (ss) sacrospinous ligament; (B) bladder; (R) rectum. **C:** Two centimeters caudal, fibers of the levator ani (*open arrow*) demarcate the superior extent of the ischiorectal fossa. The vaginal fornices (V) are asymmetric; this patient's uterus lies to the left of midline; (B) bladder. **D:** Two centimeters caudal, a section through the pubic symphysis (S) shows the bladder base (B), vagina (V), and rectum (R) enclosed by the levator ani muscle (*arrows*). A small retropubic fat space (*arrowheads*) is present, containing perivesical and uterovaginal venous plexuses.

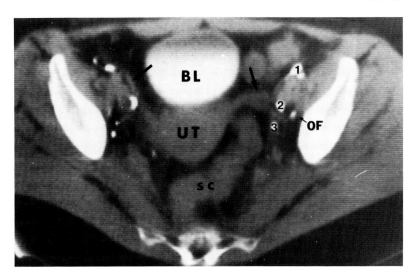

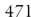

FIG. 59. Relationship of the uterus to normal lymphatics. On this image through the uterine fundus (UT), both round ligaments (*arrows*) are identified. There are three tiers of lymphatics that make up the external iliac system: (1) the lateral chain anterior to the external iliac vessels, (2) the middle chain just medial to the iliac vein, and (3) the medial chain, which is quite posterior. Note that the medial chain contains opacified nodes within fat, the obturator fossa (OF), which also contains the obturator vessels, and the obturator nerve; (sc) sigmoid colon.

FIG. 60. Parametrial tissues and associated ligaments. **A:** One centimeter cephalad, MR image through a normal cervix (CX) (TR = 500 msec, TE = 70 msec) shows the well-defined rectouterine folds (*arrows*). There is increased signal from the parametrial tissues (P) compared with muscle. Within this region is the lateral cervical (cardinal) ligament, within which courses a segment of the ureter (u); (B) bladder. **B:** One centimeter caudal, the parametrial fat (P) is shown lateral to the junction of the cervix (CX) with the vagina. The sacrospinous ligaments (*white arrows*) are evident posteriorly behind the rectum (R). The right rectouterine fold (*black arrow*) is demonstrated.

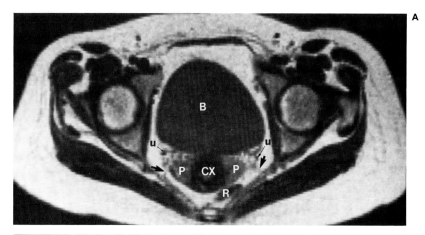

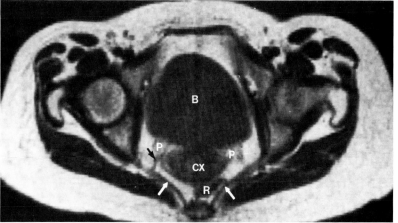

A,B

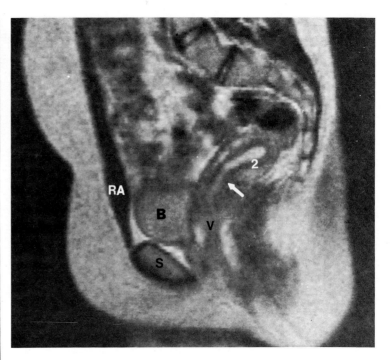

FIG. 61. A: Sagittal anatomy of the normal female pelvis. MR image (TR = 1,500 msec, TE = 70 msec) in a young woman shows the internal structure of the uterus. Intense signal is returned from the endometrial layer (1), which is surrounded by a low-intensity zone (2) reflecting a portion of the inner myometrium. An outer zone of intermediate intensity (3) corresponds to the remainder of the myometrium, a portion of which abuts the distended urinary bladder (B). The plane of this section passes through a portion of the long axis of the cervix and vagina. The central vaginal canal contains high-intensity mucus (*arrow*). **B:** Sagittal MR image in a subject with retroverted uterus (TR = 1,500 msec, TE = 70 msec) shows that the low-intensity myometrial zone (2) is continuous with a similar stripe in the cervix (*arrow*). The collapsed vaginal canal (V) is a cylindrical structure of intermediate intensity extending to the perineum; (S) symphysis pubis; (RA) rectus abdominus muscle.

a course similar to that of the vas deferens in males, ending as a fibrous cord in the labia majora. Near the attachment of the round ligament to the uterine body is the ovarian ligament and ovary. The ovaries are not closely tethered to the uterine corpus; however, they are most commonly seen in the ovarian fossa, which lies just medial to the obturator vessels and lateral to the uterine fundus near the round ligament. Finally, passing posterolaterally from the cervix are the uterosacral ligaments, which course immediately lateral to the perirectal fascia. Immediately caudal to the uterine cervix, the vagina courses in the midline to connect to the perineum. It is normally collapsed and is therefore difficult to distinguish on CT images from the periurethral tissues to which it is affixed. For this reason, a tampon usually is inserted in patients for whom determination of the anatomy of the cervicovaginal junction is important.

The complex anatomy of the female pelvis is not optimally examined in the transverse plane alone. Accordingly, ultrasound and MRI have been found to be useful in evaluating gynecologic conditions (30) (Fig. 61).

On sagittal images near the midline, T2-weighted MR images show the laminated uterine infrastructure. The deepest uterine layer is the endometrium, a high-intensity stripe approximately 5 mm in thickness. The most superficial layer is the myometrium, which has an intermediate intensity and is quite variable in thickness; in most young women it is 1 to 2 cm in breadth. Separating the two large zones is a transitional zone of low intensity measuring only a few millimeters in thickness. This has no clear anatomic correlate and may simply represent a zone of relatively high blood flow or compact myometrium.

Physiologic changes occur that alter the displayed anat-

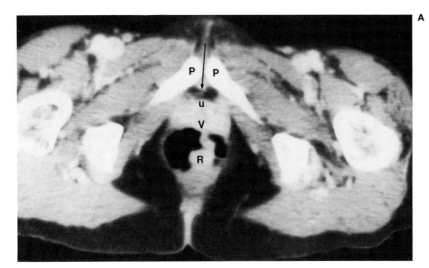

A

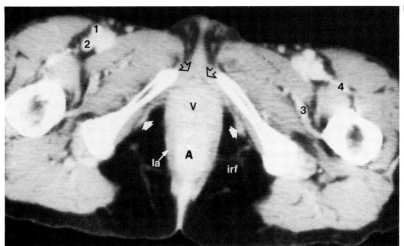

B

FIG. 62. Female perineum. **A:** The inferior rami of the pubis (P) approach the midline symphysis. Immediately posterior to their junction is a fatty triangle containing part of the perivesicular plexus (*arrow*). The enhanced urethral mucosa (u) is seen just anterior to the collapsed vagina (V). Gas and feces distend the rectum (R). **B:** One centimeter caudal, this postcontrast image allows recognition of the pudendal vessels (*arrows*) on the lateral margin of the ischiorectal fossa (irf) and the corpora cavernosa of the clitoris (*open arrows*). The femoral arteries have divided into superficial (1) and deep (2) portions. Parts of the medial (3) and lateral (4) circumflex vessels are demonstrated. There is also contrast enhancement of the mucosal surface of the anus (A) surrounded by the levator ani muscle (la). The vaginal canal (V) is collapsed.

omy of the uterine corpus; these are optimally displayed on MR images (28). The cervix is seen on sagittal images as a 3- to 4-cm cylindrical structure continuous with the uterine corpus. It passes posteroinferiorly to the bladder base. Lateral to the cervix are the parametria: zones of intermediate signal intensity that contain major uterine vessels. On axial sections, the low-intensity uterosacral ligaments are routinely observed (64).

Just caudal to the cervix is the vagina; behind the bladder base, it appears as symmetrical intermediate-intensity bands 5 to 10 mm in thickness. More caudally, the relatively higher intensity urethra is observed and lies anterior to the lower third of the vaginal canal.

The ovaries are generally identified in patients of reproductive age (19,20). On T2-weighted images, they are imaged as 2- to 3-cm oval structures of relatively high intensity. If they are displaced from the ovarian

fossa, they may be difficult to distinguish from the surrounding fat.

Female Perineum

Images obtained caudal to the pubic symphysis demonstrate the inverted-V appearance of the corpora cavernosa of the clitoris that parallel the inferior pubic ramus (Fig. 62). Posterior to the apex of these structures lie the urethra and, more posterior, the vagina. Perivaginal soft tissue extends posterolaterally into the ischiorectal fossa (Fig. 63) and contains the inferior rectal (hemorrhoidal) vessels. More caudal transaxial images will reveal the vaginal vestibule and glans clitoris immediately anterior to the anal sphincters.

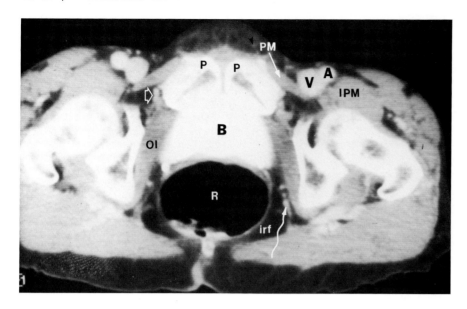

FIG. 63. Female pelvis: canals connecting the pelvis to the lower extremity. This section illustrates four major neurovascular canals: The femoral canal is marked by the femoral artery (A) and vein (V) lying anteromedial to the iliopsoas muscle (IPM) and anterolateral to the pectinus muscle (PM). The rudimentary inguinal canal is marked by the ligamentum teres uteri (round ligament) (*arrowhead*), which courses inferiorly to end in the labia. The obturator canal contains the obturator vessels (*open arrow*) and nerve lying anterolateral to the obturator internus muscle (OI). Posteriorly, along the lateral margin of the ischiorectal fossa (irf) is the pudendal canal, here marked by the pudendal vessels (*curved arrow*); (R) rectum.

REFERENCES

1. Allen KS, Siskind BN, Burrell MI. Perforation of distal esophagus with lesser sac extension: CT demonstration. *J Comput Assist Tomogr* 1986;10(4):612–614.
2. Anda S, Roysland P, Fougner R, Stovring J. CT appearance of the diaphragm varying with respiratory phase and muscular tension. *J Comput Assist Tomogr* 1986;10(5):744–745.
3. Auh YH, Rosen A, Rubenstein WA, Engel IA, Whalen JP, Kazam E. CT of the papillary process of the caudate lobe of the liver. *AJR* 1984;142:535–538.
4. Auh YH, Rubenstein WA, Markisz JA, Zirinsky K, Whalen JP, Kazam E. Intraperitoneal paravesical spaces: CT delineation with US correlation. *Radiology* 1986;159:311–317.
5. Auh YH, Rubenstein WA, Schneider M, Reckler JM, Whalen JP, Kazam E. Extraperitoneal paravesical spaces: CT delineation with US correlation. *Radiology* 1986;159:319–328.
6. Auh YH, Rubenstein WA, Zirinsky K, et al. Accessory fissures of the liver: CT and sonographic appearance. *AJR* 1984;143:565–572.
7. Baker ME, Weinecht JL, Andriani RT, Cohan RH, Dunnick NR. Lumbar hernia: diagnosis by CT. *AJR* 1987;148:565–567.
8. Balfe DM, Mauro MA, Koehler RE, et al. Gastrohepatic ligament: normal and pathologic CT anatomy. *Radiology* 1984;150:485–490.
9. Bismuth H, Houssin D, Castaing D. Major and minor segmentectomies "Reglees" in liver surgery. *World J Surg* 1982;6:10–24.
10. Boijsen E, Lin G. Lateral displacement of the right kidney by the ascending colon. *J Comput Assist Tomogr* 1983;7(2):344–346.
11. Bryan PJ, Butler HE, Nelson AD, et al. Magnetic resonance imaging of the prostate. *AJR* 1986;146:543–548.
12. Buonocore E, Hesemann C, Pavlicek W, Montie JE. Clinical and in vitro magnetic resonance imaging of prostatic carcinoma. *AJR* 1984;143:1267–1272.
13. Butch RJ, Stark DD, Wittenberg J, et al. Staging rectal cancer by MR and CT. *AJR* 1986;146:1155–1160.
14. Cooper C, Jeffrey RB, Silverman PM, Federle MP, Chun GH. Computed tomography of omental pathology. *J Comput Assist Tomogr* 1986;10(1):62–66.
15. Crass JR, Maile CW, Frick MP. Catheter drainage of the left posterior subphrenic space: a reliable percutaneous approach. *Gastrointest Radiol* 1985;10:397–398.
16. Cubillo E. Obturator hernia diagnosed by computed tomography. *AJR* 1983;140:735–736.
17. Dodds WJ, Darweesh RMA, Lawson TL, et al. The retroperitoneal spaces revisited. *AJR* 1986;147:1155–1161.
18. Dodds WJ, Foley WD, Lawson TL, Stewart ET, Taylor A. Anatomy and imaging of the lesser peritoneal sac. *AJR* 1985;144:567–575.
19. Dooms GC, Hricak H, Tscholakoff D. Adnexal structures: MR imaging. *Radiology* 1986;158:639–646.
20. Fekuda T, Ikeuchi M, Hashimoto H, et al. Computed tomography of ovarian masses. *J Comput Assist Tomogr* 1986;10(6):990–996.
21. Fried AM, Kreel L, Cosgrove DO. The hepatic interlobar fissure: combined in vitro and in vivo study. *AJR* 1984;143:561–564.
22. Gale ME. Anterior diaphragm: variations in the CT appearance. *Radiology* 1986;161:635–639.
23. Gebarski KS, Gebarski SS, Glazer GM, Samuels BI, Francis IR. The lumbosacral plexus: anatomic-radiologic-pathologic correlation using CT. *RadioGraphics* 1986;6(3):401–425.
24. Gerzof SG, Johnson WC, Robbins AH, Spechler SJ, Nabseth DC. Percutaneous drainage of infected pancreatic pseudocysts. *Arch Surg* 1984;119:888–893.
25. Grabbe E, Lierse W, Winkler R. The perirectal fascia: morphology and use in staging of rectal carcinoma. *Radiology* 1983;149:241–246.
26. Guillaumin E, Jeffrey RB, Shea WJ, Ashing CW, Goldberg HI. Perirectal inflammatory disease: CT findings. *Radiology* 1986;161:153–157.
27. Halvorsen RA, Jones MA, Rice RP, Thompson WM. Anterior left subphrenic abscess: characteristic plain film and CT appearance. *AJR* 1982;139:283–289.
28. Haynor DR, Mack LA, Soules MR, Shuman WP, Montana MA, Moss AA. Changing appearance of the normal uterus during the menstrual cycle: MR studies. *Radiology* 1986;161:459–462.
29. Hopper KD, Sherman JL, Luethke JM, Ghaed N. The retrorenal colon in the supine and prone patient. *Radiology* 1987;162:443–446.
30. Hricak H. MRI of the female pelvis: a review. *AJR* 1986;146:1115–1122.
31. Hricak H, Dooms GC, McNeal JE, et al. MR imaging of the prostate gland: normal anatomy. *AJR* 1987;148:51–58.
32. James S, Balfe DM, Lee JKT, Picus D. Small bowel disease: categorization by CT examination. *AJR* 1987;148:863–868.
33. Jeffrey RB, Federle MP, Goodman PC. Computed tomography of the lesser peritoneal sac. *Radiology* 1981;141:117–122.
34. Kuhns LR, Borlaza GS, Seigel R, Cho KJ. Localization of the head of the pancreas using the junction of the left renal vein and the inferior vena cava. *J Comput Assist Tomogr* 1978;2:170–172.
35. Kunin M. Bridging septa of the perinephric space: anatomic, pathologic, and diagnostic considerations. *Radiology* 1986;158:361–365.
36. Lanzieri CF, Hilal SK. Computed tomography of the sacral plexus and sciatic nerve in the greater sciatic foramen. *AJR* 1984;143:165–168.
37. Ling D, Lee JKT, Heiken JP, Balfe DM, Glazer HS, McClennan BL. Prostatic carcinoma and benign prostatic hyperplasia: inability

of MR imaging to distinguish between the two diseases. *Radiology* 1986;158:103–107.

38. Love L, Demos TC, Posniak H. CT of retrorenal fluid collections. *AJR* 1985;145:87–91.
39. Love L, Meyers MA, Churchill RJ, Reynes CJ, Moncada R, Gibson D. Computed tomography of extraperitoneal spaces. *AJR* 1981;136:781–789.
40. Marks WM, Collen PW. Gastroesophageal region: source of confusion on CT. *AJR* 1981;136:359–362.
41. Megibow AJ, Wagner AG. Obturator hernia. *J Comput Assist Tomogr* 1983;7(2):350–352.
42. Meziane MA, Fishman EK, Siegelman SS. Computed tomographic diagnosis of obturator foramen hernia. *Gastrointest Radiol* 1983;8:375–377.
43. Mitty HA, Cohen BA, Sprayregen S, Schwartz K. Adrenal pseudotumors on CT due to dilated portosystemic veins. *AJR* 1983;141:727–730.
44. Mueller PR, Ferrucci JT Jr, Simeone JF, et al. Lesser sac abscesses and fluid collections: drainage by transhepatic approach. *Radiology* 1985;155:615–618.
45. Nunez D, Yrizarry JM, Russell E, et al. Transgastric drainage of pancreatic fluid collections. *AJR* 1985;145:815–818.
46. Pagani JJ. Intrahepatic vascular territories shown by computed tomography. *Radiology* 1983;147:173–178.
47. Pech P, Haughton V. A correlative CT and anatomic study of the sciatic nerve. *AJR* 1985;144:1037–1041.
48. Poon PY, McCallum RW, Henkelman MM, et al. Magnetic resonance imaging of the prostate. *Radiology* 1985;154:143–149.
49. Pozniak M, Petasnick JP, Matalona TAS, Bayard WJ. Computed tomography in the differential diagnosis of pelvic and extrapelvic disease. *RadioGraphics* 1985;5(4):587–610.
50. Raptopoulos V, Kleinman PK, Marks S, Snyder M, Silverman PM. Renal fascial pathway: posterior extension of pancreatic effusions within the anterior pararenal space. *Radiology* 1986;158:367–374.
51. Rubenstein WA, Auh YH, Whalen JP, Kazam E. The perihepatic spaces: computed tomographic and ultrasound imaging. *Radiology* 1983;149:231–239.
52. Rubenstein WA, Auh YH, Zirinsky K, Kneeland JB, Whalen JP, Kazam E. Posterior peritoneal recesses: assessment using CT. *Radiology* 1985;156:461–468.
53. Schwartz AN, Goiney RC, Graney DO. Gastric diverticulum simulating an adrenal mass: CT appearance and embryogenesis. *AJR* 1986;146:553–554.
54. Sexton CC, Zeman RK. Correlation of computed tomography, sonography, and gross anatomy of the liver. *AJR* 1983;141:711–718.
55. Shapir J, Rubin J. CT appearance of the inferior mesenteric vein. *J Comput Assist Tomogr* 1984;8(5):877–880.
56. Sherman JL, Hopper KD, Greene AJ, Johns TT. The retrorenal colon on computed tomography: a normal variant. *J Comput Assist Tomogr* 1985;9(2):339–341.
57. Shin MS, Berland LL. Computed tomography of retrocrural spaces: normal, anatomic variants, and pathologic conditions. *AJR* 1985;145:81–86.
58. Silverman PM. Gastric diverticulum mimicking adrenal mass: CT demonstration. *J Comput Assist Tomogr* 1986;10(4):709–711.
59. Silverman PM, Kelvin FM, Korobkin M. Lateral displacement of the right kidney by the colon: an anatomic variation demonstrated on CT. *AJR* 1983;140:313–314.
60. Sommer FG, McNeal JE, Carrol CL. MR depiction of zonal anatomy of the prostate at 1.5 T. *J Comput Assist Tomogr* 1986;10(6):983–989.
61. Somogyi J, Cohen WN, Omar MM, Makhuli Z. Communication of right and left perirenal spaces demonstrated by computed tomography. *J Comput Assist Tomogr* 1979;3(2):270–273.
62. Thompson WM, Halvorsen RA, Williford ME, Foster WL Jr, Korobkin M. Computed tomography of the gastroesophageal junction. *RadioGraphics* 1982;2:179–193.
63. Tisnado J, Amendola MA, Walsh JW, Jordan RL, Turner MA, Krempa J. Computed tomography of the perineum. *AJR* 1981;136:475–481.
64. Togashi K, Nishimura K, Itoh K, et al. Uterine cervical cancer: assessment with high-field MR imaging. *Radiology* 1986;160:431–435.
65. Van Dyke JA, Holley HC, Anderson SD. Review of iliopsoas anatomy and pathology. *RadioGraphics* 1987;7:53–84.
66. Vibhakar SD, Bellon EM. The bare area of the spleen: a constant CT feature of the ascitic abdomen. *AJR* 1984;141:953–955.
67. Vick CW, Walsh JW, Wheelock JB, Brewer WH. Computed tomographic evaluation of parametrial extension from cervical cancer. *RadioGraphics* 1984;4(5):787–799.
68. Vick CW, Walsh JW, Wheelock JB, Brewer WH. CT of the normal and abnormal parametria in cervical cancer. *AJR* 1984;143:597–603.
69. Vincent LM, Mauro MA, Mittelstaedt CA. The lesser sac and gastrohepatic recess: sonographic appearance and differentiation of fluid collections. *Radiology* 1984;150:515–519.
70. Wechsler RJ, Schilling JF. CT of the gluteal region. *AJR* 1985;144:185–190.
71. Weinstein JB, Heiken JP, Lee JKT, et al. High resolution CT of the porta hepatis and hepatoduodenal ligament. *RadioGraphics* 1986;6(1):55–74.
72. Zirinsky K, Auh YH, Rubenstein WA, Kneeland JB, Whalen JP, Kazam E. The portacaval space: CT with MR correlation. *Radiology* 1985;156:453–460.
73. Langman J. *Medical Embryology*. 2nd ed. Baltimore: Williams & Wilkins, 1969.
74. Gardner G, Gray DJ, O'Rahilly R (eds.). *Anatomy*. 3rd ed. Philadelphia: WB Saunders, 1969.
75. Davies DV (ed.). *Gray's Anatomy*. 34th ed. London: Longmans, Green, 1967.

CHAPTER 12

Gastrointestinal Tract

Robert E. Koehler, Dennis M. Balfe, and Robert J. Stanley

Barium examination and endoscopy are the proven, time-honored primary diagnostic methods for evaluating gastrointestinal diseases. Recently, however, CT has made many contributions to the study of the gastrointestinal tract, and it is becoming an essential addition to radiological evaluation of the gastrointestinal tract. Barium studies and endoscopy both essentially are limited to examination of the surface, caliber, and contour of the bowel lumen and can provide only indirect information regarding intramural or extrinsic abnormalities. They remain the methods of choice for the initial detection of most alimentary tract disease. Although CT can also be used to evaluate the lumen, its major contribution consists of directly demonstrating the bowel wall and the adjacent tissues and organs. Being distinctly better than barium "luminography" for assessment of extraluminal abnormalities, CT is particularly useful (18) in (a) staging gastrointestinal neoplasms for planning treatment, (b) detecting and staging postoperative gastrointestinal tumor recurrence, (c) assessing tumor response to therapy, (d) evaluating possible causes for gastrointestinal organ displacement, (e) clarifying intramural and extrinsic impressions detected by barium studies or endoscopy, and (f) evaluating palpable abdominal masses.

A uniform CT staging system has been proposed for primary alimentary tract tumors and their recurrences (71):

Stage 1: Intraluminal mass without wall thickening
Stage 2: Wall thickening (focal or diffuse), with no extramural tumor extension
Stage 3: Wall thickening, with contiguous spread to adjacent tissue, with or without regional lymph node involvement
Stage 4: Distant metastatic spread

In general, stage-1 and stage-2 lesions are resectable for cure, and CT outlines the precise location and size of the tumor. Stage-3 and stage-4 lesions are unresectable for cure, and CT is used by radiation therapists for treatment planning.

Additionally, knowledge of the CT appearance of the normal alimentary tract allows discovery of previously unsuspected gastrointestinal abnormalities on images performed for other reasons. The images of the bowel loops on CT studies should be carefully evaluated, as well as the specific organs in question. Familiarity with the position, shape, and density of the normal gastrointestinal tract and its many anatomic variations seen on CT is important so as not to mistake them for masses or other abnormalities. Attention to the technique of opacifying the bowel lumen with oral contrast material is essential in dealing with the variable and ever-changing morphology of the alimentary tract. Many interpretive errors stem from lack of care in distinguishing between normal bowel and presumed intraabdominal abnormalities. A discussion of various methods for opacifying each segment of the gastrointestinal tract is given in Chapter 3, and selected comments on bowel opacification are also offered in appropriate sections of this chapter.

ESOPHAGUS

Normal Anatomy

The esophagus usually is well seen on CT images throughout its course. In all but very thin or emaciated individuals, the paraesophageal fat is visible as an interface between the esophagus and adjacent connective tissue, vascular, and cardiac structures. The cervical portion of the esophagus lies near the midline, posterior to the trachea (Fig. 1). The cervical esophagus usually does not

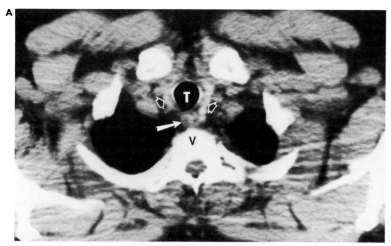

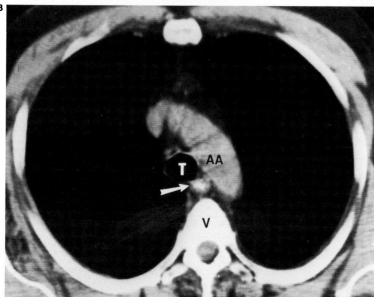

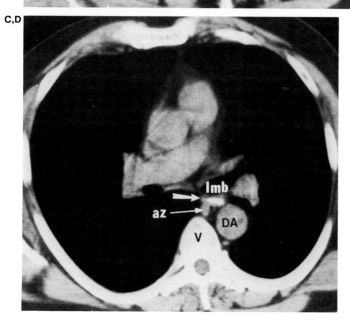

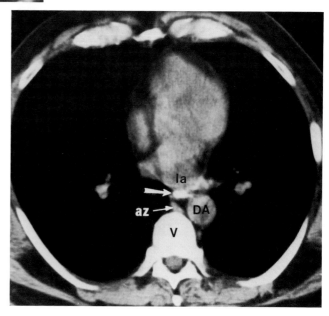

FIG. 1. Normal anatomy of intrathoracic esophagus. **A:** At the level of the thoracic inlet, the esophagus (*arrow*) occupies a relatively narrow space immediately anterior to the thoracic vertebra (V) and posterior to the trachea (T). Anterolateral to the esophageal lumen, the high-density inferior poles of the thyroid (*open arrows*) are observed. **B:** The aortic arch (AA) crosses the anterolateral surface of the barium-filled esophagus (*arrow*) on the left, and the trachea (T) lies anterior and to the right on this section. **C:** Just inferior to the carina, the esophagus (*arrow*) is abutted by the azygos vein (az) posteriorly and the descending aorta (DA) posterolaterally. The anterior surface of the esophagus contacts a long segment of the left mainstem bronchus (lmb) on this section. **D:** The left atrium (la) occupies a position immediately anterior to the distal esophagus (*arrow*); the aorta (DA) generally remains on its left posterolateral aspect.

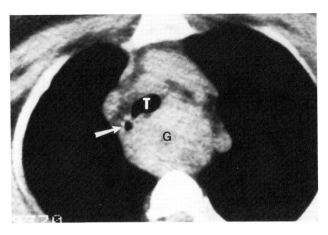

FIG. 2. Anterolateral deviation of the esophagus (*arrow*) and trachea caused by a very large goiter (G).

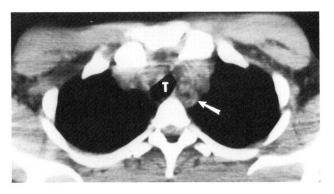

FIG. 3. Marked thickening of the esophageal wall (*arrow*) due to diffuse esophageal candidiasis in a patient with AIDS; (T) trachea.

contain air on CT images performed in the supine position. At the thoracic inlet, the esophagus lies posterior and slightly to the left of the trachea, and the fat between these two structures often is thin and invisible. Occasionally the esophagus is more lateral than usual and lies directly to the left of the trachea (13). More caudally, the esophagus is intimately related to the posterior surface of the left mainstem bronchus, separated from it by a fat plane. The esophagus pierces the diaphragm anterior to the aorta and to the left of the midline. Deviation of the esophagus from its normal course can occur whenever any of the organs adjacent to it become enlarged (Fig. 2).

Small amounts of gas are present in the thoracic esophagus in about 65% of normal patients (40). The presence of a fluid level, a fluid-filled lumen, or a luminal diameter greater than 10 mm is unusual and generally indicates the presence of an obstruction or marked esophageal dysmotility. The wall of the esophagus can easily be measured when there is either air or orally administered contrast material in the lumen. The thickness of the normal esophageal wall varies with the degree of distension. A thickness greater than 3 mm usually is abnormal when the lumen is well distended (Fig. 3). When there is a question whether or not the esophageal wall is thickened, an effervescent agent can be given orally in a small amount of water to induce esophageal distension.

It is not uncommon to see either a fat- or soft-tissue-density structure in the chest just above the esophageal hiatus, representing herniated abdominal fat or gastric cardia, respectively (Fig. 4). If such a mass causes confusion, but is thought likely to represent a hiatus hernia, a few swallows of oral contrast material can be given before rescanning to opacify the herniated stomach (Fig. 5). When there is a need to see the esophageal lumen, such as when evaluating an obstruction, a tumor, or the esophageal wall thickness, a swallow of 2% barium suspension (Esopho-CAT) given just before each image may be helpful.

Pathology

Neoplasia

The major use of CT in studying the esophagus is to evaluate known esophageal carcinoma. CT yields information on tumor size, extension, and resectability that previously could be obtained only at thoracotomy. The CT findings of carcinoma of the esophagus may include (a) an intraluminal mass (Fig. 6), (b) esophageal wall thickening, often sufficient to cause a soft-tissue mass (Fig. 7), (c) dilatation of the lumen, with or without a fluid level proximal to an obstructing tumor (Fig. 8A), (d) obliteration of the fat between the esophagus and adjacent

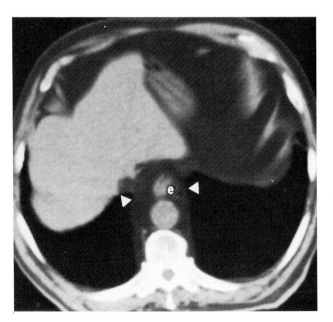

FIG. 4. In this asymptomatic patient, abdominal fat (*arrowheads*) has herniated through the abdominal hiatus to surround the distal esophagus (e).

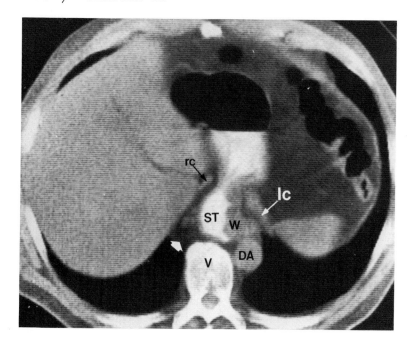

FIG. 5. Hiatal hernia. A portion of the stomach (ST), accompanied by abdominal fat (*arrow*), has herniated into the thorax through the hiatus. There is apparent thickening of the left lateral wall (W) of the intrahiatal stomach; this thickening is due to lack of distension; (rc) right diaphragmatic crus; (lc) left diaphragmatic crus; (DA) descending aorta; (V) vertebral body.

structures, such as the pericardium or aorta (Fig. 9), (e) a sinus tract or fistula to the tracheobronchial tree, (f) an irregular or eccentric lumen, and (g) metastatic disease, especially enlargement of mediastinal, retrocrural, left gastric, or celiac lymph nodes, or low-density masses in the liver (81) (Figs. 8 and 9).

Although esophagography and endoscopy remain the primary methods for the initial discovery of esophageal neoplasms, a few stage-2 carcinomas have been detected by CT in patients being imaged for other reasons. Because esophageal carcinoma usually is advanced at the time of detection, CT findings are abnormal in virtually all patients, most showing a soft-tissue mass or focal wall thickening, with an eccentric lumen. Most errors in interpretation occur in cachectic patients and in those who have had previous mediastinal surgery or radiation. Severely cachectic individuals often lack the normal fat planes around the esophagus, and surgery or radiation can alter the density of these fat planes. In all of these situations it can be difficult or impossible to be accurate in CT assessment of local mediastinal invasion of esophageal carcinoma.

The efficacy of CT in staging esophageal carcinoma is at present somewhat controversial (42,81,85,97). CT appears to be a sensitive indicator of the presence of metastatic spread to the liver and of direct invasion of the tracheobronchial tree, with an accuracy of 90% to 100% reported for each. Invasion of the descending aorta by esophageal carcinoma is somewhat more difficult to detect and has a reported accuracy of 55% to 90%. The difficulty in this area is primarily related to the fact that the esophagus normally lies in contact with the aorta in many thin patients, with no visible fat between the two structures. Thus, visualization on CT of a continuous plane of fat between tumor and aorta has proved to be a reliable in-

dicator of absence of aortic invasion, but the absence of such a plane does not reliably predict tumor invasion.

A helpful method (81) for CT assessment of the likelihood of aortic invasion by esophageal carcinoma has been described. Considering the cross section of the descending aorta as a 360° circle, the arc over which the periaortic fat is obscured by contact with the tumor can be expressed in degrees. In one study of 30 patients, aortic invasion was found in 4 of 5 patients (80%) in whom periaortic fat was obscured around 90° or more of the esophagus, and invasion was found in none of 20 patients with less than 45° of obscuration. Five patients with 60°

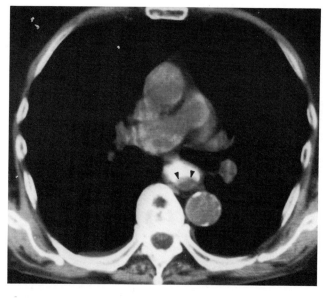

FIG. 6. Esophageal adenocarcinoma, arising in a patient with Barrett esophagus, is depicted as a discrete, chiefly intraluminal mass (*arrowheads*), with no appreciable extramural extension.

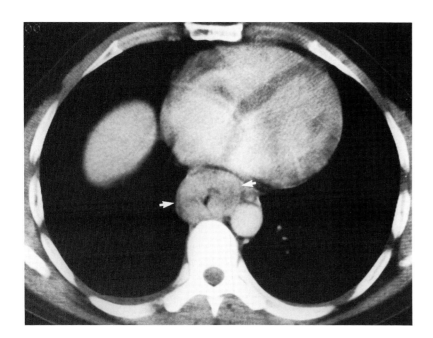

FIG. 7. Esophageal cancer. Note the marked concentric thickening of the esophageal wall (*arrows*), with concomitant luminal narrowing.

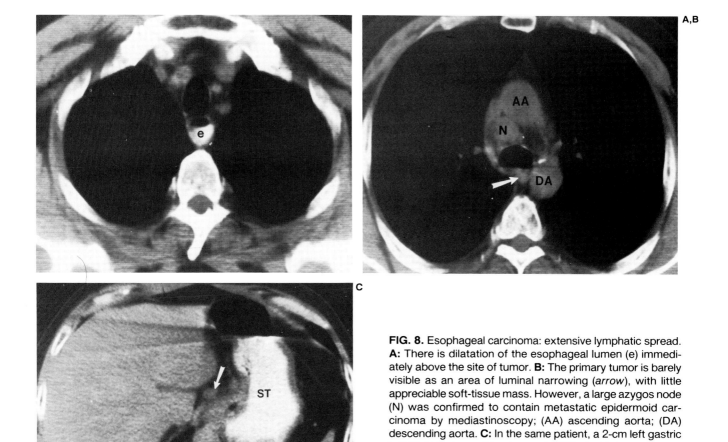

FIG. 8. Esophageal carcinoma: extensive lymphatic spread. **A:** There is dilatation of the esophageal lumen (e) immediately above the site of tumor. **B:** The primary tumor is barely visible as an area of luminal narrowing (*arrow*), with little appreciable soft-tissue mass. However, a large azygos node (N) was confirmed to contain metastatic epidermoid carcinoma by mediastinoscopy; (AA) ascending aorta; (DA) descending aorta. **C:** In the same patient, a 2-cm left gastric lymph node (*arrow*) is observed; (ST) stomach.

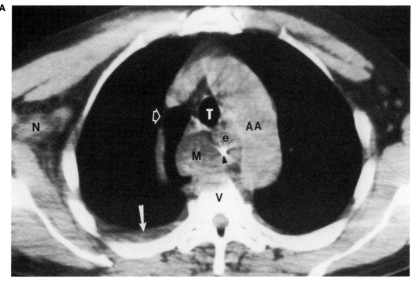

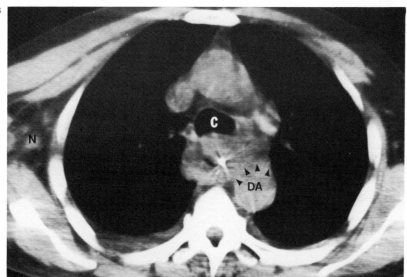

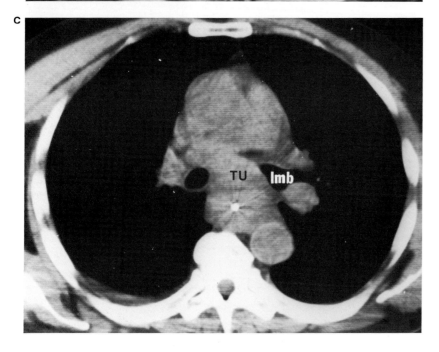

FIG. 9. Esophageal carcinoma: extensive local spread. **A:** There is marked eccentric wall thickening (M) of the proximal esophagus (e), producing displacement of a nasogastric tube within its lumen (*arrowhead*). The tumor has invaded posteriorly to involve the anterior vertebral body (V). There is also invasion of the right pleural space, producing an effusion (*arrow*). An azygos fissure (*open arrow*) is incidentally noted. Note metastatic axillary lymph nodes (N); (T) trachea; (AA) aortic arch. **B:** At the level of the carina (C), there is infiltration of the mediastinal fat on the left of the tumor. The fat plane between the descending aorta (DA) and adjacent mass has been obscured over approximately 90% of the aortic circumference (*arrowheads*), strongly suggesting aortic invasion; (N) axillary lymph nodes. **C:** The tumor (TU) bulges into the lumen of the left mainstem bronchus (lmb), distorting its contour. Tracheobronchial invasion was confirmed endoscopically.

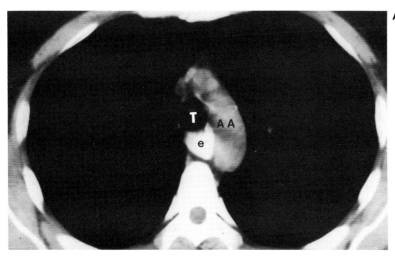

A

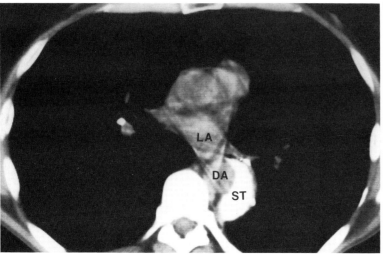

B

FIG. 10. Normal appearance after esophagogastrectomy for midesophageal carcinoma. **A:** Section at the level of the aortic arch (AA) demonstrates dilatation of the esophagus (e) immediately above the esophagogastric anastomosis; (T) trachea. **B:** The lumen of the proximal stomach (ST) is compressed by adjacent mediastinal structures, including the left atrium (LA) and descending aorta (DA).

to 75° of the aortic circumference obscured were considered indeterminate.

Least accurate of all CT assessments has been prediction of involvement of mediastinal lymph nodes. This is not surprising, because of the high frequency with which mediastinal lymph nodes of normal size are removed at the time of esophagogastrectomy, only to be found to contain microscopically visible tumor on histologic examination. CT is more useful in detecting intraabdominal lymph node involvement in patients with esophageal carcinoma, but even here the reported accuracy ranges from 75% to 85%.

Follow-up of patients treated with radiation therapy may be accomplished using CT imaging. Recurrent neoplasms may affect the mediastinal or subdiaphragmatic lymph nodes, as well as the gastric wall.

CT is useful in assessing problems that can arise after esophagogastrectomy (39,43) (Fig. 10). Standard esophagography utilizing barium or water-soluble contrast material is preferred for detection of local anastomotic recurrence (Fig. 11) or anastomotic leak (Fig. 12), but even this latter complication occasionally is detected on CT when not seen on conventional radiography following oral

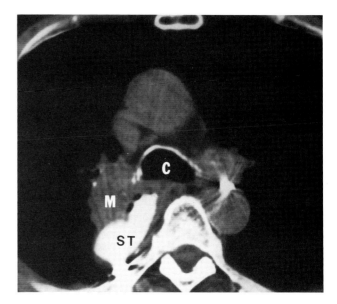

FIG. 11. Recurrent carcinoma following esophagogastrectomy. At the proximal anastomoses, the stomach (ST) normally lies to the right of the midline (ST). Immediately anterior to the stomach is a large soft-tissue mass (M) that subsequently proved to be a local recurrence; (C) carina.

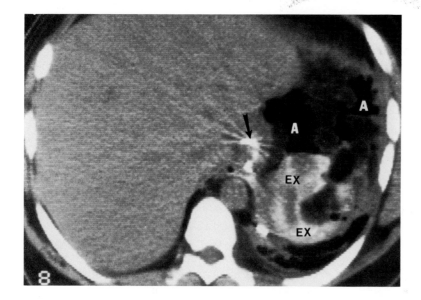

FIG. 12. Anastomotic leak following esophago-gastrectomy. CT section shows subphrenic gas (A) and dilute extravasated contrast material (EX) within an irregular subphrenic cavity. This leak was not recognized on a standard water-soluble esophagogram; (*arrow*) nasogastric tube in gastric lumen.

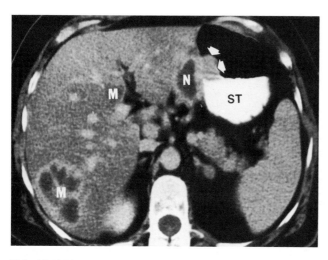

FIG. 13. Widespread recurrence after esophagogastrectomy. Section through the upper abdomen in a patient 6 months after esophageal resection shows recurrent disease in the gastric wall (*arrows*), in low-attenuation gastrohepatic lymph nodes (N), and metastates to the liver (M); (ST) stomach.

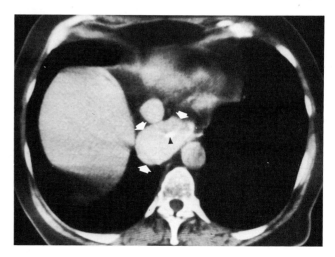

FIG. 14. Large multilobed leiomyoma (*arrows*) surrounds the esophageal lumen (*arrowhead*), producing eccentric wall thickening.

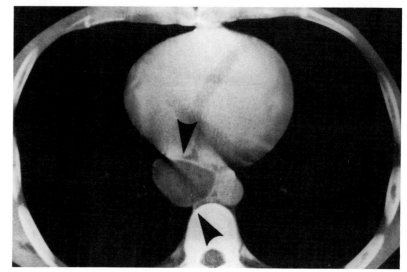

FIG. 15. Esophageal duplication cyst (*arrowheads*). Note thin smooth wall and near-water-density contents.

administration of contrast material. The real strength of CT in this setting is in detecting recurrent tumor in the adjacent mediastinum or upper abdominal lymph nodes, liver, and adrenals (Fig. 13).

Benign tumors of the esophagus may appear as intraluminal masses, focal areas of wall thickening, or discrete mediastinal masses. Most are leiomyomas and are spherical or ovoid in shape. They are of soft-tissue density and tend to be well marginated, showing no disruption of the surrounding fat (Fig. 14). Differentiation from a malignant neoplasm is not always possible. Esophageal duplication cysts appear as well-marginated, usually near-water-density spherical masses contiguous with the esophagus, with preserved surrounding fat planes (Fig. 15).

Miscellaneous Abnormalities

Varices appear as lobulated or rounded tubular densities in the distal paraesophageal and perigastric locations, especially just anterior to the esophagus as it passes through the diaphragm (Fig. 16). Serial images during an intravenous bolus of contrast material are helpful in distinguishing between varices, which are enhanced, and enlarged lymph nodes or neoplasia (14,47). When varices are suspected, careful attention should be directed toward the CT appearances of the coronary vein, splenic hilar veins, umbilical vein, and other potential portosystemic collaterals. The sizes and shapes of the liver and spleen may also give clues to the presence of cirrhosis and portal hypertension.

Striking abnormalities of the esophagus and adjacent mediastinum are visible on CT images from patients who have recently undergone endoscopic sclerotherapy for

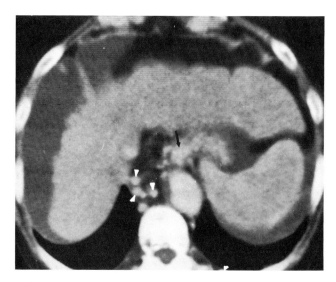

FIG. 16. Varices. Image after bolus injection of contrast material demonstrates serpentine contrast-containing tubular structures in the wall of the esophagus (*arrow*) and in dilated lesser omental collaterals (*arrowheads*). Note ascites and nodular liver surface, compatible with advanced cirrhosis.

esophageal varices (41,63). Characteristically, the wall of the lower esophagus is thickened, with a low-attenuation band of inflamed, edematous tissue between the higher-intensity inner mucosal layer and the outer muscular layer. There may be edema or effusion of the adjacent mediastinum, which can displace adjacent structures (Fig. 17). The fibrosis that results from repeated sclerotherapy for the esophagus lessens the severity of these CT abnormalities.

Esophagitis of a variety of types can cause abnormalities visible on CT (63,86). Mild-to-moderate thickening of the esophageal wall can be seen in reflux esophagitis and in moniliasis (Fig. 3). Marked esophageal thickening has been reported in esophageal intramural pseudodiverticulosis (80). Esophageal perforation may result in infected mediastinal and pleural collections containing gas and fluid.

STOMACH

Technique and Anatomy

The stomach is a distensible organ. When it is collapsed, its rugal folds become pleated and obscure the gastric lumen. Optimal examination of the stomach wall, therefore, necessitates luminal distension (Fig. 18). Most patients undergoing abdominal CT have already been given several hundred milliliters of dilute oral contrast material. An additional 200 to 300 ml of contrast material should be given orally as the imaging begins to ensure adequate gastric distension. The rate of gastric emptying varies considerably from individual to individual, and food retained in the gastric lumen may simulate a neoplasm. Therefore, when the stomach is known to be one of the organs of interest, it is useful to withhold solid food after midnight on the day preceding the examination.

The most frequent problem encountered in performing gastric CT is differentiating between pathologic wall thickening and a focal area of incomplete distension. For this purpose, gas-producing agents are practical means to achieve rapid expansion of the lumen. Rotating the patient until the segment of interest is nondependent will achieve the maximum degree of distension. Gas may be prevented from rapidly exiting the stomach by administering 0.5 mg of glucagon intravenously or 1.0 mg intramuscularly.

Examining the postoperative stomach requires techniques similar to those used in standard upper gastrointestinal studies: After the patient drinks a cup of dilute contrast material, 0.5 mg of glucagon is administered intravenously along with gas-producing granules, and the patient is slowly turned over his right side to the prone position, then over his left side to supine posture. This maneuver fills the afferent loop of a Billroth II or the proximal limb of a standard Whipple anastomosis in the majority of cases. Failure to fill these structures with air

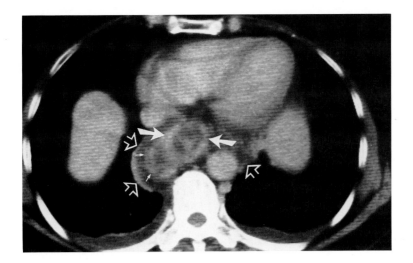

FIG. 17. Effect of variceal sclerotherapy. Postendoscopic esophageal sclerotherapy image shows enhancement of the esophageal wall (*large white arrows*). A mediastinal effusion (*open arrows*) bulges to the right; within it, there are regions of higher attenuation (*small white arrows*). Note bilateral pleural effusions. (Courtesy of Dr. Matthew Mauro, Chapel Hill, North Carolina.)

A,B

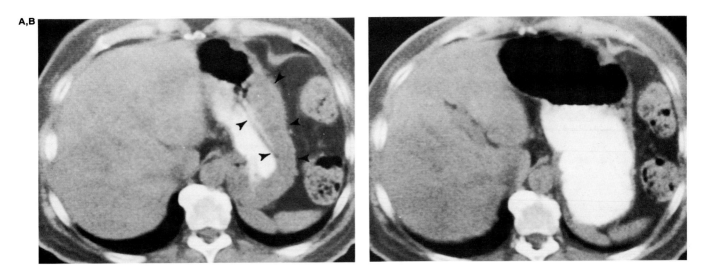

FIG. 18. Effect of distension on gastric-wall thickness. A: Image through the gastric body demonstrates apparent marked thickening of the left and posterior gastric wall (*arrowheads*). B: Image obtained immediately after administration of 300 ml of oral contrast material in same patient. Adequate distension of the lumen allows demonstration of normal wall thickness.

FIG. 19. Carcinoma infiltrating the wall of the stomach (ST). There are tumor nodules extending along the gastrosplenic ligament (*black arrow*) into the splenic hilum, and metastatic nodes within the gastrohepatic ligament (N). Tumor (*white arrow*) likewise infiltrates the gastrocolic ligament (greater omentum). Ascites (AS) is present; (S) spleen.

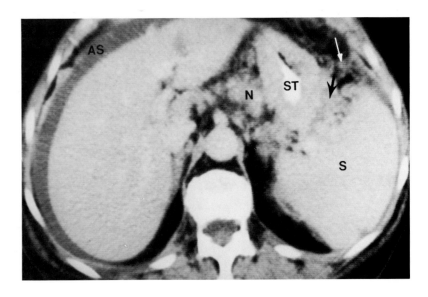

A,B

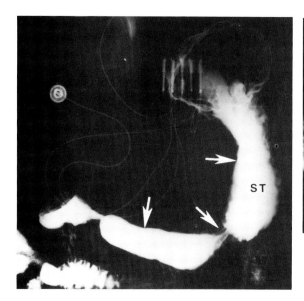

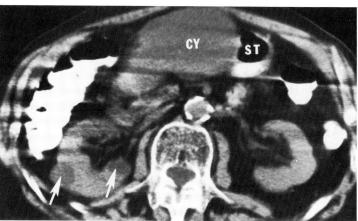

FIG. 20. Extrinsic deformity of the stomach by large hepatic cyst. **A:** Upper gastrointestinal study shows straightening and displacement of the lesser curvature (*arrows*) by a mass. **B:** CT image through the antrum (ST) shows a hepatic cyst (CY) compressing the gastric wall. Two renal cysts (*arrows*) also are present.

or contrast material may lead to confusion, because fluid-filled afferent limbs may mimic soft-tissue masses or pathologic fluid collections. Imaging is routinely performed with the patient lying in the supine position in suspended expiration. Contiguous 1-cm sections are obtained from the dome of the diaphragm throughout the stomach. Contrast material is administered intravenously if unenhanced images raise the question of vascular abnormality or of a process extending into the vessel-rich ligamentous structures attached to the stomach.

Most processes originating in the gastric wall do not rapidly cross peritoneal spaces; rather, they use attached ligaments as conduits to spread from one structure to another. In this way, carcinoma arising on the lesser curve of the stomach rarely invades the left hepatic lobe directly; instead, it proceeds along the gastrohepatic ligament into the liver hilum, where its intimate contact with the common hepatic duct may cause obstructive jaundice (Fig. 19).

Abnormalities originating from any of the viscera adjacent to the stomach can cause extrinsic deformity of the gastric wall. The most common such abnormalities are splenic masses or enlargement, hypertrophy of or metastases to the left hepatic lobe (Fig. 20), pancreatic pseudocyst or neoplasm, left renal cell carcinoma, or left adrenal carcinoma. In very thin patients, diaphragmatic slips may indent the stomach, mimicking a polyp (Fig. 21).

Pathology

Congenital Anomalies

Congenital gastric anomalies are uncommon. Duplication of the stomach accounts for approximately 4% of alimentary tract duplications. Its most common location is along the greater curve, and the cyst lumen rarely communicates with the true stomach lumen (2,25,61). The wall of the cyst is continuous with the stomach wall, and its muscular coat fuses with gastric muscle fibers. Ali-

FIG. 21. In this thin individual, a muscular slip of the diaphragm (*arrow*) indents the gastric wall, mimicking a gastric polyp; (ST) stomach.

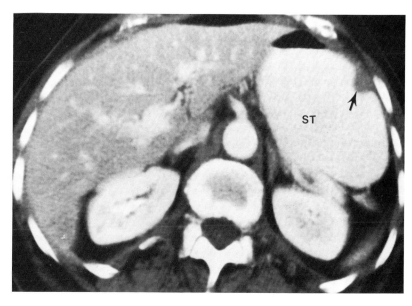

A,B

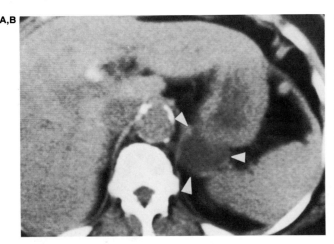
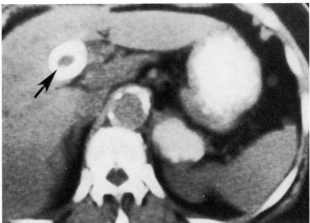

FIG. 22. Gastric diverticulum. **A:** Image through the gastric fundus shows water-attenuation mass (*arrowheads*), apparently arising posterior to the gastric wall. **B:** After contrast material was administered, the mass was clearly shown to be a gastric diverticulum. A gallstone (*arrow*) was present.

mentary epithelial lining is found internal to the cyst. On CT, a near-water-density spherical mass, indistinguishable from the wall of the stomach, is imaged. A case of lesser-curvature gastric duplication that extends into the posterior mediastinum through an esophageal hiatus has been reported (62).

Gastric diverticula characteristically arise from the posterior surface of the fundus. If oral contrast material is not administered, they may mimic adrenal or other retroperitoneal abnormalities (Fig. 22).

Neoplasms

Benign

Benign gastric tumors may be of mucosal or mesodermal origin. Generally, unless their size exceeds about 2 cm, gastric adenomas and hyperplastic polyps will not be detected by CT because they do not alter the contour of the gastric wall appreciably.

Mesodermal tumors are well imaged with CT. Leiomyomas (67) arise from the intramural smooth-muscle tissue and can expand both into and away from the gastric lumen (Fig. 23). The size of the tumor as estimated by endoscopy or upper gastrointestinal barium examination commonly is smaller than its actual size, because the tumor characteristically has a substantial extraluminal component. For this reason, CT frequently is performed prior to surgical resection to determine its effect on adjacent organs.

Lipomas need not achieve great size to be conspicuous on CT (46,69); their characteristic fat attenuation values allow definitive diagnosis of even small tumors.

Malignant

Adenocarcinoma. Gastric adenocarcinoma is the third most common gastrointestinal malignant neoplasm. Its incidence is increased in patients with pernicious anemia,

adenomatous gastric polyps, or atrophic gastritis. It is far more common in Japan than in the United States, where the incidence of the disease has been decreasing for the last two decades.

Most adenocarcinomas arise in the distal stomach. Morphologic types (Figs. 24 and 25) include exophytic, diffusely infiltrative, and ulcerating forms. Regardless of morphologic type or method of therapy, the prognosis remains dismal. Most patients in the United States present with advanced cancer; in this group, survival ranges between 4 and 18 months.

A small but important fraction of gastric cancers is discovered in patients whose initial imaging examination is CT, because it is not uncommon for stomach cancer to present with extragastric symptoms, such as jaundice, or nonspecific symptoms, such as weight loss or fatigue.

The CT findings of gastric adenocarcinoma depend on the morphologic type (4,72,83). A well-distended stomach

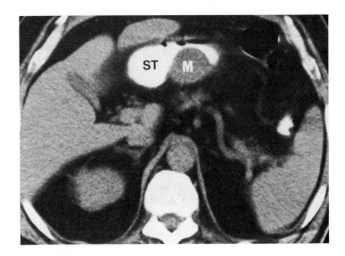

FIG. 23. Gastric leiomyoma. A smooth, homogeneous mass (M) arises from the posterior wall of the antrum (ST) in this asymptomatic patient.

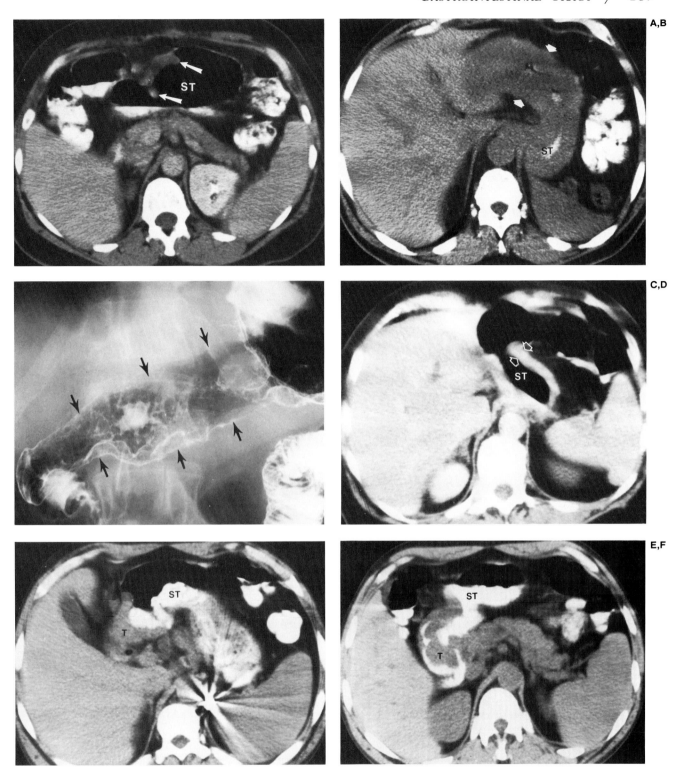

FIG. 24. Varied CT appearances of gastric adenocarcinomas. **A:** Adenocarcinoma presents as a focal plaque (*arrows*) involving the anterior surface of the prepyloric antrum; (ST) stomach. **B:** In another patient, a bulky infiltrative carcinoma produces diffuse thickening of the wall (*arrows*) of the gastric body; (ST) stomach. **C:** The barium examination from the same patient as in preceding image shows diffuse nodularity of the gastric surface (*arrows*), with loss of distensibility. **D:** In another patient with early satiety and occult gastrointestinal bleeding, the CT section shows an abrupt transition between the normally distensible, thin-walled antrum and the thick-walled body. Note the pronounced contrast enhancement of the thick gastric wall (*open arrows*) in this patient with scirrhous carcinoma (linitis plastica); (ST) stomach. **E,F:** Bulky intraluminal gastric tumor with duodenal extension. Images demonstrate lobular mass (T) originating in the gastric antrum (ST), extending to the region of the pylorus and, subsequently, 2 cm more caudal, nearly filling the duodenal lumen.

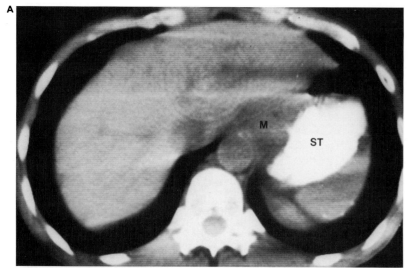

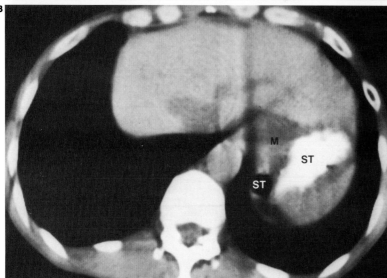

FIG. 25. Adenocarcinoma at the gastroesophageal junction. **A:** Image obtained with the patient supine shows apparent mass (M) at gastroesophageal junction. It was questioned whether or not this could represent collapsed gastric cardia within a hiatal hernia; (ST) stomach. **B:** Image performed in left lateral decubitus position at the same level shows that gas and contrast material within the lumen of the stomach (ST) outline, but do not enter, the mass (M). Surgically proven gastric adenocarcinoma, with extension into the esophagus.

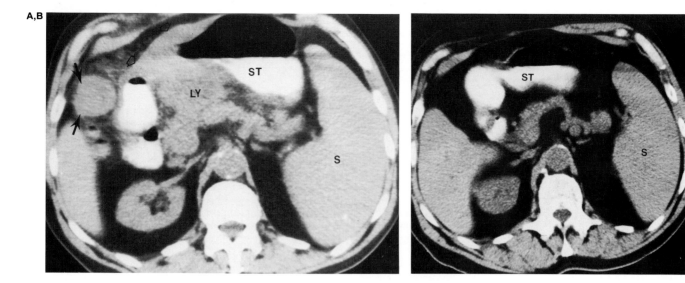

FIG. 26. Gastric lymphoma. **A:** Image through gastric antrum (ST) demonstrates bulky soft-tissue masses within the peripancreatic fat (LY), in the greater omentum (*arrows*), and intrinsic to the gastric wall (*open arrows*). Note the enlarged spleen (S). **B:** One year later, after multiple courses of chemotherapy, no abnormal soft-tissue masses remain, and the gastric wall is of normal thickness; (ST) stomach; (S) spleen.

normally demonstrates an attenuated but regular rugal-fold pattern; wall thickness is variable, but generally lies within the range 3 mm to 1 cm. Focal wall thickening and loss of the normal rugal pattern have been cited as sensitive signs of gastric abnormality, but they are not specific for gastric cancer. Linitis plastica (diffuse infiltrating gastric carcinoma) may exhibit enhancement after intravenous administration of contrast material.

The ability of CT to reveal the extent of gastric carcinoma is exceeded only by that of laparotomy (57,76). Comparing CT to direct surgical exploration, one group of investigators (17) concluded that CT routinely underestimates disease; further, the CT staging method used in that series proved inaccurate in judging resectability. The utility of CT in staging gastric carcinoma would appear to be limited to cases in which specific surgical problems are to be solved, for example, in determining whether or not metastatic lung or liver disease is present in a patient otherwise believed to be resectable for cure. Additionally, CT provides an excellent method for following patients after curative surgery has been attempted (74).

Knowledge of the precise route of spread is helpful in accurate staging of gastric cancer. Gastric carcinoma usually spreads by one of four mechanisms: (a) hematogenous spread to lungs and liver; (b) direct extension along ligamentous attachments (subperitoneal spread), such as extension to the porta hepatis via the gastrohepatic ligament, to the transverse colon via the gastrocolic ligament or (less commonly) the transverse mesocolon, or to the spleen via the gastrosplenic ligament; (c) regional nodal dissemination by way of lymphatic vessels; (d) diffuse spread throughout the peritoneal surfaces of the abdominal cavity. Intraperitoneal spread is extremely common in scirrhous carcinoma of the stomach and may exhibit a disconcertingly normal CT appearance despite the presence of widespread disease. Enhancement of the peritoneal surfaces of colon or small bowel after intravenous administration of contrast material may be a clue to the presence of peritoneal dissemination.

Lymphoma. The stomach is the most common site of gastrointestinal involvement with lymphoma, accounting for 10% of such patients. The most common cell types to involve the stomach primarily are diffuse histiocytic and poorly differentiated lymphomas (68). Gastric involvement typically is manifest by submucosal tumor spread, so that mucosal imaging, and even endoscopic biopsy, may fail to establish the diagnosis. Focal gastric-wall thickening, with distortion of the normal rugal-fold pattern, is the hallmark of gastric lymphoma on CT images (12) (Fig. 26). The majority of patients have clearly defined adenopathy in the greater omentum, gastrohepatic ligament, or gastrosplenic ligament. Some patients have widespread retroperitoneal adenopathy, indicating systemic disease.

Gastric lymphoma may be treated with chemotherapy, radiation therapy, surgery, or combinations of all three.

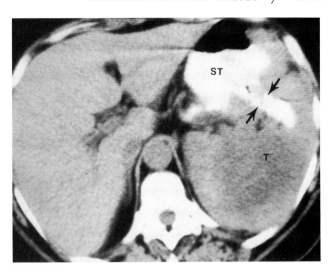

FIG. 27. Recurrent colon carcinoma after resection of a splenic flexure lesion. A large mass (T) extends into the gastrocolic ligament, invading the posterolateral wall of the stomach (ST). Tumor necrosis results in a large ulceration (arrows).

The thickness of the gastric wall generally returns to normal after successful treatment. CT imaging after treatment may show persistent nondistensibility of the stomach in a previously involved segment (60).

Leiomyosarcoma. Gastric leiomyosarcoma has rather consistent CT features. Typically there is a large, sometimes calcified, extragastric mass, often containing central necrosis. There can be low-attenuation metastases to the liver, and direct spread to adjacent viscera and/or ligamentous attachments can occur. The stretched gastric mucosa overlying the mass may be ulcerated. Gas present within the mass may help to distinguish sarcomas from other gastric tumors (88).

Metastasis. Metastatic deposits may occur in the stomach by extension to the gastric wall via a ligamentous attachment, most commonly seen in colon carcinoma (Fig. 27), by hematogenous spread (Fig. 28), and by lymphatic dissemination from carcinoma of the esophagus (31).

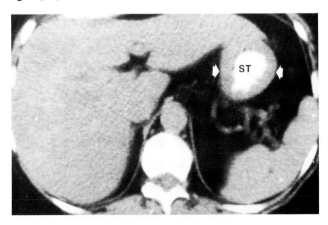

FIG. 28. Hematogenous metastases from a primary breast carcinoma have produced circumferential thickening (arrows) of the gastric body (ST).

A,B

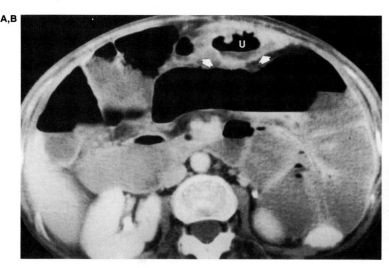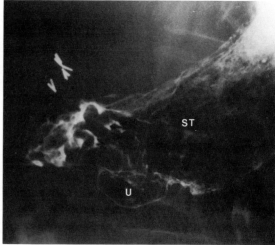

FIG. 29. Benign gastric ulcer. **A:** CT image through the gastric antrum demonstrates focal infiltration of the gastrocolic ligament (*arrows*) surrounding a large gas collection (U). **B:** Barium gastrointestinal study of the same individual shows a large benign gastric ulcer (U) extending from the greater curvature; (ST) stomach.

Inflammation

Inflammatory processes also can produce diffuse or focal wall thickening detectable on CT. Benign gastric ulcers may produce sizable deformities. Penetration of an ulcer may occur into adjacent peritoneal spaces or along ligamentous attachments (Fig. 29). The latter may simulate a malignant process. Involvement of the stomach by systemic granulomatous disease has been noted in Crohn disease, tuberculosis, sarcoidosis, and chronic granulomatous disease of childhood (53). Marked thickening of gastric rugae may be seen in Zollinger-Ellison syndrome or Menetrier disease (23). Either of these conditions may produce a picture indistinguishable from that of primary gastric lymphoma. Immunocompromised patients develop unusual infections: Cytomegalovirus and cryptosporidiosis (92) have been implicated in a case of antral narrowing, and graft-versus-host disease may likewise affect the distal stomach. These focal, circumferential thickenings may be indistinguishable from adenocarcinoma.

Varices

Patients with portal hypertension or splenic vein thrombosis may develop gastric varices. CT with bolus injection of contrast material characteristically demonstrates serpentine, brightly enhancing structures within the gastrohepatic or gastrosplenic ligaments continuous with similarly enhancing areas within the gastric wall (3,7).

Trauma

Trauma to the left hemidiaphragm may result in diaphragmatic rupture, through which the stomach may herniate (Fig. 30). Strangulation of the incarcerated stomach can occur months to years after the initial trauma and represents a surgical emergency. Rarely, gastric hematoma can occur after direct blunt trauma to the stomach wall or after incidental trauma in patients with bleeding disorders (Fig. 31).

SMALL INTESTINE

Technique and Anatomy

Achieving adequate distension of the entire small bowel represents a formidable challenge. Fortunately, in most individuals, ingestion of 600 ml of dilute water-soluble oral contrast material beginning 60 to 90 min before imaging serves to opacify most of the jejunum and ileum. The duodenum and proximal jejunum are best imaged if an additional 300 ml of contrast material is administered immediately prior to imaging. Gastric emptying is quite variable, however, and in very ill patients small-bowel motility is also reduced. In these individuals, rapid and uniform distension of the small bowel may require special techniques. One successful method is to place and subsequently inject through an enteric feeding tube. Time-release effervescent granules have been used to achieve small-intestine distension (66).

Failure to achieve adequate intestinal distension can result in troublesome artifacts: Collapse of a small-bowel segment may simulate focal wall thickening; fluid-filled segments of intestine can mimic mass lesions in the mesentery or adjacent organs.

Intravenous administration of contrast material may be helpful in judging the vascular response of a small-intestine lesion or in distinguishing mesenteric lymph nodes from mesenteric vessels.

On CT, the duodenal bulb is routinely observed posterior or posterolateral to the gastric antrum. The hepatic

A,B

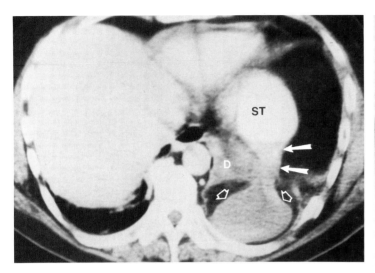

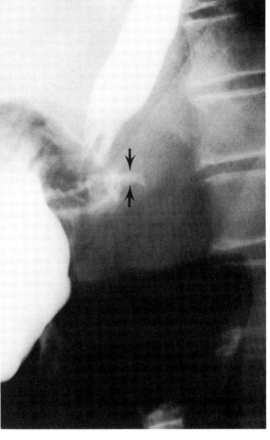

FIG. 30. Diaphragmatic tear, with incarcerated stomach, in a 44-year-old man with acute upper-quadrant pain who had had a minor auto accident 3 years previously. **A:** Image through the esophageal hiatus shows an unusual configuration of the posterior wall of the gastric fundus (*arrows*); it is narrowed posteriorly and is continuous with a fluid-containing structure (*open arrows*) that abuts the left chest wall. Note the unusual appearance of the diaphragm (D) on both sides of the narrowed area; (ST) stomach. **B:** Examination with water-soluble contrast material shows a beak-like posterior extension of contrast material (*arrows*) within the stomach. At subsequent operation, a portion of the fundus had entered a traumatic tear in the diaphragm and had become infarcted.

artery, common bile duct, and portal vein pass behind the duodenal bulb within the hepatoduodenal ligament. The postbulbar portion of the duodenum passes posteriorly to enter the retroperitoneum. More caudal sections will demonstrate the pancreaticoduodenal arcades coursing around the pancreatic head and the right gastroepiploic artery supplying this portion of the omentum. Disease processes originating in the hepatoduodenal ligament, such as cancer of the gallbladder, extend along the hepatic and gastroduodenal arteries to obscure the fat between the duodenum and pancreatic head. Immediately caudal to the gastric antrum, the duodenum and pancreas lie just posterior to the middle colic artery in the root of the transverse mesocolon; pathologic processes arising in the pancreas, stomach, or duodenum can course toward the proximal transverse colon via this route (70).

Immediately caudal to the pancreas, the duodenum turns sharply to proceed from right to left, passing between the superior mesenteric vein and artery anteriorly and the inferior vena cava and aorta posteriorly. Just to the left of the superior mesenteric artery, the duodenum turns slightly anteriorly and superiorly where it exits the retroperitoneum to become the jejunum.

Normally, the lumen of the jejunum has a somewhat feathery appearance on CT when it is well distended; the plicae circulares extend perpendicularly across the lumen in most individuals. Neither the wall nor the folds of the jejunum measure more than 3 mm in thickness in normal subjects. In most, both structures are barely perceptible on CT. Ileal loops do not normally exhibit plicae circulares. The ileocolic junction is easily recognized in many individuals by the prominent fat attenuation of the ileocecal valve.

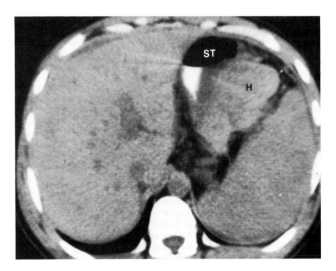

FIG. 31. Gastric hematoma. CT image from a 20-year-old hemophiliac with epigastric pain shows a large hematoma (H) within the gastric wall, extending into the gastrosplenic ligament; (ST) stomach.

A,B

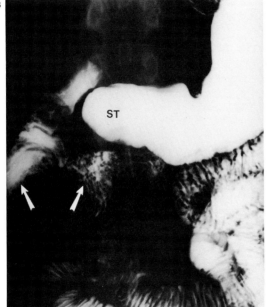

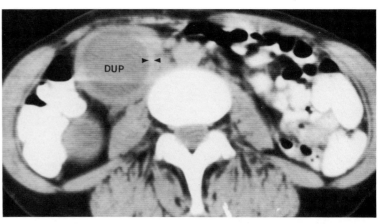

FIG. 32. Duodenal duplication. **A:** Barium upper gastrointestinal examination in a young woman with midepigastric pain shows a smooth mass (*arrows*) distorting the proximal horizontal portion of the duodenum; (ST) stomach. **B:** CT image shows near-water-attenuation mass (DUP), with thickened wall (*arrowheads*), arising from the retroperitoneum. This proved to be a duplication cyst.

Normal mesenteric fat is of the same attenuation as other body fat and contains linear branching structures that are visibly enhanced by intravenous contrast material and that can be traced to the major mesenteric vascular trunks. Mesenteric lymph nodes are difficult to detect by CT unless they are 5 to 10 mm in size. No soft-tissue structure within the mesentery exceeds 4 mm in diameter in normal individuals (48).

Congenital Abnormalities

Rotational anomalies of the small intestine are fairly common and may be clinically significant (49). "Malrotation" is the term that encompasses the whole spectrum of anomalous intestinal fixations, which range between insignificant anatomic variations and complete nonrotation. Nonrotation, the commonest form, often is asymptomatic. It is easily recognized because the duodenum fails to pass between the aorta and the superior mesenteric artery and instead lies in the right abdomen, whereas the colon is fixed on the left. Some forms of malrotation may be impossible to recognize on CT, but many predispose to intestinal volvulus. This complication of abnormal mesenteric fixation can be recognized by the CT observation of abnormally fixed, distended, edematous small-bowel loops converging to a single point of mesentery (21). In some patients, asymptomatic midgut malrotation may be exhibited by transposition of the superior mesenteric artery and vein, with the vein lying to the left of the artery (75).

Duplication cysts can occur in the small intestine and may contain ectopic gastric mucosa (Fig. 32). They are observed as water-attenuation masses lying on the nonmesenteric side of the alimentary tube.

Meckel's diverticula are remnants of the omphalomesenteric (vitelline) duct. In adults, they occur in the distal ileum, within 25 cm of the ileocecal valve. They are rarely

FIG. 33. Duodenal lipoma in a 70-year-old man with no symptoms referable to the gastrointestinal tract. Image demonstrates low-attenuation mass (*arrow*) filling the lumen of the distal descending and proximal transverse duodenum. There was no obstruction to gastric emptying.

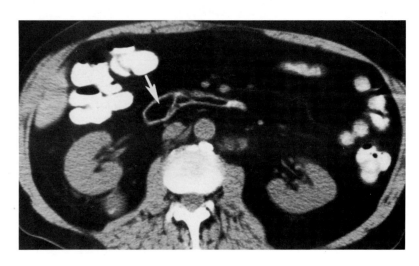

observed on CT. Stenosis and atresia of the small bowel are fairly common anomalies in the newborn, but they do not require CT for diagnosis.

Pathology

Neoplasms

Tumors of the small bowel are relatively uncommon, representing only 3% to 6% of all gastrointestinal neoplasms. Most series reflect a slight preponderance of malignant tumors over benign tumors.

Benign tumors

Leiomyomas are the most common benign neoplasms in the small intestine; they may come to clinical attention because of their tendency to ulcerate and bleed. Similar to leiomyomas elsewhere in the gastrointestinal tract, they appear on CT as smooth, homogeneous masses that are chiefly extrinsic to the lumen. Some contain amorphous calcification.

Lipomas are easily recognized by the sharp contrast between their low attenuation and that of the surrounding contrast material in the lumen (77) (Fig. 33). They are pliable, chiefly intraluminal masses that may be multiple in the proximal small bowel.

Adenomas chiefly occur proximally, in the duodenum, and may have an exuberant intraluminal extent (Fig. 34). CT demonstrates a large, soft-tissue-attenuation-value intraluminal filling defect with lobular margins.

Malignant tumors

Malignant tumors include adenocarcinoma, carcinoid, leiomyosarcoma, lymphoma, and metastatic deposits (18).

Carcinoid is the most common primary neoplasm in the small intestine (82,89). Carcinoid tumors arise from neuroendocrine cells within the submucosa, most commonly in the distal ileum (15,65) (Figs. 35 and 36). Although tumor diameters of 5 cm or more are occasionally encountered, the primary enteric carcinoid itself often is small enough to pass unnoticed on CT. Local invasion or lymphatic spread to mesenteric lymph nodes produces a peculiar thickening and retraction of the involved mesenteric fat. This retraction may secondarily produce venous or lymphatic obstruction. Lymphadenopathy in paraaortic and paracaval areas often is bulky and may mimic lymphoma. Systemic effects are produced by metastatic deposits in the liver; the tumor synthesizes vaso-

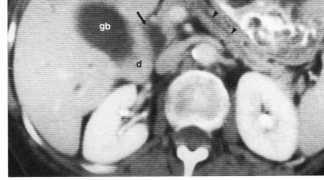

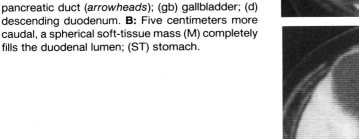

FIG. 34. Villous adenoma arising from the papilla of Vater. **A:** Image through the pancreas shows dilatation of both the common bile duct (*arrow*) and pancreatic duct (*arrowheads*); (gb) gallbladder; (d) descending duodenum. **B:** Five centimeters more caudal, a spherical soft-tissue mass (M) completely fills the duodenal lumen; (ST) stomach.

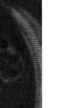

A,B

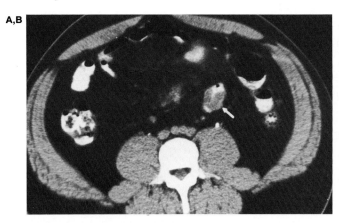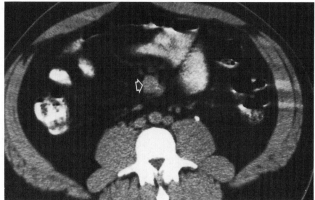

FIG. 35. Carcinoid tumor of small intestine in a 35-year-old man with vague abdominal pain. **A:** CT through midabdomen shows annular lesion of jejunum (*arrow*) producing focal luminal narrowing. **B:** One centimeter more cephalad, a large mesenteric node (*open arrow*) is demonstrated. Note slight dilatation of the proximal jejunum.

active amines capable of inducing the carcinoid syndrome, episodic flushing, headache, diarrhea, nausea, and vomiting. Metastatic deposits to liver are nearly always hypervascular.

Lymphoma, particularly the diffuse histiocytic or poorly differentiated lymphocytic subtypes, may involve the small intestine and produce a variety of morphologic appearances. Common to them is thickening of the bowel wall in diffuse or focal distribution, as well as the presence of discrete lymph node masses within the mesenteric loops supplying the involved segment (Fig. 37). American Burkitt lymphoma is an important subtype (58,87) (Fig. 38). It arises in children or young adults and shows a predilection for abdominal involvement. Bulky mesenteric masses, displacing adjacent bowel loops, and absence of retroperitoneal adenopathy have been described as typical CT findings. In all forms of lymphoma, remarkably extensive lymphomatous involvement, even with encasement of segments of the alimentary tract, may occur without appreciable obstruction.

Primary *adenocarcinoma* of the small intestine is rare; when it occurs, it generally arises in the duodenum or proximal jejunum. CT sections demonstrate focal wall thickening, with narrowing of the lumen and proximal dilatation. Regional lymph nodes may be enlarged, but widespread metastatic disease is relatively uncommon at initial presentation.

Leiomyosarcoma is the most common mesodermal malignant neoplasm arising in the small intestine. It arises in the submucosa and tends to spread radially away from the lumen. Thus, such tumors may achieve appreciable size before they produce symptoms (67). Intestinal leiomyosarcomas have a tendency to spread through the mesentery and/or peritoneal cavity. When hematogenous metastases occur to the liver, they are characteristically large and cystic in appearance.

Metastases to the small intestine undoubtedly occur far more frequently than they are imaged. Hematogenous metastases, as in patients with breast and lung carcinoma

and melanoma, appear as focal round masses originating from the antimesenteric surface of the bowel wall (Fig. 39). Intussusception can occur and is most likely when the lesion is large, as is common with melanoma. Peritoneal seeding produces metastatic nodes adherent to the small-bowel serosa, fixing one edge of the intestine and producing acute angulation and sometimes partial obstruction. This form is commonly observed in cancers of the stomach or ovary. Carcinoma of the pancreas can spread along the root of the intestinal mesentery, engulfing long segments of small bowel.

Inflammation

A number of inflammatory diseases affect the small intestine, and only the more common will be discussed here. As a generalization, inflammatory diseases arise in the mucosa or submucosa and produce mucosal irregularity or ulceration as the earliest change. CT findings may be normal in this phase. Eventually, however, edema

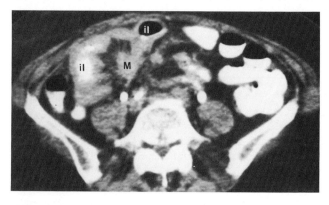

FIG. 36. Extensive carcinoid tumor. CT through the pelvic brim shows segmental thickening of the wall of the distal ileum (il) and a large mesenteric mass (M) producing retraction of adjacent ileal loops.

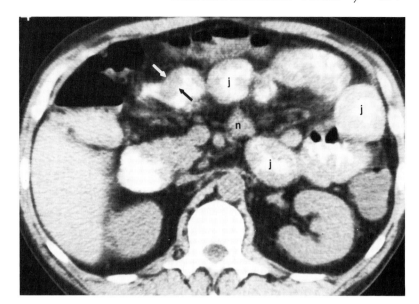

FIG. 37. Non-Hodgkin lymphoma has produced widespread thickening of the small-intestine wall (*arrows*), with adenopathy (n) in the adjacent mesentery; (j) jejunal segments.

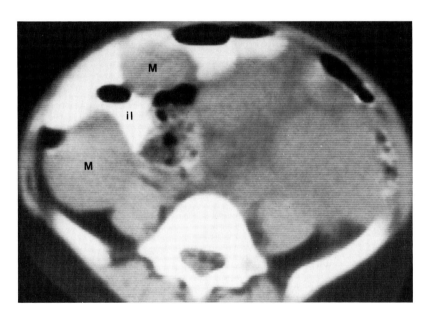

FIG. 38. Burkitt lymphoma in this young boy chiefly affects the mesentery, producing bulky mesenteric masses (M); (il) ileum.

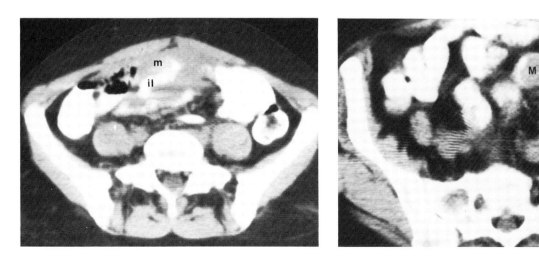

A,B

FIG. 39. Metastases to the small intestine. **A:** Peritoneally spread metastatic ovarian carcinoma (m) involves the serosal surface of the ileum (il). **B:** Hematogenous melanoma metastasis produces a spherical mass (M) in the intestinal wall.

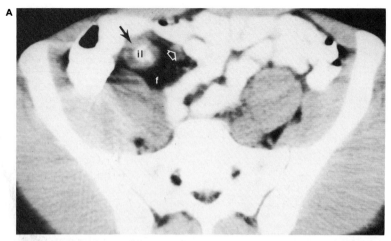

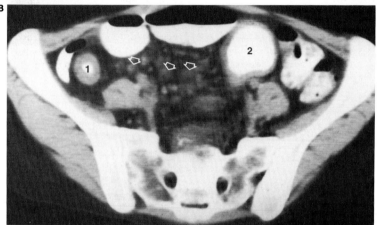

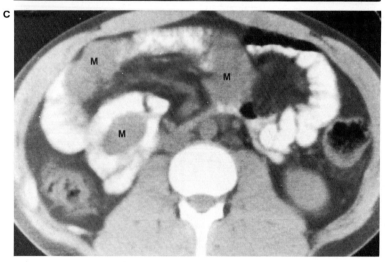

FIG. 40. Crohn disease. **A:** A 22-year-old man with right-lower-quadrant pain. Barium examination of the small intestine was performed previously and was interpreted as normal. CT shows circumferential thickening of the distal ileal wall (*arrow*); an unusual accumulation of fat (f) is seen in the adjacent mesentery, along with enlargement of a mesenteric lymph node (*open arrow*); (il) ileum. **B:** In another patient with a long history of granulomatous enteritis, there is mural thickening involving two intestinal segments (1 and 2), the more proximal of which (2) is dilated. Multiple inflammatory nodes (*open arrows*) are evident within the adjacent mesentery. **C:** Chronic inflammatory masses (M) occupy the mesentery in another patient with long-standing granulomatous enteritis.

will produce wall thickening, and localized hypervascularity will develop. In turn, the mesentery supplying the affected segment will become inflamed. In many cases, regional lymph nodes will also be enlarged. All of these manifestations can be imaged by CT. Wall thickening in inflammatory conditions rarely exceeds 1.5 cm, and abnormal mesenteric lymph nodes, if present, usually are smaller than 2 cm (48).

In the United States, Crohn's disease is the most common entity producing thickening of the wall of the small intestine. CT findings in the acute phase of Crohn's disease include circumferential wall thickening, serpiginous soft-tissue strands extending into the mesenteric fat, and enlarged lymph nodes in the same region (Fig. 40). Perforation of the intestine in Crohn's disease generally is confined and leads to a mesenteric phlegmon or some-

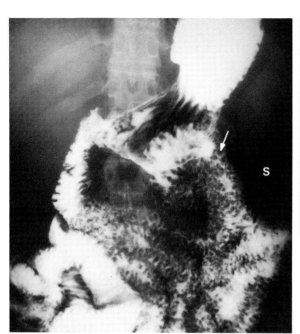

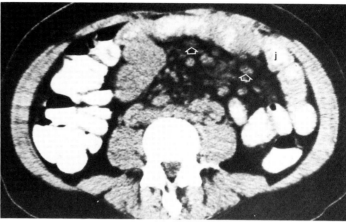

A,B

FIG. 41. *Mycobacterium intracellulare* complicating AIDS. **A:** In a 25-year-old man with AIDS and diarrhea, small-intestine examination shows nodular-fold thickening (*arrow*) throughout the small intestine, most noticeable in the proximal jejunum; (S) spleen. **B:** CT demonstrates thickened jejunal wall and multiple mesenteric lymph nodes of relatively low attenuation (*open arrow*); (j) jejunum. Paraaortic adenopathy is also present.

times a frank interloop abscess. Differentiation between a drainable abscess and a phlegmonous inflammatory mesenteric reaction may be very difficult. Gas or contrast material within a circumscribed, relatively homogeneous collection suggests abscess. The diagnosis is sometimes best confirmed by percutaneous needle aspiration.

Between acute attacks of Crohn's enteritis, the small intestine may appear quite normal on CT. Many patients have an abnormal quantity of mesenteric fat, the "creeping fat" often reported at surgical exploration, adjacent to a previously inflamed segment (26). This finding may provide a diagnostic clue. Stenotic Crohn's disease produces fixed, segmental narrowed areas with proximal small-intestine dilation in patients with long-standing disease (33,36).

Fistulas or sinus tracts may sometimes be imaged by CT as contrast-containing lines extending into the intestinal mesentery or toward the abdominal wall (34,56). The pathways of sinus tracts may be serpiginous, causing them to pass in and out of a given transverse section. For this reason, fluoroscopy usually is a simpler way to assess most fistulas, but CT may confirm the presence of extraluminal contrast material when a small tract is not fluoroscopically imaged.

Acute appendicitis produces inflammatory thickening of the distal ileum, even when no abscess is demonstrated; in this way, the CT findings of appendicitis or cecal diverticulitis may mimic those of acute granulomatous ileitis. Likewise, *Yersinia* ileitis may produce clinical and CT findings virtually indistinguishable from those of Crohn's disease.

Other acute or chronic inflammatory bowel conditions have been imaged by CT. Nonspecific jejunitis, an entity that occasionally complicates long-standing celiac disease (51), produces long segments of jejunal-wall thickening,

with edema in the adjacent mesenteric fat. Likewise, eosinophilic enteritis may result in focal wall thickening, giving rise to similar CT findings.

The recent increase in the incidence of acquired immunodeficiency syndrome (AIDS) has brought infectious enteritis to prominence. Normal individuals may become infested with *Giardia lamblia* or *Strongyloides stercoralis,* but it has been long recognized that clinical *Giardia* infestation occurs more commonly in individuals with deficiency of secretory IgA. CT is not routinely used for diagnosis in these conditions, but each can produce thickening of the duodenum and proximal jejunum, with moderate lymphadenopathy in the adjacent mesentery and evidence of hypersecretion.

Patients with AIDS or AIDS-related complex present a complicated spectrum (50). CT in those with lymphadenopathy syndrome shows mesenteric lymph node enlargement, splenomegaly, and infiltration of the rectal wall or perirectal fat. Typical enteritides occurring in these patients include cryptosporidiosis, cytomegaloviral enteritis, and involvement by *Mycoplasma avium intercellulare.* The first two generally show only nonspecific mural thickening. Mesenteric nodal enlargement may not be any greater than in AIDS patients without enteric infection. Infection with *Mycoplasma avium intercellulare* has a strong tendency to produce low-attenuation enlargement of retroperitoneal and mesenteric lymph nodes (Fig. 41). Its CT appearance and clinical presentation are strikingly similar to those in patients with Whipple disease.

Infectious granulomatous enteritis is rarely encountered in the United States. Tuberculous infection produces mural thickening of involved intestinal segments, frequently the terminal ileum, and is associated with omental and peritoneal thickening (19). Histoplasmosis, when disseminated, can have a similar appearance.

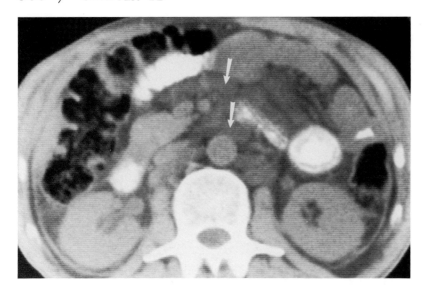

FIG. 42. Whipple disease in this patient is manifest chiefly by bulky lymphadenopathy of relatively low attenuation (*arrows*).

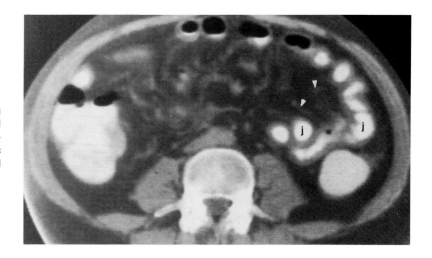

FIG. 43. Graft-versus-host disease following bone marrow transplant has produced focal wall thickening in distal jejunal segments (j) and generalized increases in the sizes of the mesenteric vessels (*arrowheads*) supplying the affected area.

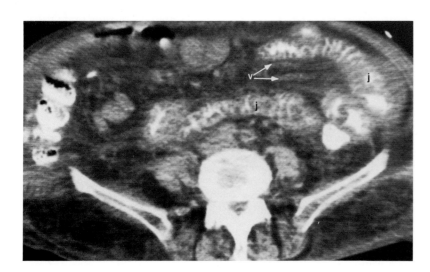

FIG. 44. Small-bowel edema, produced by profound hypoalbuminemia, is manifest on CT as fold and wall thickening and engorgement of mesenteric vessels (v); (j) jejunal segments.

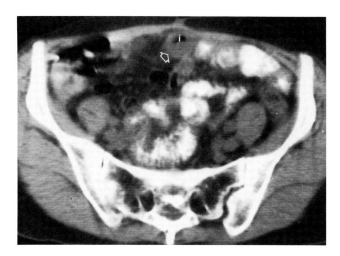

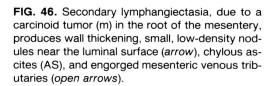

FIG. 45. Radiation effects in the small intestine (i) produce circumferential intestinal-wall thickening (*open arrow*).

Whipple's disease is produced by an unknown pathogen, thought to be a bacillus because of the presence of bacillary particles within the foamy macrophages that characterize this disease. CT shows diffuse intestinal-wall thickening, associated with large, low-attenuation mesenteric lymph nodes (Fig. 42).

Graft-versus-host disease is a condition that occasionally complicates heterotopic bone marrow transplantation (52). It is manifest by focal wall thickening, usually in the ileum, with luminal narrowing and increased mesenteric vascularity (Fig. 43).

Vasculitis and Noninflammatory Edema

Many hospitalized patients have conditions predisposing to noninflammatory edema, such as congestive heart failure and hypoalbuminemia. CT images often show modest bowel-wall thickening extending throughout the length of the alimentary tract. Fat in the mesentery commonly is edematous and therefore increased in attenuation, similar to fat elsewhere in the patient. Mesenteric vessels often are larger than normal (Fig. 44).

Focal or diffuse vasculitis also may produce mural edema. In polyarteritis nodosa, the distribution of involved segments is patchy. Radiation produces an endarteritis limited to the confines of the treatment portal (Fig. 45). CT findings include serosal thickening, increased attenuation of mesenteric fat, adhesions, and retraction of the radiated mesentery (24).

Primary intestinal lymphangiectasia is a rare congenital entity that produces dilated lacteals within intestinal villi (20). The same phenomenon results from secondary lymphangiectasia due to mesenteric tumor obstructing segmental lymphatic channels. CT demonstrates mural thickening, with characteristic low-attenuation 1- to 2-mm cystic areas within the intestinal wall (Fig. 46). Chylous ascites often is associated.

Ischemia of the small intestine may lead to frank infarction. CT findings include bowel-wall thickening and characteristic intramural gas associated with portal venous air (16,55). Thrombus and gas may be seen in the superior mesenteric artery or vein.

Bleeding into the submucosa results from a variety of disturbances of the coagulation mechanism and is observed in patients with hemophilia, Henoch-Schönlein purpura (91), bone marrow depression, thrombocytopenia, or excessive anticoagulation with dicoumarol (84) (Fig. 47). In the acute phase, bleeding produces high-attenuation, focal, submucosal intestinal-wall thickening that may produce luminal obstruction. Spontaneous resolution usually occurs in a few weeks.

Focal perforation of the small intestine occasionally occurs in a diverticulum (38). Otherwise it is uncommon,

FIG. 46. Secondary lymphangiectasia, due to a carcinoid tumor (m) in the root of the mesentery, produces wall thickening, small, low-density nodules near the luminal surface (*arrow*), chylous ascites (AS), and engorged mesenteric venous tributaries (*open arrows*).

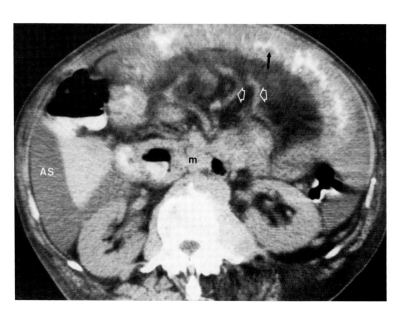

A

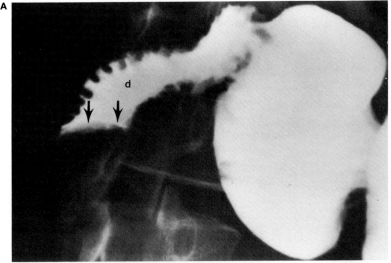

B

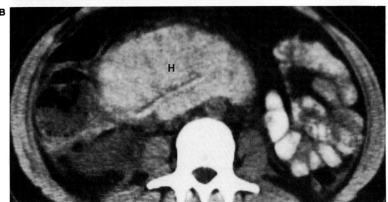

FIG. 47. Traumatic hematoma of the duodenum. Young patient with nausea and vomiting a few hours after an auto accident. **A:** Contrast examination of the upper gastrointestinal tract shows abrupt cutoff (*arrows*) in the descending duodenum (d), producing complete obstruction. **B:** CT image through the duodenum shows a large hematoma (H). The high attenuation suggests recent origin. **C:** Four days after the preceding image, the hematoma (H) has developed central low attenuation and a thick rim. Surgical decompression was necessary.

C

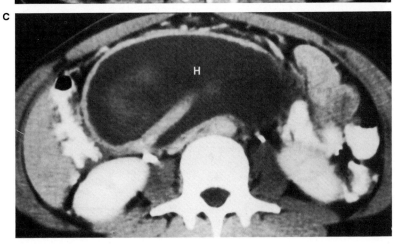

except in the duodenum, where an ulcer may penetrate into the adjacent peritoneal space. Abrupt-deceleration trauma can produce transection of the duodenum at the points that it enters or exits the retroperitoneum (32). This event characteristically leads to right-side pneumo-retroperitoneum. Intraluminal foreign bodies, most commonly toothpicks, may exit the alimentary tract in virtually any location to produce mesenteric abscesses and focal inflammatory edema (93) (Fig. 48).

Obstruction

Bowel obstruction is easily diagnosed by CT (5). Intestinal loops proximal to the obstruction are filled with fluid or dilute oral contrast material and are seen to be obviously dilated compared with the empty segments distal to an obstructing lesion (Fig. 49). After Billroth II procedures, afferent-limb obstruction is manifest by fluid of water density distending an intestinal loop in the location of the duodenum (30,94) (Fig. 50).

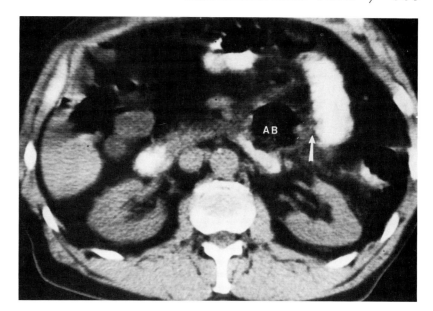

FIG. 48. Toothpick perforation of the jejunum has produced focal wall thickening (*arrow*) and a mesenteric abscess (AB), chiefly filled with gas.

Patients with scleroderma may have CT findings mimicking those of obstruction, including impressive dilatation of the small intestine (Fig. 51); the diagnosis generally is apparent clinically long before the small intestine is involved.

Hernia

A small-intestine hernia represents an abnormal protrusion through a defect in the peritoneal surface and may occur in inguinal (Fig. 52), femoral, Spiegelian (8,78), umbilical, lumbar, obturator, and paraduodenal locations. CT usually shows bowel or omentum within a hernia sac and narrowing of the small intestine and its accompanying mesentery as it passes through the peritoneal defect.

Intussusception

Enteroenteric intussusception may occur transiently in patients with celiac disease. More commonly it occurs when a focal mass within the intestinal wall becomes a lead point, carrying a segment of proximal bowel (and its attached mesentery) into the lumen of a more distal segment. CT findings (90) demonstrate a collapsed proximal segment surrounded by a fat-filled rim of mesentery lying within the opacified lumen of the distal segment (Fig. 53). When the lead mass is large, it may be directly imaged as a discrete soft-tissue mass.

COLON

The ascending and descending portions of the colon usually are well seen on CT images, being surrounded by extraperitoneal fat in the anterior pararenal space. The transverse colon lies anteriorly in the midabdomen and is distinguishable from the small intestine by its haustrations and by the bubbly appearance of its fecal contents. The transverse colon is suspended from the retroperitoneum by the transverse mesocolon, the root of which extends along the anterior surface of the pancreas from just inferior to the ampulla of Vater to a point superior to the ligament of Treitz (70). Normally, the transverse mesocolon is not visible on CT, but it may serve as a pathway along which pancreatic tumor or inflammatory disease can spread to the colon, in which case it appears as a band-like horizontal structure posterior and superior to the transverse colon. The superior surface of the transverse colon is connected to the greater curvature of the stomach by the gastrocolic ligament, which also may act as a pathway for the spread of disease. The hepatic flexure and

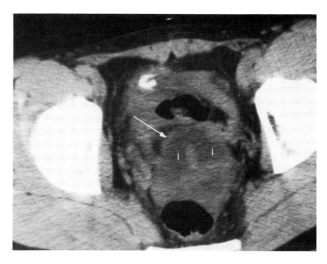

FIG. 49. Closed-loop obstruction in a young man recovering from appendectomy. Fluid-filled, thick-walled, pelvic small-bowel loops (*arrow*) mimic an abscess; (i) ileum.

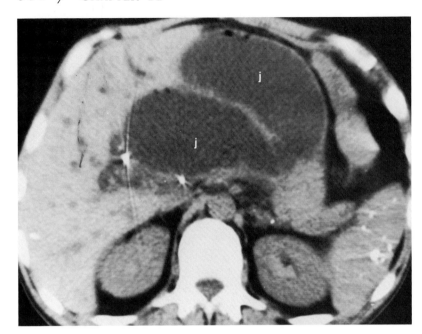

FIG. 50. Obstructed jejunal Roux-en-Y limb after choledochojejunostomy. There is marked dilatation of the jejunal biliary drainage limb (j), with mild intrahepatic biliary dilatation; the jejunal limb was obstructed by postoperative adhesions at the jejunojejunostomy site.

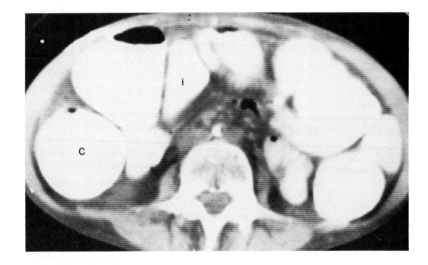

FIG. 51. Scleroderma. There is marked dilatation of both the small intestine (i) and colon (C), mimicking obstruction. Little dilution of the administered oral contrast material has occurred.

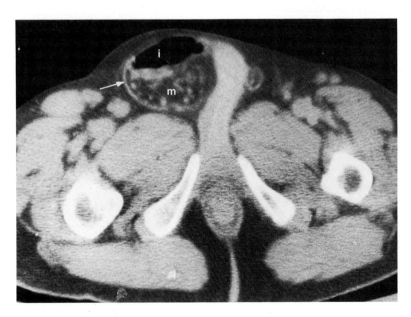

FIG. 52. A right inguinal hernia contains a gas-filled small-intestine loop (i) and mesenteric fat and vessels (m) in this asymptomatic patient.

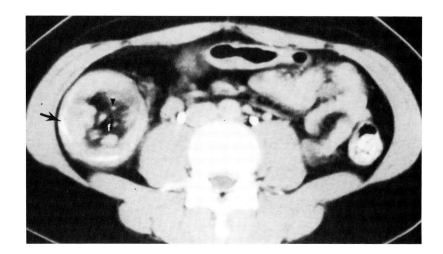

FIG. 53. Ileocolic intussusception due to non-Hodgkin lymphoma in the wall of the distal ileum has produced the characteristic "doughnut" appearance. Note oral contrast material in the lumen of the intussuscipiens (*arrow*), as well as fat (f) and dilated mesenteric vessels (*arrowhead*) that accompany the intussusception.

proximal transverse colon are closely related to the inferior surface of the liver and gallbladder and to the anterior aspect of the duodenum and upper pole of the right kidney and can be affected by direct spread of disease from these organs (70).

Gas and fluid normally are present in the colon; however, colonic distension and air–fluid levels seen on CT hold the same significance as on plain abdominal radiographs. With sufficient fluid, air, or contrast material in the lumen, the thickness of the colonic wall can be evaluated and usually is less than 3 mm (22). Often it is helpful to opacify the colonic lumen with contrast material to avoid mistaking nonopacified large bowel, particularly the sigmoid colon, for a mass lesion. This is accomplished either by administering oral contrast material well in advance of the study or, preferably, by giving an enema of dilute contrast material just prior to imaging. This is particularly important when the pelvis is the anatomic region of concern or when one suspects colonic disease.

Anatomic variations of colonic position should be kept in mind. The transverse colon, for example, can descend well into the pelvis or extend anterior and superior to the

liver. The ascending and descending portions of the colon may be suspended by a mesentery, may lack extraperitoneal fixation, and may lie more medially within the abdomen than usual. Failure of complete colonic rotation will lead to a superiorly situated cecum. Portions of the left colon fill the left renal fossa in a patient with left renal agenesis or a patient who has had left nephrectomy. A vacant right renal fossa may be filled with portions of the right colon, as well as the duodenum or liver.

Pathology

Neoplasia

Adenocarcinoma of the colon generally appears as an irregularly marginated but roughly spherical soft-tissue mass (Figs. 54–59) (64). Large tumors may show a central low-density area representing necrosis. Occasionally the primary lesion may contain gas and be indistinguishable from diverticulitis with pericolonic abscess. Lesions of the rectum and rectosigmoid are seen as asymmetrical or circumferential thickening of the bowel wall, with defor-

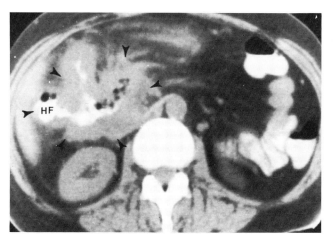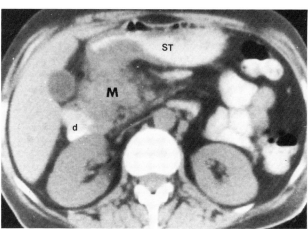

A,B

FIG. 54. Carcinoma of the hepatic flexure. **A:** Large soft-tissue mass (*arrowheads*) surrounds and distorts the hepatic flexure (HF). **B:** Four centimeters cephalad, the mass (M) is seen to extend into the head of the pancreas and the posterior surface of the gastric antrum (ST); (d) duodenum.

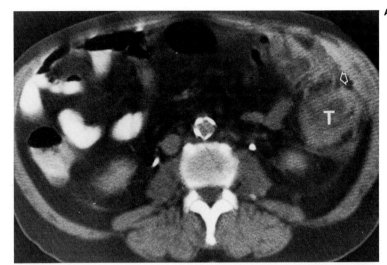

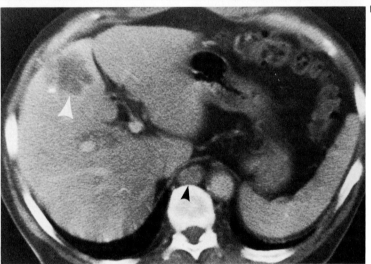

FIG. 55. Extensive carcinoma of the colon. **A:** Tumor (T) in the descending colon invades the pericolonic fat (*open arrow*) and extends to the abdominal-wall musculature. **B:** Image through the upper abdomen shows an enlarged retrocrural node (*black arrowhead*) and hepatic metastasis (*white arrowhead*).

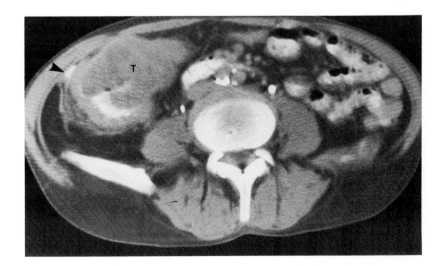

FIG. 56. Large perforated adenocarcinoma of the ascending colon (T). Note extravasation (*arrowhead*) of contrast material from the colonic lumen.

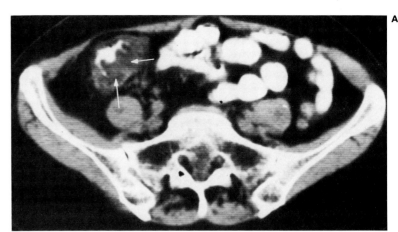

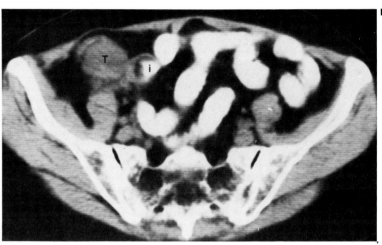

FIG. 57. Carcinoma of the colon: lymphedema and small-bowel obstruction. **A:** Section through the ascending colon shows eccentric wall thickening, with areas of low attenuation (*arrows*) pathologically corresponding to edema due to lymphatic obstruction. **B:** Tumor (T) at the ileocecal junction extends into the distal ileum (i), producing low-grade small-bowel obstruction.

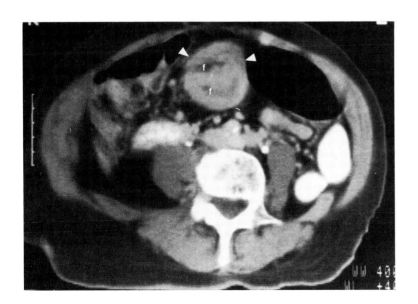

FIG. 58. Intussusception of large carcinoma originating in the proximal transverse colon. The characteristic bull's eye appearance is seen: The outer ring (*arrowheads*) is the wall of the intussuscipiens, within which lies mesocolic fat (f). The innermost circle is the wall and collapsed lumen of the intussusceptum.

A,B

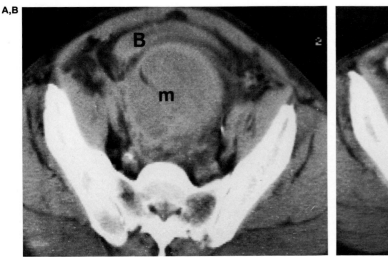 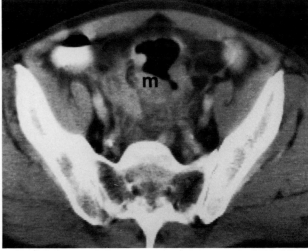

FIG. 59. Unresectable adenocarcinoma: response to treatment. A: A large mass (m) arising from the sigmoid colon compresses the posterior surface of the bladder (B). B: There is marked reduction in the size of the mass (m) after radiation and chemotherapy.

mation and narrowing of the lumen (95) (Figs. 60 and 61). Other findings may include extension of tumor into pericolonic fat, invasion of adjacent structures, lymphadenopathy, adrenal or liver metastases, hydronephrosis, ascites, and masses in the abdominal wall, omentum, or mesentery. Obscuration of the margin between the colon and an adjacent structure may indicate local extension of tumor. Common sites of local extension from rectosigmoid carcinoma include the pelvic musculature, bladder, prostate, seminal vesicles, and ovaries (95). Obliteration of the fat plane between the muscle group and the mass and enlargement of the muscle adjacent to the mass indicate muscular involvement by tumor. Spread into neighboring viscera may be difficult to predict because the tumor mass may be visually indistinguishable from a structure and yet not actually invade it (45). Direct skeletal invasion can be diagnosed when there is definite cortical disruption.

Although several studies based on the first 5 years of experience with body CT suggested that CT was an accurate method for staging carcinoma of the colon and rectum, more recent reports, in which prospective CT interpretations of all disease stages have been correlated with operative findings, are less encouraging (1,27,95,96,98,99). In its present state, CT is a poor means of determining the depth of spread of tumor in the bowel wall, and thus it cannot be used to distinguish Dukes A and Dukes B tumors. Although CT has recently been reported to have an accuracy of about 70% in predicting local extension of colorectal cancer, its sensitivity in this regard is considerably lower. Also disappointing has been the inability to use CT to detect intraperitoneal spread of malignant neoplasm. Sheets of tumor or tiny tumor nodules studding the parietal and visceral peritoneal surfaces commonly go undetected on CT. Only in the presence of visible peritoneal thickening, nodules larger than several

FIG. 60. Rectal carcinoma: stage 2. Asymmetric rectal-wall thickening (arrowheads) is present, but there is no evidence of tumor extension into adjacent pelvic structures.

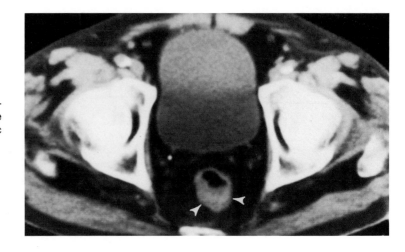

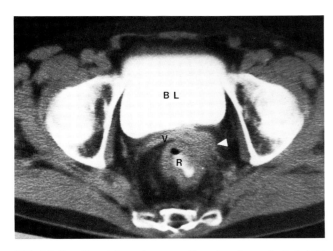

FIG. 61. Small rectal carcinoma, with extension anteriorly into left seminal vesicle (*arrowhead*) and laterally into the left pelvic sidewall; (R) rectal lumen; (V) right seminal vesicle; (BL) bladder.

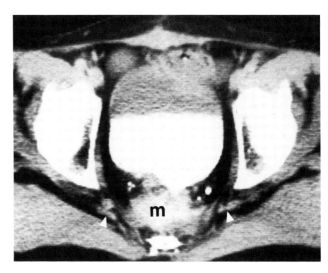

FIG. 62. Recurrence after abdominoperineal resection is depicted as a well-circumscribed presacral mass (m) that invades the posterior wall of the bladder. Note proximity of the sciatic nerves (*arrowheads*), which commonly are affected in this clinical setting.

millimeters in diameter, or increased density and thickness of the omentum is intraperitoneal spread of tumor likely to be detected on CT.

The detection of spread of colorectal carcinoma to lymph nodes has also proved problematic. Lymph nodes larger than 10 to 15 mm in size can be seen on CT in the great majority of patients and can be identified correctly as lymph nodes. However, there is relatively poor correlation between the sizes of abdominal nodes and the presence or absence of metastatic tumor within them. Using 15 mm as the upper size limit for normal abdominal lymph nodes seen on CT, a sensitivity of only 26% for detecting lymphatic spread of colorectal carcinoma has been reported (27).

Barium enema and endoscopy are of little use in detecting recurrence of tumor in patients who have undergone abdominoperineal resection for rectal carcinoma. In

these patients, CT has become the preferred method for detecting recurrence (28,45,59,73,99). Recurrent tumor in the pelvis following abdominoperineal resection usually appears as a homogeneous, globular soft-tissue mass and generally is detectable when it achieves a diameter of 1.5 cm. Invasion of the coccygeus and pyriformis muscles is common, as is encasement or displacement of the sciatic nerve, resulting in a painful leg. Recurrent tumor also may appear as a soft-tissue mass with a low-density center that may contain gas (Figs. 62–65). This appearance is not specific and can be seen in patients with abscess, uninfected hematoma, or radiation-induced necrosis. Small intestine not opacified by oral contrast material can mimic this appearance. Uncomplicated postoperative fibrosis usually appears as a streak of fibrous tissue oriented in the midsagittal plane. It does not produce a discrete mass as does recurrent neoplasm (59). However, patients with

FIG. 63. Recurrent tumor: stage 3b. A soft-tissue mass (M) anterior to the sacrum represents a recurrence after abdominoperineal resection for carcinoma of the rectosigmoid. The mass invades the posterior wall of the bladder (Bl) and the left obturator internus (oi) and pyriformis (pym) muscles and extends to the left pelvic sidewall; (gm) gluteus maximus.

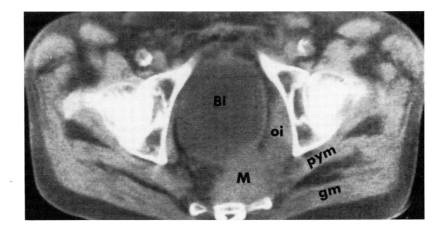

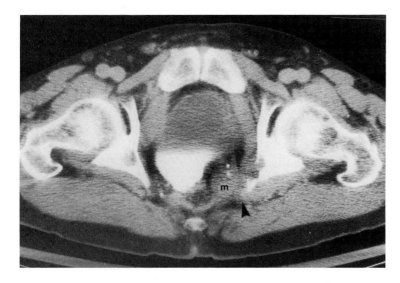

FIG. 64. Recurrent carcinoma (m) after abdominoperineal resection invades the ischium (*arrowhead*).

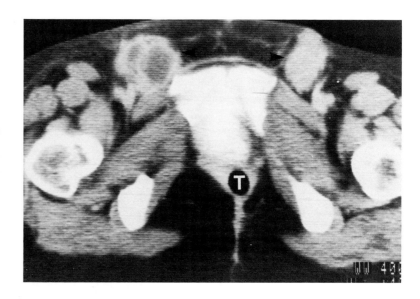

FIG. 65. Lymphatic metastases to the inguinal nodes (*arrowheads*) in a patient with recurrent squamous cell carcinoma of the anus after abdominoperineal resection. The surgical site is normal; only a thin plane of fibrous tissue is present posterior to the vagina; (T) vaginal tampon.

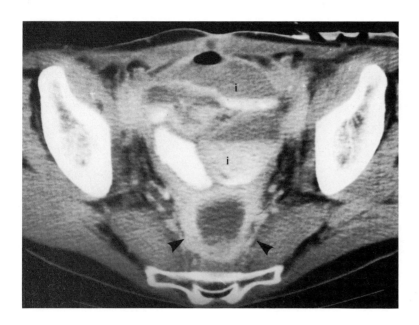

FIG. 66. Thick-walled presacral abscess (*arrowheads*) 1 month after abdominoperineal resection for rectal carcinoma. A necrotic tumor mass could have the same appearance, but would not have developed this soon. Dilated, fluid-filled small-intestine loops (i) reflect partial obstruction.

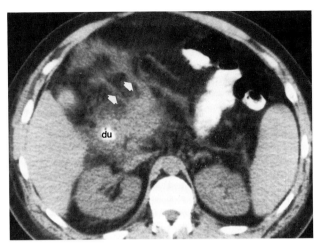
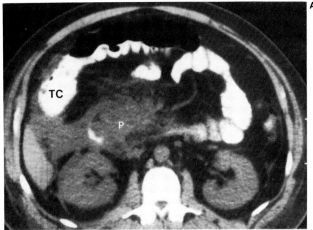

FIG. 67. Acute pancreatitis, with spread of inflammation through transverse mesocolon. **A:** There is diffuse infiltration of the wall of the duodenum (du), with extension of inflammatory strands (*arrows*) along the middle colic vessels in the root of the transverse mesocolon. **B:** Image 2 cm caudal shows transverse colon (TC) enveloped in an inflammatory reaction; (p) pancreatic head.

draining fistulas or abscesses may have soft-tissue or low-density masses (Fig. 66). CT-directed needle-aspiration biopsy can prove useful in problem cases (11). Routine postoperative images may be helpful in detecting even smaller recurrences amid the normal postoperative changes. Base-line postoperative images probably should not be performed until at least 2 to 4 months after operation to allow the morphologic changes of postoperative bleeding, inflammation, and edema to subside (54). In the first few months after this operation, a presacral mass due to benign causes is visible on CT in over half of patients.

CT also is useful in detecting recurrence of carcinoma after resection of a primary tumor located elsewhere in the colon. The entire abdomen is imaged using oral and intravenous contrast material. Tumor nodules may be seen in the liver or greater omentum or on the peritoneal surfaces. Recurrent tumor may cause enlargement of mesenteric or retroperitoneal lymph nodes. There may be ascites. False-positive interpretations usually arise from mistaking relocated pelvic organs, small-bowel loops, or postoperative fibrosis for recurrent tumor.

CT often can be helpful to differentiate a primary colonic process from a process secondarily involving the colon, such as pancreatic cancer or inflammatory disease that has extended down the transverse mesocolon (Fig. 67) or gastric carcinoma extending through the gastrocolic ligament. The sigmoid colon and ileocecal regions are common sites for metastatic intraperitoneal deposits, but other areas of the colon can be affected as well. Mural and mesenteric masses (Figs. 68 and 69) associated with stretched colonic loops can be seen.

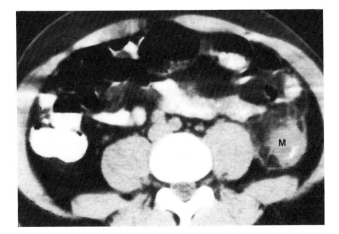

FIG. 68. An isolated metastasis (M) from a primary lung carcinoma produces eccentric thickening of the wall of the descending colon, with stranding of the pericolonic fat.

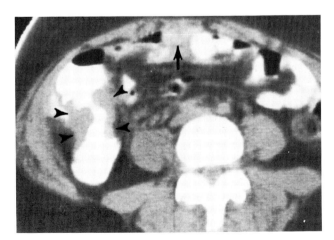

FIG. 69. Metastatic carcinoma of the breast, causing circumferential thickening (*arrowheads*) of the colonic wall. There is also an omental implant (*arrow*).

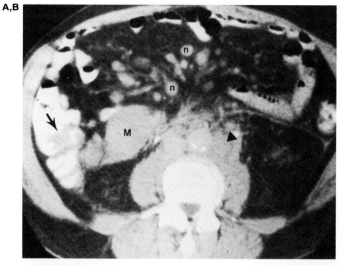
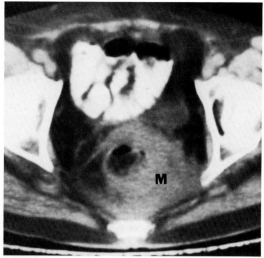

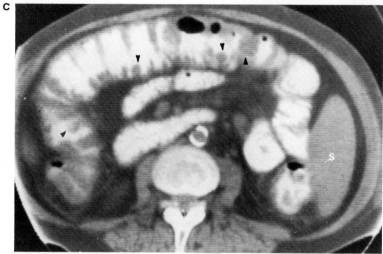

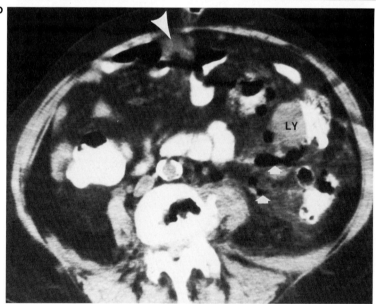

FIG. 70. Colonic lymphoma: patterns of involvement. **A:** A bulky mesenteric mass (M) is present in association with retroperitoneal adenopathy (*arrowhead*) and a small focus in the colonic wall (*arrow*); (n) enlarged mesenteric nodes. **B:** A single large rectal mass (M), with invasion of the left pelvic sidewall, is present in another patient who had no nodal involvement. **C:** Diffuse nodular infiltration of the colonic wall (*arrowheads*), resembling the pattern seen in colitis, is observed in another patient. Note the enlarged spleen (S). **D:** Focal colonic-wall mass (LY) is present in this patient who has diffuse peritoneal lymphoma. Colonic involvement produced perforation, resulting in retroperitoneal gas (*arrows*) at this site. Note omental deposit of lymphoma (*arrowhead*).

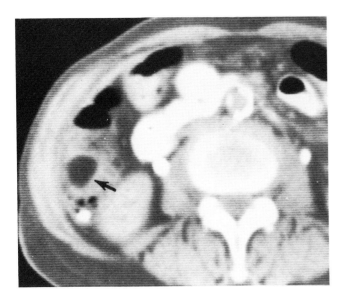

FIG. 71. Lipomatous infiltration of the ileocecal valve appears as a circumscribed cecal mass (*arrow*), with attenuation similar to that of subcutaneous fat.

Bulky masses, either single or multiple, or diffuse bowel nodularity and wall thickening can be seen with colonic lymphoma (Fig. 70). When present, splenomegaly and marked retroperitoneal or mesenteric adenopathy assist in the diagnosis.

Colonic lipomas, lipomas of the ileocecal valve, and lipomatous infiltration of the valve can be identified and classified using CT on the basis of their characteristic low CT attenuation numbers (69) (Fig. 71). Other benign colonic tumors, if visible, appear as soft-tissue-density masses.

Inflammation

CT can be useful in detecting and evaluating a variety of diffuse and focal inflammatory conditions of the colon and appendix. Pericolonic inflammation and abscess due to perforation of a colonic tumor or diverticulum or of the appendix can be well seen. The hallmark of any colonic perforation on CT is the finding of focal pericolonic inflammation, as evidenced by diffuse or streaky opacities in the pericolonic fat due to edema, hyperemia, and cellular infiltration. When the inflammation is related to diverticulitis, diverticula usually are seen, and there may be accompanying circular muscular hypertrophy. The wall of the colon usually is thickened in diverticulitis, and a frank abscess may be seen in about one-third of patients (44) (Figs. 72–75). A pericolonic diverticular abscess will appear as a mass with a thick wall of soft-tissue density and a low-density center that may contain gas or, if in communication with the lumen, contrast material. A fistula or intramural sinus tract can be seen in some patients, and the occasional finding of free intraperitoneal fluid or gas usually indicates peritonitis.

Appendicitis can also be imaged effectively with CT, and the findings can be similar to those of diverticulitis (6,9). An abscess will be identifiable in about 50% of patients, and a calcified appendicolith in about 25% (Figs. 76 and 77). In less severe appendicitis, there may be thickening and dilatation of the appendix, with surrounding inflammation, but no abscess. The sensitivities for detecting appendicitis appear to be similar for CT and contrast enema, but the former often provides a more specific indication of the nature, location, and extent of disease. CT has proved to be reliable in distinguishing phlegmon from abscess (9). In that study, patients with

A,B

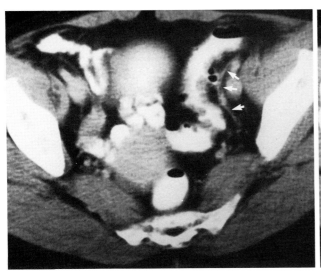
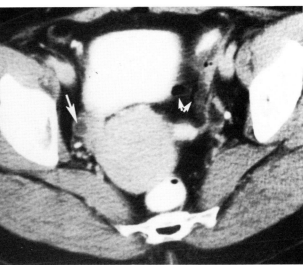

FIG. 72. Sigmoid diverticulitis. **A:** There is localized thickening of the colonic wall, with extraluminal gas adjacent to the round ligament (*arrows*). **B:** Two centimeters caudal, extraluminal gas is identified adjacent to the bladder and in the pericolonic fat (*small arrows*). No discrete abscess is present; (*large arrow*) right ovarian cyst.

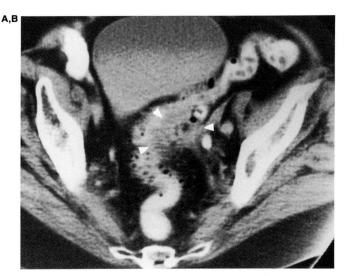 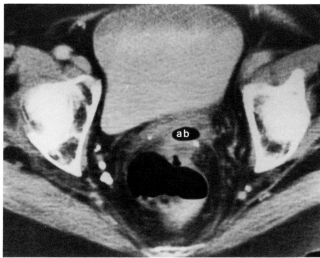

FIG. 73. Sigmoid diverticulitis, with abscess. **A:** There are numerous colonic diverticula and an ill-defined mass (*arrowheads*), producing focal eccentric sigmoid-wall thickening, with infiltration of the surrounding perisigmoid fat. **B:** Two centimeters caudal, a focal gas-containing abscess (ab) is present immediately posterior to the bladder.

large or poorly localized abscesses were treated surgically, those with well-localized abscesses were managed with CT-guided percutaneous catheter drainage, and those with purely phlegmonous inflammation responded to antibiotics alone without surgery.

Colitis is manifested on CT by a variety of abnormalities, some of which are fairly characteristic of the specific disease entity (37). In patients with ulcerative colitis, there is concentric thickening of the colonic wall (Fig. 78), averaging 8 mm in thickness. The CT attenuation of the bowel wall usually is inhomogeneous, with low-attenua-

tion areas in the wall. In the rectum, these abnormalities take on a "target" appearance, with black intraluminal air surrounded by white contrast material, which is encompassed by a dark gray layer of edematous bowel wall, in turn surrounded by a brighter, soft-tissue-attenuation layer of rectal wall. The outermost layer is a thickened layer of perirectal fat.

In patients with granulomatous colitis, the colonic wall tends to be even thicker, averaging 13 mm (Fig. 79). The CT attenuation of the wall is homogeneous. Abscesses and fistulas may be seen, and generally there is inflam-

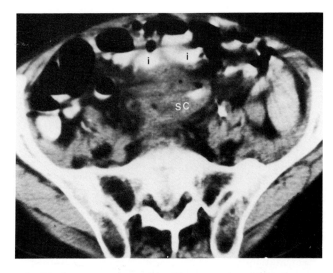

FIG. 74. Sigmoid diverticulitis. There is a focal inflammatory mass producing sigmoid-wall thickening and infiltrating the small-intestine mesentery, producing low-grade, partial small-bowel obstruction; (SC) sigmoid colon; (i) ileum.

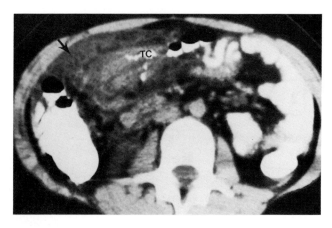

FIG. 75. Extensive omental infiltration (*arrow*) and bulky mass in the proximal transverse colon (TC) secondary to diverticulitis.

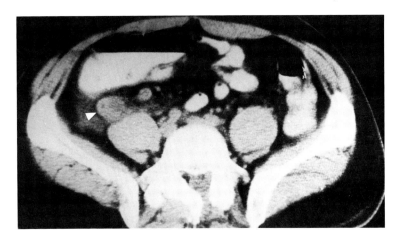

FIG. 76. Appendicitis. The appendix (*arrowhead*) is distended and has a thickened wall. Note infiltration of the surrounding fat, indicating phlegmonous reaction.

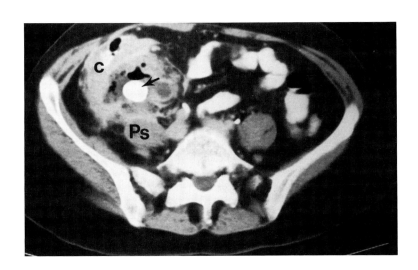

FIG. 77. Retrocecal appendicitis, with large abscess deforming the posterior cecal wall (C) and containing a large appendicolith (*arrow*); (Ps) psoas muscle.

FIG. 78. Ulcerative colitis involving the rectum (R) has produced concentric layers of differing attenuation within the colonic wall (*arrows*).

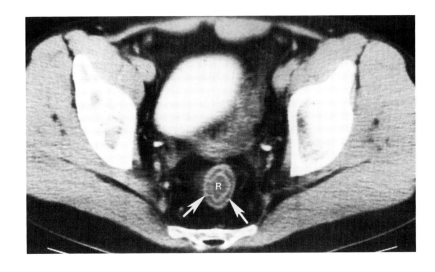

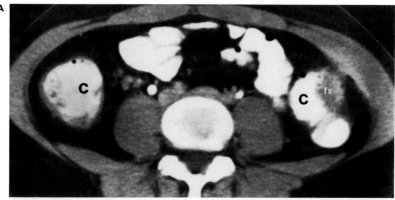

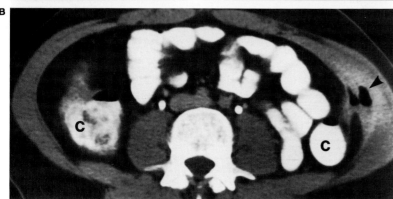

FIG. 79. Granulomatous colitis: sinus tract. **A:** There is eccentric wall thickening (fx) involving the descending colon (C); infiltration extends to the body wall. **B:** Image 2 cm caudal shows gas (*arrowhead*) within a thickened portion of the transverse abdominal and internal oblique muscles. This was documented to be a sinus tract.

FIG. 80. Granulomatous colitis: "creeping fat." There is obvious thickening (*arrow*) of the wall of the descending colon. Surrounding this segment is abundant pericolonic fat, which contains wispy strands of higher attenuation. This appearance is characteristic of chronic granulomatous colitis.

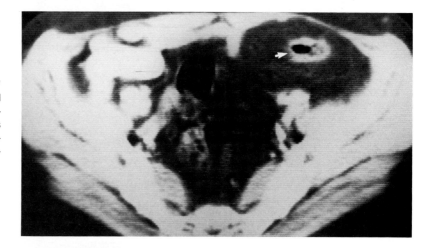

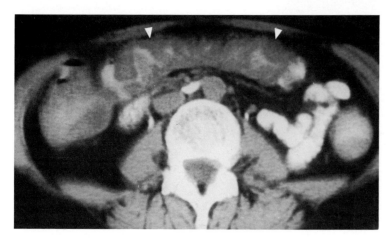

FIG. 81. Colitis due to *Salmonella* infection. There is marked thickening of the wall of the transverse colon (*arrowheads*); similar findings are present within the ascending and descending colonic segments as well.

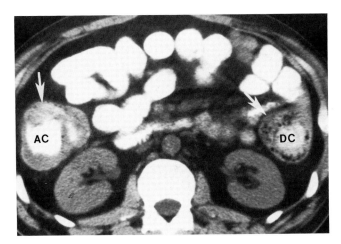

FIG. 82. There is pronounced thickening of the colonic wall (*arrows*) in a patient with antibiotic-induced pseudomembranous colitis; (AC) ascending colon; (DC) descending colon.

mation of the pericolonic fat, which appears as a diffuse, hazy increase in its CT attenuation. In some patients, the mesenteric fat in the area of the bowel involvement thickens and proliferates to the point of being mass-like, with displacement of adjacent bowel loops (Fig. 80). Not surprisingly, patients with radiographic findings on barium enema that are indeterminate for ulcerative or granulomatous colitis tend to have CT findings that are indeterminate as well.

CT abnormalities in other forms of colitis have been documented less fully. In general, CT shows abnormalities that would be predicted from the appearance on barium enema (Fig. 81). For example, in pseudomembranous colitis (10,35), CT shows marked thickening of haustral folds (Fig. 82), whereas neutropenic colitis (typhlitis) (Fig. 83) leads to severe cecal-wall thickening, with or without intramural gas (29). As might be expected, perirectal abscess

appears similar to abscess elsewhere in the body as a walled-off fluid collection, with displacement of normal structures (Fig. 84).

Miscellaneous

Ischemia

Ischemic bowel can be identified on CT by linear or punctate collections of gas in the bowel wall (Fig. 85). Gas also can extend into mesenteric and portal veins.

Radiation

The CT findings in radiation injury of the distal colon include (a) mural thickening of the irradiated segment, (b) widening of the presacral space, (c) increased perirectal fat, (d) thickening of perirectal fibrous tissue, and (e) fibrotic connections between the rectum and sacrum (28) (Fig. 86). The increased presacral space (greater than 1 cm) alone is a nonspecific finding and may be seen in normal patients. If there is a substantial increase in perirectal fat, without fibrosis or bowel-wall thickening, pelvic lipomatosis should be considered. Perirectal fibrous tissue is not seen or is barely visible in normal individuals. The symmetrical increase in perirectal fibrous tissue found after radiation helps distinguish radiation proctitis from the generally asymmetrical appearance of recurrent tumor or postoperative fibrosis. Rarely, a similar symmetric appearance can be seen in extension of prostatic cancer or following extensive perirectal inflammatory disease. After radiation, the combination of increased perirectal fat and thickened perirectal fascia can produce a "target" appearance, with the thick-walled, stenotic rectum forming the center of the target (28).

FIG. 83. Neutropenic colitis in a 17-year-old girl with acute lymphocytic leukemia. The wall of the right colon (C) is markedly thickened, and there is increased attenuation of the surrounding fat.

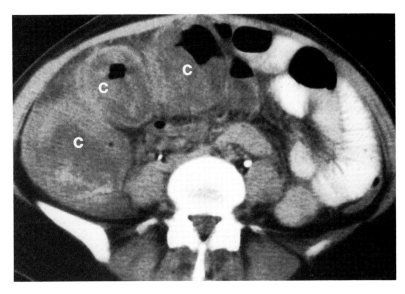

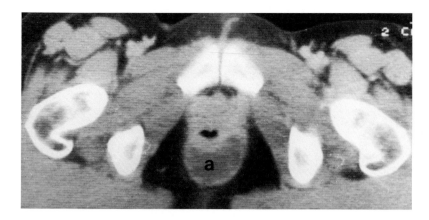

FIG. 84. Perirectal abscess (a) in a woman with leukemia. The abscess displaces the rectum anteriorly.

Obstruction

Mechanical obstruction of the colon can be identified on CT by the differential colonic distension proximal and distal to the site of obstruction. Occasionally the cause of the obstruction can be ascertained. A primary obstructing malignant neoplasm can be seen as a soft-tissue mass, with or without a narrow, irregular lumen (64). Tumors secondarily invading the colon can be seen, and their sites of origin may be determined. Ileocolic intussusception

can be identified because of its characteristic CT appearance (79,90), similar to that already described in the section on the small intestine. In adults, 50% of colonic intussusceptions are caused by malignant tumors, which are themselves occasionally imaged as soft-tissue masses within the intussuscipiens (79). A lipoma of the ileocecal valve is the most common benign tumor responsible for intussusception and occasionally may be seen as a well-defined mass within the intussuscipiens, with characteristic fatty CT attenuation values.

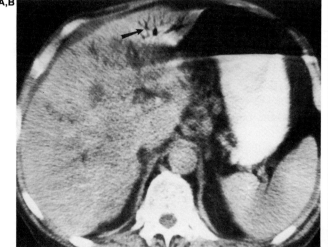

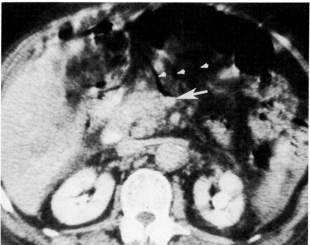

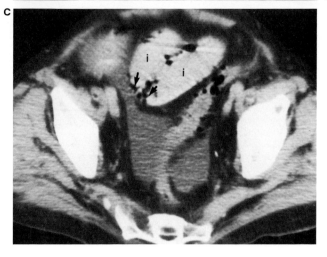

FIG. 85. CT performed to evaluate acute abdominal pain. **A:** Section through the liver shows branching, gas-containing intrahepatic portal veins (*arrow*). **B:** Image 6 cm caudal shows a contrast–air level in the superior mesenteric vein (*arrow*), as well as gas within smaller mesenteric venous tributaries (*arrowheads*). **C:** Section through the pelvis shows intramural gas (*black arrows*) within dilated intestinal loops (i). Surgical exploration revealed extensive small-intestine infarction.

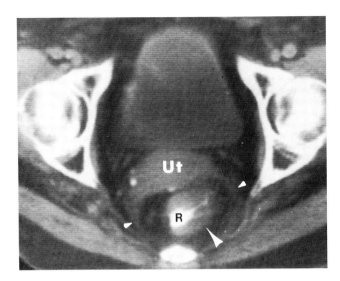

FIG. 86. Radiation proctitis. There is irregular thickening of the rectal wall (*large arrowhead*) and thickening of perirectal fascia (*small arrowheads*); (R) rectum; (Ut) uterus.

REFERENCES

1. Adalsteinsson B, Glimelius B, Graffman S, Hemmingsson A, Pahlman L. Computed tomography in staging rectal carcinoma. *Acta Radiol* 1985;26:45–50.
2. Agha FP, Gabriele OF, Abdulla FH. Complete gastric duplication. *AJR* 1981;137:406–407.
3. Baer JW, Smorzaniuk E. Gastric varices appearing as intraluminal masses on computed tomography. *Gastrointest Radiol* 1985;10:345–346.
4. Balfe DM, Koehler RE, Karstaedt N, Stanley RJ, Sagel SS. Computed tomography of gastric neoplasms. *Radiology* 1981;140:431–436.
5. Balthazar EJ, Bauman JS, Megibow AJ. CT diagnosis of closed loop obstruction. *J Comput Assist Tomogr* 1985;9:953–955.
6. Balthazar EJ, Megibow AJ, Hulnick D, Gordon RB, Nadich DP, Beranbaum ER. CT of appendicitis. *AJR* 1986;147:705–710.
7. Balthazar EJ, Megibow AJ, Naidich D, LeFleur RS. Computed tomographic recognition of gastric varices. *AJR* 1984;142:1121–1125.
8. Balthazar EJ, Subramanyam BR, Megibow AJ. Spigelian hernia: CT and ultrasonography diagnosis. *Gastrointest Radiol* 1984;9:81–84.
9. Barakos JA, Jeffrey RB, Federle MP, Wing VW, Laing FC, Hightower DR. CT in the management of periappendiceal abscess. *AJR* 1986;146:1161–1164.
10. Brunner D, Feifarek C, McNeely D, Haney P. CT of pseudomembranous colitis. *Gastrointest Radiol* 1984;9:73–75.
11. Butch RJ, Wittenberg J, Mueller PR, Simeone JF, Meyer JE, Ferrucci JT. Presacral masses after abdominoperineal resection for colorectal carcinoma: the need for needle biopsy. *AJR* 1985;144:309–312.
12. Buy J-N, Moss AA. Computed tomography of gastric lymphoma. *AJR* 1982;138:859–865.
13. Cimmino CV. The esophageal-pleural stripe: an update. *Radiology* 1981;140:609–613.
14. Clark KE, Foley WD, Lawson TL, Berland LL, Maddison FE. CT evaluation of esophageal and upper abdominal varices. *J Comput Assist Tomogr* 1980;4:510–515.
15. Cockey BM, Fishman EK, Jones B, Siegelman SS. Computed tomography of abdominal carcinoid tumor. *J Comput Assist Tomogr* 1985;9:38–42.
16. Connor R, Jones B, Fishman EK, Siegelman SS. Pneumatosis intestinalis: role of computed tomography in diagnosis and management. *J Comput Assist Tomogr* 1984;8:269–275.
17. Cook AO, Levine BA, Sirinek KR, Gaskill HV III. Evaluation of gastric adenocarcinoma: abdominal computed tomography does not replace celiotomy. *Arch Surg* 1986;121:603–606.
18. Coscina WF, Arger PH, Levine MS, et al. Gastrointestinal tract focal

mass lesions: role of CT and barium evaluations. *Radiology* 1986;158:581–587.
19. Epstein BM, Mann JH. CT of abdominal tuberculosis. *AJR* 1982;139:861.
20. Fakhri A, Fishman EK, Jones B, Kuhajda F, Siegelman SS. Primary intestinal lymphangiectasia: clinical and CT findings. *J Comput Assist Tomogr* 1985;9:767–770.
21. Fisher JK. Computed tomographic diagnosis of volvulus in intestinal malrotation. *Radiology* 1981;140:145–146.
22. Fisher JK. Normal colon wall thickness on CT. *Radiology* 1982;145:415–418.
23. Fishman EK, Magid D, Jones B, Siegelman SS. Menetrier disease. *J Comput Assist Tomogr* 1983;7:143–145.
24. Fishman EK, Zinreich ES, Jones B, Siegelman SS. Computed tomographic diagnosis of radiation ileitis. *Gastrointest Radiol* 1984;9:149–152.
25. Fitch SJ, Tonkin ILD, Tonkin AK. Imaging of foregut duplication cysts. *RadioGraphics* 1986;6:189–201.
26. Frager DH, Goldman M, Beneventano TC. Computed tomography in Crohn's disease. *J Comput Assist Tomogr* 1983;7:819–824.
27. Freeny PC, Marks WM, Ryan JA, Bolen JW. Colorectal carcinoma evaluation with CT: preoperative staging and detection of postoperative recurrence. *Radiology* 1986;158:347–353.
28. Frommhold W, Hubener KH. The role of computerized tomography in the aftercare of patients suffering from a carcinoma of the rectum. *Comput Tomogr* 1981;5:161–168.
29. Frick MP, Maile CW, Crass JR, Goldberg ME, Delaney JP. Computed tomography of neutropenic colitis. *AJR* 1984;143:763–765.
30. Gale ME, Gerzof SG, Kiser LC, et al. CT appearance of afferent loop obstruction. *AJR* 1982;138:1085–1088.
31. Glick SN, Teplick SK, Levine MS. Squamous cell metastases to the gastric cardia. *Gastrointest Radiol* 1985;10:339–344.
32. Glazer GM, Buy JN, Moss AA, Goldberg HI, Federle MP. CT detection of duodenal perforation. *AJR* 1981;137:333–336.
33. Goldberg HI, Gore RM, Margulis AR, Moss AA, Baker EL. Computed tomography in the evaluation of Crohn's disease. *AJR* 1983;140:277–282.
34. Goldman SM, Fishman EK, Gatewood OMB, Jones B, Siegelman SS. CT in the diagnosis of enterovesical fistulae. *AJR* 1985;144:1229–1233.
35. Goodman PC, Federle MP. Pseudomembranous colitis. *J Comput Assist Tomogr* 1980;4:403–404.
36. Gore RM, Cohen MI, Vogelzang RL, Neiman HL, Tsand T-K. Value of computed tomography in the detection of complications of Crohn's disease. *Dig Dis Sci* 1985;30:701–709.
37. Gore RM, Marn CS, Kirby DF, Vogelzang RL, Neiman HL. CT findings in ulcerative, granulomatous and indeterminate colitis. *AJR* 1984;143:279–282.
38. Greenstein S, Jones B, Fishman EK, Cameron JL, Siegelman SS. Small bowel diverticulitis: CT findings. *AJR* 1986;147:271–274.
39. Gross BH, Agha FP, Glazer GM, Orringer MB. Gastric interposition following transhiatal esophagectomy: CT evaluation. *Radiology* 1985;155:177–179.
40. Halber MD, Daffner RH, Thompson WM. CT of the esophagus: I. Normal appearance. *AJR* 1979;133:1047–1050.
41. Halden WJ, Harnsberger HR, Mancuso AA. Computed tomography of esophageal varices after sclerotherapy. *AJR* 1983;140:1195–1196.
42. Halvorsen RA, Thompson WM. Computed tomographic staging of gastrointestinal tract malignancies. Part I. Esophagus and stomach. *Invest Radiol* 1987;22:2–16.
43. Heiken JP, Balfe DM, Roper CL. CT evaluation after esophagogastrectomy. *AJR* 1984;143:555–560.
44. Hulnick DH, Megibow AJ, Balthazar EJ, Naidich DP, Bosniak MA. Computed tomography in the evaluation of diverticulitis. *Radiology* 1984;152:491–495.
45. Husband JE, Hodson NJ, Parsons CA. The use of computed tomography in recurrent rectal tumors. *Radiology* 1980;134:677–682.
46. Imoto T, Nobe T, Koga M, Miyamoto Y, Nakata H. Computed tomography of gastric lipomas. *Gastrointest Radiol* 1983;8:129–131.
47. Ishikawa T, Tsukune Y, Ohyama Y, Fujikawa M, Sakuyama K, Fujii M. Venous abnormalities in portal hypertension demonstrated by CT. *AJR* 1980;134:271–276.
48. James S, Balfe DM, Lee JKT, Picus D. Small bowel disease: categorization by CT examination. *AJR* 1987;148:863–867.

49. Jaramillo D, Raval B. CT diagnosis of primary small bowel volvulus. *AJR* 1986;147:941–942.

50. Jeffrey RB, Nyberg DA, Bottles K, et al. Abdominal CT in acquired immunodeficiency syndrome. *AJR* 1986;146:7–13.

51. Jones B, Bayless TM, Fishman EK, Siegelman SS. Lymphadenopathy in celiac disease: computed tomographic observations. *AJR* 1984;142:1127–1132.

52. Jones B, Fishman EK, Framer SS, et al. Computed tomography of gastrointestinal inflammation after bone marrow transplantation. *AJR* 1986;146:691–695.

53. Kenney PJ, Brinsko RE, Patel DV. Gastric involvement in chronic granulomatous disease of childhood: demonstration by computed tomography and upper gastrointestinal studies. *J Comput Assist Tomogr* 1985;9:563–565.

54. Kelvin FM, Korobkin M, Heaston DK, Grant JP, Akwari O. The pelvis after surgery for rectal carcinoma: serial CT observations with emphasis on nonneoplastic features. *AJR* 1983;141:959–964.

55. Kelvin FM, Korobkin M, Rauch RF, Rice RP, Silverman PM. Computed tomography of pneumatosis intestinalis. *J Comput Assist Tomogr* 1984;8:276–280.

56. Kerber GW, Greenberg M, Rubin JM. Computed tomography evaluation of local and extraintestinal complications of Crohn's disease. *Gastrointest Radiol* 1984;9:143–148.

57. Komaki A, Toyoshima S. CT's capability in detecting advanced gastric cancer. *Gastrointest Radiol* 1983;8:307–313.

58. Krudy AG, Dunnick NR, Magrath IT, Shawker TH, Doppman JL, Speigel R. CT of American Burkitt lymphoma. *AJR* 1981;136:747–754.

59. Lee JKT, Stanley RJ, Sagel SS, Levitt RG, McClennan BL. CT appearance of the pelvis after abdominoperineal resection for rectal carcinoma. *Radiology* 1981;141:737–741.

60. Libshitz HI, Lindell MM, Maor MH, Fuller LM. Appearance of the intact lymphomatous stomach following radiotherapy and chemotherapy. *Gastrointest Radiol* 1985;10:25–29.

61. Livingston PA, Pollock EJ, Renert WA, Seaman WB. Radiological signs in the diagnosis of enterogenous cysts. *Radiology* 1971;98:543–545.

62. Lo J, Sage MR, Paterson HS, Hamilton DW. Gastric duplication in an adult. *J Comput Assist Tomogr* 1983;7:328–330.

63. Mauro MA, Jaques PF, Swantkowski TM, Staab EV, Bozymski EM. CT after uncomplicated esophageal sclerotherapy. *AJR* 1986;146:1–5.

64. Mayes GB, Zornoza J. Computed tomography of colon carcinoma. *AJR* 1980;135:43–46.

65. McCarthy SM, Stark DD, Moss AA, Goldberg HI. Computed tomography of malignant carcinoid disease. *J Comput Assist Tomogr* 1984;8:846–850.

66. Megibow AJ, Zerhouni EA, Hulnick DH, Schumaker J, Balthazar EJ, Gordon R. Air contrast techniques in gastrointestinal computed tomography. *AJR* 1985;145:418.

67. Megibow AJ, Balthazar EJ, Hulnick DH, Naidich DP, Bosniak MA. CT evaluation of gastrointestinal leiomyomas and leiomyosarcomas. *AJR* 1985;144:727–731.

68. Megibow AJ, Balthazar EJ, Naidich DP, Bosniak MA. Computed tomography of gastrointestinal lymphoma. *AJR* 1983;141:541–547.

69. Megibow AJ, Redmond PE, Bosniak MA, Horowitz L. Diagnosis of gastrointestinal lipomas by CT. *AJR* 1979;133:743–745.

70. Meyers MA. *Dynamic radiology of the abdomen.* New York: Springer-Verlag, 1976.

71. Moss AA, Margulis AR, Schnyder P, Thoeni RF. A uniform, CT-based staging system for malignant neoplasms of the alimentary tube. *AJR* 1981;136:1251–1252.

72. Moss AA, Schnyder P, Candardjis G, Margulis AR. Computed tomography of benign and malignant gastric abnormalities. *J Clin Gastroenterol* 1980;2:401–409.

73. Moss AA, Thoeni RF, Schnyder P, Margulis AR. Value of computed tomography in the detection and staging of recurrent rectal carcinomas. *J Comput Assist Tomogr* 1981;5:870–874.

74. Mullin D, Shirkhoda A. Computed tomography after gastrectomy in primary gastric carcinoma. *J Comput Assist Tomogr* 1985;9:30–33.

75. Nichols DM, Li DK. Superior mesenteric vein rotations: a CT sign of midgut malrotation. *AJR* 1983;141:707–708.

76. Nishimura K, Togashi K, Tohdo G, et al. Computed tomography of calcified gastric carcinoma. *J Comput Assist Tomogr* 1984;8:1010–1011.

77. Ormson MJ, Stephens DH, Carlson HC. CT recognition of intestinal lipomatosis. *AJR* 1985;144:313–314.

78. Papierniak KJ, Wittenstein B, Bartizal JF, Wielgolewski JW, Love L. Diagnosis of Spigelian hernia by computed tomography. *Arch Surg* 1983;118:109–110.

79. Parienty RA, Lepreux JF, Gruson B. Sonographic and CT features of ileocolic intussusception. *AJR* 1981;136:608–610.

80. Pearlberg JL, Sandler MA, Madrazo BL. Computed tomographic features of esophageal intramural pseudodiverticulosis. *Radiology* 1983;147:189–190.

81. Picus D, Balfe DM, Koehler RE, Roper CL, Owen JW. Computed tomography in the staging of esophageal carcinoma. *Radiology* 1983;146:433–438.

82. Picus D, Glazer HS, Levitt RG, Husband JE. Computed tomography of abdominal carcinoid tumors. *AJR* 1984;143:581–584.

83. Pillari G, Weinreb J, Vernace F, et al. CT of gastric masses: image patterns and a note on potential pitfalls. *Gastrointest Radiol* 1983;8:11–17.

84. Plojoux O, Hauser H, Wettstein P. Computed tomography of intramural hematoma of the small intestine: a report of 3 cases. *Radiology* 1982;144:559–561.

85. Quint LE, Glazer GM, Orringer MB, Gross BH. Esophageal carcinoma: CT findings. *Radiology* 1985;155:171–175.

86. Reinig JW, Stanley JH, Schabel SI. CT evaluations of thickened esophageal walls. *AJR* 1983;140:931–934.

87. Rezvani L, Tully RJ, Levine C, Levine E, Rubin JM. Computed tomography in the diagnosis and followup of American Burkitt's lymphoma. *Gastrointest Radiol* 1986;11:36–40.

88. Scatarige JC, Fishman EK, Jones B, Cameron JL, Sanders RC, Siegelman SS. Gastric leiomyosarcoma: CT observations. *J Comput Assist Tomogr* 1985;9:320–327.

89. Seigel RS, Kuhns LR, Borlaza GS, McCormick TL, Simmons JL. Computed tomography and angiography in ileal carcinoid tumor and retractile mesenteritis. *Radiology* 1980;134:437–440.

90. Siegelman SS. *CT diagnosis of intussusception.* Fifth annual course of the Society of Computed Body Tomography, Tarpon Springs, Florida, 1982.

91. Siskind BN, Burrell MI, Pun H, Russo R Jr, Levin W. CT demonstration of gastrointestinal involvement in Henoch-Schönlein syndrome. *Gastrointest Radiol* 1985;10:352–354.

92. Soulen MC, Fishman EK, Scatarige JC, Hutchins D, Zerhouni EA. Cryptosporidiosis of the gastric antrum: detection using CT. *Radiology* 1986;159:705–706.

93. Strauss JE, Balthazar EJ, Naidich DP. Jejunal perforation by a toothpick: CT demonstration. *J Comput Assist Tomogr* 1985;9:812–814.

94. Swayne LC, Love MB. Computed tomography of chronic afferent loop obstruction: a case report and review. *Gastrointest Radiol* 1985;10:39–41.

95. Thoeni RF, Moss AA, Schnyder P, Margulis AR. Detection and staging of primary rectal and rectosigmoid cancer by computed tomography. *Radiology* 1981;141:135–138.

96. Thompson W, Halvorsen RA, Foster WL, Roberts L, Gibbons R. Preoperative and postoperative CT staging of rectosigmoid carcinoma. *AJR* 1986;146:703–710.

97. Thompson WM, Halvorsen RA, Foster WL, Williford ME, Postlethwait RW, Korobkin M. Computed tomography for staging esophageal and gastroesophageal cancer: reevaluation. *AJR* 1983;141:951–958.

98. Van Waes PFGM, Koehler PR, Feldberg MAM. Management of rectal carcinoma: impact of computed tomography. *AJR* 1983;140:1137–1142.

99. Zaunbauer W, Haertel M, Fuchs WA. Computed tomography in carcinoma of the rectum. *Gastrointest Radiol* 1981;6:79–84.

CHAPTER 13

Spleen

Robert E. Koehler

The spleen is well seen on computed tomography (CT) and magnetic resonance (MR) images of the abdomen in virtually every patient. Normally it appears as an oblong or ovoid organ in the left upper abdomen (Fig. 1). The contour of the superior lateral border of the spleen is smooth and convex, conforming to the shape of the adjacent abdominal wall and left hemidiaphragm (Fig. 2). The margins of the spleen are smooth, and the parenchyma is sharply demarcated from the adjacent fat. The hilum usually is directed anteromedially, and the splenic artery and vein and their branches can be seen entering the spleen in this region. The posteromedial surface of the spleen behind the hilum often is concave where it conforms to the shape of the adjacent left kidney. The medial surface anterior to the hilum is in contact with the stomach and also assumes a shallow concave shape in some patients. On images performed without intravenous injection of contrast material, the normal spleen appears homogeneous in density, with CT attenuation values equal to or slightly less than that for the normal liver.

Like the liver, the spleen ordinarily has a small area that is not covered by peritoneum, a so-called bare area (84). Smaller than the bare area of the liver, this corresponds to approximately a 2- by 3-cm portion of the spleen's surface contained between the anterior and posterior leaves of the splenorenal ligament. This area overlies the renal fascia covering the anterior aspect of the upper pole of the left kidney. Ascites and other intraperitoneal, left upper abdominal fluid collections tend to surround all surfaces of the spleen except this small area. Recognition of this feature is occasionally helpful in determining whether fluid lies in the peritoneal space or left pleural space.

The splenic vessels are seen even on non-contrast-enhanced CT images in most individuals. The splenic vein follows a fairly straight course toward the splenic hilum, running transversely along the posterior aspect of the body

and tail of the pancreas. Unlike the splenic vein, the splenic artery often is tortuous (Fig. 1), especially in older patients. On any given slice, it may appear as a single curvilinear structure, or it may wander in and out of the plane of the slice and appear as a series of round densities, each of which represents a cross-sectional image of a portion of the artery. Also in older individuals, it is common to see calcified atheromas within the wall of the splenic artery.

USE OF CONTRAST MATERIAL

It is useful to administer iodinated contrast material intravenously when examining the spleen by CT. Dynamic scans performed during a bolus injection are optimal for clarifying the nature of soft-tissue structures in the splenic hilar and retropancreatic regions that can mimic abnormalities of the pancreas or left adrenal gland, but that may, in fact, be due to normal splenic vasculature. The splenic artery and vein and their branches undergo dense contrast enhancement during bolus injection and are easily identified (Fig. 3A). Splenic parenchymal opacification also occurs and may be used to improve the detectability of focal mass lesions within the spleen. When the injection is made slowly, over a period of minutes, a uniform increase in the density of the splenic parenchyma results. However, when contrast material is given by rapid intravenous injection, most patients initially exhibit a heterogeneous pattern of splenic opacification reflecting variable blood flow patterns within different compartments of the spleen (31) (Fig. 3). Only after the passage of a minute or more does the splenic parenchyma achieve a uniform, homogeneous appearance. Care must be taken not to misinterpret this early postinjection heterogeneity of splenic density as an indication of focal abnormality.

The use of intravenously administered lipoid contrast material, such as EOE-13 (83), which is taken up by the

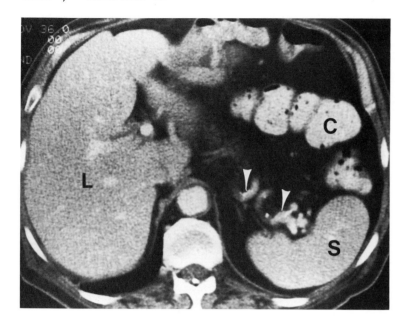

FIG. 1. CT image of normal spleen (S). The outer border is convex and conforms to the shape of the adjacent body wall. The medial surface is concave. The splenic artery (*arrowheads*) enters the hilum; (C) colon; (L) liver.

reticuloendothelial cells in the liver, spleen, and other areas, has been investigated for several years. On average, EOE-13 increases the CT attenuation of normal splenic tissue by 50 Hounsfield units (HU), while enhancing tumor tissue by an average of only 3 HU (53). Emulsified oily agents such as this are contraindicated in patients with significant pulmonary or hepatic dysfunction and can cause headache, fever, or rigors in as many as half of individuals unless steroid premedication is given. It remains to be determined whether or not a clinically acceptable agent of this type can be developed.

splenic vessels can consistently be seen without the use of intravenous contrast material.

At present, MRI does not offer any distinct advantages over CT or ultrasonography in imaging of the spleen. Therefore, MRI is relegated to a second-line status because it is more expensive and more time-consuming and has more stringent patient requirements.

MAGNETIC RESONANCE IMAGING

When examining the spleen by magnetic resonance imaging (MRI), T1-weighted images ordinarily are employed because their short repetition times allow multiple signal averages to be obtained in a reasonable period of time, with resultant decrease in respiratory-motion artifact. The MR signal intensity of splenic parenchyma is less than that of hepatic tissue and slightly greater than that of muscle (Fig. 4A). This yields an image of a dark shade of gray, much darker than surrounding fat, which is of high signal intensity. Images in the coronal and sagittal (Fig. 2) planes show the relationships of the spleen to the adjacent left kidney, adrenal, and hemidiaphragm to best advantage.

The spleen has a higher signal intensity on T2-weighted images, appearing brighter than the liver (Fig. 4B). Presently available techniques for producing T2-weighted MR images of upper abdominal structures are more susceptible to motion artifact, thereby resulting in blurring of the spleen. Because rapidly flowing blood produces little or no signal on both T1- and T2-weighted images, major

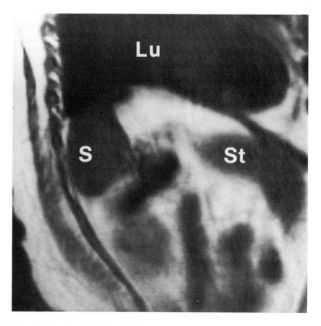

FIG. 2. Sagittal, T1-weighted MR image (TR = 300 msec, TE = 20 msec) of normal spleen (S). Note the intimate relationship of the spleen to the left hemidiaphragm and posterior body wall; (Lu) lung; (St) stomach.

A,B

![figure 3 CT images]

FIG. 3. CT appearance of the normal spleen (S) in two patients immediately after bolus intravenous injection of contrast material. **A:** Patchy pattern of splenic parenchymal enhancement. The aorta and hepatic and splenic (*arrowhead*) arteries are densely opacified. **B:** Rim-like pattern of parenchymal opacification. The heterogeneity of parenchymal opacification was transient, and the spleen appeared homogeneous on images obtained 1 min later in both patients; (K) kidney.

SPLENIC SIZE

Typically, the spleen measures about 12 cm in length, 7 cm in anteroposterior diameter, and 4 cm in thickness (64). The shape of the spleen varies so much from person to person, however, that these measurements are not of much use as a guide to normal splenic size.

A practical and more accurate approach to the assessment of splenic volume is the splenic index (45,78), which is the product of the length, width, and thickness of the spleen, each expressed in centimeters (Fig. 5). Splenic length is determined by summing the number of contiguous CT slices on which the spleen is visible. The width is the longest splenic diameter that can be drawn on any transverse image. The thickness is measured at the level of the splenic hilum and is the distance between the inner and outer (peripheral) borders of the spleen. When the thicknesses of the anterior and posterior portions of the

A,B

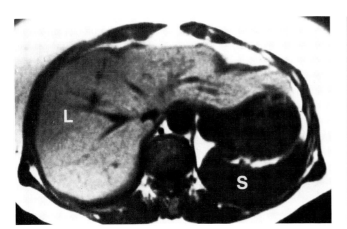
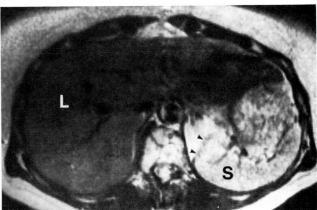

FIG. 4. MRI appearance of the normal spleen (S). **A:** On this T1-weighted image (TR = 300 msec, TE = 20 msec), the signal intensity of the spleen is less than that of the liver (L) and much less than that of the surrounding fat. **B:** On this T2-weighted MR image (TR = 1,500 msec, TE 80 msec) there is reversal of the relative signal intensities of the spleen and liver, and the spleen is sometimes difficult to distinguish from the fat surrounding it. In this image, a dark line (*arrowheads*) due to chemical-shift artifact delineates the splenic capsule medially.

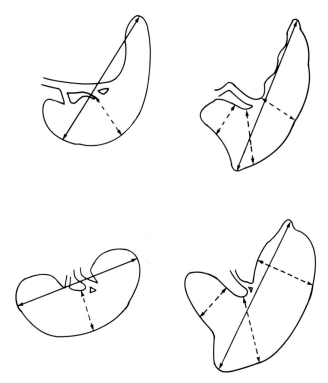

FIG. 5. Diagrammatic representation of measurements used in calculating the splenic index from transverse CT or MR images of spleens of various shapes. The width (*solid lines*) and thickness (*dashed lines*) are shown.

spleen differ significantly, two or three measurements of thickness are averaged. When determined in this way, normal splenic size corresponds to an index of 120 to 480 cm³.

The splenic index is superior to a subjective visual impression and is a more accurate criterion for splenomegaly than is extension of the spleen anterior to the aorta or below the rib cage (Fig. 6). The correlation between the splenic index, essentially a measure of splenic volume,

and the weight of the surgically excised spleen is an imperfect one. It has been demonstrated that the weight of the excised spleen averages only about half the splenic index (29,78). This is not surprising, because the size and weight of the excised spleen are affected by the amount of blood that drains from the specimen before it is weighed. The splenic index as determined by CT is probably a better indicator of splenomegaly than is the weight of the spleen as determined in the operating room or pathology laboratory.

Most accurate of all are computer programs for calculating actual splenic volume from a series of CT or MR images. However, even this method is limited in clinical usefulness, because the splenic volume varies so greatly from one normal person to another.

NORMAL VARIANTS AND CONGENITAL ANOMALIES

The shape and position of the normal spleen can vary considerably from one individual to another (Figs. 7 and 8). Commonly, there is a bulge or lobule of splenic tissue that extends medially from the visceral surface of the spleen to lie anterior to the upper pole of the left kidney (32,42,64) (Fig. 9). This can simulate the appearance of a left renal or adrenal mass on excretory urography, but is usually identifiable without difficulty by CT. Clefts between adjacent lobulations can be sharp and occasionally are as deep as 2 or 3 cm (Fig. 10). Occasionally, a lobule of splenic tissue can lie partially behind the left kidney and displace it anteriorly. In addition, the gastric fundus may indent the spleen in such a way as to simulate a tumor or other splenic defect on radionuclide examination (59). CT or MRI should readily resolve any such confusion.

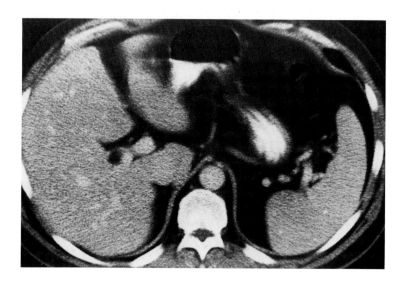

FIG. 6. Upper abdominal CT in a patient with mediastinal Hodgkin lymphoma. Whereas the CT study was initially thought to be free of signs of abdominal involvement, the vertical dimension of the spleen was 13 cm, and the splenic index was calculated to be 760. At exploratory laparotomy, the spleen contained lymphoma, with no other abdominal disease.

A,B

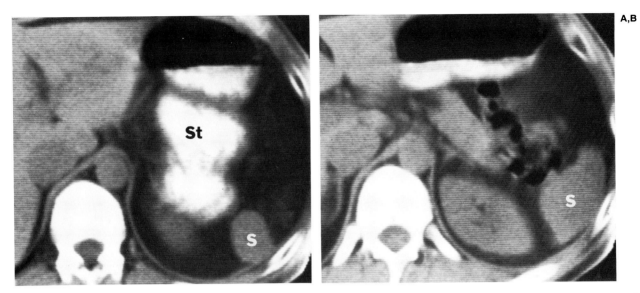

FIG. 7. Normal variation in splenic position. The spleen (S) is partially inverted, with its hilum directed medially and superiorly. **A:** Image high in the abdomen shows the upper pole as a small rounded density; (St) stomach. **B:** The spleen appears more usual in shape on a scan 2 cm lower in the abdomen.

The spleen is sufficiently soft and pliable in texture that left upper abdominal masses or organ enlargement can cause considerable displacement and deformity in its shape. When this happens, the spleen conforms to the shape of the adjacent mass, and the resulting deformity can be quite striking (Fig. 11). Likewise, changes in the position of the spleen occur when adjacent organs are surgically removed (Fig. 12A). This is particularly true in patients who have undergone left nephrectomy, in which case the spleen can occupy the left renal fossa (Fig. 12B). Occasionally, there is sufficient laxity in the ligamentous

attachments of the spleen that it lies in an unusual position in the absence of an abdominal mass or previous operation. The upside-down spleen (20,86) is a variant in which the splenic hilum is directed superiorly toward the medial, or occasionally the lateral, portion of the left hemidiaphragm.

The "wandering" spleen is another congenital variant that sometimes causes diagnostic difficulties (39). In this rare condition, most common in women, there is striking laxity of the suspensory splenic ligaments that permits the spleen to move about in the abdomen, sometimes sim-

A,B

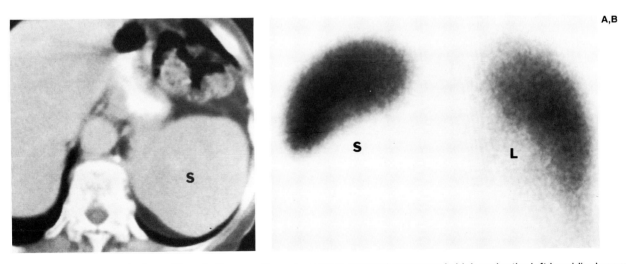

FIG. 8. Normal variation in splenic position. **A:** Because the spleen (S) is oriented transversely high under the left hemidiaphragm, it appears round and larger than normal. The craniocaudal extent was only 4 cm. **B:** Posterior view from radionuclide image confirms the normal appearance and transverse orientation; (L) liver.

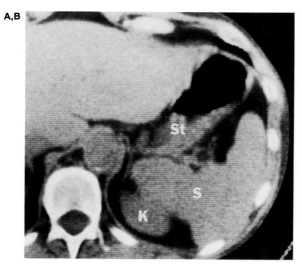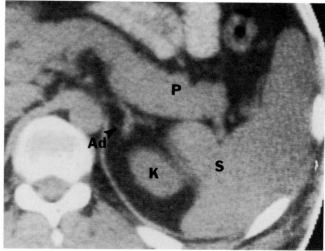

FIG. 9. Normal splenic lobulation. **A:** Prominent lobule of splenic tissue extending medially between the stomach (St) and left kidney (K). **B:** Medial lobulation of the spleen (S). Note the intimate relationship between this portion of the spleen and the adjacent kidney (K), adrenal (Ad), and pancreatic tail (P).

ulating a middle or lower abdominal neoplasm (34). The CT findings consist of an abdominal soft-tissue-density "mass" with a size appropriate for the spleen, plus the absence of a splenic shadow in the normal location (Fig. 13). It may be possible to recognize the characteristic shape of the spleen, and the density and pattern of enhancement after bolus intravenous injection of contrast material may lend additional support to the diagnosis. When there is

uncertainty whether or not the mass truly represents an ectopically located spleen, radionuclide imaging with ^{99m}Tc-sulfur colloid can resolve the dilemma. The condition usually is one of little clinical significance, but the wandering spleen can undergo torsion, with compromise of its vascular supply (39,71,75). This can lead to the development of gastric varices (76) or splenic infarction (69). If the pancreatic tail is involved in the torsion, CT may

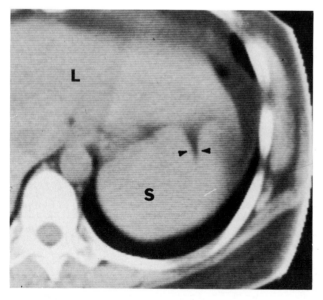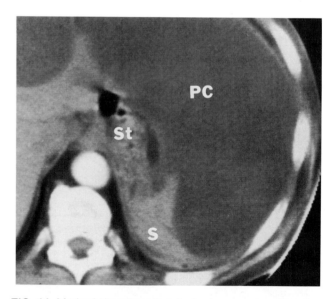

FIG. 10. Prominent cleft (*arrowheads*) between adjacent splenic lobulations. This anatomic variant can simulate an abnormality on radionuclide study, especially in patients suspected of having splenic trauma; (L) liver; (S) spleen.

FIG. 11. Marked alterations in splenic shape and position due to compression by an adjacent pancreatic pseudocyst (PC). At operation, the spleen (S) was compressed, but otherwise unaffected by the adjacent inflammatory process; (St) stomach.

A,B

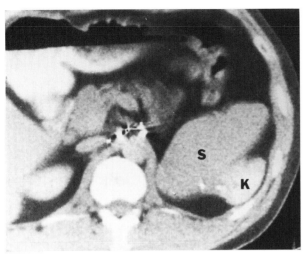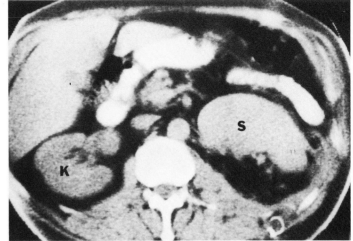

FIG. 12. Altered splenic position after left upper abdominal operation. **A:** Postoperative excretory urogram showed lateral displacement of the left kidney (K), but CT shows that this is due to shift in relative positions of spleen and kidney. **B:** In another patient, an image after left nephrectomy shows that spleen has shifted into the position formerly occupied by the left kidney. Splenic hilum is now directed posterosuperiorly.

demonstrate a whorled appearance of the pancreatic tail and adjacent fat (61).

Accessory Spleens

Accessory spleens occur in up to 40% of individuals (2,6,23) and are common findings on CT. They probably arise as a result of failure of fusion of some of the multiple buds of splenic tissue in the dorsal mesogastrium during embryonic life. They usually occur near the hilum of the spleen, but are sometimes found in its suspensory ligaments or in the tail of the pancreas. Rarely, they occur in the wall of the stomach or intestine, in the greater omentum or mesentery, or even in the pelvis or scrotum (87). In most patients they represent an incidental finding of no clinical significance.

Accessory spleens vary from microscopic deposits that

A,B

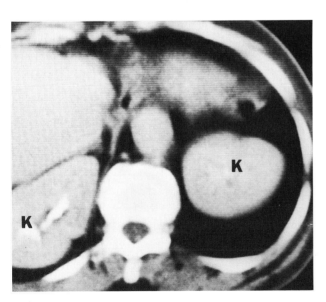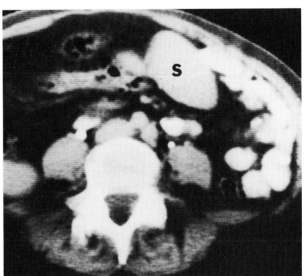

FIG. 13. Wandering spleen. **A:** No splenic shadow is seen in the left upper abdomen; (K) kidney. **B:** The spleen (S) is seen in the lower middle abdomen and mimics the appearance of an abdominal tumor.

are not visible on CT or MRI to nodules that are 2 or 3 cm in diameter (Fig. 14). Their CT attenuation and MR signal characteristics are like those of the spleen, and they have a smooth round or ovoid shape. Occasionally it is important to identify accessory splenic tissue, particularly when it is confused with a mass of another type. For instance, an accessory spleen can mimic the findings of a pancreatic, left adrenal, or other retroperitoneal mass on excretory urography (18,77). When there is uncertainty whether or not a nodule seen on CT represents an accessory spleen, one can compare the CT attenuation number of the structure in question with that of the spleen before and after intravenous injection of contrast material, because accessory splenic tissue tends to exhibit the same pattern of contrast enhancement as does the spleen itself (31,64). In problematic cases, ultrasound may be valuable to document that the vessels supplying the structure in question arise from the splenic artery and vein (79).

Another situation in which it can be important to identify accessory splenic tissue is in patients with pathologic splenic findings (Fig. 15) or those who have previously undergone splenectomy. In this situation, accessory spleens may hypertrophy and reach a size of 5 cm or more (6,40). Identification is particularly important in patients in whom the splenectomy was initially performed for a hematologic disorder resulting in hypersplenism. In these people, the growth of accessory splenic tissue may lead to a return of splenic hyperactivity, with resultant relapse (2). In such situations, radionuclide scintigraphy would generally be the radiologic method of choice for documentation.

Rare Congenital Conditions

Polysplenia is a rare combination of congenital anomalies characterized by multiple aberrant right-side splenic nodules, a central or left-side liver, absence of the gallbladder, cardiac anomalies, incomplete development of the inferior vena cava, and anomalies of other organs. When this condition is encountered on CT performed for other clinical indications, the images may demonstrate the nodules of splenic tissue in the right upper abdomen, the altered shape of the liver, and other features of the syndrome (22).

The congenital asplenia syndrome features absence of the spleen, ambiguous abdominal situs, a large transverse liver with indistinct separation of lobes, and anomalies of the biliary tract and cardiovascular system (66). Howell-Jolly bodies, which are seen in the peripheral smear in this and other conditions with diminished splenic function, may suggest the diagnosis.

PATHOLOGIC CONDITIONS

Splenomegaly

Enlargement of the spleen is detectable by a variety of means, including physical examination, and CT is rarely necessary to document the presence of splenomegaly. However, confusion sometimes arises as to whether or not a mass felt in the left upper abdomen truly represents an enlarged spleen. In such cases, CT, ultrasound, or MRI

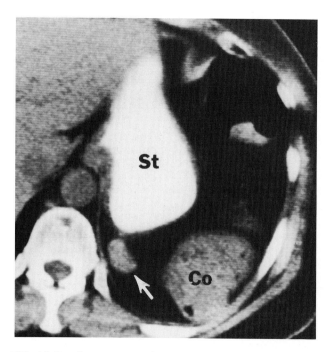

FIG. 14. Small accessory spleen (*arrow*) in a patient with prior splenectomy; (Co) colon; (St) stomach.

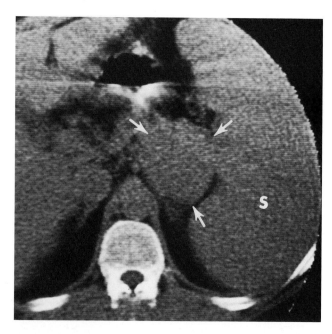

FIG. 15. Splenomegaly in a patient with lymphoma. The mass (*arrows*) in the splenic hilar region represents an enlarged accessory spleen that was also involved by the neoplasm, (S) spleen.

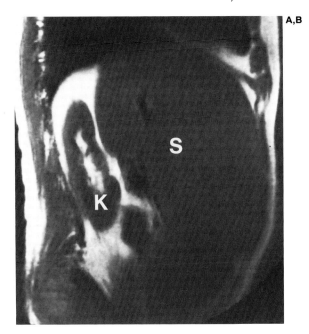

FIG. 16. Coronal (**A**) and left parasagittal (**B**) MR images (TR = 300 msec, TE = 20 msec) of an enlarged spleen (S) in a patient with Waldenström macroglobulinemia; (L) liver; (K) kidney.

can provide a definite answer as to whether the spleen is enlarged or whether there is a separate abdominal mass (11) (Fig. 16). When the spleen is enlarged, the concavity of its visceral surface often is lost as the spleen assumes a more globular shape (Fig. 17).

When splenomegaly is present, there often are CT findings that suggest the cause of the splenic enlargement. Neoplasm, abscess, or cyst can be appreciated within the spleen. Associated abdominal lymph node enlargement suggests lymphoma. Cirrhotic patients with splenomegaly on the basis of portal hypertension often show characteristic alterations in the size and shape of the liver and

prominence of the venous structures in the splenic hilum and gastrohepatic ligament (Fig. 18). There is an increase in the CT attenuation number of the spleen (as well as the liver) in some patients with hemochromatosis of either the primary or secondary type (50).

Lymphoma

The spleen often is affected in patients with lymphoma of both the Hodgkin and non-Hodgkin types (12,16). There is considerable disagreement regarding the accuracy

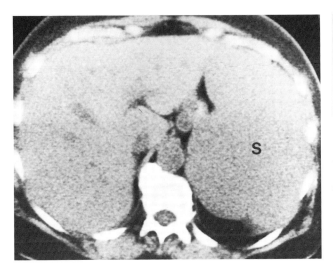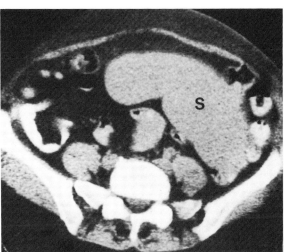

FIG. 17. Splenomegaly in a patient with chronic lymphocytic leukemia. **A:** The spleen (S) is globular in shape, and its medial border is predominantly convex. **B:** The lower pole of the spleen extends into the pelvis.

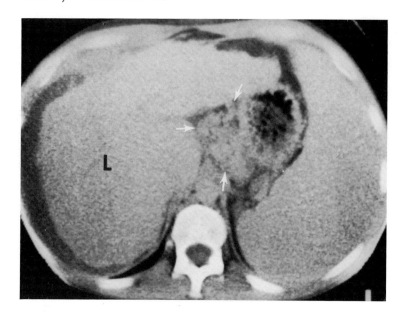

FIG. 18. Splenomegaly in a patient with cirrhosis and portal hypertension. The small nodular liver (L) and varices (*arrows*) in the gastrohepatic ligament indicate portal hypertension as the cause for splenic enlargement.

of CT as a predictor of splenic involvement with lymphoma, and reported figures for the sensitivity of CT vary from 15 to 90% (1,13,17,27,38,68,78,81).

Splenic involvement is found at staging laparotomy in about one-third of patients with previously untreated Hodgkin disease. The tumor is typically present as one or several nodules that usually are less than 1 cm in size, so-called miliary involvement. The spleen containing nodules of Hodgkin lymphoma may or may not be enlarged, and mild to moderate splenomegaly is not infrequently found in patients in whom no lymphoma is detected in the excised spleen. When splenomegaly is marked, however, it does appear to be a good predictor

of involvement by tumor in patients with Hodgkin disease. Focal nodular areas of low attenuation are occasionally seen on CT (Fig. 19), but splenomegaly alone is the most common abnormality to be detected (Fig. 6).

The non-Hodgkin lymphomas compose a heterogeneous group of lymphatic neoplasms that vary in radiological manifestations and clinical features. Splenic abnormalities are seen most often in patients with lymphoma of the diffuse histiocytic type (26,70) (Fig. 20). In patients with non-Hodgkin lymphoma, splenomegaly

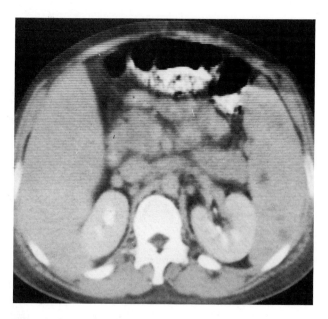

FIG. 19. Splenomegaly and multiple small splenic nodules in a patient with Hodgkin lymphoma.

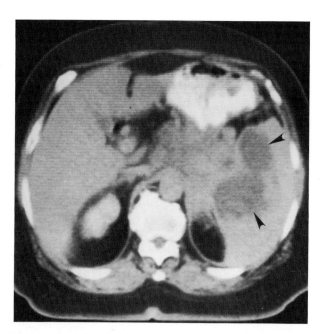

FIG. 20. Complex low-density masses (*arrowheads*) in the spleen, one of which appeared to extend into the adjacent tail of the pancreas. At operation, there were multiple foci of lymphoma in the spleen, splenic hilum, and pancreas.

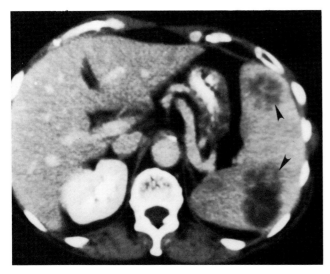

FIG. 21. Splenomegaly in a patient with diffuse histiocytic lymphoma. Two focal low-density lesions (*arrowheads*) are also noted.

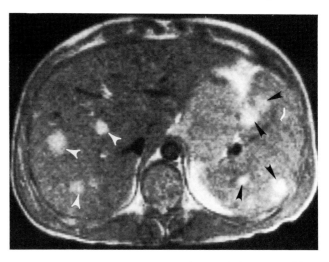

FIG. 22. Splenic and hepatic lymphoma. MR image (TR = 2,100 msec, TE = 30 msec) shows multiple hyperintense nodules in the spleen (*black arrowheads*) and liver (*white arrowheads*).

indicates a high probability of splenic involvement by tumor. In comparison with Hodgkin disease and other types of non-Hodgkin lymphoma, low-density nodules often are demonstrated by CT in patients with diffuse histiocytic lymphoma (15,27,38,44) (Fig. 21). Likewise, lymphomatous nodules can be seen on MRI. They often appear as hyperintense foci on T2-weighted images (Fig. 22).

Use of the experimental oily, emulsified agent EOE-13 increases the sensitivity of CT for detecting small splenic nodules of lymphoma of any histologic type (81).

Other Tumors

In some centers, an even more common cause of focal low-density nodules in the spleen is metastatic disease in patients with carcinomas or sarcomas originating in other areas (26,64). Malignant melanoma often is the tumor of origin (Fig. 23), but metastases can also arise from tumors of the lung, breast, and a variety of other organs (Fig. 24). Typically, CT shows one or more nodules that are 10 to 20 HU or more below the density of the surrounding splenic tissue. Metastatic nodules containing areas of necrosis and liquefaction may exhibit irregularly shaped regions within them that are even lower in density. Splenic enlargement may or may not be present.

Primary sarcomas of the spleen are rare (41,54). Most are tumors of vascular origin, such as hemangiosarcoma and hemangioendothelioma. On CT, such neoplasms generally appear as focal rounded areas of heterogeneous low attenuation (Fig. 25). Cystic and solid components may be evident within the mass (51). In some patients,

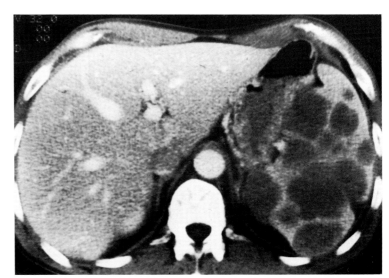

FIG. 23. Metastatic melanoma. Postcontrast CT image demonstrates multiple hypodense tumor nodules.

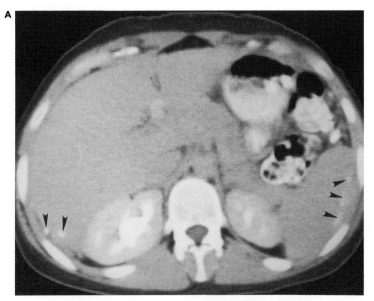

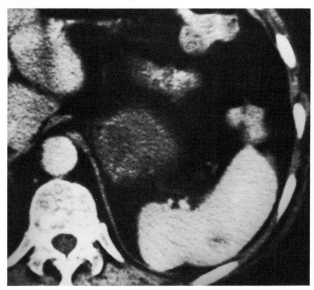

FIG. 24. Carcinoma metastatic to the spleen. **A:** Multiple small calcified metastases (*arrowheads*) are noted in the spleen, liver, and peritoneum in this patient with ovarian carcinoma. **B:** Undifferentiated carcinoma of the lung metastatic to the spleen. Note the contrast enhancement of the periphery of the lesion and patchy areas of enhancement within it. **C:** Small isolated focus of metastatic carcinoma of the breast in a male.

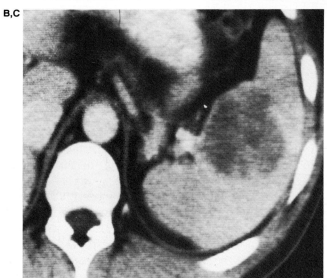

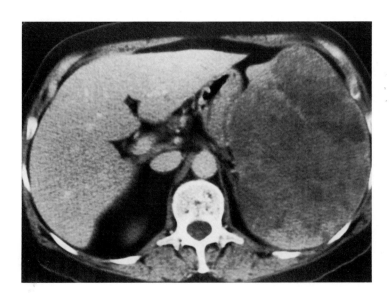

FIG. 25. Large, partially enhanced angiosarcoma of the spleen.

the development of angiosarcoma of the spleen has followed administration of Thorotrast, a colloidal suspension of thorium dioxide used until the 1950s as an angiographic contrast agent (47). In these patients, CT shows a striking increase in the attenuation of the splenic parenchyma due to chronic retention of the contrast material in reticuloendothelial cells.

Benign splenic tumors also are uncommon. Hamartomas tend to be single, spherical, and predominantly solid (55). CT or ultrasound may demonstrate small cystic areas within these tumors (14). Multiple cavernous hemangiomas may appear as myriad small, low-attenuation areas within the spleen (Fig. 26) (57). Diffuse capillary hemangiomatosis also occurs and produces splenomegaly and sometimes portal hypertension (65,80). Extensive, dense calcification can occur within the spleen involved with hemangiomatosis (37). Splenic lymphangiomatosis also presents as splenomegaly, with multiple small cystic components (82). Such benign splenic tumors can be clinically important in three ways. Rupture of a vascular splenic tumor can be a catastrophic event. Splenic capillary hemangiomatosis occasionally causes portal hypertension. Finally, the nonspecificity of the CT appearance of these tumors commonly leads to their confusion with lymphoma or other primary or secondary splenic malignancies.

Inflammatory Disease

Scattered punctate calcifications in the spleen are commonly encountered as incidental findings on CT and indicate the presence of healed granulomata (Fig. 27). In most patients in the midwestern United States, these are due to prior histoplasmosis infection. Tuberculosis can

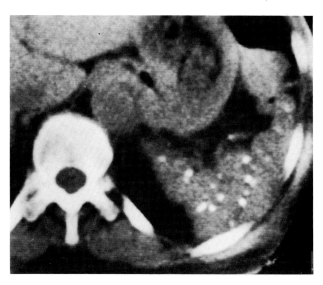

FIG. 27. Multiple calcified splenic granulomata presumed due to histoplasmosis.

also cause calcified splenic granulomata. Large, thin-rimmed, concentrically laminated calcifications have been described in splenic granulomata due to brucellosis (3).

CT can be a valuable technique for the detection of splenic abscess. In the past, this disease has involved 60% mortality, partially because it often has gone undiagnosed until the time of operation or autopsy (35,49). Earlier and more accurate detection is now available using CT. In addition, CT-guided catheter drainage of splenic abscesses is gradually becoming an accepted method of treatment (8,46) and has been successful in most reported cases.

The CT appearance of abscesses in the spleen is similar to that of abscesses in other areas (5,26,56). Typically, the abscess is a focal lesion with a density lower than that of the surrounding splenic tissue (Fig. 28). The average CT attenuation number of the abscess depends on the nature of its contents and can vary from 20 to 40 HU or more. Splenic abscesses usually are well circumscribed and often are spherical or slightly lobulated in shape (Fig. 29). They may contain gas, and there may be layering of material of different densities within the cavity. The rim of the abscess often is isodense with the surrounding spleen, but may be enhanced when iodinated contrast material is injected intravenously.

CT also provides an excellent method of detecting splenic involvement with disseminated, multifocal fungal infection (10,72). Fungal microabscesses occur in the spleen predominantly in immunosuppressed patients with lymphoma or hematologic malignancy, typically those with acute leukemia. In most instances, infection is due to *Candida,* with occasional cases due to infection with *Aspergillus* species. The CT appearance of fungal microabscesses is quite characteristic. Multiple scattered, round areas of low attenuation are seen in the spleen, and usually in the liver as well. These range from a few mil-

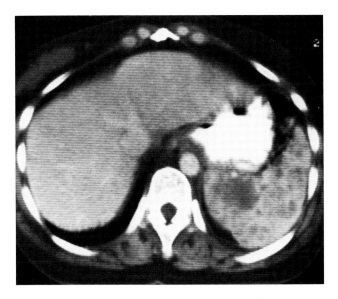

FIG. 26. Diffuse cavernous hemangiomatosis of the spleen.

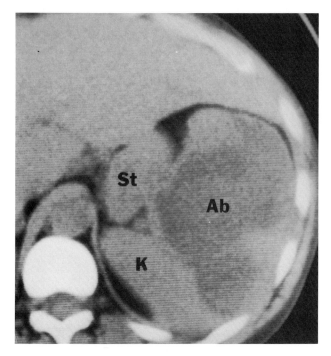

FIG. 28. Splenic abscess (Ab) in an alcoholic patient with fever. The spleen is enlarged, and the abscess appears as a lobulated, low-density region within it; (K) kidney; (St) stomach.

limeters to 2 cm in size and usually are sharply demarcated from adjacent parenchyma. CT can be used to assess the effectiveness of antifungal therapy.

Splenic abnormalities also occur in patients with pancreatitis. Fluid may collect around the spleen, particularly

laterally (Fig. 11) (85). Pseudocysts can arise in the tail of the pancreas adjacent to the splenic hilum (60) and can extend beneath the splenic capsule or even into the spleen itself. Like abscesses, pancreatic pseudocysts have low-density material within them, and the cyst wall may be enhanced after intravenous administration of contrast material.

Cysts

Three types of nonneoplastic cysts are known to occur in the spleen (19,28): parasitic cysts due to echinococcal infection, epidermoid cysts, and posttraumatic pseudocysts.

Echinococcal cysts are rare, even in patients with known echinococcal disease elsewhere in the body. They are well-circumscribed spherical lesions that enlarge the spleen and commonly contain extensive calcification within their walls.

Epidermoid cysts are congenital in origin (21,36) and usually are discovered in childhood or in the early adult years. They are much more common in females than in males. These true cysts are lined by epithelium. They are spherical, sharply circumscribed, water-density lesions, and they show no central or rim enhancement with intravenous contrast material. The wall of an epidermoid cyst will occasionally calcify (24). CT may show thin internal trabeculae.

Most splenic cysts, particularly those encountered in older individuals, are posttraumatic in origin and are thought to represent the final stage in the evolution of

A,B

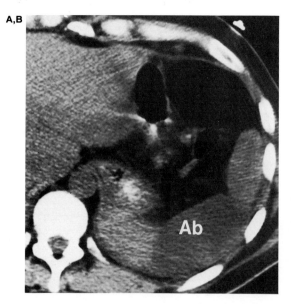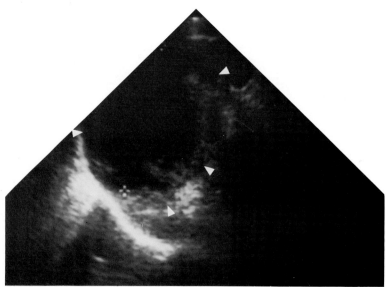

FIG. 29. Cardiac transplant patient with continued fever after drainage of left empyema. **A:** CT shows a well-demarcated low-attenuation area (Ab) in the spleen. **B:** Sonogram of the spleen (*arrowheads*) shows the lesion to be largely anechoic, with some echogenic debris within it. Needle aspirate yielded pus.

splenic hematomas. Histologically, they are not lined by epithelium and thus are referred to as pseudocysts. They may or may not calcify. Like other types of splenic cysts, they are sharply demarcated and contain fluid of a density similar to or slightly above that of water (Fig. 30). Splenic pseudocysts can also occur as a result of the trauma and fluid related to a ventriculoperitoneal shunt catheter (52).

Trauma

CT has proved to be quite useful for detecting splenic injury in patients with blunt (7) and penetrating (67) abdominal trauma. Accuracy as high as 98% has been reported for CT detection of splenic trauma (88). Injury to the spleen can take the form of subcapsular hematoma, laceration, or, less commonly, intrasplenic hematoma. Subcapsular hematomas appear as crescentic collections of fluid that flatten or indent the lateral margin of the spleen (Fig. 31). When the hematoma has been present for only 1 to 2 days, its CT attenuation value may be equal to or even greater than that of the splenic parenchyma. Over the next 10 days, the attenuation value of the fluid within the hematoma gradually decreases (43), becoming less than that of the spleen. The use of intravenous contrast material improves and may be essential for the detection of fresh subcapsular hematomas.

Splenic lacerations may occur with or without accompanying subcapsular hematoma. Findings on CT include splenic enlargement, an irregular cleft or defect in the splenic border, and the presence of blood in the peritoneal cavity (4,25) (Figs. 32 and 33). Sometimes the hematoma has a multilayered or "onion-skin" appearance. In severe cases, the spleen is shattered into small fragments (Fig. 34).

Conservative surgical management of splenic trauma is becoming more prevalent as the increased risk of serious infection is being recognized in patients who have previously undergone splenectomy. Some surgeons are now performing splenorrhaphy, suturing of splenic lacerations without removing the spleen, and CT has been found to be useful in the postoperative evaluation of these patients (30). In those who are doing well postoperatively, the spleen appears essentially normal. Subcapsular hematoma and perisplenic fluid collections can, of course, be recognized if they are present. In some centers, radiopaque Teflon felt pledgets are laid over the laceration to aid in keeping the sutures in place. These pledgets appear as focal areas of radiopacity on the splenic capsule that have a density of 85 to 100 HU (33).

Physiologic splenic activity can develop again in as many as half of patients undergoing splenectomy for trauma (62). This can be due either to growth of an accessory spleen not removed at the time of operation or to seeding of the peritoneal cavity with viable splenic tissue at the time of the initial trauma or subsequent operation, a condition known as splenosis. Although radionuclide imaging is the procedure of choice, CT can detect those foci of splenic tissue in the abdomen, particularly when liposoluble contrast material is used, and it can determine that an apparent abdominal mass represents splenosis or an accessory spleen rather than a neoplasm.

A,B

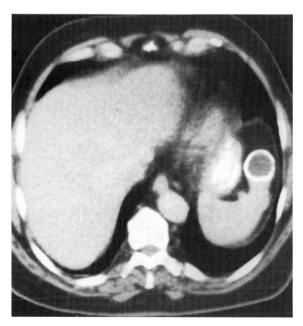 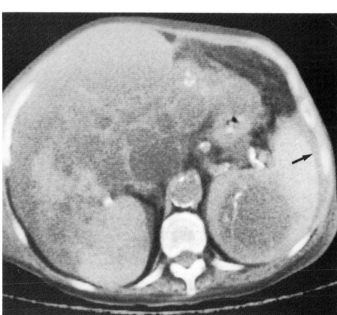

FIG. 30. Splenic cyst. **A:** The lesion is round and sharply circumscribed, with a calcified rim and low-density center. The cyst is presumed to be on a posttraumatic basis. **B:** In another patient with adult polycystic kidney disease, a large cyst with a calcified septum is seen in the spleen. Multiple cysts are also present in the liver; (arrow) ascites.

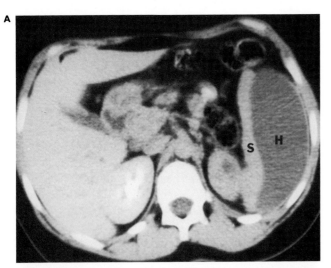

FIG. 31. Traumatic subcapsular hematoma. **A:** The low-density hematoma (H) is sharply demarcated from the adjacent spleen (S) in this postcontrast CT image. **B:** T1-weighted MR image (TR = 500 msec, TE = 30 msec). The hematoma has a lower signal intensity than the spleen. **C:** Proton-density image (TR = 1,500 msec, TE = 30 msec) shows the hematoma to have a fluid-debris level (*arrow*). The sediment has a signal intensity similar to that of the spleen.

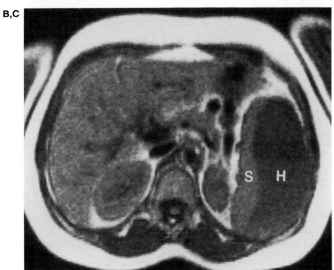

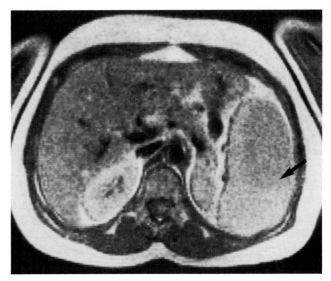

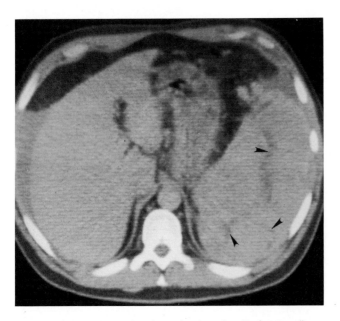

FIG. 32. Splenic laceration. Irregular, low-density fracture lines (*arrowheads*) are noted in this enlarged spleen. Blood is also present in the peritoneal cavity.

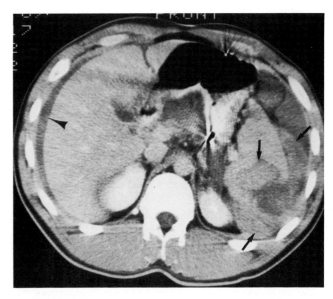

FIG. 33. Splenic trauma. Postcontrast CT image demonstrates a large defect in the posterior aspect of the spleen. Both intrasplenic and perisplenic hematomas are present (*arrows*); (*arrowheads*) hemoperitoneum.

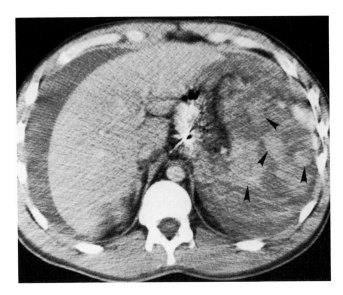

FIG. 34. Shattered spleen in an acutely traumatized patient. The spleen is broken into numerous pieces (*arrowheads*). Hemoperitoneum is also evident.

Miscellaneous Conditions

A focal low-density region in the spleen can indicate the presence of a splenic infarct (26,54) (Fig. 35). The defect may be wedge-shaped, with its base at the splenic capsule and its apex toward the hilum. Gas bubbles have been seen scattered throughout a large, nonsuppurative splenic infarct caused by transcatheter embolization of

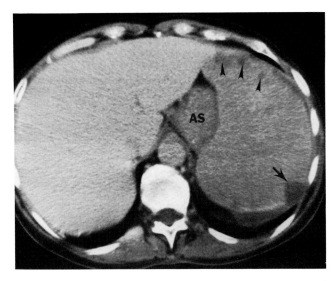

FIG. 35. Splenic infarct (*arrow*) in patient with enlargement of spleen and accessory spleen (AS) due to lymphoma. The infarct is peripheral, wedge-shaped, and lower in density than surrounding splenic parenchyma. Other low-density foci (*arrowheads*) in the spleen represent lymphomatous deposits.

the splenic arterial bed (48). When the entire spleen is infarcted, such as following occlusion or avulsion of the splenic artery, there is failure of contrast enhancement of all splenic tissue except for the parenchyma immediately subjacent to the capsule (Fig. 36). This enhancement of the periphery of the spleen, the so-called rim sign, is thought to be due to arterial supply from capsular vessels. Lack of splenic parenchymal enhancement also occurs in the setting of profound hypotension (9) and can thus mimic splenic arterial disruption after blunt abdominal trauma. Splenic infarction can also be seen with MRI. When it is hemorrhagic, it has a high signal intensity on both T1- and T2-weighted images (Fig. 37).

Patients with sickle cell anemia usually have repeated episodes of splenic infarction that eventually result in a small spleen containing diffuse microscopic deposits of calcium and iron (Fig. 38). CT has been helpful in establishing that the finding on bone scanning of a focal area of uptake of ^{99m}Tc-diphosphonate in the left upper abdomen was due to uptake in the spleen rather than in a focus of osteomyelitis in the overlying rib (63).

CLINICAL APPLICATIONS

CT and, to a lesser extent, MRI can serve many purposes and solve many problems in patients known to have or suspected of having splenic disease. Normal splenic lobulations, clefts between adjacent lobulations, and positional anomalies may present confusing appearances on radionuclide liver/spleen images, making interpretation difficult (74). When clarification is needed concerning an abnormality suspected on the basis of radionuclide imaging, CT constitutes an excellent means of clarifying the true size, shape, position, and physical integrity of a spleen.

CT, MRI, or ultrasonography can be used to document the presence or extent of splenomegaly. When the cause for splenic enlargement is not known, however, CT and MRI are the preferred techniques because they are more likely to demonstrate conditions that may be responsible for the splenomegaly, such as lymphomatous enlargement of abdominal nodes.

CT and ultrasonography are also both useful in imaging focal masses within the spleen (73). In some patients, the cystic nature of a splenic mass suspected on CT can be confirmed by ultrasonography.

At the present time, CT is the best radiologic method for screening patients who have suffered blunt abdominal trauma for the presence of splenic injury, and its use has decreased the need for abdominal arteriography and exploratory laparotomy. The sensitivity in detecting splenic injury by CT has been reported to be as high as 100% (7,88). The noninvasive nature of the examination is a clear advantage over splenic angiography, and the ability to examine the abdomen simultaneously for signs of hepatic, renal, retroperitoneal, or other trauma, as well as

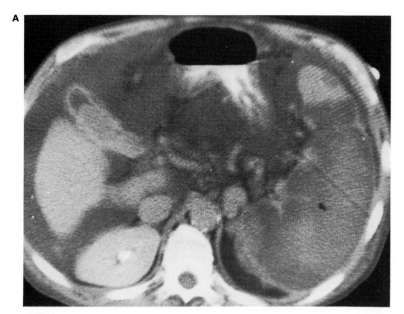

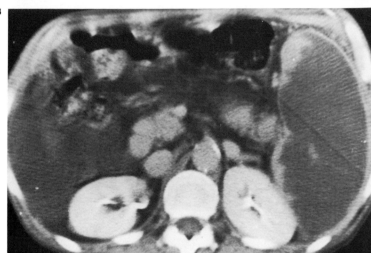

FIG. 36. A: Splenic infarction 1 week after therapeutic embolization of the splenic artery in a patient with portal hypertension and bleeding esophageal varices. There is extensive liquefactive necrosis and hemorrhage, and a tiny gas bubble, introduced during the procedure, lies near the center of the spleen. Note the rim of enhanced splenic capsule. B: Three weeks after the therapeutic infarction, the gas is gone, and the density of the hemorrhagic fluid in the spleen has decreased. Rim enhancement persists.

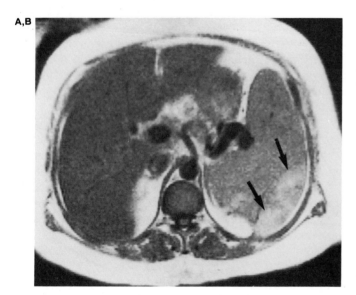
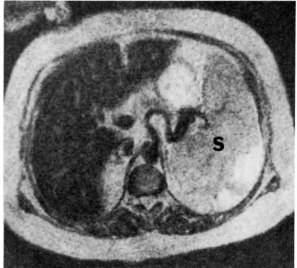

FIG. 37. Hemorrhagic splenic infarct. A: T1-weighted image (TR = 500 msec, TE = 30 msec) shows two wedge-shaped, high-intensity lesions (*arrows*) in the posterolateral aspect of the spleen. B: T2-weighted MR image (TR = 1,500 msec, TE = 90 msec). The infarcts have a higher signal intensity than the spleen (S) and fat.

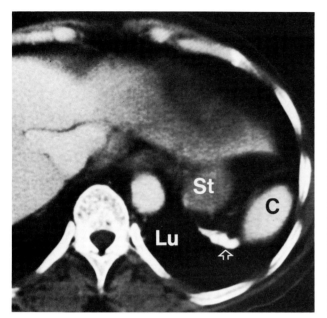 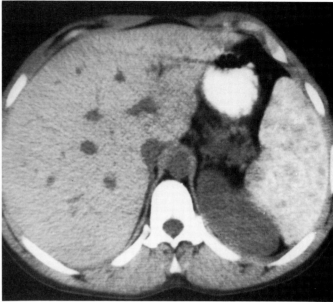

A,B

FIG. 38. A: Tiny, calcified, infarcted spleen (*open arrow*) in an adult with sickle cell anemia; (C) colon; (Lu) lung; (St) stomach. **B:** In another patient with sickle cell disease, noncontrast CT image demonstrates the spleen to be almost completely calcified, with few residual areas of normal parenchyma. This is undoubtedly due to multiple episodes of infarction.

to assess for the presence of intraperitoneal blood, constitutes a major advantage over radionuclide imaging (58). Although ultrasound can also be used to evaluate the possibility of splenic trauma, its sensitivity may not be as high (4), and it does not provide as clear a demonstration of some of the other areas of the abdomen and pelvis as can be obtained by CT. MRI at present plays little role in evaluating the acutely traumatized patient.

REFERENCES

1. Alcorn FS, Mategrano VC, Petasnick JP, Clark JW. Contribution of computed tomography in the staging and management of malignant lymphoma. *Radiology* 1977;125:721–723.
2. Ambriz P, Munoz R, Quintanar E, Sigler L, Aviles A, Pizzuto J. Accessory spleen compromising response to splenectomy for idiopathic thrombocytopenic purpura. *Radiology* 1985;155:793–796.
3. Arcomano P, Pizzolato NF, Singer R, Zucker SM. A unique type of calcification in chronic brucellosis. *AJR* 1977;128:135–137.
4. Asher WM, Parvin S, Virgilio RW, Haber K. Echographic evaluation of splenic injury after blunt trauma. *Radiology* 1976;118:411–415.
5. Balthazar EJ, Hilton S, Naidich D, Megibow A, Levine R. CT of. splenic and perisplenic abnormalities in septic patients. *AJR* 1985;144:53–56.
6. Beahrs JR, Stephens DH. Enlarged accessory spleens: CT appearance in postsplenectomy patients. *AJR* 1980;135:483–486.
7. Berger PE, Kuhn JP. CT of blunt abdominal trauma in childhood. *AJR* 1981;136:105–110.
8. Berkman WA, Harris SA, Bernardino ME. Nonsurgical drainage of splenic abscesses. *AJR* 1983;141:395–396.
9. Berland LL, Van Dyke JA. Decreased splenic enhancement of CT in traumatized hypotensive patients. *Radiology* 1985;156:469–471.
10. Berlow ME, Spirt BA, Weil L. CT follow-up of hepatic and splenic fungal microabscesses. *J Comput Assist Tomogr* 1984;8:42–45.
11. Boldt DW, Reilly BJ. Computed tomography of abdominal mass lesions in children. *Radiology* 1977;124:371–378.
12. Bragg DG, Colby TV, Ward JH. New concepts in the non-Hodgkin lymphoma: radiologic implications. *Radiology* 1986;159:289–304.
13. Breiman RS, Castellino RA, Harell GS, Marshall WH, Glatstein E, Kaplan HS. CT-pathologic correlation in Hodgkin's disease and non-Hodgkin's lymphoma. *Radiology* 1978;126:159–166.
14. Brinkley AB, Lee JKT. Cystic hamartoma of the spleen: CT and sonographic findings. *J Clin Ultrasound* 1981;9:136–138.
15. Burgener FA, Hamlin DJ. Histiocytic lymphoma of the abdomen: radiologic spectrum. *AJR* 1981;137:337–342.
16. Castellino RA. Hodgkin disease: practical concepts for the diagnostic radiologist. *Radiology* 1986;159:305–310.
17. Castellino RA, Hoppe RT, Blank N, et al. Computed tomography, lymphography, and staging laparotomy: correlations in initial staging of Hodgkin disease. *AJR* 1984;143:37–41.
18. Clark RE, Korobkin M, Palubinskas AJ. Angiography of accessory spleens. *Radiology* 1972;102:41–44.
19. Dachman AH, Ros PR, Marari PJ, Olmsted WW, Lichtenstein JE. Nonparasitic splenic cysts: a report of 52 cases with radiologic-pathologic correlation. *AJR* 1986;147:537–542.
20. D'Altorio RA, Cano JY. Upside-down spleen as cause of suprarenal mass. *Urology* 1978;11:422–424.
21. Davidson ED, Campbell WG, Hersh T. Epidermoid splenic cyst occurring in an intrapancreatic accessory spleen. *Dig Dis Sci* 1980;25:964–967.
22. DeMaeyer P, Wilms G, Baert AL. Polysplenia. *J Comput Assist Tomogr* 1981;5:104–105.
23. Eraklis AJ, Filler RM. Splenectomy in childhood: a review of 1413 cases. *J Pediatr Surg* 1972;7:382–388.
24. Favelukes HA. Calcific shadow in spleen of young man. *JAMA* 1978;239:1177–1178.
25. Federle MP, Goldberg HI, Kaiser JA, Moss AA, Jeffrey RB, Mall JC. Evaluation of abdominal trauma by computed tomography. *Radiology* 1981;138:637–644.
26. Freeman MH, Tonkin AK. Focal splenic defects. *Radiology* 1976;121:689–692.
27. Frick MP, Feinberg SB, Loken MK. Noninvasive spleen scanning in Hodgkin's disease and non-Hodgkin's lymphoma. *Comput Tomogr* 1980;5:73–80.
28. Garvin DF, King FM. Cysts of the nonlymphomatous tumors of the spleen. *Pathol Annu* 1981;16:61–80.

29. Gilbert T, Castellino RA. Critical review. *Invest Radiol* 1986;21:437–439.
30. Giuliano AE, Lim RC. Is splenic salvage safe in the traumatized patient? *Arch Surg* 1981;116:651–656.
31. Glazer GM, Axel L, Goldberg HI, Moss AA. Dynamic CT of the normal spleen. *AJR* 1981;137:343–346.
32. Gooding GAW. The ultrasonic and computed tomographic appearance of splenic lobulations: a consideration in the ultrasonic differential of masses adjacent to the left kidney. *Radiology* 1978;126:719–720.
33. Goodman PC, Federle MP. Splenorrhaphy: CT appearance. *J Comput Assist Tomogr* 1980;4:251–252.
34. Gordon DH, Burrell MI, Levin DC, Mueller CF, Becker JA. Wandering spleen—the radiological and clinical spectrum. *Radiology* 1977;125:39–46.
35. Grant E, Merens MA, Mascatello VJ. Splenic abscess: comparison of four imaging methods. *AJR* 1979;132:465–466.
36. Griscom NT, Hargreaves HK, Schwartz MZ, Reddish JM, Colodny AH. Huge splenic cyst in a newborn: comparisons with 10 cases in later childhood and adolescence. *AJR* 1977;129:889–891.
37. Halgrimson CG, Rustad DG, Zeligman BE. Calcified hemangioma of the spleen. *JAMA* 1984;252:2959–2960.
38. Harell GS. The current status of splenic computed tomography in patients with lymphoma. In: Felix R, Kazner E, Wegener OH, eds. *Contrast media in computed tomography.* Amsterdam: Excerpta Medica, 1981:237–242.
39. Isikoff MB, White DW, Diaconis JN. Torsion of the wandering spleen, seen as a migratory abdominal mass. *Radiology* 1977;123:36.
40. Joshi SN, Wolverson MK, Cusworth RB, Nair SG, Perrillo RP. Complementary use of computerized tomography and technetium scanning in the diagnosis of accessory spleen. *Dig Dis Sci* 1980;25:888–892.
41. Kishikawa T, Numaguchi Y, Tokunaga M, Matsuura K. Hemangiosarcoma of the spleen with liver metastases: angiographic manifestations. *Radiology* 1977;123:31–35.
42. Koehler RE, Evens RG. The spleen. In: Teplick JG, Haskin ME, eds. *Surgical radiology.* Philadelphia: WB Saunders, 1981:1064–1088.
43. Korobkin M, Moss AA, Callen PW, DeMartini WJ, Kaiser JA. Computed tomography of subcapsular splenic hematoma. *Radiology* 1978;129:441–445.
44. Krudy AG, Dunnick NR, Magrath IT, Shawker TH, Doppman JL, Spiegel R. CT of American Burkitt lymphoma. *AJR* 1981;136:747–754.
45. Lackner K, Brecht G, Janson R, Scherholz K, Lutzeler A, Thurn P. Wertigkeit der Computertomographic bei der Stadieneinteilung primarer Lymphknotenneoplasien. *Fortschr Roentgenstr* 1980;132:21–30.
46. Lerner RM, Spataro RF. Splenic abscess: percutaneous drainage. *Radiology* 1984;153:643–645.
47. Levy DW, Rindsberg S, Friedman AC, et al. Thorotrast-induced hepatosplenic neoplasia: CT identification. *AJR* 1986;146:997–1004.
48. Levy DW, Wasserman PI, Weiland DE. Nonsuppurative gas formation in the spleen after transcatheter splenic infarction. *Radiology* 1981;139:375–376.
49. Linos DA, Nagorney DM, McIlrath DC. Splenic abscess—the importance of early diagnosis. *Mayo Clin Proc* 1983;58:261–264.
50. Long JA, Doppman JL, Nienhaus AW, Mills SR. Computed tomographic analysis of beta-thalassemia syndromes with hemochromatosis: pathologic findings with clinical laboratory correlations. *J Comput Assist Tomogr* 1980;4:159–165.
51. Mahony B, Jeffrey RB, Federle MP. Spontaneous rupture of hepatic and splenic angiosarcoma demonstrated by CT. *AJR* 1982;138:965–966.
52. Mata J, Alegret X, Llauger J. Splenic pseudocyst as a complication of ventriculoperitoneal shunt: CT features. *J Comput Assist Tomogr* 1986;10:341–342.
53. Miller DL, Vermess M, Doppman JL, et al. CT of the liver and spleen with EOE-13: review of 225 examinations. *AJR* 1984;143:235–243.
54. Morissette JJ, Viamonte M, Viamonte M, Rolfs H. Primary spindle cell sarcoma of the spleen with angiographic demonstration. *Radiology* 1973;106:549–550.
55. Morgenstern L, McCafferty L, Rosenberg J, Michel SL. Hamartomas of the spleen. *Arch Surg* 1984;119:1291–1294.
56. Moss ML, Kirschner LP, Peereboom G, Ferris RA. CT demonstration of a splenic abscess not evident at surgery. *AJR* 1980;135:159–160.
57. Moss CN, Van Dyke JA, Koehler RE, Smedberg CT. Multiple cavernous hemangiomas of the spleen: CT appearance. *J Comput Assist Tomogr* 1986;10:338–340.
58. Nebesar RA, Rabinov KR, Potsaid MA. Radionuclide imaging of the spleen in suspected splenic injury. *Radiology* 1974;110:609–614.
59. Nov AA, Smith GR, McMillin T. Splenic "draping": clarification by gastric and splenic scintigraphy. *AJR* 1984;142:323–324.
60. Okuda K, Taguchi T, Ishihara K, Konno A. Intrasplenic pseudocyst of the pancreas. *J Clin Gastroenterol* 1981;3:37–41.
61. Parker LA, Mittelstaedt CA, Mauro MA, Mandell VS, Jaques PF. Torsion of a wandering spleen: CT appearance. *J Comput Assist Tomogr* 1984;8:1201–1204.
62. Pearson HA, Johnston D, Smith KA, Touloukian RJ. The born again spleen. Return of splenic function after splenectomy for trauma. *N Engl J Med* 1978;298:1389–1392.
63. Perlmutter S, Jacobstein JG, Kazam E. Splenic uptake of ^{99m}Tc-diphosphonate in sickle cell disease associated with increased splenic density on computerized transaxial tomography. *Gastrointest Radiol* 1977;2:77–79.
64. Piekarski J, Federle MP, Moss AA, London SS. CT of the spleen. *Radiology* 1980;135:683–689.
65. Pitlik S, Cohen L, Hadar H, Srulijes C, Rosenfeld JB. Portal hypertension and esophageal varices in hemangiomatosis of the spleen. *Gastroenterology* 1977;72:937–940.
66. Rao BK, Shore RM, Lieberman LM, Polcyn RE. Dual radiopharmaceutical imaging in congenital asplenia syndrome. *Radiology* 1982;145:805–810.
67. Rauch RF, Korobkin M, Silverman PM, Moore AV. CT detection of iatrogenic percutaneous splenic injury. *J Comput Assist Tomogr* 1983;7:1018–1021.
68. Redman HC, Glatstein E, Castellino RA, Federal WA. Computed tomography as an adjunct in the staging of Hodgkin's disease and non-Hodgkin's lymphoma. *Radiology* 1977;124:381–385.
69. Salomonowitz E, Frick MP, Lund G. Radiologic diagnosis of wandering spleen complicated by splenic volvulus and infarction. *Gastrointest Radiol* 1984;9:57–59.
70. Scully RE, Galdabini JJ, McNeely BU. Case records of the Massachusetts General Hospital, case 41-1976. *N Engl J Med* 1976;295:828–834.
71. Sheflin JR, Lee CM, Kretchmar KA. Torsion of wandering spleen and distal pancreas. *AJR* 1984;142:100–101.
72. Shirkhoda A, Lopez-Berestein G, Holbert JM, Luna MA. Hepatosplenic fungal infection: CT and pathologic evaluation after treatment with liposomal amphotericin B. *Radiology* 1986;159:349–353.
73. Shirkhoda A, McCartney WH, Staab EV, Mittelstaedt CA. Imaging of the spleen: a proposed algorithm. *AJR* 1980;135:195–198.
74. Smidt KP. Splenic scintigraphy: a large congenital fissure mimicking splenic hematoma. *Radiology* 1977;122:169.
75. Smulewicz JJ, Clement AR. Torsion of the wandering spleen. *Dig Dis* 1975;20:274–279.
76. Sorgen RA, Robbins DI. Bleeding gastric varices secondary to wandering spleen. *Gastrointest Radiol* 1980;5:25–27.
77. Stiris MG. Accessory spleen versus left adrenal tumor: computed tomographic and abdominal angiographic evaluation. *J Comput Assist Tomogr* 1980;4:543–544.
78. Strijk SP, Wagener DJT, Bogman MJJT, de Pauw BE, Wobbes T. The spleen in Hodgkin disease: diagnostic value of CT. *Radiology* 1985;154:753–757.
79. Subramanyam BR, Balthazar EJ, Horii SC. Sonography of the accessory spleen. *AJR* 1984;143:47–49.
80. Tada S, Shin M, Takashina T, et al. Diffuse capillary hemangiomatosis of the spleen as a cause of portal hypertension. *Radiology* 1972;104:63–64.
81. Thomas JL, Bernardino ME, Vermess M, et al. EOE-13 in the detection of hepatosplenic lymphoma. *Radiology* 1982;145:629–634.

82. Tuttle RJ, Leminielly JA. Splenic cystic lymphangiomatosis. *Radiology* 1978;126:47–48.

83. Vermess M, Doppman JL, Sugarbaker PH, et al. Computed tomography of the liver and spleen with intravenous lipoid contrast material: review of 60 examinations. *AJR* 1982;138:1063–1071.

84. Vibhakar SD, Bellon EM. The bare area of the spleen: a constant CT feature of the ascitic abdomen. *AJR* 1984;1412:953–955.

85. Vick CW, Simeone JF, Ferrucci JT, Wittenberg J, Mueller PR. Pancreatitis-associated fluid collections involving the spleen: sonographic and computed tomographic appearance. *Gastrointest Radiol* 1981;6:247–250.

86. Westcoll JL, Krufky EL. The upside-down spleen. *Radiology* 1972;105:517–521.

87. Wick MR, Rife CC. Paratesticular accessory spleen. *Mayo Clin Proc* 1981;56:455–456.

88. Wing VW, Federle MP, Morris JA, Jeffrey RB, Bluth R. The clinical impact of CT for blunt abdominal trauma. *AJR* 1985;145:1191–1194.

CHAPTER 14

Pancreas

Robert J. Stanley, D. Bradley Koslin, and Joseph K. T. Lee

Since the introduction of computed tomography (CT) of the body in 1975, CT has become the imaging method of choice for evaluation of the pancreas. Although other imaging methods, including ultrasound, endoscopic retrograde pancreatography, plain film radiography, and contrast examinations of the gastrointestinal tract, have definite roles in the overall evaluation of pancreatic disease, CT nevertheless provides the most reliable information when the entire spectrum of pancreatic diseases and the variety of clinical settings are all considered.

NORMAL ANATOMY

Considerable variation exists in the size, shape, and location of the normal pancreas, depending on variations in body habitus as well as the normal or abnormal size and positioning of contiguous organs. In the most common normal configuration, the long axis of the body and tail of the pancreas lies in an oblique orientation, extending from the hilum of the spleen, at its lateral and most cephalic extent, toward the midline of the body, where it passes anterior to the portal vein at its point of formation by the junction of the splenic vein and superior mesenteric vein (Fig. 1). From this point, the pancreas passes in a more vertical orientation, caudally, in a hockey-stick configuration, terminating in the most caudal extension of the pancreas, the uncinate process (Fig. 2). In addition to this basic orientation, there is also variation in the curvature of the long axis of the gland in the anteroposterior (AP) plane. For example, if the left kidney does not lie in its normal position, the body and tail of the pancreas will be oriented far more posteriorly, along with a more posterior positioning of the spleen. Alternatively, in a patient with considerable retroperitoneal fat, the pancreas may be entirely straight, remaining in the same coronal plane from the level of the pancreatic neck to the tip of the tail. More extreme variations in anatomy will be discussed

subsequently in this section under developmental anomalies.

Form

Because of improvements in CT technology resulting in shorter scanning times, as well as increased contrast and spatial resolution, the true size and shape of the pancreas can be accurately assessed. Disease of the pancreas is most often recognized because of alterations in the size, shape, or tissue density of the pancreatic parenchyma. Modern real-time ultrasound and CT both consistently show that the thickness of the normal pancreatic parenchyma, measured perpendicular to its long axis on the cross-sectional view, varies depending on whether the head, neck, body, or tail is measured. The thickness of the head averages approximately 2.0 cm; the neck of the pancreas, just anterior to the portal vein, is the thinnest portion, ranging in thickness from 0.5 to 1.0 cm; the body and tail range from 1.0 to 2.0 cm, with many normal glands tapering slightly toward the tail. The cephalocaudad dimension of the body and tail ranges from 3.0 to 4.0 cm in most individuals, whereas the cephalocaudad dimension of the head is more variable, and portions of the head can be seen over distances ranging from 3 cm to as much as 8 cm. With respect to size and shape, the most reliable indicator of a pancreatic mass is the presence of an abrupt, focal change, rather than generalized variations from the range of normal dimensions.

The surface contour of the pancreatic parenchyma can be either smooth or lobulated, the latter being more frequently seen when there is abundant peripancreatic, retroperitoneal fat (Fig. 1). Because there is no well-defined capsule to the pancreas, the lobular architecture of the pancreatic parenchyma is well defined by the interdigitating fat. Fatty replacement of much of the pancreatic substance is a common degenerative process seen in the

543

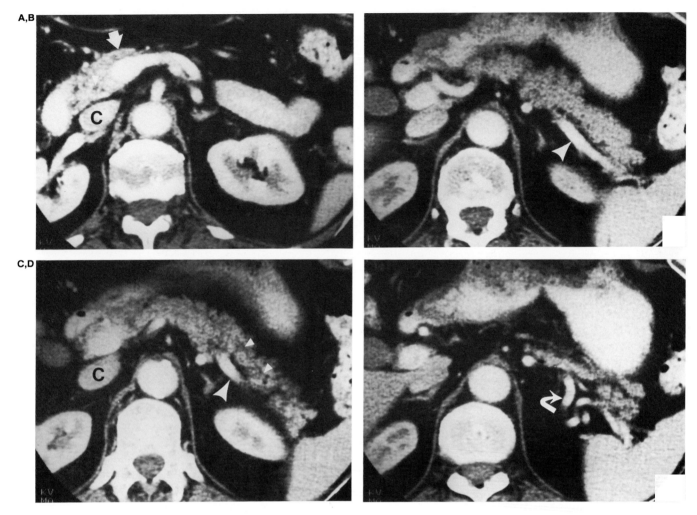

FIG. 1. A thin-section (5-mm) examination of a normal pancreas. **A–D:** The various portions of the pancreas in a caudocephalic scanning direction. Note the prominent lobulated, heterogeneous appearance of the pancreatic parenchyma of the body and tail. The neck of the pancreas (*arrow*) usually is the thinnest portion of the pancreas in the AP dimension, lying just anterior to the portal vein. The tortuous splenic artery (*curved arrow*) is visible posterior to the tail of the pancreas (**D**), whereas the straighter and wider splenic vein (*large arrowhead*) can be seen (**A–C**) as it courses toward its confluence with the superior mesenteric vein. Portions of a normal-caliber main pancreatic duct (*small arrowheads*) can be seen in the tail and head of the pancreas. **A:** Note the well-defined plane separating the posterior surface of the pancreatic head from the anterior wall of the inferior vena cava (C). The inferior aspect of the head of the pancreas and the uncinate process are not included in this figure.

elderly (Fig. 3). However, in obese individuals, marked interdigitation of peripancreatic fat can simulate this late degenerative process. As will be discussed in more detail later, fatty replacement may be associated with alterations in pancreatic function and may be a late sequel to various forms of chronic pancreatitis.

The normal main pancreatic duct can be seen in two-thirds to three-fourths of patients if high-detail CT technique is employed (Fig. 1). Thinly collimated slices in the range of 2 to 5 mm, combined with the use of intravenous contrast material to produce a greater density difference between the enhancing pancreatic parenchyma and the fluid within the duct, will increase the chances of demonstrating the main pancreatic duct, especially that seg-

ment in the body and tail of the pancreas that is lying parallel to the plane of the CT image (Fig. 4).

Anatomic Relationships

The splenic vein is a major CT landmark for identifying the body and tail of the pancreas. It lies on the dorsal surface of the body and tail of the pancreas, caudal to the splenic artery. In comparison with the more tortuous course of the splenic artery, the vein runs closely parallel to the longitudinal orientation of the pancreas (Fig. 1). A fat plane often separates the splenic vein from the pancreas and occasionally will simulate the pancreatic duct, es-

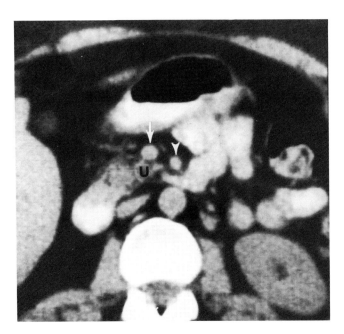

FIG. 2. Detail view of the uncinate process. The superior mesenteric vein (*arrow*), coursing parallel to and to the right of the superior mesenteric artery (*arrowhead*), lies immediately anterior to the medial tip of the uncinate process (U) of the head of the pancreas. A portion of the opacified transverse segment of the duodenum lies between the superior mesenteric artery and the aorta.

pecially if intravenous contrast material is not present to more clearly identify the nature of the splenic vein. The left adrenal gland lies posteromedial to the splenic vein and the pancreas at the junction of the body and tail.

The tail of the pancreas extends to the splenic hilum, entering the splenorenal ligament and becoming intraperitoneal for a short distance. Although generally located

anterior to the splenic vein, the tail of the pancreas occasionally may be imaged in the same plane as or even posterior to the main splenic vein or a tributary. The body and tail of the pancreas normally are located anterior or anterolateral to the left kidney. However, in a patient lacking a left kidney (surgically removed or congenitally absent) or a patient with an ectopic left kidney, the body and tail will be displaced posteromedially, lying adjacent to the spine and occupying the empty renal fossa. Usually there is an accompanying posteromedial rotation in the position of the spleen.

The body of the pancreas arches anteriorly over the superior mesenteric artery, close to its origin from the aorta, separated by a distinct fat plane in all but the leanest individuals. The superior mesenteric vein runs parallel to and to the right of the superior mesentric artery and usually is larger in diameter. At the point where the superior mesenteric vein joins the splenic vein to form the portal vein, the neck of the pancreas, the thinnest segment of the pancreas in the AP dimension, is seen to pass immediately ventral to the portal vein (Fig. 1). Generally there is no intervening fat plane between the neck of the pancreas and the portal vein.

The head of the pancreas lies medial to the second portion of the duodenum, to the right of the superior mesenteric vein, and anterior to the inferior vena cava (IVC) (Fig. 4). Generally, a thin, distinct fat plane separates the posterior surface of the head of the pancreas from the anterior surface of the IVC. The uncinate process of the pancreatic head is a curving, beak-like inferior and medial extension of the head that originates lateral to the superior mesenteric vein and curves posteriorly behind it, approximately at the level of the renal veins (Figs. 2 and 4). The normal-size common bile duct, varying in diameter from

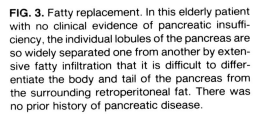

FIG. 3. Fatty replacement. In this elderly patient with no clinical evidence of pancreatic insufficiency, the individual lobules of the pancreas are so widely separated one from another by extensive fatty infiltration that it is difficult to differentiate the body and tail of the pancreas from the surrounding retroperitoneal fat. There was no prior history of pancreatic disease.

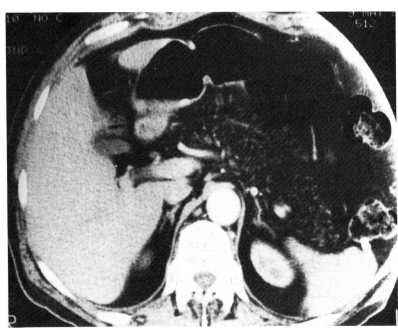

A,B

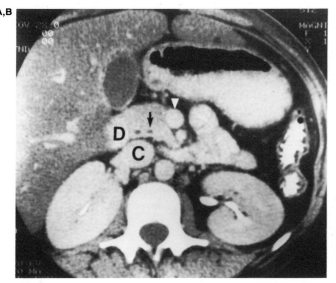 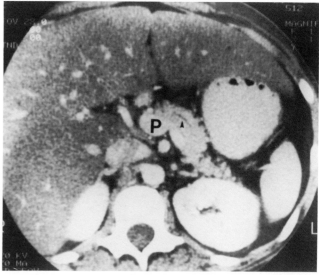

FIG. 4. Normal pancreatic anatomy. **A:** A normal-caliber distal common bile duct lies just lateral to a normal main pancreatic duct (*arrow*), both seen on end. A portion of the uncinate process extends posterior to the superior mesenteric vein (*arrowhead*); (D) duodenum; (C) inferior vena cava. **B:** Two centimeters cephalad, a portion of the body and tail of the pancreas is visible. The anterior surface of the gland is slightly lobulated. The origin of the portal vein (P) lies just posterior to the neck of the pancreas. A longitudinal segment of a normal-caliber main pancreatic duct (*arrowhead*) is visible in this thinly collimated 3-mm slice. Diffuse fatty infiltration of the liver is an incidental finding.

3 to 6 mm, can be seen in cross section within the head of the pancreas, close to its lateral and posterior surface, appearing as a circular or oval near-water-density structure. Its detectability is improved if the surrounding substance of the pancreatic parenchyma is enhanced by intravenous contrast material. Under optimal imaging conditions, the vertically oriented segment of the main pancreatic duct lying in the head can be seen running parallel to and medial to the common bile duct, ranging in diameter from 1 to 3 mm (Fig. 4).

The pancreas lies in the anterior pararenal space and is related to the second segment of the duodenum along the lateral surface of the head and to the third and fourth segments of the duodenum along the inferior surface of the head, body, and tail. The stomach lies anterior to the pancreas and is separated from it by the parietal peritoneum and the lesser sac, a potential space. The transverse mesocolon, which forms the inferior boundary of the lesser sac, is formed by the fusion of the parietal peritoneal leaves as they fuse and extend anteriorly from the ventral surface of the pancreas along its entire length. The significance of this anatomic relationship between the transverse colon and the pancreas via the transverse mesocolon becomes important in acute pancreatitis because this peritoneal communication serves as a pathway for the flow of fluids associated with pancreatitis.

When retroperitoneal, perivisceral fat is abundant, the pancreas will be well defined. However, even in lean patients, the pancreas can be accurately delineated by judicious use of ample quantities of oral contrast material to opacify the lumen of contiguous loops of bowel (Fig.

5) and intravenous contrast material to delineate the contiguous vascular structures (Fig. 6).

Developmental Variants and Anomalies

Pancreas divisum, the most common anatomic variant of the human pancreas, is defined as a completely separate pancreatic ductal system in a grossly undivided gland. It results from failure of fusion of the dorsal and ventral pancreatic ducts, which normally occurs in the second month *in utero.* The main portion of the pancreas, including the superior-anterior part of the head, the body, and the tail, is drained by the dorsal pancreatic duct through the accessory papilla. The posterior-inferior part of the head is drained by the short, narrow ventral pancreatic duct that joins the common bile duct in the ampulla. The incidence of this anatomic variant varies from 1.3% to 6.7%, as reported in different series of patients studied with endoscopic retrograde cholangiopancreatography (ERCP) (32). Pancreas divisum is considered by some to be an anatomic variant because it can be found in nearly 10% of the population. Pancreas divisum was found to occur at the same relative frequency among patients who were found to have pancreatitis as among all patients who had been evaluated with ERCP (32).

The diagnosis of pancreas divisum can be suggested with thin-section CT when an isolated ventral duct is identified or if separate dorsal and ventral pancreatic moieties can be defined. Although the overall size of the pancreas may be normal in this developmental variant,

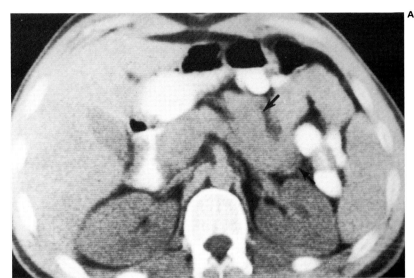

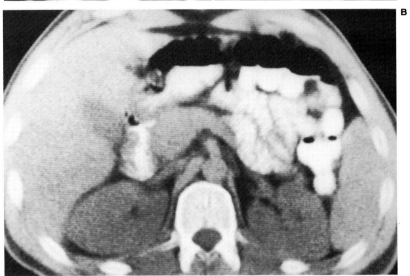

FIG. 5. Pancreatic ''pseudotumor.'' **A:** An apparent soft-tissue mass (*arrows*) is present in the region of the pancreatic tail. Is this a neoplasm or unopacified loops of bowel? **B:** Image following additional oral contrast material shows the ''mass'' to be simply proximal jejunum.

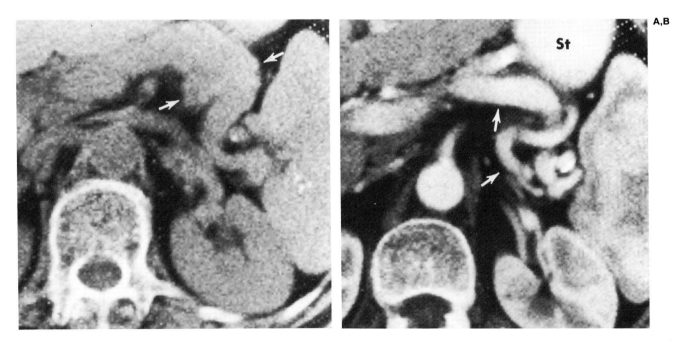

FIG. 6. Pancreatic ''pseudotumor.'' **A:** Suspicion of a mass lesion (*arrows*) in the region of the pancreatic tail. **B:** Image following intravenous bolus enhancement demonstrates the ''mass'' to be tortuous splenic vessels (*arrows*); (St) stomach.

A,B

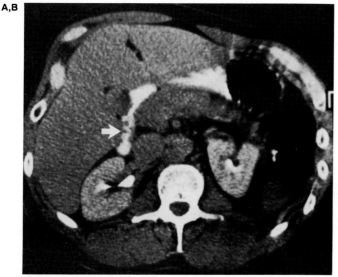

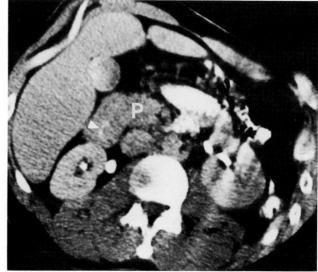

C

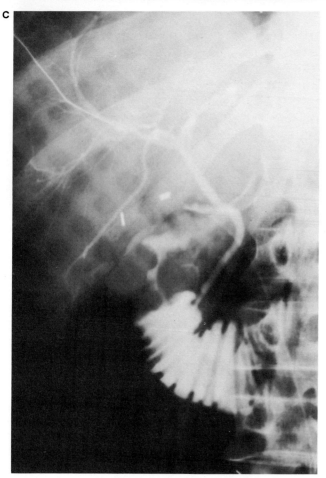

FIG. 7. Annular pancreas. **A:** At this level, the proximal portion of the duodenal loop (*arrow*) has a normal thickness to its wall as it passes lateral to the superior portion of the pancreatic head. **B:** Two centimeters caudal, the lumen of the duodenal loop (*arrowhead*) is narrowed, and the wall of the duodenum appears unusually thickened. Note that there is no plane of separation or tissue density difference between the head of the pancreas (P) and the "wall" of the duodenum. **C:** Intraoperative cholangiogram demonstrates opacification of a normal-appearing biliary tree and a classic configuration of the duodenal loop secondary to an annular pancreas. (Courtesy of Arthur Bishop, M.D., Peoria, Illinois.)

the craniocaudal extent or the AP thickness of the pancreatic head may be increased. Additionally, the ventral and dorsal pancreatic moieties may be distinctly visible, separated by a fat plane (163).

Annular pancreas, a developmental anomaly, may be suggested on CT by apparent thickening of the anterior, lateral, and posterior aspect of the descending duodenum caused by tissue having a density similar to that of the pancreatic parenchyma in the head (1,65) (Fig. 7). The diagnosis of annular pancreas on CT will be reinforced by the typical changes on an upper-gastrointestinal examination and confirmed by successful cannulation by ERCP of that portion of the pancreatic duct system within the annular component.

Agenesis of the dorsal pancreatic moiety has been reported (126). In this developmental anomaly, only the head of the pancreas is visible on CT. No pancreatic parenchyma can be identified in the expected locations of the neck, body, and tail. In contrast to pancreas divisum, dorsal pancreas agenesis is an extremely rare anomaly. A case of dorsal pancreas passing through a posterior defect in the diaphragm immediately lateral to the right crus, presenting as a mass in the right cardiophrenic angle, has been reported (24).

In a small percentage of patients, the head of the pancreas may lie in a position that is completely to the left of the aorta. Although this situation may develop because of an enlarging mass in the liver or peripancreatic area, displacing the pancreas to the left, it has also been seen in patients with no relevant abdominal disease. In these instances, despite the fact that the head of the pancreas is completely to the left of the aorta, the pancreas still bears the normal relationship to the superior mesenteric vein and artery. It has been suggested that the left-sided pancreas may be an acquired positional variation due to increasing laxity of retroperitoneal tissues occurring with age, as well as tortuosity of the abdominal aorta, causing it to swing farther to the right than usual. In one study, all the patients who had a left-sided pancreas and no associated abdominal disease were over the age of 50 years (35).

PATHOLOGIC CONDITIONS

Neoplasia

Adenocarcinoma

Adenocarcinoma, which accounts for 95% of all primary pancreatic malignant neoplasms, is currently the fourth most common cause of cancer-related mortality in the United States. There are sex and race predilections, with this neoplasm being more common in men and blacks, respectively. The risk of developing this tumor increases with age and peaks in the eighth decade (20,91,99).

CT should be the initial diagnostic procedure in any patient who is suspected of having a pancreatic neoplasm (61,99). It is approximately 95% accurate in detecting pancreatic adenocarcinoma, whereas ultrasound is able to detect approximately 80% of those located in the head or body and only approximately 40% of those located in the tail (15,20). However, in the subgroup of patients in whom CT findings are inconclusive for a pancreatic mass, sonography often is valuable in excluding or confirming its presence (103). CT also allows staging of the neoplasm and determination of resectability of the tumor.

The majority (60%) of pancreatic carcinomas occur in the head, and 15% and 5% occur in the body and tail,

respectively; 20% involve the gland diffusely (20). Because of the pancreatic head's intimate involvement with the common bile duct and duodenum, tumors that arise there tend to present clinically at an earlier stage than those that occur in the body or tail. Consequently, they tend to be smaller at the time of discovery than those in the body or tail. However, on rare occasion, very large tumors arising in the head may be present without causing jaundice.

The CT appearance of pancreatic adenocarcinomas is variable. Calcification rarely occurs in these neoplasms; however, a cancer may arise in a gland containing calcification. If intravenous contrast material is not administered, the attenuation of the tumor generally is very similar to that of normal parenchyma. Therefore, without intravenous contrast material, these tumors usually will be recognized only when they become large enough to cause a focal distortion in the expected pancreatic contour. There are several CT findings that can indicate the presence of a neoplasm when a mass is not identified. Because with aging the pancreas may become heterogeneous in density, with diffuse fatty infiltration, a focal region of homogeneous soft-tissue density within such a gland should be viewed with suspicion (88,153). Second, the presence of both a dilated common bile duct and dilated main pancreatic duct in the absence of a calculus suggests an ampullary or pancreatic head neoplasm (Fig. 8). However, this finding can be seen in benign disease (84). Third, the finding of a dilated main pancreatic duct in the body and tail, but not in the head or neck, also suggests the presence of a neoplasm (Fig. 9). A fourth suggestion of the presence of a neoplasm is the finding of rounded convex borders of both the anterior and posterior surfaces of the uncinate process (86) (Fig. 10).

Following intravenous administration of contrast material, most pancreatic adenocarcinomas are enhanced to a lesser degree than is normal parenchyma (63) (Fig. 11). This disparity in contrast enhancement may permit small masses to be identified. A further aid in the detection of small masses is the use of thinly collimated slices, i.e., 2 to 5 mm.

A carcinoma in the pancreatic head may produce changes in the body or tail that are delineated on CT. These changes include pancreatic duct dilatation (Figs. 12 and 13), cyst due to obstruction (Fig. 14), associated pancreatitis and its attendant CT findings (13,157), and atrophy (21) (Fig. 12). A dilated pancreatic duct is a sensitive indicator of pancreatic disease, but is not specific for carcinoma and can occur in pancreatitis or in duodenal inflammatory disease (14,76,84). In a patient without a history of pancreatitis, a dilated pancreatic duct implies the presence of a distal obstructing neoplasm. If the neoplasm is not identified on the CT examination, ERCP will allow further evaluation. The obstruction of the pancreatic duct may cause elevated intraductal pressure, resulting in small duct rupture and subsequent enzyme release associated with focal pancreatitis.

Text continues on page 555.

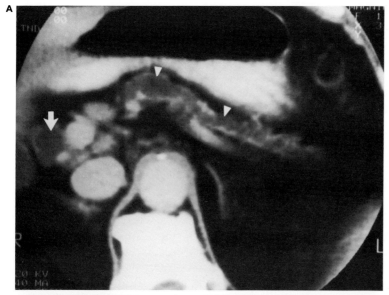

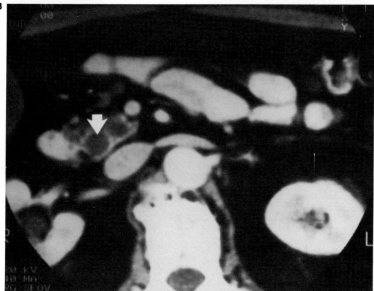

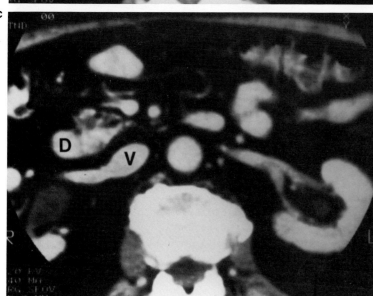

FIG. 8. Small carcinoma of the ampulla. **A:** CT image through the level of the body and tail of the pancreas shows a markedly dilated main pancreatic duct (*arrowheads*), with associated atrophy of the pancreatic parenchyma. A dilated common bile duct (*arrow*) is seen immediately lateral to the portal vein. **B:** At the level of the pancreatic head, the dilated common bile duct (*arrow*) lies parallel and lateral to the dilated main pancreatic duct, indicating a point of obstruction caudal to this. **C:** One centimeter more caudal, at the level of the uncinate process, the dilated ducts are no longer visible, indicating an abrupt obliteration of their respective lumens. No mass is discernible either in the head of the pancreas or in the adjacent duodenum (D). Note that the fat plane separating the head of the pancreas from the vena cava (V) remains intact. The absence of evidence of local invasion or hepatic metastases indicated resectability. A 1-cm-diameter carcinoma of the ampulla was found at the time of operation.

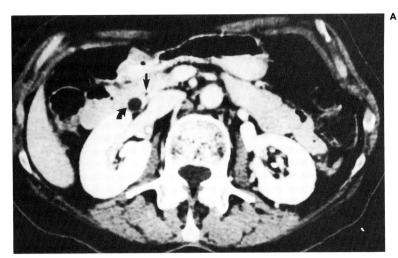

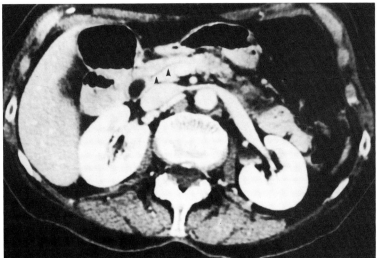

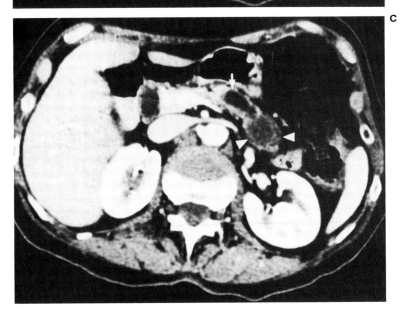

FIG. 9. Multifocal adenocarcinoma involving the body and tail. **A:** The head of the pancreas is unremarkable, and a normal-caliber main pancreatic duct (*arrow*) is visible. An incidental finding is a nonobstructed, moderately dilated distal common bile duct (*curved arrow*) in this postcholecystectomy patient. **B:** Two centimeters cephalad, the normal-caliber main pancreatic duct (*arrowheads*) extends to the region of the neck of the pancreas. **C:** At a level 1 cm cephalad to **B,** an abrupt transition in the caliber of the main pancreatic duct occurs (*white arrow*), although a discrete mass is not apparent at the point of transition. Necrotic tumor (*arrowheads*) replaces a portion of the pancreatic tail. At operation, a small focus of tumor in the neck of the pancreas obstructed the main pancreatic duct, and extensive tumor involved the remainder of the body and tail.

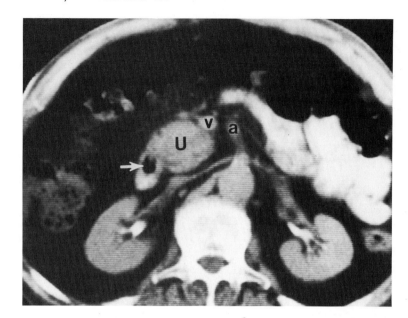

FIG. 10. Carcinoma in the uncinate process. Rounding of the normally slender hook-like configuration of the uncinate process (U) as it extends posteromedial to the superior mesenteric vein (v) indicates abnormality of this portion of the pancreatic head. Convex borders to both the anterior and posterior surfaces of the uncinate process should always be viewed with suspicion; (*arrow*) duodenum; (a) superior mesenteric artery.

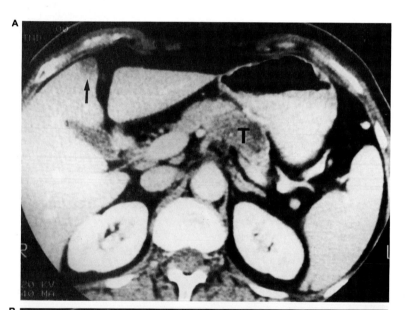

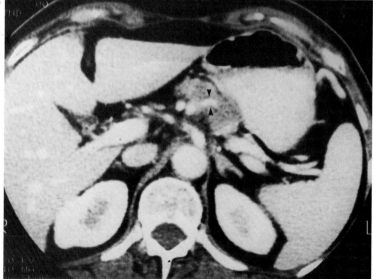

FIG. 11. Carcinoma of the body of the pancreas encasing the celiac axis. **A:** A 3-mm section through the body of the pancreas demonstrates an extensive tumor (T) involving the body of the pancreas without producing a significant enlargement in the diameter of the gland. The tumor tissue is enhanced less than the normal pancreatic parenchyma extending toward the region of the neck. The fat plane normally separating the posterior aspect of the pancreas from the celiac axis is not visible, indicating direct extension of the tumor process to the surface of the celiac axis. A subtle 1-cm metastasis is present in the anterior aspect of the medial segment of the left lobe (*arrow*). **B:** One centimeter cephalad, a portion of the tumor is seen encasing a segment of the splenic artery (*arrowheads*), a finding indicative of nonresectability.

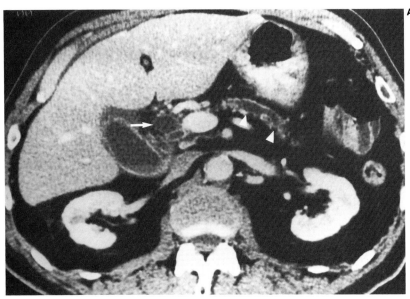

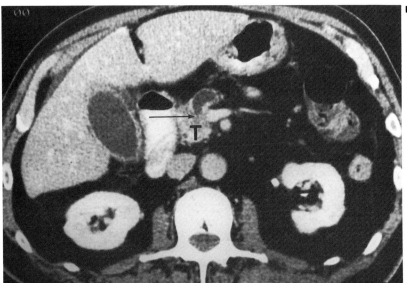

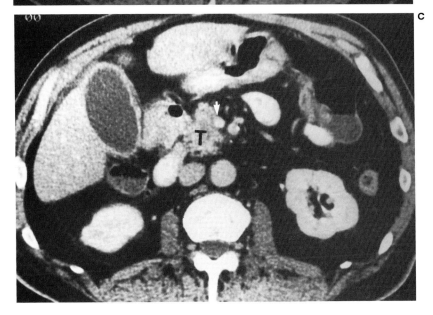

FIG. 12. Adenocarcinoma of the head of the pancreas. **A:** Dilatation of the main pancreatic duct and marked atrophy of the pancreatic parenchyma (*white arrowheads*) are apparent at this level. The common bile duct (*white arrow*) is moderately dilated, and the cystic duct is visible directly posterior to it. **B:** The point of obstruction of the main pancreatic duct (*arrow*) is visible at this level, but the common bile duct has already been obliterated by a small infiltrating tumor (T). **C:** At this level, the head of the pancreas is mostly replaced by tumor (T), which distorts the normal contour of the head of the pancreas. Because of direct contact with the superior mesenteric vein (*white arrow*), resectability of this tumor could not be confidently predicted.

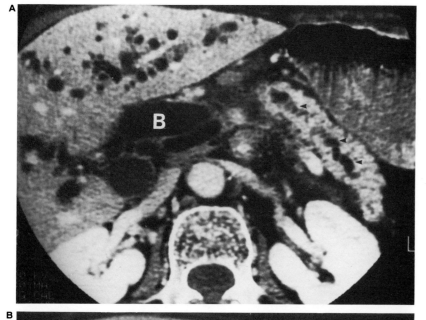

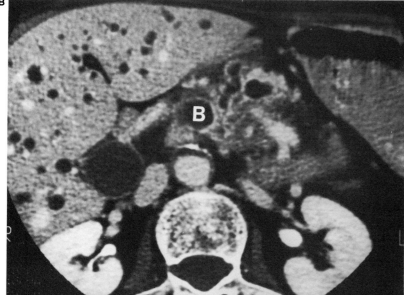

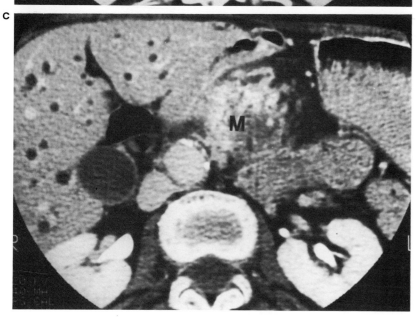

FIG. 13. Carcinoma of the head of the pancreas located entirely to the left of the aorta and to the left of midline. **A:** Marked intrahepatic and extrahepatic biliary dilatation is present. The common bile duct (B) is oriented transversely in this plane. Beaded dilatation of the main pancreatic duct (*arrowheads*) is well shown. **B:** Two centimeters caudal, the common bile duct (B) is now oriented vertically. Portions of the dilated pancreatic duct system are visible to its left. **C:** The head of the pancreas is mostly replaced by tumor mass (M), which has obliterated the lumen in both ducts. Note the position of the pancreatic head with respect to the aorta and the midline of the abdomen.

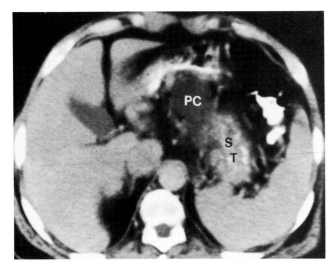
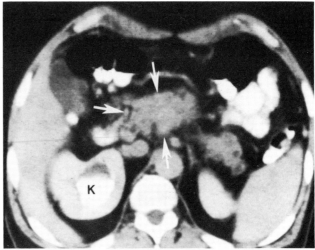

FIG. 14. Pseudocyst distal to an obstructing pancreatic carcinoma. **A:** Postcontrast CT image at the level of the porta hepatis shows a well-circumscribed pseudocyst (PC) in the body of the pancreas; (S_T) stomach. **B:** Four centimeters caudal, an irregular mass (*arrows*) is present in the pancreatic head. The mass has invaded the retropancreatic fat. Incidentally noted is a hydronephrotic right kidney (K).

Although a focal mass is the primary CT finding of a pancreatic adenocarcinoma, not all masses are carcinomas, and not all carcinomas present as masses. Differentiating between carcinoma and inflammatory disease occasionally can be difficult because the pancreas may be diffusely enlarged because of a carcinoma-induced pancreatitis and because pancreatitis can present as a focal mass (20,84,101). Secondary signs of pancreatic carcinoma, when present, may permit this distinction to be made. These secondary signs include hepatic and lymph node metastases (Figs. 12 and 15), contiguous organ invasion, and vascular encasement (12,20,76,112,158). The most common sites of metastases, in order of decreasing frequency, are liver, regional lymph nodes, peritoneum, and lungs (20). Because of the pancreas' rich lymphatic supply and lack of a capsule, metastases to regional nodes (peripancreatic, periaortic, pericaval, and periportal) tend to occur early (Figs. 14 and 15); however, lymphadenop-

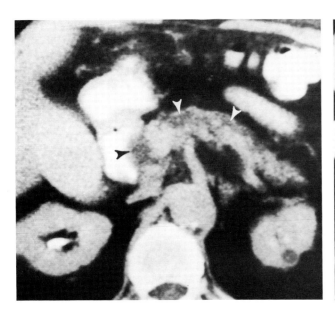
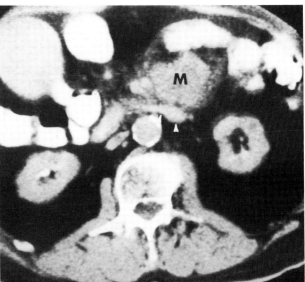

FIG. 15. Pancreatic carcinoma. **A:** A dilated common bile duct (*black arrowhead*) and an irregularly dilated main pancreatic duct (*white arrowheads*) are seen, indicating an obstructing process in the head of the pancreas. **B:** Although the primary pancreatic lesion could not be clearly defined, a large nodal metastasis (M) is seen in the root of the mesentery, anterior to the left renal vein (*arrowheads*) and caudal to and separate from the body of the pancreas, indicating a malignant cause and providing evidence for nonresectability.

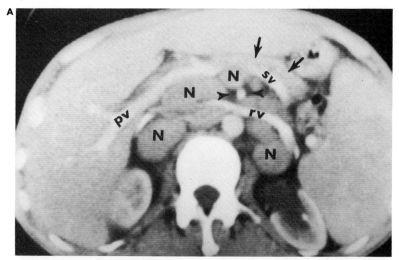

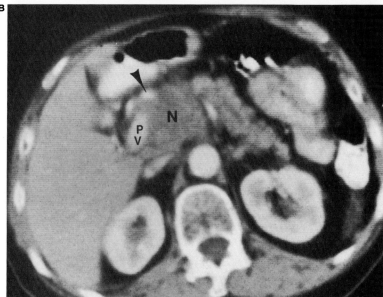

FIG. 16. Peripancreatic lymphoma. **A:** After intravenous bolus enhancement, the splenic, portal, and left renal veins are densely enhanced, and the pancreas (*arrows*) is seen to be anteriorly displaced by the lymph nodes (N) enlarged by lymphoma. Note that the fat plane surrounding the superior mesenteric artery (*arrowheads*) remains intact. This would not be the case in the presence of a similar-size adenocarcinoma of the pancreas. **B:** In another patient, postcontrast CT image shows a large nodal mass (N) in the region of the pancreatic head. It would be unusual for a pancreatic carcinoma to achieve this size without causing biliary obstruction. The pancreatic body and tail are normal; (pv) portal vein; (*arrowhead*) gastroduodenal artery; (sv) splenic vein; (rv) renal vein.

athy occasionally can be seen in patients with pancreatitis (158). Not uncommonly, peripancreatic lymphadenopathy may be indistinguishable from the pancreas and may appear as a large pancreatic mass. Differing contrast-enhancement characteristics following intravenous contrast material often will allow distinction between the nodes and pancreatic parenchyma (Fig. 16).

Encasement of the celiac axis (Figs. 11 and 17) or superior mesenteric artery (SMA) strongly suggests the presence of a neoplasm rather than benign disease. This encasement often is manifested by loss of the fat plane that separates the neck and body of the pancreas from the celiac axis and SMA. The tissue surrounding the vessels usually will be of the same density as the primary tumor. If intravenous contrast material is not administered, these encased vessels will appear thickened (Fig. 17). This thickening or increased density is thought to represent neoplastic invasion, as well as a desmoplastic response to the adenocarcinoma (96). If intravenous contrast material

is administered, the lumen of the encased vessel will appear constricted or obliterated (Figs. 11 and 17).

The appearances of the dilated common bile duct and main pancreatic duct can assist in differentiation between malignant disease and benign disease. Abrupt termination of either the common bile duct or the pancreatic duct favors the presence of malignant disease (12,112) (Figs. 8 and 12). In one large series, abrupt termination of the bile duct was seen in all patients with obstruction caused by a malignant neoplasm and in only 20% of patients with benign disease. Smooth, gradual tapering of the common bile duct was present in 80% of the patients with benign disease and in none of the patients with malignant disease (12).

Three appearances of pancreatic duct dilatation have been described (76): (a) smooth dilatation (Fig. 12), (b) beaded dilatation (Fig. 13), and (c) irregular dilatation. Smooth or beaded dilatation was seen in 85% of patients with carcinoma and 27% of patients with chronic pan-

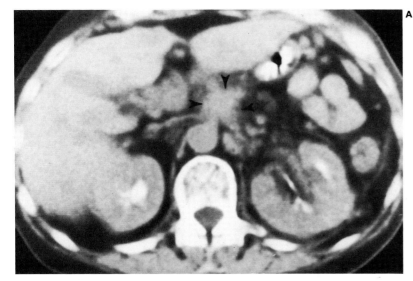

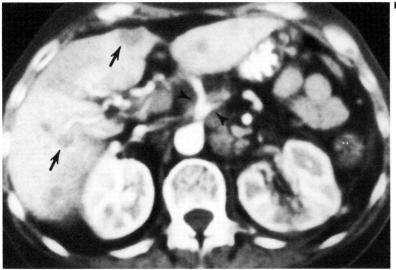

FIG. 17. Pancreatic carcinoma. **A:** A soft-tissue-density mass (*arrowheads*) surrounds the celiac trunk, indicating vascular invasion and unresectability. **B:** Image following an intravenous bolus of contrast material shows vascular encasement (*arrowheads*) of the vessels by the surrounding malignant neoplasm. Multiple hepatic metastases (*arrows*) are also shown.

creatitis. Irregular dilatation was seen in 73% of patients with chronic pancreatitis and only 15% of patients with carcinoma. When the ratio of pancreatic duct diameter to pancreatic gland width is greater than 0.5, the presence of carcinoma is favored. When the ratio is less than 0.5, benign disease is more likely. In fact, carcinoma was present approximately 90% of the time when the ratio exceeded 0.5 (76).

If secondary signs of malignant disease are not present, it may not be possible to distinguish between a carcinoma and focal pancreatitis. If the mass is thought to represent focal inflammation, follow-up studies should be performed to confirm that resolution occurs. In equivocal, nonresolving, or indeterminate cases, ERCP or direct percutaneous fine-needle aspiration can aid in diagnosis. In some cases, selective angiography may also assist in making this distinction by revealing subtle intrapancreatic vascular encasement. In a small percentage of cases, nothing short of surgically obtained histologic material will resolve the issue.

Another potentially useful aid for distinguishing between neoplastic pancreatic disease and inflammatory disease is a recently developed tumor marker, carbohydrate antigen 19-9 (CA 19-9), which frequently is elevated in patients with gastrointestinal carcinomas, especially pancreatic carcinomas. In one series (122), the CA 19-9 level was elevated in 80% of patients with carcinoma and in only 9% of patients with chronic pancreatitis. However, because the sensitivity and specificity of this marker correlate best with tumors greater than 3 cm in diameter, it is unlikely that diagnostic accuracy will be appreciably improved when the CT examination is indeterminate.

CT, in addition to its role as the initial imaging method for evaluating patients suspected of having pancreatic adenocarcinoma, plays an important role in the staging of these neoplasms and in the determination of their resectability. Pancreatic cancer tends to be disseminated at the time of diagnosis. When initially evaluated, only 14% of patients have tumor confined to the pancreas, whereas 65% of them have advanced local dissemination or distant

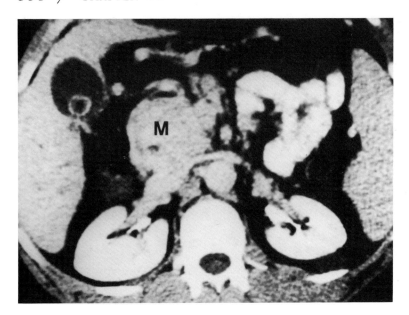

FIG. 18. Nonfunctioning islet cell tumor. A 5-cm-diameter mass (M) is present in the head of the pancreas. Despite its size, the biliary tree was not obstructed. There is nothing characteristic about this mass to allow differentiation from an adenocarcinoma, other than the lack of central necrosis. No nodal or hepatic metastases were present. A mixed-composition gallstone is noted within the gallbladder.

metastases, and the remaining 21% have localized disease, with spread to the regional lymph nodes (30). CT is able to show hepatic or other distant metastases, regional lymphadenopathy, and high-density (hemorrhagic or malignant) ascites. It is also able to reveal vascular encasement or invasion of contiguous organs. In cases of equivocal evidence of vascular encasement, selective angiography may answer this question. The neoplasm is considered unresectable if there are metastases, vascular encasement, ascites, or contiguous-organ invasion (43,46,69).

Islet Cell Tumors

It is frequently convenient to divide the rare islet cell tumors into two groups: hormonally active and quiescent. Related to their different clinical presentations, they have different CT appearances.

Hormonally quiescent islet cell tumors, which account for approximately 15% of all islet cell tumors (143), are clinically silent until they cause symptoms due to their size or to metastases. Consequently, usually they are large at the time of discovery, ranging in size from 3 to 24 cm in diameter (Fig. 18); 30% are greater than 10 cm. Following intravenous administration of contrast material, most islet cell tumors become at least partially hyperdense relative to the normal pancreatic parenchyma; hepatic metastases may be hyperdense relative to normal liver parenchyma (36) (Fig. 19).

It is important to differentiate between these neoplasms and ductal adenocarcinomas, because patients with islet cell tumors often respond favorably to specific chemotherapy and consequently have a better prognosis than patients with adenocarcinomas (87). Three features that aid in this differentiation are the presence of calcification,

the lack of vascular encasement, and the absence of central necrosis or cystic degeneration in islet cell tumors; 20% of islet cell tumors contain calcification, whereas less than 2% of adenocarcinomas do. Encasement of the celiac artery or SMA, which is commonly seen in adenocarcinomas, especially larger ones, has not been seen in islet cell tumors; however, encasement of the superior mesenteric vein (SMV) or portal vein has been reported (16,36). Islet cell tumors, even when large, rarely undergo central necrosis or cystic degeneration, because of their rich vascularity, which continues to grow as the mass grows (143). Although 60% of islet cell tumors occur in the body and

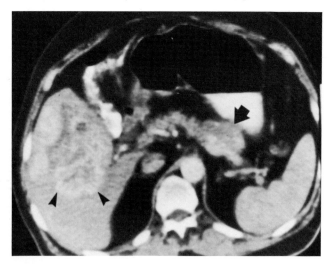

FIG. 19. Nonfunctioning islet cell carcinoma with liver metastases. A 3-cm-diameter well-defined mass arises from the pancreas at the junction of the body and tail (arrow). It is enhanced uniformly, showing no signs of central necrosis. A densely enhancing, heterogeneous-density metastasis (arrowheads) is present in the right lobe of the liver.

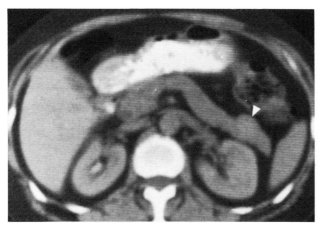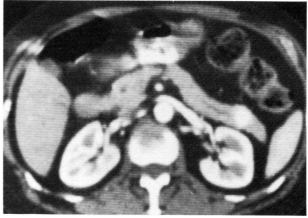

A,B

FIG. 20. Insulinoma. **A:** A subtle alteration in the contour of the anterior surface of the tail of the pancreas (*arrowhead*) is apparent in this patient suspected of having an insulinoma. **B:** Postcontrast bolus technique: A 1.5-cm densely enhancing lesion is visible in the area of contour irregularity. This pattern of enhancement is typical for an islet cell tumor.

tail, location is not a useful differentiating feature in individual cases. In summary, the diagnosis of a hormonally quiescent islet cell tumor should be considered when a large, nonuniformly enhancing, calcified pancreatic mass without cystic areas and with hyperdense areas is identified on a contrast-enhanced CT examination (36).

The presenting symptoms of a functional islet cell tumor—insulinoma, gastrinoma (57), VIPoma, glucagonoma, somatostatinoma (114)—depend on the hormone secreted. These neoplasms usually are small (90% are less than 2 cm in diameter) (42,53,54,143) and may be multiple (gastrinomas and insulinomas are multiple 60% and 10% of the time, respectively) (54,107). Because of their typically small size, they seldom alter the contour of the pancreas; therefore, intravenous contrast material must be administered as a bolus to detect them (54,80) (Fig. 20). Functioning islet cell tumors are hyperdense relative to normal pancreatic parenchyma following intravenous administration of contrast material. An additional tech-

nique to enhance the ability of CT to detect these neoplasms is to use contiguous 2- to 5-mm-thick slices through the pancreas. Calcification, which may occur in islet cell tumors, is more common in malignant than in benign neoplasms (17,159). CT is able to localize approximately 78% of functional islet cell tumors; this increases to 86% when insulinomas are excluded (82,118,139). With CT, one is able to identify about 50% of insulinomas (139). CT has not been reported to have shown these tumors when they have been in ectopic locations (stomach, duodenum, jejunum, splenic hilum) (Fig. 21). Diffuse pancreatic islet cell hyperplasia causes no discernible changes in the pancreas on CT.

In spite of these limitations and the fact that CT is not as accurate as selective angiography in the localization of functional islet cell tumors, it is nevertheless the initial radiologic test of choice because it is not invasive and is very accurate in the staging of these neoplasms. CT is able to show metastatic lymphadenopathy and hepatic metas-

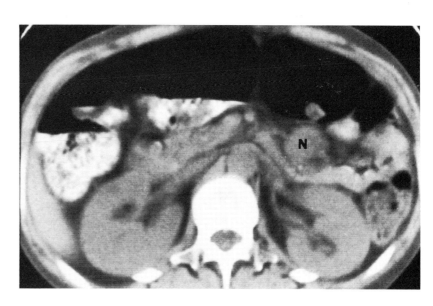

FIG. 21. Ectopic islet cell tumor. A small gastrinoma was found in the proximal jejunum at surgery in this patient with the Zollinger-Ellison syndrome. Although the primary tumor was not identified on CT, regional metastatic lymphadenopathy (N) was seen.

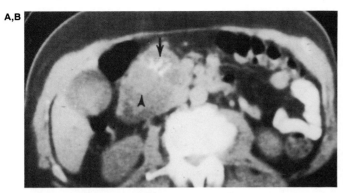
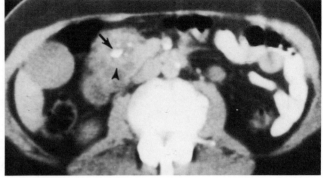

FIG. 22. Microcystic adenoma. Two serial images at a 1-cm interval show a multicystic tumor in the head of the pancreas, with central soft-tissue-density (*arrowheads*) cysts varying in size from 2 mm to 10 mm in diameter, and calcifications (*arrows*) arranged in a radial pattern.

tases even when it is not able to reveal the primary tumor. CT also allows examination of the adrenal glands for tumors, which is important because islet cell tumors can occur as part of a multiple endocrine adenomatosis syndrome. Angiography and venous sampling should be reserved for those patients who have negative or equivocal findings on CT studies.

Cystic Neoplasms

Cystic neoplasms of the pancreas are uncommon, accounting for 10% of all cystic pancreatic masses (67,165). These neoplasms are divided into two groups—microcystic adenoma (formerly termed serous cystadenoma) and macrocystic adenoma (formerly termed mucinous cystadenoma)—which have significantly different therapeutic and prognostic implications.

Microcystic adenoma has typical CT and pathologic appearances (22). This tumor is found in an elderly population (82% occur in patients 60 years or older) (47), without a strong sexual predilection (female-to-male ratio is 3 to 2) (47). The tumor can vary in size from 1 to 12 cm, with an average diameter of approximately 5 cm. It is a benign tumor with no malignant potential (47,74). These masses may occur in any part of the pancreas, but tend to predominate in the head. On CT, this neoplasm has a smooth or nodular contour, with a spectrum of appearances of the tumor tissue itself ranging from a nearly solid appearance due to the presence of innumerable minute cysts, to many small but visible cysts, to a more multilocular-appearing mass having thin septa and thin walls (Fig. 22). When there are multiple small but visible cysts, the tumor has a honeycomb appearance (67). It is not always well demarcated, as its capsule is not well developed. The soft-tissue components of this tumor are enhanced following intravenous administration of contrast material, in keeping with its angiographic hypervascular appearance (67) (Fig. 23). Occasionally a central scar is present, and its radiating beams of connective tissue may calcify in a stellate or sunburst appearance (47,67,165) (Fig. 22). At times it may be difficult from

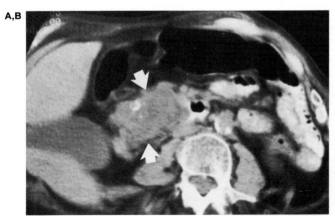
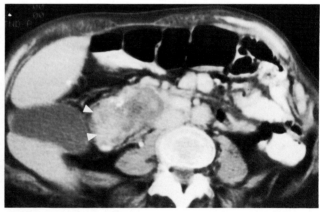

FIG. 23. Microcystic adenoma. **A:** A precontrast image shows a mass (*arrows*) of heterogeneous density in the head of the pancreas. Curvilinear calcification is present. In this case, the individual cysts are too small to be discernible. **B:** After intravenous contrast material, dense enhancement of the stroma (*arrowheads*) is apparent. Several cystic areas can now be seen in the more medial aspect of the tumor mass. (Courtesy of Dr. Arthur Bishop, Peoria, Illinois.)

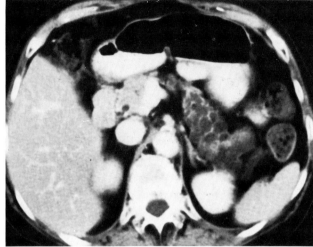

FIG. 24. Macrocystic adenoma. Two images, 2 cm apart, show a low-density mass in the body and tail of the pancreas composed of multiple cysts in the range of 1 to 2 cm in diameter, with visible septae. Because of the preponderance of cysts, minimal contrast enhancement is seen. (Courtesy of Dr. Arthur Bishop, Peoria, Illinois.)

only its CT appearance to distinguish it from other cystic pancreatic processes or, in the case of the tumor that contains innumerable minute cysts, from a solid pancreatic mass. However, on histologic examination, its cytoplasm is rich in glycogen, with little or no mucin, a distinguishing feature (22,47). When examined with ultrasound, the appearance of the tumor may range from very echogenic to a relatively hypoechoic mass that appears septated and composed of only a few cysts.

Macrocystic adenoma, the second type of cystic pancreatic neoplasm, occurs in a younger population (50% of the tumors occur in patients between the ages of 40 and 60 years) (23,47) than the microcystic adenoma and has a strong predilection for women (female-to-male ratio is 6 to 1) (47). The tumor is almost always located in the body or tail of the pancreas (23,74). These masses usually are large (mean diameter is 10 cm), encapsulated, and multiloculated (Fig. 24). Stromal elements (septa) separate

the cystic areas, which typically are greater than 2 cm in size (Fig. 25). The septae themselves are thicker than those found in microcystic adenomas and may calcify. The walls of these cystic tumors are thick and often nodular (23,67,74). The amount of stroma varies, and when small, the septae may not be apparent on CT. In that case, the tumor appears unilocular and resembles a pseudocyst. Pathologically, these neoplasms contain mucin. In contradistinction to microcystic adenomas, all macrocystic adenomas have malignant potential (Fig. 26). Therefore, if distant metastases are absent, complete excision is recommended, as this may be curative (23,47).

A possible subcategory of the macrocystic adenoma (mucinous cystadenoma) has recently been described in Japan and called the "ductectatic" type of mucinous cystadenoma (68); this tumor is believed to have the same malignant potential as the more typical macrocystic adenoma. This entity presents as localized cystic dilatation

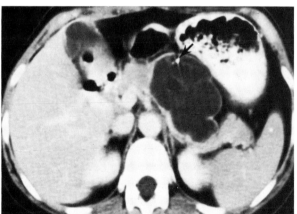
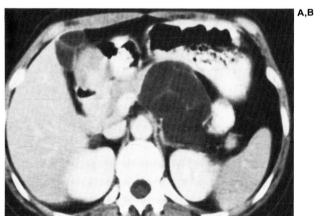

FIG. 25. Macrocystic adenoma. Two images, 2 cm apart, show a large cystic-appearing mass with minimal septation and a very sharply defined wall. A small septal calcification is noted anteriorly (arrow). As the cysts become larger in a macrocystic adenoma, it is more difficult to define the internal septal architecture on CT. (Courtesy of Dr. Arthur Bishop, Peoria, Illinois.)

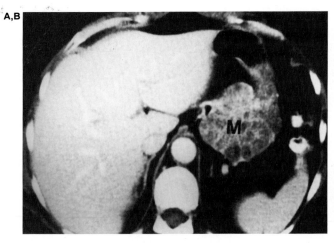
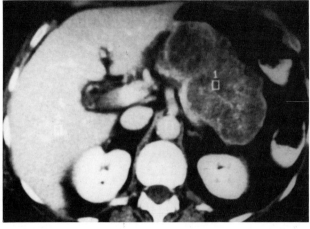

FIG. 26. Macrocystic adenocarcinoma (formerly termed mucinous cystadenocarcinoma). **A:** A large heterogeneous mass (M) with internal cysts and septations is identified in a retrogastric location. **B:** At a level 3 cm caudal to **A,** the same mass replaces the body and tail of the pancreas. The margins of the tumor are well defined, and the fat plane posterior to the pancreas is not invaded. The tumor was found to be resectable at the time of surgery. (Courtesy of Dr. Arthur Bishop, Peoria, Illinois.)

of a side branch of the main pancreatic duct lined by papillary hyperplastic epithelium with atypia, essentially indistinguishable from the epithelium seen in mucinous cystadenomas or cystadenocarcinomas. The lumen in these ectatic side branches is filled with a mucoid sub-stance, producing filling defects on ERCP. In one series of 5 cases, all lesions were located in the uncinate process, were about 3 cm in diameter, and on CT were difficult to distinguish from a simple intrapancreatic cyst such as might be found in pancreatitis. The imaging study of most

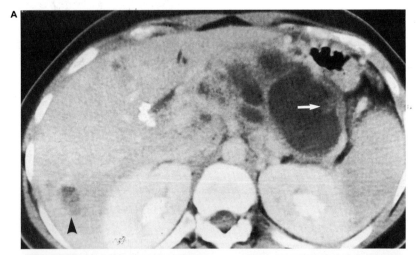
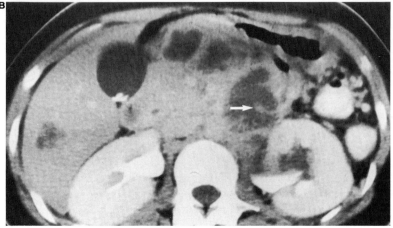

FIG. 27. Mucinous adenocarcinoma of the body and tail of the pancreas. **A,B:** Two im-ages, 3 cm apart, show a large multicystic mass occupying the area of the body and tail of the pancreas. Papillary projections (*white arrows*) arise from the thick-walled cystic portions of the tumor. One of several hepatic metastases is indicated by the *arrowhead.* Incidental gall-stones were noted in the body and neck of the gallbladder. The findings are characteristic of an extensive mucinous adenocarcinoma.

diagnostic value was ERCP, which showed localized, prominent cystic dilatation of a side branch of the main pancreatic duct, with grapelike clusters of contrast material associated with intraluminal filling defects of various sizes, located in the uncinate process.

The major pathologic entities to be differentiated from the cystic neoplasms are focal pancreatitis, with an associated pseudocyst or calcification, and a necrotic adenocarcinoma (165). A history of pancreatitis or trauma usually is present in patients with focal pancreatitis or an isolated pseudocyst; however, based on CT findings alone, it may be impossible to distinguish a cystadenoma from a pseudocyst. Necrotic adenocarcinoma characteristically has a thick irregular wall without calcification on CT. The uncommon mucinous adenocarcinoma may be difficult to distinguish from a cystadenoma (55,66,132,165) (Fig. 27). The rare pancreatic lymphangioma, a benign tumor originating from lymphatic vessels, also may be indistin-

guishable from a cystadenoma (104). Finally, cystic lesions of the pancreas associated with the von Hippel-Lindau syndrome may appear similar to pseudocysts and macrocystic adenomas.

Other Neoplastic Lesions

In addition to the previously described neoplasms, several less common neoplastic processes—solid and papillary epithelial neoplasm of the pancreas, lymphoma, metastases, and pleomorphic carcinoma—may arise in the pancreas or peripancreatic lymph nodes. Solid and papillary epithelial neoplasm of the pancreas is an uncommon low-grade malignant tumor that occurs chiefly in young women (mean age 24 years). On CT, it is seen as a large (mean 11.5 cm), sharply defined, nonhomogeneous mass that usually is located in the tail and contains areas of

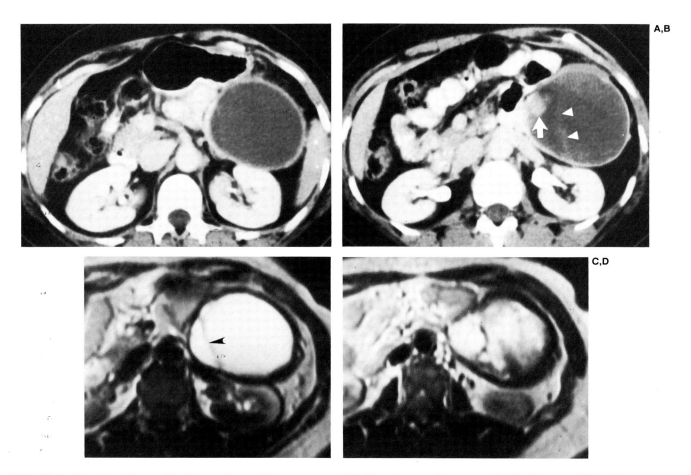

FIG. 28. Solid and papillary epithelial neoplasm of the pancreas. **A,B:** Two images, 2 cm apart, in this 41-year-old female patient with a left-upper-quadrant mass show a well-defined cystic-appearing mass with a uniformly thick wall and a papillary projection (*arrow*) arising from the medial wall. A suggestion of a septation is also seen (*arrowheads*). In this case, the most likely diagnosis would be macrocystic adenoma. However, this also falls into the spectrum of solid and papillary epithelial neoplasms. (Courtesy of Dr. Arthur Bishop.) **C:** T2-weighted MR image (SE, TR = 1,500 msec, TE = 70 msec) at a similar level as **A** shows a cystic structure with a single septation (*arrowhead*) and a thick, low-intensity wall. **D:** Three centimeters more caudal, the mass has mixed medium-to-low-signal-intensity areas representing solid components of this tumor.

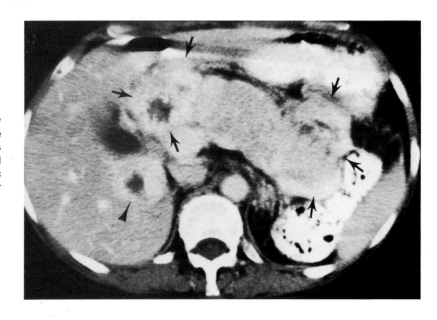

FIG. 29. Pancreatic metastases from primary renal cell carcinoma. Postcontrast CT image shows at least two hypervascular metastases (*arrows*) in the pancreas: one in the head and the other in the tail. In addition, the pancreatic body is diffusely enlarged; (*arrowhead*) liver metastasis.

cystic degeneration and necrosis (Fig. 28). The differential diagnosis includes cystic neoplasms and islet cell tumors (10,48,121). Pancreatic metastases, which are rarely diagnosed clinically, most commonly arise from melanoma and carcinomas of the breast, lung, kidney, prostate, and gastrointestinal tract. Isolated metastases to the pancreas from primary bone tumors have also been reported (119). When multiple masses are present in the pancreas in a patient with a known primary carcinoma, metastases can be presumed (Fig. 29); however, when solitary, it may be indistinguishable from primary pancreatic carcinoma (104,120).

Pleomorphic carcinoma is an uncommon malignant neoplasm that has a fulminant clinical course. It metastasizes to the liver, lung, adrenal, kidney, thyroid, and bone. This tumor shows irregular enhancement after intravenous contrast material, and it may be cystic, with thick irregular walls and a lobulated contour. The presence of extensive retroperitoneal lymphadenopathy helps differentiate it from adenocarcinoma (160).

Although lymphoma can involve the pancreas and peripancreatic lymph nodes and can be confused with a primary pancreatic neoplasm, usually it is a systemic disease, with retroperitoneal and mesenteric lymphadenopathy also present (Fig. 30). The two best signs to distinguish peripancreatic lymphadenopathy from a primary neoplasm are intact fat planes between the nodes and the pancreas and anterior displacement of the pancreas (Fig. 16); however, these signs are seen less than half the time (164). Lymphoma often is larger than adenocarcinoma. In one study it was reported that no adenocarcinoma was larger than 10 cm, and 60% were between 4 and 6 cm (142).

Inflammation

Acute Pancreatitis

Since the advent of CT, our understanding of the various inflammatory diseases affecting the pancreas has increased by a level of magnitude unsurpassed by that for any of the other disease processes within the abdomen. With regard to acute pancreatitis, we are now able to show the morphologic changes in this disease, ranging from minimal edema of the pancreatic parenchyma in interstitial inflammation to the extensive phlegmon, fluid collections, hemorrhage, and necrosis that develop in fulminant necrotizing hemorrhagic pancreatitis.

Acute pancreatitis frequently is associated with exudation of fluid into the interstitium of the pancreas and subsequent leakage of this fluid containing activated proteolytic enzymes into the surrounding tissue spaces. The pancreatic enzyme trypsin is suspected to be the agent in the ensuing coagulative necrosis (29,33,85). Although much has been learned concerning the pathophysiology of pancreatitis, the pathogenetic mechanism of autodigestion remains unclear (49,95).

The diagnosis of uncomplicated acute pancreatitis generally is established by the clinical presentation and biochemical tests without the need for diagnostic imaging. However, biochemical abnormalities are not always evident at the time of initial presentation. The serum amylase level may initially be normal in up to one-third of patients clinically suspected of having acute pancreatitis associated with alcohol abuse who have CT or ultrasound findings consistent with pancreatitis (136). However, one must recognize that CT changes indicative of subacute or

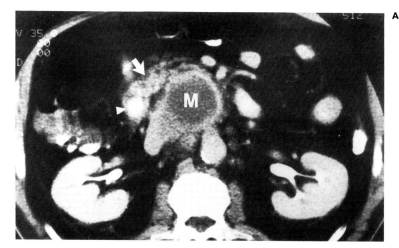

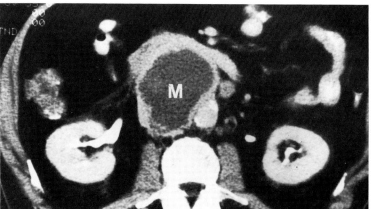

FIG. 30. Peripancreatic lymphoma. **A,B:** A large, centrally hypodense mass (M) displaces the uncinate process (*arrow*) and the duodenum (*arrowhead*) anterolaterally. A mass with this appearance and location could simulate a pseudocyst of the pancreas. **C,D:** Posttherapy 6-month follow-up study shows marked reduction in the overall size of the mass (M), with a nearly normal appearance to the region of the uncinate process (*arrow*), but persistence of a mass posterior to the duodenum. A preaortic node (N) has doubled in diameter during the interval.

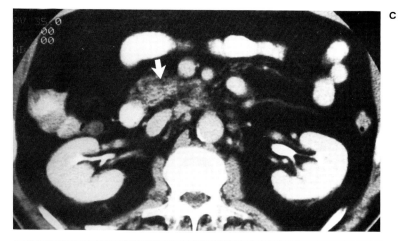

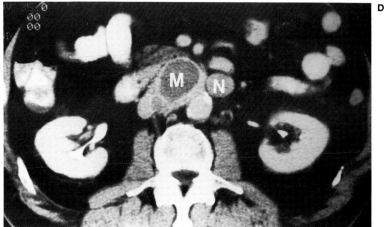

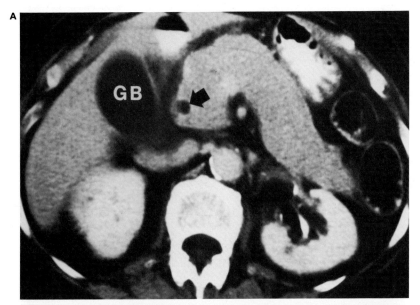

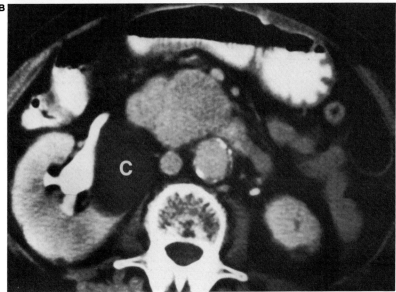

FIG. 31. Acute pancreatitis with a 9-month follow-up. **A,B:** Marked swelling of the entire pancreas is seen on this examination. The homogeneous appearance of the pancreatic parenchyma, with little, if any, change in the peripancreatic fat, is unusual in acute pancreatitis; (*arrow*) common bile duct; (GB) gallbladder; (C) parapelvic renal cyst. **C** and **D** on *facing page*.

chronic pancreatitis do not prove the existence of the acute form of the disease (81).

Thus, although CT is not necessary in all cases of acute pancreatitis, it is quite valuable when the diagnosis has not been firmly established clinically or when complications are suspected. Ultrasound and CT imaging should be used to evaluate for pancreatitis in acutely ill patients with excruciating abdominal pain, hypotension, and leukocytosis (58,98). In former years, exploratory laparotomy was performed on many such patients to exclude a ruptured viscus, vascular occlusion, or other abdominal catastrophe. The mortality among such patients after unnecessary surgery varied from 20% to 80% (6).

In some patients, the inflammatory process in acute pancreatitis results in no more than transient edema of the gland, followed by full recovery. CT will show a normal-appearing gland in one-third or more of patients with acute pancreatitis (33,98,130). The changes of acute pan-

creatitis recognizable with CT include diffuse (Fig. 31) or focal glandular enlargement, contour irregularity, focal irregular areas of decreased attenuation presumably secondary to edema or focal necrosis, and changes in the peripancreatic areolar tissues, fat, and parietal peritoneal planes (33,98,129,130).

The initial changes that are shown by CT include blurring of the outline of a swollen-appearing pancreas by edematous and inflammatory changes in the contiguous peripancreatic fat (Fig. 32). Changes will also be recognizable in the anterior pararenal space because of dissection of fluid, initially limited in quantity, into the left lateral extent of this space, resulting in the appearance of thickening of the anterior perinephric fascia (Gerota's fascia) (Fig. 33). As the inflammatory and exudative process continues, the space fills with fluid, spreading superiorly and inferiorly in this anterior compartment of the retroperitoneum. Small fluid collections can develop within

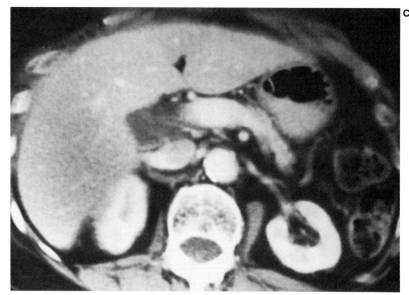

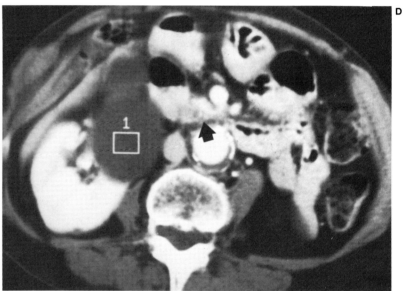

FIG. 31. (*Continued.*) Parts **A** and **B** on *facing page.* **C,D:** Comparable levels from a 9-month follow-up examination show a complete return to normal size of the pancreas. The uncinate process (*arrow*) now no longer displaces the mesenteric vessels anteriorly, compared with the earlier study. No clinically apparent sequelae were evident.

the pancreas as well as in the immediate peripancreatic space. These fluid collections do not warrant the term "pseudocyst," because they usually are poorly encapsulated and transient.

Early in the evolution of complicated acute pancreatitis, the barrier provided by the parietal peritoneum overlying the pancreas may be disrupted, and inflammatory fluid will enter the lesser sac (Fig. 34). From this location the fluid may enter the main peritoneal cavity through the foramen of Winslow or may enter directly by disrupting the peritoneum in the anterior surface of the lesser sac (Fig. 32). In complicated pancreatitis, generally there is an inverse relationship between the degree of autodigestion of the gland and the volume of the peripancreatic fluid (129). Large collections of fluid often are accompanied by relative preservation of the pancreas, whereas cases involving severe parenchymal damage, including

pancreatic necrosis, are more apt to be associated with lesser amounts of peripancreatic fluid.

Originally, on the basis of accepted anatomic concepts and earlier-generation CT images, it was believed that the posterior pararenal space was also commonly involved in the inflammatory process of extensive complicated pancreatitis. However, a more recent study has shown that the posterior collections actually represent extension of pancreatitis from the anterior pararenal space to a potential space between the laminae of the posterior renal fascia (111). Among 40 patients with posterior extension of pancreatic effusion or phlegmon, interfascial involvement was observed in all 40, and was bilateral in 9 (23%). True involvement of the posterior pararenal space was uncommon, as was extension into the perirenal space. These investigators noted that the posterior renal fascia was thicker than the anterior and had at least two layers that

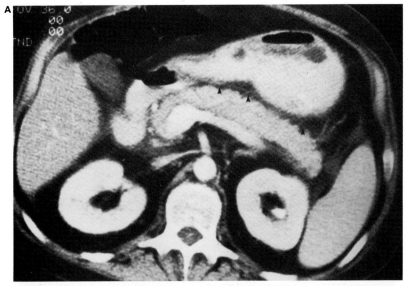

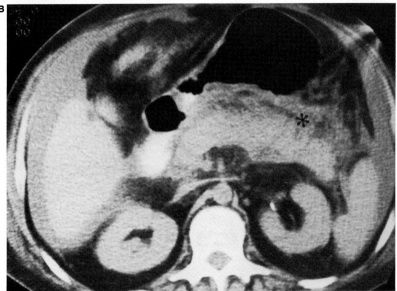

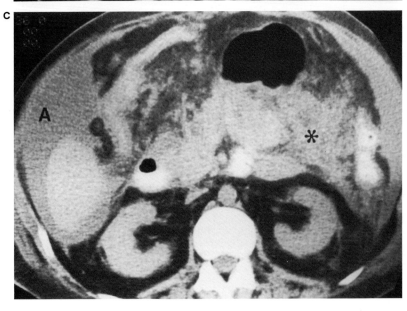

FIG. 32. Worsening pancreatitis. **A:** Image of the pancreas in a cardiac transplant patient with clinical signs of acute pancreatitis. Slight blurring of the anterior margin of the pancreas is seen, and an increase in the density of the peripancreatic fat (*arrowheads*) can be seen. The findings would be consistent with mild changes of pancreatitis. **B,C:** Eighteen-day follow-up study, performed without intravenous contrast material, shows a marked worsening in the appearance of the pancreas and peripancreatic tissues. Extensive fluid and phlegmonous changes are present in the anterior pararenal space (asterisk), and a large amount of high-density ascites (A) has also developed in the interim. This finding frequently indicates the presence of blood within the ascitic fluid. Note that the posterior wall of the stomach has been obscured by the contiguous inflammatory process.

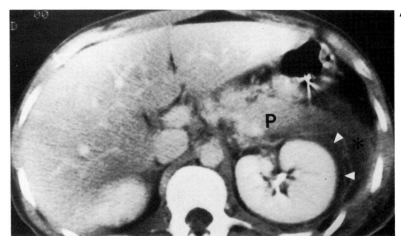

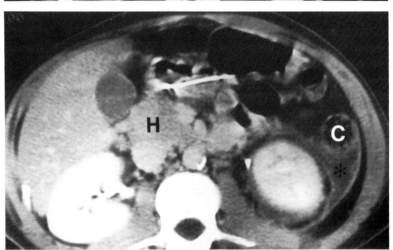

FIG. 33. Acute pancreatitis extending into the leaves of the posterior perinephric fascia. **A:** At the level of the body of the pancreas (P), the margins are blurred, and peripancreatic fluids and phlegmonous changes (asterisk) extend laterally and posteriorly into the region of the lateral conal fascia. Some increase in the density of the perinephric fat (*arrowheads*) is evident at this level. **B:** The lateral extent of the anterior pararenal space is clearly defined by the extension of the peripancreatic fluid (asterisk) into the left colic gutter. Note that there are no obvious inflammatory changes surrounding the head (H) of the pancreas. The beginning of dissection between the lamina of the posterior perinephric fascia can be appreciated on this image; (C) descending colon.

could be easily separated. The lateroconal fascia was shown to be continuous with the posterior lamina of the posterior renal fascia (Fig. 33), thereby serving to direct the inflammatory exudate between the fascial layers, producing an appearance that simulated extension into the posterior pararenal space.

Pathways of dissection commonly followed by the peripancreatic fluid include the gastrohepatic (Figs. 35 and 36), gastrosplenic, and gastrocolic ligaments. Fluid will also dissect into the transverse mesocolon (Fig. 37) and along the root of the mesentery. Large extrapancreatic fluid collections can extend superiorly into the medias-

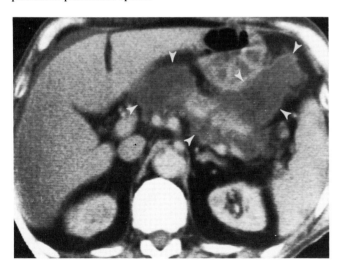

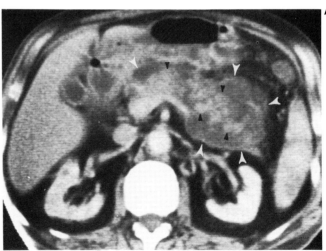

FIG. 34. Fluid collections associated with acute pancreatitis. **A:** A fluid collection (*arrowheads*) is seen extending into the lesser sac. **B:** On an image 2 cm caudad, the fluid collection (*white arrowheads*) surrounds the lobules of pancreatic tissue (*black arrowheads*). A small amount of ascites is present.

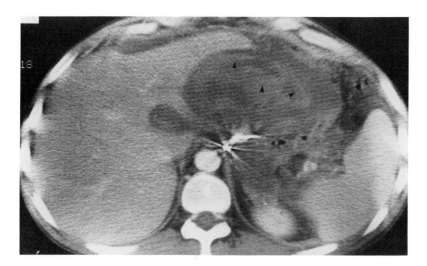

FIG. 35. Hemorrhagic complications in acute pancreatitis. Layers of higher-density blood clot (*arrowheads*) are visible within a large peripancreatic fluid collection that has dissected into the region of the gastrohepatic ligament. Intrapancreatic and peripancreatic hemorrhages are more frequently recognized on CT examinations than is clinically suspected.

tinum (Fig. 36) and even into the pericardial space (89,93). Following the pathways provided by the root of the mesentery and the anterior pararenal space, large collections can extend to and around segments of the cecum, ascending colon, and descending colon, as well as extending inferiorly into the lumbar, pelvic, and inguinal regions (70). A more destructive inflammatory process resulting in a phlegmon can also extend along the same pathways (Fig. 38). Involvement of the ascending or descending colon in the phlegmon of acute pancreatitis can be severe enough to lead to hemorrhage, necrosis, perforation, and stricture formation (141). A pancreatic inflammatory mass

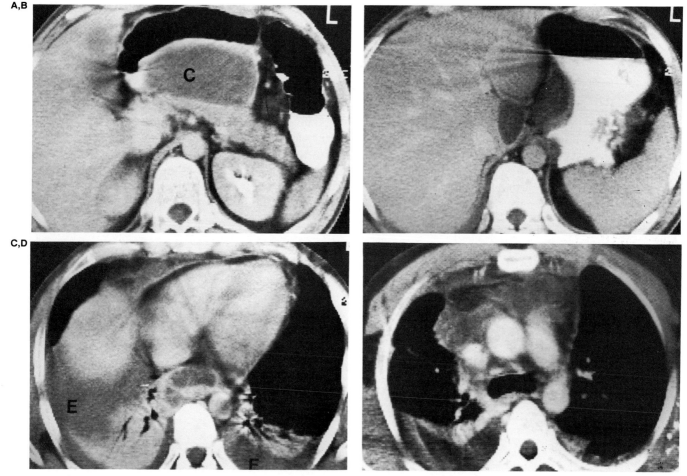

FIG. 36. Mediastinal dissection of a pancreatic pseudocyst. Four imaging levels track a pancreatic pseudocyst (C) from its original lesser-sac location (**A**) into the region of the gastrohepatic ligament (**B**), through the diaphragmatic hiatus (**C**), and superiorly into the superior anterior mediastinum (**D**). Bilateral pleural effusions (E) and lower-lobe atelectasis are also present.

involving the colon may be difficult to distinguish from a primary colonic neoplasm with local spread, based on the CT images alone (Fig. 39). Clues to the neoplastic nature of such a process include the relatively high density of the mass and the normal appearance of the retroperitoneal fat immediately contiguous with the mass.

As was mentioned in the section on anatomy, a fat plane is generally seen separating the posterior surface of the body of the pancreas from the SMA. In complicated acute pancreatitis, an increase in the density of the peripancreatic fat is commonly observed (Fig. 40). However, for reasons not fully understood, a cylindrical envelope of fat surrounding the SMA and SMV usually remains unaltered by the inflammatory process. In some complex cases this observation may be helpful in the distinction between inflammatory and neoplastic diseases.

The extensive pancreatic and peripancreatic fluid collections that are frequently seen in complicated acute pancreatitis are not considered pseudocysts. These fluid collections are dynamic by nature, changing in size, shape, and location depending on the persistence of the source. They commonly maintain a communication with the pancreatic duct system, and an equilibrium may be established between the quantity of fluid being extravasated and the absorption taking place in the peritoneal or retroperitoneal space; 20% to 25% of such fluid collections will completely resolve over a period of weeks (85). In contrast, pseudocysts are more permanent in nature; a pseudocyst has a thick, well-defined capsule composed of dense fibrous connective tissue and usually is round or oval in shape. Pseudocysts are more often associated with subacute or chronic pancreatitis. Many can be shown to communicate with the pancreatic duct system by ERCP or operative pancreatic ductography. However, they manifest none of the dynamism of the acute fluid collections discussed earlier. Usually the fluid in a pseudocyst is homogeneous in density and of near-water attenuation value. When the contents of a pseudocyst are either heterogeneous or uniformly increased in density, intracystic hemorrhage or infection may be present. If discrete areas of high-density material can be seen within a pseudocyst, clot formation secondary to hemorrhage should be strongly suspected (Fig. 41). These same changes can occur in peripancreatic fluid collections secondary to hemor-

Text continues on page 575.

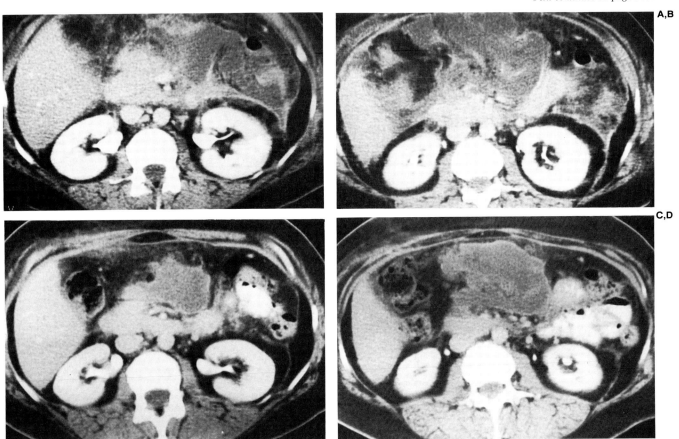

FIG. 37. Complicated acute pancreatitis, with partial resolution at 6 weeks. **A,B:** Extensive phlegmonous changes of complicated pancreatitis are noted at the levels of the pancreatic head and transverse portion of the duodenum, respectively. The phlegmonous process extends throughout the anterior pararenal space (**A**), into the root of the mesentery (**B**), reaching the anterior abdominal wall. **C,D:** Images from comparable levels on a 6-week follow-up examination following nonsurgical, supportive management. The margins of more homogeneous fluid collections are now better defined, and the adjacent fat shows less inflammatory change. Overall, there has been a significant reduction in the extent of the retroperitoneal phlegmon.

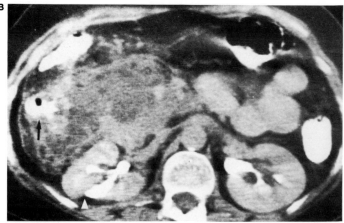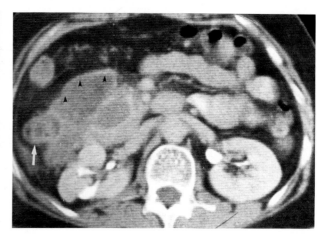

FIG. 38. Evolution of peripancreatic phlegmon. **A:** CT image at the level of the middle ascending colon (*arrow*) shows an extensive phlegmon dissecting through the mesentery, encircling and distorting the contour of the lumen of the ascending colon. Note the classic scar of atrophic pyelonephritis (*white arrowhead*) in the right kidney. **B:** Follow-up image at the same level following 5 weeks of medical therapy shows significant reduction in size, more clear definition, and development of discrete walls (*arrowheads*) surrounding this cystic, phlegmonous process. Note that the process abuts only the most medial aspect of the ascending colon (*arrow*) at this time.

A,B

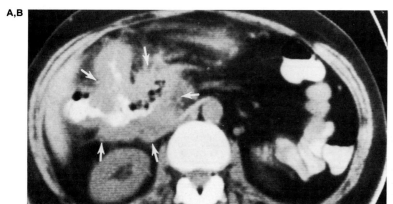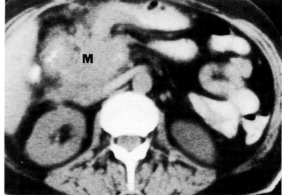

FIG. 39. Colon carcinoma simulating complicated pancreatitis. **A:** An extensive circumferential soft-tissue mass (*arrows*) is present, distorting the hepatic flexure. **B:** Image 1 cm cephalad shows the mass (M) involving the region of the pancreatic head. At presentation, this patient had biochemical evidence of pancreatitis, and the CT examination was interpreted as showing a pancreatic phlegmon involving the colon. After follow-up images showed no improvement, the presence of a malignant neoplasm was suggested. At operation, a large hepatic-flexure carcinoma was present, infiltrating the pancreatic bed.

A

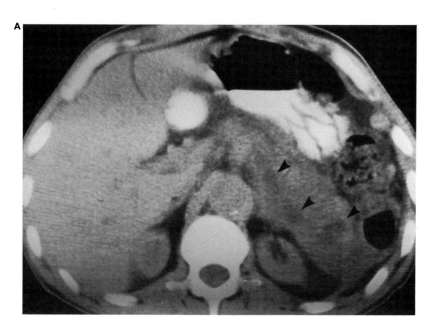

FIG. 40. Acute pancreatitis in a renal transplant patient with a 1-month follow-up study. **A,B** (*facing page*): Noncontrast images at the level of the pancreas show marked enlargement of the body and tail of the pancreas, low-density fluid loculations (*arrowheads*), and extension of the phlegmonous process into the retropancreatic area (*arrows*). Note that the sleeve of fat normally surrounding the superior mesenteric artery (*curved arrow*) is partially obscured. Such a change is infrequently seen in pancreatitis and is more commonly seen in the presence of an invasive carcinoma. Parts **C** and **D** on *facing page*.

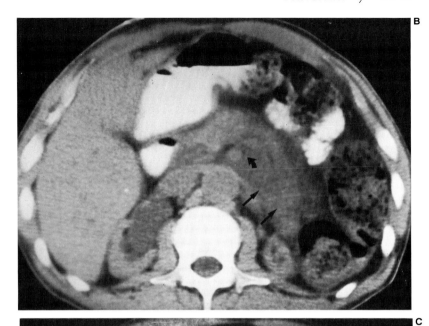

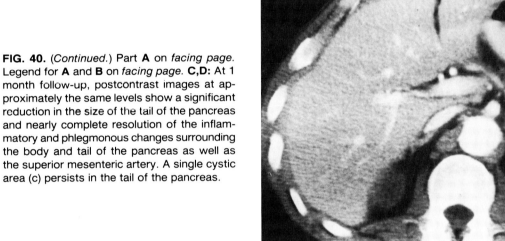

FIG. 40. (*Continued.*) Part **A** on *facing page.* Legend for **A** and **B** on *facing page.* **C,D:** At 1 month follow-up, postcontrast images at approximately the same levels show a significant reduction in the size of the tail of the pancreas and nearly complete resolution of the inflammatory and phlegmonous changes surrounding the body and tail of the pancreas as well as the superior mesenteric artery. A single cystic area (c) persists in the tail of the pancreas.

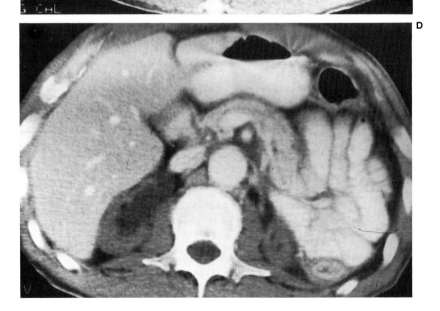

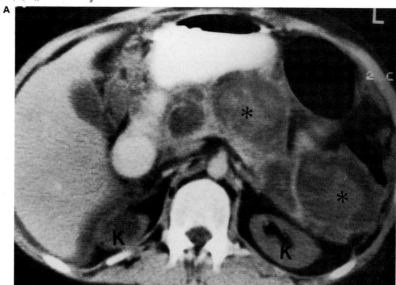

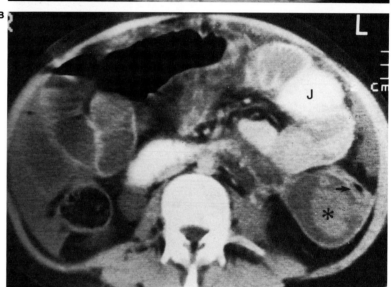

FIG. 41. Hemorrhagic pancreatitis in a renal transplant patient. **A,B:** Large collections of fluid containing high-density, suspended blood clot (asterisk) are noted in the bed of the pancreas and extending laterally in the anterior pararenal space. Note the compressed descending colon (*arrow*) and a dilated proximal jejunal loop (J). The bilaterally atrophic kidneys (K) reflect the end-stage renal disease.

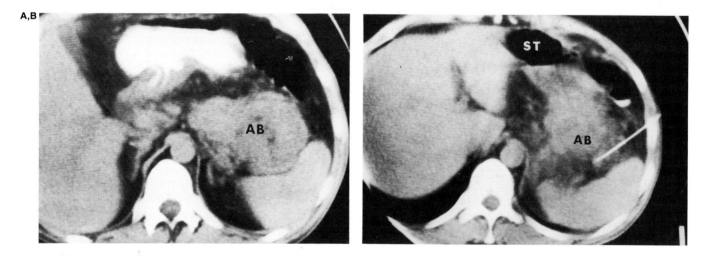

FIG. 42. Pancreatic abscess. **A:** Inhomogeneous mass (AB) occupying the left anterior pararenal space and lesser sac in a febrile patient with acute pancreatitis. **B:** CT-guided thin-needle aspiration revealed pus; (ST) stomach; (AB) abscess.

rhage within the substance of the pancreas or secondary to erosion of an extrapancreatic blood vessel (58) (Fig. 35).

Pseudocysts in the bowel wall have been reported in the duodenum, stomach, and colon. The rarity of intramural pseudocysts suggests that the bowel wall is a relatively strong barrier to proteolytic pancreatic enzymes. However, once the barrier is crossed, expansion of the pseudocysts within the wall is capable of producing obstruction of the bowel lumen, most typically involving the posterolateral wall of the second portion of the duodenum (94). Two CT features distinctive of the intramural location are (a) the extension of the pseudocyst along the wall of the duodenum, resulting in a tubular shape conforming to the course of the duodenum, and (b) abrupt flattening of the otherwise tubular or spherical pseudocyst at the border of the duodenal lumen. Circumferential involvement of the duodenum may occur.

The term "phlegmon" was first applied to pancreatic disease in 1973 (83), and it was defined pathologically as "a solid mass of indurated pancreas and adjacent retroperitoneal tissues due to edema, infiltration by inflammatory cells, and tissue necrosis" (83,151). A phlegmon secondary to pancreatitis is a frequent finding when complicated pancreatitis is evaluated with CT. Its spread in the retroperitoneum is similar to the spread of peripancreatic fluid. Generally, the attenuation value of the phlegmon is greater than that of the low-density fluid and may be heterogeneous because of the inclusion of necrotic tissue, fragmented retroperitoneal fat, and hemorrhage (Figs. 32 and 38). In contrast to the transient character of much of the peripancreatic fluid, phlegmonous changes in the retroperitoneum evolve very slowly and sometimes result in the development of abscess.

Pancreatic Abscess

An occasional sequel to a phlegmon is the development of a pancreatic or peripancreatic abscess (37). In addition to evolving from a phlegmon, a pancreatic abscess can occur where there is secondary infection of pancreatic or extrapancreatic fluid collections. Pancreatic abscess continues to be a lethal complication of acute pancreatitis, with mortality of 40% in large surgical series (2,28).

The extrapancreatic abscesses spread along fascial planes similar to other extrapancreatic collections. The attenuation value of an abscess is quite variable, but generally is higher than those of sterile fluid collections or pseudocysts (100). Gas within such a collection is a strong indicator of abscess formation, but it was present in only one-third to two-thirds of cases in several reported series (39,98,161). Often a pancreatic abscess appears as a poorly defined, inhomogeneous mass or fluid collection displacing adjacent structures. In the appropriate clinical setting, CT-directed or ultrasound-directed percutaneous needle aspiration of the collection is indicated to differentiate between sterile and infected processes (39,62,97,161) (Fig. 42).

Although gas within a collection is highly suggestive of abscess, extraluminal gas can develop secondary to spontaneous or surgical communications of the fluid collection or pseudocyst with the gastrointestinal tract (64,79,97). In rare instances, gas may accumulate within the pancreas or within a region of phlegmon without the presence or subsequent development of an abscess (155). In general, the presence of scattered bubbles of gas throughout the collection almost always indicates an abscess (Fig. 43), whereas a larger collection of gas or a gas–fluid level may be related to bland communication with the lumen of the gut, as well as to a real abscess. Clinical correlation and percutaneous needle aspiration are necessary in this setting.

As greater experience has been gained in the percutaneous management of intraabdominal abscesses, these interventional techniques have been more frequently applied in the management of complicated pancreatitis (50,149). From the standpoint of interventional management, pancreatitis can be classified into four distinct entities: (a) a sterile pancreatic pseudocyst that, when uncomplicated, is initially managed medically, but it may require internal drainage when persistent beyond 6 weeks; (b) an infected pancreatic pseudocyst that requires external drainage, either operative or percutaneous; (c) a sterile pancreatic phlegmon; (d) an infected pancreatic phlegmon (pancreatic abscess) (50). The latter requires operative drainage and debridement of infected necrotic debris, whereas the response of an infected pseudocyst to percutaneous drainage is equivalent to the response of an intraperitoneal abscess of nonpancreatic origin (50). However, success is infrequently achieved in percutaneous drainage of sterile pseudocysts that are still in communication with the pancreatic duct system.

Determination of Prognosis

In acute pancreatitis, frequently it is difficult to predict a patient's outcome based on the initial presentation. Surprising swings in a patient's condition are fairly commonplace. Of the many protocols that have been developed to assess prognosis, one that is widely used is that described by Ranson, which involves assessment of 11 prognostic signs; 5 are determined at the time of admission, and the remaining 6 within the first 48 hr of hospitalization (109). The 5 initial prognostic signs are age greater than 55 years, blood glucose level exceeding 200 mg/dl, leukocyte count exceeding 16,000/mm^3, serum aspartate transaminase level greater than 250 U per liter, and serum lactic dehydrogenase level greater than 350 IU per liter. The 6 signs that have prognostic significance during the first 48 hr are a decrease in hematocrit greater than 10 percentage points, a serum calcium level less than 8 mg/dl, arterial PO$_2$ less than 60 mm Hg, an increase in

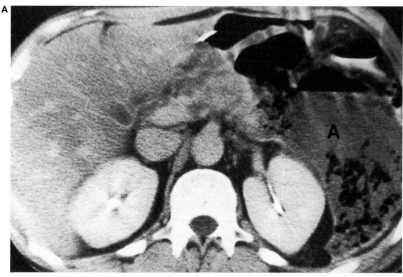

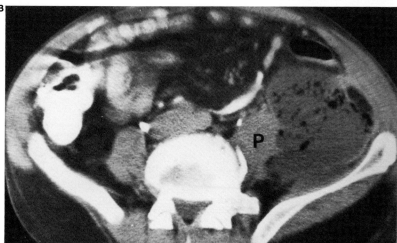

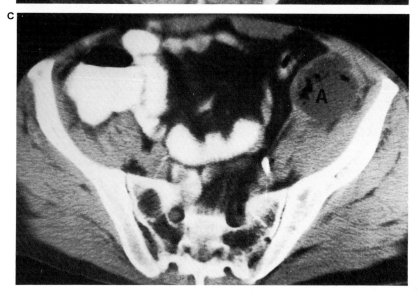

FIG. 43. Abscess complicating pancreatitis. **A:** A high-density fluid collection with numerous bubbles and an air–fluid level grossly distends the anterior pararenal space in this septic patient with complicated necrotizing pancreatitis; (A) abscess. **B:** At the level of the aortic bifurcation, the abscess has tracked inferiorly and is now contiguous with the left psoas muscle (P). **C:** The abscess (A) continues to track inferiorly within or adjacent to the fascial compartment of the iliopsoas muscle group. This abscess spontaneously exited on the anterior aspect of the patient's proximal thigh.

blood urea nitrogen greater than 5 mg/dl, a base deficit greater than 4 mEq/liter, and fluid sequestration greater than 6 liters. Ranson attributed no prognostic significance to the degree of amylase elevation. In Ranson's experience, mortality was approximately 1% among patients with less than three signs, 15% if three or four signs were positive, 40% if five or six signs were positive, and 100% if seven or more signs were positive.

Several recent studies have shown that there is a correlation between the clinical severity of pancreatitis, as defined by Ranson's criteria, and the spectrum of morphologic changes in pancreatitis, as demonstrated by CT (7,9,102,110,124,135,150). In general, for patients with clinically diagnosed acute pancreatitis whose CT images appeared either normal or showed only edematous changes of the pancreas on the initial CT evaluation, their clinical courses were benign, and few, if any, complications developed. In contrast, up to 25% of patients who showed evidence of spread of the disease to one or more extrapancreatic locations, or who were found to have evidence of a pancreatic and peripancreatic phlegmon, developed major complications. Prolonged hospital stays and death as a direct result of complications of pancreatitis were confined to the latter groups. The correlation is not always exact, in that some patients with mild pancreatitis according to Ranson's clinical criteria will nevertheless develop severe complications (9,102,110,135).

An important CT criterion is to determine whether or not pancreatic ischemia or necrosis is present. The systemic hypotension that frequently follows the tremendous outpouring of fluids in pancreatitis may cause stasis within the microcirculation of the pancreas, leading to intensification of the pancreatic inflammation and ultimate ischemia and necrosis. In order to determine if necrosis is present, several investigators have used the relative degree of enhancement of the pancreatic parenchyma following a large intravenous bolus of contrast material as a determinant of the presence of ischemia or necrosis (78,124,125). In one study of 58 patients with alcohol-induced acute pancreatitis, all 36 patients with uncomplicated pancreatitis showed increased or normal contrast enhancement during the first 2 min following an intravenous bolus of contrast material, whereas all those with fulminant pancreatitis (22 patients with hemorrhagic necrotizing pancreatitis proved at laparotomy) showed decreased contrast enhancement of the pancreas (124). The patients with three or more prognostic signs (modified Ranson's criteria) showed lower enhancement values than those with fewer prognostic signs, but the prognostic signs did not correlate as well with the clinical course as did the degree of contrast enhancement.

In a separate retrospective review of 22 patients with surgical documentation of pancreatic and peripancreatic necrosis, the noncontrast CT findings indicating necrosis varied with the developmental stage of the necrotizing process (154). In the acute phase of disease, considerable morphologic overlap existed between necrosis and pancreatic phlegmon. More characteristic findings were seen in the subacute and chronic stages, including diffuse enlargement of the gland, with largely decreased, heterogeneous central density. A thick, smooth surrounding rim produced a characteristic sac-like configuration. Four of these patients were percutaneously aspirated for suspected superinfection, and in 2 patients the aspirate confirmed the presence of superinfecting microorganisms.

Association of Acute Pancreatitis with End-Stage Renal Disease

Various reports in the literature have suggested an association between acute pancreatitis and end-stage renal disease (ESRD), including patients on maintenance dialysis (11,51,115). The association of acute pancreatitis with renal transplantation also has been emphasized (25,40,45,73,106,147) (Figs. 40 and 41). Because the patients are compromised hosts, they have an increased risk of morbidity and mortality from the disease. Furthermore, acute pancreatitis may be underdiagnosed in this category of patients, in whom elevated serum amylase levels are of limited diagnostic value. Abdominal pain in patients with ESRD should signal the possibility of acute pancreatitis and the need for appropriate imaging studies (147).

Association of Acute Pancreatitis with Pancreas Divisum

Although some investigators consider pancreas divisum as nothing more than an anatomic variant of no clinical significance (32), others believe that it has a higher-than-expected association with idiopathic recurrent pancreatitis (26,52). The latter postulate that the association of pancreas divisum with pancreatitis occurs because most of the functioning pancreatic tissue coming from the dorsal pancreas has to discharge its exocrine secretions into the duodenum through the relatively small orifice at the minor papilla.

Chronic Pancreatitis

Chronic pancreatitis may not simply be the end result of repeated attacks of acute pancreatitis. Rather, it is believed by many to be a separate and distinct disease entity. The average age of onset for acute pancreatitis (51 years) is 13 years greater than that for chronic calcifying pancreatitis (38 years) (123). Most cases of true acute pancreatitis, such as recurring bouts of acute pancreatitis secondary to biliary disease, do not result in chronic pancreatitis. There is a strong association of alcohol abuse with chronic pancreatitis. It is postulated that when the first bout of clinical pancreatitis occurs in patients who are alcoholics of 6 years' duration or greater, the pancreas is already diffusely scarred, and the initial bout of alcoholic pancreatitis actually heralds the onset of chronic pancreatitis (108,123).

In support of the concept that acute pancreatitis and chronic pancreatitis are separate diseases, a long-term follow-up of 27 patients who were treated with conservative surgery for necrohemorrhagic pancreatitis showed that almost complete recovery of exocrine function was achieved within 4 years after discharge, whereas about

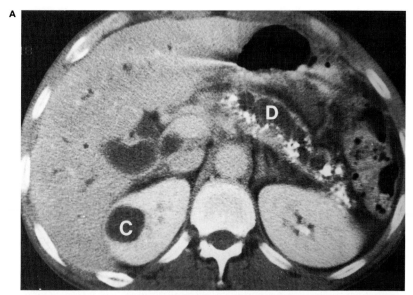

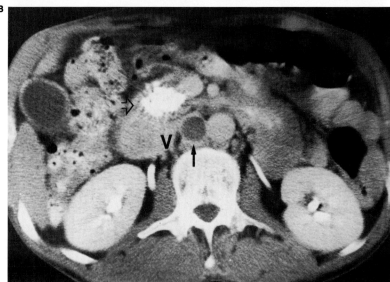

FIG. 44. Chronic pancreatitis and pseudocyst formation. **A:** Marked dilatation of the main pancreatic duct (D) and multiple periductal calculi are present in this patient with a history of chronic pancreatitis. An incidental renal cyst (C) is present. **B:** A 2-cm-diameter pseudocyst (*arrow*) displaces the poorly defined vena cava (V) slightly to the right. Dense calcification is present in the head of the pancreas (*open arrow*), associated with the marked pancreatic duct dilatation.

half of these patients still showed abnormal endocrine function (3). The morphologic sequelae remained relatively unchanged during the follow-up period, and the data appear to exclude an evolution of necrotizing hemorrhagic pancreatitis toward chronic pancreatitis. Laboratory tests showed defective pancreatic secretion in 40% of the patients at the first control, but in only 7% at the second control. Assessment of endocrine function, however, showed an increased incidence of diabetes at the time of the follow-up evaluation, from 11% initially to 47% of subjects after 4 years. The clinical correlation agreed with the laboratory data in that during the 4 years of the follow-up, none of the 27 patients complained of symptoms suspicious for chronic recurrent pancreatitis (3).

In addition to chronic alcoholic pancreatitis, chronic pancreatitis is found with familial occurrence in kindreds with hyperlipidemia, hyperparathyroidism, cystic fibrosis, and cholelithiasis (77). Additionally, there is a distinct group of patients with a familial form of pancreatitis in whom precipitating factors are not identified. This form of familial pancreatitis, termed hereditary pancreatitis, is thought to be inherited as an autosomal dominant, with variable penetrance. The typical clinical features include an early age of onset, with varying degrees of abdominal pain and disability. Complications of endocrine and exocrine pancreatic insufficiency, pseudocyst formation, and adenocarcinoma of the pancreas may develop. The hallmark finding in this form of pancreatitis is the presence of very large calculi within dilated pancreatic ducts, visible on plain radiographs of the abdomen in childhood (77,116).

In an earlier series of patients with chronic pancreatitis, the CT findings were considered entirely normal in approximately 16% of patients, whereas advanced cases showed an atrophic gland, with or without fatty replacement (41). A more recent retrospective analysis of contrast-enhanced, current-generation CT examinations

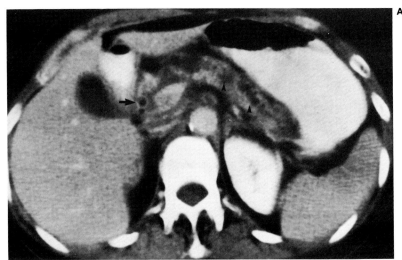

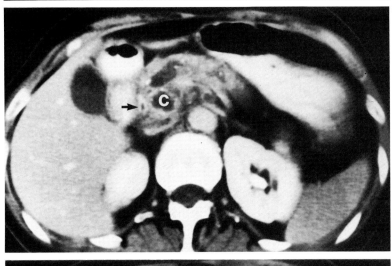

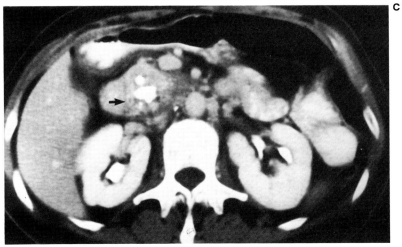

FIG. 45. Chronic pancreatitis. **A:** The main pancreatic duct (*arrowheads*) is irregularly dilated. A normal-caliber common bile duct with slightly enhancing wall (*arrow*) is visible. **B:** Small calculi are present along the course of the main pancreatic duct, and a 1.5-cm pseudocyst (C) is present in the head of the pancreas just medial to the normal-caliber common duct (*arrow*). **C:** At the level of the distal main pancreatic duct, a large intraductal calculus is present, as are several smaller calculi. The unaffected common bile duct (*arrow*) can still be seen immediately proximal to the ampulla.

showed dilatation of the main pancreatic duct (66%), parenchymal atrophy (54%), pancreatic calcifications (50%), pseudocysts (34%), focal pancreatic enlargement (32%), biliary ductal dilatation (29%), and alterations in peripancreatic fat or fascia (16%) (Fig. 44). In only 7% of the patients were no abnormalities detected. Also lacking, compared with earlier descriptions, was generalized pancreatic enlargement (90).

As stated previously, smooth or beaded dilatation of the main pancreatic duct is most commonly associated with carcinoma, whereas irregular dilatation is more frequently seen in chronic pancreatitis. Furthermore, a ratio of duct width to total gland width less than 0.5 favors the diagnosis of chronic pancreatitis (76) (Fig. 45). Chronic pancreatitis occasionally can present as a focal, noncalcified mass that by all CT criteria would be indistinguish-

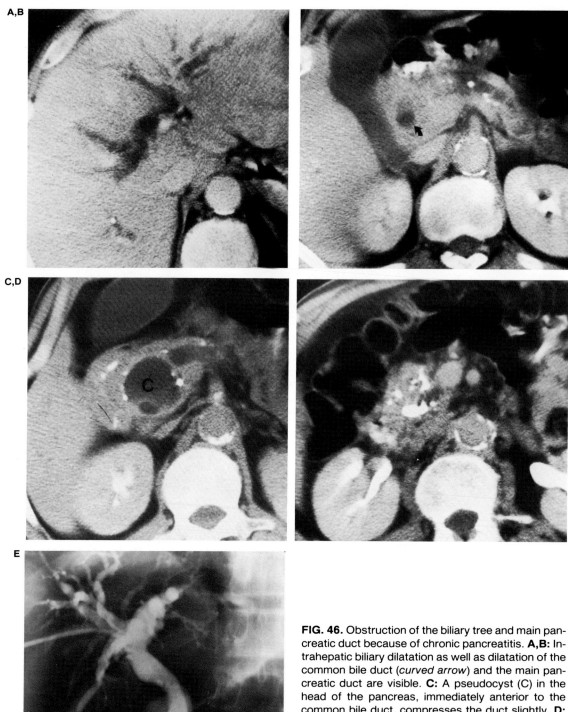

FIG. 46. Obstruction of the biliary tree and main pancreatic duct because of chronic pancreatitis. **A,B:** Intrahepatic biliary dilatation as well as dilatation of the common bile duct (*curved arrow*) and the main pancreatic duct are visible. **C:** A pseudocyst (C) in the head of the pancreas, immediately anterior to the common bile duct, compresses the duct slightly. **D:** However, intraductal pancreatic calculi and fibrotic changes in the head are the primary causes for ductal dilatation. **E:** Cholangiogram via a decompressing catheter with its tip in the duodenal lumen shows the tapered narrowing of the common bile duct secondary to the chronic inflammatory changes in the pancreatic head.

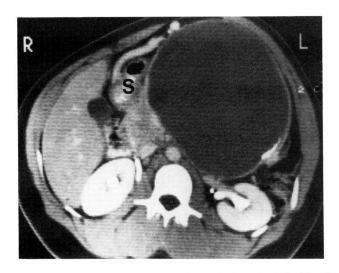

FIG. 47. A huge pancreatic pseudocyst bulges the left side of the anterior abdominal wall, displacing the stomach (S) anteriorly and to the right. Note the low-density, homogeneous nature of the cyst fluid. A section of mural calcification is present on the posterolateral wall of the cyst. Out of the clinical context, this could not be differentiated from a single-chamber macrocystic adenoma.

able from a carcinoma (84,101). Despite appropriate follow-up periods and the performance of transhepatic cholangiography and/or ERCP and percutaneous needle biopsy, many of these cases remain indeterminate, and direct surgical assessment is required.

Chronic pancreatitis can also be associated with obstruction of the biliary tree. In most instances, the lumen of the obstructed common bile duct tapers gradually (Fig. 46), in contrast to an abrupt transition commonly associated with neoplasm. In an analysis of 51 patients with chronic alcoholic pancreatitis and common-duct obstruction, an elevated serum alkaline phosphatase level was the most frequent abnormal laboratory finding (4). The elevation in serum bilirubin level was never progressive; a rising-and-falling pattern was most often encountered. The combination of CT evaluation and cholangiography by either the percutaneous or endoscopic route, correlated with the clinical and laboratory findings, generally will permit differentiation of this type of bile duct obstruction secondary to fibrosis from that due to neoplasm.

Pseudocysts can occur in both acute pancreatitis and chronic pancreatitis (Figs. 47 and 48). When pseudocysts

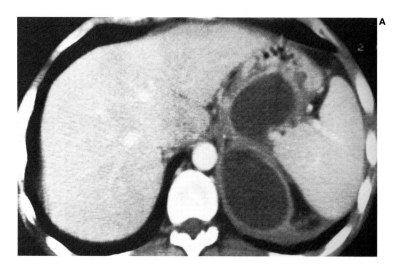

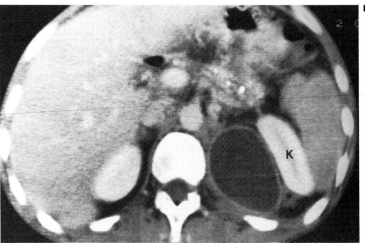

FIG. 48. Pancreatic pseudocyst. **A:** A biloculated pseudocyst displaces the spleen laterally and the stomach anteriorly. The uniform low density of the fluid and the well-defined wall are characteristic of a mature pseudocyst. **B:** The inferior extension of the posterior component of the pseudocyst displaces and compresses the left kidney (K) between itself and the spleen. Flecks of calcification are present within the body of the pancreas, consistent with the patient's known chronic pancreatitis.

are found in association with ductal dilatation and intraductal calcification, chronic pancreatitis is the underlying disease (Fig. 49). Along with hemorrhage and superinfection, as previously discussed, another major complication of pseudocyst formation is spontaneous rupture. Pseudocysts may rupture into the peritoneal cavity (with the development of ascites), into the extraperitoneal spaces, or into the gastrointestinal tract (152). When communication with the lumen of the bowel is established, gas may be seen within the pseudocyst and will not necessarily be an indication of a gas-forming infection (97,98,145).

Pseudocysts can be confused with cystic (Fig. 47) or necrotic tumors, a markedly dilated and tortuous pancreatic duct, or a true or false aneurysm of an intrapancreatic or peripancreatic artery (75). Cystic tumors usually occur in patients without a history of pancreatitis and may show some characteristic CT findings, as described previously. Necrotic tumors generally have thick and irregular walls that rarely, if ever, calcify, compared with the uniform, occasionally calcified walls of pseudocysts. Aneurysms or false aneurysms characteristically will be enhanced following an intravenous bolus of contrast material. Even prior to administration of contrast material, the similarity between the density of the fluid within the false aneurysm and the density of the blood within the aorta or vena cava will be a clue to its nature. Aneurysms

or false aneurysms can also be diagnosed by magnetic resonance imaging (MRI) and pulsed Doppler ultrasound without the use of intravenous contrast agents.

Chronic pancreatitis frequently results in pancreatic insufficiency of both the exocrine and endocrine functions. However, some patients may initially present in a state of pancreatic insufficiency without a clear cause being apparent in the patient's prior medical history. In one retrospective review of patients diagnosed as having pancreatic insufficiency, CT was found to be a key diagnostic tool in understanding the cause of the problem. Previously undiagnosed carcinoma, classic changes of chronic pancreatitis, confirmation of complete surgical removal, and evidence of complete idiopathic atrophy were some of the diagnostic findings described. Because pancreatic insufficiency often is a difficult clinical diagnostic problem, CT should be used if abdominal radiographs or sonograms are nondiagnostic (128).

Pancreatic Changes in Cystic Fibrosis and Associated Diseases

Complete fatty replacement of the pancreatic parenchyma has been shown both by CT and by ultrasound to

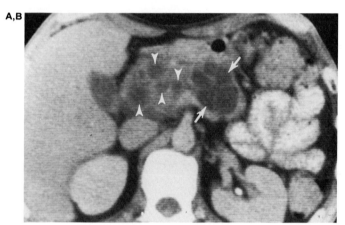
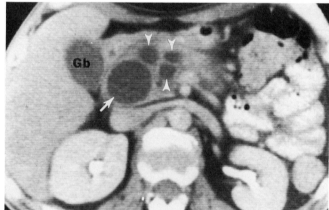
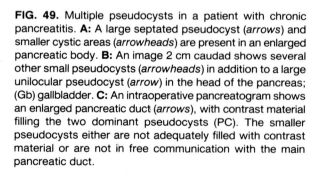
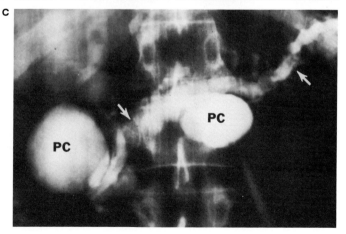

FIG. 49. Multiple pseudocysts in a patient with chronic pancreatitis. **A:** A large septated pseudocyst (*arrows*) and smaller cystic areas (*arrowheads*) are present in an enlarged pancreatic body. **B:** An image 2 cm caudad shows several other small pseudocysts (*arrowheads*) in addition to a large unilocular pseudocyst (*arrow*) in the head of the pancreas; (Gb) gallbladder. **C:** An intraoperative pancreatogram shows an enlarged pancreatic duct (*arrows*), with contrast material filling the two dominant pseudocysts (PC). The smaller pseudocysts either are not adequately filled with contrast material or are not in free communication with the main pancreatic duct.

occur in cystic fibrosis (31,105). A less common manifestation of cystic fibrosis has been complete replacement of the pancreas by multiple macroscopic cysts. This form of pancreatic cystosis is considered an inflammatory process in which complete cystic transformation of the pancreas occurs, possibly related to ductal protein hyperconcentration, inspissation, and ductal ectasia (19,60).

The Schwachman-Diamond syndrome is considered second only to cystic fibrosis as a cause of exocrine pancreatic insufficiency in children. The absence of abnormal sweat electrolytes and the tendency toward improvement distinguishes this disease from cystic fibrosis. On CT examination in this disease, the pancreas commonly is totally replaced by fat. Lipomatosis of the pancreas is the typical pathologic feature of this syndrome (113).

Pancreatic Trauma

Because of its relatively fixed extraperitoneal location just anterior to the spine, the pancreas occasionally is affected in blunt upper abdominal trauma. Either blunt or sharp abdominal trauma may cause pancreatic ductal disruption, with subsequent escape of pancreatic enzymes and the potential for development of the entire spectrum of acute pancreatitis. The appearances of traumatic pancreatitis on CT are the same as with a nontraumatic cause (144).

Complete transection of the pancreas can be diagnosed by CT. The two ends of the transected gland generally are separated by a variable quantity of low-density fluid that will remain relatively confined to the anterior pararenal space in the immediate postinjury period (5) (Fig. 50). Intraoperative injury of the pancreas occasionally will be seen following splenectomy. The diagnosis can be established by CT in the early postoperative period (8).

Postoperative Evaluation

In patients who have had either partial or total pancreatectomy, most often for neoplastic disease, frequently it is difficult to opacify, with oral contrast material, those segments of bowel used for the anastomosis to the biliary tree or remaining segment of pancreas, because of the direction of flow in these Roux-en-Y loops. Administration of glucagon prior to CT imaging facilitates opacification of the afferent jejunal loop with oral contrast material, thus helping to define the structures in the right upper quadrant and to distinguish the unopacified loop of bowel from possible recurrent tumor in the region of the head of the pancreas (59) (Fig. 51). In postoperative patients, the lymph-node-bearing region between the aorta and the SMV and SMA, previously occupied by the un-

cinate process of the pancreas, is an important area to evaluate for tumor recurrence. Because radical pancreatectomy usually leaves this area free of tissue having the attenuation value of either pancreatic tissue or lymph nodes, tumor recurrence will be readily detectable by CT.

Pancreas Transplantation

Pancreas transplantation is performed in only a few medical centers in this country and usually is done in conjunction with a renal transplant. The pancreas transplants usually are anastomosed to either the right or left common iliac vessels, resulting in a soft-tissue mass in the upper pelvis slightly to the right or left of midline. The major value of CT in the assessment of pancreas transplantation is in the identification and management of perigraft abdominal fluid collections in transplant patients with abdominal pain and fever. The fluid represents the exocrine secretion of the transplant. During the initial development of techniques for performing pancreas transplantation, either the pancreas was allowed to drain openly into the peritoneum or else the pancreatic duct was ligated, injected with polymers, or internally drained via a Roux-en-Y pancreaticojejunostomy. A more recent surgical technique has been to anastomose a cuff of accompanying duodenum to the dome of the urinary bladder, allowing drainage of pancreatic secretions into the lumen of the bladder. In such cases, good CT technique, with complete opacification of the bowel lumen, as well as precise knowledge of the surgical technique employed, is necessary for adequate evaluation of these complex cases. CT has not been particularly valuable in determining the presence or absence of transplant rejection (92), but it can be helpful in revealing subtle anastomotic leaks.

Accuracy

The overall accuracy of CT in diagnosing pancreatic diseases has ranged from 83% to 94% (56,88,127,137). The sensitivity of CT in pancreatic carcinoma ranges from 88% to 94%, compared with 56% to 90% in pancreatitis (38,86). Although fewer than 10% of symptomatic patients with pancreatic carcinoma have normal CT findings, a normal-appearing gland occasionally is seen in acute pancreatitis. The likelihood of a normal-appearing gland being present in chronic pancreatitis is considerably less.

In an attempt to eliminate some of the statistical flaws apparent in earlier studies, a prospective cooperative study was performed to assess the relative efficacy of CT and ultrasound in detecting and identifying pancreatic lesions (61). Of the 279 patients, all of whom were studied with both CT and ultrasound, 146 were found to have normal pancreas, and 133 had abnormal pancreas. After excluding the data from the technically suboptimal ultrasound ex-

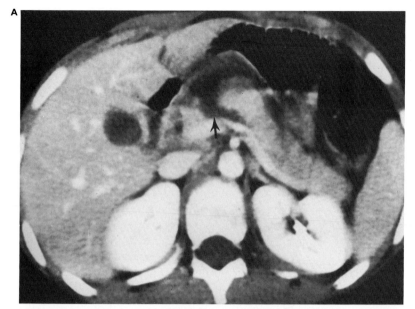

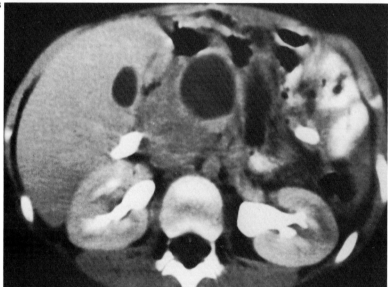

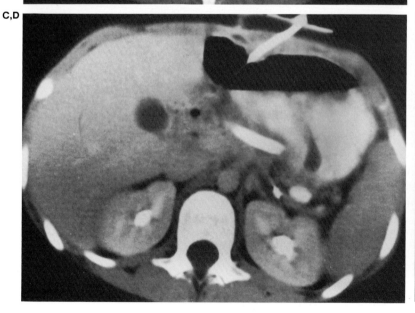

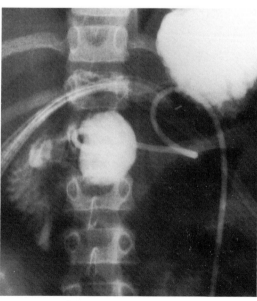

FIG. 50. Posttraumatic transection of the body of the pancreas. This 8-year-old child sustained blunt trauma to the midabdomen and developed peritoneal signs within 24 hr. **A:** A CT image at the level of the junction of the neck and body of the pancreas shows complete transection of the pancreatic parenchyma at this point, with a small accumulation of fluid at the site of transection (*arrow*). **B:** CT study on the 16th postoperative day shows a 4-cm-diameter fluid collection at the site of the resection of the body and tail of the pancreas, despite the presence of drainage catheters in the operative bed. **C:** Following percutaneous transgastric placement of a drainage catheter, complete collapse of the infected fluid collection is achieved. **D:** Transcatheter "abscessogram" shows the position of the cavity on an AP radiograph of the abdomen. Following 2 weeks of drainage, the catheter was removed, without further sequelae. (Courtesy of Dr. Javier Casillas, University of Miami, Miami, Florida.)

A,B

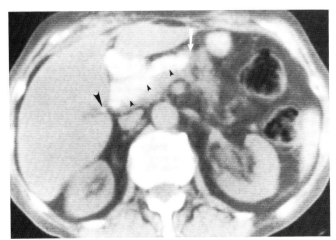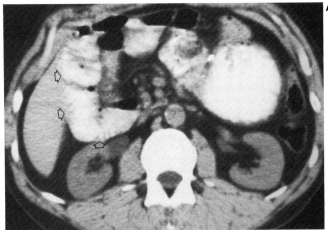

FIG. 51. Normal post-Whipple CT appearance. **A:** Pancreaticojejunal anastomosis (*white arrow*) is seen anterior to the SMA at the level of the splenic vein. Jejunal loop filled with oral contrast material (*small arrowheads*) courses rightward to porta hepatis, where contrast material has refluxed into the common hepatic duct (*large arrowhead*). **B:** CT images from a different patient who was given intravenous glucagon prior to imaging. The afferent jejunal loop (*arrows*) has filled with oral contrast material, probably as a result of paralysis of antegrade peristalsis. (From ref. 59.)

aminations (15.7%), CT had a sensitivity of 0.87 and a specificity of 0.90 in detecting abnormal pancreas, whereas ultrasound had a sensitivity of 0.69 and a specificity of 0.82. In the further differentiation between malignant and inflammatory lesions, CT was shown to have a sensitivity of 0.84, and ultrasound 0.56. Therefore, CT was recommended as the method of choice for detecting a pancreatic lesion, establishing a cause, and evaluating its extent.

MRI

The normal pancreas has been one of the most difficult organs to image by MRI because respiratory motion and bowel peristalsis create image unsharpness in the upper abdomen that limits spatial resolution, even for relatively immobile retroperitoneal structures (133). The lack of optimal oral contrast agents to opacify the gastrointestinal tract also has made it difficult to differentiate pancreas from adjacent small-bowel loops. This is a problem particularly in patients with a paucity of retroperitoneal fat. However, it is now possible to delineate the entire pancreas in a majority of cases using a medium-field-strength imaging system (138,146). Anatomic detail can further be improved by the use of a surface coil (131).

The normal pancreas has a medium signal intensity, similar to that of the liver, on both T1- and T2-weighted sequences (Figs. 52 and 53). If there is fatty replacement of the pancreas, a common degenerative process seen in the elderly, the pancreas has a high signal intensity similar

A,B

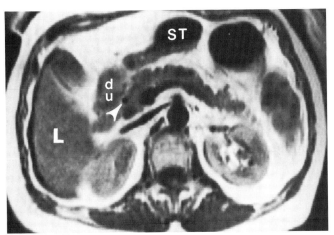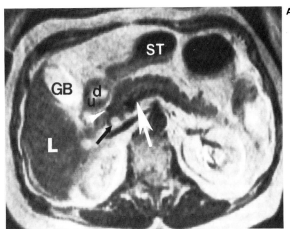

FIG. 52. Normal pancreas: MRI appearance. **A:** Proton-density weighted image (SE, TR = 2,100 msec, TE = 35 msec) shows a normal pancreas with a lobulated contour in this patient with abundant retroperitoneal fat. **B:** A slightly dilated distal common bile duct (*black arrow*) is better seen on this T2-weighted image (SE, TR = 2,100 msec, TE = 90 msec). The pancreas has a signal intensity similar to that of the liver (L); (*arrowhead*) gastroduodenal artery; (*white arrow*) confluence of splenic vein and superior mesenteric vein; (GB) gallbladder; (ST) stomach; (du) duodenum.

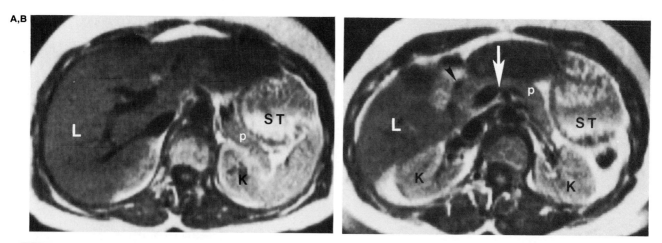

FIG. 53. Normal pancreas: MRI appearance. **A,B:** Proton-density weighted images (SE, TR = 2,100 msec, TE = 35 msec), 1 cm apart, show that the pancreas (p) has a smooth contour in this patient who has relatively sparse retroperitoneal fat; (L) liver; (ST) stomach; (K) kidney; (arrow) junction between splenic vein and superior mesenteric vein; (arrowhead) gastroduodenal artery.

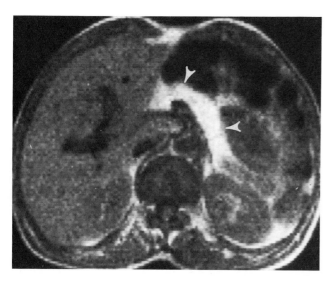

FIG. 54. Fatty replacement of the pancreas in a 75-year-old asymptomatic woman. T1-weighted image (SE, TR = 500 msec, TE = 30 msec) shows that the signal intensity of this entire pancreas (arrowheads) is similar to that of fat.

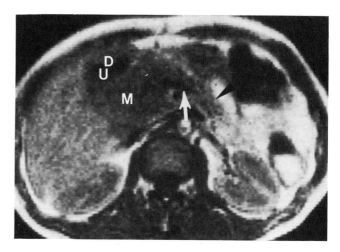

FIG. 55. Pancreatic carcinoma. T1-weighted image (SE, TR = 500 msec, TE = 30 msec) shows an irregular medium-intensity mass in the pancreatic head (M). Note that the pancreatic body (arrowhead) is normal in size; (DU) duodenum; (arrow) splenic vein.

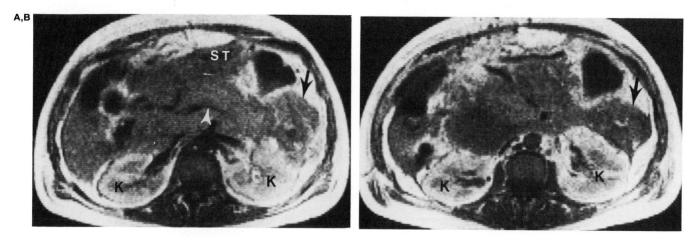

FIG. 56. Acute pancreatitis. **A,B:** Transaxial MR images (SE, TR = 900 msec, TE = 30 msec), 1 cm apart, show a diffusely enlarged pancreas, with inflammatory changes extending into the retropancreatic area as well as into the anterior pararenal space (arrow); (K) kidney; (ST) stomach; (arrowhead) splenic vein.

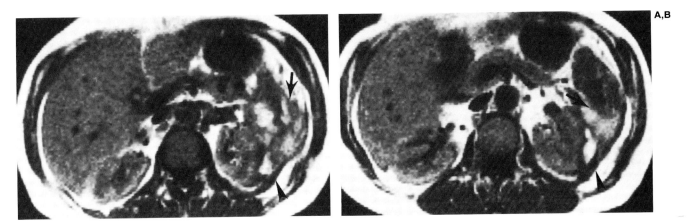

FIG. 57. Hemorrhagic pancreatitis. **A,B:** T1-weighted images (SE, TR = 500 msec, TE = 30 msec), 1 cm apart, show a normal-size pancreas and a large pancreatic effusion (*arrow*) in the left anterior pararenal space. The high intensity of this collection on a T1-weighted sequence is compatible with subacute hemorrhage; (*arrowhead*) thickened posterior renal fascia.

to that of fat (Fig. 54). The contour of the pancreatic parenchyma can be either smooth or lobulated, the latter being more frequently seen in patients with abundant retroperitoneal and peripancreatic fat (Figs. 52 and 53). Because of the "flow-void" phenomenon, major vessels such as the celiac axis, the SMA, the splenic vein, and the SMV can be easily distinguished from the pancreatic parenchyma.

Both neoplastic and inflammatory diseases of the pancreas can be detected by MRI using morphological criteria analogous to those of CT. Whereas pancreatic carcinoma usually presents as a focal, irregular mass (Fig. 55), pancreatitis often affects the entire organ (Fig. 56). Furthermore, hemorrhagic pancreatitis can be differentiated from nonhemorrhagic pancreatitis because subacute hemorrhage has a high signal intensity on a T1-weighted sequence (Fig. 57), whereas nonhemorrhagic pancreatic effusions have a low-to-medium signal intensity. Pancreatic pseudocysts appear as well-defined masses with low-to-

medium signal intensity on T1-weighted images and a high signal intensity on T2-weighted images (Fig. 58). Although most pathologic processes affecting the pancreas (neoplasm, inflammation, transplant rejection) cause prolongation of pancreatic T1 and T2 values, it has not been possible to use either the relaxation times or MR signal intensities to differentiate reliably between normal and diseased pancreatic tissue or to distinguish between neoplasm and inflammation (72,146,148). Furthermore, small calcifications that often are present in patients with chronic pancreatitis are difficult to detect on MRI. At present, MRI offers no distinct advantage over CT in imaging the pancreas (140). However, MRI may be helpful in delineating the pancreas in patients with multiple surgical clips, which often degrade the quality of CT studies (146). Rarely, MRI may be helpful in delineating the cause of an apparent enlargement of the pancreas seen on CT (Fig. 59) or in confirming the presence of a vascular abnormality (Fig. 60).

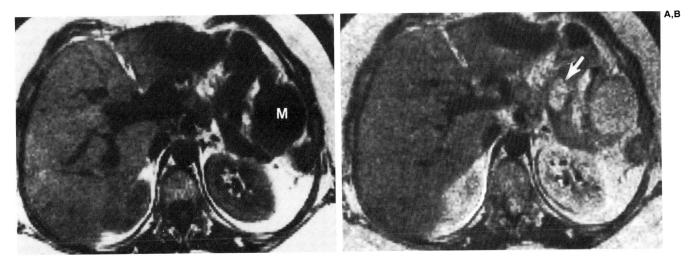

FIG. 58. Pancreatic pseudocyst. **A:** T1-weighted image (SE, TR = 500 msec, TE = 35 msec) shows a round, low-intensity mass (M) near the pancreatic tail. **B:** T2-weighted image (SE, TR = 1,500 msec, TE = 90 msec) at the same level shows an additional smaller pseudocyst (*arrow*) at the junction of pancreatic body and tail.

Clinical Applications

CT is a highly accurate noninvasive method of evaluating pancreatic disease. Its value lies not only in the diagnosis of inflammatory or neoplastic disease but also in the evaluation of the extent of carcinoma or the detection of complications of pancreatitis (162). Because CT can image other upper abdominal structures simultaneously, the detection of unsuspected additional or related abnormalities that may be responsible for clinical symptoms is also possible. For example, CT not only can show changes of acute pancreatitis but also can demonstrate the presence of cholelithiasis, cholecystitis, or choledocholithiasis as associated and possibly etiologic factors (134).

The high sensitivity of CT in detecting carcinoma of the pancreas is in part due to the relatively advanced nature of the disease at clinical presentation. There is little evidence to indicate that the improvement in the time of diagnosis related to CT has had a noticeably favorable influence on the mortality associated with this disease. Nevertheless, there are definable social as well as medical benefits to be derived by a more timely diagnosis. For example, combining CT with percutaneous biopsy and

biliary drainage has, at times, obviated an operation and shortened the hospital stay.

As discussed earlier, indeterminate pancreatic masses remain a problem despite optimal CT imaging. Appropriate use of needle-aspiration biopsy, direct contrast imaging of the biliary and pancreatic duct systems, and, in rare circumstances, selective angiography may be of value in clarifying a diagnostic dilemma.

CT and ultrasound technologies continue to improve, and the relative roles of these imaging methods are still evolving (71). However, there remains a consistent number of patients in whom ultrasound will be technically suboptimal, with part or all of the gland obscured by overlying bowel gas. One study comparing CT and ultrasound in the evaluation of 54 patients suspected of having pseudocysts, a lesion considered especially well suited for evaluation by ultrasound, confirmed CT's superiority (156). This study concluded that CT was more accurate than ultrasound in both diagnosing and demonstrating the extent of pseudocysts of the pancreas.

ERCP is of value in patients with a high clinical suspicion of pancreatic disease when the CT findings are normal, equivocal, or technically unsatisfactory because

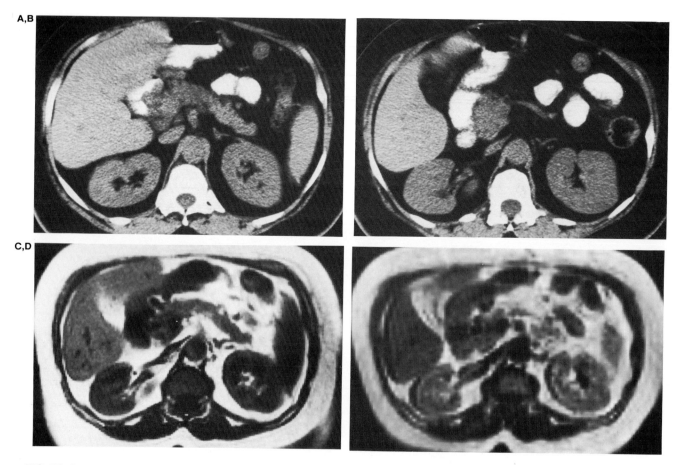

FIG. 59. Peripancreatic venous collaterals simulating pancreatic mass. **A,B:** Noncontrast CT images, 1 cm apart, show enlarged pancreatic head and uncinate process, suspicious for a neoplasm. **C,D:** Corresponding MR images demonstrate multiple collateral vessels surrounding the pancreatic head and uncinate process, accounting for the apparent enlargement on CT. An occluded splenic vein was shown at another level.

A,B

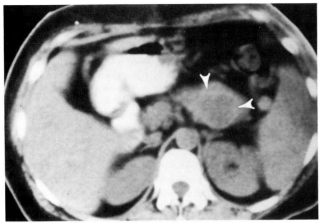
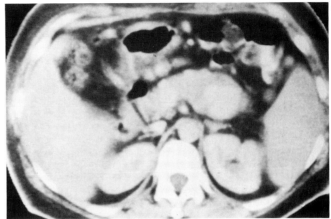

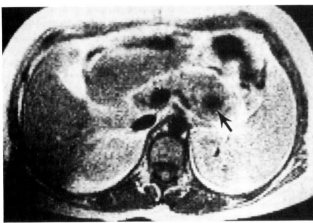

C

FIG. 60. Splenic artery pseudoaneurysm. **A:** Precontrast CT image demonstrates a pancreatic mass with a faintly calcified rim (*arrowheads*). The center of the mass has an attenuation value between those of water and paraspinal muscle. **B:** Post-contrast image shows moderate enhancement of the mass. **C:** MR image (SE, TR = 900 msec, TE = 30 msec) shows a signal void (*arrow*) in the center of the mass, compatible with flowing blood.

of, for example, the presence of multiple surgical clips in the area of interest. Despite ERCP's sensitivity and accuracy for pancreatic carcinoma when used alone, the combined use of ERCP and CT increases the accuracy in carcinoma detection compared with either technique alone. By using ERCP, one can also evaluate the duodenal mucosa, the periampullary region, and biliary tree and obtain pancreatic secretions for cytology (27). However, ERCP is a more invasive technique than CT and is heavily dependent on the technical ability of the endoscopist.

As mentioned earlier, ultrasound- or CT-guided percutaneous thin-needle aspiration of the pancreas, a technique with low morbidity, is of value in nonoperative establishment of a diagnosis of cancer as well as in making the distinction between sterile and infected fluid collections. Percutaneous transhepatic cholangiography is extremely valuable in a patient with an obstructed biliary tree when it is necessary to delineate precisely the abnormal biliary anatomy, especially if biliary enteric bypass surgery is contemplated. It also serves as the initial step in percutaneous biliary decompression.

Selective angiography is infrequently used for evaluation of pancreatic adenocarcinoma or pancreatitis. In instances of massive upper gastrointestinal hemorrhage associated with pancreatitis, angiography not only may be of great diagnostic value but also may play a therapeutic role if embolization or occlusion of the source of hem-

orrhage is indicated. Pseudoaneurysms of pancreatic and peripancreatic blood vessels are recognized complications of severe pancreatitis. Although CT is quite good for the prediction of surgical resectability, angiography occasionally may be indicated to detect previously unsuspected vessel encasement, as well as to provide a vascular road map (69). Angiography remains the primary radiographic method for evaluation of islet cell tumors that are too small to be detected with CT (44,117). Percutaneous transhepatic transportal pancreatic venous sampling also is helpful in the detection of small functioning islet cell tumors or islet cell hyperplasia. However, this technique is not in widespread use (18,34). As stated previously, the role of MRI in imaging the pancreas is limited.

REFERENCES

1. Ahmed A, Chan KF, Song IS. Annular pancreas. *J Comput Assist Tomogr* 1982;6:409–411.
2. Altmeier WA, Alexander JW. Pancreatic abscess: a study of 32 cases. *Arch Surg* 1963;87:80–89.
3. Angelini G, Pederzoli P, Caliari S, et al. Long-term outcome of acute necrohemorrhagic pancreatitis: a 4-year follow-up. *Digestion* 1984;30:131–137.
4. Aranha GV, Prinz RA, Freeark RJ, Greenlee HB. The spectrum of biliary tract obstruction from chronic pancreatitis. *Arch Surg* 1984;119:595–600.
5. Baker LP, Wagner EJ, Brotman S, Whitley NO. Transection of the pancreas. *J Comput Assist Tomogr* 1982;6:411–412.

6. Baker RJ. Acute surgical diseases of the pancreas. *Surg Clin North Am* 1972;52:239–256.
7. Balthazar EJ. Prognostic value of CT in acute pancreatitis: is the early CT examination indicated? (letter). *Radiology* 1987;162:876–878.
8. Balthazar EJ, Megibow A, Rothberg M, Lefleur RS. CT evaluation of pancreatic injury following splenectomy. *Gastrointest Radiol* 1985;10:139–144.
9. Balthazar EJ, Ranson JHC, Naidich DP, Megibow AJ, Caccavale R, Cooper MM. Acute pancreatitis: prognostic value of CT. *Radiology* 1985;156:767–772.
10. Balthazar EJ, Subramanyam BR, Lefleur RS, Barone CM. Solid and papillary epithelial neoplasm of the pancreas: radiographic, CT, sonographic, and angiographic features. *Radiology* 1984;150:39–40.
11. Barcenas CG, Gonzalez-Molina M, Hull AR. Association between acute pancreatitis and malignant hypertension with renal failure. *Arch Intern Med* 1978;138:1254–1256.
12. Baron RL, Stanley RJ, Lee JKT, Koehler RE, Levitt RG. Computed tomographic features of biliary obstruction. *AJR* 1983;140:1173–1178.
13. Berk T, Friedman LS, Goldstein SD, Marks GP, Rosato FE. Relapsing acute pancreatitis as the presenting manifestation of an ampullary neoplasm in a patient with familial polyposis coli. *Am J Gastroenterol* 1985;80:627–629.
14. Berland LL, Lawson TL, Foley WD, Geenen JE, Stewart ET. Computed tomography of the normal and abnormal pancreatic duct: correlation with pancreatic ductography. *Radiology* 1981;141:715–724.
15. Bernardino ME, Barnes PA. Imaging the pancreatic neoplasm. *Cancer* 1982;50:2681–2688.
16. Bok EJ, Cho KJ, Williams DM, Brady TM, Weiss CA, Forrest ME. Venous involvement in islet cell tumors of the pancreas. *AJR* 1984;142:319–322.
17. Breatnach ES, Han SY, Rahatzad MT, Stanley RJ. CT evaluation of glucagonomas. *J Comput Assist Tomogr* 1985;9:25–29.
18. Burcharth F, Stage JG, Stadil F, Jensen LI, Fischermann K. Localization of gastrinomas by transhepatic portal catheterization and gastrin assay. *Gastroenterology* 1979;77:444–450.
19. Churchill RJ, Cunningham DG, Henkin RE, Reynes CJ. Macroscopic cysts of the pancreas in cystic fibrosis demonstrated by multiple radiological modalities. *JAMA* 1981;245:72–74.
20. Clark LR, Jaffe MH, Choyke PL, Grant EG, Zeman RK. Pancreatic imaging. *Radiol Clin North Am* 1985;23:489–501.
21. Cohen DJ, Fagelman D. Pancreas islet cell carcinoma with complete fatty replacement: CT characteristics. *J Comput Assist Tomogr* 1986;10:1050–1051.
22. Compagno J, Oertel JE. Microcystic adenomas of the pancreas (glycogen-rich cystadenomas). *Am J Clin Pathol* 1978;69:289–298.
23. Compagno J, Oertel JE. Mucinous cystic neoplasms of the pancreas with overt and latent malignancy (cystadenocarcinoma and cystadenoma): a clinicopathologic study of 41 cases. *Am J Clin Pathol* 1978;69:573–580.
24. Coral A, Jones SN, Lees WR. Dorsal pancreas presenting as a mass in the chest. *AJR* 1987;149:718–720.
25. Corrodi P, Knoblauch M, Binswanger U, Scholzel E, Largiander F. Pancreatitis after renal transplantation. *Gut* 1975;16:285–289.
26. Cotton PB. Congenital anomaly of pancreas divisum as cause of obstructive pain and pancreatitis. *Gut* 1980;21:105–114.
27. Cotton PB, Lees WR, Vallon AG, Cottone M, Croker JR, Chapman M. Gray-scale ultrasonography and endoscopic pancreatography in pancreatic diagnosis. *Radiology* 1980;134:453–459.
28. Crass RA, Meyer AA, Jeffrey RB, et al. Pancreatic abscess: impact of computerized tomography on early diagnosis and surgery. *Am J Surg* 1985;150:127–131.
29. Creutzfelt W, Schmidt H. Aetiology and pathogenesis of pancreatitis. *Scand J Gastroenterol* 1970;5:47–62.
30. Cubilla AL, Fitzgerald PJ. Cancer of the pancreas (nonendocrine): a suggested morphologic clarification. *Semin Oncol* 1979;6:285–297.
31. Daneman A, Gaskin K, Martin DJ, Cutz E. Pancreatic changes in cystic fibrosis: CT and sonographic appearances. *AJR* 1983;141:653–655.
32. Delhaye M, Engelholm L, Cremer M. Pancreas divisum: Congenital anatomic variant or anomaly? Contribution of endoscopic retrograde dorsal pancreatography. *Gastroenterology* 1985;89:951–958.
33. Donovan PJ, Sanders RC, Siegelman SS. Collections of fluid after pancreatitis: evaluation by computed tomography and ultrasonography. *Radiol Clin North Am* 1982;20:653–665.
34. Doppman JL, Brennan MF, Dunnick NR, Kahn CR, Gorden P. The role of pancreatic venous sampling in the localization of occult insulinomas. *Radiology* 1981;138:557–562.
35. Dunn GD, Gibson RN. The left-sided pancreas. *Radiology* 1986;159:713–714.
36. Eelkema EA, Stephens DH, Ward EM, Sheedy PF II. CT features of nonfunctioning islet cell carcinoma. *AJR* 1984;143:943–948.
37. Evans FC. Pancreatic abscess. *Am J Surg* 1969;117:537–540.
38. Fawcitt RA, Forbes C, Isherwood I. Computed tomography in pancreatic disease. *Br J Radiol* 1978;51:1–4.
39. Federle MP, Jeffrey RB, Crass RA, van Dalsem V. Computed tomography of pancreatic abscesses. *AJR* 1981;136:879–882.
40. Fernandez JA, Rosenberg JC. Post-transplantation pancreatitis. *Surg Gynecol Obstet* 1976;143:795–798.
41. Ferrucci JT, Wittenberg J, Black EB, Kirkpatrick RH, Hall DA. Computed body tomography in chronic pancreatitis. *Radiology* 1979;130:175–182.
42. Fink IJ, Krudy AG, Shawker TH, Norton JA, Gorden P, Doppman JL. Demonstration of an angiographically hypovascular insulinoma with intraarterial dynamic CT. *AJR* 1985;144:555–556.
43. Freeny PC, Ball TJ. Endoscopic retrograde cholangiopancreatography (ERCP) and percutaneous transhepatic cholangiography (PTC) in the evaluation of suspected pancreatic carcinoma: diagnostic limitations and contemporary roles. *Cancer* 1981;47:1666–1678.
44. Freeny PC, Ball TJ, Ryan J. Impact of new diagnostic imaging methods on pancreatic angiography. *AJR* 1979;133:619–624.
45. Freeny PC, Lawson TL. *Radiology of the pancreas.* New York: Springer-Verlag, 1982:170–171.
46. Freeny PC, Marks WM, Ryan JA, Traverso LW. Pancreatic ductal adenocarcinoma: diagnosis and staging with dynamic CT. *Radiology* 1988;166:125–133.
47. Friedman AC, Lichtenstein JE, Dachman AH. Cystic neoplasms of the pancreas: radiological-pathological correlation. *Radiology* 1983;149:45–50.
48. Friedman AC, Lichtenstein JE, Fishman EK, Oertel JE, Dachman AH, Siegelman SS. Solid and papillary epithelial neoplasm of the pancreas. *Radiology* 1985;154:333–337.
49. Geokas MC, Baltaxe HA, Banks PA, Silva J Jr, Frey CF. Davis conference. Acute pancreatitis. *Ann Intern Med* 1985;103:86–100.
50. Gerzof SG, Johnson WC, Robbins AH, Spechler SJ, Nabseth DC. Percutaneous drainage of infected pancreatic pseudocysts. *Arch Surg* 1984;119:888–893.
51. Gilboa N, Largent JA, Urizar RE. Acute pancreatitis in an anephric child maintained on chronic hemodialysis. *Int J Pediatr Nephrol* 1980;1:64–65.
52. Gold RP, Berman H, Fakhry J, Heier S, Rosenthal W, DelGuercio L. Pancreas divisum with pancreatitis and pseudocyst. *AJR* 1984;143:1343–1344.
53. Günther RW, Klose KJ, Rückert K, Beyer J, Kuhn F-P, Klotter H-J. Localization of small islet-cell tumors. Preoperative and intraoperative ultrasound, computed tomography, arteriography, digital subtraction angiography, and pancreatic venous sampling. *Gastrointest Radiol* 1985;10:145–152.
54. Günther RW, Klose KJ, Rückert K, et al. Islet-cell tumors: detection of small lesions with computed tomography and ultrasound. *Radiology* 1983;148:485–488.
55. Gustafson KD, Karnaze GC, Hattery RR, Scheithauer BW. Pseudomyxoma peritonei associated with mucinous adenocarcinoma of the pancreas: CT findings and CT-guided biopsy. *J Comput Assist Tomogr* 1984;8:335–338.
56. Haaga RJ, Alfidi RJ, Havrilla TR, et al. Definitive role of CT scanning of the pancreas. *Radiology* 1977;124:723–730.
57. Harmon JW, Norton JA, Collin MJ, et al. Removal of gastrinomas for control of Zollinger-Ellison syndrome. *Ann Surg* 1984;200:396–404.
58. Hashimoto BE, Laing FC, Jeffrey RB Jr, Federle MP. Hemorrhagic pancreatic fluid collections examined by ultrasound. *Radiology* 1984;150:803–808.
59. Heiken JP, Balfe DM, Picus D, Scharp DW. Radical pancreatectomy: Postoperative evaluation by CT. *Radiology* 1984;153:211–215.

60. Hernanz-Schulman M, Teele RL, Perez-Atayde A, et al. Pancreatic cystosis in cystic fibrosis. *Radiology* 1986;158:629–631.

61. Hessel SJ, Siegelman SS, McNeil BJ, et al. A prospective evaluation of computed tomography and ultrasound of the pancreas. *Radiology* 1982;143:129–133.

62. Hill MC, Dach JL, Barkin J, Isikoff MB, Morse B. The role of percutaneous aspiration in the diagnosis of pancreatic abscess. *AJR* 1983;141:1035–1038.

63. Hosoki T. Dynamic CT of pancreatic tumors. *AJR* 1983;140:959–965.

64. Hughes JJ, Blunck CE. CT demonstration of gastropancreatic fistula due to penetrating gastric ulcer. *J Comput Assist Tomogr* 1987;11:709–711.

65. Inamoto K, Ishikawa Y, Itoh N. CT demonstration of annular pancreas: case report. *Gastrointest Radiol* 1983;8:143–144.

66. Itai Y, Kokubo T, Atomi Y, Kuroda A, Haraguchi Y, Terano A. Mucin-hypersecreting carcinoma of the pancreas. *Radiology* 1987;165:51–55.

67. Itai Y, Moss AA, Ohtomo K. Computed tomography of cystadenoma and cystadenocarcinoma of the pancreas. *Radiology* 1982;145:419–425.

68. Itai Y, Ohhashi K, Nagai H, et al. "Ductectatic" mucinous cystadenoma and cystadenocarcinoma of the pancreas. *Radiology* 1986;161:697–700.

69. Jafri SZH, Aisen AM, Glazer GM, Weiss CA. Comparison of CT and angiography in assessing resectability of pancreatic carcinoma. *AJR* 1984;142:525–529.

70. Jeffrey RB, Federle MP, Laing FC. Computed tomography of mesenteric involvement in fulminant pancreatitis. *Radiology* 1983;147:185–188.

71. Jeffrey RB Jr, Laing FC, Wing VW. Extrapancreatic spread of acute pancreatitis: New observations with real-time US. *Radiology* 1986;159:707–711.

72. Jenkins JPR, Braganza JM, Hickey DS, Isherwood I, Machin M. Quantitative tissue characterisation in pancreatic disease using magnetic resonance imaging. *Br J Radiol* 1987;60:333–341.

73. Johnson WC, Nabseth DC. Pancreatitis in renal transplantation. *Ann Surg* 1970;171:309–314.

74. Kalmar JA, Merritt CRB, Matthews CC. CT demonstration of cystadenocarcinoma of the pancreas with calcified lymphadenopathy. *South Med J* 1983;76:1042–1044.

75. Kaplan JO, Isikoff MB, Barkin J, Livingstone AS. Necrotic carcinoma of the pancreas: "the pseudo-pseudocyst." *J Comput Assist Tomogr* 1980;4:166–167.

76. Karasawa E, Goldberg HI, Moss AA, Federle MP, London SS. CT pancreatogram in carcinoma of the pancreas and chronic pancreatitis. *Radiology* 1983;148:489–493.

77. Kattwinkel J, Lapey A, DiSant'Agnese PA, Edwards WA, Jufty MP. Hereditary pancreatitis: three new kindreds and a critical review of the literature. *Pediatrics* 1973;51:55–69.

78. Kivisaari L, Somer K, Standertskjöld-Nordenstam C-G, Schröder T, Kivilaakso E, Lempinen M. A new method for the diagnosis of acute hemorrhagic-necrotizing pancreatitis using contrast-enhanced CT. *Gastrointest Radiol* 1984;9:27–30.

79. Kolmannskog F, Kolbenstvedt A, Aakhus T. Computed tomography in inflammatory mass lesions following acute pancreatitis. *J Comput Assist Tomogr* 1981;5:169–172.

80. Kolmannskog F, Schrumpf E, Valnes K. Computed tomography and angiography in pancreatic apudomas and cystadenomas. *Acta Radiol Diagn* 1982;23:365–372.

81. Kressel HY. Pancreatitis: through the looking glass (editorial). *Dig Dis Sci* 1984;29:285–286.

82. Krudy AG, Doppman JL, Jensen RT, et al. Localization of islet cell tumors by dynamic CT: comparison with plain CT, arteriography, sonography, and venous sampling. *AJR* 1984;143:585–589.

83. Kune GA, King R. The late complications of acute pancreatitis: pancreatic swelling, cyst and abscess. *Med J Aust* 1973;1:1241–1246.

84. Lammer J, Herlinger H, Zalaudek G, Hofler H. Pseudotumorous pancreatitis. *Gastrointest Radiol* 1985;10:59–67.

85. Lawson TL. Acute pancreatitis and its complications: computed tomography and sonography. *Radiol Clin North Am* 1983;21:495–513.

86. Lee JKT, Stanley RJ, Melson GL, Sagel SS. Pancreatic imaging by ultrasound and computed tomography. *Radiol Clin North Am* 1979;16:105–117.

87. Letourneau JG, Day DL, Crass JR, Goldberg ME, Drake DG. Abdominal case of the day. *AJR* 1987;148:1043–1047.

88. Levitt RG, Stanley RJ, Sagel SS, Lee JKT, Weyman PJ. Computed tomography of the pancreas: 3 second scanning vs 18 second scanning. *J Comput Assist Tomogr* 1982;6:259–267.

89. Louie S, McGahan JP, Frey C, Cross CE. Pancreatic pleuropericardial effusions: fistulous tracts demonstrated by computed tomography. *Arch Intern Med* 1985;145:1231–1234.

90. Luetmer PH, Stephens DH, Ward EM. Chronic pancreatitis: reassessment with current CT (abstract). In *Syllabus of the Society of Gastrointestinal Radiologists,* Seventeenth Annual Meeting and Postgraduate Course, January 16–20, 1988, Nassau, Bahamas, p. 32.

91. Macdonald JS, Gunderson LL, Cohn I Jr. Cancer of the pancreas. In: DeVita VT Jr, Hellman S, Rosenberg SA, eds. *Cancer. Principles and practice of oncology.* Philadelphia: JB Lippincott, 1982:563–589.

92. Maile CW, Crass JR, Frick MP, Feinberg SB, Goldberg ME, Sutherland DER. CT of pancreas transplantation. *Invest Radiol* 1985;20:609–612.

93. McCarthy S, Pellegrini CA, Moss AA, Way LW. Pleuropancreatic fistula: endoscopic retrograde cholangiopancreatography and computed tomography. *AJR* 1984;142:1151–1154.

94. McCowin MJ, Federle MP. Computed tomography of pancreatic pseudocysts of the duodenum. *AJR* 1985;145:1003–1007.

95. Mechanism of pancreatic auto digestion (editorial). *N Engl J Med* 1970;283:487–488.

96. Megibow AJ, Bosniak MA, Ambos MA, Beranbaum ER. Thickening of the celiac axis and/or superior mesenteric artery: a sign of pancreatic carcinoma on computed tomography. *Radiology* 1981;141:449–453.

97. Mendez G Jr, Isikoff MB. Significance of intrapancreatic gas demonstrated by CT: a review of nine cases. *AJR* 1979;132:59–62.

98. Mendez G, Isikoff MB, Hill MC. CT of acute pancreatitis: interim assessment. *AJR* 1980;135:463–469.

99. Moossa AR. Pancreatic cancer: approach to diagnosis, selection for surgery and choice of operation. *Cancer* 1982;50:2689–2698.

100. Moss AA, Kressel HY. Computed tomography of the pancreas. *Dig Dis* 1977;22:1018–1027.

101. Neff CC, Simeone JF, Wittenberg J, Mueller PR, Ferrucci JT Jr. Inflammatory pancreatic masses: problems in differentiating focal pancreatitis from carcinoma. *Radiology* 1984;150:35–38.

102. Nordestgaard AG, Wilson SE, Williams RA. Early computerized tomography as a predictor of outcome in acute pancreatitis. *Am J Surg* 1986;152:127–132.

103. Ormson MJ, Charboneau JW, Stephens DH. Sonography in patients with a possible pancreatic mass shown on CT. *AJR* 1987;148:551–555.

104. Pandolfo I, Scribano E, Gaeta M, Fiumara F, Longo M. Cystic lymphangioma of the pancreas: CT demonstration. *J Comput Assist Tomogr* 1985;9:209–213.

105. Patel S, Bellon EM, Haaga J. Fat replacement of the exocrine pancreas. *AJR* 1980;135:843–845.

106. Penn I, Durst AL, Machado, M, et al. Acute pancreatitis and hyperamylasemia in renal homograft recipients. *Arch Surg* 1972;105:167–172.

107. Price J, Cockram CS, McGuire LJ, Crofts TJ, Stewart IET, Metreweli C. Uptake of ^{99m}Tc-methylene diphosphonate by pancreatic insulinoma. *AJR* 1987;149:69–70.

108. Ranson JHC. Acute pancreatitis—where are we? *Surg Clin North Am* 1981;61:55–70.

109. Ranson JHC. Etiological and prognostic factors in human acute pancreatitis: a review. *Am J Gastroenterol* 1982;77:633–638.

110. Ranson JHC, Balthazar E, Caccavale R, Cooper M. Computed tomography and the prediction of pancreatic abscess in acute pancreatitis. *Ann Surg* 1985;201:656–665.

111. Raptopoulos V, Kleinman PK, Marks S Jr, Snyder M, Silverman PM. Renal fascial pathway: posterior extension of pancreatic effusions within the anterior pararenal space. *Radiology* 1986;158:367–374.

112. Reiman TH, Balfe DM, Weyman PJ. Suprapancreatic biliary obstruction: CT evaluation. *Radiology* 1987;163:49–56.

113. Robberecht E, Nachtegaele P, Van Rattinghe R, Afschrift M, Kunnen M, Verhaaren R. Pancreatic lipomatosis in the Shwachman Diamond syndrome: identification by sonography and CT-scan. *Pediatr Radiol* 1985;15:348–349.

114. Roberts L Jr, Dunnick NR, Foster WL Jr, et al. Somatostatinoma of the endocrine pancreas: CT findings. *J Comput Assist Tomogr* 1984;8:1015–1018.

115. Robinson DO, Alp MH, Grant AK, Lawrence JR. Pancreatitis and renal disease. *Scand J Gastroenterol* 1977;12:17–20.

116. Rohrmann CA, Surawicz CM, Hutchinson D, Silverstein FE, White TT, Marchioro TL. The diagnosis of hereditary pancreatitis by pancreatography. *Gastrointest Endosc* 1981;27:168–173.

117. Rosch J, Keller FS. Pancreatic arteriography, transhepatic pancreatic venography, and pancreatic venous sampling in diagnosis of pancreatic cancer. *Cancer* 1981;47:1679–1684.

118. Rossi P, Baert A, Passariello R, Simonetti G, Pavone P, Tempesta P. CT of functioning tumors of the pancreas. *AJR* 1985;144:57–60.

119. Rubin E, Dunham WK, Stanley RJ. Pancreatic metastases in bone sarcomas: CT demonstration. *J Comput Assist Tomogr* 1985;9:886–888.

120. Rumancik WM, Megibow AJ, Bosniak MA, Hilton S. Metastatic disease to the pancreas: evaluation by computed tomography. *J Comput Assist Tomogr* 1984;8:829–834.

121. Rustin RB, Broughan TA, Hermann RE, Grundfest-Broniatowski SF, Petras RE, Hart WR. Papillary cystic epithelial neoplasms of the pancreas: a clinical study of four cases. *Arch Surg* 1986;121:1073–1076.

122. Sakahara H, Endo K, Nakajima K, et al. Serum CA 19-9 concentrations and computed tomography findings in patients with pancreatic carcinoma. *Cancer* 1986;57:1324–1326.

123. Sarles H. Chronic calcifying pancreatitis—chronic alcoholic pancreatitis. *Gastroenterology* 1974;66:604–616.

124. Schröder T, Kivisaari L, Somer K, Standertskjöld-Nordenstam C-G, Kivilaakso E, Lempinen M. Significance of extrapancreatic findings in computed tomography (CT) of acute pancreatitis. *Eur J Radiol* 1985;5:273–275.

125. Schröder T, Kivisaari L, Standertskjöld-Nordenstam C-G, Somer K, Kivilaakso E, Lempinen M. The clinical significance of contrast enhanced computed tomography in acute pancreatitis. *Ann Chir Gynaecol* 1984;73:268–272.

126. Shah KK, DeRidder PH, Schwab RE, Alexander TJ. CT diagnosis of dorsal pancreas agenesis. *J Comput Assist Tomogr* 1987;11:170–171.

127. Sheedy PF, Stephens DH, Hattery RR, MacCarty RL, Williamson B. Computed tomography of the pancreas. *Radiol Clin North Am* 1977;15:349.

128. Shuman WP, Carter SJ, Montana MA, Mack LA, Moss AA. Pancreatic insufficiency: role of CT evaluation. *Radiology* 1986;158:625–627.

129. Siegelman SS, Copeland BE, Saba GP, Cameron JL, Sanders RC, Zerhouni EA. CT of fluid collections associated with pancreatitis. *AJR* 1980;134:1121–1132.

130. Silverstein W, Isikoff MB, Hill MC, Barkin J. Diagnostic imaging of acute pancreatitis: prospective study using CT and sonography. *AJR* 1981;137:497–502.

131. Simeone JF, Edelman RR, Stark DD, et al. Surface coil MR imaging of abdominal viscera. Part III: The pancreas. *Radiology* 1985;157:437–441.

132. Smith E, Matzen P. Mucus-producing tumors with mucinous biliary obstruction causing jaundice: diagnosed and treated endoscopically. *Am J Gastroenterol* 1985;80:287–289.

133. Smith FW, Reid A, Hutchison JMS, Mallard JR. Nuclear magnetic resonance imaging of the pancreas. *Radiology* 1982;142:677–680.

134. Somer K, Kivisaari L, Standertskjöld-Nordenstam C-G, Kalima TV. Contrast-enhanced computed tomography of the gallbladder in acute pancreatitis. *Gastrointest Radiol* 1984;9:31–34.

135. Sostre CF, Flournoy JG, Bova JG, Goldstein HM, Schenker S. Pancreatic phlegmon. Clinical features and course. *Dig Dis Sci* 1985;30:918–927.

136. Spechler SJ, Dalton JW, Robbins AH, et al. Prevalence of normal serum amylase levels in patients with acute alcoholic pancreatitis. *Dig Dis Sci* 1983;28:865–869.

137. Stanley RJ, Sagel SS, Levitt RG. Computed tomographic evaluation of the pancreas. *Radiology* 1977;124:715–722.

138. Stark DD, Moss AA, Goldberg HI, Davis PL, Federle MP. Magnetic resonance and CT of the normal and diseased pancreas: a comparative study. *Radiology* 1984;150:153–162.

139. Stark DD, Moss AA, Goldberg HI, Deveney CW. CT of pancreatic islet cell tumors. *Radiology* 1984;150:491–494.

140. Stark DD, Moss AA, Goldberg HI, Deveney CW, Way L. Computed tomography and nuclear magnetic resonance imaging of pancreatic islet cell tumors. *Surgery* 1983;94:1024–1027.

141. Strax R, Toombs BD, Rauschkolb EN. Correlation of barium enema and CT in acute pancreatitis. *AJR* 1981;136:1219–1220.

142. Teefey SA, Stephens DH, Sheedy PF II. CT appearance of primary pancreatic lymphoma. *Gastrointest Radiol* 1986;11:41–43.

143. Thompson NW, Eckhauser FE, Vinik AI, Lloyd RV, Fiddian-Green RG, Strodel WE. Cystic neuroendocrine neoplasms of the pancreas and liver. *Ann Surg* 1984;199:158–164.

144. Toombs BD, Lester RG, Ben-Menachem Y, Sandler CM. Computed tomography in blunt trauma. *Radiol Clin North Am* 1981;19:17–35.

145. Torres WE, Clements JL, Sones PJ, Knopf DR. Gas in the pancreatic bed without abscess. *AJR* 1981;137:1131–1133.

146. Tscholakoff D, Hricak H, Thoeni R, Winkler ML, Margulis AR. MR imaging in the diagnosis of pancreatic disease. *AJR* 1987;148:703–709.

147. Van Dyke JA, Rutsky EA, Stanley RJ. Acute pancreatitis associated with end-stage renal disease. *Radiology* 1986;160:403–405.

148. Vahey TN, Glazer GM, Francis IR, et al. MR diagnosis of pancreatic transplant rejection. *AJR* 1988;150:557–560.

149. van Sonnenberg E, Wittich GR, Casola G, et al. Complicated pancreatic inflammatory disease: diagnostic and therapeutic role of interventional radiology. *Radiology* 1985;155:335–340.

150. Vernacchia FS, Jeffrey RB Jr, Federle MP, et al. Pancreatic abscess: predictive value of early abdominal CT. *Radiology* 1987;162:435–438.

151. Warshaw AL. Inflammatory masses following acute pancreatitis: phlegmon, pseudocyst, and abscess. *Surg Clin North Am* 1974;54:621–636.

152. Weiner SN, Das K, Gold M, Stollman Y, Bernstein RG. Demonstration of an internal pancreatic fistula by computed tomography. *Gastrointest Radiol* 1984;9:123–125.

153. Weyman PJ, Stanley RJ, Levitt RG. Computed tomography in evaluation of the pancreas. *Semin Roentgenol* 1981;16:301–311.

154. White EM, Wittenberg J, Mueller PR, et al. Pancreatic necrosis: CT manifestations. *Radiology* 1986;158:343–346.

155. White M, Simeone JF, Wittenberg J. Air within a pancreatic inflammatory mass: not necessarily a sign of abscess. *J Clin Gastroenterol* 1983;5:173–175.

156. Williford ME, Foster WL Jr, Halvorsen RA, Thompson WM. Pancreatic pseudocyst: comparative evaluation by sonography and computed tomography. *AJR* 1983;140:53–57.

157. Wise RH Jr, Stanley RJ. Carcinoma of the ampulla of Vater presenting as acute pancreatitis. *J Comput Assist Tomogr* 1984;8:158–161.

158. Wittenberg J, Simeone JF, Ferrucci JT Jr, Mueller PR, van Sonnenberg E, Neff CC. Non-focal enlargement in pancreatic carcinoma. *Radiology* 1982;144:131–135.

159. Wolf EL, Sprayregen S, Frager D, Rifkin H, Gliedman ML. Calcification in an insulinoma of the pancreas. *Am J Gastroenterol* 1984;79:559–561.

160. Wolfman NT, Karstaedt N, Kawamoto EH. Pleomorphic carcinoma of the pancreas: computed-tomographic, sonographic, and pathologic findings. *Radiology* 1985;154:329–332.

161. Woodard S, Kelvin FM, Rice RP, Thompson WM. Pancreatic abscess: importance of conventional radiology. *AJR* 1981;136:871–878.

162. Yankaskas BC, Staab EV, Rudnick SA, Fletcher RH. The radiologic diagnosis of pancreatic cancer: the effect of new imaging techniques. *Invest Radiol* 1985;20:73–78.

163. Zeman RK, McVay L, Silverman PM, et al. Thin section CT of pancreas divisum (abstract). In *Syllabus of the Society of Gastrointestinal Radiologists,* Seventeenth Annual Meeting and Postgraduate Course, January 16–20, 1988, Nassau, Bahamas, p. 31.

164. Zeman RK, Schiebler M, Clark LR, et al. The clinical and imaging spectrum of pancreaticoduodenal lymph node enlargement. *AJR* 1985;144:1223–1227.

165. Zirinsky K, Abiri M, Baer JW. Computed tomography demonstration of pancreatic microcystic adenoma. *Am J Gastroenterol* 1984;79:139–142.

CHAPTER 15

Liver and Biliary Tract

Lincoln Berland, Joseph K. T. Lee, and Robert J. Stanley

In the past 15 years the radiologic diagnosis of liver disease has evolved remarkably. Whereas at one time diagnosticians were limited to using a few invasive methods, there is now an abundance of imaging techniques. These new techniques combine ease of performance with much greater accuracy in a wide spectrum of clinical circumstances, and the technology continues to evolve, particularly in ultrasound and magnetic-resonance imaging (MRI).

The lack of controlled trials comparing state-of-the-art imaging methods and techniques makes the choice of imaging studies difficult. This chapter will highlight the use of computed tomography (CT) and MRI in diagnosing focal and diffuse liver disease and biliary tract abnormalities. We shall also provide general guidelines to aid in appropriately selecting imaging tests.

TECHNIQUE

Noncontrast CT

Although noncontrast imaging of the liver is still performed in some centers as an adjunct to a contrast-enhanced study, most have eliminated the noncontrast part of the examination when possible, unless there is a specific indication, such as in patients suspected of having metastases from vascular tumors that may become isodense on contrast studies. The noncontrast study is also done in patients who cannot safely receive iodinated contrast material intravenously. The accuracy of this method is good, but less than that for other techniques described in more detail later.

Contrast-Enhanced CT

Dynamic incremental CT is the preferred *routine* technique for examining the liver when searching for lesions (20). With this technique, a large amount of contrast material (about 150–180 ml of 60% contrast material for an average-size patient) is injected intravenously either by hand or by an automatic power injector. Contrast material must be injected rapidly enough (in 2 min or less) to achieve satisfactory vascular and tissue enhancement. Images are obtained at a rate of approximately 4 to 10 per minute after beginning the injection so as to allow the contrast material to circulate into the portal venous system. If properly performed, dynamic incremental CT can detect virtually all lesions greater than 2 cm and a smaller percentage of lesions less than 2 cm (93,107) (Fig. 1). This technique also provides valuable information regarding the enhancement patterns of lesions and of extrahepatic abnormalities (6,88).

Routine imaging during a slow infusion of contrast material is the worst of all methods to examine the liver. The slow infusion only mildly enhances the liver image and permits lesions to take up enough contrast material to become isodense and obscured. This technique is inferior even to noncontrast imaging in sensitivity, and it exposes the patient to the risk of intravenous contrast material while actually decreasing the value of the examination.

Delayed CT

If findings on a dynamic contrast-enhanced CT study are equivocal or negative (when strong clinical suspicion exists), delayed images about 4 hr after the contrast injection may be helpful (28). Small lesions may be missed on dynamic images because they take up contrast material during the dynamic injection and therefore become isodense with the liver (Fig. 2). The rationale for delayed CT is based on the fact that normal hepatocytes excrete 1% to 2% of the iodine load into the biliary system, whereas focal hepatic lesions do not. The peak of hepatocellular excretion of contrast material occurs approximately 4 hr

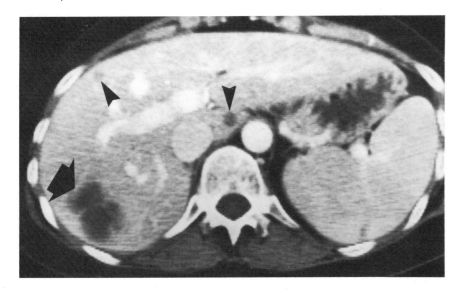

FIG. 1. Dynamic incremental CT. In addition to the large metastases in the posterior right lobe (*arrow*), CT shows two smaller lesions (*arrowheads*) in the anterior right lobe and in the caudate lobe. In this patient, CT findings precluded the possibility of partial hepatic resection.

after injection, during which time normal liver is densely enhanced, whereas focal lesions appear as hypodense areas. This technique has been shown to be slightly more sensitive for detecting liver lesions than is dynamic imaging, but should not be considered a substitute for dynamic imaging (28).

CT Angiography

Although it is a more complex and invasive procedure than those described earlier, CT angiography has been shown to be the most sensitive CT technique for detecting focal liver lesions. The method involves placement of an arterial catheter in either the hepatic or superior mesenteric artery and infusion of contrast material during dynamic imaging (90,92,197). Hepatic arterial injections often produce dense enhancement of the lesions themselves, because most hepatic tumors are supplied by the hepatic artery. Injection via the superior mesenteric artery produces dense enhancement of the portal venous blood, and thus the arterially supplied lesions stand out as negative defects. We prefer injection into the superior mesenteric artery, rather than the hepatic artery, because the latter route causes more streaky artifacts in the liver.

Up to 100 ml of 60% contrast material may be injected at a rate of 0.5 to 2 ml/sec, with a delay of 20 to 30 sec between the beginning of the injection and the beginning of imaging. This technique is reserved for those patients who have been identified as having neoplastic lesions limited to one lobe and are being considered for partial hepatic resection, and it often detects additional lesions as small as a few millimeters (Fig. 3).

FIG. 2. Delayed CT 4 hr after intravenous administration of contrast material. The increased liver density is caused by excretion of contrast material by hepatocytes. Note the normal splenic density in comparison. A liver metastasis in the right lobe is easily identified as a low-attenuation defect because the contrast material that caused it to be enhanced during dynamic imaging has already completely diffused out of the vascular system.

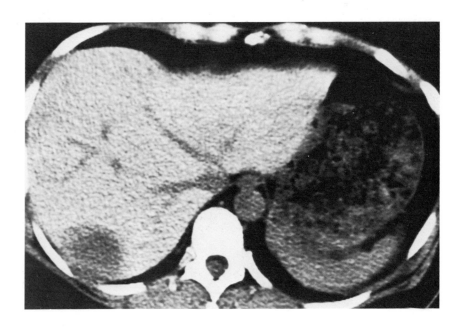

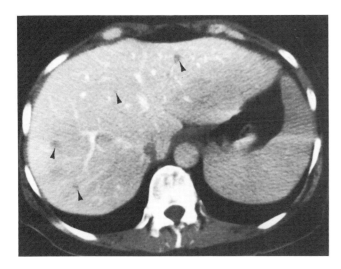

FIG. 3. CT angiogram performed with the catheter placed in the superior mesenteric artery. Multiple hypodense lesions (*arrowheads*) are seen in both lobes of the liver in this patient with metastatic leiomyosarcoma. The smallest lesion detected measured 2 mm in size. Note dense opacification of portal vein branches with this technique.

MRI

The liver usually is imaged at 1-cm intervals with a 1-cm slice thickness, without respiratory or cardiac gating. Transverse views are obtained in all cases; direct coronal and sagittal images are obtained in selected cases to define the relationships between hepatic masses and the diaphragm and to evaluate lesions involving the inferior vena cava or right atrium. Although infinite numbers of pulse sequences are available for hepatic imaging, spin-echo (SE) techniques with a short TR (<500 msec) and short TE (<20 msec) or a long TR (>1,500 msec) and long TE (>80 msec) are the most commonly used sequences. The short-TR, short-TE sequence is T1-weighted; it provides excellent anatomic detail and is less affected by motion artifact (Fig. 4A). The long-TR, long-TE sequence provides T2 weighting and is useful for differentiating cysts and cavernous hemangiomas from benign and malignant neoplasms (101,203,256). However, T2-weighted images generally are more "noisy" and more susceptible to motion artifacts (Fig. 4B). Both T1- and T2-weighted sequences are needed for lesion identification and tissue characterization.

Because the conventional SE technique is insensitive for detecting fatty infiltration of the liver, we have used a proton spectroscopic imaging method to evaluate patients suspected of having focal or diffuse fatty liver. This technique is a simple modification of the conventional SE technique and is based on the difference in precessional frequency between water protons and fat protons. The details of this technique are described in Chapter 4.

An inversion-recovery (IR) technique with either an intermediate (TI = 400 msec) or short (TI = 100 msec) inversion time is also useful for detecting hepatic lesions (45,115,117,189). The use of a short TI results in suppression of the subcutaneous fat signal and reduces motion artifacts. However, the IR technique has a poorer signal-to-noise ratio than the SE technique and has not been widely used.

Techniques that use a very short TR (15–50 msec) and a reduced flip angle (<90°) have been developed. Variously called FLASH, GRASS, SRPS, and other names,

A,B

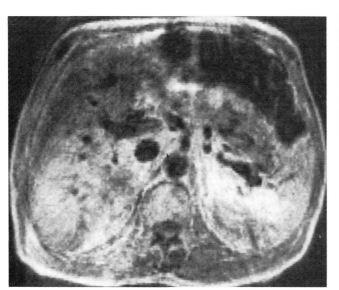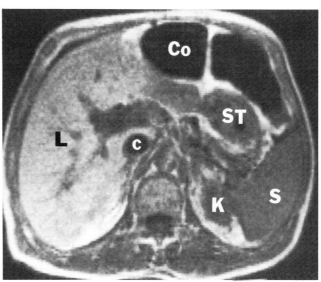

FIG. 4. Normal liver: effect of short-TR/TE sequence. **A:** Transverse MR image (TR = 3,000 msec, TE = 35 msec). The image is blurred because of respiratory motion. The liver and other intraabdominal organs appear inhomogeneous. **B:** Repeat image in the same patient with TR = 300 msec and TE = 15 msec shows marked improvement in image quality. The liver (L) and spleen (S) appear homogeneous. The colon (Co) and stomach (ST) are also clearly delineated; (c) inferior vena cava; (K) kidney.

these allow imaging of a single section in as little time as 2 sec (71). Artifacts related to respiratory motion can be eliminated, and the entire liver can be examined in just a few minutes. However, this method is more susceptible to magnetic-field inhomogeneity and ferromagnetic artifacts than is the conventional SE technique. Clinical studies are underway to assess the full potential of this method for hepatic imaging.

NORMAL ANATOMY

Gross Morphology

The liver is the largest organ in the abdomen, and it has considerable individual variations in size and shape (206,229,239,287). The right lobe usually is larger than the left, which may be quite small. The caudal extent of the right hepatic lobe usually is anterior, being indented posteriorly by the contents of the right renal fossa. Riedel's lobe, generally found in women, is an infrequently encountered caudal bulbous extension of the right lobe. In this variation, the right lobe tapers normally moving inferiorly, but then shows a bulbous widening on more caudad images.

The left lobe is particularly inconsistent in size, shape, and location. It may remain entirely on the right of the abdomen or may extend across the midline to varying degrees, even as far as the left lateral wall of the upper abdomen. The most lateral portion of the left lobe may even wrap around and be contiguous with the spleen. Knowledge of this variation may be important, because pathological processes arising in this portion of the left lobe may be mistaken for diseases originating within the spleen or stomach.

Although the liver normally is adjacent to the inner portion of the anterior abdominal wall, in some cases portions of the colon may be interposed between the liver and abdominal wall. A variation that may be confusing is indentation of the liver by leaves of the diaphragm as they insert on the ribs. These indentations are more prominent on images obtained during suspended inspiration and may be so prominent as to be misinterpreted as intrahepatic lesions (see Fig. 112, Chapter 7).

The liver is directly adherent to the diaphragm posteriorly in a cephalad and medial location. Because of the absence of a potential peritoneal space at this "bare area of the liver," fluid found posterior to the liver at this location must be either beneath the liver capsule or, more likely, within the pleural space (229).

Density measurements of the liver vary because of patient-to-patient differences and technical inaccuracies in CT attenuation determinations. On images obtained without contrast material, the liver appears slightly more dense than the other intraabdominal organs. However, after intravenous administration of contrast material, the liver often appears slightly lower in density than the other intraabdominal organs, depending on the volume and method of administration of contrast material.

The porta hepatis is the hilum of the liver through which the hepatic arteries, portal veins, and bile ducts pass. The gallbladder neck, cystic duct, nerves, and lymphatic vessels are also present in this region, and normal-size lymph nodes frequently are seen. The anatomy of the porta hepatis is highly variable and often confusing (287).

The caudate process is an inferior extension of the caudate lobe. On transaxial images, a portion of the caudate process occasionally appears to be separate from the remaining liver and thus can be mistaken for an enlarged lymph node. Conversely, enlarged nodes contiguous to

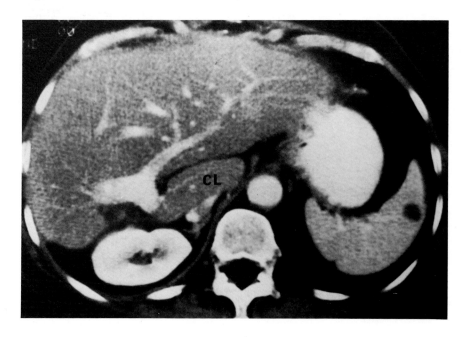

FIG. 5. CT image from a patient who previously had resection of the right hepatic lobe. Note the distortion of the normal vascular anatomy. The remaining left and caudate lobes (CL) regenerated to form a liver comparable to the preoperative size.

the caudate lobe may be mistaken for a part of this caudate process.

After partial hepatic resection, liver tissue may regenerate quite rapidly, even returning to normal volume within several months (Fig. 5). After right-lobe resection, the left lobe enlarges toward the right and may take on an elliptical appearance. Left-lobe resection tends to lead to a more rounded configuration of the remaining right lobe.

Wedge resection of the liver often produces residual scars and focal irregularities. Small persistent fluid collections or granulomas may be seen at the point of resection. The distorted position of the portal vein in hepatic resection after regeneration may be confusing, particularly on noncontrast images. Because of its unusual position, the portal vein may be mistaken for a recurrent intrahepatic lesion.

Segmental and Venous Anatomy

The liver is divided primarily into the right and left hepatic lobes. Each of these has two segments, with the left lobe having medial and lateral segments, and the right lobe anterior and posterior segments (Fig. 6). Additionally, there is a separate, smaller caudate lobe that is anatomically distinct because it derives its arterial supply from both the right and left hepatic arteries, and hepatic venous blood from the caudate lobe drains directly into the inferior vena cava (206). The medial segment of the left hepatic lobe has previously been termed the quadrate lobe, which should not be confused with the caudate lobe. Students first learning segmental hepatic anatomy often become confused about differentiating the medial and lateral segments of the left lobe. This is because in many patients the medial segment is actually located lateral to the lateral segment when the left lobe is entirely to the right of the patient's midline. The correct terminology may be remembered by conceptualizing the left hepatic lobe as an entirely left-side organ, in which case the medial segment is indeed more medial.

Three fissures help define the segmentation of the liver. The interlobar fissure is an incomplete structure that defines the inferior margin of the separation between the right and left lobes. Although a portion of this fissure contains fat in many patients, this fissure is generally difficult to identify. It is oriented on a vertical plane from the gallbladder fossa inferiorly to the middle hepatic vein superiorly (239).

The left intersegmental fissure defines the inferior boundary between the medial and lateral segments of the left hepatic lobe. This is also termed the fissure for the ligamentum teres (Fig. 6C). The ligamentum teres passes through this fissure and usually is surrounded by a small amount of fat. When the ligamentum passes out of the liver ventrally, it is located in the free edge of the falciform

ligament, a peritoneal reflection arising from the anterosuperior surface of the left lobe.

The third fissure is present at the point of contact between the lateral segment of the left hepatic lobe and the caudate lobe. This is the fissure for the ligamentum venosum, which is in continuity with the fissure for the ligamentum teres (Fig. 6B). However, the fissure for the ligamentum venosum has a right–left orientation on cross-sectional view, whereas the fissure for the ligamentum teres is anteroposterior. The fissure for the ligamentum venosum usually is best seen in images taken cephalad to the fissure for the ligamentum teres. All of these fissures and the associated boundaries between hepatic segments are oriented in vertical (cephalocaudad) anatomic planes. Therefore, the fissures are seen in the same location on contiguous axial images, and where fissures are no longer visible on contiguous images, imaginary lines usually may be drawn in the expected location of the fissures to help extrapolate and define segmental boundaries.

Intrahepatic portal triads include branches of the portal vein, hepatic arteries, and bile ducts (Fig. 6B). These structures course through the central portions of lobes and segments. By contrast, the hepatic veins are unaccompanied by other structures, and these veins are found between adjacent lobes and segments (Fig. 6A). The portal vein is primarily divided into right and left branches, with further branches traveling to each segment. Although the branches of the portal vein supply the central portion of each segment, a short portion of the left portal vein is found in the fissure for the ligamentum teres that separates the medial and lateral segments of the left lobe. This portal vein branch passes this location as it extends to supply the central portion of the lateral segment of the left lobe. The most superior visible boundary between the medial and lateral segments of the left lobe is the left hepatic vein. At a more caudad level, a portion of the left portal vein lies between the segments; further caudad, fat within the fissure is visible.

As mentioned earlier, the main hepatic veins are found between hepatic segments. The three main hepatic veins are the right, middle, and left, and cephalad the veins merge into the inferior vena cava (IVC) at nearly the same level. The right hepatic vein lies between the anterior and posterior segments of the right lobe, the middle hepatic vein lies between the right and left lobes, and the left hepatic vein is between the medial and lateral segments of the left lobe. Vertical (cephalocaudad) anatomic planes drawn through these main hepatic veins roughly demarcate the main hepatic segments. A line drawn through the middle hepatic vein superiorly and the gallbladder fossa inferiorly connected by a vertical plane will define the margin between the right and left lobes.

Most commonly, the middle and left hepatic veins merge with one another within about 1 cm of their junction with the IVC. However, they may enter the IVC separately. The right hepatic vein usually enters the IVC sep-

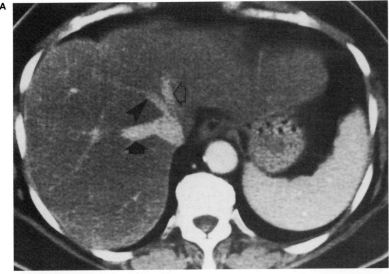

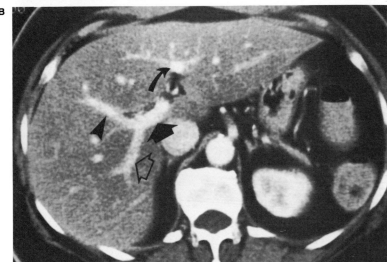

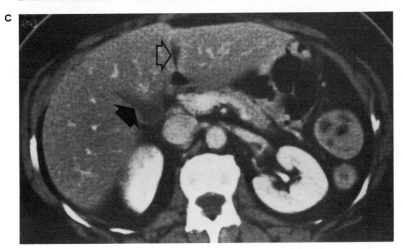

FIG. 6. Normal hepatic anatomy. A: Image through the superior aspect of the liver demonstrates the right (*arrow*), middle (*arrowhead*), and left (*open arrow*) hepatic veins. The right hepatic vein forms the margin between the anterior and posterior segments of the right lobe. The middle hepatic vein forms the border between the right and left lobes. The left hepatic vein passes between the medial and lateral segments of the left lobe. B: Image 5 cm caudal to A. The right portal vein (*black arrow*) lies anterior to the inferior vena cava. The anterior (*arrowhead*) and posterior (*open arrow*) branches of the right portal vein drain the central portions of these lobar segments. At this level, a cross section of the left portal vein is identified within the fissure for the ligamentum teres (*curved arrow*), which forms the margin between the medial and lateral segments of the left lobe. C: Image 4 cm caudal to B. The gallbladder (*arrow*) is seen within the interlobar fissure. The fissure for the ligamentum teres (*open arrow*) is well seen.

arately. Accessory hepatic veins are common. They may enter the IVC separately from the three main veins, but still within the same imaging slice, which creates a confusing appearance when attempting to determine hepatic

segmentation. An additional accessory hepatic vein may be seen in lower slices in other patients (Fig. 7).

Hepatic veins draining the caudate lobe enter the IVC separate from the main hepatic veins, and the arterial

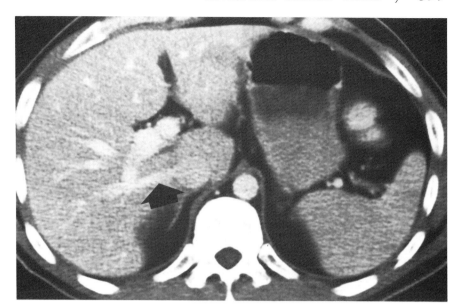

FIG. 7. Variations in hepatic venous anatomy. An accessory right hepatic vein (*arrow*) enters the IVC at a lower level than usual.

supply to the caudate lobe is derived from both the right and left hepatic arteries, leading to the description of the caudate lobe as a separate hepatic segment. These veins usually are too small to identify as discrete structures, even with good contrast enhancement (206).

In the cephalad portions of the liver, the IVC is largely encompassed by hepatic tissue, and the IVC is said to be "intrahepatic." At more caudad levels, beginning near the level of the caudate lobe, the IVC emerges from hepatic tissue. Depending on the relative densities of the blood and liver, the IVC may in some cases present a confusing appearance and can be mistaken for an intrahepatic lesion. Another important anatomic feature identifying the position of the caudate lobe and caudate process is that they are located between the IVC and the portal vein.

Arterial and Biliary Anatomy

The arteries and ducts within the liver travel with the portal vein radicles, which are normally larger. Intrahepatic arteries are best visualized soon after rapid intravenous injection of contrast material. Arteries then rapidly fade to isodensity with the adjacent portal veins as the portal venous circulation begins to accumulate contrast material.

Within the porta hepatis, the hepatic artery may be seen anterior and slightly medial to the main portal vein, whereas the common hepatic duct is generally anterior and slightly lateral to the portal vein (Fig. 8). However, variations in orientation are frequent. An anomalous right

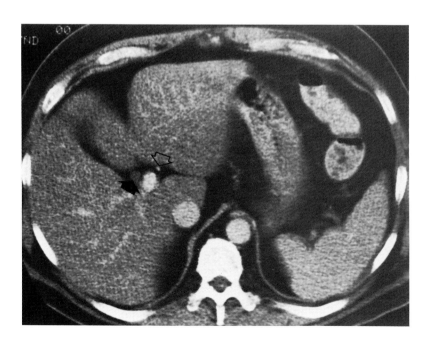

FIG. 8. Normal porta hepatis: CT. A normal-size common hepatic duct (*arrow*) is seen anterolateral to the enhanced portal vein. A small section of the hepatic artery (*open arrow*) is also seen anteromedial to the vein.

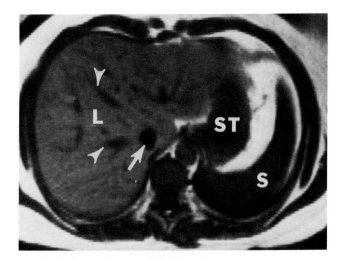

FIG. 9. Normal liver: MR image (TR = 300 msec, TE = 15 msec). The liver parenchyma (L) has a homogeneous medium signal intensity higher than that for the spleen (S). Note that the IVC (*arrow*) and hepatic vein branches (*arrowheads*) appear as areas of "signal void"; (ST) stomach.

hepatic artery is also commonly seen and may travel behind, rather than anterior to, the portal vein.

Normal-size intrahepatic bile ducts may be seen centrally near the bifurcation of the common hepatic duct into the right and left branches (287). The common hepatic and common bile ducts usually are visualized within the hepatoduodenal ligament. They are better seen when dynamic imaging with intravenous contrast enhancement has been used, because the bile duct walls are enhanced.

It may be difficult to distinguish between the central intrahepatic bile ducts and a small amount of fat within the fissures in this location. However, when low-attenuation structures are seen more peripherally within the liver with contrast enhancement, they usually indicate dilated bile ducts.

Gallbladder

The gallbladder is an oval or elliptical structure of near water density usually located at the inferior surface of the liver between the right and left lobes (Fig. 6C). A thin wall often is seen in normal patients, particularly when intravenous contrast material is used.

The gallbladder neck often is folded, and a portion of it may be seen cut in cross section. Particularly if intravenous contrast material is used, this small circular portion of the gallbladder neck with an enhanced wall may be mistaken for a gallstone. The cystic artery may also be brightly enhanced with the use of dynamic imaging with intravenous contrast material and may also occasionally be mistaken for a gallstone.

The gallbladder may project beyond the margin of the liver parenchyma or may be located in an ectopic, intra-

hepatic location. When in an "ectopic" location, the gallbladder may invaginate deeply into the interlobar fissure.

MRI

With MRI, the normal liver appears as an organ of homogeneous medium intensity (Fig. 9). The signal intensity of the liver is similar to that of the pancreas on both T1- and T2-weighted images. It has a higher signal intensity on T1-weighted images, but a lower signal intensity on T2-weighted images, than does the spleen. Normal hepatic vessels are clearly shown as signal-free structures. Both slow blood flow and thrombus may produce signal, but they can be differentiated from one another by comparing the signal intensities on the first and second echoes of a dual-echo sequence (83). The signal intensity due to slow blood flow often increases from the first to the second echo, whereas the absolute intensity of a thrombus invariably diminishes on the second-echo image. The hepatic veins, the portal veins, and the intrahepatic portion of the IVC are seen in almost every case. The hepatic artery is seen less frequently (83) (Fig. 10).

Normal intrahepatic biliary radicles are not visible, whereas the normal extrahepatic common bile duct can be seen in up to 50% of cases (253). When seen, the common bile duct has a low signal intensity on a T1-weighted sequence and a high signal intensity on a T2-weighted sequence (Fig. 11). The MRI appearance of normal gallbladder varies with the state of fasting. When imaged after

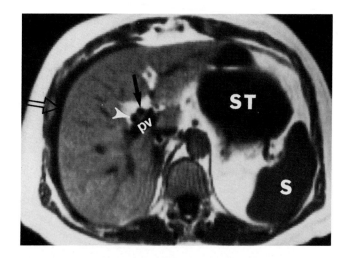

FIG. 10. Normal porta hepatis: MR image (TR = 300 msec, TE = 30 msec). The fat in the ligamentum venosum and ligamentum teres has a high signal intensity, and the liver parenchyma has a homogeneous medium signal intensity. The portal vein (pv) and hepatic artery (*arrow*) yield low signal intensities because of the "flow-void" phenomenon. The common hepatic duct (*arrowhead*) also has a low signal intensity on this T1-weighted image because of the long T1 of bile. A small amount of ascites is present (*open arrow*); (ST) stomach; (S) spleen.

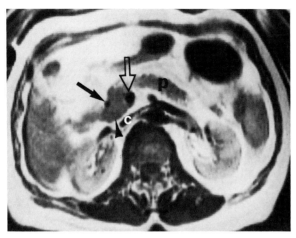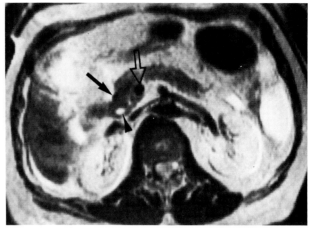

FIG. 11. Normal distal common bile duct. **A:** Balanced MR image (TR = 2,100 msec, TE = 35 msec). The distal common bile duct (*arrowhead*) is almost isointense with the pancreas (p); (*arrow*) gastroduodenal artery; (*open arrow*) superior mesenteric vein; (c) IVC. **B:** T2-weighted MR image (TR = 2,100 msec, TE = 90 msec). The distal common bile duct (*arrowhead*) has a much higher signal intensity and can be easily differentiated from the pancreas. Note that both the superior mesenteric vein (*open arrow*) and the gastroduodenal artery (*arrow*) still appear as areas of "flow void."

prolonged fasting (>14 hr), the normal gallbladder has a high signal intensity on T1-weighted images because of the presence of concentrated bile (123). In contradistinction, gallbladders containing dilute bile have a low signal intensity on T1-weighted images (Fig. 12). The periportal fat and fat in the ligamentum teres are seen as high-intensity structures.

Image Degradation and Artifacts

Radiating streaks from an air–fluid level within the stomach often obscure a portion of the left hepatic lobe or even the central liver (19). This artifact, consisting of alternating radiating bands of bright and dark streaks, is caused by the abrupt density differences between contrast material and air within the stomach and by the slight fluid waves present within this air–fluid level during the period of imaging. It is less conspicuous on newer-model scanners and can be minimized by using intravenous contrast material properly to increase contrast within liver tissue, by reducing the density of the oral contrast material, or by changing the patient's orientation to project the streak artifacts away from liver parenchyma.

A similar type of artifact is found at the thoracoabdominal junction. One may see a vague area of altered atten-

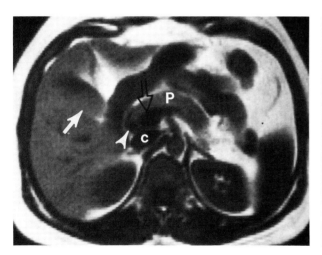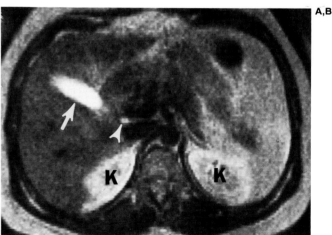

FIG. 12. Normal gallbladder. **A:** T1-weighted MR image (TR = 300 msec, TE = 15 msec). The dependent portion of the gallbladder (*arrow*) has a medium signal intensity similar to that of the liver, whereas the top layer has a lower signal intensity. Note that the distal common bile duct (*arrowhead*) has a similar low signal intensity; (P) pancreas; (c) IVC; (*open arrow*) superior mesenteric vein. **B:** T2-weighted MR image (TR = 2,100 msec, TE = 90 msec). Both the gallbladder (*arrow*) and distal common bile duct (*arrowhead*) have high signal intensities; (K) kidney.

uation or faint parallel streaks within the dome of the liver. These artifacts are caused by the abrupt attenuation differences between the liver and lung tissue and slight degrees of motion caused by transmission of cardiac pulsations and slight degrees of breathing during imaging. Again, these artifacts are less apparent on images obtained with sub-5-sec scanners. Misinterpretation may be avoided by careful review of adjacent images and reimaging when necessary.

At any point within the liver, breathing may cause artifactual areas of abnormal attenuation or create a "ghost" contour to the liver margin that may be mistaken for a small amount of extrahepatic fluid. Comparison with adjacent images and reimaging may be helpful to avoid misinterpretation.

Another artifact, focal low-density areas near ribs, is caused by slight geometric inconsistencies in the X-ray projections and by hardening of the X-ray beam as it passes through the higher-density ribs. For a given scanner, it is difficult to eliminate such rib artifacts. However, potential misinterpretation can be minimized by appreciating their presence.

An additional artifact related to hardening of the X-ray beam is the cupping artifact. Because the X-ray beam is hardened to a greater degree when passing through the central portions, as compared with the peripheral portions, of the body, the computed reconstruction may not be able to fully compensate for this effect, leading to the appearance of relatively higher attenuation in the periphery of the liver. Such an artifact may lead to misinterpretation of apparent regional variations in liver attenuation that are not actually present.

Volume-averaging artifacts are frequent sources of misinterpretation. Such artifacts are formed by inclusion of two different types of tissue within the thickness of the imaged slice. The most frequent locations of such artifacts are the renal fossa, the gallbladder fossa, and the cardiac apex. Careful review of contiguous images usually can resolve questions about possible lesions in these areas.

PATHOLOGY

Diseases of the Hepatic Parenchyma

Neoplasms

The expectations among clinicians regarding imaging studies of the liver have increased because of the additional information such studies are known to produce. Previously, diagnostic examinations might be called on only to reveal the presence or extent of hepatic abnormalities. Examinations are now expected to accomplish these tasks with greater accuracy and further to help differentiate between benign and malignant lesions and even differentiate lesions of differing histology from one another.

Many imaging techniques have been used to evaluate the liver (20,23,28,42,54,88,90). Controversy exists as to which noninvasive imaging method should be used as the initial choice for detecting focal liver lesions. Although it is generally agreed that a well-performed CT study is superior to ultrasound and radionuclide scintigraphy for detecting hepatic neoplasms (2,20), several investigators have recently advocated the use of MRI as the initial procedure, especially in the case of metastases, because of its slightly higher sensitivity (222,260). However, we continue to use CT as the primary procedure, because in imaging oncologic patients, the liver is only one of the many organs that need to be assessed, and CT is more accurate than MRI for examining the retroperitoneum and other intraabdominal organs. Furthermore, CT is more readily available, has less stringent patient requirements, and can be carried out much more rapidly.

More invasive diagnostic studies, such as hepatic arteriography and CT angiography, are restricted to patients who are being considered for partial hepatic resection for their primary or metastatic neoplasms. Surgery may be obviated if small additional lesions are found. Such studies usually are not indicated in patients who are scheduled to receive chemotherapy.

Published reports regarding the appearance of lesions and the accuracy of detecting lesions often are controversial and confusing. In some cases, studies may be accurate, yet not applicable. For example, much of the literature from Japan (69,70,126,127,131,152,197) regarding primary hepatic neoplasms describes a different typical presentation than is seen in America. Therefore, the conclusions from such studies cannot be applied uniformly to American and European populations.

Hepatocellular carcinoma

Hepatocellular carcinoma (hepatoma), a primary malignant neoplasm arising from hepatocytes, is much more common in Africa and Asia than in Europe and America (154). In the United States, a patient with hepatocellular carcinoma (HCC) often presents with pain, weight loss, and/or a palpable abdominal mass. Alpha-fetoprotein levels usually are markedly elevated. In Japan and other countries with high incidences of hepatoma, the majority of cases occur in patients with cirrhosis (166). However, in the United States, the majority of cases occur de novo.

About three-fourths of patients with HCC have extrahepatic spread of the disease, with local extension being the most common occurrence (154). Most hepatomas are unresectable when first detected (154). Areas of involvement include the pancreatic bed, liver capsule and adjacent abdominal wall and diaphragm, regional lymph nodes, omentum, and mesentery. Pancreatic bed involvement, from retrograde extension through the portal vein, and regional lymph node invasion account for some reported cases in which the hepatoma has initially presented

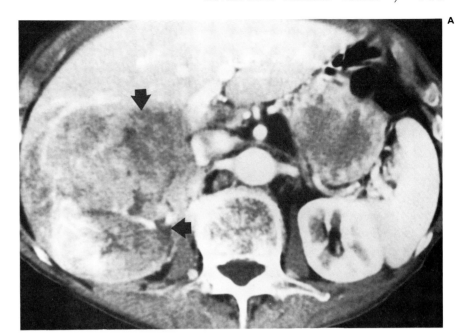

A

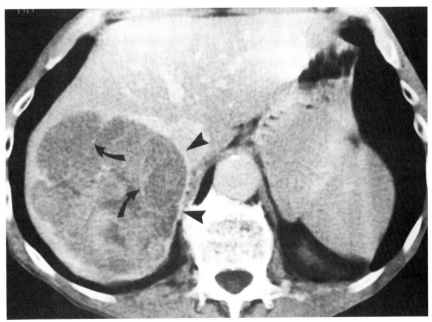

B

FIG. 13. Hepatoma. **A:** CT image during an intravenous bolus of contrast material. Note the areas of marked enhancement and inhomogeneity within this well-demarcated lesion. Scattered areas of necrosis (*arrows*) extend to the lesion periphery. **B:** Image through nearby area done about 10 min after **A,** but after an additional bolus. The inhomogeneity is less marked, but an enhancing capsule (*arrowheads*) is seen, and vessels (*curved arrows*) are identified deep within the lesion.

as an extrahepatic mass, even without apparent liver involvement (166). HCC occasionally metastasizes distantly to lung, brain, bone, and spleen.

CT. Hepatoma may appear as a solitary mass, a dominant mass with one or more smaller "satellite" lesions (Fig. 13), or diffuse involvement. When presenting as a solitary or dominant mass with satellite metastases, the hepatoma often is hypodense or isodense on noncontrast images, with a circumferential, well-defined narrow circular zone of lower density (127). Such lesions often protrude beyond the hepatic surface and may even be pedunculated. Hepatomas calcify in only about 10% of cases (127).

Hepatomas often exhibit transient, intense, but heterogeneous contrast enhancement. Large vascular channels and scattered areas of low attenuation often extend to the peripheral zone. Portal vein invasion (Fig. 14) occurs in about one-third of cases (154); invasion of the IVC and hepatic arteries and veins is also common.

Vascular involvement by hepatoma often leads to redistribution of hepatic blood flow. Arterioportal shunts cause early and prolonged portal vein enhancement and transiently increased attenuation of contralateral lobes or segments (131). This latter effect apparently is caused by arterioportal shunting, with partial or complete obstruction of the portal vein branch to the involved segment.

A,B

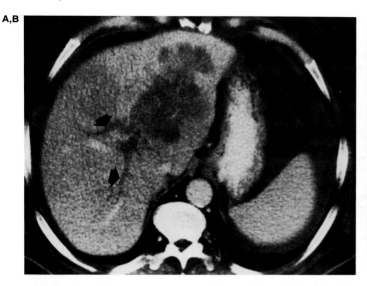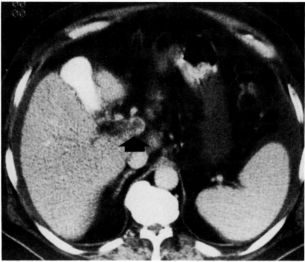

FIG. 14. Hepatoma invading the portal vein. A: Postcontrast CT image demonstrates a large mass in the left lobe. The tubular low-density structures (*arrows*) represent thrombosed portal vein radicles caused by invasion and obstruction by the liver mass. B: Image 4 cm below A. Note the thrombus within the main portal vein (*arrow*). There is a small amount of ascites, and the gallbladder is enhanced because of prior administration of contrast material.

Thus, overall portal flow is increased, but directed away from the lobe or segment containing the tumor. One may also see dilated, abnormal intrahepatic vessels, irregular enhancing areas, and wedge-shaped areas of enhancement peripheral to the tumor (131,197). Alterations in the patterns of enhancement depend on the location of the tumor and the particular complex combination of venous obstruction and arterioportal shunting. Although such altered flow patterns occur more commonly with HCC than with other focal hepatic abnormalities, shunting may also be seen in trauma and cirrhosis. Additionally, other conditions may create peculiar, transient patterns of enhancement caused by altered blood flow. Hepatic veno-occlusive disease and congestive hepatomegaly caused by

cardiac disease may produce patchy and lobular patterns of enhancement that may be confused with shunting or other focal diseases.

Although HCC commonly presents as a mass with a well-defined capsule, tumor margins may be more ill-defined in some cases (Fig. 15), making distinction from metastases more difficult. Also, particularly in patients with cirrhosis, the tumor often spreads diffusely and is more difficult to separate from the background of diffuse liver abnormality. A lesion may also be mistaken for a regenerating nodule, or vice versa.

Although the radiographic findings often strongly suggest the proper diagnosis, tissue diagnosis usually is required. If percutaneous biopsy is performed, one must be

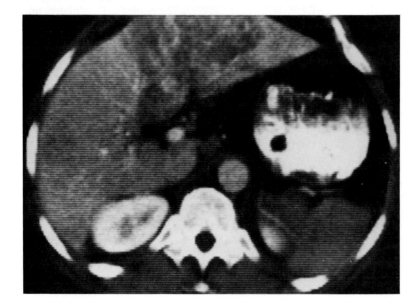

FIG. 15. Hepatoma. The margins are not well defined. The lesion only mildly deforms the contour of the liver, indicating that this lesion is more infiltrative.

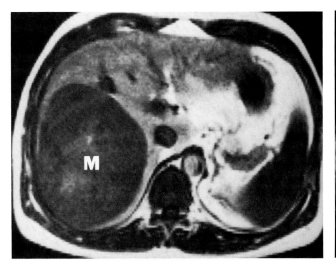 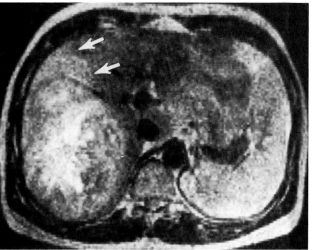

A,B

FIG. 16. Hepatoma. **A:** T1-weighted MR image (TR = 300 msec, TE = 15 msec) shows a well-circumscribed, predominantly hypointense mass (M) occupying nearly the entire right lobe. High-signal-intensity foci within the tumor correspond to areas of hemorrhage. **B:** T2-weighted MR image (TR = 2,100 msec, TE = 90 msec) shows the tumor to be hyperintense relative to normal liver. The tumor margin is less distinct. The liver parenchyma adjacent to the tumor (*arrows*) also has a slightly higher signal intensity and is believed to be secondary to congestion.

cautious because of the highly vascular nature of these lesions. The differential diagnosis of masses suspected to be hepatomas covers a broad range, including metastatic disease, benign adenoma, abscess, and other types of liver masses (127).

MRI. Compared with adjacent normal liver parenchyma, hepatomas usually appear as masses of lower signal intensity on T1-weighted images and of higher signal intensity on T2-weighted images (Fig. 16). Although the relaxation characteristics of hepatomas are not tissue-specific, T1 values for small hepatomas have been found to roughly parallel the amount of fibrosis and fat contained within the tumor. Whereas hepatomas with fibrosis have long T1 values, those with steatosis have short T1 values (70). A low-intensity rim, which corresponds to a fibrous pseudocapsule, has been observed on T1-weighted images of nearly half of the hepatomas in Japan (70,133) (Fig. 17). Displacement and invasion of portal and hepatic veins are well seen with MRI (Fig. 18). Tumor thrombus appears as an area of increased signal within a normally signal-free vessel.

MRI is equal in accuracy to CT for detecting hepatomas. In one study, MRI correctly identified 98% of hepatomas greater than 2 cm and 33% of those less than 2 cm (70). MRI is superior to CT for demonstrating the pseudocapsule, internal architecture, margin of the tumor, and venous invasion, but it is inferior to CT for detecting calcifications (70,133,189,283).

Metastases

Most small, solitary lesions in patients with no known primary malignant neoplasms are benign, most com-

monly hemangiomas or cysts. Because these types of benign lesions may be multiple, the presence of numerous small lesions must not be assumed to indicate metastases, even if the patient has a known primary malignancy. Depending on the clinical circumstances, follow-up examination, rather than immediate further evaluation of uncertain cases, is often appropriate. The factors one must consider in determining the appropriate approach include the natural course of the known or suspected disease, the likelihood of involvement of other organs, the likelihood of response to therapy, the growth rate of the suspected

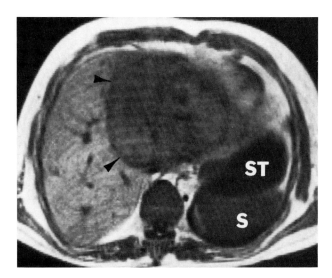

FIG. 17. Hepatoma. T1-weighted MR image (TR = 300 msec, TE = 15 msec) shows a low-intensity rim (*arrowheads*) surrounding a left-lobe hepatoma; (ST) stomach; (S) spleen.

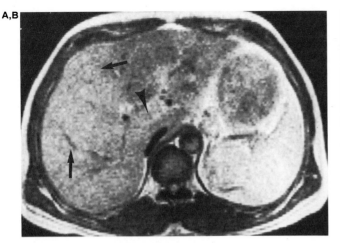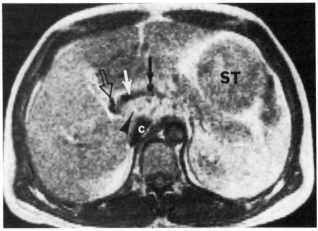

FIG. 18. Hepatoma invading the portal vein. **A:** MR image (TR = 1,500 msec, TE = 30 msec) shows an ill-defined mass (*arrows*) with a signal intensity slightly higher than that of normal liver in the anterior portion of the right lobe. Note a medium-signal-intensity mass (*arrowhead*) in the region of normal portal vein. **B:** Image 1 cm caudal to **A**. The anterior portion of the portal vein (*white arrow*) appears black, indicating rapid blood flow within the residual lumen. Tumor thrombus (*arrowhead*) within the portal vein is again noted; (*black arrow*) hepatic artery; (*open arrow*) common hepatic duct; (ST) stomach; (c) IVC.

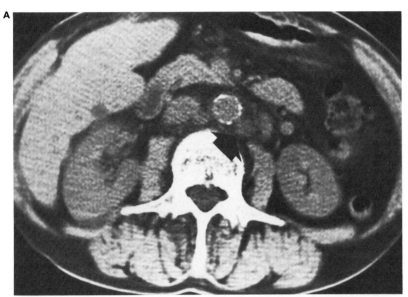

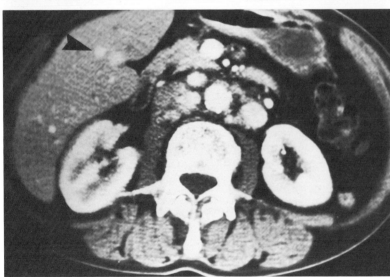

FIG. 19. Metastatic thyroid carcinoma. **A:** Noncontrast CT image shows enlarged retroperitoneal lymph nodes (*arrow*) and an incidental liver cyst. **B:** After bolus injection of contrast material, CT shows an unusually marked degree of enhancement of these nodes. Enhancing liver metastases (*arrowhead*) are also seen. Such enhancing metastases are uncommon. Because of the propensity of vascular metastases to take up contrast material, some such lesions may be obscured with the dynamic imaging technique.

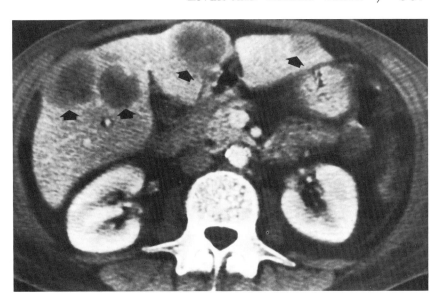

FIG. 20. Typical CT appearance of metastases from colon carcinoma. There are multiple lesions (*arrows*) of similar sizes. Note a fine rim of enhancement and the internal inhomogeneity that is not found in hemangioma.

lesion, and whether or not aggressive treatment is being contemplated (1,82,125,147,170,200,270). For example, it is more appropriate to perform thorough diagnostic testing for a patient who is a candidate for a partial hepatic resection than for a patient for whom chemotherapy is contemplated and the purpose of the study is solely for base-line determination of disease extent.

It is now common practice to diagnose metastases without biopsy confirmation when both clinical findings and imaging evidence indicate a very high probability. However, percutaneous biopsy under ultrasound or CT

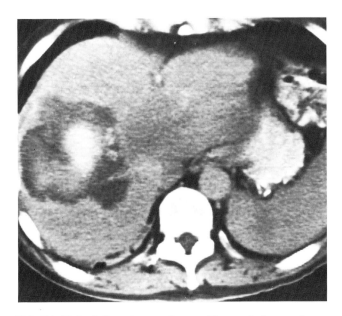

FIG. 21. Metastatic colon carcinoma. The central amorphous density represents calcification, which occurs in a minority of metastases.

guidance is a rapid, relatively innocuous way to obtain cytologic or histologic confirmation (174).

CT. Metastases vary in their CT appearance (54,248). Borders may be sharp, ill-defined, or nodular. The shape may be round, ovoid, or irregular. Attenuation usually is lower than that for the surrounding liver both before and after intravenous administration of contrast material. However, lesions occasionally are isodense or hyperdense (Fig. 19) relative to liver. There may be concentric bands of variable attenuation, with the lowest central density representing tumor necrosis. Peripheral ring enhancement also occurs frequently (Fig. 20) and should be distinguished from the characteristic enhancement pattern of hemangioma, which will be described later. Depending on the primary histology, metastases may have punctate or psammomatous calcifications (234) (Figs. 21 and 22). Leiomyosarcomas metastasize to the liver more commonly than to other organs, with liver spread discovered in 37% of cases in one series (181). Such metastases frequently are markedly necrotic and do not contain calcifications (Fig. 23).

If a study is performed approximately 10 to 20 min following intravenous administration of a large volume of contrast material, some metastases develop an appearance of somewhat increased central attenuation relative to a decreased-attenuation peripheral band (193) (Fig. 24). This is a pattern found in metastases, but not hemangiomas or most other lesions.

Diffuse involvement of the liver by metastases may be difficult to recognize. Dynamic imaging may help demonstrate the parenchymal inhomogeneity and distortion of vascular pattern. A truly diffuse pattern of involvement often is seen in carcinoma of the breast (295) (Fig. 25), but only rarely in colon or lung tumors.

It is also more difficult to detect metastases in a fatty liver in which the decreased attenuation of the liver may

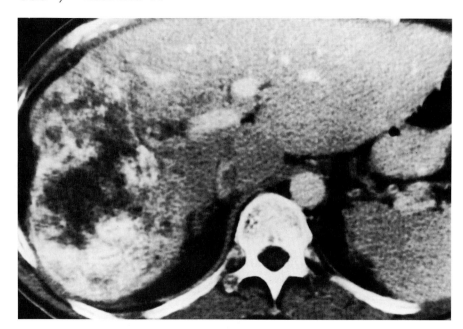

FIG. 22. Unusually densely calcified metastasis in the right lobe from colon carcinoma. Some mucinous colon tumors contain psammomatous calcification.

match the attenuation of the lesion (Fig. 26). In addition, some small vascular metastases may be difficult to see because contrast material is taken up as rapidly in the lesions as it is within the liver tissue (37). One study showed that 39% of cases of metastases from vascular primary tumors such as carcinoid, islet cell tumor, pheochromocytoma, and renal cell carcinoma became isodense or nearly so during dynamic imaging (37). Noncontrast or delayed images help detect lesions in such cases.

The differential diagnosis of multiple hepatic lesions must consider hemangiomas, pyogenic abscesses, fungal microabscesses, and rarely multicentric hepatomas. Even when HCC appears as a dominant mass with multiple satellite nodules, it may still be distinguished from metastases by several findings (127). Metastases commonly

present as multiple lesions of varying sizes. Even when one lesion can be selected as the dominant or largest lesion, others of substantial size usually are present elsewhere in the liver. This differs from the appearance of hepatoma with satellite lesions, in that the satellite nodules usually are small and relatively close to the primary mass. Calcifications are more common in metastases than in hepatomas. Metastases, particularly from colon carcinoma, commonly show a gradual decrease in attenuation toward the center, or a doughnut configuration with nodular or ill-defined enhancing peripheral margins, a rare finding in HCC. Metastases rarely protrude prominently from the liver surface. Whereas most hepatomas are highly vascular, most metastases are not, although the peripheral zone may be enhanced as described.

FIG. 23. Metastatic leiomyosarcoma. Postcontrast CT image shows two large metastases. The centers of these lesions have attenuation values near that for water, representing areas of necrosis.

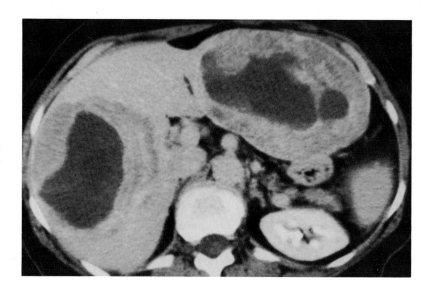

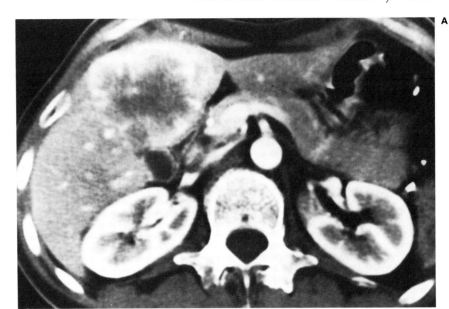

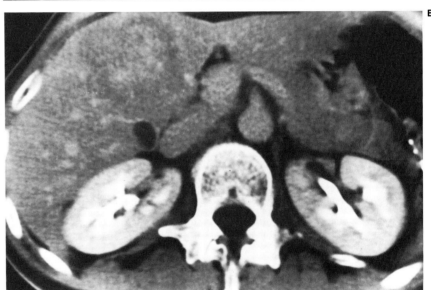

FIG. 24. Peripheral halo in liver metastasis. A: There is an enhancing rim on this lesion. Note, however, that it does not have the nodular appearance seen in the hemangioma shown in Fig. 30. There is also a gradation of attenuation from the periphery to the center, rather than a relatively homogeneous central low attenuation as seen early in dynamic imaging of the hemangiomas. B: CT image obtained 10 min after A. The central area of the lesion is somewhat increased in attenuation relative to its periphery. This pattern of enhancement is found in metastases, but not hemangiomas.

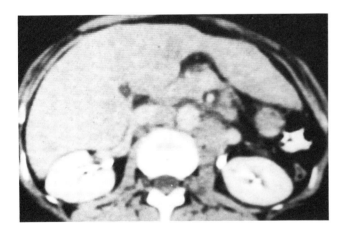

FIG. 25. Diffuse hepatic metastases from carcinoma of the breast. Postcontrast CT image demonstrates subtle inhomogeneity of the entire liver, representing diffuse metastases. Subtle abnormalities like this often can be accentuated by narrowing the window settings.

MRI. The T1 and T2 values for metastases are generally longer than those for normal hepatic tissue (Figs. 27 and 28), but not as long as those for hepatic cysts (67,189,250).

MRI has an accuracy similar to or greater than that of CT for detecting hepatic metastases (100,115,189, 222,260). The detection rate by MRI varies depending on the type of imager and pulsing parameters used. Whereas some have shown T1-weighted images with TE values less than 20 msec to be the most sensitive (260), we have found T1- and T2-weighted sequences to be equally important. We have encountered cases in which lesions were seen on T2-weighted images, but not on T1-weighted images (Fig. 29).

Although a hyperintense halo, which is present in up to 25% of metastases, has been reported to be specific for metastases, there are no absolute MRI criteria to distinguish metastases from primary hepatic neoplasm (80).

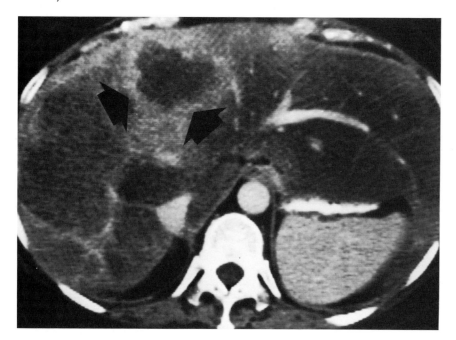

FIG. 26. A large metastatic lesion is seen in the right lobe in this patient with co-existing fatty infiltration of the liver. Metastasis can be differentiated from a geographic pattern of focal fatty infiltration because of the rounded enhancing borders (*arrows*) on one ill-defined lesion. Also, there are no normal-appearing blood vessels traversing the large inhomogeneous area in the right lobe.

Ancillary findings such as the number, size, and location of the lesions often are used to distinguish these two entities.

Hemangioma

Hemangioma is the most common hepatic neoplasm (140,243). Variations in size are extreme. Whereas hemangioma is solitary in the majority of cases, a significant percentage of patients have multiple lesions (130). Cavernous hemangiomas constitute the most common form, but capillary lesions have also been described.

Large lesions or moderate-size lesions located superficially or adjacent to the IVC may produce right-upper-quadrant discomfort or pain (130,140). Most lesions are harmless, but may bleed when they grow to large size, are traumatized, or are superficial.

Despite their usual benign behavior, hepatic hemangiomas frequently cause diagnostic problems because they can be confused with a malignant neoplasm. Numerous methods are commonly applied to making this distinction, including CT, ultrasound, radionuclide studies, and angiography (243).

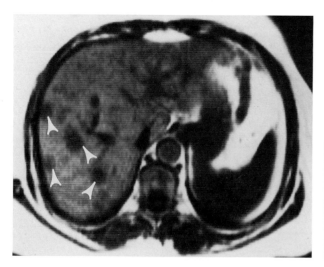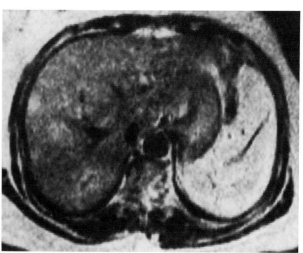

A,B

FIG. 27. Hepatic metastases from primary breast carcinoma. **A:** T1-weighted MR image (TR = 300 msec, TE = 15 msec) shows multiple hypointense lesions (*arrowheads*) in the right lobe of the liver. Note absence of left breast. **B:** T2-weighted MR image (TR = 2,100 msec, TE = 90 msec) demonstrates that metastases are hyperintense relative to normal liver because of their longer T2 value. More metastases were shown on a T1-weighted sequence in this patient.

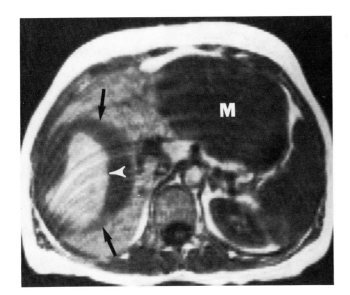

FIG. 28. Metastatic hepatic leiomyosarcomas. T1-weighted MR image (TR = 300 msec, TE = 15 msec) shows two large metastases: one in the left lobe (M) and the other in the right lobe (*arrows*). The left-lobe lesion is uniformly hypointense, whereas the right-lobe lesion contains a central hyperintense area representing hemorrhage (*arrowhead*).

CT. A definitive CT diagnosis of hemangioma can be made by obtaining dynamic, serial images at a single level after administration of no less than 75 ml of 60% contrast material as a rapid intravenous bolus (36,91). Although a definitive diagnosis of hemangioma may be suggested based on findings from an incremental dynamic study, the disadvantage of this technique is that each level is seen only once during the examination, and thus the charac-

teristic pattern of change over time cannot be appreciated. Studies from several centers (12,127,140) suggest that with the proper criteria, hemangiomas can be diagnosed with both high sensitivity and specificity. However, a recent study done at the Mason Clinic found that only 54% of hemangiomas had a "typical" pattern (91), but the criteria used in that study were not the generally accepted criteria.

On noncontrast images, hemangiomas usually are discrete and homogeneous and of decreased attenuation relative to the liver (36,91,140). Calcifications are uncommon. On dynamic imaging, hemangiomas demonstrate brightly enhanced nodular or corrugated borders (140) (Fig. 30). Early during the examination, the nodular border usually does not form a continuous rim, but rather has the appearance of bright papillary projections pointing toward the center of the lesion. Enhancement then progresses slowly for 2 to 10 min or even longer from the periphery of the lesion toward the center, depending on the size of the lesion. Although other lesions such as colon metastases also show progressive enhancement from the periphery toward the center, the progression usually is more rapid initially until enhancement reaches the necrotic center of the tumor, and the rim is of relatively lower attenuation when compared with adjacent contrast-enhanced vessels.

In many cases there is eventually a complete or nearly complete fill-in of the entire lesion with contrast material over several minutes (36,91), sometimes resulting in positive enhancement of the lesion with respect to the liver parenchyma. A central focus or cleft of low density representing fibrosis often is seen in hemangiomas, particularly larger ones (235). The specificity of isodensity may be overemphasized in the literature, because many small and moderate-size metastases also become isodense with

A,B

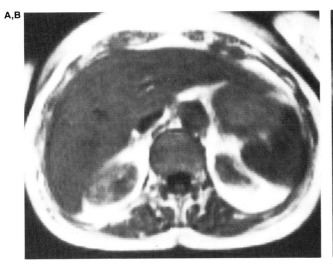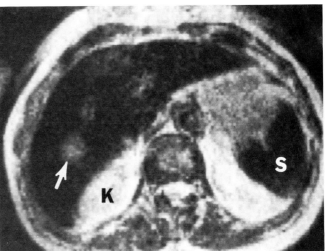

FIG. 29. Hepatic metastases from oat cell carcinoma of the lung. **A:** T1-weighted MR image (TR = 300 msec, TE = 15 msec) shows no focal hepatic lesion. **B:** T2-weighted MR image (TR = 2,100 msec, TE = 90 msec). In spite of poorer signal-to-noise ratio with this sequence, a 1.5-cm hyperintense metastasis is clearly demonstrated in the right lobe of the liver (*arrow*); (K) kidney; (S) spleen.

A,B

C,D

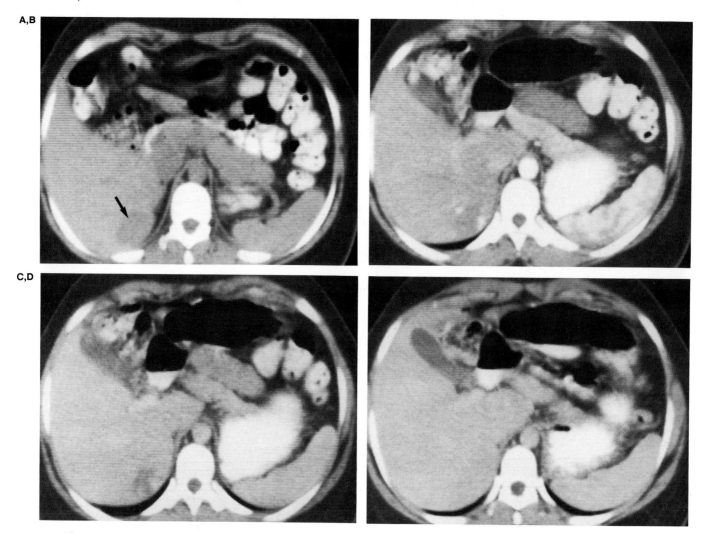

FIG. 30. Cavernous hemangioma: typical enhancement pattern. **A:** Noncontrast CT image demonstrates a 3-cm hypodense lesion (*arrow*) in the posterior aspect of the right lobe. **B:** Fifteen seconds after initiation of an intravenous bolus injection of contrast material, clusters of contrast material are noted around the periphery of the lesion. **C:** Forty-five seconds after the bolus, clusters of contrast material have diffused from the periphery toward the center of the lesion. **D:** Five minutes after the bolus, the lesion is no longer visible because it is now isodense with adjacent liver parenchyma.

liver parenchyma. However, persistent uniform hyperdensity relative to surrounding liver after several minutes does indeed suggest hemangioma, although some vascular metastases may become hyperdense transiently during the arterial phase of the dynamic injection. A pattern of central density exceeding peripheral density several minutes after bolus injection also indicates that the lesion is not a hemangioma. This pattern is found in some metastases with necrotic centers in which the contrast material transiently enhances a peripheral ring of viable tumor; as contrast material diffuses out of the vascularized periphery, it diffuses into the space within the central area of necrosis.

Some hemangiomas demonstrate atypical features such as cystic areas, probably caused by hemorrhage or thrombosis (264). Other lesions simply fail to demonstrate the typical pattern well enough to confirm the diagnosis.

There are several possible pitfalls in the diagnosis of hemangioma. As mentioned earlier, peripheral enhance-

ment alone is a feature common to many lesions. Small lesions may be difficult to diagnose because they fill in quickly after contrast material is administered. Large lesions may be difficult to evaluate because of bizarre patterns of enhancement, exceptionally slow fill-in, and areas of fibrosis and partial thrombosis (235) (Fig. 31). Multiple lesions may be difficult to evaluate because it is not possible to perform dynamic imaging simultaneously in multiple areas of the liver.

MRI. Cavernous hemangiomas most often appear as homogeneous, rounded, subcapsular, sharply marginated masses (101,134,256). They are of lower signal intensity than normal liver on T1-weighted images and higher signal intensity on T2-weighted images. Although the intensity of a hemangioma on a T1-weighted image will overlap the intensities of other hepatic neoplasms, its signal intensity on a T2-weighted image will be significantly higher than those of other tumors (101,203,256) (Figs. 32 and

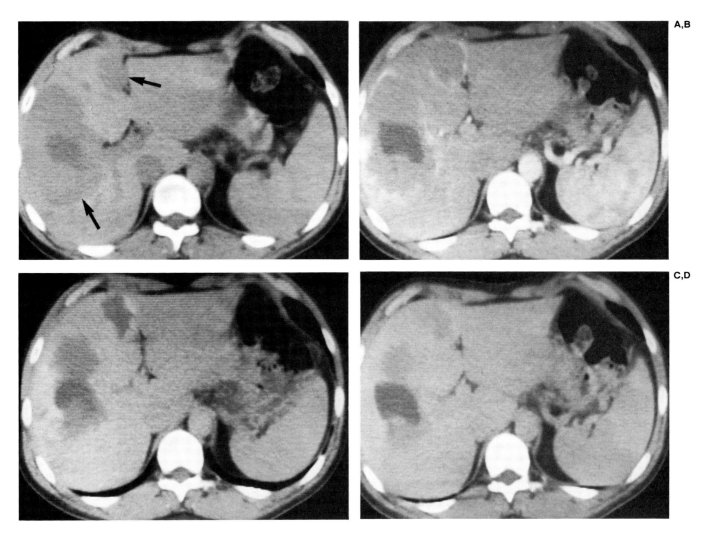

FIG. 31. Cavernous hemangioma: atypical enhancement pattern. **A:** Precontrast CT image demonstrates two hypodense lesions (*arrows*). **B:** Immediately following a bolus injection of contrast material, dense peripheral enhancement is noted in both lesions. **C:** CT image obtained 2 min after contrast administration shows gradual fill-in of both lesions. **D:** Image obtained 20 min after contrast administration demonstrates the center of the large lesion to be persistently hypodense, whereas the peripheral portion has become isodense. The central low density often is seen in large hemangiomas and is secondary to fibrosis and thrombosis.

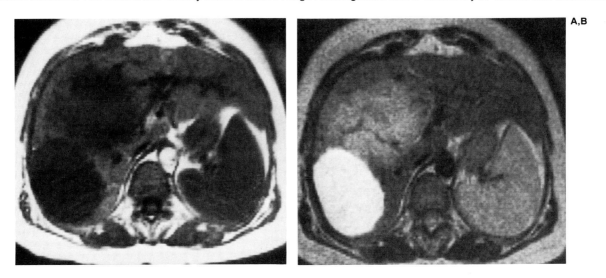

FIG. 32. Differentiation between hepatoma and cavernous hemangioma. **A:** T1-weighted MR image (TR = 500 msec, TE = 15 msec) shows two hypointense lesions in the liver. The anterior lesion (hepatoma) has an irregular border, whereas the posterior lesion (hemangioma) has a smooth contour. However, the signal intensities for these two lesions are similar in this sequence. **B:** T2-weighted MR image (TR = 2,100 msec, TE = 90 msec). Although both lesions are hyperintense relative to normal liver, cavernous hemangioma has a much higher signal intensity than does hepatoma because of its longer T2.

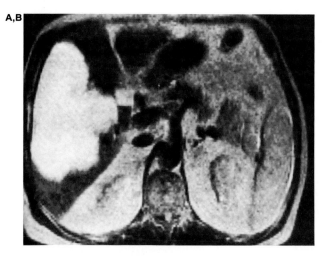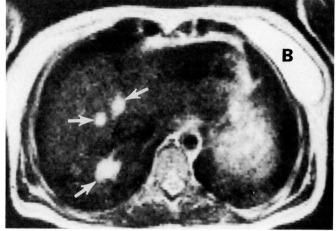

FIG. 33. Hepatic cavernous hemangioma in 2 patients. **A:** T2-weighted MR image (TR = 2,100 msec, TE = 90 msec) shows a large, lobulated, markedly hyperintense lesion in the right lobe of the liver. **B:** T2-weighted MR image (TR = 1,500 msec, TE = 90 msec) demonstrates three hyperintense lesions (*arrows*) in this patient with a left-breast implant (B).

33). The high intensity of a hemangioma will persist even on an image obtained with a TE of 180 msec, reflecting its relatively long T2 value. In one study, 15 of 18 hemangiomas had T2 values greater than 80 msec, whereas only 1 of 20 malignant neoplasms under 3 cm had such a value (134).

The appearance of cavernous hemangiomas on noncontrast MR images is by no means pathognomonic. Simple hepatic cysts may give a similar high signal on T2-weighted images. Although hepatic cysts usually can be distinguished from hemangiomas because the former have even longer T1 and T2 values, the distinction between small cysts and hemangiomas (<1.5 cm) may be difficult because of the effect of partial-volume averaging. Necrotic or very vascular metastases may yield a very high signal similar to that from hemangiomas, but they tend to be inhomogeneous. In addition, fibrotic or thrombosed hemangiomas may not have a typical MRI appearance and can be confused with other neoplasms (256).

Cavernous hemangiomas may exhibit a typical contrast-enhancement pattern (205). After intravenous administration of gadolinium DTPA (Gd-DTPA), a paramagnetic contrast agent whose pharmacokinetics are similar to those of iodinated contrast material, high-intensity foci first appear around the periphery of the lesion on T1-weighted images. This is followed by gradual fill-in of the rest of the lesion on delayed images. In one study, this enhancement pattern was seen in 5 of 7 hemangiomas, but none of the 29 malignant neoplasms (205).

Although the numbers of hemangiomas studied with MRI have been small, several groups have reported that MRI is superior to CT and radionuclide scintigraphy for detecting hemangiomas less than 3 cm in size (101,134,245,256). Although those retrospective studies suffered from small data bases and inconsistent CT tech-

niques, they nevertheless illustrated the difficulty in using CT for the diagnosis of hemangiomas. We have also encountered cases in which small hemangiomas were initially missed on routine bolus-infusion CT studies (Fig. 34).

Clinical Application. The following principles are suggested as providing a logical and cost-effective approach to the diagnosis of hemangiomas. However, these principles must be considered in light of specific clinical circumstances, the availability of the equipment, and the experience of the radiologist with that particular technology. Lesions incidentally discovered on CT or ultrasound that are solitary and typical of hemangioma in patients with no history of primary malignant tumor may be ignored or reexamined in several months with the same imaging technique to determine if there is any change in size. Lesions that have atypical features on the initial CT should be examined with another imaging test. We prefer radionuclide scintigraphy if the lesion is greater than 3 cm, and ultrasound if the lesion is smaller than 3 cm. However, radionuclide studies with single-photon-emission CT have been shown to provide improved results over conventional planar techniques and can be used to evaluate lesions as small as 1 cm (274). MRI is another reasonable alternative in institutions where it is available. If after the performance of a second test, such as ultrasound, the diagnosis still is not certain, one must consider what is indicated next: more imaging studies, biopsy, or follow-up. If the lesion is most likely to represent a hemangioma and a definitive answer is not urgently needed, follow-up usually is satisfactory. In cases in which the patient or clinician is not willing to accept the uncertainty, another imaging test such as an angiogram is preferred to biopsy of a likely hemangioma. If lesions are found in a patient in whom determining the presence of a neoplasm

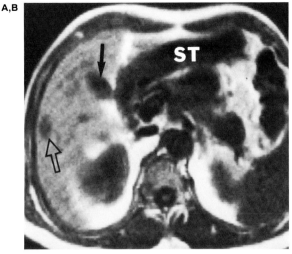
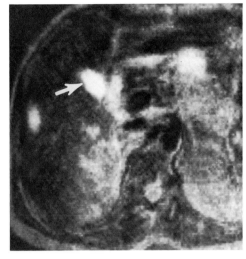

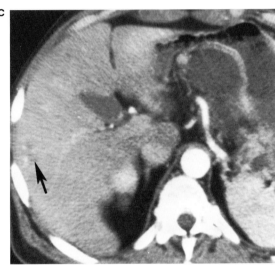

FIG. 34. Hepatic cavernous hemangioma: MRI versus CT. **A:** T1-weighted MR image (TR = 300 msec, TE = 15 msec) shows a 1-cm hypointense lesion (*open arrow*) near the periphery of the liver; (*arrow*) gallbladder; (ST) stomach. **B:** T2-weighted MR image (TR = 2,100 msec, TE = 90 msec). The lesion has a high signal intensity similar to that of the gallbladder (*arrow*). **C:** CT image obtained immediately after bolus administration of contrast material confirms the lesion to be a cavernous hemangioma, with typical nodular, peripheral enhancement (*arrow*) that was completely filled in on a later image. This lesion was not seen on a prior CT image obtained with a bolus infusion technique.

will greatly affect management, then biopsy may be indicated.

Focal nodular hyperplasia vs. adenoma

These benign lesions occur in similar populations of patients and in many cases have similar imaging features (8,225). However, there is a need to distinguish these lesions from one another because they are managed quite differently.

Hepatic adenomas are found in young adult women in about 95% of cases and have a strong association with the use of birth-control pills (176). These lesions present with acute abdominal pain and hepatomegaly, as well as spontaneous hemorrhage in up to 50% of cases (176,288). They should be removed because of the possibilities of severe hemorrhage and malignant degeneration (288).

Focal nodular hyperplasia (FNH) also affects young women, but about 10% to 20% of cases occur in men (176,225). Many consider FNH to be unassociated with

the use of birth-control pills, but one study reported their use in 81% of 21 cases (176), whereas another study reported their use in only 11% (225). About one-half of patients are symptomatic, usually presenting with right-upper-quadrant discomfort. Hemorrhage is rare unless the lesions have been traumatized. These have no malignant potential, and they need not be surgically removed (51).

CT. Hepatic adenoma typically presents as a discrete mass or masses that experience homogeneous, rapid, transient enhancement on dynamic CT (Fig. 35), except in areas with acute or remote hemorrhage. Occasionally these lesions are hypovascular. Hemorrhage is identified as areas of heterogeneous attenuation with high-density components when bleeding has been recent (Fig. 36). It has previously been suggested that on radionuclide sulfur colloid scintigraphy, they show no uptake, because adenomas contain no reticuloendothelial cells (84,288). However, a recent study showed that Kupffer cells were present in 13 cases of pathologically proven hepatic adenomas (167). Furthermore, uptake occurred in 3 of these

A,B

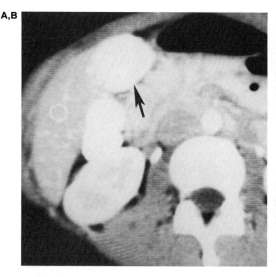 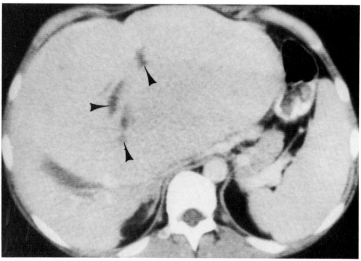

FIG. 35. Hepatic adenomas in two different women, both of whom had been on birth-control pills. **A:** CT image obtained immediately after bolus injection of contrast material shows the adenoma (*arrow*) to be uniformly hyperdense relative to the normal liver parenchyma. **B:** Postcontrast CT image in a different woman shows the lesion to be only slightly hyperdense relative to normal parenchyma. Several nonenhancing areas (*arrowheads*) representing necrosis are noted within the mass. The gallbladder is compressed between the mass and right hepatic lobe.

13, indicating that this traditional method of differentiating hepatic adenoma and FNH may not be infallible.

FNH lesions may be single or multiple and usually are discrete (51). However, they often experience a characteristic homogeneous intense contrast enhancement (Fig. 37). A small central stellate area of decreased attenuation is seen in up to 60% (288). The blood supply often radiates from the center of FNH, and the presence of transiently increased attenuation of the central focus on dynamic images suggests FNH (176). Usually no hemorrhage is identified. In about 50% of patients there is uptake of sulfur colloid particles within the lesion to the same degree or to a greater degree than within the normal surrounding liver (225).

Differentiation between FNH and adenoma may be difficult with any one imaging test. If lesions are less than 3 cm in diameter and are without evidence of hemorrhage, distinction between these two entities may be impossible using any combination of imaging techniques (176).

MRI. There have been few reports concerning the MRI appearances of FNH and adenoma. In one report, two cases of hepatic adenomas were described to have an MRI appearance indistinguishable from that of primary HCC (189). In contradistinction, a majority of FNH cases reported to date have had characteristic features. With the exception of a central scar, these lesions were homogeneous and nearly isointense with adjacent liver parenchyma on all pulse sequences (43,178). The margins of the lesions were either ill-defined or not visible. The central scar that was seen in over half of the reported cases was hypointense on T1-weighted images and hyperintense on T2-weighted images. The hyperintensity of the central scar

on T2-weighted images was attributed to the presence of bile duct and arterial and venous channels (178). This is in contradistinction to the persistent low signal intensity of the central scar seen on all sequences in some fibrolamellar HCC.

Clinical Application. If a lesion that is less than 3 cm and is without evidence of hemorrhage is discovered in an asymptomatic patient, birth-control pills, if in use, should be stopped, and the lesion followed with subsequent imaging studies. If the lesion is larger than 3 cm and has evidence of hemorrhage, it is most likely an adenoma and should be removed. If a lesion is larger than 3 cm and has no obvious hemorrhage, then it should be studied further by radionuclide scintigraphy to help determine whether it is FNH or adenoma (176).

Cysts

Hepatic cysts are common and often multiple (11). They usually are asymptomatic, unless very large. Multiple liver cysts are found in over 50% of patients with polycystic kidney disease (Fig. 38). Complications of cysts in this disease are rare, but tumor, infection, and biliary obstruction have been described (163). Liver function impairment also is uncommon, but when present, it is usually related to the foregoing complications.

CT. Cysts characteristically have sharp margins, with thin walls or no definable walls (11). They usually are not perfectly spherical or ovoid. They usually contain a homogeneous central area of near water density and show no significant change in attenuation after intravenous ad-

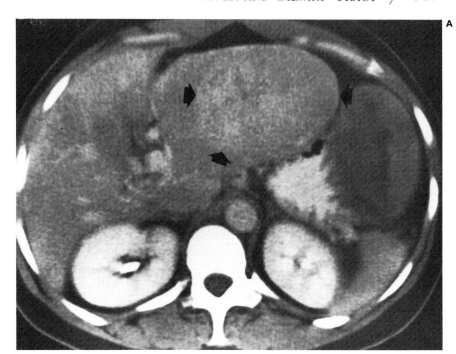

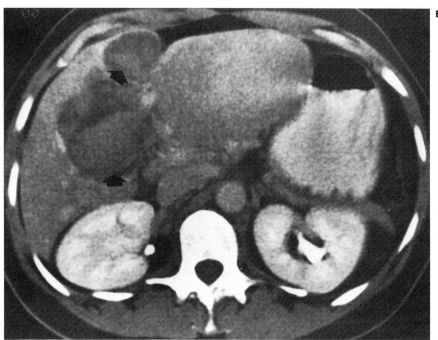

FIG. 36. Hemorrhage within hepatic adenomas. **A:** An adenoma (*arrows*) is seen in the left lobe. Additionally, there is an area of hemorrhage to the left. **B:** Further areas of hemorrhage (*arrows*) in the right lobe are identified by their characteristic relatively high density.

ministration of contrast material (Fig. 39). Cysts may demonstrate a slight change in attenuation between precontrast and postcontrast images that represents artifactual density changes, usually due to the marked change in density of surrounding tissue caused by the contrast material.

Several pitfalls can be encountered in the diagnosis of liver cysts. Very small cysts are difficult to differentiate from solid liver lesions because of the difficulty in obtaining accurate attenuation numbers, because of volume averaging (Fig. 40). In such cases, ultrasound usually is

diagnostic. Ultrasound is also helpful in clarifying the nature of the lesions that are identified on poor-quality images or images in which there are some atypical features, such as septations, apparent mural nodules, high-density fluid, or a thick wall (78).

Bile collections or bile lakes that are caused as a result of biliary obstruction or injury may have an appearance nearly identical with that for simple liver cysts. They may be single or multiple and may vary in size. An intravenous contrast agent excreted into the bile (e.g., Cholografin) may be used to determine if the bile cysts communicate

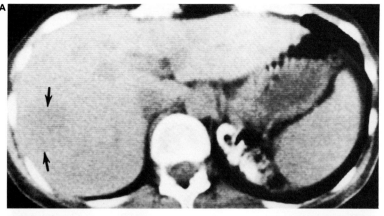

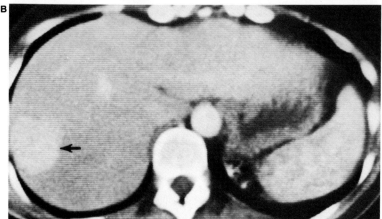

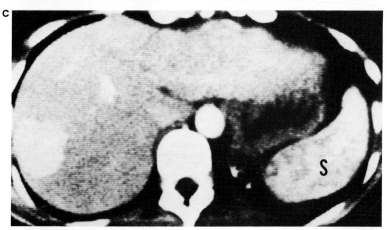

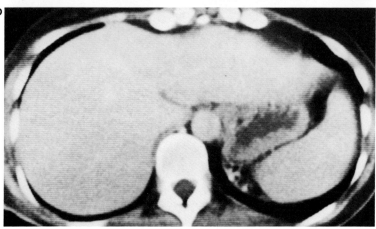

FIG. 37. FNH. **A:** On this precontrast image, the nearly isodense focal defect (*arrows*) is barely perceptible. **B,C:** Images of the lesion made with standard and narrow window settings early after bolus injection of contrast medium show the dense, homogeneous, transient enhancement of this vascular benign lesion (*arrow*). The level of these images was not through the center of the tumor, and therefore they do not show the central, nonenhancing stellate scar characteristic of FNH and present in this lesion when examined pathologically. Note the typical nonuniform early enhancement pattern of the spleen (S). **D:** At the same level as **B** and **C,** and 30 sec later in the sequence, the lesion is now isodense with the surrounding hepatic parenchyma and virtually imperceptible. This enhancement pattern is similar to what would be seen with a hepatic adenoma. Without evidence of a fresh intratumoral hemorrhage, common with adenomas, the two lesions would be difficult to differentiate. This lesion probably would not have been detectable if the early image after the bolus injection of contrast material had not been obtained or if the infusion technique had been used.

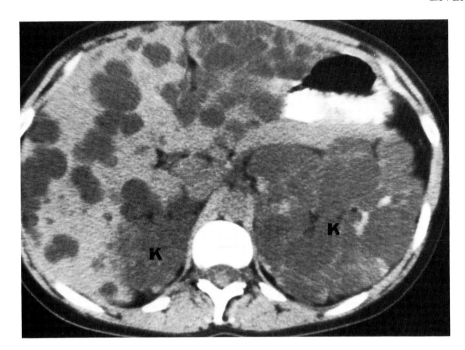

FIG. 38. Polycystic liver disease. The liver contains numerous cysts in this patient with adult polycystic kidney disease. Note that both kidneys (K) are almost entirely replaced with cysts. Some of the cysts in the left kidney have calcified walls.

with the biliary tree. Biliary radiopharmaceuticals can also be used to differentiate communicating and noncommunicating cysts.

Abscesses and neoplasms may have cystic components (78); however, features atypical of cysts usually are identified, such as a thick wall, mural nodules, increased attenuation, inhomogeneity, or fluid–fluid levels.

MRI. Hepatic cysts usually are spherical and show sharply defined margins on MRI. They are of homoge-

neous low intensity on T1-weighted images and high intensity on T2-weighted images. They can be easily distinguished from most benign and malignant neoplasms because of their extremely long T1 and T2 values (250,256). However, as stated previously, it may be difficult to distinguish between small cysts and small hemangiomas because of partial-volume averaging. Hemorrhagic cysts have a high signal intensity on T1-weighted images and thus can be distinguished from uncomplicated

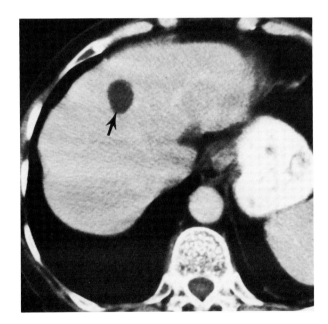

FIG. 39. Benign hepatic cyst. Postcontrast CT image shows a sharply defined, water-density, homogeneous mass (*arrow*) near the dome of the liver. The mass had an identical appearance on a noncontrast image.

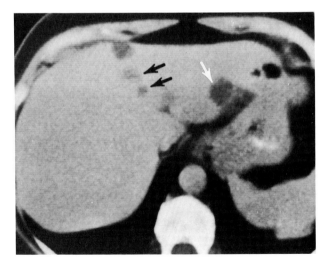

FIG. 40. A spectrum of densities is shown here, related to the sizes of these multiple benign hepatic cysts. The smaller cysts (*black arrows*) have an attenuation value midway between those for water and normal hepatic parenchyma, primarily reflecting volume averaging and resulting in falsely high values. The largest cyst (*white arrow*), which occupies the full thickness of the slice, measures correctly near the attenuation value of water.

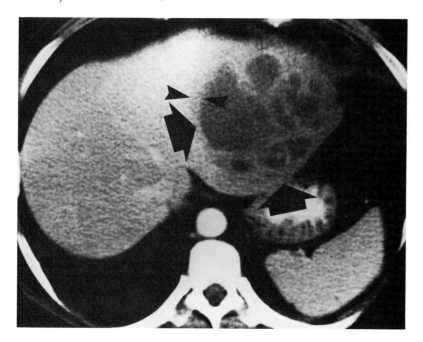

FIG. 41. Hepatic abscess. A large lesion (*arrows*) is present in the lateral segment of the left lobe. There are numerous septations, a well-defined peripheral zone of intermediate attenuation (*arrowheads*), and a relatively homogeneous center of near water attenuation. Despite the presence of septations, such lesions often are satisfactorily drained with a single percutaneously placed catheter. (Courtesy of Dr. Robert Simpson, Selma, Ala.)

cysts (290). The high signal intensity of hemorrhagic cysts on T1-weighted images is due to the shortening of T1 by methemoglobin (34).

Abscesses

Pyogenic abscesses

Patients with pyogenic abscesses usually are symptomatic, with symptoms varying in severity. There is often an association with predisposing conditions. Such conditions as recent surgery, biliary disease, diverticulitis, Crohn disease, and alcoholism predispose to hepatic abscess (30,268). However, the liver abscess may present clinically before the underlying cause of the abscess is evident.

CT. A characteristic CT feature of most abscesses is a peripheral rim or capsule that is enhanced following intravenous contrast material. Occasionally a relatively narrow transition zone of slightly decreased attenuation is encountered between the peripheral rim and the central area of uniformly lower attenuation (268) (Figs. 41 and 42). Most abscesses have sharp, although irregular, external margins, especially on contrast-enhanced images. Internal septations or papillary projections are usual features, and extrahepatic inflammatory changes may occur around the lesion if one border abuts the margin of the liver. Some pyogenic abscesses are multiple, but even in such cases, one of the lesions usually is significantly larger than the remainder. Gas bubbles may be present within the lesion in about 20% of cases, indicating the presence of a gas-forming organism. Uncommonly, an air–fluid level or fluid–debris level is also detected. A large air–fluid level

may indicate communication with the gastrointestinal tract (136).

Cystic, necrotic metastases, as are seen with leiomyosarcoma or ovarian carcinoma, can simulate a hepatic abscess because of the central low attenuation and peripheral rim enhancement (268) (Fig. 43). The necrotic area of a neoplastic lesion may occasionally become infected.

About 90% to 95% of pyogenic hepatic abscesses are successfully treated with a combination of antibiotics and percutaneous drainage (56). Even when abscesses appeared loculated, drainage with one catheter was successful in 11 of 12 cases because septations were incomplete

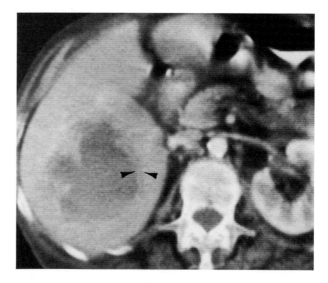

FIG. 42. Hepatic abscess. A large hypodense lesion with irregular borders is seen in the posterior right lobe. A peripheral zone of intermediate attenuation (*arrowheads*) is best seen along its medial border.

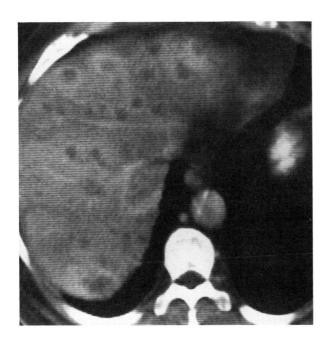

FIG. 43. Infected metastases. Multiple metastases in the liver have a somewhat unusually brightly enhancing border. These proved to be superinfected with a pyogenic organism.

(27,136). When abscesses appear multiple, draining the dominant lesion or lesions usually is satisfactory, because the smaller, remote lesions often resolve following antibiotic therapy. Although some patients may require subsequent surgery to correct the predisposing cause of the abscess or to drain a persistent collection, a trial of percutaneous drainage prior to surgery still is advisable in most cases, rather than simultaneous surgical drainage with correction of the underlying cause of the abscess. If the patient is septic, the improvement in the patient's condition effected by percutaneous drainage may improve the operative risk (96,97).

MRI. There has not yet been a report on MRI for pyogenic hepatic abscesses. However, data from *in vitro* evaluations of different types of body fluids indicate that a large overlap exists in the T1 and T2 values of abscess contents and other fluid collections (40). Therefore, it is unlikely that MRI will increase the diagnostic specificity of the existing imaging methods. In most cases of suspected hepatic abscesses, percutaneous needle aspiration still will be required to firmly establish such a diagnosis.

Nonpyogenic abscesses

Amebic Abscesses. Amebic abscesses most commonly occur in tropical or subtropical climates, and they present with acute pain in about 85% of cases. Patients may also have fever, weight loss, nausea and vomiting, diarrhea, and anorexia. One series included about 80% solitary lesions, with the remaining patients having up to five lesions (156). They have a propensity to peripheral locations, of-

ten invading the diaphragm. Generally, these lesions respond well to medical therapy, with very low mortality.

On CT, they have many features similar to those of pyogenic abscesses. The narrow transition zone of density described with pyogenic abscesses is also seen with amebic lesions (Fig. 44). However, the collections usually are unilocular, and the proper diagnosis may be suggested when this finding is present. Percutaneous drainage, when done because of a presumed pyogenic abscess, usually is uneventful.

Fungal Microabscesses. Fungal microabscesses are most often found in immunocompromised patients, usually with leukemia (26,46,118,244). *Candida albicans* is the most common organism, although *Aspergillus* and *Cryptococcus* are sometimes found. Typically, numerous small, low-density lesions are distributed evenly throughout the liver (Fig. 45). They may also involve the spleen. Some of these lesions may have a small central density zone, so-called target lesions, representing collections of hyphae. Multiple metastases and, rarely, lymphoma or focal fatty infiltration of the liver may simulate fungal microabscesses.

Changes in the sizes of these lesions may correspond to the effectiveness of treatment (26,244). These lesions sometimes resolve completely with treatment, but in other cases may persist or calcify even though the causative organism has been eradicated.

Echinococcal Infection. *Echinococcus granulosus* causing hydatid cysts usually is found in endemic areas and may involve many organs (17,143). However, in the liver, it is usually manifested as an intrahepatic multicystic lesion, often with a capsule (Fig. 46). Daughter cysts are peripherally arranged within the larger cyst, and CT shows decreased attenuation relative to the remaining fluid. Calcification may occur centrally or in the cyst rim (143). A low-signal-intensity rim that probably corresponds to the fibrous capsule (pericyst) of the lesion may aid in its diagnosis by MRI (119). Treatment is surgical removal, and they recur in about one-fourth of cases (142).

Echinococcus alveolaris (multilocularis) differs in radiographic appearance and geographic distribution, being found in Europe, the USSR, and North America (61). Lesions typically are heterogeneous and hyperdense, with irregular contours and indistinct margins. Calcification is found in the majority of lesions. Hepatic hilar lymph node involvement and biliary dilatation are common. The nonspecific appearance of these lesions makes confusion with metastasis likely.

Schistosomiasis Infestations. Schistosomiasis japonica occurs in endemic areas in China, Taiwan, and the southern Philippines and is associated with an increased incidence of HCC (5). Peripheral hepatic or capsular calcification is a hallmark of this disease. Gross pseudoseptations occur in the liver, with geographic bands of calcification and notches in the liver margin. Prominent periportal low-density may also be present (5,109).

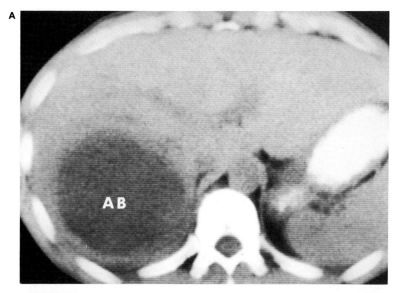

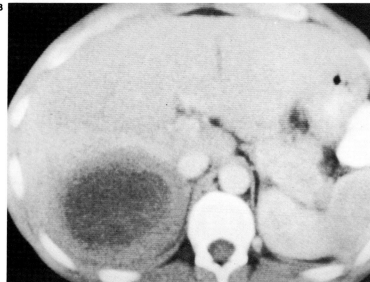

FIG. 44. Amebic abscess. **A:** A large, well-defined, low-density mass (25 HU) (AB) is shown in the posterior aspect of the right lobe, a very common location for solitary abscesses. The patient's history and clinical course were suggestive of an amebic abscess. **B:** Following a rapid infusion of contrast material, a ''halo'' effect is obtained as the perimeter of the abscess appears to enhance slightly compared with the nonenhancing center, consisting of ''anchovy paste'' debris.

FIG. 45. Fungal microabscesses. The association of numerous, widespread small lesions in both the liver and spleen is characteristic of fungal microabscesses, usually in an immunocompromised patient. However, such an appearance can also be seen in metastases from such tumors as melanoma.

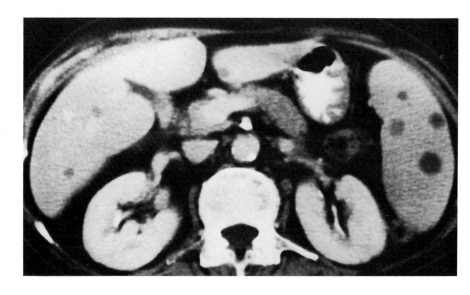

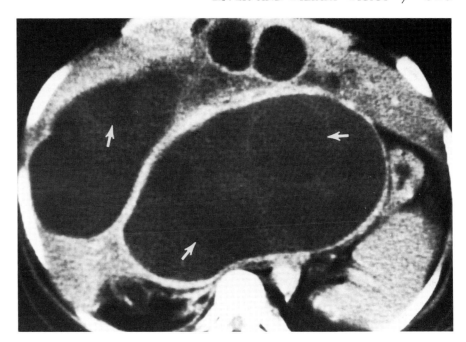

FIG. 46. Hydatid cysts. Note the numerous lower-attenuation daughter cysts (*arrows*) typical of hydatid disease. (Courtesy of Dr. M. A. Rudwan, Ibn Sina Hospital, Kuwait.)

The mansoni variety is endemic to Egypt and appears as low-density, rounded foci, with linear, branching bands encompassing the portal tracts. These bands of fibrosis are enhanced following intravenous contrast material. These lesions do not calcify and should not be confused with metastases, which do not have the branching pattern described (74).

Other Hepatic Lesions

Hepatic adenomatosis

Hepatic adenomatosis appears to be an entity distinct from hepatic adenoma or FNH. Men are affected about as often as women, and the disease is unrelated to contraceptive use. Abnormal liver function tests usually are encountered (85). The CT appearance usually is of an extensive process of many focal lesions that may have an appearance similar to that of multiple adenomas.

Acquired immunodeficiency syndrome

Acquired immunodeficiency syndrome (AIDS) is sometimes manifested within the liver. Lymphoma commonly occurs with AIDS and has a somewhat different manifestation than in a non-AIDS patient. There is an increased likeiihood of focal lesions in the liver, as compared with non-AIDS lymphoma (201). There also is an increased incidence of fungal microabscesses (139).

Angiosarcoma

Angiosarcoma is a rare malignant neoplasm that may arise primarily in the liver. Although these lesions have vascular channels that become brightly enhanced similar to benign cavernous hemangiomas, they usually do not have discrete borders in the entire periphery and generally are larger and more bizarre in appearance (279). This neoplasm has been reported to rupture (169). Use of the older contrast agent Thorotrast is associated with induction of hepatic angiosarcoma (220,246), as is Fowler's solution, containing arsenic, once used as treatment for psoriasis (157).

Nodular regenerative hyperplasia

Nodular regenerative hyperplasia (NRH), also known as nodular transformation, is characterized histologically by diffuse involvement of the liver by hyperplastic nodules composed of cells resembling normal hepatocytes (58). No significant fibrosis is found in or around the nodules, an important feature distinguishing NRH from cirrhosis and FNH. Unlike FNH, NRH may bleed, may be associated with portal hypertension in one-half of cases, and often is associated with a systemic disease such as a myeloproliferative or lymphoproliferative disorder. They often are hypodense on CT, without significant contrast enhancement simulating metastases.

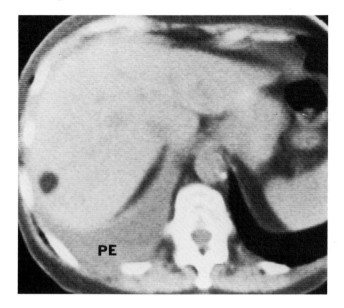

FIG. 47. Hepatic lipoma. Note that the lesion has an attenuation value similar to that of subcutaneous fat. Soft-tissue septae are faintly visible; (PE) pleural effusion.

Bile duct hamartoma

Bile duct hamartoma may be associated with polycystic liver disease. These lesions are composed of proliferating ducts lined by epithelium within a fibrous stroma. They present as numerous small, low-density liver lesions (72).

Fibrolamellar hepatocellular carcinoma

This uncommon variety of hepatocellular carcinoma appears to be an entity distinct from the more common hepatoma. This disease occurs in a younger population, having a mean age of 20 years. Although it is malignant, it has a somewhat better prognosis, with about 25% of patients having resectable lesions, and a mean survival of 32 months for those with unresected lesions (94). Small central calcifications occur in about one-third of patients, and when seen in a young patient, they should suggest the proper diagnosis. Enhancement patterns may be similar to those for FNH or hepatic adenoma. These lesions may even be confusing histologically, especially when only small tissue samples are available.

Hereditary hemorrhagic telangiectasia

These multiple focal liver lesions are associated with enlarged, tortuous hepatic arteries. There is hepatic-arterial-to-hepatic-venous shunting, without clear visualization of discrete enhancing lesions (116).

Lipomas

Hepatic lipomas occur in approximately 10% of patients with renal angiomyolipoma (224). However, hepatic lipomas do not occur exclusively in association with these renal lesions (121). Hepatic lipomas appear as they do elsewhere in the body, as discrete areas of fatty attenuation, sometimes with fine soft-tissue-density septae (Fig. 47).

The MRI appearances of hepatic lipomas have been reported (135). As expected, the signal intensity for hepatic lipoma is identical with that for subcutaneous fat on all pulse sequences. A hepatic lipoma can be easily distinguished from a fat-containing hepatoma because the latter has a very inhomogeneous MRI appearance (135).

Thorotrast

Injection of Thorotrast has been associated with secondary hepatic neoplasms such as angiosarcoma, hepatoma, and cholangiocarcinoma (220,246). Prior to the development of such malignancies, the contrast material, which is taken up by the reticuloendothelial cells of the body, may show a reticular appearance resulting from migration of the contrast material into lymphatics. Both the spleen and, to a lesser degree, the liver have extremely high attenuation values on CT images (Fig. 48).

FIG. 48. Effect of prior Thorotrast administration. Noncontrast CT image demonstrates that the spleen and, to a lesser extent, the liver have abnormally high attenuation values. Multiple high-density lymph nodes are also noted in the hepatic hilus and peripancreatic region. Also noted is an enlarged retrocrural node (*arrow*).

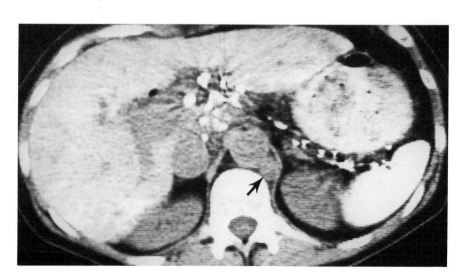

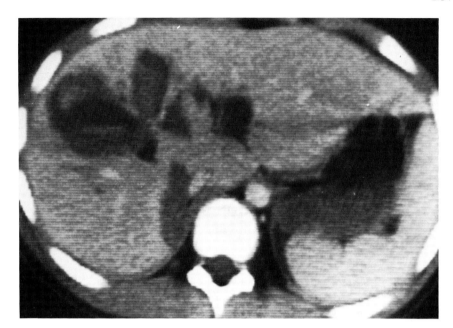

FIG. 49. Traumatic liver fracture. Note the scattered areas of higher attenuation, representing acute intrahepatic hemorrhage, within the irregular-shaped, well-circumscribed lower-density lesion.

Trauma

Blunt trauma, penetrating trauma, and iatrogenic trauma, such as that due to surgery, percutaneous biopsies, and other procedures, may cause hepatic injury (75,79,110,275). Reports vary widely regarding the mortality associated with significant liver injury from blunt trauma. Older studies suggested mortality in the range of 15% to 45% (75).

CT is the best method to determine the presence and extent of liver injury and often is the definitive method for helping to properly direct patient management (75,77,110,185). A feature common to most liver injuries is intrahepatic blood (Fig. 49). Hemorrhage often has a characteristic layered or inhomogeneous pattern caused by successive bleeding and clotting. A portion of the hepatic hematoma usually is in contact with some part of the liver surface (233). Fresh clot must be discriminated from enhancement if intravenous contrast material has been given. Rarely, gas may be present within a traumatic lesion, even though there is no infection or communication with bowel or air, possibly caused by the products of acute tissue necrosis (207).

Intraperitoneal blood may also be present with liver injuries extending to the liver surface. Although other sources of fluid, such as urine, preexisting ascites, or peritoneal lavage fluid, are possibilities, high-density fluid strongly suggests recent bleeding (75,110).

Whereas most intrahepatic hematomas and contusions resolve spontaneously within weeks to several months, posttraumatic cysts or pseudoaneurysms may develop in some cases (110,233,263) (Fig. 50). Focal fatty infiltration is another possible late effect of hepatic trauma (208), possibly related to local vascular injury.

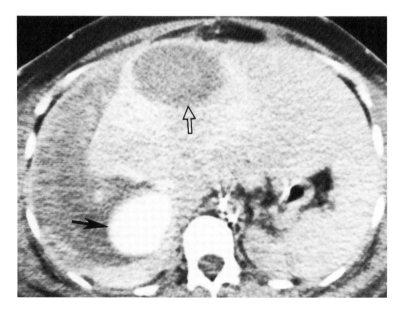

FIG. 50. Posttraumatic hepatic artery pseudoaneurysm in a 45-year-old woman who had blunt trauma to the upper abdomen several months earlier. CT image obtained during infusion of contrast material through a celiac artery catheter shows a pseudoaneurysm (*black arrow*) in the posterior right lobe of the liver. A large intraparenchymal hematoma (*open arrow*) is also present.

A,B

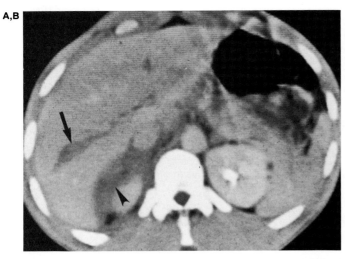
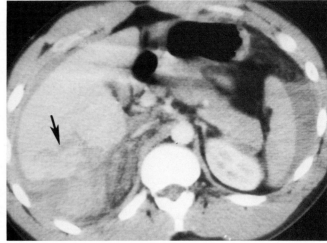

FIG. 51. Liver lacerations. **A:** Postcontrast CT image demonstrates a linear fracture (*arrow*) along the plane of the right posterior portal vein. Blood is present in the Morison pouch (*arrowhead*). **B:** In another patient, a more irregularly shaped fracture is seen in the posterior right lobe (*arrow*). Blood is also present in the greater peritoneal cavity.

Another form of liver injury is laceration or fracture, including the stellate or burst-type fracture (273) (Fig. 51). Large hematomas near the IVC–hepatic-vein junction may indicate a major hepatic vein laceration, and failure to recognize such a finding may result in rapid exsanguination at laparotomy.

Bilomas or bile pseudocysts usually are subcapsular or perihepatic in location (153,190). They are caused by iatrogenic, spontaneous, or traumatic performation of the extrahepatic biliary system (75,79). They usually present as large, homogeneous, thin-walled fluid collections markedly displacing the liver (Fig. 52). These collections sometimes may be treated with percutaneous drainage alone, but surgical repair often is necessary.

Hepatic lobar necrosis may occur, which may be recognized by low attenuation and absence of enhancement. If there is a large amount of devitalized tissue, an abscess may develop (110,233). Another complication of such a lesion is late rebleeding (233).

Subcapsular hematomas and bile leaks may be caused by liver biopsy or other iatrogenic procedures and usually are small collections of no clinical significance (75,275). Patients presenting with acute intraabdominal hemorrhage may be found to have neoplastic liver masses such

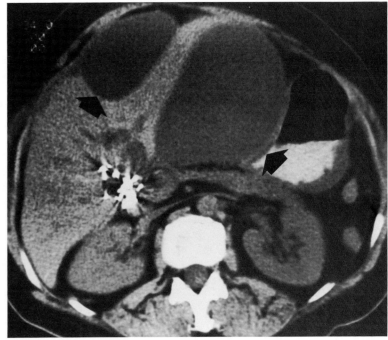
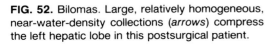

FIG. 52. Bilomas. Large, relatively homogeneous, near-water-density collections (*arrows*) compress the left hepatic lobe in this postsurgical patient.

A,B

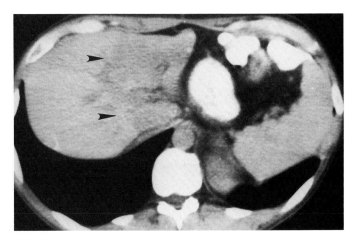 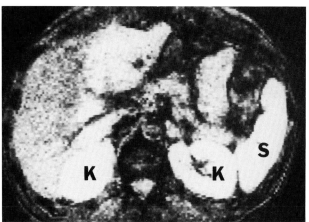

FIG. 53. Radiation hepatitis in 60-year-old man who had received radiation treatment for distal esophageal carcinoma 2 years earlier. **A:** Noncontrast CT image. The medial portion of the liver has a lower attenuation value than the lateral portion. The demarcation between the two areas is straight (*arrowheads*) and corresponds to the prior radiation port. **B:** Proton spectroscopic image (TR = 1,500 msec, TE = 40 msec) at a lower level than **A**. The medial portion of the liver has a higher signal intensity than the lateral portion, reflecting its higher water content. Note the sharp border between the two areas; (K) kidney; (S) spleen.

as hepatoma, adenoma, or metastasis that have bled from relatively minor trauma (57).

Radiation effects

Radiation usually is not applied to the liver for therapeutic purposes, but often the liver is incidentally irradiated to encompass tumors in other organs. The effects of radiation may appear on imaging studies within weeks after the radiation course has been initiated (138,150). Local pain may be experienced that resolves over several months.

A band or zone of low attenuation, caused by some fatty infiltration in the distribution of the radiation port, may be seen (Fig. 53). The cause of the zone of altered attenuation may be suspected because the area of involvement bridges normal anatomic segments. Over a period of weeks, the initially sharp borders of the zone may become more irregular as adjacent areas of parenchyma regenerate. The irradiated area eventually becomes atrophic. Rarely, increased attenuation within the radiation port may occur, presumably because of more severe diffuse fatty infiltration involving the normal portions of the liver (Fig. 54). Another effect of radiation seen soon after completion of a course of radiation has been patchy congestion that may simulate tumor nodules (251).

The MRI appearance of radiation hepatitis has been reported (277). The irradiated area has a uniformly lower signal intensity than normal liver parenchyma on T1-weighted images and a higher signal intensity on T2-weighted or proton spectroscopic images (Fig. 53B). These changes have been attributed to the increase in water content. Although the changes in signal intensity in the irradiated liver are nonspecific and also can be seen in neoplastic disease, the sharply demarcated interface between

normal and abnormal regions seen in radiation hepatitis would be unusual for a neoplastic process.

Miscellaneous

Several other lesions may affect the liver: hepatic lymphangiomatosis (262), mesenchymal hamartoma (99,226), and plasmacytoma (175), as well as others. However, these abnormalities are rare and usually do not have specific CT appearances.

Diffuse Diseases

Neoplasm

Tumors that diffusely involve the liver parenchyma include lymphoma, metastatic breast cancer (Fig. 26), melanoma, and hepatoma in patients with cirrhosis. Several other types of tumors may metastasize to the liver in an extensive pattern. Features of diffuse hepatic neoplasm include hepatomegaly, diffuse liver inhomogeneity, and decreased attenuation on noncontrast images or decreased enhancement on postcontrast examinations. Compression and distortion of normal vascular anatomy may also be present.

Fatty metamorphosis

Fatty metamorphosis is also known as fatty infiltration or fatty change. It occurs in association with numerous disorders and conditions, including obesity, Cushing disease or syndrome, chemotherapy, hyperalimentation, alcoholism, and diabetes (164). Fatty infiltration is caused

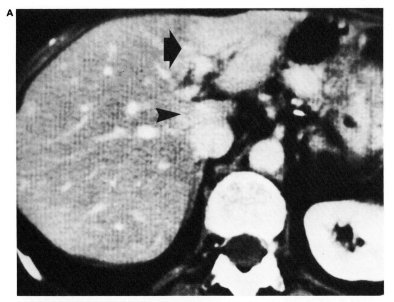

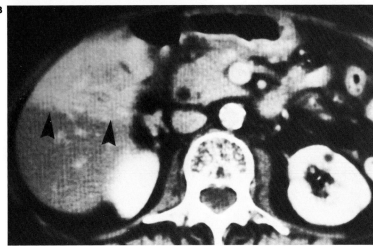

FIG. 54. Radiation effect on the liver. **A:** The liver shows fatty infiltration except within the small left lobe (*arrow*) and caudate lobe (*arrowhead*). These margins formed the lateral boundary of an anterior radiation port. **B:** At a lower level in the same patient there is a horizontal boundary (*arrowheads*) through the right hepatic lobe. The more dense area was within a lateral radiation port. The radiation effect apparently prevented fatty metamorphosis from involving these areas of the liver. Normally, radiation causes relatively decreased attenuation rather than increased density as in this case.

by an accumulation of triglycerides within hepatocytes (108,164).

CT. Although the normal attenuation values for the liver vary from about 50 to 75 Hounsfield units (HU), the difference in attenuation between the liver and spleen is relatively constant, with the liver averaging 8 HU greater than the spleen (212). However, the spleen may appear transiently higher in density when using large doses of intravenous contrast material injected rapidly (25). Therefore, fatty infiltration may be diagnosed on noncontrast images when the liver appears lower in density than the spleen. The diagnosis is more difficult with mild degrees of change when only enhanced images are used.

Fatty infiltration may be focal (Fig. 55) or diffuse (Fig. 6), may appear and be reversed quickly, and may change its pattern of distribution (16,86,164). The diffuse form of fatty infiltration involves hepatomegaly and lower attenuation for the liver tissue (164,249). The liver may become so infiltrated with fat that its natural density appears lower than that for nonenhanced blood vessels. The

measured attenuation value for the liver may be similar to that for water, although the tissue actually produces a combination of soft-tissue density and fatty density.

Focal fatty infiltration may have a spectrum of appearances, from involvement of only one small area of the liver to involvement of nearly the entire liver, with only a small area spared (146,164). The distribution of fatty changes may be lobar or segmental or may involve scattered areas throughout the liver. There may be patchy involvement, with margins that are discrete or vague, at times producing a bizarre geographic distribution (266).

Rarely, fatty infiltration can present as small discrete nodules (9,293) (Fig. 56), some with a central nidus of increased density that may mimic multiple fungal abscesses (293). Larger lesions may also show central areas of increased attenuation (86). Involved areas of the liver can show a mass effect, but usually not as marked as with neoplasms (108). Rather, fatty infiltration often is characterized by a relative absence of a mass effect for the size of the lesion. Blood vessels usually are seen passing

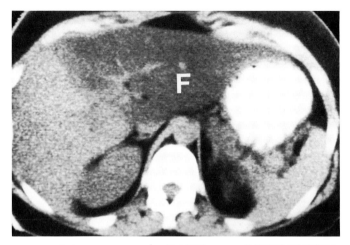

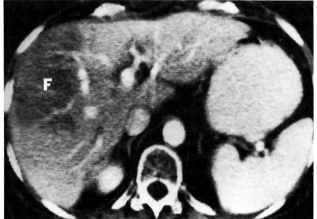

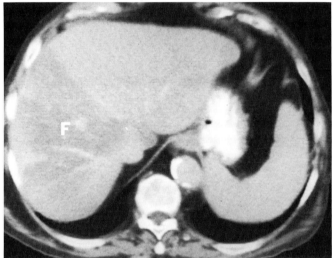

FIG. 55. Three cases of focal fatty infiltration (F). In **A**, the distribution is primarily lobar, whereas in **B** and **C** only a portion of the right lobe is affected by the process.

through the affected area in a normal pattern. In cirrhosis, focal fatty changes may correspond to architectural changes related to fibrosis (266).

Fatty infiltration of the liver sometimes can obscure dilated bile ducts and other liver lesions (164,216). Segmental lucent defects from vascular compromise can be confused with simple fatty changes. Amyloidosis may take on the appearance of fatty change with hepatomegaly, diffuse decreased attenuation, and decreased enhancement. If there are large areas of varied attenuation on CT, but there is normal uptake on liver-spleen scintigraphy, fatty infiltration is more probable than are multiple neoplastic masses (237).

MRI. Conventional spin-echo and inversion-recovery techniques have proved to be insensitive for detection of fatty infiltration of the liver (67,255,257). In experimental models, the signal intensity for the liver was shown to increase only minimally despite massive increases in liver triglyceride content (255). It is certainly rare for even lobar fatty infiltration to be clearly visible as an area of high signal intensity on spin-echo (SE) sequences (289) (Fig. 57).

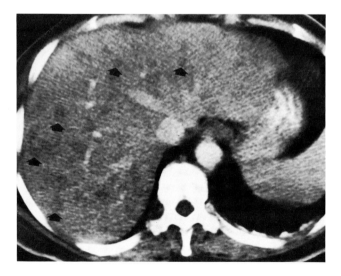

FIG. 56. Unusual appearance of focal fatty infiltration of the liver. There are numerous small rounded foci (*arrows*) of decreased attenuation. These lesions would be compatible with fungal microabscesses on CT alone. Multiple biopsies demonstrated focal fatty infiltration.

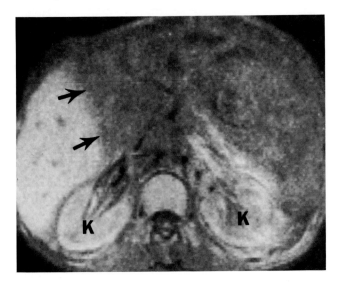

FIG. 57. Lobar fatty infiltration: MR image (TR = 500 msec, TE = 30 msec). The lateral portion of the liver has a high signal intensity corresponding to an area of fatty infiltration on CT. The medial portion of the liver (*arrows*) is of normal signal intensity; (K) kidney.

In contradistinction to conventional SE sequences, proton spectroscopic imaging is a sensitive method for detecting fatty infiltration of the liver. With this technique, diffuse and focal fatty liver can be distinguished from normal liver both visually and quantitatively (114,159). On an opposed image in which pixel brightness is a net difference between water and fat magnetizations, normal liver has an intermediate signal intensity greater than that of muscle, whereas fatty liver generally has a lower signal intensity, equal to or less than that of muscle (Fig. 58). In normal liver, the lipid signal fraction is less than 10%, whereas in fatty liver, it is greater than 10% and usually exceeds 20%. This technique is particularly helpful in dif-

ferentiating between focal fatty infiltration and metastases, because such a distinction occasionally can be difficult with CT (Fig. 59). In addition, proton spectroscopic imaging may be more sensitive than CT or conventional SE techniques for detecting hepatic metastases in patients with associated fatty infiltration (160,261) (Fig. 60).

Cirrhosis

CT. Hepatic cirrhosis involves chronic fibrosis of portal vein sinusoids, leading to redistribution of the blood supply within the liver and abdomen. Characteristic features of advanced cirrhosis include decreased sizes of the right hepatic lobe and medial segment of the left lobe, with corresponding increased sizes of the lateral segment of the left lobe and the caudate lobe (272) (Figs. 61 and 62). Liver margins often are irregular, with inhomogeneous and decreased enhancement after intravenous administration of contrast material. Hepatic and portal vein radicles within the liver are compressed and often difficult to visualize on CT.

A ratio comparing the sizes of the caudate lobe and the right lobe may be helpful in identifying patients with cirrhosis. The caudate is measured transversely from the medial aspect of the caudate to the lateral aspect of the main portal vein. The right lobe is measured from this same point at the portal vein to the right lateral margin of the liver. A caudate-to-right-lobe ratio greater than 0.65 provides 96% confidence in the diagnosis of cirrhosis. A caudate-to-right-lobe ratio less than 0.6 makes cirrhosis unlikely, whereas a ratio of 0.37 is the average for normal livers (111). Several other findings commonly seen in patients with cirrhosis include splenomegaly, ascites, and varices in numerous locations.

MRI. Although early studies with 0.08- to 0.15-T systems showed moderate-to-marked prolongation of T1

A,B

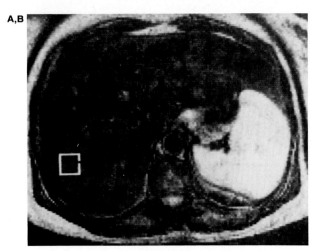 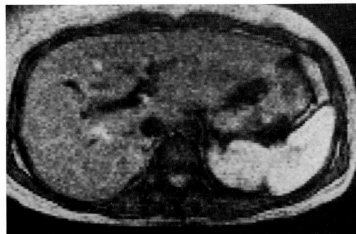

FIG. 58. Demonstration of fatty infiltration by proton spectroscopic imaging (TR = 1,500 msec, TE = 40 msec). **A:** Fatty liver. Note the signal intensity of the liver to be lower than that of paraspinal muscle using this pulse sequence. **B:** Normal liver. The signal intensity of normal liver is higher than that of paraspinal muscle.

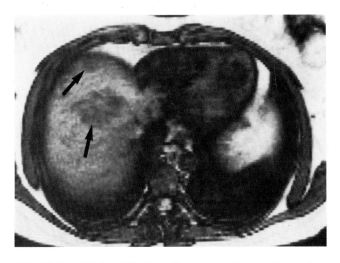

FIG. 59. Focal fatty infiltration. Proton spectroscopic imaging (TR = 1,500 msec, TE = 40 msec) shows two lesions (*arrows*) near the dome of the liver, both of which have a signal intensity lower than that of paraspinal muscle, compatible with focal fatty infiltration. If these were metastases, they would appear as high-signal-intensity areas. Because of the small size of these lesions, a prior CT study was not able to distinguish between these two entities.

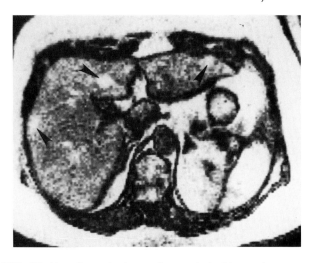

FIG. 60. Hepatic metastases demonstrated by proton spectroscopic imaging (TR = 1,500 msec, TE = 40 msec). Several discrete hyperintense metastases approximately 1 cm in diameter (*arrowheads*) are seen in both lobes of the liver in this patient with a history of breast carcinoma. The findings on CT examination were negative.

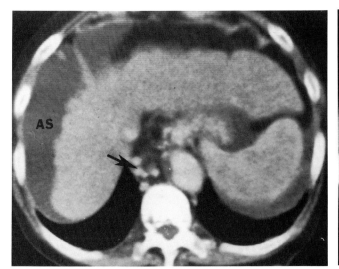
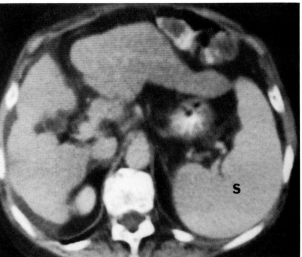

A,B

FIG. 61. Advanced cirrhosis. **A:** Postcontrast CT image demonstrates a small nodular liver. Extensive esophageal and paraesophageal varices (*arrow*) are present; (AS) ascites. **B:** Image 4 cm caudal to **A.** The lateral segment of the left lobe is unusually large compared with the right lobe, a feature commonly seen in advanced cirrhosis. The spleen (S) is enlarged.

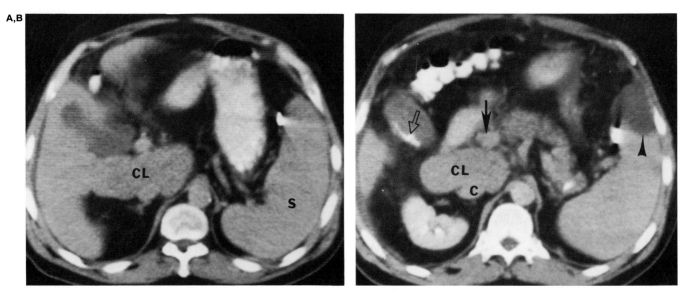

FIG. 62. Advanced cirrhosis. **A:** Both the caudate lobe (CL) and the spleen (S) are enlarged. **B:** Image 3 cm caudal to **A**. The inferior extension of the enlarged caudate lobe (CL) is seen as a discrete mass between the IVC (C) and the portal vein (*arrow*); this should not be confused with a mass of the pancreatic head. Incidentally noted are a splenic infarct (*arrowhead*) and gallstones (*open arrow*).

values, with resultant decreased signal intensities on T1-weighted images, in cirrhosis (41,67,250), more recent investigations using 0.35-T systems have failed to demonstrate any appreciable alterations in MRI characteristics in pure hepatic fibrosis (102). The morphologic changes associated with advanced cirrhosis, however, can be detected by MRI. These include a nodular appearance of the liver, hypertrophy of the caudate lobe, dilated collateral vessels, splenomegaly, and ascites. In patients in whom there are contraindications to administration of iodinated contrast material for CT, MRI is helpful in confirming

the patency of the portal venous system and the presence of collateral vessels (204) (Figs. 63 and 64). In addition, MRI is an accurate method for determining the patency of surgically created portal systemic shunts (29) (Fig. 65).

Hemochromatosis

In primary hemochromatosis, iron accumulates in numerous organs, including the liver, causing increased attenuation. Cirrhosis and portal hypertension occur, and

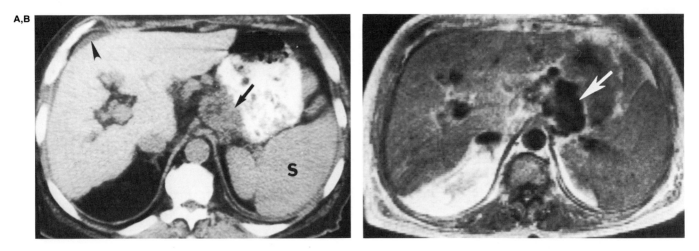

FIG. 63. Esophageal varices in a 70-year-old woman who presented with splenomegaly of unknown cause. **A:** Noncontrast CT image shows a soft-tissue mass in the gastrohepatic ligament (*arrow*) that could represent celiac lymphadenopathy or varices. The spleen (S) is moderately enlarged. A small amount of ascites (*arrowhead*) is present. **B:** MR image (TR = 500 msec, TE = 35 msec) at the same level shows the mass (*arrow*) to be vascular in nature, compatible with varices.

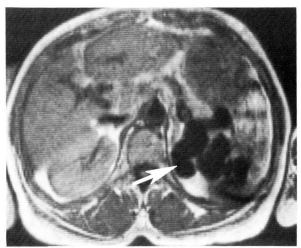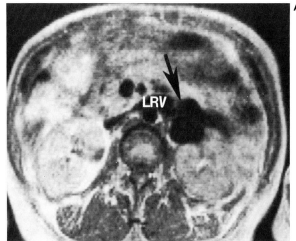

FIG. 64. Spontaneous splenorenal shunt. **A:** MR image (TR = 500 msec, TE = 35 msec) shows a dilated and markedly tortuous vessel (*arrow*) originating from the splenic hilum. **B:** MR image (TR = 2,100 msec, TE = 35 msec) 5 cm caudal demonstrates the junction between collateral vessel (*arrow*) and the left renal vein (LRV).

congestive heart failure may ensue because of myocardial deposition.

Secondary hemochromatosis results from iron overload and deposition of iron within the reticuloendothelial system, thus increasing densities for both liver and spleen on CT (Fig. 66A).

Hemochromatosis, either primary or secondary to such conditions as thalassemia or hemosiderosis, results in a dramatic reduction in hepatic MRI signal intensity (31,35,161,231,255) (Fig. 66B). Tissue iron is detected by MRI not because it creates a signal but because it is paramagnetic and decreases the relaxation times of nearby hydrogen nuclei (39,259). It has been shown that ferric ions cause shortening of both T1 and T2 values, although the T2 effect predominates at a concentration greater than 15 mmol/liter. The marked shortening of T2 by ferric ions accounts for the extreme low signal intensity in the liver in patients with iron-overload disease.

Although the diagnosis of hemochromatosis by MRI is easy, quantitative assay of iron levels using clinical imaging systems has been difficult because of the fairly broad range of normal values for both T1 and T2 in the liver (39). Similarly, because the T1 and T2 values for a normal liver fluctuate with time, and the degree of this variation is fairly large relative to the expected changes due to iron deposition in the tissue, the potential for use of MRI in monitoring the treatment of patients with iron load is also doubtful (39).

Amiodarone toxicity

Amiodarone is an antiarrhythmic medication that may cause markedly elevated liver density, usually without a marked change in splenic attenuation, a feature that distinguishes it from hemochromatosis. The cause of the increased density relates to the accumulation within hepatocytes of the drug or its metabolites, which contain iodine. The density change may itself provide an index for the degree of toxicity, which primarily manifests itself as a diffuse interstitial lung disease (173).

Glycogen storage disease

This entity involves accumulation of glycogen within liver cells. The density of glycogen itself leads to an elevated liver density in many patients with this disease (65). However, some patients have concomitant fatty infiltration that moderates the increased attenuation or actually

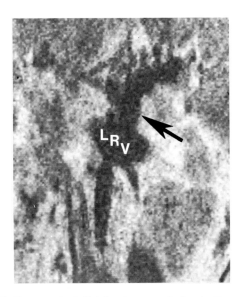

FIG. 65. Postsurgical distal splenorenal shunt. Coronal MR image (TR = 500 msec, TE = 70 msec) shows a patent distal splenorenal shunt (*arrow*) and a dilated left renal vein (LRV).

A,B

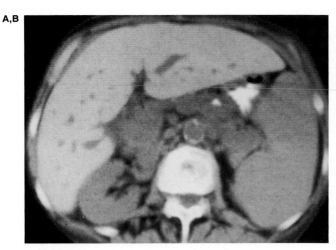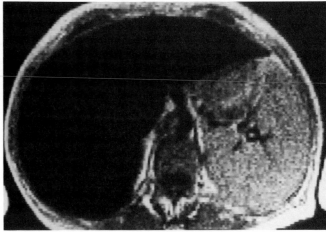

FIG. 66. Hemochromatosis. **A:** Noncontrast CT image shows the liver to have a much higher attenuation value than the visceral organs. **B:** MR image (TR = 500 msec, TE = 30 msec). The liver is extremely low in signal intensity.

causes a density lower than normal. There is an increased incidence of primary hepatic tumors in glycogen storage disease, and these must be distinguished from areas of focal fatty infiltration.

Gold storage

Gold preparations injected for treatment of rheumatoid arthritis accumulate in the reticuloendothelial system, leading to a markedly increased liver density (59).

Miscellaneous

Other conditions such as Dubin-Johnson syndrome (230), hemophilia (141), and Wilson disease (53,62) may affect liver attenuation measurements. However, in these diseases, the degree of overlap with the normal range is

too great to make attenuation measurements diagnostically useful.

Disorders of Hepatic Vessels

Portal Vein Thrombosis

CT. Partial or complete thrombosis of the portal venous system may be caused by hypercoagulable states such as occur in polycythemia vera, other hematologic disorders, various malignant neoplasms, or infections. Extrinsic compression or invasion by tumor or trauma may lead to thrombosis of part or all of the portal venous system (183) (Fig. 67). This entity often produces a clinical enigma, because patients present with acute or subacute nonspecific abdominal pain. In the past, this condition

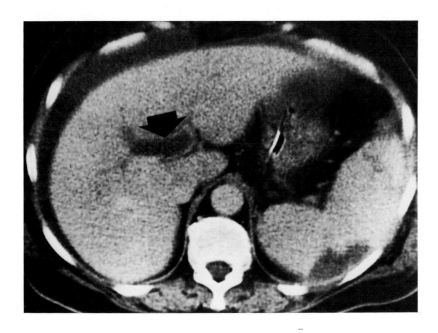

FIG. 67. Spontaneous portal vein thrombosis. Note the low attenuation within the central portal vein (*arrow*). There are also scattered low-attenuation areas in the spleen representing infarcts. Ascites is present.

A,B

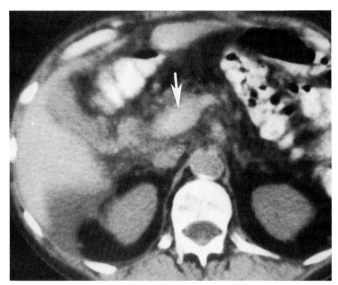
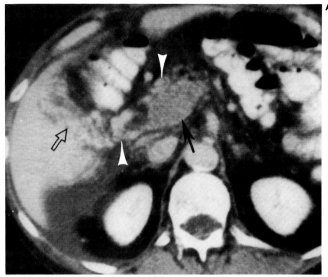

FIG. 68. Cavernous transformation of the portal vein in a 55-year-old man with no history of prior illness who presented with acute abdominal pain. **A:** Noncontrast CT image shows a hyperdense thrombus in the portal vein (*arrow*). **B:** Postcontrast image demonstrates extensive collaterals (*arrowheads*) around the thrombosed portal vein (*arrow*), as well as in the gallbladder fossa (*open arrow*). Note that the portal vein was not enhanced after contrast material was given.

often went unrecognized, but it is now readily diagnosed with CT and ultrasound.

Portal vein thrombosis usually is best seen with the incremental dynamic imaging technique (183). Acutely, the involved vessels enlarge. The vessel wall may appear somewhat thickened and enhanced, or there may be a small amount of contrast material passing around the thrombus. The vessel has a relatively low central density, and there may be regional alterations of the contrast-enhancement pattern within the liver (177,265). Serial CT

examinations may demonstrate a change in the location or extent of thrombus, recanalization of part of the vessel, or retraction of the intravascular thrombus, perhaps with collateral vein enlargement (177). Portal vein thrombosis may cause extensive periportal collaterals to dilate markedly, which has been termed "cavernous transformation of the portal vein" or "portal cavernoma" (177,223) (Fig. 68).

MRI. Tumoral or nontumoral thrombi produce intraluminal signals (Fig. 69) and usually can be differentiated

A,B

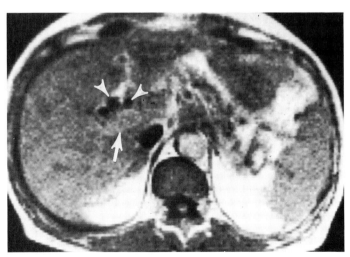
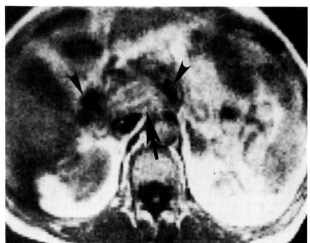

FIG. 69. Portal vein thrombosis. **A:** MR image (TR = 500 msec, TE = 30 msec). The main portal vein (*arrow*) contains medium-intensity signal, whereas the hepatic artery branches (*arrowheads*) appear as areas of signal void. **B:** Three centimeters caudal, the thrombosed portal vein (*arrow*) is surrounded by clusters of signal-void structures (*arrowheads*); the latter represent collateral vessels or portal cavernoma.

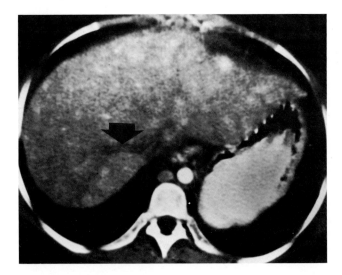

FIG. 70. Hepatic veno-occlusive disease. There is inhomogeneous enhancement of the liver, with contrast pooling around small hepatic arterial branches. A small, thrombosed right hepatic vein is seen (*arrow*).

from slow flow by comparing the signal intensities on the first and second echoes or by using phase-sensitive imaging sequences (73,122). However, in patients with portal hypertension, distinction between these two entities may be difficult (291). Demonstration of periportal collaterals ("portal cavernoma") often aids in the diagnosis of portal vein occlusion (227).

Hepatic Veno-occlusive Disease (Budd-Chiari Syndrome)

Hepatic veno-occlusive disease can lead to abdominal pain and has multiple causes. For example, neoplasm, medications, paroxysmal nocturnal hemoglobinuria, polycythemia vera, systemic lupus erythematosus, and trauma have been associated with this disorder (112,228), and it may occur in infancy.

CT. The CT appearance is characterized by hepatomegaly and ascites. The hepatic veins usually are not clearly visualized (Fig. 70). Early during dynamic imaging there is patchy increased attenuation centrally near the IVC. Later, this enhancement changes to decreased attenuation, with general hepatic inhomogeneity. One often sees enhanced lobules of the liver, with progressive spread of this appearance from the caval area outward (112,194,228,292). In chronic cases, the caudate lobe is enlarged.

A similar CT appearance of the liver, consisting of lobulation and patchy inhomogeneity, is seen in patients with congestive heart failure (Figs. 71 and 72). The pathophysiologies are similar. However, the appearance differs from that of Budd-Chiari syndrome in that in patients with congestive failure, the hepatic veins are patent and enlarged, rather than thrombosed or obliterated (120).

MRI. Specific features of Budd-Chiari syndrome that can be demonstrated on MRI include reduction of caliber or complete absence of the hepatic veins, multiple "comma-shaped," signal-void foci representing intrahepatic collateral vessels, and/or marked constriction of the

A,B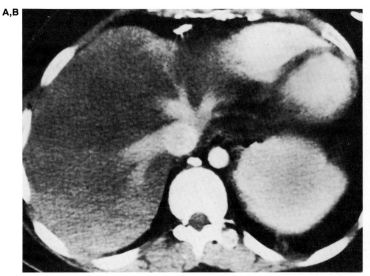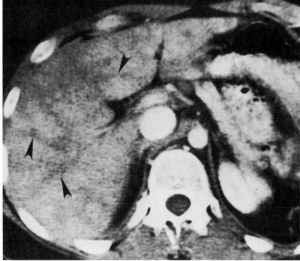

FIG. 71. Liver enhancement pattern in a patient with severe, chronic congestive heart failure. **A:** At the beginning of dynamic imaging, the liver shows less than usual enhancement because of a very slow circulation time. Also, contrast material injected in the arm has refluxed through the right atrium into the IVC and hepatic veins. **B:** Later during imaging the hepatic enhancement has taken a lobulated pattern, with apparent poorly enhancing septae (*arrowheads*). Subsequently, the liver eventually became homogeneously enhanced.

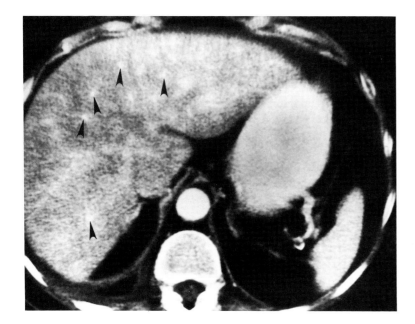

FIG. 72. Early phase of enhancement in a patient with congestive heart failure. There is a punctate type (*arrowheads*) of enhancement that represents enhancement of small hepatic artery branches and the immediately surrounding parenchyma.

intrahepatic IVC (95,258) (Fig. 73). Nonspecific findings such as ascites and hepatomegaly likewise can be seen. Although compression and distortion of hepatic veins also can be seen in patients with end-stage cirrhosis, a patient with acute or treated Budd-Chiari syndrome usually has a smooth, normal-size liver without extrahepatic varices, in contradistinction to a small nodular liver seen in end-stage cirrhosis.

Arterial Abnormalities

Arterial enlargement is seen in conditions in which the portal venous flow is compromised, such as cirrhosis, or in which hepatic arterial flow is increased by arterioportal shunting, such as may occur with hepatoma. After trauma, a posttraumatic false aneurysm or an arteriovenous fistula may form (87) (Figs. 50 and 74).

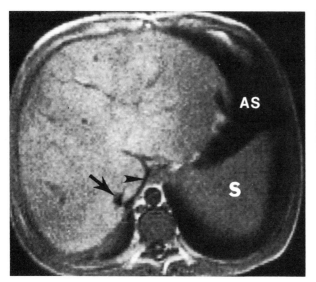
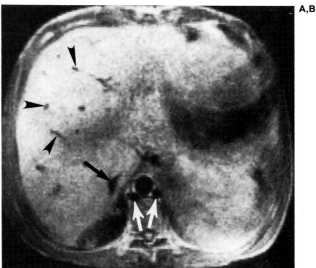

A,B

FIG. 73. Budd-Chiari syndrome. **A:** T1-weighted MR image (TR = 300 msec, TE = 15 msec). The liver is large and diffusely inhomogeneous in signal intensity. The IVC (*arrow*) is small, and normal hepatic veins are not visible; (S) spleen; (AS) ascites; (*arrowhead*) ascites surrounding the caudate lobe. **B:** Proton-density image (TR = 2,100 msec, TE = 35 msec) demonstrates multiple comma-shaped signal-void areas representing intrahepatic collateral vessels (*arrowheads*). The IVC (*black arrow*) is compressed; the azygos and hemiazygos veins (*white arrows*) are dilated.

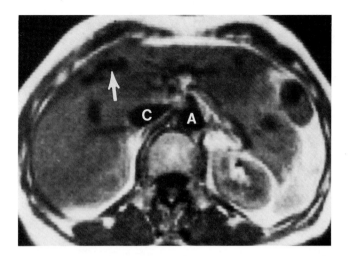

FIG. 74. Arterial venous fistula secondary to prior liver biopsy. MR image (TR = 1,500 msec, TE = 35 msec) shows a serpiginous signal-void area (*arrow*) in the periphery of the quadrate lobe (the site of a prior liver biopsy); (C) IVC; (A) aorta.

If hepatic arterial branches are occluded, hepatic infarcts may develop, with subsequent atrophy of the involved lobe (Fig. 75). Hepatic infarcts may present confusing appearances, because the lesions may be round or oval and centrally located, rather than wedge-shaped and peripheral. They may be poorly demarcated, low-density areas that progress to become confluent, with distinct margins (162). Infarcts may also contain gas and therefore be mistaken for abscesses (162). Bile lakes caused by disruption of biliary radicles may also be seen (211) (Fig. 76).

Segmental Density Alterations

Lobar segmental or subsegmental regions of altered density may appear as a result of arterioportal shunting or venous compression/occlusion. In the case of arterioportal shunting, segmental areas of increased enhancement are seen transiently early after a bolus injection because of the dual rapid flow of both arterial and portal flows into the affected areas (199) (Fig. 77). An arterioportal shunt may result from cirrhosis, as well as primary or metastatic tumor, in which portal vein invasion causes such shunting (132,198). A posttraumatic arteriovenous fistula, such as may be caused by percutaneous biopsy, can also cause such shunting.

In the case of venous compression or occlusion, the affected area has a lower attenuation value on noncontrast images and can be confused with focal fatty infiltration. It is postulated that the lower attenuation value seen in this condition may be caused by glycogen depletion (66). Both portal and hepatic vein occlusions may cause this effect, because both processes divert blood from the affected areas. Chronic portal vein occlusion may also lead to lobar or segmental atrophy (265) (Fig. 77).

Liver Transplantation

CT is useful for evaluating patients prior to liver transplantation (158) and for following possible complications of the surgery (238). Because no anastomosis of lymphatics is performed during liver transplantation, early after transplantation there is accumulation of lymphatic fluid within the liver in a characteristic pattern. This is repre-

A,B

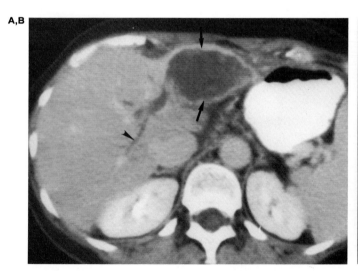 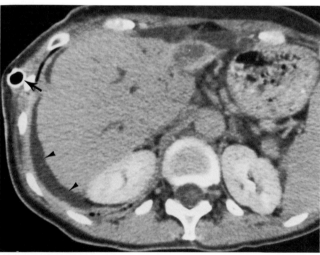

FIG. 75. Hepatic infarct secondary to intraarterial chemotherapy. **A:** Postcontrast CT image demonstrates no enhancement of the lateral segment except its peripheral border (*arrows*); (*arrowhead*) dilated intrahepatic biliary radicles. **B:** Follow-up CT image several months after **A**. Note marked diminution in the size of the lateral segment, which is not enhanced in this postcontrast image. A thoracostomy tube (*arrow*) and ascites (*arrowheads*) are also present.

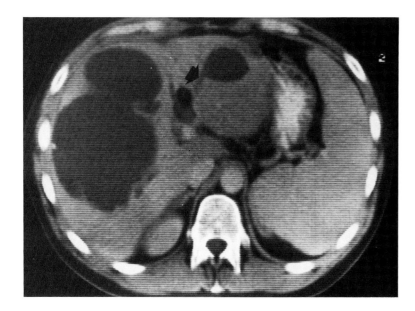

FIG. 76. Bile lakes. Postcontrast CT image demonstrates several large, low-attenuation lesions within the liver. This patient had been undergoing hepatic arterial infusion chemotherapy, with resolution of visible colonic carcinoma metastases. These large lesions developed over a 2-month period and represent bile lakes rather than recurrent metastases. Mild biliary dilatation was caused by hepatic arterial infusion chemotherapy. Note the dilated bile duct (arrow) leading into the smaller collection. Bile lakes probably result from biliary obstruction, and they are difficult to distinguish from simple hepatic cysts except by history and the identification of biliary obstruction.

sented as a halo of decreased density surrounding the IVC and portal venous radicles (172) (Fig. 78). Interestingly, a similar pattern of apparent lymphatic obstruction and dilatation occurs in patients with Budd-Chiari syndrome and congestive heart failure, as well as conditions that can directly affect the draining lymphatic pathways, such as malignant lymph node enlargement or hematomas compressing the cisterna chyli or thoracic duct secondary to trauma.

In hepatic transplants, lobar areas of inhomogeneous low attenuation are highly suggestive of partial or complete hepatic artery obstruction with ischemia (238) (Fig. 78B). Such occurrences may require retransplantation for survival. Other transplant complications, such as bilomas, abscesses, and hematomas, are well diagnosed by CT. Although CT is essential to evaluate patients suspected of having complications of liver transplants, CT must be supplemented by other examinations such as arteriography and Doppler ultrasound to assess vascular patency.

Diseases of the Biliary Tract

By appropriate utilization of a variety of laboratory tests of liver function, combined with the pertinent historical and physical findings, the clinician is able to determine the correct cause in the majority of patients presenting with clinical or biochemical evidence of jaundice. Despite their high predictive ability, it is now common practice to make use of the noninvasive imaging capabilities of ultrasound and CT to confirm or correct the clinical impression rapidly. In addition to demonstrating the presence or absence of morphologic changes that will be indicative of obstructive jaundice (extrahepatic cholestasis), both CT and ultrasound can show the precise level and, in many cases, the actual cause of obstruction (15,149,184,210,240).

Techniques

With the exception of occasionally being able to define the main right and left hepatic ducts, the normal-caliber intrahepatic biliary tree is not visible, except when air is

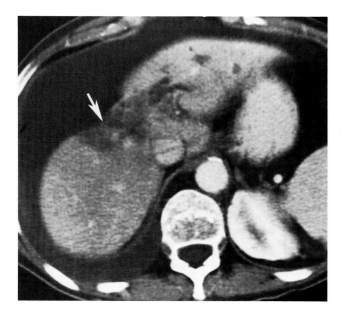

FIG. 77. Lobar attenuation difference due to metastatic breast carcinoma. The metastatic disease (arrow) has diminished in size since a previous image, accounting for the indentation in the liver margin. However, the left lobe has been enhanced more by intravenous contrast material than has the right lobe. Such a finding may be caused by shunting of blood through neoplastic fistulas between hepatic artery and portal vein branches, or by increased arterial perfusion compensating for focal portal venous obstruction. Ascites is also present.

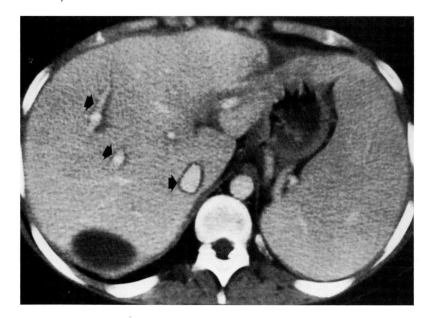

FIG. 78. Liver transplant. There are fine hypodense areas (*arrows*) encompassing the IVC and adjacent to portal vein radicles. These represent lymphatic congestion, which tends to disappear after several months. This patient also has splenomegaly and a small perihepatic fluid collection posteriorly.

present (Fig. 79). The techniques of examination for biliary disease generally are the same as the techniques for evaluating focal and diffuse liver disease. Intravenous iodinated contrast material is necessary to detect minimal dilatation of the intrahepatic biliary tree with confidence. Enhancement of the hepatic parenchyma and vasculature causes the nonenhancing branches of the biliary tree to become more visible. The use of intravenous contrast material also greatly assists in evaluation of the extrahepatic portion of the biliary tree by enhancing the contiguous vascular structures and the pancreatic parenchyma,

causing the normal or dilated common duct to be much more detectable in its cross-sectional, end-on appearance. It has been reported that the normal-caliber extrahepatic common duct, ranging in diameter from 2 to 6 mm, can be identified in approximately 50% of patients (55,89) (Fig. 80). However, this figure probably will be substantially higher with consistent use of dynamic imaging during contrast enhancement, especially when thin collimation (4–5 mm) and smaller fields of reconstruction are used.

Opacification of parts of the biliary tract with oral or intravenous cholangiographic agents is also possible (105,215). However, these agents have not achieved widespread acceptance or utility in CT evaluation of the biliary tree.

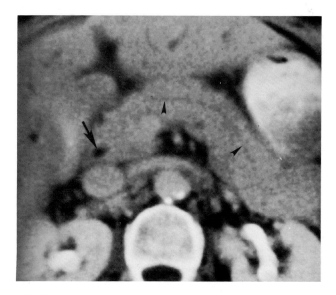

FIG. 79. Numerous branching gas collections (*arrowheads*) within the liver representing intrabiliary air. This patient previously had a biliary bypass procedure. Gas within the biliary tree tends to accumulate ventrally. However, the flow of bile often prevents the gas from extending to the extreme liver periphery, as may be seen with portal venous gas.

FIG. 80. Normal common bile duct (*arrow*) and pancreatic duct (*arrowheads*) are clearly seen on this postcontrast image obtained with 5-mm collimation.

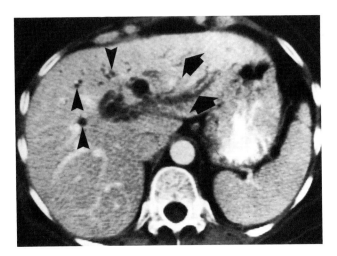

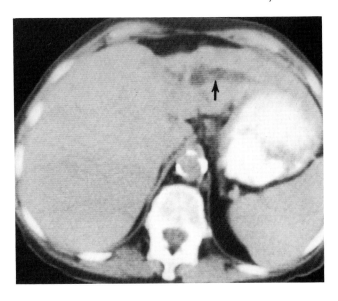

FIG. 81. Moderate biliary dilatation of the left hepatic lobe secondary to a postsurgical stricture. Dilated ducts are seen both in longitudinal section (*arrows*) and cross section (*arrowheads*). Ductal dilatation generally differs from venous thrombosis in appearance because the ducts tend to be more tortuous and irregular in caliber.

FIG. 82. Isolated dilatation of the left hepatic duct system (*arrow*) in this patient was associated with atrophy of the left hepatic lobe secondary to a vascular injury, rather than actual obstruction of the ducts.

In most cases, contiguous 1-cm-thick sections are imaged from the dome of the liver to the level of the third duodenum. By proceeding in this sequential fashion, one can trace the entire biliary system, measure the length of the dilated common duct proximal to the point of obstruction, and predict whether the junctional, suprapancreatic, intrapancreatic, or ampullary portion of the duct is the site of the obstructing lesion (15,210). Additional information often can be gained by using high-resolution techniques with thinner collimation (4–5 mm) and magnification CT techniques (19,55), which are especially helpful in evaluating the porta hepatis.

Jaundice, Biliary Obstruction, Choledocholithiasis

CT. The CT diagnosis of biliary obstruction is based on demonstration of dilated intrahepatic or extrahepatic bile ducts. Dilated intrahepatic bile ducts will be apparent as linear, branching, or circular structures of near water density, enlarging as they approach the junction of the left and right hepatic ducts in the porta hepatis (Fig. 81). Rarely, infiltrating periductal neoplasms may mimic biliary dilatation (187). There may be a predilection for more severe dilatation involving the left lobe than the right lobe, even when the cause of obstruction is extrahepatic in location (44).

Although it may be difficult to appreciate mild-to-moderate biliary dilatation without the use of intravenous contrast material, it is still possible with good-quality scans. Whereas the portal veins normally are lower in attenuation than the hepatic parenchyma on noncontrast images, the bile ducts are still lower in attenuation. Therefore, it may be possible to discriminate between the

near water density of the dilated biliary system and the blood density of the portal venous system.

Segmental dilatation of only a portion of the intrahepatic biliary tree, with the remainder of the intrahepatic and extrahepatic biliary tree appearing normal, can be demonstrated with CT (7) (Fig. 82). In these patients, the serum bilirubin level may be normal, and the clue to biliary tract disease may be an elevated serum alkaline phosphatase. Intrahepatic focal obstruction may be caused by neoplasm, inflammation, trauma (196), stricture, or stones. Chronic obstruction may lead to focal hepatic atrophy (Fig. 83).

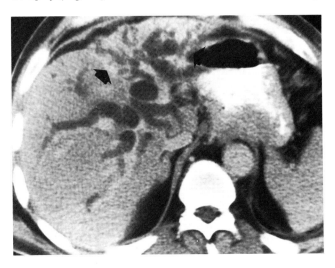

FIG. 83. Marked biliary dilatation in a patient with cancer of the pancreatic head. There is marked atrophy of the left lobe of the liver (*arrows*), with resultant crowding of the dilated ducts. This feature may also be found in some patients with cholangiocarcinoma.

A,B

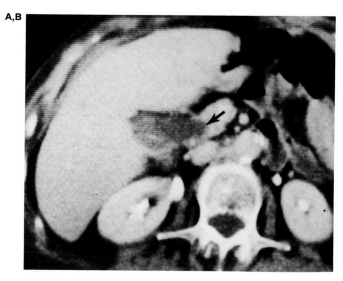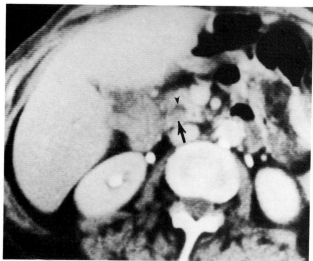

FIG. 84. A: No detectable intrahepatic biliary dilatation was present in this patient with a mildly dilated (10 mm), obliquely oriented common duct (*arrow*) at the point where it enters the head of the pancreas. **B:** Two centimeters caudad, a tissue-density calculus (*arrow*) nearly fills the lumen of the distal common bile duct, leaving a crescent of bile (*arrowhead*) as a clue to the presence of this intraluminal filling defect. This crescent sign should be carefully sought when common duct stones are suspected and an obvious calcified stone is not initially detected. (From ref. 64.)

The extrahepatic bile duct is considered unequivocally dilated if it is 9 mm or more in diameter (15,191). Ducts of 7 or 8 mm are of borderline size and raise the suspicion of obstruction. Those less than 7 mm are considered normal in caliber. These size criteria should apply equally to postcholecystectomy patients. One study has shown that there is no consistent increase in the caliber of the common bile duct following cholecystectomy (191). If the duct is normal in caliber prior to cholecystectomy and measures larger subsequently, some element of obstruction should be suspected.

Unfortunately, there is not always a direct relationship between the caliber of the biliary tree and the presence or absence of clinically significant obstruction. In patients with significant dilatation of the biliary tree in whom the obstruction is later relieved surgically or by spontaneous passage of a calculus, the bile duct may remain somewhat more dilated than normal for the remainder of the patient's life. In such patients, CT findings can falsely suggest the presence of biliary obstruction. In patients with little or no clinical or biochemical evidence for biliary obstruction in whom CT shows a dilated bile duct but no tumor, calculus, or other obstructing lesion, one must be skeptical about the presence of obstruction. In this situation, percutaneous cholangiography can be used to determine how readily bile passes from the dilated bile duct into the duo-

A,B

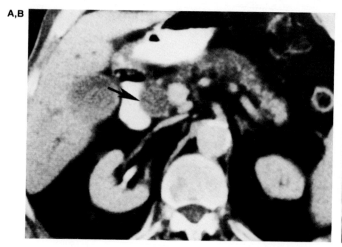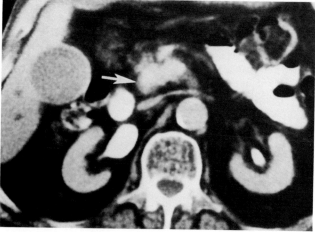

FIG. 85. Biliary obstruction due to pancreatic carcinoma. **A:** A dilated common bile duct (*arrow*) is noted in the pancreatic head. **B:** One centimeter caudal to **A**, the common bile duct is not visible. This type of abrupt termination of a dilated common duct is highly suggestive of a malignant process. A small tumor was found in the uncinate process (*arrow*) at surgery.

denum and whether or not a stricture is present in the distal common bile duct. Radionuclide imaging using imidodiacetic acid derivatives, i.e., technetium-HIDA, may provide similar functional evaluation.

Isolated dilatation of the extrahepatic bile ducts, without intrahepatic biliary duct dilatation, has been well documented in patients with proven biliary obstruction (15,210,240) (Fig. 84). Also, a normal-caliber bile duct can be present with a surgically correctable cause of jaundice (192,240). Intermittently obstructing calculi and subtle strictures of the extrahepatic ducts may be present when overall duct caliber is normal. When the clinical course, including liver function tests, suggests the possibility of an intermittent or low-grade obstruction, while CT or ultrasound examination demonstrates a duct of "normal" caliber, cholangiography by the percutaneous or endoscopic route may be necessary to provide more precise anatomic details.

Evidence of main pancreatic duct dilatation would help to localize the level of obstruction to the pancreatic or ampullary segment (22,210). By careful attention to the appearance of the transition point from dilated to narrowed (or obliterated), one can make further predictions

concerning the nature of the obstruction. For example, an abrupt transition from dilated to obliterated would be most characteristic of neoplasm (Fig. 85), whereas a gradual continuous tapering of the common duct into and through the pancreatic segment would be far more characteristic of narrowing due to chronic pancreatitis (Fig. 86). In such an instance, the pancreas and peripancreatic areas should be carefully evaluated for additional signs of pancreatitis, such as thickening of renal fascia and pancreatic pseudocysts. When present, pancreatic pseudocysts may appear to cause, but usually do not by themselves cause, biliary obstruction. Rather, the associated fibrotic changes in the pancreatic head in chronic pancreatitis are likely to cause the typical long-tapered obstruction (284).

The combination of abrupt termination and absence of a mass may be caused by either a common duct stone (137) or a small tumor (13). The degree of ductal dilatation is not necessarily diagnostic regarding the nature of the process. However, malignant obstructions tend to cause more severe degrees of dilatation (14).

The detection of a common bile duct stone by CT is dependent on its composition. When a common bile duct stone is calcified (Fig. 87), its identification is easy if nar-

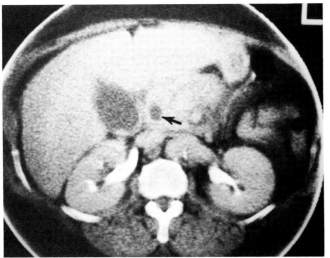

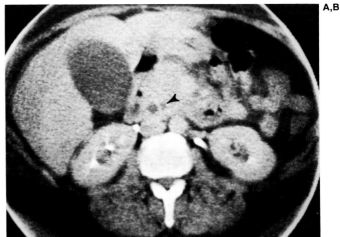

A,B

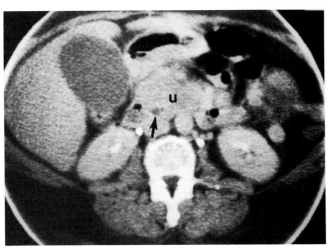

C

FIG. 86. Biliary obstruction due to pancreatitis. **A:** Postcontrast CT image at the level of the pancreatic head shows a mildly dilated common bile duct (*arrow*). **B:** One centimeter caudal, the common bile duct is less dilated at this level; (*arrowhead*) pancreatic duct. **C:** One centimeter more caudal, the uncinate process (U) is enlarged, and there is further reduction in the caliber of the common bile duct (*arrow*). The gradual tapering of the dilated common duct is characteristic of a benign process.

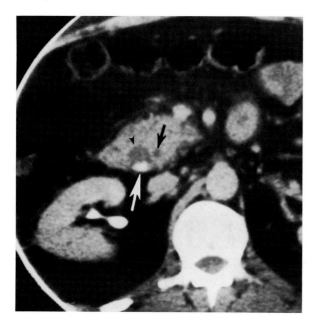

FIG. 87. In this patient with intermittent pain and fluctuating serum bilirubin concentrations, moderate dilatation of the common bile duct (*arrowhead*) and slight dilatation of the pancreatic duct (*black arrow*), shown here at the level of the uncinate process of the pancreas, were due to impaction of a small calcium bilirubinate stone in the ampulla. Several other stones (*white arrow*) are seen layered in a dependent position just proximal to the point of obstruction. Although they may not be visible on a radiograph, some stones found within the gallbladder and biliary tree will contain sufficient calcium to be seen on CT.

sound is generally used first to evaluate the biliary system (81,98,179). CT is reserved for patients in whom (a) sonographic abnormalities indicate ductal dilatation, but do not clearly establish the level and cause of the obstruction, (b) sonographic findings are equivocal, or (c) there is strong clinical suspicion of biliary obstruction despite apparently normal findings on sonography. In patients who are obese and in those with prior biliary-enteric bypass procedures, one can anticipate the likelihood of an unsatisfactory sonographic examination, and in these patients, CT is the optimal initial procedure. We currently reserve percutaneous cholangiography or endoscopic retrograde cholangiography for patients in whom both CT and ultrasound findings are equivocal or unsatisfactory, or for patients in whom a fluoroscopically guided biliary drainage procedure is planned. In selected patients with ductal obstruction high in the porta hepatis, we also employ percutaneous cholangiography to help the surgeon decide if a surgical biliary-enteric bypass procedure is feasible.

MRI. Image blurring and ghosting due to respiratory motion are major problems in evaluating the biliary system. Although MRI is capable of demonstrating dilated intrahepatic and extrahepatic bile ducts, as well as determining the extent of obstruction (63), it offers no advantage compared with ultrasound and CT. As in the case of a normal biliary system, dilated bile ducts usually have a low signal intensity on T1-weighted images and high signal intensity on T2-weighted images.

row scanning intervals and collimation of 4 to 5 mm are used. If noncalcified, it may appear as an intraluminal soft-tissue density, with lower-density bile surrounding it, creating what is called a "target sign," or as a soft-tissue density in the dependent part of the bile duct, with a "crescent" of lower-density bile anteriorly (Figs. 84B and 88).

Intrahepatic ductal calculi are uncommon in Western countries. These may form spontaneously or may be found in Caroli disease or proximal to stenosis of a previous surgical anastomosis (182). Because intrahepatic calculi often are of soft-tissue density, CT tends to miss cases of intrahepatic calculi or underestimate the number of stones present (7,52,182). Also, calcified hepatic granulomas can be mistaken for intrahepatic calculi.

CT has proved to be useful and accurate in establishing a diagnosis of biliary obstruction. In one study, obstruction was correctly identified in 96% of cases (15). Accuracy rates for CT in determining the level of obstruction have been reported as high as 90% (98), and for the cause of biliary obstruction, up to 70% (13). However, it remains controversial whether CT or ultrasound is more sensitive for determining the exact level and cause of obstruction and determining the resectability of tumors (15,81,98,155,202). Because of its lower cost, absence of ionizing radiation, and relatively high accuracy, ultra-

Cholangiocarcinoma

Cholangiocarcinoma is a primary malignancy of bile ducts, usually adenocarcinoma, that develops in some pa-

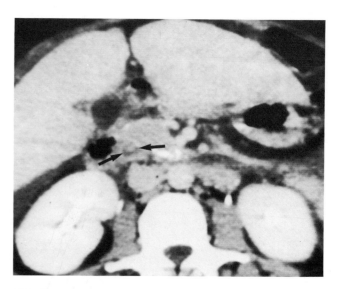

FIG. 88. Noncalcified common bile duct stone. A rim of bile (*arrows*) surrounds a noncalcified common duct stone, creating a target-like appearance.

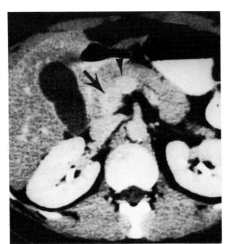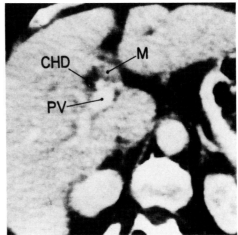

A,B

FIG. 89. Cholangiocarcinoma: CT appearances. **A:** In this patient with cholangiocarcinoma of the distal common bile duct, the tumor (*arrow*) is enhanced almost to the same degree as the superior mesenteric vein (*arrowhead*). (Courtesy of Dr. Arthur Bishop, Peoria, Ill.) **B:** In another patient, the tumor (M) is enhanced to a lesser degree than the portal vein (PV). If it were not for the dense opacification of the blood vessel and the narrow slice collimation (4 mm), the mass would not have been detected; (CHD) dilated common hepatic duct.

tients with gallstones, liver fluke infestation, biliary papillomas, and chronic ulcerative colitis complicated by sclerosing cholangitis. Cholangiocarcinoma may also arise within a choledochal cyst. About half of cholangiocarcinomas are located at the ductal bifurcation or distal common duct, causing bilobar biliary obstruction. They may also occur peripherally within the liver (128). The usually small, stricturing cholangiocarcinoma arising at the junction of the right and left hepatic ducts is known as a Klatskin tumor (48). Patients with cholangiocarcinoma present with jaundice and weight loss in over three-fourths of cases (271). Occasionally a peripheral cholangiocarcinoma is resectable for cure when it does not involve the caudate lobe, IVC, or lymph nodes in the porta hepatis (48). Central tumors are almost always unresectable.

CT. A minority of cholangiocarcinomas will be enhanced on dynamic images, but when they are not, the primary tumor may be difficult to identify (64,128) (Fig. 89). Biliary obstruction may be the most prominent CT feature. Because often such tumors arise in the central intrahepatic biliary system, one must suspect cholangiocarcinoma when intrahepatic biliary dilatation is associated with a normal-size extrahepatic biliary system. When a cholangiocarcinoma is located more peripherally, it may simply present as an intrahepatic mass and simulate hepatocellular carcinoma or metastases (271) (Fig. 90). Disparities between the degrees of biliary dilatation in the left and right lobes may occur despite the central location of the obstruction (48), with a tendency for the left-lobe biliary system to dilate more than the right-lobe system. Klatskin tumors may more completely obstruct one hepatic duct than the other.

Some patients with cholangiocarcinoma may have lobar atrophy, with dilated, crowded ducts. This may be a result of concomitant venous obstruction. Although this sign has been described as occurring in cases of cholangiocarcinoma (48,280), it may also occur in other instances of chronic focal biliary obstruction.

The appearance of rounded cystic masses with internal papillary projections has been described as a characteristic feature of some cholangiocarcinomas in Japan, but these observations have not been reported from other populations (128).

One study of over 104 cases of primary sclerosing cholangitis found 13 examples of progression to cholangiocarcinoma (168). These cases of malignant degeneration were characterized by more marked biliary dilatation, progressive dilatation on follow-up, progressive stricturing, and more frequent occurrence of intraductal polypoid masses on direct cholangiography.

MRI. Cholangiocarcinomas may appear as soft-tissue masses that are either slightly hypointense or isointense with the liver on T1-weighted images and hyperintense with the liver on T2-weighted images (Fig. 91). Although well-differentiated adenocarcinomas often exhibit marked hyperintensity on T2-weighted images, the scirrhous subtype is only slightly higher in intensity than normal liver parenchyma. This is because the scirrhous subtype is partly composed of fibrous stroma, which characteristically has a short T2 value (64). Encasement of the adjacent vessels and contiguous and distant metastases likewise can be shown on MRI. In one study, MRI was superior to CT in demonstrating the extent of the tumor, but CT was better in showing intrahepatic bile duct dilatation (64). It is presumed that MRI will not be able to differentiate between primary sclerosing cholangitis and cholangiocarcinoma unless secondary signs such as metastases to the liver or lymph nodes are present.

A,B

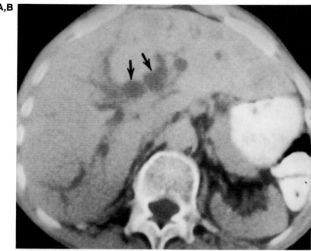 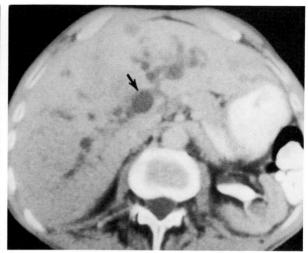

C

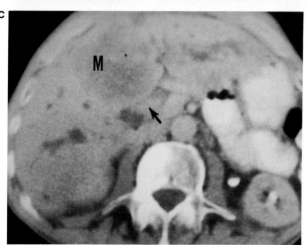

FIG. 90. Cholangiocarcinoma, with obstruction of the common hepatic duct and metastasis to the liver. **A:** The left and right hepatic ducts (*arrows*) and their tributaries are grossly dilated. **B:** At the level of the proximal common hepatic duct (*arrow*), the diameter of the duct measures 18 mm. **C:** Two centimeters caudad, the lumen of the common hepatic duct is obliterated, and in its expected location, only a small soft-tissue density (*arrow*) is present. A large metastatic lesion (M) replaces and enlarges the medial segment of the left lobe. The study confirms the presence and level of biliary obstruction and strongly suggests the cause and stage of the malignant process based on the CT findings alone. (From ref. 64.)

Biliary Cystadenoma and Cystadenocarcinoma

The categorization of these neoplasms under the biliary system is somewhat arbitrary. Although these rare tumors apparently arise from biliary tissue, they usually present in adults as large intraparenchymal lesions. They have a multilocular, cystic appearance and vary in size from 3.5 to 25 cm in diameter (254) (Figs. 92 and 93); 85% grow from intrahepatic ducts, and the remainder from the extrahepatic biliary system. These masses usually have a higher density than simple cysts, and the masses may have fluid–fluid levels, mural nodules, or septations. Although these lesions usually do not have the typical features of benign cysts, abscesses, or echinococcal (hydatid) cysts, they may be confused with cystic hepatic metastases.

Sclerosing Cholangitis

Primary sclerosing cholangitis may occur unassociated with prior medical conditions, but often it is seen in patients with preexisting conditions, such as ulcerative co-

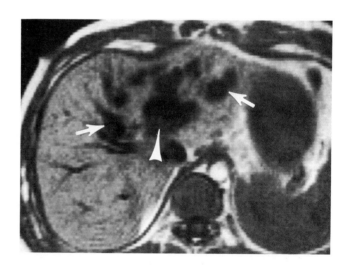

FIG. 91. Biliary obstruction secondary to cholangiocarcinoma. T1-weighted MR image (TR = 300 msec, TE = 15 msec) shows marked dilatation of left intrahepatic ducts (*arrows*). A mass (*arrowhead*) with signal intensity intermediate between those for liver and bile is seen near the origin of the left hepatic duct.

A,B

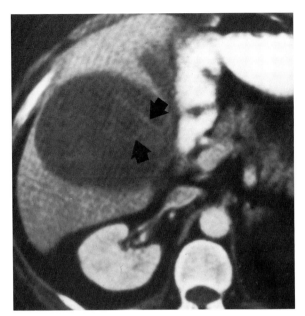 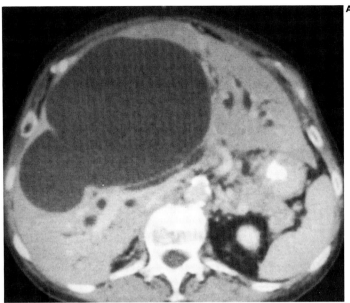

FIG. 92. Biliary cystadenoma. **A:** Well-defined cystic lesion within the liver. This differs from most other benign liver cysts in that several septations (*arrows*) are clearly seen. **B:** Postcontrast CT image in another patient shows a large multiloculated cystic mass in the liver causing proximal biliary obstruction.

litis, retroperitoneal fibrosis, and Riedel's struma (242). Sclerosing cholangitis may progress to produce cirrhosis and portal hypertension (3,50,217). Secondary sclerosing cholangitis is caused by prior biliary surgery, biliary stones, carcinoma, or prior infection.

Sclerosing cholangitis usually leads to nonuniform biliary dilatation, with segmentation and beading of ducts

(Fig. 94). Focal discontinuous areas of minimal dilatation help differentiate this disease from other causes of biliary dilatation, such as tumor, stone, or an inflammatory mass. Such a pattern of discontinuous dilatation can also be seen in a diffuse form of cholangiocarcinoma (217). Thickening of the bile duct wall is another finding in sclerosing cholangitis (50).

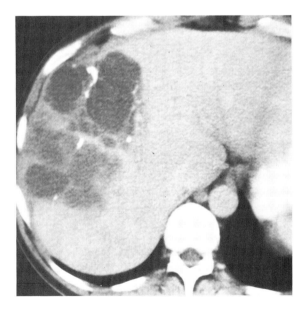 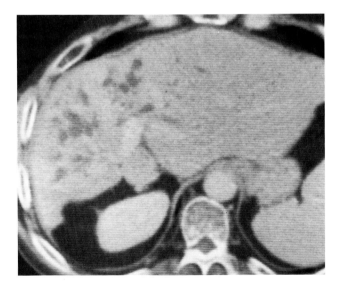

FIG. 93. Biliary cystadenocarcinoma. Postcontrast CT image demonstrates a complex cystic mass with multiple calcifications and soft-tissue septae in the right lobe of the liver. The mass was reported to be present at surgery 30 years ago and had increased in size during the last 2 years.

FIG. 94. Sclerosing cholangitis. Postcontrast CT image shows nonuniform dilatation of intrahepatic bile ducts, with focal areas of narrowing and dilatation. This type of beaded appearance is characteristic of sclerosing cholangitis. In addition, there is atrophy of the right lobe, with compensatory hypertrophy of the left lobe.

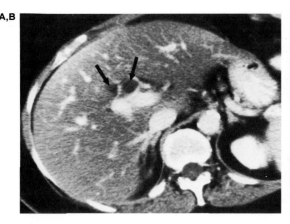
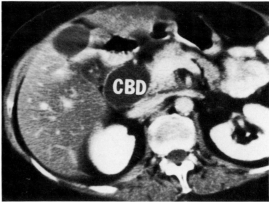

FIG. 95. Choledochal cyst, Alonso-Lej type I. A: The right and left hepatic ducts (arrows) are mildly enlarged on this postcontrast CT image. The more peripheral branches are not dilated. B: Four centimeters caudal, a markedly dilated common bile duct (CBD), measuring 5 cm in maximum diameter, and a normal-size gallbladder are noted. The duct tapered rapidly below this point to a normal caliber at the ampulla. The findings in this case are diagnostic of a choledochal cyst.

Infectious Cholangitis

Infectious cholangitis may be caused by many organisms, usually of gastrointestinal origin. However, *Candida* or parasites may also infect the biliary tree (219). Features of infectious cholangitis include gas within the biliary tree, common bile duct wall thickening, and dilated ducts. There has also been a reported case of portal vein gas associated with pyogenic cholangitis (60). However, these findings are not specific and can be found in other conditions.

Cystic Diseases of the Biliary Tree

Several diseases may affect the biliary tree by causing cystic changes. One entity is the choledochal cyst, which usually involves focal dilatation of the common bile duct alone or may be associated with proximal intrahepatic biliary dilatation (104,221) (Fig. 95). There may be widespread ductal dysplasia, with multiple areas of dilatation within the liver, and an abnormal pancreatic duct. The common duct dilatation may be disproportionately large for the degree of intrahepatic dilatation, and chronic ulcerations may occur within the dilated common duct, leading to strictures or cholangiocarcinoma. Surgical resection may be indicated.

Another condition is the choledochocele, in which the wall of the common bile duct herniates into the duodenum and is demonstrated as a cystic mass contiguous with the distal common bile duct (38,214). A common bile duct diverticulum may be demonstrated as a focal outpouching of the common duct.

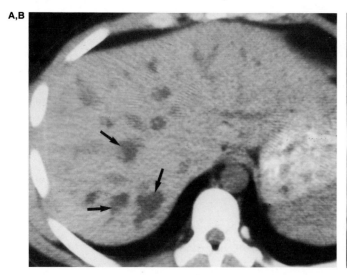
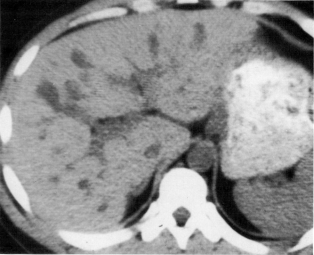

FIG. 96. Caroli disease. A: A cluster of near-water-density cystic-appearing areas (arrows) is noted in the right lobe of the liver. B: Three centimeters caudal, several of the cystic areas appear to be arranged in a branching pattern similar to that of bile ducts, suggesting the diagnosis of Caroli disease.

Caroli disease causes marked segmental dilatation of intrahepatic bile ducts, with numerous liver cysts scattered throughout the liver (195,252) (Fig. 96). This may initially be difficult to differentiate from polycystic liver disease; however, most of the cysts in Caroli disease are arranged in a branching pattern. The use of an intravenous cholangiographic agent with delayed images can confirm communication of the large cyst cavities with the biliary system, which does not occur with simple cysts. Administration of radiopharmaceuticals that are concentrated in the biliary system may also be diagnostic.

Mirizzi Syndrome

The Mirizzi syndrome involves extrinsic compression of the common hepatic duct in patients with cholecystitis and cholelithiasis (124). This usually is caused by extrusion of stones through the gallbladder or cystic duct to compress and involve the common hepatic duct, causing obstruction (148,209). It is clinically important to recognize this prior to attempted treatment, because it may lead to unrewarding exploration of the common duct, followed by postoperative persistence of obstruction because the extraluminal obstructing process is unappreciated. Alternatively, a cavity with edema and inflammation can be formed by the erosion of a stone through the wall of the cystic duct or gallbladder that may appear to be gallbladder itself; consequently, the common hepatic duct is mistaken for the cystic duct leading from it. This confusing anatomic appearance at surgery may lead to inadvertent ligation and transection of the common duct, followed by jaundice or fistula formation (124).

The CT appearance of Mirizzi syndrome includes widening at the gallbladder neck, calculi outside the gallbladder, an irregular cavity near the gallbladder neck, and suprapancreatic obstruction of the extrahepatic common duct (24,209).

Oriental Cholangiohepatitis

This disease has several names, including oriental cholangiohepatitis, recurrent pyogenic cholangitis, and simply a non-Western pattern of biliary stones (76,236,278). The entity is found in endemic areas in Japan, China, Indonesia, Hong Kong, and South Africa, as well as in immigrants to the United States from these areas. Clinically, the disease presents with recurrent cholangitis, with jaundice, hepatosplenomegaly, and abdominal pain. The disease is found in individuals of low socioeconomic status and may be related to diets very low in protein and fat. However, infection with enteric organisms such as *Escherichia coli* is often documented, as is infestation with the Chinese liver fluke or *Ascaris lumbricoides*.

CT will reveal gross dilatation of intrahepatic and ex-

trahepatic ducts, with the presence of sludge and casts known as "biliary mud," stones, concretions, and strictures (76). Treatment consists in removal of as much of the intraductal matter as possible, but this is always difficult and often unsuccessful, and recurrence is the rule, with frequent fatalities.

Hepatic Arterial Infusion Pump

Many patients on hepatic-arterial infusion-pump (HAIP) chemotherapy develop jaundice, sometimes transiently. Although some develop obstruction caused by progression of metastatic tumor, many develop a 1- to 3-cm tapering stricture near the bifurcation of the common hepatic duct (4,32,113,213,241). This probably is caused by the toxicity of the chemotherapy infusion on the wall of the bile duct (4,113). On CT, wispy soft-tissue strands may be seen at the site of obstruction. On direct cholangiography, this may be mistaken for extrinsic compression. This process usually causes only mild-to-moderate diffuse intrahepatic biliary dilatation (Fig. 97), although it can also be focal and may be seen in patients without any symptoms. In the latter patients, serum alkaline phosphatase may be elevated.

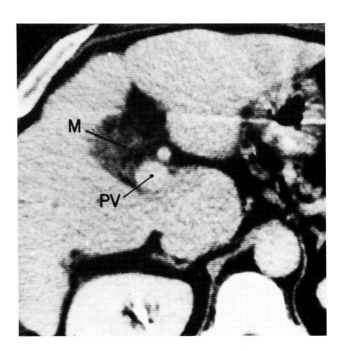

FIG. 97. Biliary obstruction secondary to HAIP chemotherapy. Amorphous soft-tissue strands (M) are noted in the porta hepatis surrounding the common hepatic duct in this patient who had received 5-FU treatment via an indwelling intraarterial catheter for colon metastases. Mild intrahepatic ductal dilatation was present on a higher image (not shown). Surgical biopsy of amorphous strands yielded only fibrosis.

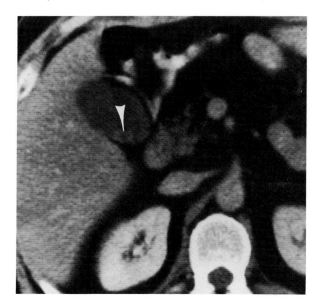

FIG. 98. Faintly calcified gallstones (*arrowhead*).

Gallbladder

Calculi

CT is inferior to ultrasound for detection of gallstones (10). However, CT may reveal unsuspected cholelithiasis during studies performed for other reasons. Densely or faintly calcified stones compose the pattern most often found. In some cases there is a rim of calcification sur-

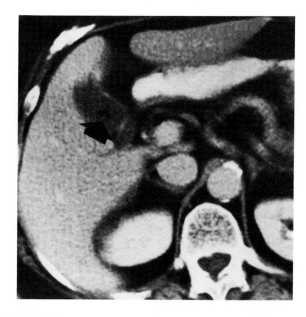

FIG. 99. Triradiate low-attenuation structure (*arrow*) within the gallbladder represents gas within a cholesterol stone. This is the CT appearance of the Mercedes-Benz sign, so called because of its resemblance to the auto insignia. The stone itself is difficult to see because the cholesterol component of the stone is isodense with bile.

rounding an otherwise low-density stone (Fig. 98). Cholesterol stones may be recognized because they are of lower attenuation than surrounding bile. We have also seen examples of the so-called Mercedes-Benz sign, in which a triradiate cleft in a cholesterol stone fills with gas (Fig. 99). Stones that tend to be missed on CT are cholesterol stones that are isodense with bile (10,18).

On MRI, the majority of gallstones produce no signal because of the lack of mobile protons (Fig. 100). Some gallstones, usually the mixed type, may emit a measurable signal from the center (186,188). This central signal is thought to originate from water in clefts or pores within the stone (186).

Inflammatory conditions

CT. Cholecystitis may cause visible gallbladder-wall thickening and nodularity. Gallstones, poor definition of the wall, gallbladder dilatation, and increased bile density may also be seen (144). Chemical cholecystitis may be associated with HAIP (49).

Severe cholecystitis, gangrenous cholecystitis, or gallbladder empyema may be included under the common name of complicated cholecystitis. Pathologically, there may be wall thickening, with an inhomogeneous texture of the gallbladder wall; bile, pericholecystic fluid, and inflammatory changes in fat may be present adjacent to the gallbladder. Although CT can demonstrate these changes (247) (Fig. 101), it tends to underestimate the degree of wall thickening (267). Also, even with gallbladder empyema, the attenuation of bile may not exceed 20 HU. Gallstones were seen with CT in only 65% in the preceding series, but were present at pathological examination in all but one of the remainder. Gas may be present within the

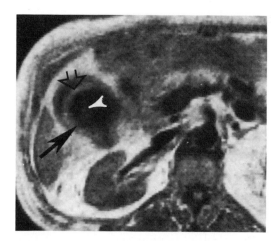

FIG. 100. MRI appearance of a gallstone (TR = 2,100 msec, TE = 35 msec). The stone (*arrow*) appears as an area of extreme low signal intensity, with stronger signal originating from its center (*arrowhead*); (*open arrow*) a crescent of bile in the gallbladder.

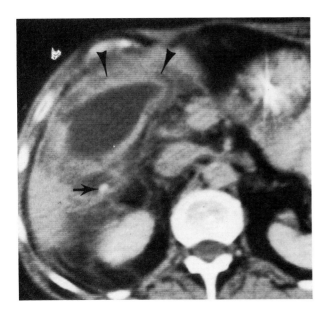

FIG. 101. Complicated cholecystitis. Postcontrast CT image demonstrates a distended gallbladder with a thickened wall. A well-defined halo (*arrowheads*) surrounds the anteromedial aspect of the gallbladder, whereas amorphous soft-tissue densities are seen adjacent to its posterolateral border. There is also infiltration of the pericholecystic and perirenal fat. At surgery, a gangrenous gallbladder with pericholecystic inflammation was found; (*arrow*) gallstone.

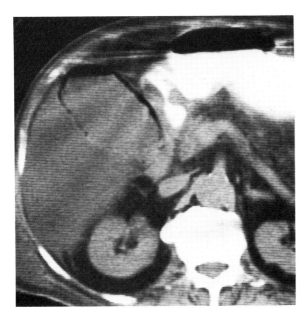

FIG. 102. Emphysematous cholecystitis in a diabetic man. Air is present in the wall, as well as in the lumen of the gallbladder.

gallbladder or gallbladder wall in some cases of empyema (144) (Fig. 102).

In about one-fifth of patients, this CT appearance of complicated cholecystitis may be missed. In others, the CT findings may precede severe symptoms, leading to skepticism on the part of the patient's clinicians regarding the severity of the illness. In the series discussed earlier (267), a gallbladder cause for the patient's symptoms was the most likely initial clinical diagnosis in only 7 of 23 patients.

MRI. The MR signal intensity of bile in the gallbladder has been used to diagnose cholecystitis (123,180). In one study, gallbladder bile was shown to be hyperintense compared with the liver in healthy volunteers and in patients with asymptomatic gallstones on images obtained after 12 hr of fasting using a TR of 500 msec and TE of 56 msec. In contradistinction, 5 of 8 patients with symptomatic cholecystitis had hypointense bile in the gallbladder (180). This hypointensity persisted with prolongation of TR and TE parameters. However, *in vitro* MRI evaluation of gallbladder bile obtained from normal subjects as well as patients with either acute or chronic cholecystitis showed significant overlap in mean T1 and T2 values among all three groups (165). It is uncertain at present what role, if any, MRI will play in the evaluation of patients suspected of having gallbladder disease.

Other Inflammatory Conditions

Xanthogranulomatous cholecystitis causes irregular thickening of the gallbladder wall, with a poorly defined border. The size of the gallbladder may be large or contracted. Localized calcifications may be present, with a poorly defined interface with the liver. The appearance may be so bizarre as to mimic cancer of the gallbladder (68).

High-density bile or milk-of-calcium bile may be seen in cystic duct obstruction or chronic cholecystitis (276). Adenomyomatosis is another condition that may be suggested by its CT appearance. It may be possible to identify the intramural diverticula representing Rokitansky-Aschoff sinuses in this disease (33).

Fistulas between the gallbladder and duodenum usually are caused by cholelithiasis or peptic ulcer disease (106). However, malignancy such as pancreatic carcinoma may cause such fistulas (218).

Gallbladder Neoplasms

Cancer of the gallbladder is uncommon in the United States, but is frequent in populations with a high incidence of gallstones and cholecystitis, such as Central and South American Indians. Cancer of the gallbladder is characterized by a mass filling and replacing the gallbladder, a

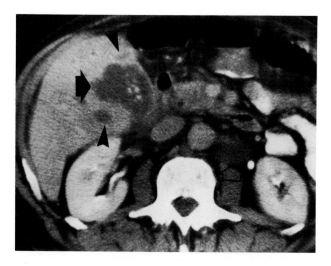

FIG. 103. Carcinoma of the gallbladder. The gallbladder contains several calcified stones. The lateral margin (*arrow*) of the apparent gallbladder is ill-defined, and other low-attenuation areas (*arrowheads*) are seen adjacent to the gallbladder. Retroperitoneal adenopathy (*open arrow*) is also present.

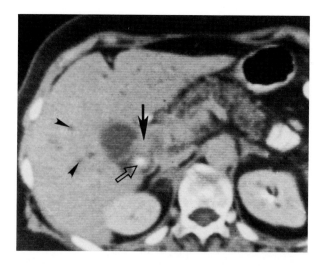

FIG. 104. Gallbladder carcinoma causing proximal biliary obstruction. Postcontrast CT image shows a soft-tissue mass (*arrow*) along the medial wall of the gallbladder, extending into the portocaval space. There is dilatation of intrahepatic radicles (*arrowheads*), but not the extrahepatic duct, indicating a proximal obstruction; (*open arrow*) calcified gallstone.

mass protruding into the gallbladder lumen, or focal thickening of the gallbladder walls (Figs. 103 and 104). Sometimes there is invasion of the adjacent liver, with bulging of the quadrate lobe, fistula formation to adjacent organs, proximal biliary dilatation, and retroperitoneal or liver metastases (18,129,285,294). Gallstones are found in nearly all patients, and the survival rate is poor. On CT, metastatic nodes to the region of the pancreatic head may be mistaken for a primary pancreatic cancer.

Metastases to the gallbladder from other primary tumors are uncommon. In our experience they have most commonly been caused by melanoma (Fig. 105).

Gallbladder-Wall Thickening

Thickening of the gallbladder wall is a nonspecific finding that may occur with hypoproteinemia, hepatitis, pancreatitis, cholecystitis, or other conditions. At times, this thickening can be mistaken for apparent pericholecystic fluid (103).

Porcelain Gallbladder

Calcification may occur within the gallbladder wall, termed porcelain gallbladder (Fig. 106). This condition is recognized by diffuse or focal dense or faint calcification of the gallbladder wall. It is possible to confuse the presence of a large stone with a calcified rim within a contracted gallbladder for a porcelain gallbladder. One small study of patients found a 33% incidence of gallbladder carcinoma (145).

Hemobilia

Hemobilia may occur secondary to trauma (e.g., iatrogenic), with either a hepatic artery or portal vein fistula to the biliary system. Hemobilia may be identified by the high density of bile contents. There may be a laminated appearance of blood clots within the gallbladder caused by successive episodes of bleeding and clotting (21,151).

Pneumobilia

Gas within the gallbladder or biliary tree is not a specific finding and can be caused by biliary-enteric bypass, a biliary drainage catheter, an incompetent sphincter of Oddi, sphincterotomy, cholecystoduodenal fistula, cholangitis, or cholecystic infection with a gas-forming organism (218). At times it is difficult to recognize the presence of gas within the gallbladder because an air–fluid level in this area may resemble a simple air–fluid level within a loop of bowel.

HEPATIC CONTRAST AGENTS FOR CT AND MRI

CT

Several different types of intravenous contrast agents have been tested or are currently under evaluation. One of these agents is EOE-13. This has been found to be useful because the agent is taken up by normal reticuloendothelial cells, but not by neoplasms, leading to a marked

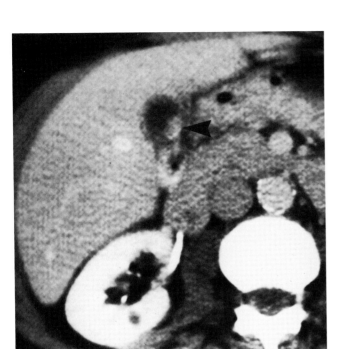

FIG. 105. Metastatic melanoma to the gallbladder. Enhancing mass (*arrowhead*) is seen attached to the gallbladder wall.

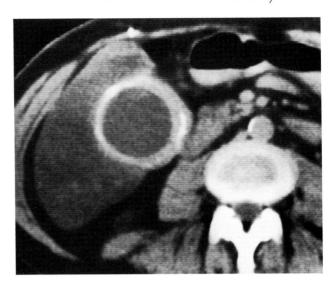

FIG. 106. Porcelain gallbladder. The gallbladder wall is thickened and contains calcification.

improvement in contrast between normal background liver and lesions (222,269,281,282). However, because of nonstability and multiple side effects, this material is unsuitable for general clinical use; slightly modified chemical agents are now being tested.

Other hepatic contrast agents that are under evaluation include cholesterol iopanoate, which is a lipid-soluble agent, and perfluoroctyl bromide. The latter agent has been shown to have the effect of enhancing the boundaries of liver lesions on both CT and sonographic examinations. Development of such agents may significantly improve the ability of CT to detect focal liver lesions in the future.

MRI

The rationale for developing hepatic MRI contrast agents is to improve detection rates for hepatic neoplasms and to reduce overall imaging time. In general, MRI contrast agents affect tissue signal intensity by altering its T1 and T2 values. It is hoped that by using an appropriate contrast agent, more time-efficient T1-weighted sequences can replace the time-consuming T2-weighted sequence. Although many agents with different pharmacokinetic and magnetic properties have been investigated, Gd-DTPA is the only agent that is currently available for human investigations. The pharmacokinetic and biodistribution properties of Gd-DTPA are essentially analogous to those for conventional iodinated contrast agents used for CT (286). The predominant effect of Gd-DTPA is that of T1

shortening at low concentration and T2 shortening at high concentration. Early clinical trials of Gd-DTPA-enhanced liver MRI for detection of liver metastases were disappointing because images were obtained essentially in the "equilibrium phase" (45). Images obtained immediately after administration of contrast material (1–2 min) using a short-TR/TE SE technique have shown significant improvement in liver–tumor contrast (232). The use of Gd-DTPA also has allowed a more specific diagnosis of cavernous hemangiomas (171,205).

Another type of liver contrast agent under investigation is the superparamagnetic ferrite iron oxide particle (Fe_2O_3) (80). Ferrite particles are taken up by reticuloendothelial cells and cause a marked reduction in hepatic signal by selective shortening of T2 values, similar to the effect of ferric ion in hemochromatosis. Because tumors contain no reticuloendothelial cells, they appear as masses of relatively high intensity against a low-intensity liver on T1-weighted images. If a suitable compound can be developed for clinical use, it will significantly improve the ability of MRI to detect focal liver disease.

REFERENCES

1. Adson MA. Hepatic metastases in perspective. *AJR* 1983;140:695–700.
2. Alderson PO, Adams DF, McNeil BJ, et al. Computed tomography, ultrasound and scintigraphy of the liver in patients with colon or breast carcinoma: a prospective comparison. *Radiology* 1983;149:225.
3. Ament AE, Haaga JR, Wiedenmann SD, Barkmeier JD, Morrison SC. Primary sclerosing cholangitis: CT findings. *J Comput Assist Tomogr* 1983;7:795–800.
4. Anderson SD, Holley HC, Berland LL, Van Dyke JA, Stanley RJ. Causes of jaundice during hepatic artery infusion chemotherapy. *Radiology* 1986;161:439–442.
5. Araki T, Hayakawa K, Okada J, Hayashi S, Uchiyama G, Yamada

K. Hepatic schistosomiasis japonica identified by CT. *Radiology* 1985;157:757–760.

6. Araki T, Itai Y, Furui S, Tasaka A. Dynamic CT densitometry of hepatic tumors. *AJR* 1980;135:1037–1043.
7. Araki T, Itai Y, Tasaka A. Computed tomography of localized dilatation of the intrahepatic bile ducts. *Radiology* 1981;141:733–736.
8. Atkinson GO Jr, Kodroff M, Sones PJ, Gay BB Jr. Focal nodular hyperplasia of the liver in children: a report of three new cases. *Radiology* 1980;137:171–174.
9. Baker ME, Silverman PM. Nodular focal fatty infiltration of the liver: CT appearance. *AJR* 1985;145:79–80.
10. Barakos JA, Ralls PW, Lapin SA, et al. Cholelithiasis: evaluation with CT. *Radiology* 1987;162:415–418.
11. Barnes PA, Thomas JL, Bernardino ME. Pitfalls in the diagnosis of hepatic cysts by computed tomography. *Radiology* 1981;141:129–133.
12. Barnett PH, Zerhouni EA, White RI Jr, Siegelman SS. Computed tomography in the diagnosis of cavernous hemangioma of the liver. *AJR* 1980;134:439–447.
13. Baron RL. Common bile duct stones: reassessment of criteria for CT diagnosis. *Radiology* 1987;162:419–424.
14. Baron RL, Stanley RJ, Lee JKT, Koehler RE, Levitt RG. Computed tomographic features of biliary obstruction. *AJR* 1983;140:1173–1178.
15. Baron RL, Stanley RJ, Lee JKT, et al. A prospective comparison of the evaluation of biliary obstruction using computed tomography and ultrasonography. *Radiology* 1982;145:91–98.
16. Bashist B, Hecht HL, Harley WD. Computed tomographic demonstration of rapid changes in fatty infiltration of the liver. *Radiology* 1982;142:691–692.
17. Beggs I. The radiology of hydatid disease. *AJR* 1985;145:639–648.
18. Berk RN, Ferrucci JT, Fordtran JS, Cooperberg PL, Weissmann HS. The radiological diagnosis of gallbladder disease. *Radiology* 1981;141:49–56.
19. Berland LL. *Practical CT: technology and techniques.* New York: Raven Press, 1987.
20. Berland LL. Screening for diffuse and focal liver disease: the case for hepatic computed tomography. *J Clin Ultrasound* 1984;12:83–89.
21. Berland LL, Doust BD, Foley WD. Acute hemorrhage into the gallbladder diagnosed by computerized tomography and ultrasonography. *J Comput Assist Tomogr* 1980;4:260–262.
22. Berland LL, Lawson TL, Foley WD, Geenen JE, Stewart ET. Computed tomography of the normal and abnormal pancreatic duct: correlation with pancreatic ductography. *Radiology* 1981;141:715–724.
23. Berland LL, Lawson TL, Foley WD, Melrose BL, Chintapalli KN, Taylor AJ. Comparison of pre- and post-contrast CT in hepatic masses. *AJR* 1982;138:853–858.
24. Berland LL, Lawson TL, Stanley RJ. CT appearance of Mirizzi syndrome. *J Comput Assist Tomogr* 1984;8:165–166.
25. Berland LL, Van Dyke JA. Decreased splenic enhancement on CT in traumatized hypotensive patients. *Radiology* 1985;156:469–471.
26. Below ME, Spirt BA, Weil L. CT follow-up of hepatic and splenic fungal microabscesses. *J Comput Assist Tomogr* 1984;8:42–45.
27. Bernardino ME, Berkman WA, Plemmons M, Sones PJ Jr, Price RB, Casarella WJ. Percutaneous drainage of multiseptated hepatic abscess. *J Comput Assist Tomogr* 1984;8:38–41.
28. Bernardino ME, Erwin BC, Steinberg HV, Baumgartner BR, Torres WE, Gedgaudas-McClees RK. Delayed hepatic CT scanning: increased confidence and improved detection of hepatic metastases. *Radiology* 1986;159:71–74.
29. Bernardino ME, Steinberg HV, Pearson TC, Gedgaudas-McClees RK, Torres WE, Henderson JM. Shunts for portal hypertension: MR and angiography for determination of patency. *Radiology* 1986;158:57–61.
30. Bertel CK, Van Heerden JA, Sheedy PF. Treatment of pyogenic hepatic abscesses. *Arch Surg* 1986;121:554–558.
31. Borkowski GP, Buonocore E, George CR, Go RT, O'Donovan PB, Meaney TF. Nuclear magnetic resonance (NMR) imaging in the evaluation of the liver: a preliminary experience. *J Comput Assist Tomogr* 1983;7:768–774.
32. Botet JF, Watson RC, Kemeny N, Daly JM, Yeh S. Cholangitis complicating intraarterial chemotherapy in liver metastases. *Radiology* 1985;156:335–337.
33. Boukadoum M, Siddiky MA, Zerhouni EA, Stitik RP. CT demonstration of adenomyomatosis of the gallbladder. *J Comput Assist Tomogr* 1984;8:177–180.
34. Bradley WG, Schmidt PG. Effect of methemoglobin formation on the MR appearance of subarachnoid hemorrhage. *Radiology* 1985;156:99–103.
35. Brasch RC, Wesbey GE, Gooding CA, Koerper MA. Magnetic resonance imaging of transfusional hemosiderosis complicating thalassemia major. *Radiology* 1984;150:767–771.
36. Bree RL, Schwab RE, Neiman HL. Solitary echogenic spot in the liver: is it diagnostic of a hemangioma? *AJR* 1983;140:41–45.
37. Bressler EL, Alpern MB, Glazer GM, Francis IR, Ensminger WD. Hypervascular hepatic metastases: CT evaluation. *Radiology* 1987;162:49–51.
38. Brodey PA, Fisch AE, Fertig S, Roberts GS. Computed tomography of choledochocele. *J Comput Assist Tomogr* 1984;8:162–164.
39. Brown DW, Henkelman RM, Poon PY, Fisher MM. Nuclear magnetic resonance study of iron overload in liver tissue. *Magnetic Resonance Imaging* 1985;3:275–282.
40. Brown JJ, van Sonnenberg E, Gerber KH, Strich G, Wittich GR, Slutsky RA. Magnetic resonance relaxation times of percutaneously obtained normal and abnormal body fluids. *Radiology* 1985;154:727–731.
41. Buonocore E, Borkowski GP, Pavlicek W, Ngo F. NMR imaging of the abdomen: technical considerations. *AJR* 1983;141:1171–1178.
42. Burgener FA, Hamlin DJ. Contrast enhancement of hepatic tumors in CT: comparison between bolus and infusion techniques. *AJR* 1983;140:291–295.
43. Butch RJ, Stark DD, Malt RA. MR imaging of hepatic focal nodular hyperplasia. *J Comput Assist Tomogr* 1986;10:874–877.
44. Buxton-Thomas M, Chisholm R, Dixon AK. Intrahepatic bile duct dilatation shown by computed tomography—predilection for the left lobe? *Br J Radiol* 1985;58:499–502.
45. Bydder GM, Steiner RE, Blumgart LH, Khenia S, Young IR. MR imaging of the liver using short TI inversion recovery sequences. *J Comput Assist Tomogr* 1985;9:1084–1089.
46. Callen PW, Filly RA, Marcus FS. Ultrasonography and computed tomography in the evaluation of hepatic microabscesses in the immunosuppressed patient. *Radiology* 1980;136:433–434.
47. Carr DH, Graif M, Niendorf HP, et al. Gadolinium-DTPA in the assessment of liver tumours by magnetic resonance imaging. *Clin Radiol* 1986;37:347–353.
48. Carr DH, Hadjis NS, Banks LM, Hemingway AP, Blumgart LH. Computed tomography of hilar cholangiocarcinoma: a new sign. *AJR* 1985;145:53–56.
49. Carrasco CH, Freeny PC, Chuang VP, Wallace S. Chemical cholecystitis associated with hepatic artery infusion chemotherapy. *AJR* 1983;141:703–706.
50. Carroll BA, Oppenheimer DA. Sclerosing cholangitis: sonographic demonstration of bile duct wall thickening. *AJR* 1982;139:1016–1018.
51. Casarella WJ, Knowles DM, Wolff M, Johnson PM. Focal nodular hyperplasia and liver cell adenoma: radiologic and pathologic differentiation. *AJR* 1978;131:393–402.
52. Chang T-M, Passaro E. Intrahepatic stones: the Taiwan experience. *Am J Surg* 1983;146:241–244.
53. Chen XR, Shen TZ, Li NZ, Liu DK. Computed tomography in hepatolenticular degeneration (Wilson's disease). *Computerized Radiol* 1983;7:361–364.
54. Clark RA, Matsui O. CT of liver tumors. *Semin Roentgenol* 1983;18:149–162.
55. Co CS, Shea WJ, Goldberg HI. Evaluation of common bile duct diameter using high resolution computed tomography. *J Comput Assist Tomogr* 1986;10:424–427.
56. Conter RL, Pitt HA, Tompkins RK, Longmire WP Jr. Differentiation of pyogenic from amebic hepatic abscesses. *Surg Gynecol Obstet* 1986;162:114–120.
57. Cook DE, Walsh JW, Vick CW, Brewer WH. Upper abdominal trauma: pitfalls in CT diagnosis. *Radiology* 1986;159:65–69.
58. Dachman AH, Ros PR, Goodman ZD, Olmsted WW, Ishak KG. Nodular regenerative hyperplasia of the liver: clinical and radiologic observations. *AJR* 1987;148:717–722.

59. DeMaria M, DeSimone G, Laconi A, Mercadante G, Pavone P, Rossi P. Gold storage in the liver: appearance on CT scans. *Radiology* 1986;159:355–356.

60. Dennis MA, Pretorius D, Manco-Johnson ML, Bangert-Burroughs KB. CT detection of portal venous gas associated with suppurative cholangitis and cholecystitis. *AJR* 1985;145:1017–1018.

61. Didier D, Weiler S, Rohmer P, et al. Hepatic alveolar echinococcosis: correlative US and CT study. *Radiology* 1985;154:179–186.

62. Dixon AK, Walshe JM. Computed tomography of the liver in Wilson disease. *J Comput Assist Tomogr* 1984;8:46–49.

63. Dooms GC, Fisher MR, Higgins CB, Hricak H, Goldberg HI, Margulis AR. MR imaging of the dilated biliary tract. *Radiology* 1986;158:337–341.

64. Dooms GC, Kerlan RK Jr, Hricak H, Wall SD, Margulis AR. Cholangiocarcinoma: imaging by MR. *Radiology* 1986;159:89–94.

65. Doppman JL, Cornblath M, Dwyer AJ, Adams AJ, Girton ME, Sidbury J. Computed tomography of the liver and kidneys in glycogen storage disease. *J Comput Assist Tomogr* 1982;6:67–71.

66. Doppman JL, Dwyer AD, Vermess M, et al. Segmental hyperlucent defects in the liver. *J Comput Assist Tomogr* 1984;8:50–57.

67. Doyle FH, Pennock JM, Banks LM, et al. Nuclear magnetic resonance imaging of the liver: initial experience. *AJR* 1982;138:193–200.

68. Duber C, Storkel S, Wagner P-K, Muller J. Xanthogranulomatous cholecystitis mimicking carcinoma of the gallbladder: CT findings. *J Comput Assist Tomogr* 1984;8:1195–1198.

69. Ebara M, Ohto M, Shinagawa T, et al. Natural history of minute hepatocellular carcinoma smaller than three centimeters complicating cirrhosis. *Gastroenterology* 1986;90:289–298.

70. Ebara M, Ohto M, Watanabe Y, et al. Diagnosis of small hepatocellular carcinoma: correlation of MR imaging and tumor histologic studies. *Radiology* 1986;159:371–377.

71. Edelman R, Hahn PF, Buxton R, Wittenberg J, Ferrucci JT, Jr., Saini S, Brady TJ. Rapid MR imaging with suspended respiration: clinical application in the liver. *Radiology* 1986;161:125–131.

72. Eisenbert D, Hurwitz L, Yu AC. CT and sonography of multiple bile-duct hamartomas simulating malignant liver disease (case report). *AJR* 1986;147:279–280.

73. Edman WA, Weinreb JC, Cohen JM, Buja LM, Chaney C, Peshock RM. Venous thrombosis: clinical and experimental MR imaging. *Radiology* 1986;161:233–238.

74. Fataar S, Bassiony H, Satyanath S, et al. CT of hepatic schistosomiasis mansoni. *AJR* 1985;145:63–66.

75. Federle M. CT of abdominal trauma. *CRC Crit Rev Diagnostic Imaging* 1981;19:257–316.

76. Federle M, Cello JP, Laing FC, Jeffrey RB Jr. Recurrent pyogenic cholangitis in Asian immigrants. *Radiology* 1982;143:151–156.

77. Federle MP, Crass RA, Jeffrey RB, Trunkey DD. Computed tomography in blunt abdominal trauma. *Arch Surg* 1982;117:645–650.

78. Federle MP, Filly RA, Moss AA. Cystic hepatic neoplasms: complementary roles of CT and sonography. *AJR* 1981;136:345–348.

79. Federle MP, Goldberg GI, Kaiser JA, Moss A, Jeffrey RB, Mall JC. Evaluation of abdominal trauma by computed tomography. *Radiology* 1981;138:637–644.

80. Ferrucci JT. MR imaging of the liver. *AJR* 1986;147:1103–1116.

81. Ferrucci JT, Adson MA, Mueller PR, Stanley RJ, Stewart ET. Advances in the radiology of jaundice: a symposium and review. *AJR* 1983;141:1–20.

82. Finlay IG, Meek DR, Gray HW, Duncan JG, McArdle CS. Incidence and detection of occult hepatic metastases in colorectal carcinoma. *Br Med J* 1982;284:203–205.

83. Fisher MR, Wall SD, Hricak H, McCarthy S, Kerlan RK. Hepatic vascular anatomy on magnetic resonance imaging. *AJR* 1985;144:739–746.

84. Fishman EK, Farmlett E, Kadir S, Siegelman SS. Computed tomography of benign hepatic tumors. *J Comput Assist Tomogr* 1982;6:472–481.

85. Flejou JF, Barge J, Menu Y, et al. Liver adenomatosis: an entity distinct from liver adenoma? *Gastroenterology* 1985;89:1132–1138.

86. Flournoy JG, Potter JL, Sullivan BM, Gerza CB, Ramzy I. CT appearance of multifocal hepatic steatosis. *J Comput Assist Tomogr* 1984;8:1192–1194.

87. Foley WD, Berland LL, Lawson TL, Maddison FE. Computed tomography in the demonstration of hepatic pseudoaneurysm with hemobilia. *J Comput Assist Tomogr* 1980;4:863–865.

88. Foley WD, Berland LL, Lawson TL, Smith DF, Thorsen MK. Contrast enhancement technique for dynamic hepatic computed tomographic scanning. *Radiology* 1983;147:797–803.

89. Foley WD, Wilson CR, Quiroz FA, Lawson TL. Demonstration of the normal extrahepatic biliary tract with computed tomography. *J Comput Assist Tomogr* 1980;4:48–52.

90. Freeny PC, Marks WM. Hepatic perfusion abnormalities during CT angiography: detection and interpretation. *Radiology* 1986;159:685–691.

91. Freeny PC, Marks WM. Patterns of contrast enhancement of benign and malignant hepatic neoplasms during bolus dynamic and delayed CT. *Radiology* 1986;160:613–618.

92. Freeny PC, Marks WM. Computed tomographic arteriography of the liver. *Radiology* 1983;148:193–197.

93. Freeny PC, Marks WM, Ryan JA, Bolen JW. Colorectal carcinoma evaluation with CT: preoperative staging and detection of postoperative recurrence. *Radiology* 1986;158:347–353.

94. Friedman AC, Lichtenstein JE, Goodman Z, Fishman EK, Siegelman SS, Dachman AH. Fibrolamellar hepatocellular carcinoma. *Radiology* 1985;157:583–587.

95. Friedman AC, Ramchandani P, Black M, Caroline DF, Radecki PD, Heeger P. Magnetic resonance imaging diagnosis of Budd-Chiari syndrome. *Gastroenterology* 1986;91:1289–1295.

96. Gerzof SG, Robbins AH, Birkett DH, Johnson WC, Pugatch RD, Vincent ME. Percutaneous catheter drainage of abdominal abscesses guided by ultrasound and computed tomography. *AJR* 1979;133:1–8.

97. Gerzof SG, Robbins AH, Johnson WC, Birkett DH, Nasbeth DC. Percutaneous catheter drainage of abdominal abscesses: a five-year experience. *N Engl J Med* 1981;305:653–657.

98. Gibson RN, Yeung E, Thompson JN, et al. Bile duct obstruction: radiologic evaluation of level, cause, and tumor resectability. *Radiology* 1986;160:43–47.

99. Giyanani VL, Meyers PC, Wolfson JJ. Mesenchymal hamartoma of the liver: computed tomography and ultrasonography. *J Comput Assist Tomogr* 1986;10:51–54.

100. Glazer GM, Aisen AM, Francis IR, Gross BH, Gyves JW, Ensminger WD. Evaluation of focal hepatic masses: a comparative study of MRI and CT. *Gastrointest Radiol* 1986;11:263–268.

101. Glazer GM, Aisen AM, Francis IR, Gyves JW, Lande I, Adler DD. Hepatic cavernous hemangioma: magnetic resonance imaging. Work in progress. *Radiology* 1985;155:417–420.

102. Goldberg HI, Moss AA, Stark DD, McKerrow J, Engelstad B, Brito A. Hepatic cirrhosis: magnetic resonance imaging. *Radiology* 1984;153:737–739.

103. Goldstein RB, Wing VW, Lanning FC, Jeffrey RB. Computed tomography of thick-walled gallbladder mimicking pericholecystic fluid. *J Comput Assist Tomogr* 1986;10:55–56.

104. Goodman A, Harries-Jones EP, Lipinski JK. Two unusual cases of jaundice with similar ultrasound and CT findings. *J Comput Assist Tomogr* 1984;8:1110–1113.

105. Greenberg M, Rubin JM, Greenberg BM. Appearance of the gallbladder and biliary tree by CT cholangiography. *J Comput Assist Tomogr* 1983;7:788–794.

106. Grumbach K, Levine MS, Wexler JA. Gallstone ileus diagnosed by computed tomography. *J Comput Assist Tomogr* 1986;10:146–148.

107. Gunven P, Makuuchi M, Takayasu K, Moriyama N, Yamasaki S, Hasegawa H. Preoperative imaging of liver metastases. *Ann Surg* 1985;202:573–579.

108. Halvorsen RA, Korobkin M, Ram RC, Thompson WM. CT appearance of focal fatty infiltration of the liver. *AJR* 1982;139:277–281.

109. Hamada M, Ohta M, Yasuda Y, et al. Hepatic calcification in schistosomiasis japonica. *J Comput Assist Tomogr* 1982;6:76–78.

110. Haney PJ, Whitley NO, Brothman S, Cunat JS, Whitley J. Liver injury and complications in the postoperative trauma patient: CT evaluation. *AJR* 1982;139:271–275.

111. Harbin WP, Robert NJ, Ferrucci JT. Diagnosis of cirrhosis based on regional changes in hepatic morphology. *Radiology* 1980;135:273–283.

112. Harter LP, Gross BH, Hilaire JS, Filly RA, Goldberg HI. CT and

sonographic appearance of hepatic vein obstruction. *AJR* 1982;139:176–178.

113. Haq MM, Valdes LG, Peterson DF, Gourley WK. Fibrosis of extrahepatic biliary system after continuous hepatic artery infusion of floxuridine through an implantable pump (Infusaid pump). *Cancer* 1986;57:1281–1283.

114. Heiken JP, Lee JKT, Dixon WT. Fatty infiltration of the liver: evaluation by proton spectroscopic imaging. *Radiology* 1985;157:707–710.

115. Heiken JP, Lee JKT, Glazer HS, Ling D. Hepatic metastases studied with MR and CT. *Radiology* 1985;156:423–427.

116. Henderson JM, Liechty EJ, Jahnke RW. Liver involvement in hereditary hemorrhagic telangiectasis. *J Comput Assist Tomogr* 1981;5:773–776.

117. Henkelman RM, Hardy P, Poon PY, Bronskill MJ. Optimal pulse sequence for imaging hepatic metastases. *Radiology* 1986;161:727–734.

118. Ho B, Cooperberg PL, Li DK, Mach L, Naiman SC, Grossman L. Ultrasonography and computed tomography of hepatic candidiasis in immunosuppressed patients. *J Ultrasound Med* 1982;1:157–195.

119. Hoff FL, Aisen AM, Walden ME, Glazer GM. MR imaging in hydatid disease of the liver. *Gastrointest Radiol* 1987;12:39–42.

120. Holley HC, Koslin DB, Berland LL, Anderson SD, Stanley RJ. Striated hepatic enhancement pattern seen on contrast-enhanced dynamic CT scanning secondary to passive liver congestion. Presented at RSNA, Chicago, 1986.

121. Honda H, Watanabe K, Mihara K, Hoshi H, Sakihama M. Lipoma of the hepatic falciform ligament. *J Comput Assist Tomogr* 1983;7:170.

122. Hricak H, Amparo EG, Fisher MR, Crooks LE, Higgins CB. Abdominal venous system: assessment using MR. *Radiology* 1985;156:415–422.

123. Hricak H, Filly RA, Margulis AR, Moon KL, Crooks LE, Kaufman L. Work in progress: nuclear magnetic resonance imaging of the gallbladder. *Radiology* 1983;147:481–484.

124. Htoo MM. Surgical implications of stone impaction in the gallbladder neck with compression of the common hepatic duct (Mirizzi's syndrome). *Clin Radiol* 1983;3:651–655.

125. Ihde DC, Dunnick NR, Johnston-Early A, Bunn PA, Cohen MH, Minna JD. Abdominal computed tomography in small cell lung cancer: assessment of extent of disease and response to therapy. *Cancer* 1982;49:1485–1490.

126. Inamoto K, Tanaka S, Yamazaki H, Okamoto E. Computed tomography in the detection of small hepatocellular carcinomas. *Gastrointest Radiol* 1983;8:321–326.

127. Itai Y, Araki T, Furui S, Tasaka A. Differential diagnosis of hepatic masses on computed tomography, with particular reference to hepatocellular carcinoma. *J Comput Assist Tomogr* 1981;5:834–842.

128. Itai Y, Araki T, Furui S, Yashiro N, Ohtomo K, Lio M. Computed tomography of primary intrahepatic biliary malignancy. *Radiology* 1983;147:485–490.

129. Itai Y, Araki T, Yoshikawa K, Furui S, Yashiro N, Tasaka A. Computed tomography of gallbladder carcinoma. *Radiology* 1980;137:713–718.

130. Itai Y, Furui S, Araki T, Tashiro N, Tasaka A. Computed tomography of cavernous hemangioma of the liver. *Radiology* 1980;137:149–155.

131. Itai Y, Furui S, Ohtomo K, Kokubo T, Yamauchi T, Minami M, Tashiro N. Dynamic CT features of arterioportal shunts in hepatocellular carcinoma. *AJR* 1986;146:723–727.

132. Itai Y, Moss AA, Goldberg HI. Transient hepatic attenuation difference of lobar or segmental distribution detected by dynamic computed tomography. *Radiology* 1982;144:835–839.

133. Itai Y, Ohtomo K, Furui S, Minami M, Yoshikawa K, Yashiro N. MR imaging of hepatocellular carcinoma. *J Comput Assist Tomogr* 1986;10:963–968.

134. Itai Y, Ohtomo K, Furui S, Yamauchi T, Minami M, Yashiro N. Noninvasive diagnosis of small cavernous hemangioma of the liver: advantage of MRI. *AJR* 1985;145:1195–1199.

135. Itai Y, Ohtomo K, Kokubo T, et al. CT and MR imaging of fatty tumors of the liver. *J Comput Assist Tomogr* 1987;11:253–257.

136. Jaques P, Mauro MA, Safrit H, Yankaskas B, Piggott B. CT features of intraabdominal abscesses: prediction of successful percutaneous drainage. *AJR* 1986;146:1041–1045.

137. Jeffrey RB, Federle MP, Laing FC, Wall S, Rego J, Moss AA. Computed tomography of choledocholithiasis. *AJR* 1983;140:1179–1183.

138. Jeffrey RB, Moss A, Quivey JM, Federle MP, Wara WM. CT of radiation-induced hepatic injury. *AJR* 1980;135:445–448.

139. Jeffrey RB, Nyberg DA, Bottles K, et al. Abdominal CT in acquired immunodeficiency syndrome. *AJR* 1986;146:7–13.

140. Johnson CM, Sheedy PF, Stanson AW, Stephens DH, Hattery RR, Adson MA. Computed tomography and angiography of cavernous hemangiomas of the liver. *Radiology* 1981;138:115–121.

141. Johnson RJ, Zhu XP, Isherwood I, et al. Computed tomography: qualitative and quantitative recognition of liver disease in hemophilia. *J Comput Assist Tomogr* 1983;7:1000–1006.

142. Kalovidouris A, Gouliamos A, Demou L, Vassilopoulos P, Vlachos L, Papavassiliou K. Postsurgical evaluation of hydatid disease with CT: diagnostic pitfalls. *J Comput Assist Tomogr* 1984;8:1114–1119.

143. Kalovidouris A, Pissiotis C, Pontifex G, Gouliamos A, Pentea A, Papavassiliou C. CT characterization of multivesicular hydatid cysts. *J Comput Assist Tomogr* 1986;10:428–431.

144. Kane RA, Costello P, Duszlak E. Computed tomography in acute cholecystitis: new observations. *AJR* 1983;141:697–701.

145. Kane RA, Jacobs R, Katz J, Costello P. Porcelain gallbladder: ultrasound and CT appearance. *Radiology* 1984;152:137–141.

146. Kawashima A, Suehiro S, Murayama S, Russell WJ. Focal fatty infiltration of the liver mimicking a tumor: sonographic and CT features. *J Comput Assist Tomogr* 1986;10:329–331.

147. Kemeny MM, Ganteaume L, Goldberg DA, Hogar JM, Terz JJ. Preoperative staging with computerized axial tomography and biochemical laboratory tests in patients with hepatic metastases. *Ann Surg* 1986;203:169–172.

148. Koehler RE, Melson GL, Lee JKT, Long J. Common hepatic duct obstruction by cystic duct stone: Mirizzi syndrome. *AJR* 1979;132:1007–1009.

149. Koehler RE, Stanley RJ. Computed tomography of the gallbladder and bile ducts. In: Berk RN, Ferrucci JT, Leopold GR, eds. *Radiology of the gallbladder and bile ducts: diagnosis and intervention.* Philadelphia: WB Saunders, 1983.

150. Kolbenstvedt A, Kjølseth I, Klepp O, Kolmannskog F. Postirradiation changes of the liver demonstrated by computed tomography. *Radiology* 1980;135:391.

151. Krundy AG, Doppman JL, Bissonette MB, Girton M. Hemobilia: computed tomographic diagnosis. *Radiology* 1983;148:785–789.

152. Kudo M, Hirasa M, Takakuwa H, et al. Small hepatocellular carcinomas in chronic liver disease: detection with SPECT. *Radiology* 1986;159:697–703.

153. Kuligowska E, Schlesinger A, Miller KB, Lee VW, Grosso D. Bilomas: a new approach to the diagnosis and treatment. *Gastrointest Radiol* 1983;8:237–243.

154. LaBerge JM, Laing FC, Federle MP, Jeffrey RB Jr, Lim RC Jr. Hepatocellular carcinoma: assessment of resectability by computed tomography and ultrasound. *Radiology* 1984;152:485–490.

155. Laing FC, Jeffrey RB Jr, Wing VW, Nyberg DA. Biliary dilatation: defining the level and cause by real-time US. *Radiology* 1986;160:39–42.

156. Landay MJ, Setaiwan H, Hirsch G, Christensen EE, Conrad MR. Hepatic and thoracic amebiasis. *AJR* 1980;135:449–454.

157. Lander JJ, Stanley RJ, Summer HW, Boswell DC, Aach RD. Angiosarcoma of the liver associated with Fowler's solution (potassium arsenite). *Gastroenterology* 1975;68:1582–1586.

158. Ledesma-Medina J, Dominguez R, Bowen A, Young LW, Bron KM. Pediatric liver transplantation (part I). *Radiology* 1985;157:335–338.

159. Lee JKT, Dixon WT, Ling D, Levitt RG, Murphy WA Jr. Fatty infiltration of the liver: demonstration by proton spectroscopic imaging. Preliminary observations. *Radiology* 1984;153:195–201.

160. Lee JKT, Heiken JP, Dixon WT. Detection of hepatic metastases by proton spectroscopic imaging. Work in progress. *Radiology* 1985;156:429–433.

161. Leung AW-L, Steiner RE, Young IR. NMR imaging of the liver in two cases of iron overload. *J Comput Assist Tomogr* 1984;8:446–449.

162. Lev-Toaff AS, Friedman AC, Cohen LM, Radecki PD, Caroline DF. Hepatic infarcts: new observations by CT and sonography. *AJR* 1987;149:87–90.

163. Levine E, Cook LT, Grantham JJ. Liver cysts in autosomal-dom-

inant polycystic kidney disease: clinical and computed tomographic study. *AJR* 1985;145:229–233.

164. Lewis E, Bernardino ME, Barnes PA, Parvey HR, Soo C-S, Chuang VP. The fatty liver: pitfalls in the CT and angiographic evaluation of metastatic disease. *J Comput Assist Tomogr* 1983;7:235–241.

165. Loflin TG, Simeone JF, Mueller PR, et al. Gallbladder bile in cholecystitis: in vitro MR evaluation. *Radiology* 1985;157:457–459.

166. Longmaid HE, Seltzer SE, Costello P, Gordon P. Hepatocellular carcinoma presenting as primary extrahepatic mass on CT. *AJR* 1986;146:1005–1009.

167. Lubbers PR, Ros PR, Goodman ZD, Ishak KG. Accumulation of technetium-99m sulfur colloid by hepatocellular adenoma: scintigraphic–pathologic correlation. *AJR* 1987;148:1105–1108.

168. MacCarty RL, LaRusso NF, May GR, et al. Cholangiocarcinoma complicating primary sclerosing cholangitis: cholangiographic appearances. *Radiology* 1985;156:43–46.

169. Mahony B, Jeffrey RB, Federle MP. Spontaneous rupture of hepatic and splenic angiosarcoma demonstrated by CT. *AJR* 1982;138:965–966.

170. Malt RA. Surgery for hepatic neoplasms. *N Engl J Med* 1985;313:1591–1596.

171. Mano I, Yoshida H, Nakabayashi K, Yashiro N, Iio M. Fast spin echo imaging with suspended respiration: gadolinium enhanced MR imaging of liver tumors. *J Comput Assist Tomogr* 1987;11:73–80.

172. Marincek B, Barbier PA, Becker CD, Mettler D, Ruchti C. CT appearance of impaired lymphatic drainage in liver transplants. *AJR* 1986;147:519–523.

173. Markos J, Veronese ME, Nicholson MR, McLean S, Shevland JE. Value of hepatic computerized tomographic scanning during amiodarone therapy. *Am J Cardiol* 1985;56:89–92.

174. Martino CR, Haaga JR, Bryan PJ, LiPuma JP, El Yousef SJ, Alfidi RJ. CT-guided liver biopsies: eight years' experience. *Radiology* 1984;152:755–757.

175. Mathieu D, Elouaer-Blanc L, Divine M, Rene E, Vasile N. Hepatic plasmocytoma: sonographic and CT findings. *J Comput Assist Tomogr* 1986;10:144–145.

176. Mathieu D, Bruneton JN, Drouillard J, Pointreau CC, Vasile N. Hepatic adenomas and focal nodular hyperplasia: dynamic CT study. *Radiology* 1986;160:53–58.

177. Mathieu D, Vasile N, Grenier P. Portal thrombosis: dynamic CT features and course. *Radiology* 1985;154:737–741.

178. Mattison GR, Glazer GM, Quint LE, Francis IR, Bree RL, Ensminger WD. MR imaging of hepatic focal nodular hyperplasia: characterization and distinction from primary malignant hepatic tumors. *AJR* 1987;148:711–715.

179. Matzen P, Malchow-Moller A, Brun B, et al. Ultrasonography, computed tomography, and cholescintigraphy in suspected obstructive jaundice—a prospective comparative study. *Gastroenterology* 1983;84:1492–1497.

180. McCarthy S, Hricak H, Cohen M, et al. Cholecystitis: detection with MR imaging. *Radiology* 1986;158:333–336.

181. McLeod AJ, Zornosa J, Shirkhoda A. Leiomyosarcoma: computed tomographic findings. *Radiology* 1984;152:133–136.

182. Menu Y, Lorphelin J-M, Scherrer A, Grenier P, Nahum H. Sonographic and computed tomographic evaluation of intrahepatic calculi. *AJR* 1985;145:579–583.

183. Miller VE, Berland LL. Pulsed Doppler duplex sonography and CT of portal vein thrombosis. *AJR* 1985;145:73–76.

184. Mitchell SE, Clark RA. A comparison of computed tomography and sonography in choledocholithiasis. *AJR* 1984;142:729–733.

185. Moon KL Jr, Federle MP. Computed tomography in hepatic trauma. *AJR* 1983;141:309–314.

186. Moon KL Jr, Hricak H, Margulis AR, et al. Nuclear magnetic resonance imaging characteristics of gallstones in vitro. *Radiology* 1983;148:753–756.

187. Morehouse H, Leibman AJ, Biempica L, Hoffman J. Infiltrating periductal neoplasm mimicking biliary dilatation on computed tomography. *J Comput Assist Tomogr* 1983;7:721–723.

188. Moriyasu F, Ban N, Nishida O, et al. Central signals of gallstones in magnetic resonance imaging. *Am J Gastroenterol* 1987;82:139–142.

189. Moss AA, Goldberg HI, Stark DB, et al. Hepatic tumors: magnetic resonance and CT appearance. *Radiology* 1984;150:141–147.

190. Mueller PR, Ferrucci JT Jr, Simeone JF, et al. Detection and drainage of bilomas: special considerations. *AJR* 1983;140:715–720.

191. Mueller PR, Ferrucci JT Jr, Simeone JF, et al. Post cholecystectomy bile duct dilatation: Myth or reality? *AJR* 1981;136:355–358.

192. Muhletaler CA, Gerlock AJ Jr, Fleischer AC, James AE Jr. Diagnosis of obstructive jaundice with nondilated bile ducts. *AJR* 1980;134:1149–1152.

193. Muramatsu Y, Takayasu K, Moriyama N, et al. Peripheral low-density area of hepatic tumors: CT-pathologic correlation. *Radiology* 1986;160:49–52.

194. Murphy FB, Steinberg HV, Shires GT, Martin LG, Bernardino ME. The Budd-Chiari syndrome: a review. *AJR* 1986;147:9–15.

195. Musante F, Derchi LE, Bonati P. CT cholangiography in suspected Caroli's disease. *J Comput Assist Tomogr* 1982;6:482–485.

196. Myracle MR, Stadalnik RC, Blaisdell FW, Farkas JP, Martin P. Segmental biliary obstruction: diagnostic significance of bile duct crowding. *AJR* 1981;137:169–171.

197. Nakao N, Miura K, Takayasu Y, Wada Y, Miura T. CT angiography in hepatocellular carcinoma. *J Comput Assist Tomogr* 1983;7:780–787.

198. Nakayama T, Hiyama Y, Ohnishi K, et al. Arterioportal shunts on dynamic computed tomography. *AJR* 1983;140:953–957.

199. Nishikawa J, Itai Y, Tasaka A. Lobar attenuation difference of the liver on computed tomography. *Radiology* 1981;141:725–728.

200. Norton JA, Doppman JL, Gardner JD, et al. Aggressive resection of metastatic disease in selected patients with malignant gastrinoma. *Ann Surg* 1986;203:352–359.

201. Nyberg DA, Jeffrey RB Jr, Federle MP, Bottles K, Abrams DI. AIDS-related lymphomas: evaluation by abdominal CT. *Radiology* 1986;159:59–63.

202. O'Connor KW, Snodgrass PJ, Swonder JE, et al. A blinded prospective study comparing four current noninvasive approaches in the differential diagnosis of medical versus surgical jaundice. *Gastroenterology* 1983;84:1498–1504.

203. Ohtomo K, Itai Y, Furui S, Yashiro N, Yoshikawa K, Iio M. Hepatic tumors: differentiation by transverse relaxation time (T2) of magnetic resonance imaging. *Radiology* 1985;155:421–423.

204. Ohtomo K, Itai Y, Makita K, et al. Portosystemic collaterals on MR imaging. *J Comput Assist Tomogr* 1986;10:751–755.

205. Ohtomo K, Itai Y, Yoshikawa K, et al. Hepatic tumors: dynamic MR imaging. *Radiology* 1987;163:27–31.

206. Pagani JJ. Intrahepatic vascular territories shown by computed tomography (CT). *Radiology* 1983;147:173–178.

207. Panicek DM, Paquet DJ, Clark KG, Urrutia EJ, Brinsko RE. Hepatic parenchymal gas after blunt trauma. *Radiology* 1986;159:343–344.

208. Pardes JG, Haaga JR, Borkowski G. Focal hepatic fatty metamorphosis secondary to trauma. *J Comput Assist Tomogr* 1982;6:769–771.

209. Pedrosa CS, Casanova R, Torre SDE, Villacorta J. CT findings in Mirizzi syndrome. *J Comput Assist Tomogr* 1983;7:419–425.

210. Pedrosa CS, Casanova R, Lezana AH, Fernandex MC. Computed tomography in obstructive jaundice. Part II: the cause of obstruction. *Radiology* 1981;139:635–645.

211. Peterson IM, Neumann CH. Focal hepatic infarction with bile lake formation. *AJR* 1984;142:1155–1156.

212. Piekarski J, Goldberg HI, Royal SA, Axel L, Moss AA. Difference between liver and spleen CT numbers in the normal adult: its usefulness in predicting the presence of diffuse liver disease. *Radiology* 1980;137:727–729.

213. Pien EH, Zeman RK, Benjamin SB, et al. Iatrogenic sclerosing cholangitis following hepatic arterial chemotherapy infusion. *Radiology* 1985;156:329–330.

214. Pollack M, Shirkhoda A, Charnsangavej C. Computed tomography of choledochocele. *J Comput Assist Tomogr* 1985;9:360–362.

215. Pretorius DH, Gosink BB, Olson LK. CT of the opacified biliary tract: use of calcium ipodate. *AJR* 1982;138:1073–1075.

216. Quint LE, Glazer GM. CT evaluation of the bile ducts in patients with fatty liver. *Radiology* 1984;153:755–756.

217. Rahn NH III, Koehler RE, Weyman PJ, Truss CD, Sagel SS, Stanley RJ. CT appearance of sclerosing cholangitis. *AJR* 1983;141:549–552.

218. Radin DR, Santiago EM. Cholecystoduodenal fistula due to pancreatic carcinoma: CT diagnosis. *J Comput Assist Tomogr* 1986;10:149–150.

219. Radin DR, Vachon LA. CT findings in biliary and pancreatic ascariasis. *J Comput Assist Tomogr* 1986;10:508–509.

220. Rao BK, Brodell GK, Haaga JR, Whitlatch S, Chiu LC. Visceral CT findings associated with thorotrast. *J Comput Assist Tomogr* 1986;10:57–61.

221. Rattner DW, Schapiro RH, Warshaw AL. Abnormalities of the pancreatic and biliary ducts in adult patients with choledochal cysts. *Arch Surg* 1983;118:1068–1073.

222. Reinig JW, Dwyer AJ, Miller DL, et al. Liver metastasis detection: comparative sensitivities of MR imaging and CT scanning. *Radiology* 1987;162:43–47.

223. Reinig JW, Sanchez FW, Vujic I. Hemodynamics of portal blood flow shown by CT portography. *Radiology* 1985;154:473–476.

224. Roberts JL, Fishman EK, Hartman DS, Sanders R, Goodman Z, Siegelman SS. Lipomatous tumors of the liver: evaluation with CT and US. *Radiology* 1986;158:613–617.

225. Rogers JV, Mack LA, Freeny PC, Johnson ML, Sones PJ. Hepatic focal nodular hyperplasia: angiography, CT, sonography and scintigraphy. *AJR* 1981;137:983–990.

226. Ros PR, Goodman ZD, Ishak KG, et al. Mesenchymal hamartoma of the liver: radiologic–pathologic correlation. *Radiology* 1986;158:619–624.

227. Ros PR, Viamonte M Jr, Koila K, Sheldon JJ, Tobias J, Bohen B. Demonstration of cavernomatous transformation of the portal vein by magnetic resonance imaging. *Gastrointest Radiol* 1986;11:90–92.

228. Rossi P, Sposito M, Simonetti G, Sposato S, Cusumano G. CT diagnosis of Budd-Chiari syndrome. *J Comput Assist Tomogr* 1981;5:366–369.

229. Rubenstein WA, Auh YH, Whalen JP, Kazam E. The perihepatic spaces: computed tomographic and ultrasound imaging. *Radiology* 1983;149:231–239.

230. Rubinstein ZJ, Seligsohn U, Modan M, Shani M. Hepatic computerized tomography in the Dubin-Johnson syndrome: increased liver density as a diagnostic aid. *Computerized Radiol* 1985;9:315–318.

231. Runge VM, Clanton JA, Smith FW, et al. NMR of iron and copper disease states. *AJR* 1983;141:943–948.

232. Saini S, Stark DD, Brady TJ, Wittenberg J, Ferrucci JT Jr. Dynamic spin-echo MRI of liver cancer using gadolinium-DTPA: animal investigation. *AJR* 1986;147:357–362.

233. Savolaine ER, Grecos GP, Howard J, White P. Evolution of CT findings in hepatic hematoma. *J Comput Assist Tomogr* 1985;9:1090–1096.

234. Scatarige JC, Fishman EK, Saksouk FA, Siegelman SS. Computed tomography of calcified liver masses. *J Comput Assist Tomogr* 1983;7:83–89.

235. Scatarige JC, Kenny JM, Fishman EK, Herlong FH, Siegelman SS. CT of giant cavernous hemangioma. *AJR* 1987;149:83–85.

236. Schulman A. Non-western pattern of biliary stones and the role of ascariasis. *Radiology* 1987;162:425–430.

237. Scott WW Jr, Sanders RC, Siegelman SS. Irregular fatty infiltration of the liver: diagnostic dilemmas. *AJR* 1980;135:67–71.

238. Segel MC, Zajko AB, Bowen A, et al. Hepatic artery thrombosis after liver transplantation: radiologic evaluation. *AJR* 1986;146:137–141.

239. Sexton CC, Zeman RK. Correlation of computed tomography, sonography and gross anatomy of the liver. *AJR* 1983;141:711–718.

240. Shanser JD, Korobkin M, Goldberg HI, Rohlfing BM. Computed tomographic diagnosis of obstructive jaundice in the absence of intrahepatic ductal dilatation. *AJR* 1978;131:389–392.

241. Shea WJ Jr, Demas BE, Goldberg HI, Horn DC, Ferrell LD, Kerlan RK. Sclerosing cholangitis associated with hepatic arterial FUDR chemotherapy: radiographic–histologic correlation. *AJR* 1986;146:717–721.

242. Sherlock S. Liver in infections and in ulcerative colitis. In: *Diseases of the liver and biliary system*. Philadelphia: FA Davis, 1968:589–650.

243. Sherlock S, Dick D. The impact of radiology on hepatology. *AJR* 1986;147:1116–1122.

244. Shirkhoda A, Lopez-Berestein G, Holbert JM, Lunga MA. Hepatosplenic fungal infection: CT and pathologic evaluation after treatment with liposomal amphotericin B. *Radiology* 1986;159:349–353.

245. Sigal R, Lanir A, Atlan H, et al. Nuclear magnetic resonance imaging of liver hemangiomas. *J Nucl Med* 1985;26:1117–1122.

246. Silverman PM, Ram PC, Korobkin M. CT appearance of abdominal Thorotrast deposition and Thorotrast-induced angiosarcoma of the liver. *J Comput Assist Tomogr* 1983;7:655–658.

247. Smathers R, Lee JKT, Heiken JP. Differentiation of complicated cholecystitis from gallbladder carcinoma by computed tomography. *AJR* 1984;143:255–259.

248. Smevik B, Kolmannskog F, Aakhus T. Computed tomography and angiography in carcinoid liver metastases. *Acta Radiol Diagn* 1983;24:189–193.

249. Smevik B, Swensen T, Kolbenstvedt A, Trygstad O. Computed tomography and ultrasonography of the abdomen in congenital generalized lipodystrophy. *Radiology* 1982;142:687–689.

250. Smith FW, Mallard JR. NMR imaging in liver disease. *Br Med Bull* 1984;40:194–196.

251. Sonoda T, Reynolds RD, Galey WT. The computerized tomographic appearance of patchy liver congestion due to irradiation. *Computerized Radiol* 1983;7:135–140.

252. Sorensen KW, Glazer GM, Francis IR. Diagnosis of cystic ectasia of intrahepatic bile ducts by computed tomography. *J Comput Assist Tomogr* 1982;6:486–489.

253. Spritzer C, Kressel HY, Mitchell D, Axel L. MR imaging of normal extrahepatic bile duct. *J Comput Assist Tomogr* 1987;11:248–252.

254. Stanley J, Vujic I, Schabel SI, Gobien RP, Reines HD. Evaluation of biliary cystadenoma and cystadenocarcinoma. *Gastrointest Radiol* 1983;8:245–248.

255. Stark DD, Bass NM, Moss AA, et al. Nuclear magnetic resonance imaging of experimentally induced liver disease. *Radiology* 1983;148:743–751.

256. Stark DD, Felder RC, Wittenberg J, et al. Magnetic resonance imaging of cavernous hemangioma of the liver: tissue-specific characterization. *AJR* 1985;145:213–222.

257. Stark DD, Goldberg HI, Moss AA, Bass NM. Chronic liver disease: evaluation by magnetic resonance. *Radiology* 1984;150:149–151.

258. Stark DD, Hahn PF, Trey C, Clouse ME, Ferrucci JT Jr. MRI of the Budd-Chiari syndrome. *AJR* 1986;146:1141–1148.

259. Stark DD, Moseley ME, Bacon BR, et al. Magnetic resonance imaging and spectoscopy of hepatic iron overload. *Radiology* 1985;154:137–142.

260. Stark DD, Wittenberg J, Edelman RR, et al. Detection of hepatic metastases: analysis of pulse sequence performance in MR imaging. *Radiology* 1986;159:365–370.

261. Stark DD, Wittenberg J, Middleton MS, Ferrucci JT Jr. Liver metastases: detection by phase-contrast MR imaging. *Radiology* 1986;158:327–332.

262. Steenbergen WV, Joosten E, Marchal G, et al. Hepatic lymphangiomatosis. Report of a case and review of the literature. *Gastroenterology* 1985;88:1968–1972.

263. Sugimoto T, Yoshioka T, Sawada Y, Sugimoto H, Maemura K. Post-traumatic cyst of the liver found on CT scan—a new concept. *J Trauma* 1982;22:797–800.

264. Takayasu K, Moriyama N, Shima Y, et al. Atypical radiographic findings in hepatic cavernous hemangioma: correlation with histologic features. *AJR* 1986;146:1149–1153.

265. Takayasu K, Muramats Y, Shima Y, Moriyama N, Yamada T, Mukuuchi M. Hepatic lobar atrophy following obstruction of the ipsilateral portal vein from hilar cholangiocarcinoma. *Radiology* 1986;160:389–393.

266. Tang-Barton P, Vas W, Weissman J, Salimi Z, Patel R, Morris L. Focal fatty liver lesions in alcoholic liver disease: a broadened spectrum of CT appearances. *Gastrointest Radiol* 1985;10:133–137.

267. Terrier F, Becker CD, Stoller C, Triller JK. Computed tomography in complicated cholecystitis. *J Comput Assist Tomogr* 1984;8:58–62.

268. Terrier F, Becker CD, Triller JK. Morphologic aspects of hepatic abscesses at computed tomography and ultrasound. *Acta Radiol Diagn* 1983;24:129–137.

269. Thomas JL, Bernardino ME, Vermess M, et al. EOE-13 in the detection of hepatosplenic lymphoma. *Radiology* 1982;145:629–634.

270. Thompson WM, Halvorsen RA, Foster WL Jr, Roberts L, Gibbons R. Preoperative and postoperative CT staging of rectosigmoid carcinoma. *AJR* 1986;146:703–710.

271. Thorsen MK, Quiroz F, Lawson TL, Smith DF, Foley WD, Stewart

ET. Primary biliary carcinoma: CT evaluation. *Radiology* 1984;152: 479–483.

272. Torres WE, Whitmire LF, Gedgaudas-McClees K, Bernardino ME. Computed tomography of hepatic morphologic changes in cirrhosis of the liver. *J Comput Assist Tomogr* 1986;10:47–50.

273. Toombs BD, Sandler CM, Rauschkolb EN, Strax R, Harle TL. Assessment of hepatic injuries with computed tomography. *J Comput Assist Tomogr* 1982;1:72–75.

274. Tumeh SS, Benson C, Nagel JS, English RJ, Holman BL. Cavernous hemangioma of the liver: detection with single-photon emission computed tomography. *Radiology* 1987;164:353–356.

275. Tylen U, Hoevels J, Nilsson U. Computed tomography of iatrogenic hepatic lesions following percutaneous transhepatic cholangiography and portography. *J Comput Assist Tomogr* 1981;5:15–18.

276. Ueda J, Hara K, Ohishi H, Uchida H. High density bile in the gallbladder observed by computed tomography. *J Comput Assist Tomogr* 1983;7:801–804.

277. Unger EC, Lee JKT, Weyman PW. CT and MR imaging of radiation hepatitis. *J Comput Assist Tomogr* 1987;11:264–268.

278. van Sonnenberg E, Casola G, Cubberley DA, et al. Oriental cholangiohepatitis: diagnostic imaging and interventional management. *AJR* 1986;146:327–331.

279. Vasile N, Larde D, Zafrani ES, Berard H, Mathieu D. Hepatic angiosarcoma. *J Comput Assist Tomogr* 1983;7:899–901.

280. Vazquez JL, Thorsen MK, Dodds WJ, Foley WD, Lawson TL. Atrophy of the left hepatic lobe caused by a cholangiocarcinoma. *AJR* 1985;144:547–548.

281. Vermess M, Doppman JL. CT of the liver with intravenous lipoid contrast material: review of the current status. *Semin Roentgenol* 1983;18:102–105.

282. Vermess M, Doppman JL, Sugarbaker PH, et al. Computed tomography of the liver and spleen with intravenous lipoid contrast material: review of 60 examinations. *AJR* 1982;138:1063–1071.

283. Vermess M, Leung AW-L, Bydder GM, Steiner RE, Blumgart LH,

284. Warshaw AL, Rattner DW. Facts and fallacies of common bile duct obstruction by pancreatic pseudocysts. *Ann Surg* 1980;192: 33–37.

285. Weiner SN, Koenigsberg M, Morehouse H, Hoffman J. Sonography and computed tomography in the diagnosis of carcinoma of the gallbladder. *AJR* 1984;142:735–739.

286. Weinman HJ, Brasch RC, Press WR, Wesbey GE. Characteristics of gadolinium-DTPA complex: a potential NMR contrast agent. *AJR* 1984;142:619–624.

287. Weinstein JB, Heiken JP, Lee JKT, et al. High resolution CT of the porta hepatis and hepatoduodenal ligament. *RadioGraphics* 1986;6:55–74.

288. Welch TJ, Sheedy PF II, Johnson CM, et al. Focal nodular hyperplasia and hepatic adenoma: comparison of angiography, CT, US, and scintigraphy. *Radiology* 1985;156:593–595.

289. Wenker JC, Baker MK, Ellis JH, Glant MD. Focal fatty infiltration of the liver: demonstration by magnetic resonance imaging. *AJR* 1984;143:573–574.

290. Wilcox DM, Weinreb JC, Lesh P. MR imaging of a hemorrhagic hepatic cyst in a patient with polycystic liver disease. *J Comput Assist Tomogr* 1985;9:183–185.

291. Williams DM, Cho KJ, Aisen AM, Eckhauser FE. Portal hypertension evaluated by MR imaging. *Radiology* 1985;157:703–706.

292. Yang PJ, Glazer GM, Bowerman RA. Budd-Chiari syndrome: computed tomographic and ultrasonographic findings. *J Comput Assist Tomogr* 1983;7:148–150.

293. Yates CK, Streight RA. Focal fatty infiltration of the liver simulating metastatic disease. *Radiology* 1986;159:83–88.

294. Yeh H-C. Ultrasonography and computed tomography of carcinoma of the gallbladder. *Radiology* 1979;133:167–173.

295. Zeman RK, Paushter DM, Schiebler ML, Choyke PL, Jaffe MH, Clark LR. Hepatic imaging: current status. *Radiol Clin North Am* 1985;23:473–487.

Young IR. MR imaging of the liver in primary hepatocellular carcinoma. *J Comput Assist Tomogr* 1985;9:749–754.

CHAPTER 16

Abdominal Wall and Peritoneal Cavity

Jay P. Heiken

ABDOMINAL WALL

Normal Anatomy

The anterior abdominal wall is composed of several layers: skin, superficial fascia, subcutaneous fat, anterolateral and midline (rectus) muscle groups, transversalis fascia, extraperitoneal fat, and peritoneum. Most adults have sufficient body fat to allow identification of the subcutaneous fat layer and individual muscles on computed tomography (CT) (Fig. 1) (34). In very thin or muscular individuals, the three anterolateral muscles (external oblique, internal oblique, and transversus) may appear as a single muscle mass. The aponeuroses of the anterolateral muscles unite at the lateral border of the rectus muscle to form the Spigelian fascia, which splits to become the anterior and posterior rectus sheaths. The paired rectus muscles are joined in the midline by the junction of these fascial sheaths to form the linea alba, which is 4 to 6 mm in width. The inguinal canal begins at the level of the anterior superior iliac spine and extends medially and inferiorly to the pubic tubercle. The anterior wall of the canal is formed by the aponeurosis of the external oblique muscle and the posterior wall by the transversalis fascia (Fig. 2) (128). The primary muscles composing the posterior abdominal wall include the latissimus dorsi and the paraspinal muscle groups.

Pathologic Conditions

Hernias

Although the diagnosis of hernia almost always can be established clinically, CT may be useful in selected instances in differentiating between a hernia and a mass within the abdominal cavity or abdominal wall. In addition, CT may identify clinically unsuspected incisional hernias in patients undergoing postoperative CT exami-

nations (38). Herniation of intraperitoneal fat and bowel through fascial defects in the abdominal wall is easily demonstrated on CT images. A ventral hernia is produced when the linea alba is disrupted and fat and bowel herniate anteriorly through the defect (Fig. 3). A Spigelian hernia results from weakness in the internal oblique and transversus aponeuroses, allowing peritoneal contents to herniate beneath an intact external oblique muscle. CT can establish the diagnosis by demonstrating a peritoneal and muscular defect at the lateral border of the rectus sheath (7) (Fig. 4). Lumbar hernias can occur at two weak points in the posterolateral abdominal wall (73,160). The lower of the two weak points, called the inferior lumbar triangle, or Petit's triangle, lies just above the iliac crest between the external oblique and latissimus dorsi muscles (6,73). The larger superior lumbar triangle, or Grynfelt's triangle, is bounded by the 12th rib, the serratus posticus muscle, the internal oblique muscle, and the erector spinae muscles. These rare posterior abdominal-wall hernias may contain intraperitoneal or extraperitoneal contents.

The inguinal hernia, the most common type of external abdominal hernia, results from herniation of peritoneal contents through the deep inguinal ring (Fig. 2). If sufficiently large, the hernia sac may extend into the scrotum in men or into the labium majus in women. A femoral hernia results when peritoneal contents enter the femoral canal adjacent to the femoral artery and vein. In this type of hernia, the sac protrudes lateral to the inguinal canal between the external oblique muscle insertion on the superior pubic ramus and the superior pubic ramus itself (128).

Masses

Hematoma

Abdominal-wall hematomas occur most commonly within the sheath of the rectus abdominis muscle and are most often secondary to anticoagulant therapy, although

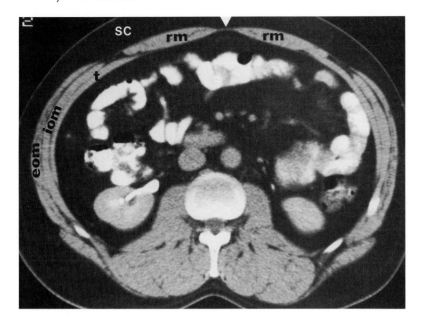

FIG. 1. Normal anatomy of the anterior abdominal wall. The subcutaneous fat layer and individual muscles of the anterolateral muscle group are identified. The rectus muscles are joined in the midline by the linea alba (*arrowhead*); (sc) subcutaneous fat; (eom) external oblique muscle; (iom) internal oblique muscle; (t) transversus muscle; (rm) rectus muscle.

they may result from blunt or penetrating abdominal trauma. Clinical findings that suggest an abdominal-wall hematoma include acute onset of abdominal pain in association with a palpable mass, discoloration of the skin overlying the mass, and a decreasing hematocrit. CT may be performed to corroborate the diagnosis, to assess the extent of hematoma, and to determine if a concomitant intraabdominal or retroperitoneal hematoma is present.

The CT appearance of abdominal-wall hematoma is that of an abnormal mass, often elliptical or spindle-shaped, within one or more layers of the abdominal wall, enlarging, obliterating, or displacing normal structures (Fig. 5). Rectus sheath hematomas usually are limited to one side of the abdomen by the linea alba. However, large hematomas may dissect inferiorly along fascial planes and extend into the pelvis, compressing viscera and crossing to the contralateral side (113). An acute abdominal-wall hematoma has a density equal to or greater than the density of the abdominal muscles (Fig. 5) because of the high protein content of hemoglobin. Seventy-five percent of body-wall hematomas imaged within the first 2 weeks after hemorrhage are hyperdense, and they often are inhomogeneous (137). On occasion, a fluid–fluid level can be seen because of the settling of cellular elements within the hematoma ("the hematocrit effect"). As the hematoma matures, the progressive breakdown and removal of protein within red blood cells reduces the hematoma's attenuation value (104). The process of clot lysis often occurs in a centripetal fashion, producing a low-attenuation halo at the periphery that widens as lysis progresses. By 2 to 4 weeks after the initial bleeding episode, the density of the hematoma may approach that of serum (20–30 Hounsfield units, HU) and then remain at serum density for the duration of its existence (Fig. 6A). With time, a fibroblastic and vascular membrane (pseudocapsule) grows around the hematoma, producing a dense rim on CT images (Fig. 6A). On occasion, the periphery of a chronic hematoma (seroma) may calcify.

The magnetic resonance imaging (MRI) appearance of abdominal-wall hematoma is similar to that seen on CT.

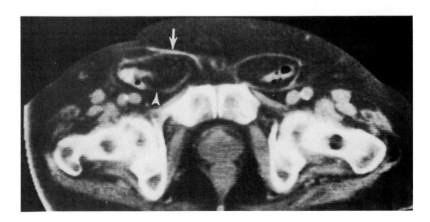

FIG. 2. Bilateral inguinal hernias. Bowel opacified with oral contrast material has herniated into both inguinal canals. The aponeurosis of the external oblique muscle (*arrow*) forms the anterior wall, and the aponeurosis of the transversus muscle (*arrowhead*) forms the posterior wall of the canal.

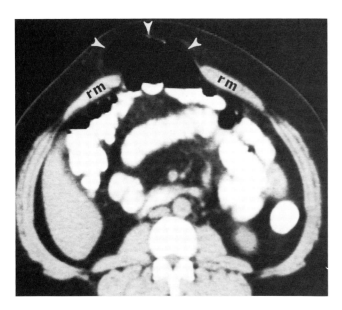

FIG. 3. Ventral hernia. Air-filled bowel has herniated anteriorly through a defect in the linea alba (*arrowheads*); (rm) rectus muscle.

However, in addition to age, the MRI appearance of a hematoma depends on the magnetic-field strength at which it is imaged. The signal intensity of an acute hematoma imaged at low magnetic-field strength (0.15–0.5 T) is less than that of muscle on T1-weighted images (28,136). In contradistinction, when examined at high magnetic-field strength (1.5 T), an acute hematoma has a signal intensity similar to that of muscle on T1-weighted images, with marked hypointensity on T2-weighted images (120). The prominent hypointensity on T2-weighted images implies preferential T2 proton-relaxation enhancement, which is more pronounced at higher field strength (41). It has been proposed that the high concentration of Fe^{2+}-deoxyhemoglobin inside intact red blood cells creates slowly varying local heterogeneity of magnetic susceptibility, resulting in preferential T2 proton-relaxation enhancement in acute hematomas (41). Large acute hematomas may demonstrate a fluid–fluid level on MR images, similar to that seen on CT. On CT, the dependent portion of the hematoma is high in attenuation. On T1-weighted MR images obtained at low magnetic-field

FIG. 4. Spigelian hernia. **A:** A defect (*arrow*) in the aponeuroses of the internal oblique and transversus muscles allows intraperitoneal fat to herniate into the abdominal wall beneath an intact external oblique muscle (*arrowhead*); (rm) rectus muscle. **B:** The hernia becomes more pronounced during a Valsalva maneuver, accounting for a right-lower-quadrant "mass" detected by the patient.

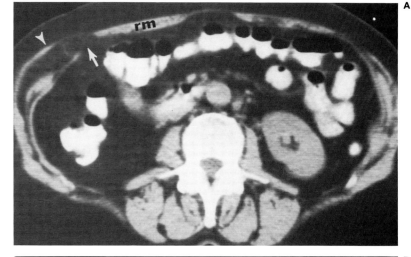

A

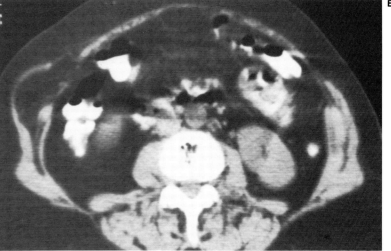

B

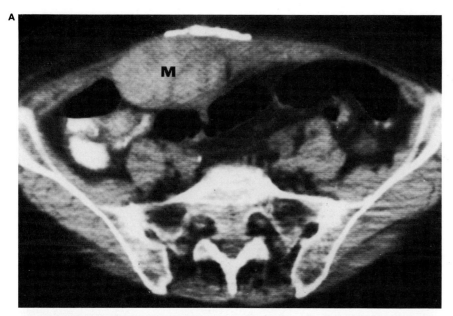

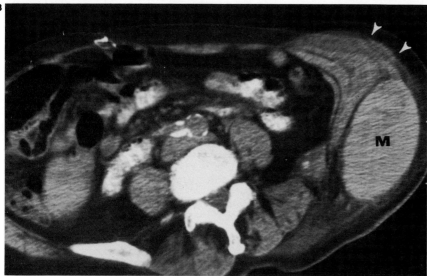

FIG. 5. Acute abdominal-wall hematomas. **A:** An inhomogeneous high-attenuation mass (M) enlarges the right rectus abdominis muscle, beneath a surgically inserted Teflon mesh. **B:** An elliptical high-attenuation mass (M) enlarges the left lateral abdominal wall and dissects along fascial planes into the anterolateral muscles (*arrowheads*).

strength (0.15–0.5 T), the dependent portion is hyperintense compared with the supernatant, whereas on T2-weighted images, this signal-intensity relationship is reversed (47).

Subacute hematomas (older than 1 week) have a more characteristic MRI appearance, consisting of a medium-signal-intensity (slightly greater than muscle) central area, surrounded by a high-intensity (similar to fat) ring that in turn is surrounded by a rim of very low signal intensity (47,120,141) (Fig. 6B and C). This appearance is best seen on T1-weighted images. On T2-weighted images, the signal intensity of the central core increases relative to that for the peripheral zone. The rim remains very low in signal intensity. The central medium-signal-intensity area corresponds to the high-attenuation area on CT, and the peripheral hyperintense zone corresponds to the area of low attenuation on CT (141). The high signal intensity of subacute hematomas is due to T1 shortening, which parallels

the formation of methemoglobin resulting from oxidative denaturation of hemoglobin (12).

Inflammation/infection

Inflammation within the abdominal wall is most often the result of postoperative wound infection (158). Other less common causes include trauma, direct extension from intraabdominal inflammatory processes, and altered host defense. Clinical diagnosis of an abdominal-wall abscess often is difficult, especially in early postoperative or obese patients. CT can be useful for differentiating between abscess and cellulitis, diagnosing or excluding abscess in patients with postoperative wound tenderness, delineating the size and extent of an abscess when present, and determining whether or not the peritoneal cavity is involved.

The CT findings of abdominal-wall inflammation are nonspecific and include streaky soft-tissue densities, loss

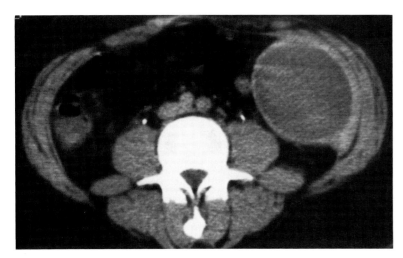
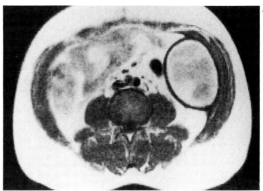
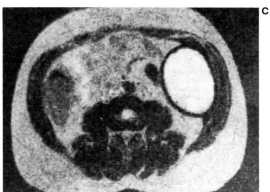

FIG. 6. Chronic abdominal-wall hematoma 3 months after a knife wound. **A:** On CT, the mass is largely of near-water attenuation value, with some central, relatively higher-density material and a soft-tissue-density rim. **B:** A T1-weighted (TR = 500 msec, TE = 30 msec) MR image shows some peripheral areas of high signal intensity within a rim of virtual absence of signal. The central area of decreased signal intensity corresponds to the area of relatively higher density on CT. **C:** On a T2-weighted (TR = 1,500 msec, TE = 90 msec) MR image, the mass appears higher in signal intensity compared with the surrounding tissues. The heterogeneity of the hematoma is less well appreciated. (From ref. 141.)

of normal intermuscular fat planes, enlargement of abdominal-wall muscles, localized masses of varying densities, and masses that dissect along fascial planes. An abdominal-wall abscess appears as an abnormal mass that frequently has a low-attenuation central zone (Fig. 7). The peripheral zone or wall of the abscess may be enhanced after intravenous administration of iodinated contrast material. Occasionally, gas, resulting from gas-producing organisms, may be present within an abdominal-wall abscess. However, the presence of gas within the abdominal wall is not a specific sign of abscess, because gas in a partially open abdominal wound or gas in a fistula connecting bowel to the skin surface may have a similar appearance. Because the CT appearance of abscess is not specific, needle aspiration may be necessary to confirm the diagnosis.

Neoplasm

Both primary and secondary neoplasms can involve the abdominal wall. Although large masses generally are discovered by inspection and palpation, small tumors may be difficult to detect clinically, particularly in obese patients or in those with surgical scars or indurated tissue. CT is capable of demonstrating small abdominal-wall tumors and may be valuable in defining the extent of palpable lesions for the purpose of placing radiotherapy ports and assessing the effectiveness of chemotherapy. CT is also helpful in detecting tumor recurrence after surgical excision (28).

Benign masses involving the abdominal wall include cysts, desmoids, and endometriomas. Desmoid tumors are locally aggressive, benign fibrous-tissue neoplasms that occur most commonly in the rectus muscle and sheath. Approximately three-fourths of desmoids occur in women, predominantly during the childbearing years (13). On precontrast CT images, desmoids have an attenuation

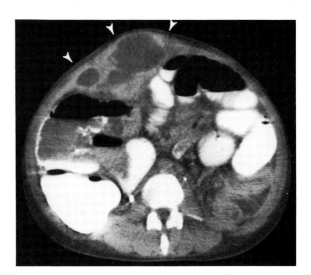

FIG. 7. Abdominal-wall abscess. A mass within the anterior abdominal wall (*arrowheads*), containing several areas of near-water attenuation value, displaces air- and oral-contrast-filled bowel loops posteriorly.

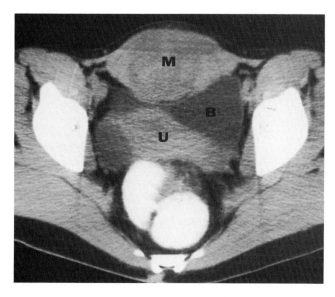

FIG. 8. Desmoid tumor 15 months after colectomy in a woman with Gardner's syndrome. A soft-tissue-density mass (M) involving the rectus abdominus muscles indents the anterior wall of the bladder (B); (U) uterus.

value similar to that for muscle (Fig. 8), but they may be enhanced on postcontrast CT images to become hyperdense relative to muscle (55). Abdominal-wall endometriomas almost always occur in a preexisting surgical scar or in the umbilicus (135). Of those involving surgical scars, nearly half occur after cesarean section. The CT appearance of abdominal-wall endometrioma is nonspecific, consisting of a soft-tissue-density mass enlarging the rectus abdominis muscle (4).

The most common primary malignant neoplasms of the abdominal wall are sarcomas, followed in frequency by lymphomas. Hematogenously spread metastases may involve either the abdominal-wall muscles or the subcutaneous fat. Metastatic involvement of muscle produces enlargement of the muscle, often with an associated decrease in attenuation value (Fig. 9). Subcutaneous metastases usually are nodular (Fig. 10). Direct spread to the abdominal wall by an intraabdominal neoplasm appears as a thickening of the muscles, with loss of the intermuscular and perimuscular fat planes (112) (Fig. 11). Malignant neoplasms that spread intraperitoneally, such as ovarian and gastrointestinal carcinoma, have a tendency to involve the umbilical region, producing periumbilical masses (Fig. 12). Differentiation between abdominal-wall neoplasm and abscess or hematoma may not be possible using CT criteria alone, and clinical correlation is usually necessary. Percutaneous needle biopsy under CT guidance may be required to differentiate among these entities.

PERITONEAL CAVITY

Anatomy

The peritoneal cavity contains a series of communicating but compartmentalized potential spaces that are not visualized on CT images unless they are distended by fluid. Knowledge of the anatomy of these spaces and of the ligaments that define them is important in understanding pathologic processes involving the peritoneal cavity.

The walls of the peritoneal cavity, as well as the abdominal and pelvic organs contained within, are lined with *peritoneum,* an areolar membrane covered by a single

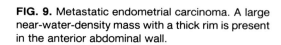

FIG. 9. Metastatic endometrial carcinoma. A large near-water-density mass with a thick rim is present in the anterior abdominal wall.

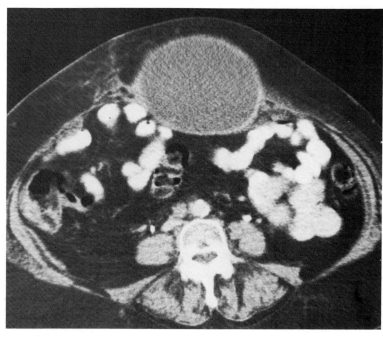

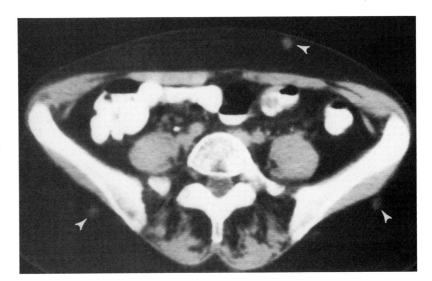

FIG. 10. Subcutaneous metastatic melanoma. Multiple small soft-tissue-density nodules (*arrowheads*) are seen within the subcutaneous fat.

row of mesothelial cells (44). Folds of peritoneum, called *ligaments,* connect and provide support for structures within this cavity. The name of a particular ligament usually reflects the two major structures that it joins; e.g., the gastrocolic ligament extends between the greater curvature of the stomach and the transverse colon. A ligament connecting the stomach to another structure is called an *omentum.* The greater omentum joins the greater curvature of the stomach to the colon, and then continues downward anterior to the small bowel. The lesser omentum (also called the gastrohepatic ligament) joins the lesser curvature of the stomach to the liver. A *mesentery* is a fold of peritoneum connecting either the small bowel or portions of the colon to the posterior abdominal wall. Normally, these peritoneal folds are not directly imaged by CT, but fat, lymph nodes, and vessels contained within them can be identified (132). However, when the peritoneal folds become thickened by edema, inflammation, or neoplastic infiltration, they can be directly visualized on CT images.

The major barrier dividing the peritoneal cavity is the transverse mesocolon, which separates the cavity into supramesocolic and inframesocolic compartments (94). An understanding of the anatomy of the supramesocolic compartment is aided by familiarity with the embryologic development of this space (see Chapter 11).

Supramesocolic Compartment

In the following discussion, the left and right peritoneal spaces are arbitrarily divided into a number of subspaces. Although these spaces freely communicate, they often become separated by fibrous adhesions formed by the inflammatory or neoplastic cause of the fluid collections

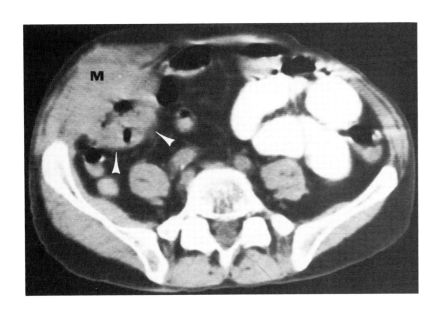

FIG. 11. Recurrent colon carcinoma, with direct spread to the abdominal wall. A soft-tissue mass (*arrowheads*) involving the right colon extends directly into the abdominal-wall muscles (M).

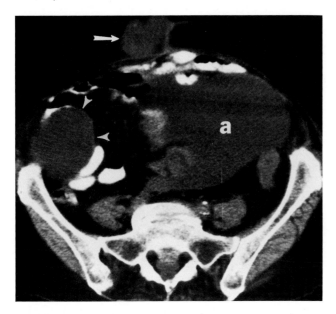

FIG. 12. Periumbilical metastasis. A lobulated mass (*arrow*) occupies the right periumbilical region in a patient with metastatic colon cancer. Ascites (a) is also present. Note the displacement of adjacent bowel loops by an area of loculated ascites (*arrowheads*).

filling these spaces. (For a complete discussion of the anatomy of the peritoneal spaces, see Chapter 11.)

Left peritoneal space

The left peritoneal space can be divided into anterior and posterior perihepatic spaces and anterior and posterior subphrenic spaces. The *left anterior perihepatic space* can be affected by pathologic processes emanating from the left lobe of the liver or the anterior wall of the body and antrum of the stomach. In addition, it may be involved

by extension of pathologic processes from other portions of the left peritoneal space.

The *left posterior perihepatic space* is also referred to as the gastrohepatic recess. This space may be affected by pathologic processes arising in any of the structures to which it is closely related, including the left lobe of the liver, the lesser curvature of the stomach, the anterior wall of the duodenal bulb, and the anterior wall of the gallbladder (147) (Fig. 13).

The *left anterior subphrenic space* is in direct continuity with the left anterior perihepatic space inferomedially and with the left posterior subphrenic space dorsally (55,135) (Fig. 14). Fluid collections in this region may result from perforation of the splenic flexure of the colon or of the fundus or upper body of the stomach (Fig. 15). In addition, collections in the left anterior subphrenic space may result from extension of disease processes involving the left perihepatic spaces or the left posterior subphrenic space.

The *left posterior subphrenic (perisplenic) space* is the posterior continuation of the anterior subphrenic space (Fig. 14). Common sources of pathologic processes involving the left posterior subphrenic space include splenic surgery (i.e., postoperative abscess or hematoma), splenic trauma, and extension of disease processes involving the anterior subphrenic space (Figs. 16 and 17). In addition, pathologic processes involving the tail of the pancreas can affect the left subphrenic space. Uncommonly, disease processes arising in retroperitoneal organs such as the left kidney or left adrenal gland can extend into this peritoneal space.

Right peritoneal space

The right peritoneal space includes both the lesser sac and the right portion of the greater peritoneal space sur-

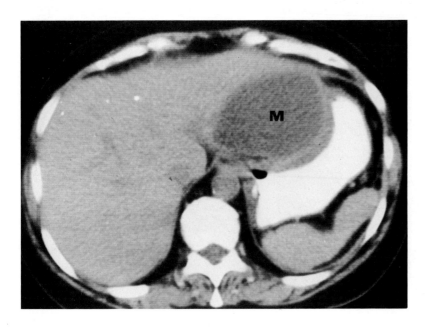

FIG. 13. Abscess of left posterior perihepatic space secondary to gallbladder perforation. Adjacent to the left lobe of the liver, a relatively low-density mass (M) with a higher-attenuation-value rim displaces the contrast-filled stomach posteriorly.

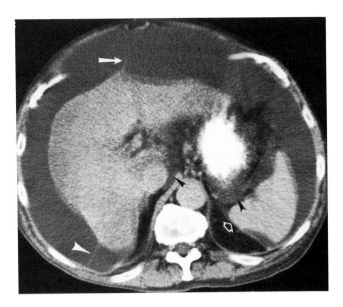

FIG. 14. Ascites in a patient with cirrhosis. A large amount of ascitic fluid fills the right and left greater peritoneal spaces, with only a very small amount in the lesser sac (*black arrowheads*). The falciform ligament (*arrow*) separates the right and left peritoneal spaces anteriorly. The triangular ligament (*white arrowhead*) separates fluid in the right subphrenic space from a small amount of fluid in the superior recess of the right subhepatic space medially. Note the continuity of the anterior perihepatic, anterior subphrenic, and posterior subphrenic (perisplenic) spaces on the left. Along the posterior border of the spleen, fluid is limited medially by the spleen's peritoneal reflection (the "bare area" of the spleen) (*open arrow*).

rounding the liver, i.e., the right perihepatic space. These two spaces communicate via the epiploic foramen (foramen of Winslow).

Right Perihepatic Space. The right perihepatic space consists of a subphrenic space and a subhepatic space, which are partially separated by the right coronary ligaments. The posterior subhepatic space projects cephalad into the recess between the liver and the right kidney. This recess, known as the hepatorenal fossa or Morison's pouch, is the most dependent part of the subhepatic space when the body is in the supine position and is therefore important in the spread and localization of intraperitoneal fluid collections. Common sources of pathologic processes causing fluid collections in the right perihepatic space include the gallbladder, the descending portion of the duodenum (Fig. 18), the right lobe of the liver, and the right colon. Another important cause of a right perihepatic fluid collection is cephalad extension of pelvic fluid via the right paracolic gutter. Occasionally, retroperitoneal disease processes arising in the right kidney, right adrenal gland, or head of the pancreas can extend into the right perihepatic space.

Lesser Sac. The lesser sac communicates with the remainder of the right peritoneal space through a narrow inlet between the inferior vena cava and the free margin of the hepatoduodenal ligament called the epiploic foramen (foramen of Winslow). However, in patients with intraperitoneal inflammation, this foramen may seal, separating the lesser sac from the greater peritoneal cavity (94). A prominent fold of peritoneum, elevated from the posterior abdominal wall by the left gastric artery, divides the lesser sac into two compartments: a large lateral compartment on the left and a smaller medial compartment on the right (94) (Fig. 19). The medial compartment con-

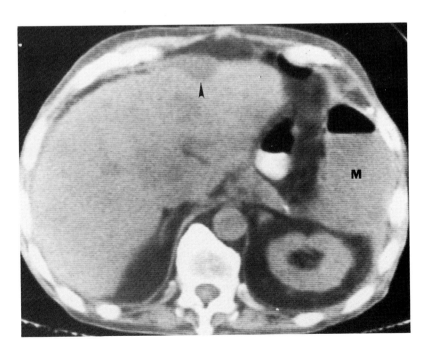

FIG. 15. Left anterior subphrenic abscess. A mass (M) of less than soft-tissue density, with an air–fluid level, occupies the left anterior subphrenic space. Liver metastases and a small amount of loculated ascites (*arrowhead*) are also present.

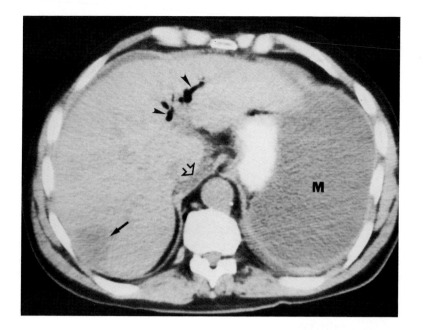

FIG. 16. Left subphrenic seroma 2 weeks after splenectomy and total pancreatectomy for pancreatic carcinoma. A large near-water-density mass (M) fills the left subphrenic space and displaces the contrast-filled stomach medially. A small amount of fluid is also present in the superior recess of the medial compartment of the lesser sac (*open arrow*). The low-density lesion in the liver (*arrow*) proved to be a cavernous hemangioma. Note the air in the biliary tree (*arrowheads*).

FIG. 17. Left subphrenic abscess. A near-water-density mass (M) with a soft-tissue-density rim occupies the left posterior subphrenic space; (*arrowhead*) atelectatic lung.

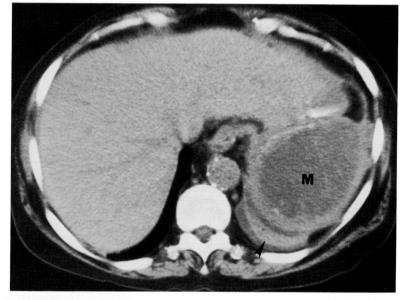

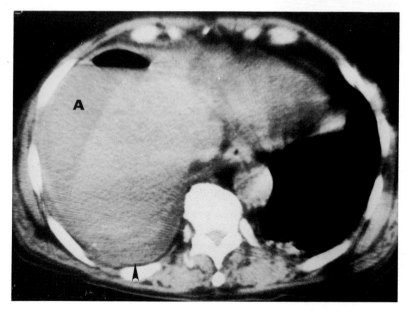

FIG. 18. Abscess of right perihepatic space secondary to a perforated duodenal ulcer. A near-water-density collection (A) with an air–fluid level is present in the right perihepatic (subphrenic) space. A right pleural effusion (*arrowhead*) is also identified.

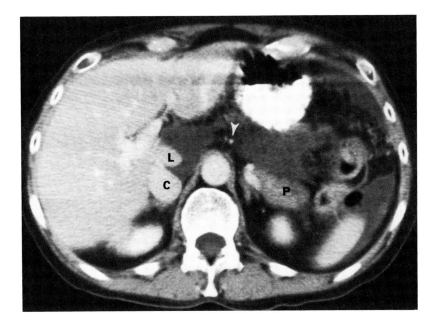

FIG. 19. Lesser-sac ascites in a patient with metastatic endometrial carcinoma. The left gastric artery (*arrowhead*) partially separates the lesser-sac fluid into medial and lateral compartments. The superior recess of the medial compartment abuts the caudate lobe of the liver (L) and the inferior vena cava (C); (P) tail of pancreas.

tains a superior recess that wraps around the caudate lobe of the liver (Figs. 20 and 21).

Disease processes involving the pancreas, transverse colon, posterior wall of the stomach, posterior wall of the duodenum, and caudate lobe of the liver can produce pathologic changes within the lesser sac (Figs. 20–22). The most common lesser-sac collection is ascites (27). Whereas patients with benign, transudative ascites tend to have large greater-sac collections, with little fluid in the lesser sac, patients with peritoneal carcinomatosis often have proportional fluid volumes in the two spaces (42). The largest fluid collections to occupy the lesser sac occur in patients with disease processes involving organs directly bordering this space, the most common being pancreatitis. Fluid collections involving the lateral compartment displace the stomach anteriorly and sometimes medially, whereas medial-compartment collections may cause lateral displacement of the stomach. Collections extending below the level of the pancreatic body displace the transverse colon and mesocolon caudally. Less commonly, a lesser-sac collection may extend ventral and caudal to the transverse colon because of a persistent inferior lesser-sac recess within the leaves of the greater omentum (27). Occasionally, inflammation involving the medial compartment may extend via the aortic or diaphragmatic hiatus into the lower mediastinum (27).

A,B

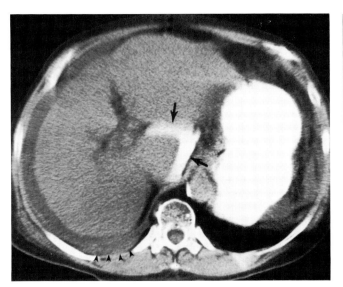 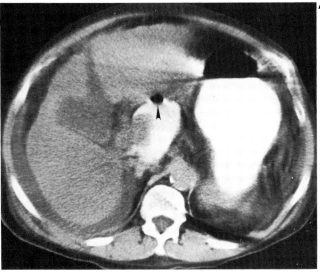

FIG. 20. Extravasation of oral contrast material into the lesser sac from a perforated antral ulcer. **A:** Oral contrast material in the superior recess of the medial compartment of the lesser sac (*arrows*) wraps around the caudate lobe of the liver. Peritoneal fluid borders the liver. A small right pleural effusion is also present (*small arrowheads*). **B:** A more caudal image demonstrates gas (*arrowhead*) within the lesser-sac fluid.

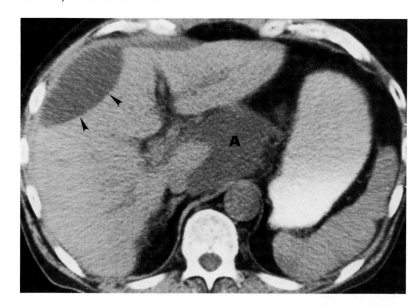

FIG. 21. Pancreatic ascites. Peritoneal fluid fills the superior recess of the medial compartment of the lesser sac (A). Loculated fluid is also present in the right greater peritoneal space (*arrowheads*).

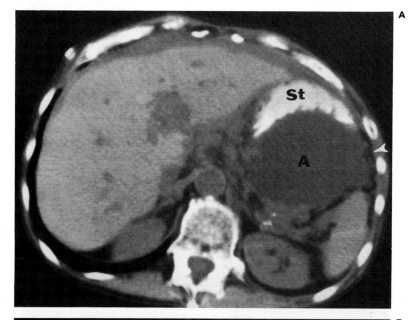

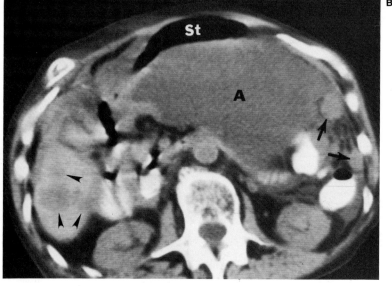

FIG. 22. Lesser-sac ascites in a patient with ovarian carcinoma. **A:** Fluid (A) within the lateral recess of the lesser sac displaces the fundus of the stomach (St) anteriorly and the gastrosplenic ligament (*arrowhead*) laterally. A smaller amount of fluid in the greater peritoneal space surrounds the anterior surface of the liver. **B:** At a more caudal level, the lesser-sac fluid displaces the air-filled gastric antrum (St) anteriorly. Liver metastases (*arrowheads*) and peritoneal tumor implants (*arrows*) are also identified.

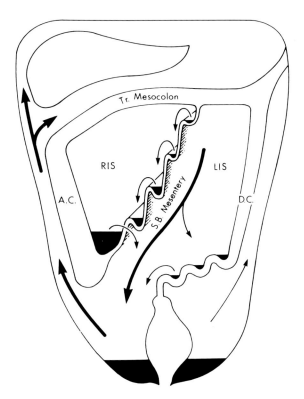

FIG. 23. Schematic diagram of the inframesocolic compartment of the peritoneal cavity. The small-bowel mesentery divides the inframesocolic compartment into two unequal spaces. *Arrows* indicate the natural flow of ascites within the peritoneal cavity; (RIS) right infracolic space; (LIS) left infracolic space; (A.C.) ascending colon; (D.C.) descending colon.

Inframesocolic Compartment

The inframesocolic compartment is divided into two unequal spaces by the obliquely oriented small-bowel mesentery (Fig. 23). The smaller right infracolic space is restricted inferiorly by the junction of the distal small-bowel mesentery with the cecum, whereas the larger left infracolic space is open to the pelvis inferiorly except where it is bounded by the sigmoid mesocolon.

The paracolic gutters are located lateral to the attachments of the peritoneal reflections of the ascending and descending colon. The right paracolic gutter is continuous superiorly with the right perihepatic space. On the left, however, the phrenicocolic ligament forms a partial barrier between the left paracolic gutter and the left subphrenic space. The most dependent portion of the peritoneal cavity in both the erect and supine positions is the pelvis, which consists of lateral paravesical spaces and the midline pouch of Douglas (rectovaginal space in women, rectovesical space in men).

The natural flow of intraperitoneal fluid is directed by gravity and variations in intraabdominal pressure due to respiration along pathways determined by the anatomic compartmentalization of the peritoneal cavity (94) (Fig. 23). Abscesses usually form and metastases usually grow

in sites where natural flow permits infected fluid or malignant ascites to pool.

Fluid within the inframesocolic compartment rapidly seeks the pelvis, where it first fills the pouch of Douglas and then the lateral paravesical fossae. Fluid in the right infracolic space flows along the recesses of the small-bowel mesentery until it pools at the confluence of the mesentery with the colon near the ileocecal junction, with subsequent overflow into the pouch of Douglas (Fig. 24). Fluid in the left infracolic space frequently is arrested by the sigmoid mesocolon before descending into the pelvis. From the pelvis, fluid can ascend both paracolic gutters with changes in intraabdominal pressure during respiration. Flow along the left paracolic gutter is slow and weak, and cephalad extension usually is limited by the phrenicocolic ligament (91,92). The major flow is along the right paracolic gutter into the right subhepatic space, particularly the posterior extension of this space, Morison's pouch (91). From the right subhepatic space, fluid may ascend farther into the right subphrenic space. Direct spread from the right subphrenic space across the midline to the left subphrenic space is prevented by the falciform ligament.

The most common sites for pooling of infected peritoneal fluid, and thus for abscess formation, are the pelvis, right subhepatic space, and right subphrenic space (94). Similarly, the most common sites for pooling of malignant ascites and subsequent fixation and growth of peritoneal metastases are the pouch of Douglas, the lower small-bowel mesentery near the ileocecal junction, the sigmoid mesocolon, and the right paracolic gutter (93).

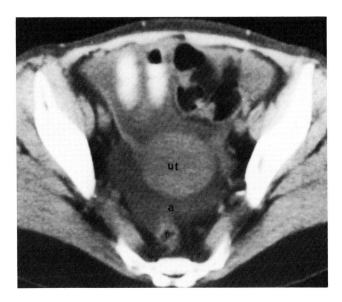

FIG. 24. Ascites in the pouch of Douglas. Ascites (a) fills the cul-de-sac between the uterus (ut) and rectum (r). Fluid is also present anterior to the uterus.

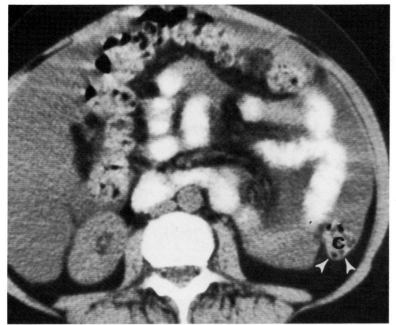

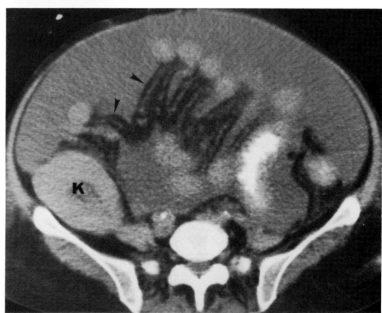

FIG. 25. Ascites. The retroperitoneal fat posterior to the descending colon is preserved (*arrowheads*).

FIG. 26. Massive ascites. The small-bowel loops are located centrally within the abdomen. The pleated nature of the small-bowel mesentery can be appreciated as fluid outlines several of the mesenteric leaves (*arrowheads*); (K) transplant kidney.

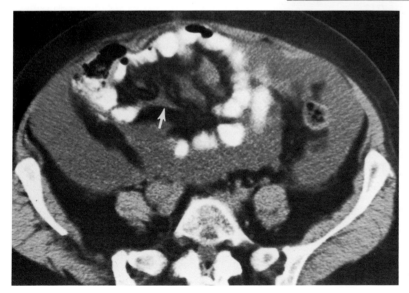

FIG. 27. Ascites in a patient with metastatic ovarian carcinoma. Fluid accumulating between leaves of the small-bowel mesentery takes on a triangular configuration (*arrow*).

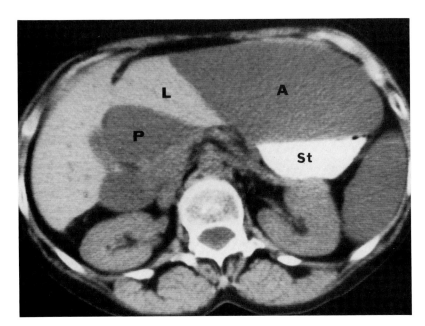

FIG. 28. Loculated ascites in a patient with metastatic ovarian carcinoma. Fluid loculated within the left anterior perihepatic space (A) compresses the stomach (St) and the left lobe of the liver (L). A smaller collection of loculated fluid is present in the left posterior perihepatic space (P).

Pathologic Conditions

Ascites

Ascites is the accumulation of fluid within the peritoneal cavity resulting from either increased fluid production or impaired removal. The causes of ascites include hypoalbuminemia, inflammation, and venous or lymphatic obstruction. CT can accurately demonstrate and localize even small amounts of free peritoneal fluid. Localized collections of ascites frequently are seen in the right perihepatic space, Morison's pouch, or the pouch of Douglas. Peritoneal fluid in the paracolic gutter is easily distinguished from retroperitoneal fluid by the preservation of the retroperitoneal fat posterior to the ascending or descending colon (61,64) (Fig. 25). When a large amount of ascites is present, the small-bowel loops usually are located centrally within the abdomen (Fig. 26), and fluid often accumulates in triangular configurations within the leaves of the small-bowel mesentery or adjacent to bowel loops (121) (Fig. 27). Loculated ascites, secondary to postoperative, inflammatory, or neoplastic adhesions, may appear as a well-defined fluid-attenuation mass that displaces adjacent structures (Figs. 12 and 28).

The attenuation of ascitic fluid generally ranges from 0 to 30 HU, but may be higher in cases of exudative ascites, the density of the fluid increasing with increasing protein content (16). However, attenuation values of ascitic fluid are nonspecific, and infected or malignant ascites cannot reliably be distinguished from uncomplicated transudative ascites on the basis of attenuation value alone. Relatively acute intraperitoneal hemorrhage can be distinguished from other fluid collections because it usually results in peritoneal fluid with an attenuation value greater than 30 HU (33).

The distribution of ascitic fluid within the peritoneal cavity may suggest the nature of the fluid. Patients with benign transudative ascites tend to have large greater-sac collections, with little fluid in the lesser sac, whereas patients with malignant ascites often have proportional volumes of fluid in these peritoneal spaces (19). However, these CT features are not specific, and needle aspiration may be necessary to differentiate transudative and exudative ascites.

MRI can also be used to evaluate intraabdominal fluid collections. Transudative ascites is low in signal intensity on T1-weighted images, where it is seen best, and high in signal intensity on T2-weighted images because of its long T1 and T2 relaxation values (19,149) (Fig. 29). T1 relaxation values for fluid collections decrease with increasing protein concentration (139). Thus, exudative fluid collections demonstrate intermediate to short T1 values and long T2 values. These collections are best seen on T2-weighted images, where they appear high in signal intensity (19). Although MRI holds potential for distinguishing among different types of intraabdominal fluid collections, the MRI appearance and relaxation times are not specific enough to obviate diagnostic needle aspiration. In addition, the lack of a reliable gastrointestinal contrast agent for MRI makes it difficult to distinguish small extraluminal fluid collections from dilated fluid-filled bowel loops. Additionally, lesser-sac collections are more difficult to demonstrate on MR images, possibly because of the effect of peristaltic- and respiratory-motion artifacts (19).

A,B

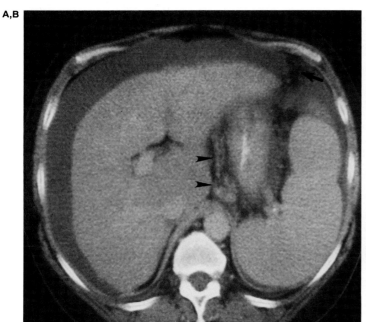

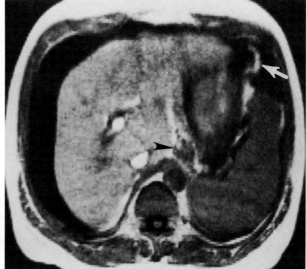

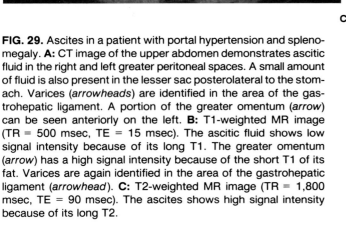

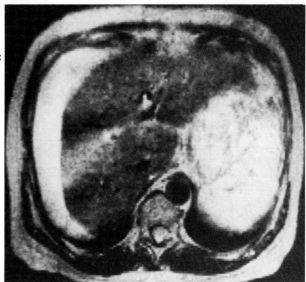

C

FIG. 29. Ascites in a patient with portal hypertension and spleno-megaly. **A:** CT image of the upper abdomen demonstrates ascitic fluid in the right and left greater peritoneal spaces. A small amount of fluid is also present in the lesser sac posterolateral to the stomach. Varices (*arrowheads*) are identified in the area of the gastrohepatic ligament. A portion of the greater omentum (*arrow*) can be seen anteriorly on the left. **B:** T1-weighted MR image (TR = 500 msec, TE = 15 msec). The ascitic fluid shows low signal intensity because of its long T1. The greater omentum (*arrow*) has a high signal intensity because of the short T1 of its fat. Varices are again identified in the area of the gastrohepatic ligament (*arrowhead*). **C:** T2-weighted MR image (TR = 1,800 msec, TE = 90 msec). The ascites shows high signal intensity because of its long T2.

Intraperitoneal Abscess

The epidemiology of intraabdominal abscess has changed in recent decades. In the first half of the 20th century, perforated ulcer, appendicitis, and biliary tract disease were the most common causes (31,109). However, over the past several decades, intraabdominal abscess has occurred most commonly after surgery, particularly surgery involving the stomach, biliary tract, and colon (49,123,129,150). Despite advances in surgical technique and antimicrobial therapy, intraabdominal abscess remains a serious diagnostic and therapeutic problem. Even with treatment, mortality can reach 30% (115).

Although most patients present with fever, leukocytosis, and abdominal pain, patients with chronic, walled-off abscesses may present with few overt clinical signs or symptoms. Furthermore, some symptoms may be masked by the administration of antibiotics or corticosteriods (3).

CT provides an accurate method for diagnosing in-

traabdominal abscess. When examining a patient for a suspected abscess, careful attention to technique is crucial for correct diagnosis. The entire abdomen, from the diaphragm to the pubic symphysis, should be imaged, and adequate oral contrast material should be administered to avoid mistaking a fluid-filled bowel loop for an abscess.

The CT appearance of an abscess is variable, depending on its age and location. In its earliest stage, an abscess consists of a focal accumulation of neutrophils in a tissue or organ seeded by bacteria and thus appears as a mass with an attenuation value near that of soft tissue (Fig. 30). As the abscess matures, it undergoes liquefactive necrosis. At the same time, highly vascularized connective tissue proliferates around the central necrotic region. At this stage, the abscess has a central region of near-water attenuation surrounded by a higher-attenuation rim that usually is enhanced after intravenous administration of contrast material (5) (Figs. 13 and 31). Approximately one-third of abscesses contain variable amounts of air,

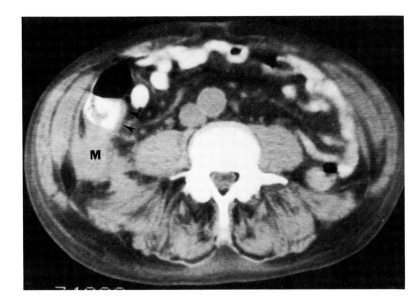

FIG. 30. Appendiceal abscess. A mass (M) of soft-tissue attenuation value abuts the cecum and extends irregularly into the adjacent mesenteric and retroperitoneal fat. The wall of the cecum (*arrowheads*) is thickened.

appearing on CT images either as multiple small bubbles or as an air–fluid level (5,17,48,59,70,156) (Figs. 31 and 32). The presence of a long air–fluid level suggests communication with the gastrointestinal tract (59). Ancillary findings include displacement of surrounding structures, thickening or obliteration of adjacent fascial planes, and increased density of adjacent mesenteric fat (Fig. 31). Whereas most abscesses are round or oval in shape, those adjacent to solid organs, such as the liver, may have a crescentic or lenticular configuration (Fig. 18).

In some cases, the CT appearance of an abscess can suggest its cause. A low-density right-lower-quadrant mass containing a round calcific density is highly suggestive of an appendiceal abscess with an appendicolith. Elsewhere in the abdomen, a low-density mass containing a high-density object suggests a foreign-body abscess (Fig. 32).

Although these CT findings are highly suggestive of abscess, they are not specific. Other masses that can have a central low attenuation value include cyst, pseudocyst, hematoma, urinoma, lymphocele, biloma, loculated as-

cites, thrombosed aneurysm, and necrotic neoplasm. In addition, normal structures such as unopacified bladder, stomach, and bowel can mimic the appearance of an abscess (Fig. 33). Thickening of adjacent fascial planes is also nonspecific and can be seen with intraabdominal hematoma and neoplastic infiltration. Even the presence of gas within a mass is nonspecific for abscess, because a necrotic noninfected neoplasm and a mass that communicates with bowel can also contain gas. Because a specific diagnosis of abscess based on CT findings alone is not possible, correlation with clinical history is important. Percutaneous needle aspiration may be necessary to make a definitive diagnosis. In this regard, CT can be very helpful in identifying a plane of access for aspiration that is both safe and free of contamination from bowel. The presence or absence of an abscess can be established by obtaining a specimen for Gram stain and culture. In most instances, if an abscess is present, a catheter can be inserted percutaneously for definitive drainage (134,144). Although it was originally thought that only well-defined, unilocular

FIG. 31. Appendiceal abscess. A low-attenuation mass (M) with an air–fluid level is present in the right lower quadrant. The mass is surrounded by a higher-attenuation rim and streaky soft-tissue densities extending into the adjacent mesenteric fat; (P) right psoas muscle.

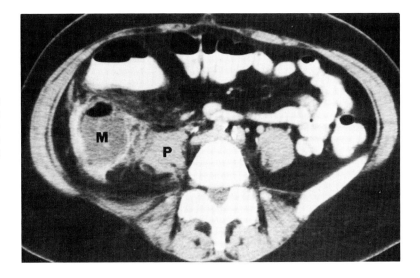

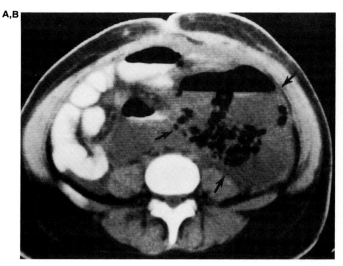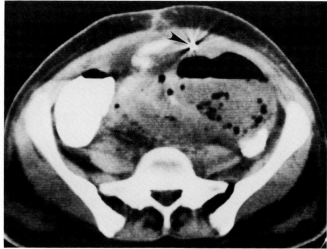

FIG. 32. Foreign-body abscess. **A:** Large, relatively low-attenuation mass (*arrows*) containing multiple air bubbles and a long air–fluid level occupies the left lower quadrant of the abdomen. **B:** At a more caudal level, a metallic foreign body (*arrowhead*) that had perforated through the gastrointestinal tract is identifed.

abscesses with safe drainage routes should be drained percutaneously, the criteria for percutaneous drainage have been expanded to include ill-defined and multiseptated abscesses, as well as those communicating with the gastrointestinal tract or located deep to major abdominal organs (37,100). Even potentially complicated abscesses such as appendiceal, diverticular, and interloop abscesses secondary to Crohn disease can be drained without complications (8,63,103,107,122,143). In the case of periappendiceal abscesses, percutaneous drainage may completely eliminate the need for surgery (8,63,107,143), whereas percutaneous drainage of diverticular abscesses often converts complex two- or three-stage surgical procedures to safer one-stage colonic resections (103). The

only factor of value in predicting the eventual outcome of percutaneous drainage is location, subphrenic and hepatic abscesses being more likely to have a successful outcome than those in other locations (59). Because no specific CT features of an abscess (other than location) provide predictive value, all intraabdominal abscesses should be considered candidates for percutaneous drainage (37,59). The technical details of CT-guided abscess drainage are described in Chapter 5.

The MRI appearance of intraabdominal abscess is also nonspecific. Because of its short or intermediate T1 and long T2, an abscess demonstrates intermediate to high signal intensity on T1-weighted images and high signal intensity on T2-weighted images (19,149). It usually is best seen on T1-weighted images (19,149). In a study of percutaneously obtained normal and abnormal body fluids, the mean T1 value for abscess contents was found to be significantly shorter, and the mean T2 value significantly longer, than those for bile, ascitic fluid, urine collections, cysts, pseudocyst fluid, and pleural fluid (15). However, although MRI may potentially provide useful information about the nature of intraabdominal fluid collections, the MRI appearances and relaxation times for various types of collections do not appear specific enough to eliminate the need for aspiration to establish a diagnosis.

Accuracy of CT in intraperitoneal abscess

The accuracy of CT in detecting intraabdominal abscess is approximately 95% (5,46,48,69–71,124,156). Most false-positive diagnoses are due to mistaking unopacified fluid-filled stomach, bowel, or bladder for an abscess. If a question exists as to the nature of a fluid-filled structure, additional oral, rectal, or intravenous contrast material can be administered.

FIG. 33. Closed-loop obstruction simulating an abscess. An inhomogeneous low-attenuation mass (M) displaces the rectosigmoid colon laterally.

Comparison of CT and other imaging techniques

Other imaging techniques have also been shown to be accurate in the detection of intraabdominal abscess, particularly ultrasound and radionuclide imaging. In a number of published studies, sensitivity and overall accuracy for ultrasound have ranged from 90% to 96% (71,84,138), although one study reported an accuracy of only 44% (82). Ultrasound images can be obtained in multiple anatomic planes, and a thorough examination can be performed in a relatively short period of time. In addition, if a patient is too unstable to be moved, an ultrasound study can be done at the patient's bedside. The areas of the abdomen best suited to ultrasound diagnosis of abscess are the right and left upper quadrants and the pelvis (145). In these areas, the liver, spleen, and distended urinary bladder can be used as acoustic windows for transmission of the ultrasonic beam into the abdomen. However, abscesses located in the midabdomen may be difficult to detect with ultrasound because of interruption of the ultrasonic beam by bowel gas and mesenteric fat (14). In addition, other patient factors, such as obesity or the presence of open wounds, drainage tubes, and large dressings, may hamper the ultrasound examination. In comparison with the potential limitations of ultrasound, CT is capable of providing high-quality images of all areas of the abdomen and pelvis, including the retroperitoneum, regardless of body habitus and despite the presence of open wounds, drainage tubes, overlying dressings, and large amounts of bowel gas. CT is thus better able to detect and define the extent of intraabdominal fluid collections and to aid in the planning of either percutaneous or surgical abscess drainage by clearly delineating the relationships of the abscess to surrounding structures.

Radionuclide imaging using leukocytes labeled with gallium 67 citrate (^{67}Ga) or indium 111 (^{111}In) has also been effective in detecting and localizing intraabdominal abscesses. Various studies have reported sensitivities ranging from 80% to 92% (71,75,89). The major advantage of radionuclide scintigraphy is that it provides images of the entire body, thus occasionally displaying unsuspected extraabdominal sites of infection (125). The major disadvantage of ^{67}Ga imaging is that 48 to 72 hr frequently are required before the study can be properly interpreted (69). In addition, uptake of ^{67}Ga is nonspecific in that it accumulates in certain tumors, postsurgical beds, healing wounds, and other areas of simple inflammation (69,75). Because it is excreted by the colon, difficulty can be encountered in differentiating between an abdominal abscess and normal colonic activity (71). ^{111}In imaging avoids some of the problems of ^{67}Ga imaging, because it does not take as long, is not excreted by the colon, and does not accumulate in tumors. However, ^{111}In is a cyclotron-produced isotope whose preparation requires care to maintain the function of the leukocytes (69). In addition,

the distribution of the labeled leukocytes and their accumulation at sites of inflammation may be altered by splenectomy, bone marrow radiation, hyperalimentation, hemodialysis, hyperglycemia, and antibiotic therapy (69). Furthermore, a chronic abscess may have a well-defined wall without significant inflammatory response and therefore may not be detected by ^{111}In-leukocyte studies (69). Other limitations include obscuration of upper abdominal abscesses by activity in the liver and spleen and nonspecific uptake of ^{111}In-leukocytes by other inflammatory and some noninflammatory processes (87). Another limitation of radionuclide imaging for evaluation of a suspected abdominal abscess is that when an abnormal accumulation of radiotracer is identified, an additional imaging study usually is needed to provide more specific anatomic localization.

Approach to imaging a suspected intraabdominal abscess

In patients who are acutely ill or who have localized clinical findings, CT is the initial imaging procedure of choice for detecting and defining the extent of intraabdominal abscesses. If the findings on CT examination are equivocal, ultrasound may provide valuable information. Ultrasound can be used as the initial examination if a right-upper-quadrant, left-upper-quadrant, or pelvic abscess is suspected. However, a negative result on ultrasound examination should be followed by CT, because ultrasound does not optimally evaluate the middle abdomen and retroperitoneum. If the findings on CT examination of the entire abdomen and pelvis are unequivocally normal, abscess can be confidently excluded.

In patients suspected of having abdominal abscesses who are not acutely ill and who have no localizing signs, radionuclide imaging with ^{67}Ga-citrate- or ^{111}In-labeled leukocytes can be considered as the initial screening technique. If the findings on radionuclide examination are normal, usually no further radiologic evaluation is indicated. If the examination demonstrates one or more areas of increased activity, a CT or ultrasound examination is then performed to document and further evaluate the area of possible abscess. MRI, because of its limited availability, stringent patient requirements, relatively high cost, and relatively long examination time, plays only a limited role in the detection of intraabdominal abscesses.

Other Intraperitoneal Fluid Collections

Intraperitoneal hemorrhage may result from excessive anticoagulation, bleeding diathesis, trauma to the liver, spleen, or mesentery, or spontaneous rupture of a vascular neoplasm, hemorrhagic cyst, or ectopic pregnancy. CT is highly sensitive and specific for diagnosing hemoperitoneum (33), the diagnosis being based on the high atten-

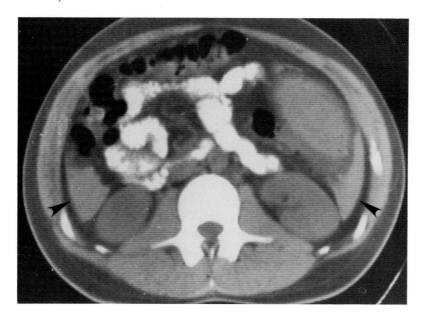

FIG. 34. Acute intraperitoneal hemorrhage secondary to splenic rupture. Peritoneal fluid with an attenuation value slightly higher than that for muscle is present in both paracolic gutters (*arrowheads*).

uation value of the peritoneal fluid (Figs. 34 and 35). The CT appearance of intraperitoneal hemorrhage depends on the location, age, and extent of the bleeding. Immediately after hemorrhage, intraperitoneal blood has the same attenuation value as circulating blood. However, within hours, attenuation increases as hemoglobin is concentrated during clot formation (104,105). In most cases, the attenuation value begins to decrease within several days as clot lysis takes place (10). The attenuation value decreases steadily with time and often approaches that of water (0–20 HU) after 2 to 4 weeks (72) (Fig. 36). During the hyperdense phase, the attenuation value of intraperitoneal blood ranges from 20 to 90 HU (33,77,137,155). In one large study, all patients with hemoperitoneum less than 48 hr old had fluid collections containing areas that showed attenuation values greater than 30 HU (33). The morphologic characteristics of recent intraperitoneal hemorrhage are variable. The fluid collection may be homogeneously hyperdense or may be inhomogeneous, with nodular or linear areas of high attenuation surrounded by lower-attenuation fluid. The inhomogeneity may result from irregular clot resorption or intermittent bleeding (155). In most cases, intraperitoneal blood contains focal areas of clot that have higher attenuation values than the free intraperitoneal blood. These localized clots are helpful in determining the bleeding site, because they usually form adjacent to the organ from which the hemorrhage originated (33). Occasionally, fresh blood within a hematoma or confined within a peritoneal space may show a "hematocrit effect," with sedimented erythrocytes producing a dependent layer of high attenuation. The most common site of blood accumulation seen on CT images after upper abdominal trauma is Morison's pouch (33,85). The right paracolic gutter is another common site of blood collection, even in cases of splenic trauma. With extensive hemorrhage, large collections of blood may fill the pelvis,

with little blood in upper abdominal sites. Therefore, it is important to include the pelvis in any CT examination performed for suspected intraabdominal hemorrhage, particularly in patients who have sustained blunt abdominal trauma (33).

If a CT image without intravenous contrast material has been obtained, viewing the images with a narrow window width is helpful to accentuate the density difference between the fresh blood and the adjacent soft tissues. However, in most cases, a precontrast CT examination is unnecessary, and one can begin the study with intravenous contrast material administered as a bolus, followed by a rapid infusion. The contrast enhancement helps to dem-

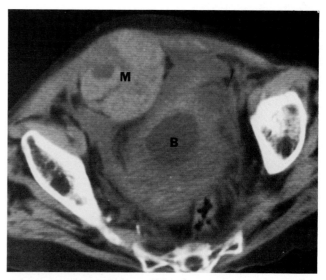

FIG. 35. Hemoperitoneum and rectus hematoma. Peritoneal fluid within the pelvis, with an attenuation value near that of muscle, surrounds the bladder (B). A large inhomogeneous mass (M) of density higher than that for muscle within the right rectus muscle represents an acute hematoma.

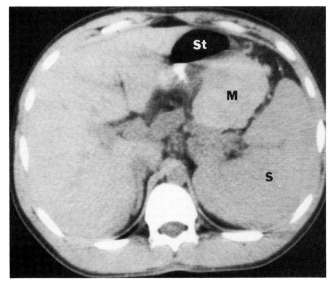

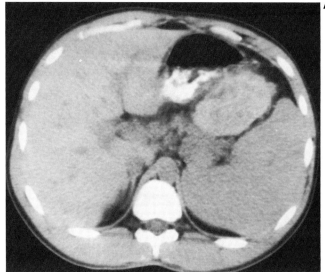

A,B

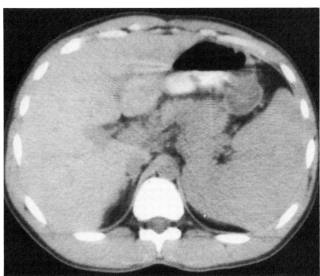

C

FIG. 36. Hemorrhage within the gastrosplenic ligament in a patient with hemophilia. **A:** Large homogeneous mass (M) with an attenuation value similar to that of muscle is present posterior to the body of the stomach (St). The spleen (S) is enlarged. **B:** Three days later, the mass has become inhomogeneous. **C:** Two months later, the mass has become smaller, with an attenuation value near that of water.

onstrate injuries to the liver, spleen, and kidneys and makes intraperitoneal fluid collections more apparent by increasing the density of the surrounding tissues. Before beginning the examination, adequate oral contrast material should be administered to opacify all abdominal and pelvic bowel loops. Images of the upper abdomen should be obtained at 1-cm intervals to allow adequate visualization of the liver, spleen, and kidneys. Below the kidneys, images may be obtained at 2-cm intervals to the pubic symphysis. If a pelvic abnormality is demonstrated or if a pelvic fracture is suspected, a more detailed examination of the pelvis can be performed.

MRI can also be used to demonstrate intraperitoneal hemorrhage. However, many patients referred for suspected intraabdominal hemorrhage are unstable and require extensive monitoring and supportive equipment, making MRI impractical. In addition, a hematoma less than 48 hr old may have a nonspecific signal intensity (141).

Intraperitoneal bile accumulation (biloma) is caused by iatrogenic, traumatic, or spontaneous rupture of the biliary tree (146). The bile elicits a low-grade inflammatory response that generally walls off the collection by formation of a thin capsule or inflammatory adhesions within the mesentery and omentum (81,146). Most bilomas appear round or oval and have attenuation values less than 20 HU. Those complicated by hemorrhage or infection may be higher in density. Bilomas usually are confined to the upper abdomen. Although most are located in the right upper quadrant, left-upper-quadrant bilomas are not uncommon, occurring in approximately 30% of cases (101,146) (Fig. 37). Because the CT appearance is not specific, biloma cannot be distinguished from other abdominal fluid collections, and usually either needle aspiration or biliary scintigraphy is required to establish the diagnosis. Most bilomas can be treated successfully with percutaneous catheter drainage (101,146).

Intraabdominal collections of urine may result from

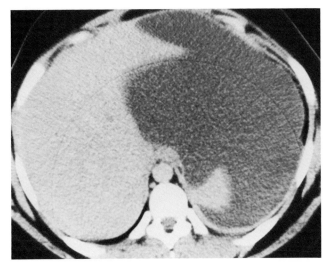

FIG. 37. Biloma 3 weeks after cholecystectomy. A large peritoneal fluid collection occupies the left peritoneal spaces.

urinary tract obstruction or from surgery or trauma involving the kidney, ureter, or bladder. Free intraperitoneal urine usually is the result of traumatic rupture of the bladder dome. CT images from patients with intraperitoneal bladder rupture performed after cystography or intravenous administration of contrast material will show high-density fluid freely filling the peritoneal spaces (Fig. 38). Although localized collections of urine (urinomas) usually occur within the perirenal space, an intraperitoneal urinoma can occur if the anatomic boundaries of the retroperitoneum have been disrupted by trauma or prior surgery (54). On CT images obtained without intravenous contrast material, the attenuation value of a urinoma is less than 20 HU. After intravenous administration of contrast material, however, the attenuation can increase because of extravasation of opacified urine into the fluid collection. Thus, delayed CT images may be helpful in establishing the diagnosis of urinoma.

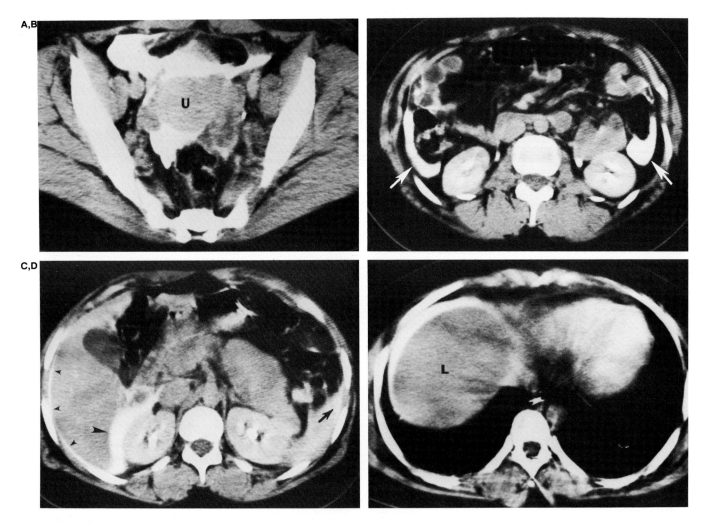

FIG. 38. Intraperitoneal bladder rupture. **A:** Extravasated iodinated contrast material from a cystogram fills the peritoneal spaces surrounding the uterus (U). **B:** At a more cephalad level, the contrast material is identified in both paracolic gutters (*white arrows*). **C:** More cephalad, contrast material fills Morison's pouch (*large arrowhead*) and the right perihepatic space (*small arrowheads*). A small amount of fluid is also present in the left peritoneal space (*arrow*). **D:** Contrast material in the right subphrenic space outlines the dome of the liver (L).

Lymphoceles are abnormal accumulations of lymphatic fluid, usually resulting from operative disruption of lymphatic vessels. The most common procedures to cause lymphoceles are renal transplantation and retroperitoneal lymph node dissection. Although most lymphoceles are confined to the retroperitoneum, intraperitoneal lymphoceles do occur. The more common manifestation of intraperitoneal lymph leakage, however, is chylous ascites, usually resulting from lymphatic obstruction by tumor (116). A lymphocele has a nonspecific appearance and cannot be distinguished from other abdominal fluid collections by its CT or MRI features alone. Similarly, chylous ascites cannot be differentiated from other types of ascitic fluid, although occasionally the diagnosis may be suggested if negative Hounsfield numbers, due to the high fat content of lymph, are detected. The diagnosis of lymphocele can be established by percutaneous aspiration (116,151).

Mesentery

Normal anatomy

The small-bowel mesentery is a broad, fan-shaped fold of peritoneum that connects the jejunum and ileum to the posterior abdominal wall (44). It originates at the duodenojejunal flexure just to the left of the spine and extends obliquely to the ileocecal junction. Within its two fused layers are contained the intestinal branches of the superior mesenteric artery and vein, lymphatic vessels, lymph nodes, nerves, and variable amounts of fat. On CT, the mesentery appears as a fat-containing area central to the small-bowel loops, within which the jejunal and ileal vessels can be identified as distinct round or linear densities (132) (Fig. 39). Normal lymph nodes less than 1 cm in diameter are occasionally identified. The normal mesenteric fat is similar to the subcutaneous fat in attenuation (−100 to −160 HU) (131). In patients with a large amount of ascites, the pleated nature of the mesentery can be appreciated as fluid outlines the mesenteric folds (Fig. 26).

The transverse mesocolon, which extends from the anterior surface of the pancreas to the transverse colon, contains the middle colic arteries and veins (Fig. 40). On the right, the root of the mesocolon is continuous with the duodenocolic ligament and thus the posterior aspect of the hepatic flexure. Medially it crosses the descending duodenum and head of pancreas, extending along the lower anterior edge of the body and tail of the pancreas. On the left it is continuous with the phrenicocolic and splenorenal ligaments (97). In most patients, the transverse mesocolon is readily identified on CT as a fat-containing area extending from the pancreas, particularly at the level of the uncinate process, to the margin of the colonic wall (62). However, in thin patients, the transverse mesocolon may be difficult to identify because of lack of mesenteric fat and the steeply oblique orientation of the mesentery in such patients. Nevertheless, the middle colic branches of the transverse mesocolon can be identified in nearly all patients (132). The root of the small-bowel mesentery at its origin near the duodenojejunal flexure is continuous with the root of the transverse mesocolon (95). The sigmoid mesocolon, extending from the posterior pelvic wall and containing the sigmoid and hemorrhoidal vessels, usually can be identified deep within the pelvis (Fig. 41).

Pathologic conditions involving the mesentery and peritoneum

Mesenteric abnormalities are readily identified on CT in all but the leanest patients because of the abundance of fat present within the normal mesentery. Various pathologic processes, both benign and malignant, may infiltrate the mesentery, causing an increase in attenuation of the mesenteric fat, distortion of the mesenteric architecture, and obscuration of the mesenteric vessels. Some of these processes may also cause thickening of the peri-

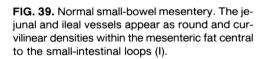

FIG. 39. Normal small-bowel mesentery. The jejunal and ileal vessels appear as round and curvilinear densities within the mesenteric fat central to the small-intestinal loops (I).

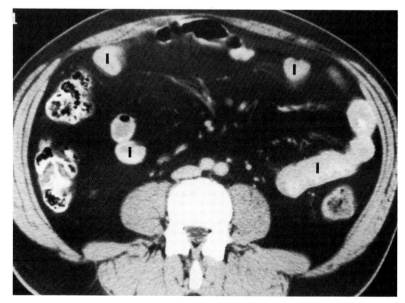

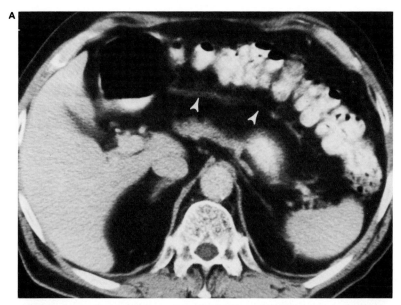

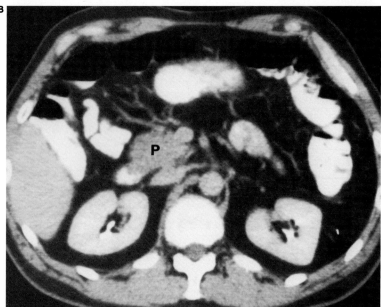

FIG. 40. Normal transverse mesocolon. **A:** The middle colic vessels (*arrowheads*) are easily identifiable within the fat posterior to the transverse colon. **B:** The fat and vessels within the transverse mesocolon often are easiest to identify at the level of the uncinate process of the pancreas (P).

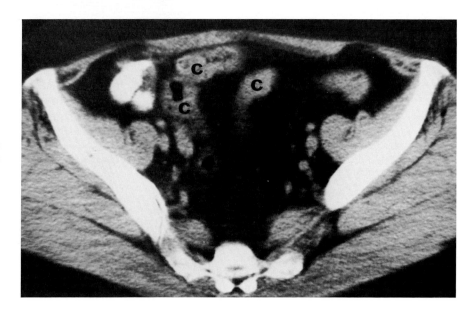

FIG. 41. Normal sigmoid mesocolon. The vessels of the sigmoid mesocolon are identified within the fat extending between the sacrum and the sigmoid colon (C).

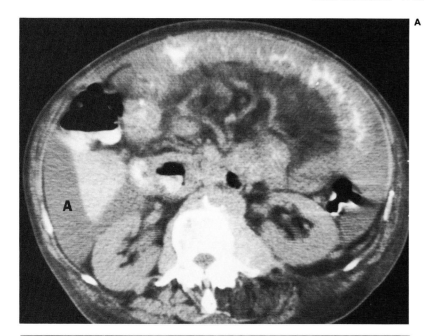

A

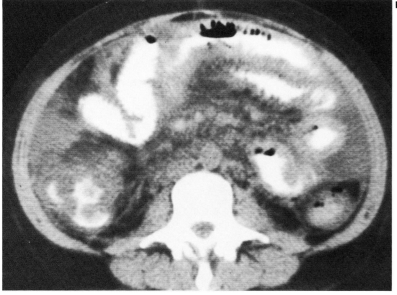

B

FIG. 42. Mesenteric edema in two patients. **A:** The small-bowel mesentery is increased in density, and the segmental mesenteric vessels are poorly defined in a patient with intestinal lymphangiectasis. The small-bowel loops are diffusely thickened, and chylous ascites (A) surrounds the right lobe of the liver. **B:** Patient with mesenteric ischemia secondary to systemic lupus erythematosus. The mesenteric fat is increased in density, and the mesenteric vessels are poorly defined. Diffuse bowel-wall thickening and ascites are also present.

toneal lining. Detection of mesenteric abnormalities requires rigorous attention to CT technique. It is particularly important to opacify the gastrointestinal tract with oral contrast material so that unopacified bowel will not be mistaken for a mesenteric mass. Conversely, a small mesenteric mass can be obscured if surrounded by unopacified bowel loops. Approximately 500 ml of an oral contrast agent should be given at least 1 hr prior to the examination in order to opacify the distal small bowel. Another 500 ml of contrast material should be given 15 min before the examination to opacify the stomach and proximal small bowel. If bowel cannot confidently be distinguished from a mesenteric mass, additional contiguous images through the suspicious area can be obtained after additional oral contrast material has been administered. Occasionally it is helpful to opacify the colon per rectum with a dilute

contrast solution to differentiate between a redundant sigmoid colon and a pelvic mass.

MRI is not as valuable as CT for detecting, characterizing, and delineating mesenteric abnormalities. Peristaltic- and respiratory-motion artifacts can degrade MR images and limit spatial resolution in the region of the mesentery. In addition, lack of a reliable oral contrast agent for MRI makes it difficult to differentiate mesenteric masses and bowel loops in many cases.

Edema. Diffuse mesenteric edema is most commonly the result of hypoalbuminemia, usually caused by either cirrhosis or the nephrotic syndrome. Mesenteric ischemia and mesenteric venous or lymphatic obstruction are less common causes. The CT findings characteristic of mesenteric edema include increased density of the mesenteric fat, poor definition of segmental mesenteric vessels, rel-

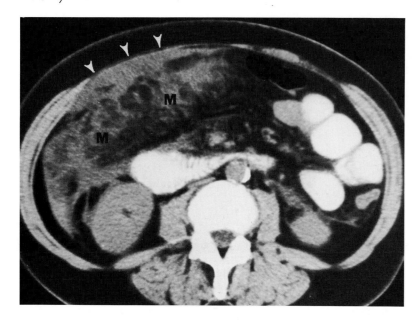

FIG. 43. Inflammation of the transverse meso-colon in a patient with acute pancreatitis. The transverse mesocolon (M) is diffusely increased in density, with irregular areas of soft-tissue attenuation. The greater omentum (*arrowheads*) is also involved.

ative sparing of the retroperitoneal fat, and association with subcutaneous edema (131) (Fig. 42). Bowel-wall thickening is also present in some patients. When this pattern is identified, careful evaluation of the root of the mesentery should be made to exclude a focal tumor mass obstructing mesenteric vessels and creating secondary edema (131). Although diffuse infiltration of the mesentery by metastatic tumor may have an appearance similar to that of mesenteric edema, it usually can be distinguished from edema by the rigidity of the mesenteric leaves. Lateral decubitus or prone images may be helpful in demonstrating the mesenteric fixation.

Pancreatitis. The transverse mesocolon is affected by dissection of pancreatic enzymes in a small percentage of patients with a clinical diagnosis of acute pancreatitis (90,133). However, in patients with fulminant pancreati-

tis, the mesocolon is involved approximately one-third of the time (62). The small-bowel mesentery is involved much less commonly. The main CT finding in patients with mesenteric inflammation related to pancreatitis is increased density of the mesenteric fat. Diffuse inflammation results in ill-defined streaks of soft-tissue density within the fat (Fig. 43). When a phlegmon is present, the involved mesentery has a more homogeneous soft-tissue density. Mesenteric fluid collections appear as water-density masses. The presence of air bubbles within a mesenteric fluid collection indicates either an abscess or communication with the gastrointestinal tract (Fig. 44). Patients with mesenteric involvement demonstrated by CT have higher morbidity and mortality than patients without CT evidence of mesenteric spread (62).

Crohn Disease. Crohn disease is a chronic granulo-

FIG. 44. Abscess in the transverse mesocolon secondary to acute pancreatitis. An elongated soft-tissue mass containing multiple air bubbles (*arrowheads*) occupies the fat posterior to the transverse colon.

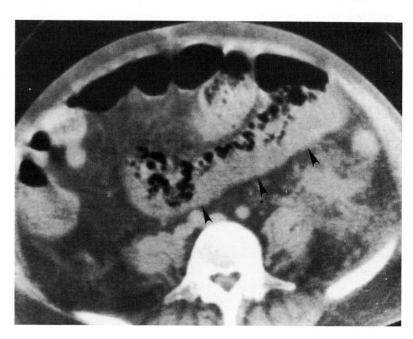

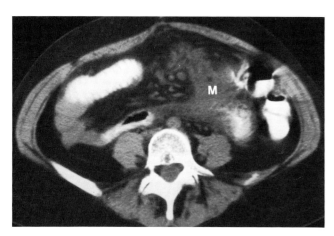

FIG. 45. Mesenteric inflammatory mass in a patient with Crohn disease. An ill-defined soft-tissue-density mass (M) extends into the small-bowel mesentery from a thickened small-bowel loop.

matous disease of the alimentary tract that most commonly involves the small intestine or colon. The major benefit of CT imaging in patients with Crohn disease is to identify and characterize the extramucosal abnormalities that cause separation of bowel loops on barium studies (40). Most important, CT is helpful in differentiating mesenteric abscess from fibro-fatty proliferation or diffuse inflammatory reaction of the mesentery. Fibro-fatty mesenteric proliferation, the most common cause of bowel-loop separation, is characterized by increased density of the fat between the separated loops (−70 to −90 HU) and lack of a soft-tissue mass or fluid collection in the affected region (35,40). A diffuse inflammatory reaction of the mesentery produces a similar increase in density of the

mesenteric fat, but with no clearly defined borders. An abscess can be confidently diagnosed when a well-marginated near-water-density mass is identified. Occasionally, the mass may contain air and oral contrast material, indicating communication with bowel (40,67). CT can also be helpful in identifying and defining the extent of sinus tracts and fistulae. In cases in which a mesenteric mass has an attenuation value near that of soft tissue, it may be difficult to differentiate between an abscess and an inflammatory mass (67) (Fig. 45). Occasionally, identification of fibro-fatty proliferation of the mesentery on CT can be helpful in establishing a diagnosis of Crohn disease when a patient's inflammatory bowel disease is difficult to classify clinically, because mesenteric fat proliferation does not appear to be a feature of ulcerative colitis (43).

Diverticulitis. The most common CT finding in patients with diverticulitis is inflammation of the pericolonic fat, characterized by poorly defined soft-tissue density and fine linear strands within the fat adjacent to the involved colon (56,80) (Fig. 46). Although the barium-enema examination has long served as the primary imaging test for diagnosing diverticulitis, it does not delineate the extracolonic extent of disease. The advantage of CT is that it clearly delineates the extracolonic extent of disease, including any complicating pericolic abscess (Fig. 47), while not requiring direct distension of the colon with contrast material. In addition, because CT images the entire abdomen, it is useful in demonstrating other complications of diverticulitis, such as bladder involvement, ureteral obstruction, and distant abscesses. In one study, CT demonstrated the extracolonic extent and complications of diverticulitis more accurately than contrast-enema examination in 41% of cases (56). The association of colon-

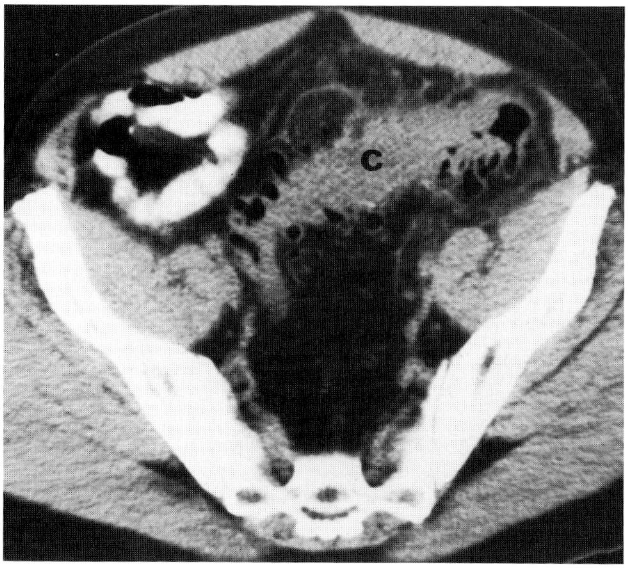

FIG. 46. Diverticulitis. The wall of the sigmoid colon (C) is thickened, and strands of soft-tissue density extend into the adjacent mesenteric fat. Multiple air-filled diverticula can be identified along the wall of the colon.

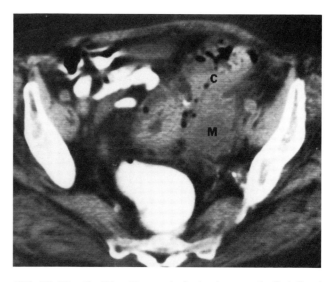

FIG. 47. Diverticulitis with a pericolonic abscess. An ill-defined near-water-density mass (M) abuts the thickened sigmoid colon (C).

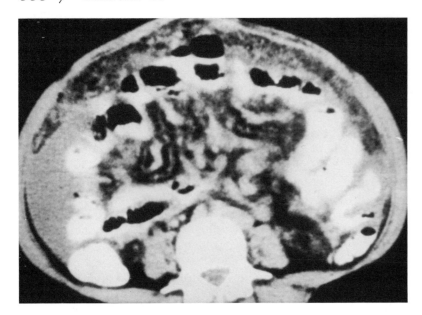

FIG. 48. Tuberculous peritonitis. High-density ascites is present. The omentum and mesentery are thickened, and several mildly enlarged mesenteric lymph nodes can be identified. (Courtesy of Rodney Reznek, M.D., London, England.)

wall thickening and pericolonic inflammatory changes is not pathognomonic for diverticulitis and can be mimicked by perforated colon carcinoma, pelvic inflammatory disease, appendicitis, endometriosis, Crohn disease, and other forms of colitis.

Peritonitis. Peritonitis is an inflammation of the peritoneum that can result from numerous causes and can be either localized or diffuse. The major types of peritonitis include bacterial, granulomatous, and chemical (115). Although bacterial peritonitis is sometimes primary, it usually results secondarily from perforation of an abdominal viscus. Common causes include appendicitis, diverticulitis, perforated ulcer, perforated carcinoma, acute cholecystitis, pancreatitis, salpingitis, and abdominal surgery (115). With diffuse peritonitis, the CT findings consist of thickening of the mesentery, increased density of the mesenteric fat, and ascites (152). This CT appearance is nonspecific and can also be seen in patients with metastatic cancer or peritoneal mesothelioma.

Tuberculous peritonitis has become a relatively rare disease. It is believed to occur by direct extension (ruptured lymph nodes or perforation of a tuberculous lesion in the gastrointestinal or genitourinary tract) or by lymphatic or hematogenous spread (140). The CT appearance of tuberculous peritonitis is varied. The most common CT feature is lymphadenopathy, predominantly in the mesenteric and peripancreatic areas (57). A central low density within the enlarged lymph nodes, presumably due to caseation necrosis, is seen in approximately 40% of patients (30,57). High-density ascites (20–45 HU) is another char-

FIG. 49. Mesenteric panniculitis. The transverse mesocolon is increased in density, with multiple strands of linear soft-tissue density (*arrowheads*).

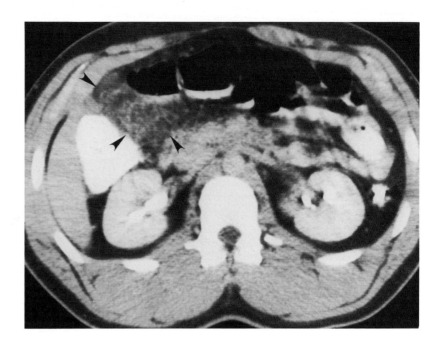

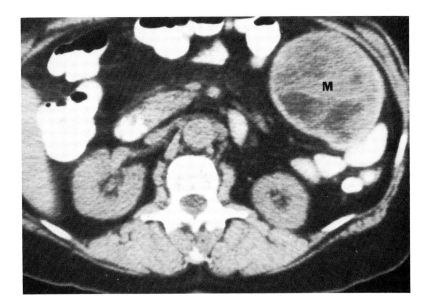

FIG. 50. Mass-like intraabdominal panniculitis. A large, well-defined mass (M) containing mixed soft-tissue- and fat-density material displaces bowel loops on the left side of the abdomen. The mass arose within the transverse mesocolon. (From ref. 66.)

acteristic feature of tuberculous peritonitis, the increased density being related to the high protein content of the fluid (24,30,51,57). Additional CT findings include thickening and nodularity of peritoneal surfaces, mesentery, and omentum (24,30,57) (Fig. 48). Although these CT features are highly suggestive of tuberculous peritonitis, they are not pathognomonic, and other diseases, such as nontuberculous peritonitis, lymphoma, metastatic carcinoma, peritoneal mesothelioma, and pseudomyxoma peritonei, should be included in the differential diagnosis.

Mesenteric Panniculitis. Intraabdominal panniculitis or fat necrosis (also called lipodystrophy) is an inflammatory condition of adipose tissue that can affect the mesentery, omentum, or retroperitoneum (68,110). The association of fat necrosis and acute pancreatitis is well recognized (36). Intraabdominal fat necrosis unassociated with pancreatitis usually is idiopathic, although some cases have been associated with infection, recent surgery, or a foreign body (66). The CT appearance of fat necrosis depends on whether the involvement is diffuse or nodular.

Diffuse panniculitis produces a generalized increase in the density of the involved adipose tissue, which usually contains multiple strands of linear soft-tissue density (Fig. 49). Nodular or mass-like fat necrosis results in lesions that have well-defined walls and contain areas of fat density interspersed with areas of near-water or soft-tissue density (53,66) (Fig. 50). The higher-attenuation areas represent edema, inflammatory infiltrate, and fibrosis (66). Calcification in the necrotic central portion may also be detected (52). In some cases, the CT appearance of mass-like fat necrosis may not be distinguishable from that of a liposarcoma or a fat-containing teratoma.

Mesenteric Cysts. Mesenteric cysts appear on CT as well-defined, near-water-density abdominal masses that sometimes contain thin higher-density septa (50) (Fig. 51). In some cases, a thin wall can be identified peripherally. Mesenteric cysts are benign masses containing either serous or chylous fluid (142). Their etiology is poorly understood. They usually present as asymptomatic abdominal masses, but can cause chronic abdominal pain or

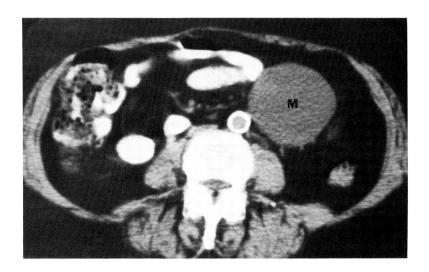

FIG. 51. Mesenteric cyst. A well-defined near-water-density mass (M) is present within the small-bowel mesentery.

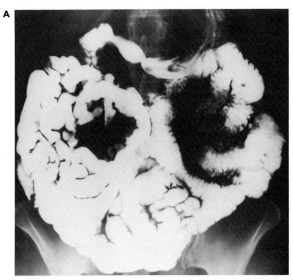

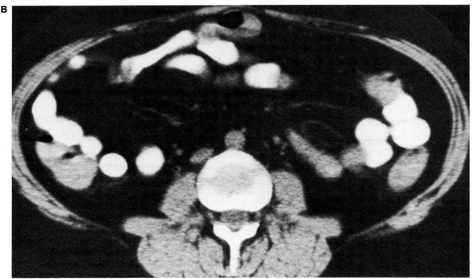

FIG. 52. Pseudotumoral mesenteric lipomatosis. **A:** Barium small-bowel examination demonstrates displacement of small-bowel loops in the middle abdomen. **B:** CT image through the middle abdomen shows that the displacement of bowel loops is due to a large amount of fat within the small-bowel mesentery.

acute pain secondary to a complication such as torsion, rupture, hemorrhage, or gastrointestinal obstruction. The most common location of a mesenteric cyst is in the small-bowel mesentery, with the mesocolon and omentum being less common sites of origin (50,127). The cysts usually are single, but they can be multiple and vary widely in size. In children, the cysts may fill most of the abdomen (50). Although the cyst content usually is of water density, cysts containing mucinous fluid or hemorrhage can have higher CT numbers (152).

Other Nonneoplastic Processes Involving the Mesentery. Mesenteric hemorrhage, similar to hemorrhage elsewhere in the peritoneum, has a varied appearance depending on the age and extent of the bleeding. Acute mesenteric hemorrhage may produce localized, well-defined, soft-tissue masses adjacent to bowel loops or larger "cake-like" masses that displace the bowel loops (152). With diffuse involvement, the mesenteric fat is obliterated. The

attenuation of the hematoma is initially high, with a gradual decrease in attenuation over a period of weeks, followed by gradual resorption of the remaining seroma. After complete resorption, the mesentery may return to a normal appearance or may contain residual fibrosis (152).

Pseudotumoral lipomatosis of the mesentery consists of excessive proliferation of normal mesenteric fat. This benign condition can be idiopathic or can be seen in association with obesity, Cushing syndrome, or steroid therapy (78). On contrast studies of the gastrointestinal tract, mesenteric lipomatosis may displace bowel loops, simulating an abdominal mass or ascites. CT can exclude the presence of neoplasm by showing that the displacement is due to either diffuse or focal accumulation of normal fat (20,78,130) (Fig. 52).

Systemic amyloidosis is characterized by diffuse extracellular tissue deposition of an amorphous eosinophilic protein-polysaccharide complex (22). Amyloidosis can

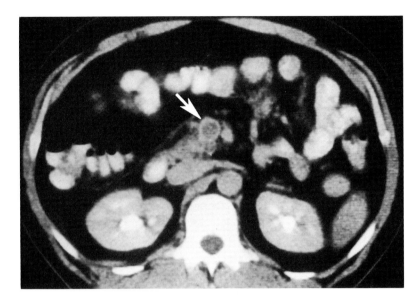

FIG. 53. Thrombosis of the superior mesenteric vein (SMV). The SMV (*arrow*) is enlarged and contains a central low density, surrounded by a higher-density wall.

occur as a primary process or in association with chronic inflammatory disease or multiple myeloma. Involvement of the mesentery, when extensive, is easily demonstrated by CT (2). The CT appearance, consisting of increased density of mesenteric fat, with encasement of mesenteric vessels, is indistinguishable from those of other disease processes causing diffuse mesenteric infiltration, including peritonitis, metastatic carcinoma, and peritoneal mesothelioma.

The most commonly recognized radiographic manifestation of Whipple disease is thickening of the valvulae conniventes of the small bowel. However, CT is capable of demonstrating some of the less well recognized extraintestinal manifestations of the disease, including low-density retroperitoneal and mesenteric lymphadenopathy and sacroileitis (79,118) (see Chapter 17, Fig. 44). The enlarged

lymph nodes in Whipple disease may be low in attenuation secondary to deposition of neutral fat and fatty acids within the nodes (79).

Mesenteric venous thrombosis is responsible for 5% to 15% of cases of intestinal ischemia (45). The superior mesenteric vein (SMV), which is involved in 95% of these cases, is easily imaged by CT. The typical appearance of chronic SMV thrombosis consists of enlargement of the vein, with a central low density surrounded by a higher-density wall (119) (Fig. 53). The wall of the vein is enhanced after intravenous administration of contrast material, possibly because of enhancement of the arterially supplied vasa vasorum (160). The thrombus may show a higher attenuation value than soft tissue when SMV thrombosis is acute (Fig. 54). In some cases, mesenteric venous thrombosis is associated with increased density of

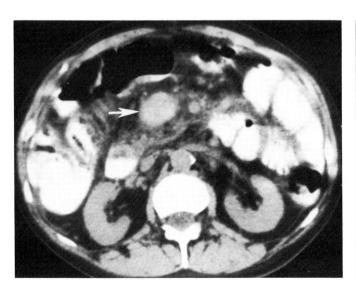
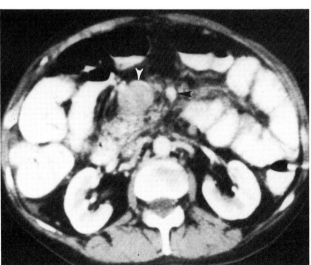

A,B

FIG. 54. Acute SMV thrombosis. **A:** Before intravenous administration of contrast material, the SMV (*arrow*) is enlarged and higher in attenuation value than muscle. **B:** After intravenous contrast material, the SMV is not enhanced. A collateral vessel (*white arrowhead*) crosses anterior to the SMV; (*black arrowhead*) superior mesenteric artery.

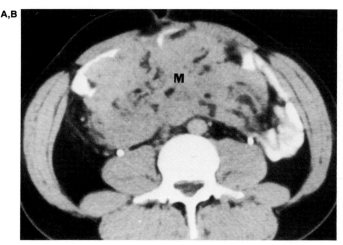
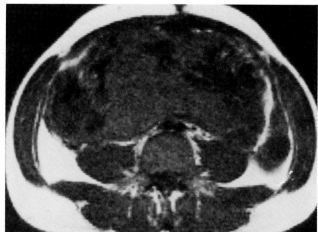
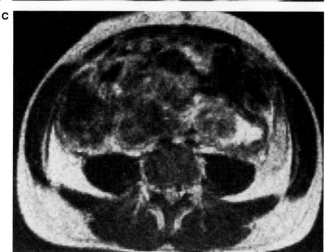

FIG. 55. Mesenteric desmoid tumor in a patient with Gardner's syndrome. **A:** Large, soft-tissue-density mass (M) diffusely infiltrates the mesentery and displaces adjacent small-bowel loops. The colon has been resected. **B:** Relatively T1-weighted MR image (TR = 500 msec, TE = 35 msec). The mass has a low signal intensity similar to that of muscle. **C:** T2-weighted MR image (TR = 2,100 msec, TE = 90 msec). The mass remains low in signal intensity, reflecting the short T2 of fibrous tissue.

the mesenteric fat and poor definition of segmental mesenteric vessels, because of mesenteric edema (131). Thickening of the bowel wall may also be present. If the mesenteric ischemia is severe enough to cause bowel infarction, intramural, portal vein, or mesenteric vein gas may also be identified (32).

Primary Neoplasms. Primary neoplasms of the peritoneum are rare and generally are of mesenchymal origin. The mesenteric desmoid tumor is a nonencapsulated, locally invasive form of fibromatosis (102). It occurs predominantly in patients with Gardner's syndrome who have undergone abdominal surgery, although it occasionally occurs as an isolated abnormality (9,83,102). On CT, a desmoid tumor appears as a soft-tissue mass displacing adjacent visceral structures (9) (Fig. 55). Although the mass may appear well circumscribed, it often has irregular margins reflecting its infiltrative nature (Fig. 56). Attenuation values range from 40 to 60 HU (9,83). Other neoplasms such as mesenteric metastases and lymphoma can present a similar CT appearance. On MRI, a desmoid tumor has a low signal intensity on T1-weighted images and remains relatively low in intensity on T2-weighted images, reflecting its largely fibrous composition (Fig. 55B and C).

Lipomatous tumors, which occur predominantly in the retroperitoneum, rarely involve the peritoneal cavity. Benign lipomas (Fig. 57) and lipogenic sarcomas show predominantly a fat density, the sarcomas being distinguishable because they contain components of higher-density tissue. Myxoid liposarcomas usually are of intermediate density, ranging from near-water density to that of muscle (148). A myxoid liposarcoma may be difficult to differentiate from a necrotic neoplasm or from mass-like intraabdominal panniculitis.

The MR signal characteristics of benign lipomas are similar to those of normal body fat. However, myxoid liposarcomas, because of their significant content of non-fatty tissue, have a variable appearance on MR images.

Benign primary peritoneal tumors other than desmoids and lipomas are extremely rare, but can arise from any of the mesenchymal tissue elements. Mesenteric Castleman tumor (angiomatous lymphoid hamartoma), an idiopathic massive enlargement of lymph nodes, has been reported to appear on CT as a well-circumscribed, homogeneous soft-tissue-density mass, with moderate contrast enhancement (58).

Mesothelioma is a rare malignant neoplasm arising from the serosal lining of the pleura, peritoneum, and

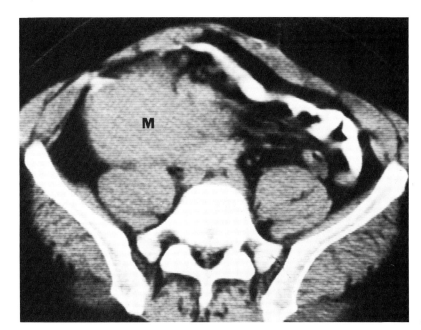

FIG. 56. Mesenteric desmoid tumor. A large soft-tissue-density mass (M) displaces adjacent small-bowel loops. The anterior and medial borders of the mass are irregular, reflecting its infiltrative nature. (Courtesy of Dr. Janet E. Husband, London, England.)

pericardium. Peritoneal involvement may occur, either alone or in combination with pleural involvement (88). CT findings in patients with peritoneal mesothelioma include peritoneal thickening that may appear irregular or nodular, omental and mesenteric thickening, and ascites (117,154) (Fig. 58). The mesenteric involvement may produce a "stellate" appearance due to thickening of the perivascular bundles by tumor (154). The CT appearance of peritoneal mesothelioma may be indistinguishable from that of peritoneal carcinomatosis or, rarely, lymphoma. Benign disease processes such as tuberculous peritonitis may also have a similar appearance.

Secondary Neoplasms. The most common malignant neoplasms involving the peritoneum are metastatic carcinoma and lymphoma. Metastases usually arise from the stomach, colon, or ovary, and less commonly from the

pancreas, biliary tract, or uterus (1,25). Prior to the availability of CT, peritoneal metastases were not detectable radiographically until they were large enough to displace adjacent organs or cause intestinal obstruction. Now, with the availability of CT, peritoneal metastases as small as 1 cm in diameter can be detected before they are large enough to cause symptoms. Rigorous attention to technique is important in detecting small mesenteric and omental tumor implants.

Metastatic neoplasm can disseminate through the peritoneal cavity by four pathways: direct spread along mesenteric and ligamentous attachments, intraperitoneal seeding, lymphatic extension, and embolic hematogenous dissemination (96). Many neoplasms metastasize predominantly by one particular route, producing characteristic CT findings (74).

FIG. 57. Benign mesenteric lipoma. A well-defined mass (M) of homogeneous fat density is present in the mesentery anterior to the ascending colon.

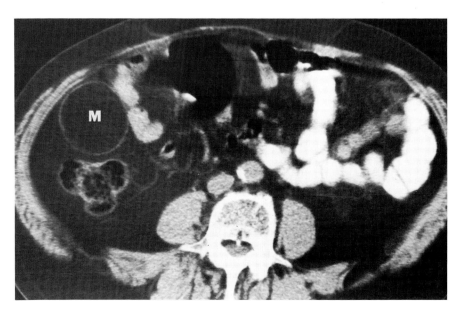

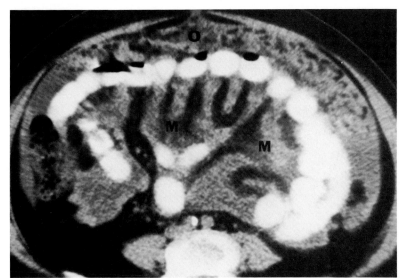

FIG. 58. Peritoneal mesothelioma. The CT findings include ascites and thickening of the mesentery (M) and omentum (O).

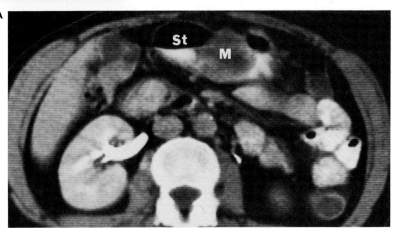

A

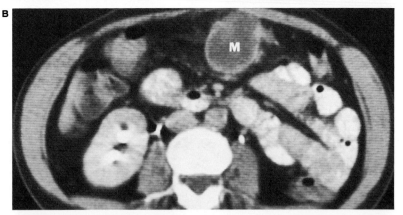

B

FIG. 59. Direct spread of gastric adenocarcinoma to the transverse colon along the gastrocolic ligament. **A:** A mass (M) involving the antrum of the stomach (St) is identified. **B:** Several centimeters caudad, the low-attenuation mass (M) extends along the gastrocolic ligament. **C:** Slightly more caudad, the mass (M) invades the transverse colon (*arrowheads*).

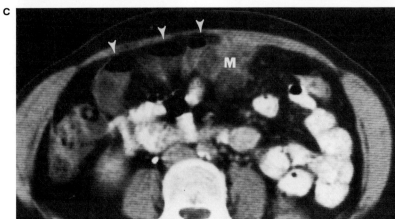

C

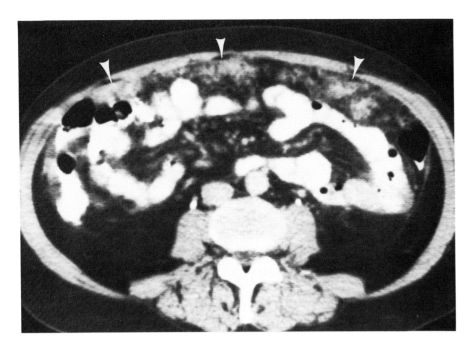

FIG. 60. Omental infiltration by metastatic neoplasm. The fat anterior to the colon and small bowel is thickened by multiple irregular soft-tissue-density masses (*arrowheads*).

Direct Spread Along Peritoneal Surfaces. Malignant neoplasms of the stomach, colon, pancreas, and ovary that have penetrated beyond the borders of these organs can spread directly along the adjacent visceral peritoneal surfaces to involve other peritoneal structures. Neoplastic spread along peritoneal pathways can also involve bowel at some distance from the primary tumor. The transverse mesocolon serves as a major route for spread from the stomach, colon, and pancreas. The gastrocolic ligament (greater omentum) is another important pathway between stomach and colon. Gastric malignancies can also extend along the gastrosplenic ligament to the spleen, and neoplasms in the tail of the pancreas may spread via the phrenicocolic ligament to involve the anatomic splenic flexure of the colon (97). Biliary neoplasms often spread along the gastrohepatic and hepatoduodenal ligaments. Ovarian carcinoma spreads diffusely along all adjacent mesothelial surfaces. The CT appearance of direct peritoneal extension of tumor depends on the degree of spread. Early peritoneal infiltration produces an increase in the density of the fat adjacent to the neoplasm. More advanced spread results in a mass that is contiguous with the primary neoplasm and often extends along the expected course of the ligamentous attachment to involve adjacent organs (111) (Fig. 59). Because of their continuity with the retroperitoneum, the peritoneal ligaments, in addition to serving as the avenues for intraperitoneal tumor spread, serve as conduits for spread of disease processes between the peritoneum and retroperitoneum (97).

Neoplastic infiltration of the greater omentum can produce a distinctive CT appearance ranging from small nodules or strands of soft tissue that increase the density of the fat anterior to the colon or small intestine (Fig. 60) to large masses that separate the colon or small intestine from the anterior abdominal wall ("omental cakes") (21,76) (Figs. 61 and 62). Extensive neoplastic infiltration of the omentum is produced most frequently by metastatic ovarian carcinoma, but it can occur with other neoplasms. Occasionally, omental metastases from ovarian carcinoma calcify (Fig. 62). Inflammatory thickening of the omentum, such as that produced by peritonitis, may be indistinguishable from neoplastic infiltration of the omentum (21) (Fig. 48).

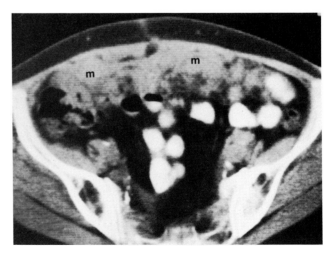

FIG. 61. Omental metastases in a patient with ovarian carcinoma. Confluent soft-tissue masses (m) separate the colon and small bowel from the anterior abdominal wall.

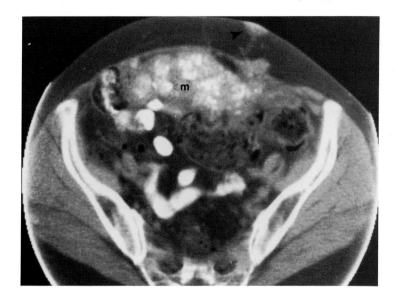

FIG. 62. Involvement of the abdominal wall by neoplasm. Calcified "omental cake" (m) due to metastatic ovarian carcinoma separates bowel from the abdominal wall and grows into an incisional scar (*arrowhead*).

Involvement of the small-bowel mesentery by carcinoid tumor often produces a characteristic CT appearance (Fig. 63). The presence of a soft-tissue mass in the mesentery of the right lower quadrant, displacing surrounding bowel loops, with or without lymphadenopathy and/or liver metastases, is highly suggestive of carcinoid tumor (18,114). Radiating soft-tissue strands due to reactive desmoplasia often surround the mass. Many patients have liver metastases at the time of diagnosis.

Intraperitoneal Seeding. Intraperitoneal seeding of neoplasm depends on the natural flow of fluid within the peritoneal cavity, which is governed by the compartmentalization of the peritoneal spaces, in combination with the effects of gravity and changes in intraabdominal pressure caused by respiration (93). The most common sites for pooling of ascites and subsequent fixation and growth of peritoneal metastases are the pouch of Douglas, the

lower small-bowel mesentery near the ileocecal junction, the sigmoid mesocolon, and the right paracolic gutter (93). The primary neoplasms that most commonly spread by this route are adenocarcinomas of the ovary, colon, stomach, and pancreas. On CT images, seeded metastases appear as soft-tissue masses, frequently associated with ascites, at one or more of the sites of normal pooling (60) (Fig. 64). In some cases, the peritoneum is diffusely thickened (Fig. 65). If a moderate amount of ascites is present, peritoneal implants less than 1 cm in diameter can be identified (Fig. 66). If the metastases are very small, ascites may be the only sign of intraperitoneal seeding. When little or no ascites is present, the only CT manifestation of intraabdominal carcinomatosis may be replacement of the normal mesenteric fat density with soft-tissue density. MRI can also be used to identify peritoneal metastases, although inferior spatial resolution and difficulty in iden-

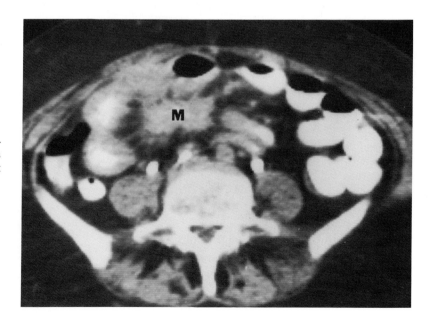

FIG. 63. Carcinoid tumor. A mesenteric soft-tissue mass (M) is surrounded by radiating strands of soft-tissue density. The wall of an adjacent small-bowel loop is thickened.

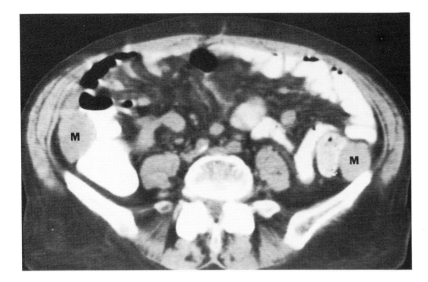

FIG. 64. Peritoneal metastases in a patient with fallopian tube carcinoma. Soft-tissue masses in both paracolic gutters (M) displace the ascending and descending colon medially. The mesentery is thickened, and several enlarged mesenteric lymph nodes are present.

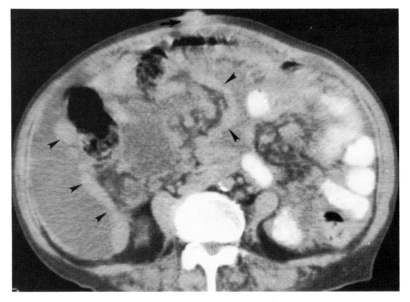

FIG. 65. Peritoneal metastases in a patient with ovarian carcinoma. The peritoneum is diffusely thickened by tumor (*arrowheads*). A periumbilical metastasis (*arrow*) and ascites are also present.

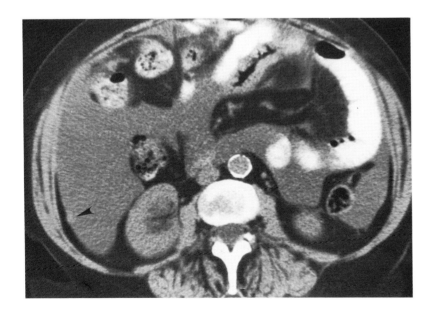

FIG. 66. Small peritoneal implant. When a substantial amount of ascites is present, peritoneal tumor implants as small as 1 cm (*arrowhead*) can be identified with CT.

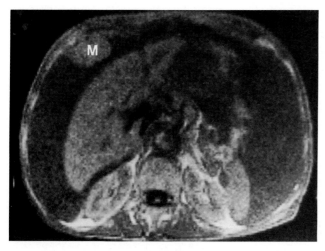

FIG. 67. Peritoneal metastasis from colon carcinoma. T1-weighted MR image (TR = 500 msec, TE = 30 msec). An intermediate-signal-intensity mass (M) is well outlined by the low-signal-intensity ascites.

tifying bowel limit its value in this regard compared with CT. The best contrast between tumor implants and ascites is obtained with T1-weighted images (Fig. 67).

The small-bowel mesentery and the greater omentum frequently are involved by intraperitoneally disseminated tumor. Four general CT patterns of mesenteric involvement have been described: rounded masses, cake-like masses, ill-defined masses, and a stellate pattern (153). Rounded masses are seen most commonly with non-Hodgkin lymphoma (due primarily to lymphadenopathy rather than intraperitoneal seeding) (11,153) (Fig. 68), but can also be seen with other metastatic tumors (Fig. 69). Irregular ill-defined and cake-like masses are seen most often with ovarian carcinoma, although non-Hodgkin

lymphoma (Fig. 70) and metastatic carcinoma (Fig. 71) sometimes produce a similar appearance. Cystic mesenteric masses are occasional manifestations of ovarian carcinoma (Fig. 72). The stellate pattern, consisting of a radiating pattern of the mesenteric leaves, can be produced by a number of metastatic carcinomas, including ovarian, pancreatic, colonic, and breast (Fig. 73). This pattern results from diffuse mesenteric tumor infiltration, causing thickening and rigidity of the perivascular bundles (76). These mesenteric patterns, although characteristic of metastatic involvement, are by no means specific and can be mimicked by primary peritoneal neoplasms, such as mesothelioma, and by inflammatory processes, such as pancreatitis and tuberculous peritonitis (Fig. 48).

A distinctive CT appearance is produced by pseudomyxoma peritonei, in which the peritoneal surfaces become diffusely involved with large amounts of mucinous material. This condition results from rupture of a mucinous cystadenocarcinoma or cystadenoma, usually of the ovary or appendix. CT findings can include low-attenuation masses, which may be surrounded by discrete walls, or diffuse intraperitoneal low-attenuation material that may contain septations and often causes scalloping of the liver margin (23,86,106,126,159) (Fig. 74). Occasionally the walls or septations contain calcification (86). If the walls of the cystic masses are thin, the CT appearance may be similar to that produced by loculated ascites. Scalloping of the liver margin by extrinsic pressure of the gelatinous masses, and failure of bowel loops to float up toward the anterior abdominal wall, may be useful in differentiating pseudomyxoma peritonei and ascites (126).

Lymphatic Dissemination. Lymphatic extension plays a minor role in the intraperitoneal dissemination of metastatic carcinoma (94), but it is the primary mode of spread of lymphoma to mesenteric lymph nodes. At the time of presentation, approximately 50% of patients with non-Hodgkin lymphoma have mesenteric lymph node involvement, whereas only 5% of patients with Hodgkin disease have mesenteric disease at presentation (39).

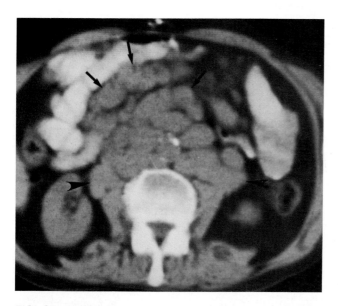

FIG. 68. Non-Hodgkin lymphoma. Multiple enlarged lymph nodes are present in the mesentery (*arrows*) and retroperitoneum (*arrowheads*).

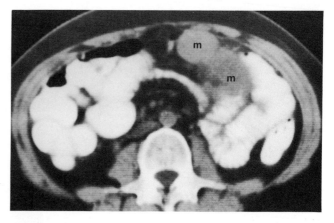

FIG. 69. Mesenteric metastases from uterine leiomyosarcoma. Mesenteric soft-tissue masses (m) are outlined by mesenteric fat and adjacent small-bowel loops.

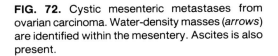

FIG. 70. Lymphoma involving the peritoneum and mesentery. **A:** Peritoneal soft-tissue mass (*arrowheads*) is outlined by ascites in the right perihepatic space. **B:** Image 8 cm caudad shows lymphoma infiltrating the mesentery (*arrows*) and compressing the third duodenum (du). Ascites (a) within the hepatorenal fossa and infiltration of the omentum by lymphoma (*arrowheads*) are also seen.

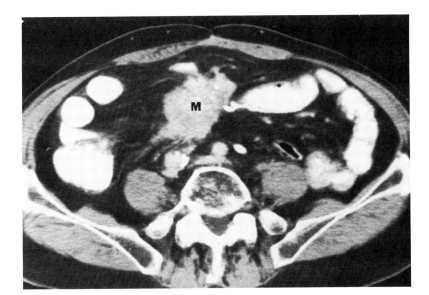

FIG. 71. Mesenteric metastasis from colon cancer. An irregular soft-tissue-attenuation mass (M) is seen within the mesenteric fat.

FIG. 72. Cystic mesenteric metastases from ovarian carcinoma. Water-density masses (*arrows*) are identified within the mesentery. Ascites is also present.

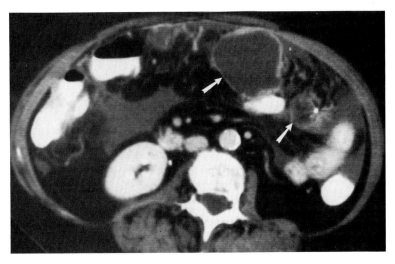

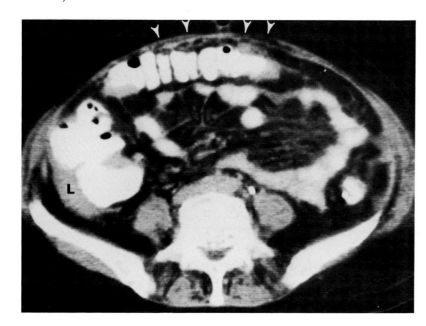

FIG. 73. Mesenteric metastases from breast carcinoma. The mesentery is thickened and appears fixed because of infiltration of the perivascular bundles by tumor. Mild thickening of the greater omentum (*arrowheads*) is also seen; (L) liver.

Identification of mesenteric lymph node disease is extremely important, because it almost always indicates the need for chemotherapy, sometimes in combination with radiation therapy (74).

On CT, the appearance of mesenteric lymph node involvement by lymphoma ranges from small round or oval masses within the mesenteric fat (Fig. 75) to large confluent masses displacing adjacent bowel loops (11,76,153) (Fig. 76). Large confluent masses of lymphomatous nodes may surround the superior mesenteric artery and veins, producing a "sandwich-like" appearance (99) (Fig. 77). Occasionally, the earliest CT sign of mesenteric lymphoma is an increased number of normal-size (<1 cm) lymph nodes within the mesentery. However, mild mesenteric lymphadenopathy is a nonspecific finding and does not always represent lymphoma. Nonneoplastic causes of mesenteric lymphadenopathy include infiltrative and inflammatory disease, such as Crohn disease (26), sarcoidosis, Whipple disease (79,118), sprue (65), giardiasis, tuberculous peritonitis (57), mastocytosis (26), and acquired immune-deficiency syndrome (AIDS) (98,108). Occasionally, enlarged mesenteric vessels oriented perpendicular to the plane of the CT section may simulate mesenteric lymphadenopathy. Enhancement of mesenteric vessels after intravenous administration of contrast material easily distinguishes them from lymph nodes. Alternatively, MRI can distinguish vessels from lymph nodes by virtue of the signal void produced within vessels by

FIG. 74. Pseudomyxoma peritonei. Multiple low-attenuation intraperitoneal masses cause scalloping of the liver margin. Many of the masses contain septations and mural calcification. (Courtesy of Dr. Mark E. Baker, Durham, North Carolina.)

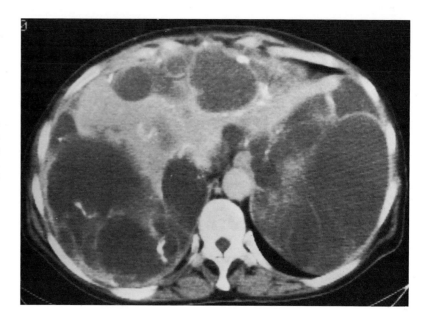

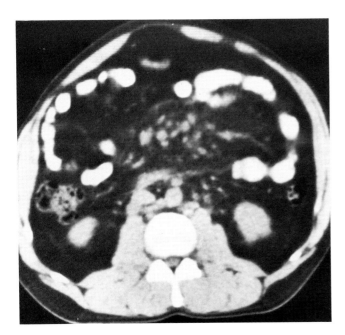

FIG. 75. Mesenteric lymphadenopathy. Multiple small, round mesenteric and retroperitoneal masses are present in a patient with lymphoma.

flowing blood. When lymphoma disseminates to peritoneal surfaces other than the mesentery, the CT appearance may be indistinguishable from that of metastatic carcinoma (74) (Fig. 70).

Embolic Metastases. Tumor emboli may be spread via the mesenteric arteries to the antimesenteric border of bowel, where the cells implant and subsequently grow into intramural tumor nodules (96). On CT, these embolic metastases may produce thickening of the mesenteric leaves or focal bowel-wall thickening, occasionally with recognizable ulceration. The most common neoplasms to

spread in this manner are melanoma and carcinoma of the breast or lung.

Relationship of CT to Other Techniques for Evaluating Neoplasms of the Peritoneal Cavity. CT is the initial imaging procedure of choice for evaluating patients known to have or suspected of having peritoneal or mesenteric neoplasms. Conventional barium studies of the gastrointestinal tract provide only indirect signs of peritoneal and mesenteric disease. Abnormal findings on CT examination often eliminate the need for a barium study, although CT demonstration of a bowel-centered process or a process causing significant extrinsic involvement of the bowel can help direct further appropriate diagnostic evaluation, i.e., barium enema or small-bowel series. However, normal findings on abdominal CT examination certainly do not eliminate the need for a barium examination of the gastrointestinal tract if the clinical findings suggest involvement.

In patients with large amounts of ascites, ultrasound is capable of demonstrating superficial peritoneal and omental tumor nodules as small as 2 to 3 mm because of the acoustic window provided by the peritoneal fluid (157). However, it is difficult to detect peritoneal masses with ultrasound in patients with little or no ascites. Furthermore, centrally located tumors are poorly imaged by ultrasound because of the acoustic impedance of bowel gas and mesenteric fat (14).

Although MRI of the peritoneal cavity offers superior tissue contrast as compared with CT, the spatial resolution of peritoneal and mesenteric structures obtainable with current MR imagers is inferior to that provided by CT scanners, mainly because of respiratory- and peristaltic-motion artifacts associated with MRI. In addition, lack of a reliable gastrointestinal contrast agent for MRI makes it difficult to distinguish between mesenteric masses and normal bowel loops in many cases.

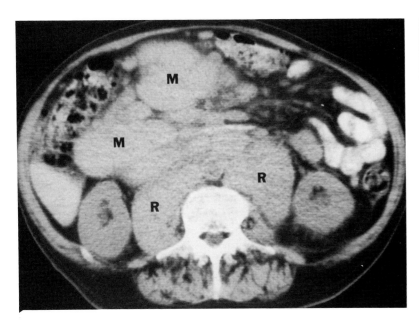

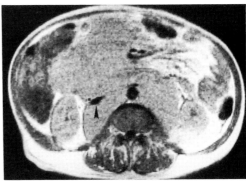

A,B

FIG. 76. Massive mesenteric and retroperitoneal lymphadenopathy. A: CT image demonstrates large confluent lymph node masses in the mesentery (M) and retroperitoneum (R). B: MR image (TR = 900 msec, TE = 30 msec) at the same level demonstrates the lymph node masses in addition to anterior displacement of the inferior vena cava (arrowhead).

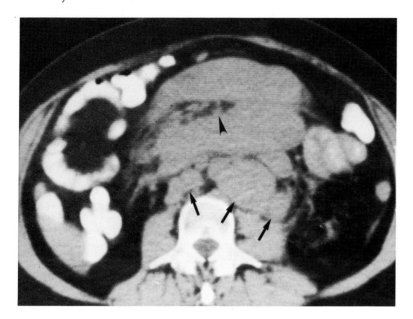

FIG. 77. Massive mesenteric lymphadenopathy. Large confluent masses of lymphomatous nodes surround the superior mesenteric artery (*arrowhead*) and veins, producing a "sandwich-like" appearance. Retroperitoneal lymphadenopathy is also present (*arrows*).

REFERENCES

1. Ackerman LV. *Atlas of tumor pathology. Fascicles 23 and 24: Tumors of the retroperitoneum, mesentery and omentum.* Washington, DC: Armed Forces Institute of Pathology, 1954.
2. Allen HA III, Vick CW, Messmer JM, Parker GA. Diffuse mesenteric amyloidosis: CT, sonographic, and pathologic findings. *J Comput Assist Tomogr* 1985;9:196–198.
3. Altemeier WA, Culbertson WR, Fullen WD, Shook CD. Intra-abdominal abscess. *Am J Surg* 1973;125:70–79.
4. Amato M, Levitt R. Abdominal wall endometrioma: CT findings. *J Comput Assist Tomogr* 1984;8:1213–1214.
5. Aronberg DJ, Stanley RJ, Levitt RG, Sagel SS. Evaluation of abdominal abscess with computed tomography. *J Comput Assist Tomogr* 1978;2:184–187.
6. Baker ME, Weinerth JL, Andriani RT, Cohan RH, Dunnick NR. Lumbar hernia: diagnosis by CT. *AJR* 1987;148:565–567.
7. Balthazar EJ, Subramanyam BR, Megibow A. Spigelian hernia: CT and ultrasonography diagnosis. *Gastrointest Radiol* 1984;9:81–84.
8. Barakos JA, Jeffrey RB Jr, Federle MP, Wing VW, Laing FC, Hightower DR. CT in the management of periappendiceal abscess. *AJR* 1986;146:1161–1164.
9. Baron RL, Lee JKT. Mesenteric desmoid tumors: sonographic and computed-tomographic appearance. *Radiology* 1981;140:777–779.
10. Bergström M, Ericson K, Levander B, Svendsen P, Larsson S. Variation with time of the attenuation values of intracranial hematomas. *J Comput Assist Tomogr* 1977;1:57–63.
11. Bernardino ME, Jing BS, Wallace S. Computed tomography diagnosis of mesenteric masses. *AJR* 1979;132:33–36.
12. Bradley WG Jr, Schmidt PG. Effect of methemoglobin formation on the MR appearance of subarachnoid hemorrhage. *Radiology* 1985;156:99–103.
13. Brasfield RD, Das Gupta TK. Desmoid tumors of the anterior abdominal wall. *Surgery* 1969;65:241–246.
14. Bree RL, Schwab RE. Contribution of mesenteric fat to unsatisfactory abdominal and pelvic ultrasonography. *Radiology* 1981;140:773–776.
15. Brown JJ, van Sonnenberg E, Gerber KH, Strich G, Wittich GR, Slutsky RA. Magnetic resonance relaxation times of percutaneously obtained normal and abnormal body fluids. *Radiology* 1985;154:727–731.
16. Bydder GM, Kreel L. Attenuation values of fluid collections within the abdomen. *J Comput Assist Tomogr* 1980;4:145–150.
17. Callen PW. Computed tomographic evaluation of abdominal and pelvic abscesses. *Radiology* 1979;131:171–175.
18. Cockey BM, Fishman EK, Jones B, Siegelman SS. Computed tomography of abdominal carcinoid tumor. *J Comput Assist Tomogr* 1985;9:38–42.
19. Cohen JM, Weinreb JC, Maravilla KR. Fluid collections in the intraperitoneal and extraperitoneal spaces: comparison of MR and CT. *Radiology* 1985;155:705–708.
20. Cohen WN, Seidelmann FE, Bryan PJ. Computed tomography of localized adipose deposits presenting as tumor masses. *AJR* 1977;128:1007–1011.
21. Cooper CR, Jeffrey RB, Silverman PM, Federle MP, Chun GH. Computed tomography of omental pathology. *J Comput Assist Tomogr* 1986;10:62–66.
22. Cryer PE, Kissane J. Infiltrative gastrointestinal disease. *Am J Med* 1974;57:127–134.
23. Dachman AH, Lichtenstein JE, Friedman AC. Mucocele of the appendix and pseudomyxoma peritonei. *AJR* 1985;144:923–929.
24. Dahlene DH Jr, Stanley RJ, Koehler RE, Shin MS, Tishler JMA. Abdominal tuberculosis: CT findings. *J Comput Assist Tomogr* 1984;8:443–445.
25. Daniel O. The differential diagnosis of malignant disease of the peritoneum. *Br J Surg* 1951;39:147–156.
26. Deutch SJ, Sandler MA, Alpern MB. Abdominal lymphadenopathy in benign disease: CT detection. *Radiology* 1987;163:335–338.
27. Dodds WJ, Foley WD, Lawson TL, Stewart ET, Taylor A. Anatomy and imaging of the lesser peritoneal sac. *AJR* 1985;144:567–575.
28. Dooms GC, Fisher MR, Hricak H, Higgins CB. MR of intramuscular hemorrhage. *J Comput Assist Tomogr* 1985;9:908–913.
29. Dunnick NR, Schaner EG, Doppman JL. Detection of subcutaneous metastases by computed tomography. *J Comput Assist Tomogr* 1978;2:275–279.
30. Epstein BM, Mann JH. CT of abdominal tuberculosis. *AJR* 1982;139:861–866.
31. Faxon HH. Subphrenic abscess. *N Engl J Med* 1940;222:289–299.
32. Federle MP, Chun G, Jeffrey RB, Raynor R. Computed tomographic findings in bowel infarction. *AJR* 1984;142:91–95.
33. Federle MP, Jeffrey RB Jr. Hemoperitoneum studied by computed tomography. *Radiology* 1983;148:187–192.
34. Fisch AE, Brodey PA. Computed tomography of the anterior ab-

dominal wall: normal anatomy and pathology. *J Comput Assist Tomogr* 1981;5:728–733.

35. Frager DH, Goldman M, Beneventano TC. Computed tomography in Crohn disease. *J Comput Assist Tomogr* 1983;7:819–824.

36. Gedgaudas RK, Rice RP. Radiologic evaluation of complicated pancreatitis. *CRC Crit Rev Diagn Imaging* 1981;15:319–367.

37. Gerzof SG, Johnson WC, Robbins AH, Nabseth DC. Expanded criteria for percutaneous abscess drainage. *Arch Surg* 1985;120: 227–232.

38. Ghahremani GG, Jiminez MA, Rosenfeld M, Rochester D. CT diagnosis of occult incisional hernias. *AJR* 1987;148:139–142.

39. Goffinet DR, Castellino RA, Kim H, et al. Staging laparotomies in unselected previously untreated patients with non-Hodgkin's lymphoma. *Cancer* 1973;32:672–681.

40. Goldberg HI, Gore RM, Margulis AR, Moss AA, Baker EL. Computed tomography in the evaluation of Crohn disease. *AJR* 1983;140:277–282.

41. Gomori JM, Grossman RI, Goldberg HI, Zimmerman RA, Bilaniuk LT. Intracranial hematomas: imaging by high-field MR. *Radiology* 1985;157:87–93.

42. Gore RM, Callen PW, Filly RA. Lesser sac fluid in predicting the etiology of ascites: CT findings. *AJR* 1982;139:71–74.

43. Gore RM, Marn CS, Kirby DF, Vogelzang RL, Neiman HL. CT findings in ulcerative, granulomatous and indeterminate colitis. *AJR* 1984;143:279–284.

44. Goss CM, ed. *Gray's Anatomy of the Human Body*. 29th American ed. Philadelphia: Lea & Febiger, 1973.

45. Grendell JH, Ockner RK. Mesenteric venous thrombosis. *Gastroenterology* 1982;82:358–372.

46. Haaga JR, Alfidi RJ, Havrilla TR, et al. CT detection and aspiration of abdominal abscesses. *AJR* 1977;128:465–474.

47. Hahn PF, Saini S, Stark DD, Papanicolaou N, Ferrucci JT Jr. Intraabdominal hematoma: the concentric-ring sign in MR imaging. *AJR* 1987;148:115–119.

48. Halber MD, Daffner RH, Morgan CL, et al. Intraabdominal abscess: current concepts in radiologic evaluation. *AJR* 1979;133:9–13.

49. Halliday P, Halliday H. Subphrenic abscess: a study of 241 patients at the Royal Prince Edward Hospital, 1950–1973. *Br J Surg* 1976;63:352.

50. Haney PJ, Whitley NO. CT of benign cystic abdominal masses in children. *AJR* 1984;142:1279–1281.

51. Hanson RD, Hunter TB. Tuberculous peritonitis: CT appearance. *AJR* 1985;144:931–932.

52. Hayashi S, Oyama K, Hirakawa K, Oda M, Kogure T. Mesenteric panniculitis—case report and its radiological diagnosis including CT. *Rinsho Hoshasen* 1982;27:143–146.

53. Haynes JW, Brewer WH, Walsh JW. Focal fat necrosis presenting as a palpable abdominal mass: CT evaluation. *J Comput Assist Tomogr* 1985;9:568–569.

54. Healy ME, Teng SS, Moss AA. Uriniferous pseudocyst: computed tomographic findings. *Radiology* 1984;153:757–762.

55. Hudson TM, Vandergriend RA, Springfield DS, et al. Aggressive fibromatosis: evaluation by computed tomography and angiography. *Radiology* 1984;150:495–501.

56. Hulnick DH, Megibow AJ, Balthazar EJ, Naidich DP, Bosniak MA. Computed tomography in the evaluation of diverticulitis. *Radiology* 1984;152:491–495.

57. Hulnick DH, Megibow AJ, Naidich DP, Hilton S, Cho KC, Balthazar EJ. Abdominal tuberculosis: CT evaluation. *Radiology* 1985;157:199–204.

58. Iida E, Kohno A, Mikami T, Kumekawa H, Akimoto S, Hamano K. Mesenteric Castleman tumor. *J Comput Assist Tomogr* 1983;7: 338–340.

59. Jaques P, Mauro M, Safrit H, Yankaskas B, Piggott B. CT features of intraabdominal abscess: prediction of successful percutaneous drainage. *AJR* 1986;146:1041–1045.

60. Jeffrey RB Jr. CT demonstration of peritoneal implants. *AJR* 1980;135:323–326.

61. Jeffrey RB. Computed tomography of the peritoneal cavity and mesentery. In: Moss AA, Gamsu G, Genant HK, eds. *Computed tomography of the body*. Philadelphia: WB Saunders, 1983.

62. Jeffrey RB, Federle MP, Laing FC. Computed tomography of mesenteric involvement in fulminant pancreatitis. *Radiology* 1983;147: 185–188.

63. Jeffrey RB Jr, Tolentino CS, Federle MP, Laing FC. Percutaneous drainage of periappendiceal abscesses: review of 20 patients. *AJR* 1987;149:59–62.

64. Jolles H, Coulam CM. CT of ascites: differential diagnosis. *AJR* 1980;135:315–322.

65. Jones B, Bayless TM, Fishman EK, Siegelman SS. Lymphadenopathy in celiac disease: computed tomographic observations. *AJR* 1984;142:1127–1132.

66. Katz ME, Heiken JP, Glazer HS, Lee JKT. Intraabdominal panniculitis: clinical, radiographic, and CT features. *AJR* 1985;145: 293–296.

67. Kerber GW, Greenberg M, Rubin JM. Computed tomography evaluation of local and extraintestinal complications of Crohn's disease. *Gastrointest Radiol* 1984;9:143–148.

68. Kipfer RE, Moertel CG, Dahlin DC. Mesenteric lipodystrophy. *Ann Intern Med* 1974;80:582–588.

69. Knochel JQ, Koehler PR, Lee TG, Welch DM. Diagnosis of abdominal abscesses with computed tomography, ultrasound, and ^{111}In leukocyte scans. *Radiology* 1980;137:425–432.

70. Koehler PR, Moss AA. Diagnosis of intra-abdominal and pelvic abscesses by computerized tomography. *JAMA* 1980;244:49–52.

71. Korobkin M, Callen PW, Filly RA, Hoffer PB, Shimshak RR, Kressel HY. Comparison of computed tomography, ultrasonography, and gallium-67 scanning in the evaluation of suspected abdominal abscess. *Radiology* 1978;129:89–93.

72. Korobkin M, Moss AA, Callen PW, DeMartini WJ, Kaiser JA. Computed tomography of subcapsular splenic hematoma: clinical and experimental studies. *Radiology* 1978;129:441–445.

73. Lawdahl RB, Moss CN, VanDyke JA. Inferior lumbar (Petit's) hernia. *AJR* 1986;147:744–745.

74. Levitt RG. Abdominal wall and peritoneal cavity. In: Lee JKT, Sagel SS, Stanley RJ, eds. *Computed body tomography*. New York: Raven Press, 1983.

75. Levitt RG, Biello DR, Sagel SS, et al. Computed tomography and ^{67}Ga citrate radionuclide imaging for evaluating suspected abdominal abscess. *AJR* 1979;132:529–534.

76. Levitt RG, Sagel SS, Stanley RJ. Detection of neoplastic involvement of the mesentery and omentum by computed tomography. *AJR* 1978;131:835–838.

77. Lewin JR, Patterson EA. CT recognition of spontaneous intraperitoneal hemorrhage complicating anticoagulant therapy. *AJR* 1980;134:1271–1272.

78. Lewis VL, Shaffer HA Jr, Williamson BRJ. Pseudotumoral lipomatosis of the abdomen. *J Comput Assist Tomogr* 1982;6:79–82.

79. Li DKB, Rennie CS. Abdominal computed tomography in Whipple's disease. *J Comput Assist Tomogr* 1981;5:249–252.

80. Lieberman JM, Haaga JR. Computed tomography of diverticulitis. *J Comput Assist Tomogr* 1983;7:431–433.

81. Lorenz R, Beyer D, Peters PE. Detection of intraperitoneal bile accumulations: significance of ultrasonography, CT, and cholescintigraphy. *Gastrointest Radiol* 1984;9:213–217.

82. Lundstedt C, Hederstrom E, Holmin T, Lunderquist A, Navne T, Owman T. Radiologic diagnosis in proven intra-abdominal abscess formation. *Gastrointest Radiol* 1983;8:261–266.

83. Magid D, Fishman EK, Jones B, Hoover HC, Feinstein R, Siegelman SS. Desmoid tumors in Gardner's syndrome: use of computed tomography. *AJR* 1984;142:1141–1145.

84. Maklad NF, Doust BD, Baum JK. Ultrasonic diagnosis of postoperative intra-abdominal abscess. *Radiology* 1974;113:417–422.

85. Mall JC, Kaiser JA. CT diagnosis of splenic laceration. *AJR* 1980;134:265–269.

86. Mayes GB, Chuang VP, Fisher RG. CT of pseudomyxoma peritonei. *AJR* 1981;136:807–808.

87. McAfee JG, Samin A. In-111 labeled leukocytes: a review of problems in image interpretation. *Radiology* 1985;155:221–229.

88. McDonald AD, Harper A, El Attar OA, McDonald JC. Epidemiology of primary malignant mesothelial tumors in Canada. *Cancer* 1970;26:914–919.

89. McDougall IR, Baumert JE, Lantiere RL. Evaluation of ^{111}In leukocyte whole body scanning. *AJR* 1979;133:849–854.

90. Mendez G Jr, Isikoff MB, Hill MC. CT of acute pancreatitis: interim assessment. *AJR* 1980;135:463–469.

91. Meyers MA. Roentgen significance of the phrenicocolic ligament. *Radiology* 1970;95:539–545.

92. Meyers MA. The spread and localization of acute intraperitoneal effusions. *Radiology* 1970;95:547–554.

93. Meyers MA. Distribution of intra-abdominal malignancy seeding: dependency on dynamics of flow of ascitic fluid. *AJR* 1973;119: 198–206.

94. Meyers MA. *Dynamic radiology of the abdomen: normal and pathologic anatomy.* 2nd ed. New York: Springer-Verlag, 1982.

95. Meyers MA, Evans JA. Effects of pancreatitis on the small bowel and colon: spread along mesenteric planes. *AJR* 1973;119:151–165.

96. Meyers MA, McSweeney J. Secondary neoplasms of bowel. *Radiology* 1972;105:1–11.

97. Meyers MA, Oliphant M, Berne AS, Feldberg MAM. The peritoneal ligaments and mesenteries: pathways of intraabdominal spread of disease. *Radiology* 1987;163:593–604.

98. Moon KL, Federle MP, Abrams DI, Volberding P, Lewis BJ. Kaposi sarcoma and lymphadenopathy syndrome: limitations of abdominal CT in acquired immunodeficiency syndrome. *Radiology* 1984;150: 479–483.

99. Mueller PR, Ferrucci JT Jr, Harbin WP, Kirkpatrick RH, Simeone JF, Wittenberg J. Appearance of lymphomatous involvement of the mesentery by ultrasonography and body computed tomography: the "sandwich sign." *Radiology* 1980;134:467–473.

100. Mueller PR, Ferrucci JT Jr, Simeone JF, et al. Lesser sac abscesses and fluid collections: drainage by transhepatic approach. *Radiology* 1985;155:615–618.

101. Mueller PR, Ferrucci JT Jr, Simeone JF, et al. Detection and drainage of bilomas: special considerations. *AJR* 1983;140:715–720.

102. Naylor EW, Gardner EJ, Richards RC. Desmoid tumors and mesenteric fibromatosis in Gardner's syndrome. *Arch Surg* 1979;114:1181–1185.

103. Neff CC, van Sonnenberg E, Casola G, et al. Diverticular abscesses: percutaneous drainage. *Radiology* 1987;163:15–18.

104. New PF, Aronow S. Attenuation measurements of whole blood and blood fractions in computed tomography. *Radiology* 1976;121:635–640.

105. Norman D, Price D, Boyd D, Fishman R, Newton TH. Aspects of computed tomography of the blood and cerebrospinal fluid. *Radiology* 1977;123:335–338.

106. Novetsky GJ, Berlin L, Epstein AJ, Lobo N, Miller SH. Pseudomyxoma peritonei. *J Comput Assist Tomogr* 1982;6:398–399.

107. Nunez D Jr, Huber JS, Yrizarry JM, Mendez G, Russell E. Nonsurgical drainage of appendiceal abscess. *AJR* 1986;146:587–589.

108. Nyberg DA, Federle MP, Jeffrey RB, Bottles K, Wofsy CB. Abdominal CT findings of disseminated *Mycobacterium avium intracellulare* in AIDS. *AJR* 1985;145:297–299.

109. Ochsner A, Graves AM. Subphrenic abscess: an analysis of 3372 collected and personal cases. *Ann Surg* 1933;98:961–990.

110. Ogden WW II, Bradburn DM, Rives JD. Mesenteric panniculitis. Review of 27 cases. *Ann Surg* 1965;161:864–875.

111. Oliphant M, Berne AS. Computed tomography of the subperitoneal space: demonstration of direct spread of intraabdominal disease. *J Comput Assist Tomogr* 1982;6:1127–1137.

112. Pandolfo I, Blandino A, Gaeta M, Racchiusa S, Chirico G. CT findings in palpable lesions of the anterior abdominal wall. *J Comput Assist Tomogr* 1986;10:629–633.

113. Pastakia B, Horvath K, Kurtz D, Udelsman R, Doppman JL. Giant rectus sheath hematomas of the pelvis complicating anticoagulant therapy: CT findings. *J Comput Assist Tomogr* 1984;8:1120–1123.

114. Picus D, Glazer HS, Levitt RG, Husband JE. Computed tomography of abdominal carcinoid tumors. *AJR* 1984;143:581–584.

115. Pitt HA. Peritonitis, intraabdominal abscess, and retroperitoneal abscess. In: Shackelford RT, Zuidema GD, eds. *Surgery of the alimentary tract, volume 5.* 2nd ed. Philadelphia: WB Saunders, 1986.

116. Press OW, Press NO, Kaufman SD. Evaluation and management of chylous ascites. *Ann Intern Med* 1982;96:358–364.

117. Reuter K, Raptopoulos V, Reale F, et al. Diagnosis of peritoneal mesothelioma: computed tomography, sonography, and fine-needle aspiration biopsy. *AJR* 1983;140:1189–1194.

118. Rijke AM, Falke THM, de Vries RRP. Computed tomography in Whipple disease. *J Comput Assist Tomogr* 1983;7:1101–1102.

119. Rosen A, Korobkin M, Silverman PM, Dunnick NR, Kelvin FM. Mesenteric vein thrombosis: CT identification. *AJR* 1984;143:83–86.

120. Rubin JI, Gomori JM, Grossman RI, Gefter WB, Kressel HY. High-field MR imaging of extracranial hematomas. *AJR* 1987;148: 813–817.

121. Rust RJ, Kopecky KK, Holden RW. The triangle sign: a CT sign of intraperitoneal fluid. *Gastrointest Radiol* 1984;9:107–113.

122. Safrit HD, Mauro MA, Jaques PF. Percutaneous abscess drainage in Crohn's disease. *AJR* 1987;148:859–862.

123. Sanders RC. The changing epidemiology of subphrenic abscess and its clinical and radiological consequences. *Br J Surg* 1970;57:449–455.

124. Schneekloth G, Terrier F, Fuchs WA. Computed tomography of intraperitoneal abscesses. *Gastrointest Radiol* 1982;7:35–41.

125. Seabold JE, Wilson DG, Lieberman LM, Boyd CM. Unsuspected extra-abdominal sites of infection: scintigraphic detection with indium-111-labeled leukocytes. *Radiology* 1984;151:213–217.

126. Seshul MB, Coulam CM. Pseudomyxoma peritonei: computed tomography and sonography. *AJR* 1981;136:803–806.

127. Shackelford GD, McAlister WH. Cysts of the omentum. *Pediatr Radiol* 1975;3:152–155.

128. Shackelford RT, Grose WE. Groin hernia. In: Shackelford RT, Zuidema GD, eds. *Surgery of the alimentary tract, volume 5.* 2nd ed. Philadelphia: WB Saunders, 1986.

129. Sherman JJ, Davis JR, Jeseph JE. Subphrenic abscess: a continuing hazard. *Am J Surg* 1969;117:117–123.

130. Shin MS, Ferrucci JT Jr, Wittenberg J. Computed tomographic diagnosis of pseudoascites (floating viscera syndrome). *J Comput Assist Tomogr* 1978;2:594–597.

131. Silverman PM, Baker ME, Cooper C, Kelvin F. CT appearance of diffuse mesenteric edema. *J Comput Assist Tomogr* 1986;10:67–70.

132. Silverman PM, Kelvin FM, Korobkin M, Dunnick NR. Computed tomography of the normal mesentery. *AJR* 1984;143:953–957.

133. Silverstein W, Isikoff MB, Hill MC, Barkin J. Diagnostic imaging of acute pancreatitis: prospective study using CT and sonography. *AJR* 1981;137:497–502.

134. Sones PJ. Percutaneous drainage of abdominal abscesses. *AJR* 1984;142:35–39.

135. Steck CW, Helwig EB. Cutaneous endometriosis. *Clin Obstet Gynecol* 1966;9:373–383.

136. Swensen SJ, Keller PL, Berquist TH, McCleod RA, Stephens DH. Magnetic resonance imaging of hemorrhage. *AJR* 1985;145:921–927.

137. Swensen SJ, McLeod RA, Stephens DH. CT of extracranial hemorrhage and hematomas. *AJR* 1984;143:907–912.

138. Taylor KJW, Sullivan DC, Wasson JF, Rosenfield AT. Ultrasound and gallium for the diagnosis of abdominal and pelvic abscesses. *Gastrointest Radiol* 1978;3:281–286.

139. Terrier F, Revel D, Pajannen H, Richardson M, Hricak H, Higgins CB. MR imaging of body fluid collections. *J Comput Assist Tomogr* 1986;10:953–962.

140. Thoeni RF, Margulis AR. Gastrointestinal tuberculosis. *Semin Roentgenol* 1979;14:283–294.

141. Unger EC, Glazer HS, Lee JKT, Ling D. MRI of extracranial hematomas: preliminary observations. *AJR* 1986;146:403–407.

142. Vanek VW, Phillips AK. Retroperitoneal, mesenteric, and omental cysts. *Arch Surg* 1984;119:838–842.

143. van Sonnenberg E, Wittich GR, Casola G, et al. Periappendiceal abscesses: percutaneous drainage. *Radiology* 1987;163:23–26.

144. van Sonnenberg E, Mueller PR, Ferrucci JT Jr. Percutaneous drainage of 250 abdominal abscesses and fluid collections. Part I: results, failures, and complications. *Radiology* 1984;151:337–341.

145. van Sonnenberg E, Mueller PR, Wittenberg J, et al. Comparative utility of ultrasound and computed tomography in suspected abdominal abscesses. Presented at the 66th Scientific Assembly and Annual Meeting of the Radiological Society of North America, Dallas, Texas, November 1980.

146. Vazquez JL, Thorsen MK, Dodds WJ, et al. Evaluation and treatment of intraabdominal bilomas. *AJR* 1985;144:933–938.

147. Vincent LM, Mauro MA, Mittelstaedt CA. The lesser sac and gastrohepatic recess: sonographic appearance and differentiation of fluid collections. *Radiology* 1984;150:515–519.

148. Waligore MP, Stephens DH, Soule EH, McLeod RA. Lipomatous tumors of the abdominal cavity: CT appearance and pathologic correlation. *AJR* 1981;137:539–545.

149. Wall SD, Hricak H, Bailey GD, Kerlan RK Jr, Goldberg HI, Higgins

CB. MR of pathologic abdominal fluid collections. *J Comput Assist Tomogr* 1986;10:746–750.

150. Wang SM, Wilson SE. Subphrenic abscess: the new epidemiology. *Arch Surg* 1977;112:934–936.

151. White M, Mueller PR, Ferrucci JT Jr, et al. Percutaneous drainage of postoperative abdominal and pelvic lymphoceles. *AJR* 1985;145: 1065–1069.

152. Whitley NO. Mesenteric disease. In: Meyers MA, ed. *Computed tomography of the gastrointestinal tract.* New York: Springer-Verlag, 1986.

153. Whitley NO, Bohlman ME, Baker LP. CT patterns of mesenteric disease. *J Comput Assist Tomogr* 1982;6:490–496.

154. Whitley NO, Brenner DE, Antman KH, Grant D, Aisner J. CT of peritoneal mesothelioma: analysis of eight cases. *AJR* 1982;138: 531–535.

155. Wolverson MK, Crepps LF, Sundaram M, Heiberg E, Vas WG, Shields JB. Hyperdensity of recent hemorrhage at body computed tomography: incidence and morphologic variation. *Radiology* 1983;148:779–784.

156. Wolverson MK, Jagannadharao B, Sundaram M, Joyce PF, Riaz MA, Shields JB. CT as a primary diagnostic method in evaluating intraabdominal abscess. *AJR* 1979;133:1089–1095.

157. Yeh HC. Ultrasonography of peritoneal tumors. *Radiology* 1979;133:419–424.

158. Yeh H-C, Rabinowitz JG. Ultrasonography and computed tomography in inflammatory abdominal wall lesions. *Radiology* 1982;144:859–863.

159. Yeh H-C, Shafir MK, Slater G, Meyer RJ, Cohen B, Geller SA. Ultrasonography and computed tomography of pseudomyxoma peritonei. *Radiology* 1984;153:507–510.

160. Zerhouni EA, Barth KA, Siegelman SS. Demonstration of venous thrombosis by computed tomography. *AJR* 1980;134:753–758.

161. Zimmerman LM, Anson BJ. *Anatomy and surgery of hernia.* 2nd ed. Baltimore: Williams & Wilkins, 1967.

CHAPTER 17

Retroperitoneum

Joseph K. T. Lee

The retroperitoneum, bounded anteriorly by the parietal peritoneum and posteriorly by the transversalis fascia, extends from the diaphragm superiorly to the level of pelvic viscera inferiorly. At the level of the kidneys, the retroperitoneal space is divided into three compartments: the perirenal space surrounded by the anterior and posterior pararenal spaces. Two types of viscera exist in the retroperitoneal space: the true embryonic retroperitoneal organs (i.e., the adrenal glands, kidneys, ureters, and gonads), and those structures closely attached to the posterior abdominal wall and only partly covered by the peritoneum (i.e., aorta, inferior vena cava, pancreas, portions of the duodenum, colon, lymph nodes, and nerves).

In the past, the evaluation of most retroperitoneal structures by conventional radiography has been difficult. Since the advent of computed tomography (CT) and, more recently, magnetic resonance imaging (MRI), direct noninvasive demonstration of normal and pathologic retroperitoneal anatomy has become possible with a high level of clarity (83,136) (Fig. 1). Diagnostic images can be obtained in almost all but the leanest patients because there is normally sufficient fat in the retroperitoneum to profile the normal structures. In this chapter, discussion will be limited to diseases involving the great vessels, lymph nodes, and psoas muscle, as well as primary retroperitoneal neoplasms. Diseases related to other solid retroperitoneal organs, such as the kidneys, the adrenals, and the pancreas, are covered in other chapters. Inflammatory diseases (i.e., abscesses) will be dealt with in Chapter 16.

TECHNIQUE

CT

As in other parts of the body, careful patient preparation and attention to technical details are essential to the optimal conduct of CT evaluation of the retroperitoneum. A survey examination of the retroperitoneum is routinely performed with 1-cm slice collimation at 2-cm intervals. In some cases, contiguous slices may be used to clarify some equivocal findings. A large amount of oral contrast material (dilute barium suspension or iodinated water-soluble contrast material), usually in excess of 1,000 ml, is given to the patient at least 1 hr before the examination in order to opacify the colon and distal small-bowel loops. An additional 300 to 500 ml of contrast material is given approximately 15 min before the study to opacify the stomach and proximal small-bowel loops. In most Americans, normally there is abundant fat in the retroperitoneum, profiling the normal structures, so that the retroperitoneum can be adequately studied without the use of intravenous contrast material. Although intravenous contrast material is used in every case in some institutions, we reserve its use for cases in which distinction between a vascular structure and a nonvascular structure is essential, or sometimes to determine the effect of a retroperitoneal mass on the urinary tract or to corroborate a lesion in another abdominal organ. For the initial indication, a bolus injection of approximately 20 g of iodine is given, followed by serial dynamic imaging at the level(s) of interest. A rapid infusion of 150 to 200 cc of 60% iodine solution after a priming bolus is used in cases in which a large area needs to be examined. Thorough bowel opacification, coupled with judicious use of intravenous contrast material, allows detection of retroperitoneal abnormalities even in the leanest patients (Fig. 2).

MRI

The retroperitoneum can likewise be successfully examined with MRI. Both T1- and T2-weighted sequences are required for lesion detection and characterization. Whereas transverse images are obtained in all patients, usually with 1 cm collimation and at 2-cm intervals, coronal and sagittal images are obtained in selected patients to better define abnormalities of the aorta, inferior vena cava, and psoas muscle.

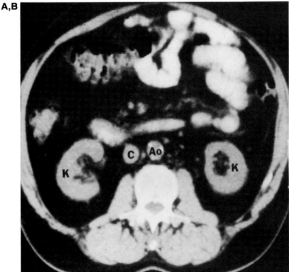

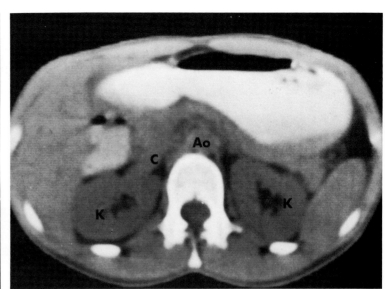

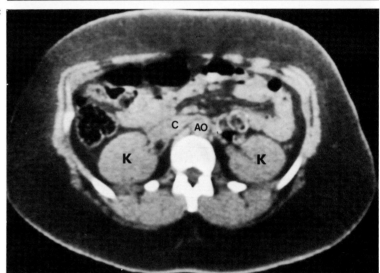

FIG. 1. CT images of the normal retroperitoneum in patients with variations in body habitus. **A:** Abundant intraabdominal fat, making identification of normal retroperitoneal structures easy. **B:** With scant intraabdominal fat present in a thin patient, the retroperitoneal and intraperitoneal structures are crowded together, and delineation of each individual organ is less distinct. However, with proper opacification of bowel loops with oral contrast material, and occasionally intravenous contrast material as well, retroperitoneal disease still can be discerned or excluded with a high degree of certainty. **C:** Obese woman in whom fat is almost exclusively deposited in the subcutaneous tissue, with little retroperitoneal fat present. This distribution of body fat is almost always seen in women, especially with large weight gain after puberty; (AO) aorta; (C) inferior vena cava; (K) kidneys.

AORTA

Normal Anatomy

CT

The abdominal aorta begins at the hiatus in the diaphragm and usually extends along the ventral aspect of the lumbar spine to the level of the fourth lumbar vertebra, where it divides into the two common iliac arteries. On CT images, the aorta appears as a circular soft-tissue density in a prevertebral location. The caliber of the abdominal aorta decreases as it progresses distally toward the bifurcation. The major branches arising from the abdominal aorta that can be seen on the CT image include the celiac trunk, the superior mesenteric artery, and renal arteries. Although the origin of the inferior mesenteric artery can be identified on CT images in over 90% of cases, it rarely can be traced more than 1 cm beyond its origin.

The noncalcified aortic wall cannot be distinguished from its intraluminal blood on precontrast images except in anemic patients. Whereas the attenuation value of the blood in the aortic lumen ranges from 50 to 70 Hounsfield units (HU) in normal subjects, it is considerably less in patients with a markedly reduced hematocrit. Thus, a visible, noncalcified aortic wall is a clue to the presence of anemia. Following intravenous administration of water-soluble iodinated contrast material, the attenuation value of the aortic lumen can rise as high as +400 HU after a bolus injection.

MRI

Because blood flowing at normal velocities (>10 cm/sec) usually produces no signal, the aorta and its major branches appear as areas of "signal void" (73). These arteries can be easily distinguished on both T1- and T2-weighted images from the surrounding retroperitoneal fat, which displays a high signal intensity, and adjacent muscle, which has a low signal intensity (Fig. 3). When transaxial images are obtained with a multislice technique, the aorta often demonstrates signal on the most cranial slice

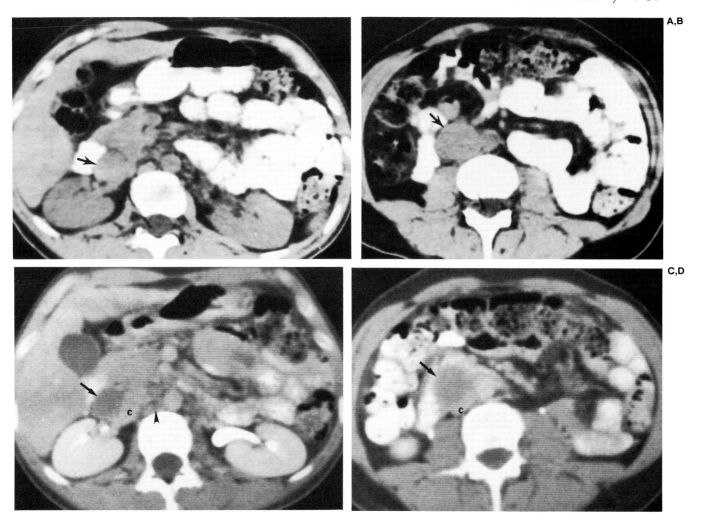

FIG. 2. Value of intravenous contrast material in a 25-year-old man with right testicular seminoma. **A,B:** Non-contrast-enhanced CT images demonstrate apparent enlargement of the inferior vena cava (*arrow*), a finding not uncommonly seen during a Valsalva maneuver. **C,D:** Repeat images after intravenous administration of contrast material show an enlarged, low-density lymph node (*arrow*) compressing the contrast-enhanced inferior vena cava (c). Additional lymph nodes (*arrowhead*) are noted between the aorta and the cava.

FIG. 3. Normal abdominal aorta. **A:** Coronal MR image (TR = 500 msec, TE = 30 msec). A portion of the abdominal aorta, both renal arteries (*arrows*), and common iliac arteries are well delineated in this section. **B:** Sagittal MR image of a different patient (TR = 500 msec, TE = 30 msec). The origin of the celiac axis (*arrowhead*) and the superior mesenteric artery (*open arrow*) are clearly seen; (c) inferior vena cava; (pv) portal vein.

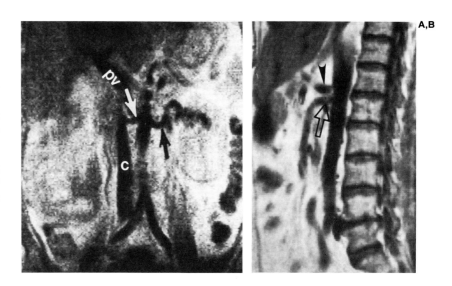

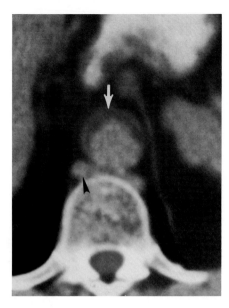

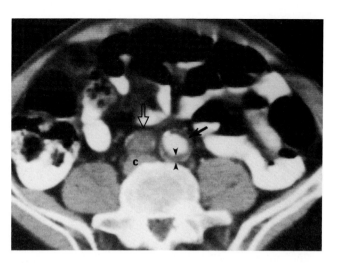

FIG. 4. Atheromatous plaque in a normal-size aorta. The atheroma (*arrow*) has a lower attenuation value and is clearly differentiated from the aortic lumen on this postcontrast CT image; (*arrowhead*) azygos vein.

FIG. 5. Complete occlusion of right common iliac artery. Postcontrast CT image demonstrates an enhanced, ectatic left common iliac artery (*arrow*). There is no enhancement of right common iliac artery (*open arrow*); (c) inferior vena cava; (*arrowheads*) atheromatous plaque.

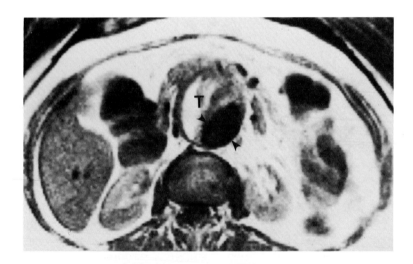

FIG. 6. Atheromatous plaques in an aortic aneurysm. Transverse MR image (TR = 500 msec, TE = 30 msec). The aortic lumen (*arrowheads*) contains no signal and can be easily differentiated from adjacent thrombus (T), which contains a mixture of high and medium signal intensities. Fresh thrombi usually have higher signal intensity than chronic thrombi.

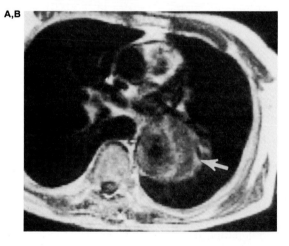

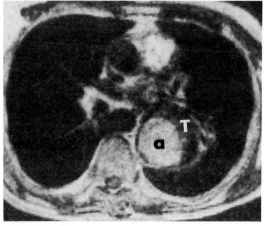

FIG. 7. Differentiation between slow flow and atheromatous thrombus in a descending thoracic aortic aneurysm. **A:** Transverse MR image (TR = 500 msec, TE = 30 msec) shows an aneurysmal descending aorta (*arrow*). The lumen size cannot be accurately discerned on this image. **B:** On second-echo image (TR = 500 msec, TE = 60 msec) there is an increase in signal intensity in the aortic lumen (a) that is related to slow flow. The thrombus (T), which shows decrease in signal intensity, can therefore be easily distinguished from the aortic lumen. (From ref. 62.)

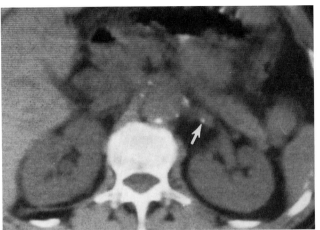
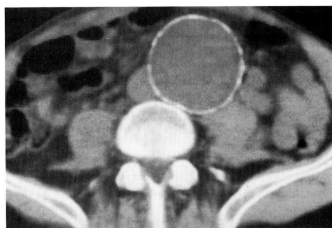
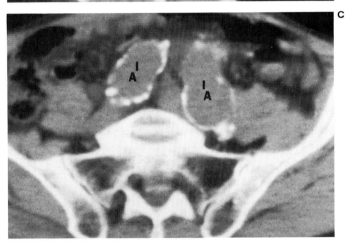

FIG. 8. Infrarenal aortic aneurysm with involvement of both iliac arteries. **A:** The aorta is normal in size at the level of the left renal artery (*arrow*). **B:** Five centimeters caudal to **A,** the aorta is calcified and markedly dilated. **C:** Scan obtained 2 cm caudal to **B** shows dilatation of both proximal common iliac arteries (IA).

of the imaged volume because of a flow-related enhancement effect (14). The thin wall of the normal aorta is not always clearly identified as a separate structure, because of its low signal intensity.

Pathologic Conditions

Atherosclerosis

CT

Atherosclerotic changes of the aorta can be detected on CT images. These include calcification in the wall, mild ectasia, and increased tortuosity. Although the aorta is usually located in a prevertebral position, it may be parallel to the spine or even lie to the right of the vertebral column in patients with severe atherosclerosis. An atheromatous plaque or a thrombus may have a lower attenuation value than the flowing blood; it is best appreciated on postcontrast images (Fig. 4). Complete occlusion of a vessel can likewise be demonstrated on postcontrast images (Fig. 5).

MRI

Atherosclerotic changes of the aorta also can be seen on magnetic resonance (MR) images. Calcification of the aortic wall appears as an arc or circumferential rim of low signal intensity. Both atheromatous plaques and thrombus produce intraluminal signals of various intensities (5,72,91) and can be differentiated easily from the

aortic lumen, which usually appears as an area of signal void (Fig. 6). However, slow blood flow may result in intraluminal signal. The signal from slow flow can be distinguished from that of atheromatous plaques and thrombus by comparing the signal intensities on first- and second-echo images. Slow flow shows an increase in the absolute signal intensity on the second or even echo, whereas the signal produced by thrombus and the atheromatous plaque decreases in intensity on the second echo (Fig. 7). This increase in signal strength in blood vessels with slow flow has been described as an even-echo rephasing effect (14).

Aortic Aneurysms

CT

In the United States, abdominal aortic aneurysms are mostly due to atherosclerosis. Syphilitic or traumatic causes are uncommon. Aneurysms can be detected and differentiated from a tortuous aorta by CT regardless of the presence or absence of aortic-wall calcification. Measurements obtained on CT correlate precisely with those found at surgery (6,8,65,114,116). The lumen size can be differentiated from the adjacent atheroma/thrombus following intravenous injection of contrast agents (99). The origin and the length of an aneurysm, as well as its relationship to renal and iliac arteries, can be traced on serial cephalic and caudad scans (Fig. 8).

The diagnosis of ruptured abdominal aortic aneurysm is based on demonstration of obscuration or anterior displacement of the aneurysm by an irregular high-density (approximately +70 HU) mass or collection that extends into one or both perirenal spaces, and less commonly pararenal spaces (Fig. 9). Additional findings include anterior displacement of the kidney by the hematoma, enlargement or obscuration of the psoas muscle, and a focally indistinct aortic margin that corresponds to the site of rupture (56,120).

In comparison with acute rupture, a chronic aortic pseudoaneurysm (false aneurysm) appears as a well-defined, usually round mass with an attenuation value similar to or lower than that of the native aorta on noncontrast images. On postcontrast images, the lumina of both aneurysms as well as their communication may be enhanced (Fig. 10). A mycotic aneurysm usually has a saccular appearance (Fig. 11) and can be diagnosed by CT if gas is seen within the wall of the aorta (117). Additional features that often aid in the diagnosis include splenic infarcts and lack of atherosclerotic changes in the other vessels. In chronic forms, erosion of an adjacent vertebral body and a paravertebral soft-tissue mass may be identified (7). An infected atherosclerotic aortic aneurysm can likewise be seen on CT (Fig. 12).

Dissection of the aorta usually originates in the thoracic cavity, but sometimes extends into the abdomen. Its diagnosis is based on demonstration of displaced intimal calcifications, or the presence of an intimal flap with enhancement of both the true and false lumina after intravenous administration of contrast material (41,67,68,86)

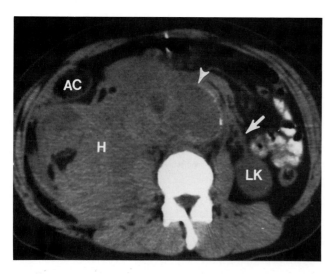

FIG. 9. Leaking aortic aneurysm. Non-contrast-enhanced CT image demonstrates a large irregular mass, with heterogeneous attenuation value in right abdomen. Portion of the mass has an attenuation value compatible with acute hematoma. The hematoma (H) expands the right perinephric space and obscures the inferior vena cava, right psoas muscle, and right lateral wall of the aortic aneurysm (arrowhead). A small amount of hemorrhage (arrow) extends into left perinephric space; (AC) ascending colon; (LK) left kidney.

(Fig. 13). In addition, hyperdensity of the aortic wall at multiple levels has been reported to be specific for acute aortic dissection (71). However, CT may be unable to differentiate dissection from a fusiform aneurysm when the false lumen does not fill with contrast material.

MRI

MRI is an accurate method for demonstrating abdominal aortic aneurysms (5,47,54,91). It can accurately depict the size of an aneurysm, its relationship to the origin of the renal arteries, and the status of the iliac arteries in all patients (Fig. 14). Although only transaxial images are needed to determine the presence and size of an abdominal aortic aneurysm, sagittal sections more directly display the cephalocaudad extent of the aneurysm and its relationship to the visceral arteries (Fig. 15). Coronal images are of limited value, because usually only a portion of the aorta is seen on any one section because of the tortuosity of the aorta and the normal lordosis of most patients (91).

Because of its relatively long imaging time and because of the difficulty in monitoring critically ill patients, MRI has not been used to evaluate patients suspected of having rupture of abdominal aortic aneurysms. Furthermore, MRI cannot distinguish acute hematoma from other fluid collections, because of their similar signal intensities.

MRI is as accurate as CT and arteriography in the detection of aortic dissection (4,33,58,62). The MRI diagnosis of an aortic dissection requires the demonstration of an intimal flap, which can be easily identified when both the true and false lumina appear as signal-void areas (Fig. 16). On occasion, intraluminal signal may appear in the false channel because of slow blood flow or thrombus. As stated previously, slow flow can be differentiated from thrombus by comparing the signal intensities on the first- and second-echo images. In general, the false channel is more likely than the true channel to show evidence of slow blood flow and thrombus.

The inability of MRI to consistently demonstrate small calcifications is not of clinical significance in most patients. However, in the rare case of complete thrombosis of the false channel, detection of an intimal flap by MRI may not be possible. In these patients, CT can more easily diagnose an aortic dissection if inward displacement of intimal calcification can be demonstrated.

Postoperative Complications

CT

Aortic grafts are performed for replacing aneurysms and bypassing occlusive vascular disease. The CT appearance of an aortic graft depends on the type of surgery performed (82,101). There are three common configurations for the

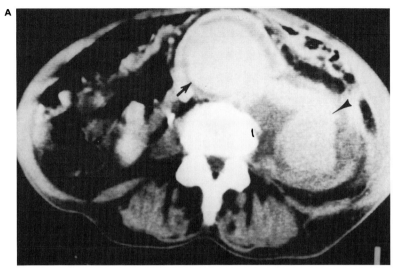

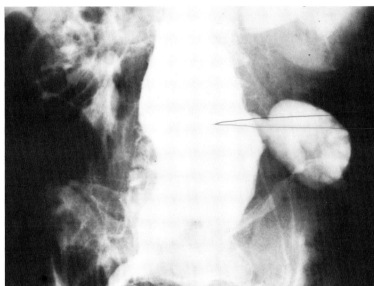

FIG. 10. Aortic aneurysm and associated chronic pseudoaneurysm. **A:** Postcontrast CT image demonstrates a large abdominal aortic aneurysm, extending posterolaterally into left paravertebral area. Note the centrally enhanced lumen in both the true (*arrow*) and false aneurysm (*arrowhead*). The lower-density periphery represents either an atheroma or thrombus. The left psoas muscle is obscured secondary to the pseudoaneurysm. **B:** The abdominal arteriogram shows findings similar to those on CT study.

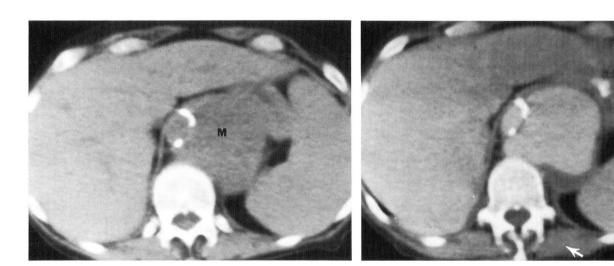

FIG. 11. Mycotic aortic aneurysm. **A:** Non-contrast-enhanced CT image shows a large soft-tissue mass (M) adjacent to the calcified descending aorta. This could be confused with lymphadenopathy. **B:** Postcontrast image demonstrates enhancement of this mass to the same degree as the aorta, thus establishing its vascular nature.

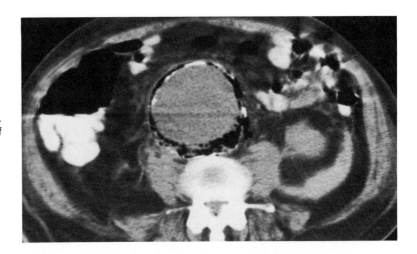

FIG. 12. Infected atherosclerotic aortic aneurysm. Numerous air bubbles are seen within the wall of this fusiform aneurysm.

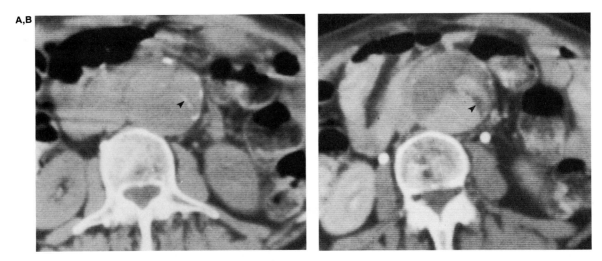

FIG. 13. Acute dissection in a preexisting aortic aneurysm. **A:** Precontrast CT image shows inward displacement of intimal calcifications (*arrowhead*). **B:** Postcontrast image demonstrates equal enhancement of both lumina, with clear delineation of the nonenhancing intimal flap (*arrowhead*) and a large atheromatous plaque.

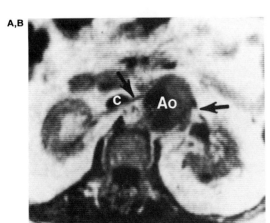

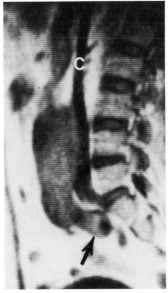

FIG. 14. Transrenal aortic aneurysm, with involvement of iliac artery. **A:** Transverse MR image (TR = 900 msec, TE = 30 msec) at the level of origin of both renal arteries (*arrows*). The aorta (Ao) measured 4.5 cm in its widest diameter. **B:** Sagittal MR image (TR = 500 msec, TE = 30 msec) shows cephalocaudal extent of the aortic aneurysm. A dilated right common iliac artery (*arrow*) is also noted; (C) inferior vena cava.

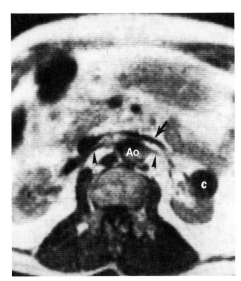 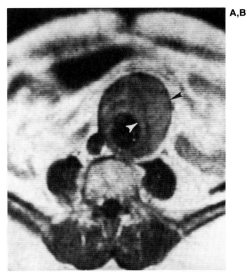

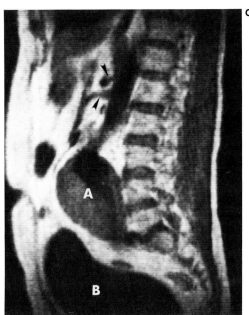

FIG. 15. Infrarenal aortic aneurysm. A: Transverse MR image (TR = 900 msec, TE = 30 msec). The aorta (Ao) is of normal caliber at the level of the renal arteries (*arrowheads*); (*arrow*) left renal vein; (C) renal cyst. B: Eight centimeters caudad to A, the aorta is markedly aneurysmal, measuring 6 cm in its widest diameter. Note that the thrombus (*arrowheads*) has a higher signal intensity than does the aortic lumen. C: Sagittal MR image (TR = 500 msec, TE = 30 msec) shows the relationship between the aneurysm (A) and the visceral arteries; (*lower arrowhead*) superior mesenteric artery; (*upper arrow*) celiac axis; (B) urinary bladder. (From ref. 91.)

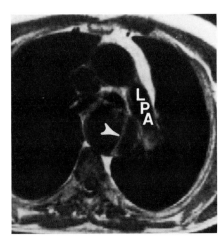 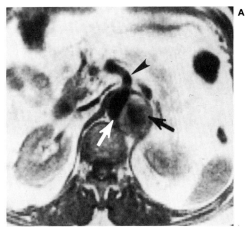

FIG. 16. Dissecting aortic aneurysm. A: Transverse MR image (TR = 500 msec, TE = 30 msec) at the level of the left pulmonary artery (LPA) shows an intimal flap (*arrowhead*) separating the true and false lumina. Both lumina appear as areas of signal void due to rapid blood flow. B: Transverse MR image at the level of the origin of the superior mesenteric artery (*arrowhead*) demonstrates signal within the false lumen (*black arrow*), presumably secondary to slower blood flow. The true lumen (*white arrow*) still emits no signal.

A,B

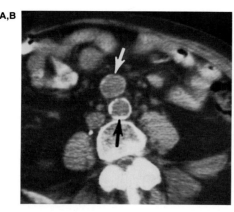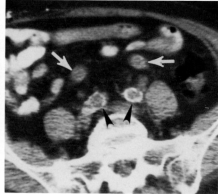

FIG. 17. CT appearance of normal aortoiliac graft with end-to-side anastomosis. **A:** The aortic graft (*white arrow*) lies anterior to the native, calcified aorta (*black arrow*). **B:** The iliac artery grafts (*arrows*) lie several centimeters anterior to the native vessels (*arrowheads*).

proximal anastomosis in these grafts: (a) end-to-side anastomosis, (b) end-to-end anastomosis, and (c) end-to-end anastomosis within the sac of an aneurysm.

In the case of an end-to-side anastomosis, the graft is seen ventral to the native aorta (Fig. 17). The iliac branches of the graft are seen as two dense circular structures anterior to the calcified native iliac arteries, which are commonly thrombosed. The bifurcation of the graft usually is located 2 to 3 cm cephalad to the native aortic bifurcation. The CT appearance of end-to-end anastomosis differs from that of end-to-side anastomosis in its complete interruption of the native aorta at the anastomotic site. Therefore, the distal native aorta is not opacified on postcontrast images. In patients who have had end-to-end anastomosis within the sac of an aneurysm, a collection of serous fluid often can be identified between the synthetic graft and the native aortic wall, which is used to wrap around the graft (Fig. 18).

Postoperative complications of abdominal aortic graft surgery that can be diagnosed by CT include hemorrhage and false aneurysm formation, major vessel or graft limb occlusion, infection, and aortoenteric fistula (31,74, 82,100). When acute hemorrhage is suspected, a noncontrast CT image often is helpful for appreciation of the increased attenuation of fresh blood. False aneurysms occur at the suture line and are more common in the femoral area than in the region of the aortoiliac system. They appear as paragraft fluid collections that may be enhanced to the same degree as the native aorta/graft on postcontrast images.

The diagnosis of graft occlusion is based on the demonstration of a low-density lumen representing thrombus, with lack of enhancement following administration of contrast material. When grafts become infected, irregular, septate fluid collections often are present around the prosthesis, sometimes associated with small pockets of

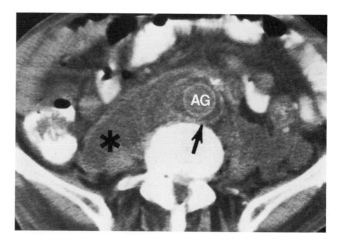

FIG. 18. CT appearance of normal aortoiliac graft: end-to-end anastomosis within an aneurysmal sac. A layer of fluid (*) with near water density is present between the native aortic wall (*arrow*) and the synthetic graft (*measuring cursor*).

FIG. 19. Infected aortic graft. Non-contrast-enhanced CT image demonstrates several fluid collections (*) surrounding the aortic graft (AG). A thin layer of fluid collection is also seen between the graft and the native aortic wall (*arrow*), a finding present in many normal postgraft patients. Culture of needle aspirate from the larger collection yielded mixed flora.

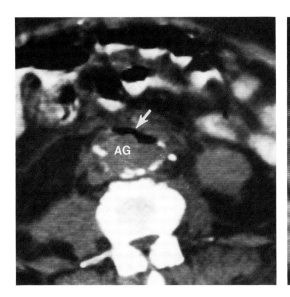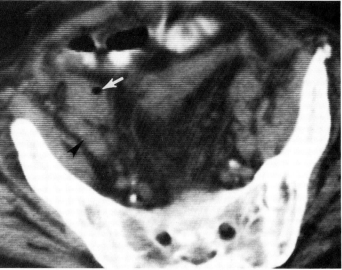

A,B

FIG. 20. Infected aortoiliac graft. **A:** An elongated gas bubble (*arrow*) is noted between the aortic graft (AG) and the calcified, native aortic wall. **B:** At the level of the external iliac artery, the right iliac graft is obscured by a fluid collection that contains a single air bubble (*arrow*); (*arrowhead*) native external iliac artery and vein.

gas (Figs. 19 and 20). These gas collections usually are multiple in number and posterior in location and most often occur more than 10 days after the initial surgery (69). This is in contradistinction to "normal" gas collections seen in the immediate postoperative period, which usually are single in number and anterior in location. Because gas occurs in only a small percentage of perigraft infections, and because gas may be a normal finding in the immediate postoperative period, needle aspiration of any suspicious perigraft fluid collection is advised in any patient suspected of having infection.

MRI

There has been limited experience with MRI for patients following placement of aortoiliofemoral grafts. The prosthetic graft itself does not produce any signal and therefore cannot be delineated as a separate structure if blood flow within the graft is rapid enough to produce a signal void (81). Any signal detected along the periphery of the graft is more likely to be related to the native wall of the aorta or possibly the development of a perigraft fibrous capsule. In patients who have had end-to-end anastomosis within the sac of an aneurysm, a collection of serous fluid that shows relatively low signal intensity on T1-weighted images and high signal intensity on T2-weighted images often develops between the graft and the native aortic wall (Fig. 21).

On MRI, perigraft abscesses may show higher signal intensity than an uncomplicated postoperative seroma (81). Although a perigraft abscess may have a signal intensity similar to that of an acute hematoma, usually it can be differentiated from a subacute hematoma because the latter has a higher signal intensity on T1-weighted

images. A significant limitation of MRI is its inability to detect small collections of air. In addition, MRI cannot reliably differentiate between a collection of air and a small cluster of calcifications.

Clinical Application

Although both CT and MRI can detect the presence and the size of aortic aneurysms and their internal character with a high degree of accuracy (5,8,65,91,116), ultrasound still remains the procedure of choice in patients suspected of having abdominal aortic aneurysms because of its ease of performance, absence of ionizing radiation,

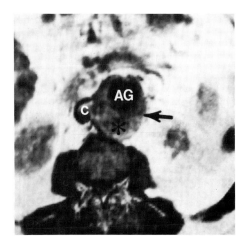

FIG. 21. MRI appearance of a normal aortic graft: end-to-end anastomosis within an aneurysmal sac. Note the presence of a large fluid collection (*) between the native aortic wall (*arrow*) and the synthetic graft (AG); (c) inferior vena cava.

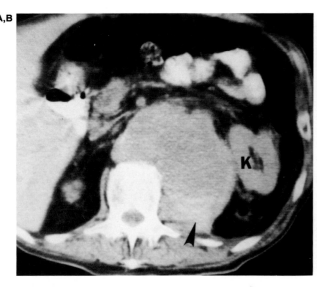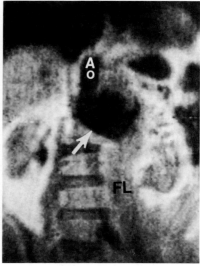

FIG. 22. Ruptured mycotic aneurysm in a 70-year-old man with bilateral renal calculi who presented with back pain and leukocytosis. **A:** Non-contrast-enhanced CT image demonstrates a large retroperitoneal soft-tissue mass obscuring the aortic silhouette and displacing the left kidney (K) laterally. The posterior portion of the mass (*arrowhead*) appears to be of higher attenuation value, suggesting acute hemorrhage. Intravenous contrast material could not be given because of patient's high serum creatinine level. **B:** Coronal MR image shows a large saccular aneurysm (*arrow*) at the level of CT abnormality. A large fluid collection (FL), found to be a mixture of blood and pus at surgery, is present in the left perinephric space; (Ao) normal proximal aorta. (From ref. 91.)

lower cost, and portability. For patients in whom the findings on sonographic examination have been negative or equivocal, because of postsurgical scar tissue, obesity, or abundant bowel gas, either CT or MRI study may be performed. However, in most cases, we prefer CT to MRI. On some occasions, optimal CT evaluation of the abdominal aorta requires intravenous administration of contrast material, e.g., differentiation between a pseudoaneurysm and paraaortic lymphadenopathy. Thus, in patients who have a contraindication to the use of iodinated contrast material, it is advantageous to perform MRI rather than a CT examination (Figs. 22 and 23).

In our experience, CT has been superior to ultrasound and MRI for detecting infected aortic grafts and leaking abdominal aortic aneurysms because of its superior ability to demonstrate small collections of air, its proven ability to diagnose recent hemorrhage, and the ease with which patients can be monitored during the study.

Although not universally accepted, MRI can be performed as the initial imaging study in a clinically stable patient who is suspected of having a dissecting aortic aneurysm. MRI can accurately detect aortic dissections and define their superior and inferior extents. Although CT is also highly accurate in the diagnosis of an aortic dissection (141), CT diagnosis of a dissection usually requires administration of iodinated contrast material, which is clinically important if additional angiographic studies are contemplated. If MRI or CT shows a type A dissection, angiography may be needed to evaluate the status of the coronal arteries and aortic valve.

INFERIOR VENA CAVA AND ITS TRIBUTARIES

Normal Anatomy

CT

The inferior vena cava is formed by the two common iliac veins at the level of the fifth lumbar vertebra. From this point it ascends along the vertebral column to the right of the aorta to the level of the diaphragm and enters the chest, terminating in the right atrium. Although it is in close proximity to the lumbar vertebral bodies in its most caudal position, it assumes a more ventral position at its cephalic end.

The shape, which may be round or flat, and the size of the inferior vena cava vary from patient to patient and even in the same patient at different levels. Performance of a Valsalva maneuver usually results in more distension of the inferior vena cava. The renal veins, which are located ventral to the renal arteries, often can be seen in their entirety entering the vena cava. The left renal vein usually is longer than the right and passes across the midline between the abdominal aorta and the superior mesenteric artery. The main hepatic veins and their tributaries converge into the vena cava near the diaphragm.

The inferior vena cava, the iliac veins, and the renal veins can easily be seen even on noncontrast CT images. The main hepatic veins and their tributaries also can be seen on noncontrast images because they have a slightly lower attenuation value than the normal hepatic paren-

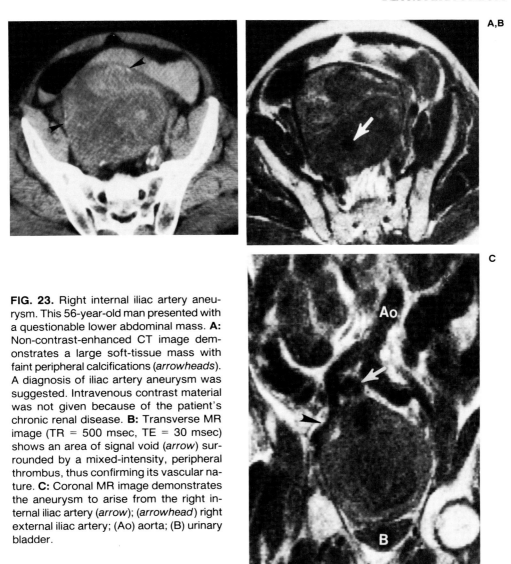

FIG. 23. Right internal iliac artery aneurysm. This 56-year-old man presented with a questionable lower abdominal mass. **A:** Non-contrast-enhanced CT image demonstrates a large soft-tissue mass with faint peripheral calcifications (*arrowheads*). A diagnosis of iliac artery aneurysm was suggested. Intravenous contrast material was not given because of the patient's chronic renal disease. **B:** Transverse MR image (TR = 500 msec, TE = 30 msec) shows an area of signal void (*arrow*) surrounded by a mixed-intensity, peripheral thrombus, thus confirming its vascular nature. **C:** Coronal MR image demonstrates the aneurysm to arise from the right internal iliac artery (*arrow*); (*arrowhead*) right external iliac artery; (Ao) aorta; (B) urinary bladder.

chyma. Normal-caliber gonadal veins cannot be identified reliably on CT images. Occasionally they are enlarged in multiparous women and in men with varicoceles and thus will be apparent on CT images (Fig. 24).

The attenuation value of the lumen of the inferior vena cava is similar to that of the abdominal aorta and thus varies with the hematocrit of the individual patient. However, in comparison to the aortic wall, the wall of the inferior vena cava is thin and rarely visible as a discrete structure even in severely anemic patients.

MRI

The inferior vena cava and its tributaries are well delineated by MRI because of the excellent contrast between vascular structures with flowing blood and adjacent soft tissue. The normal inferior vena cava demonstrates no intraluminal signal (Fig. 25); however, as in the aorta, a flow-related enhancement effect can produce a signal in the inferior vena cava when transverse images are obtained. Unlike the situation for the aorta, the flow-related signal is observed on the most caudal slice of the imaged volume because of the opposite direction of the flow of blood. The wall of the inferior vena cava occasionally can be identified as a structure of relatively low intensity, easily distinguishable from the high-intensity pericaval fat.

Normal Variations (Congenital Anomalies)

Precise knowledge of the various developmental anomalies of the venous system and recognition of their CT and MRI appearances are of paramount importance lest they be misinterpreted as pathologic abnormalities, possibly leading to unnecessary surgical evaluation.

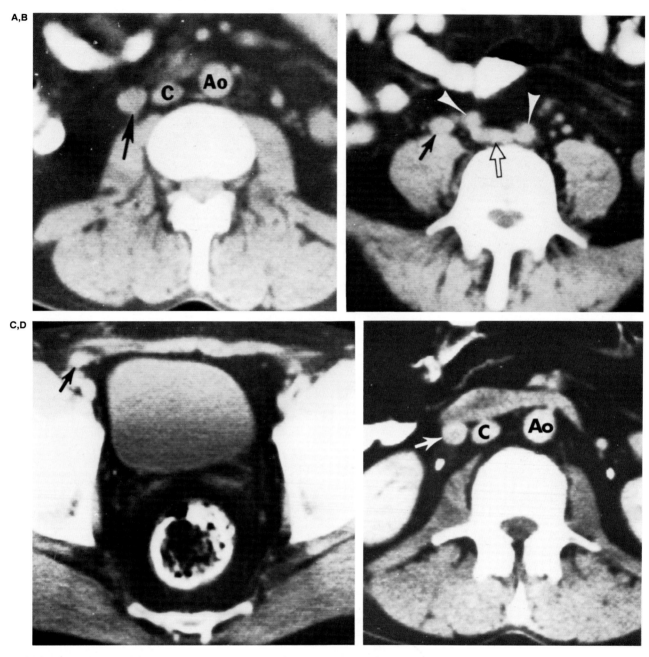

FIG. 24. An enlarged right gonadal vein in a man with an asymptomatic varicocele. **A:** Precontrast CT image just below both kidneys shows an oval soft-tissue density (*arrow*) lateral to the inferior vena cava (C). **B:** At the level of the common iliac artery (*arrowheads*), an extra soft-tissue density (*arrow*) lies anterior to the psoas muscle and lateral to the iliac artery; (*open arrow*) confluence of the common iliac vein. **C:** At the level of acetabula, the soft-tissue density (*arrow*) is seen near the internal (deep) inguinal ring. The presence of such a soft-tissue density over several images indicates that this is a tubular structure. **D:** Postcontrast image at a level slightly above **A** demonstrates the previously noted soft-tissue structure (*arrow*) to enhance to a similar degree as the adjacent inferior vena cava (C), thus documenting its vascular nature. Scrutiny of sequential images and intravenous administration of contrast material often are needed to clarify such complex venous anomalies; (Ao) aorta; (C) inferior vena cava.

The inferior vena cava is formed by the successive development and regression of three paired veins (26,27,122) (Fig. 26). Early in embryogenesis, the posterior supracardinal and more anterior subcardinal veins are formed. Later, the most caudal segment of the right supracardinal vein becomes the infrarenal vena cava. The middle segment joins with part of the right subcardinal vein to form the renal portion of the inferior vena cava. The cephalic portion of the inferior vena cava is formed from the efferent veins of the liver. The portion of the right supracardinal vein cephalad to the kidneys becomes the azygos vein; similarly, that portion on the left forms the hemi-

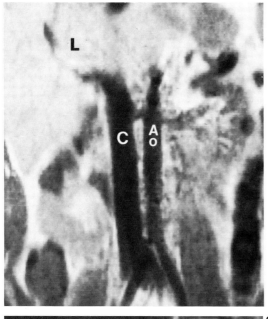
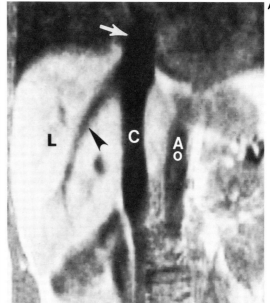

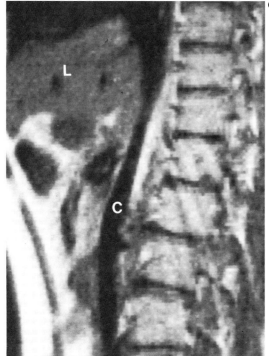

C

FIG. 25. Normal inferior vena cava. **A,B:** Coronal MR images (TR = 500 msec, TE = 15 msec) show the entire course of a normal inferior vena cava (C) in the abdomen. **C:** Sagittal MR image (TR = 500 msec, TE = 30 msec) in another patient; (L) liver; (*arrowhead*) right hepatic vein; (*arrow*) junction between inferior vena cava and right atrium; (Ao) abdominal aorta.

azygos system. The rest of the left cardinal system undergoes involution.

Interruption of normal regression of any of these venous structures results in different anomalies. Azygos vein continuation is an anomaly of the suprarenal segment. Circumaortic venous rings and retroaortic left renal vein involve the renal segment. Circumcaval ureter, transposition, and duplication of the inferior vena cava involve the infrarenal segment. Schematic representations of these various anomalies are shown in Fig. 27. Most of these venous anomalies can be diagnosed with confidence on

noncontrast CT images by tracing their courses on contiguous slices. If some confusion persists regarding noncontrast CT images, the vascular nature of these structures can be proved by intravenous administration of contrast material.

MRI can accurately demonstrate venous anomalies without the use of intravenous contrast material (29, 53,129). The absence of intraluminal signal allows the venous channels to be readily differentiated from retroperitoneal fat, muscle, and enlarged lymph nodes. Transverse images are the most helpful for defining anomalous

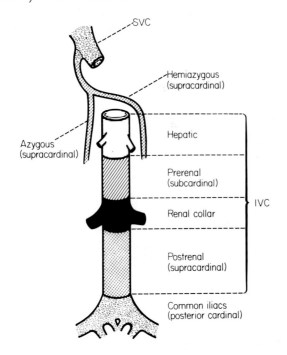

FIG. 26. Schematic diagram showing the precursors of different segments of the inferior vena cava.

venous anatomy. Sagittal and coronal images, in general, do not provide any additional information.

Interrupted Inferior Vena Cava with Azygos/Hemiazygos Continuation

When the subcardinal vein fails to connect with the hepatic veins during the sixth fetal week, blood returns to the heart from the postrenal segment through the azygos/hemiazygos system, and the hepatic veins drain directly into the right atrium (26,27,59). This anomaly usually occurs as an isolated lesion, but occasionally can be associated with cardiac abnormalities or other visceral anomalies such as the asplenia and polysplenia syndromes.

On transverse CT or MRI study, a normal inferior vena cava is seen from the confluence of common iliac veins to the level of both kidneys. An intrahepatic segment of the inferior vena cava, lying anterior to the right diaphragmatic crus and posterior to the caudate lobe of the liver, is absent. However, an enlarged azygos vein, and often a hemiazygos vein as well, can be seen in the retrocrural space on both sides of the aorta. The azygos vein can be further traced on more cephalic images to the level

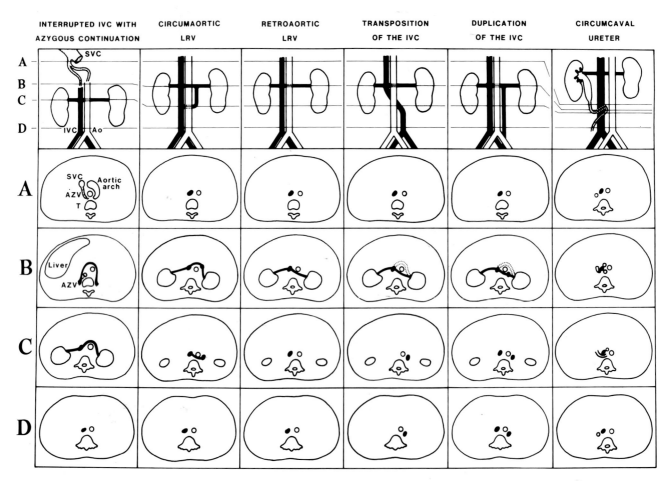

FIG. 27. Diagram showing relationships of aorta, inferior vena cava, and left renal vein in various congenital venous anomalies. (Adapted from ref. 122.)

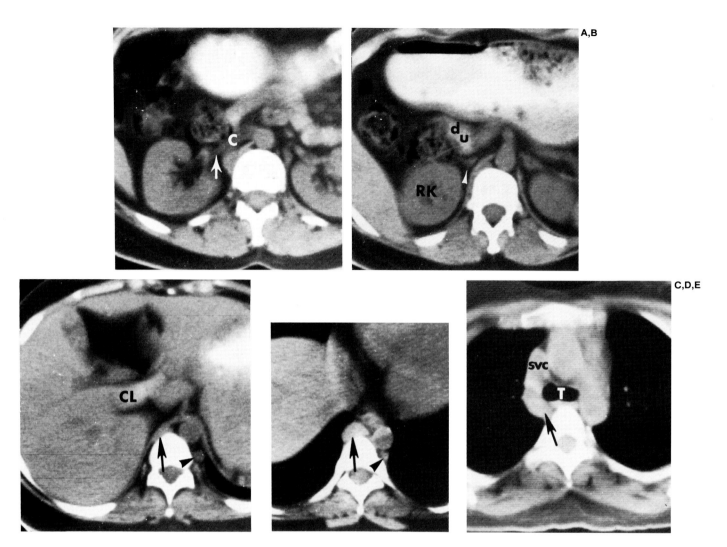

FIG. 28. Interrupted inferior vena cava with azygos/hemiazygos continuation: CT appearance. **A:** At the level of renal hilum, the right renal vein (*white arrow*) drains into the inferior vena cava (C). **B:** Image through the upper pole of the right kidney (RK) shows absence of an inferior vena cava. Note that the right adrenal gland (*white arrowhead*) lies directly posterior to the descending duodenum (du). **C:** At the level of the hepatic hilus, enlarged azygos (*arrow*) and hemiazygos (*arrowhead*) veins can be seen in the retrocrural space. An intrahepatic segment of the inferior vena cava, which normally is situated posterior to the caudate lobe of the liver (CL), is not present in this case. **D:** A more cephalic image, again demonstrating abnormally enlarged azygos (*arrow*) and hemiazygos (*arrowhead*) veins. **E:** At the level of tracheal bifurcation (T), the enlarged azygos vein (*arrow*) drains into the superior vena cava (svc).

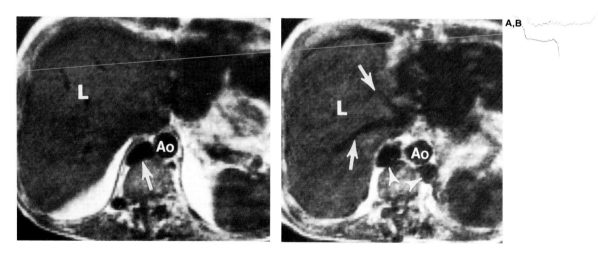

FIG. 29. Interrupted inferior vena cava with azygos/hemiazygos continuation: MR appearance (TR = 500 msec, TE = 30 msec). **A:** The intrahepatic portion of the inferior vena cava is absent, and the azygos vein (*arrow*) is enlarged. **B:** Two centimeters cephalad to **A,** the right and middle hepatic veins (*arrows*) drain directly into the right atrium. Both azygos and hemiazygos veins (*arrowheads*) are enlarged at this level; (Ao) aorta; (L) liver.

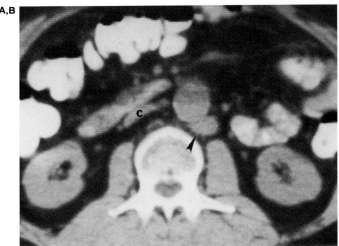

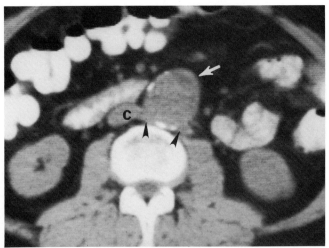

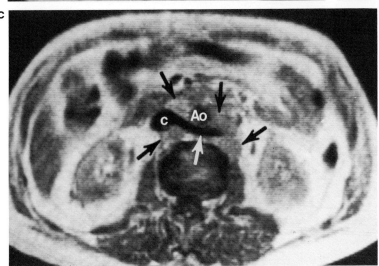

FIG. 30. Retroaortic left renal vein. **A,B:** Two consecutive CT images showing the course of the retroaortic left renal vein (*arrowheads*) in this patient with an aortic aneurysm (*arrow*); (C) inferior vena cava. **C:** MR image (TR = 900 msec, TE = 30 msec) in a patient with metastatic lymphadenopathy (*arrows*) from prostatic carcinoma demonstrates drainage of a retroaortic left renal vein (*white arrow*) into the inferior vena cava (C); (Ao) aorta. (**C** from ref. 89.)

where it arches anteriorly to join the superior vena cava or just below the level of the aortic arch (Figs. 28 and 29).

Circumaortic Left Renal Vein

There is a true vascular ring about the aorta in this anomaly. The preaortic left renal vein crosses from the left kidney to the inferior vena cava at the expected level of the renal veins. The additional retroaortic left renal vein or veins connect to the inferior vena cava by descending caudally and crossing the spine behind the aorta, usually one or two vertebrae below the level of the preaortic left renal vein (122). On a CT or MRI study, a normal, albeit somewhat diminutive, left renal vein can be seen in its preaortic position. The anomalous retroaortic left renal vein is identified in a more caudal position.

Retroaortic Left Renal Vein

In this anomaly, the anterior subcardinal veins regress completely, and only the retroaortic supracardinal veins remain to connect the left kidney to the inferior vena cava

(122,142). The retroaortic left renal vein (Fig. 30) can be seen either at the same level as a normal left renal vein or in a more caudal position, sometimes as low as the confluence of iliac veins.

Transposition of the Inferior Vena Cava

Anomalous regression of the right cardinal veins and persistence of the left cardinal system result in transposition of the inferior vena cava (26,122). In this entity, a single inferior vena cava ascends on the left side of the spine and crosses either anterior or posterior to the aorta at the level of the renal veins to ascend farther to the right atrium on the right side of the spine (Fig. 31). The characteristic appearance on CT or transverse MRI examination is a single inferior vena cava to the right of the aorta at levels above the renal vein, a vascular structure crossing either anterior or posterior to the aorta at the level of the renal veins, and a large single inferior vena cava to the left of the spine at levels below the renal veins.

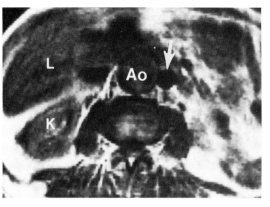

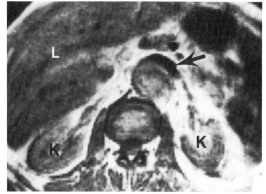

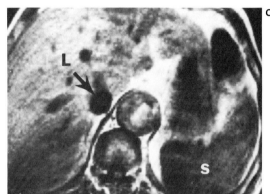

FIG. 31. Transposition of the inferior vena cava. **A:** MR image below the level of the renal vein shows the inferior vena cava (*arrow*) on the left side of a dilated aorta (Ao). **B:** At the level of the renal veins, the inferior vena cava (*arrow*) crosses anterior to the aorta toward the right side. **C:** Cephalad to the level of the renal veins, the inferior vena cava (*arrow*) lies on the right side of the aorta; (K) kidney; (L) liver; (S) spleen.

Duplication of the Inferior Vena Cava

In duplication of the inferior vena cava there is an inferior vena cava, albeit smaller than usual in size, along the right side of the spine (26,48,122). In addition, a left-side inferior vena cava ascends to the level of the renal veins to join the right-side inferior vena cava through a vascular structure that may pass either anterior or posterior to the aorta at the level of the renal veins. Either vena cava can be the predominant vessel, or they can be of equal size. On a CT or MRI study, a single right-side inferior vena cava is seen at levels above the renal veins. A vascular structure crossing either anterior or posterior to the aorta is seen at the level of the renal veins, and two venae cavae, one on each side of the aorta, are present below the level of the renal veins (Fig. 32). A duplicated left inferior vena cava can be differentiated from a dilated left gonadal vein by following its course to the more caudal images. Whereas a duplicated left inferior vena cava ends at the level of common iliac veins, a dilated left gonadal vein can be traced farther inferiorly to the level of the inguinal canal (122).

Circumcaval Ureter

Embryologically, circumcaval ureters result from anomalous regression of the most caudal segment of the supracardinal vein and the persistence of the subcardinal vein. Consequently, the ureter passes behind and around the medial aspect of the inferior vena cava as it courses to the bladder. As in other types of vena caval anomalies, circumcaval ureter may be discovered as an incidental radiographic finding. However, patients with this condition sometimes present with signs and symptoms related to right ureteral obstruction. Whereas asymptomatic patients or patients with minimal caliectasis require only occasional follow-up, patients with significant renal obstruction often require surgical correction.

Inasmuch as circumcaval ureter has a characteristic appearance on excretory urography (medial deviation of the upper one-third of the ureter, with a sharp turn toward the pedicle of the third or fourth lumbar vertebra, producing a reverse-J configuration), a definitive diagnosis by conventional imaging methods often requires concomitant opacification of the ureter and inferior vena cava, e.g., inferior vena cavography in conjunction with retrograde ureteral pyelography. CT can eliminate the need for vena cavography in corroborating the diagnosis should this be considered necessary. With CT, the proximal right ureter can be seen coursing medially behind and then anteriorly around the inferior vena cava so as to encircle it partially (Fig. 33). The distal ureter may be better distended and delineated with the aid of a lower abdominal compression device (57).

A,B

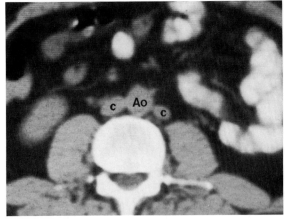 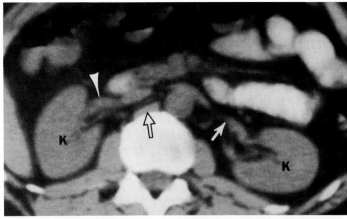

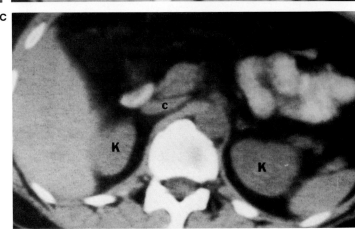

C

FIG. 32. Duplication of the inferior vena cava. **A:** CT image below the level of the renal veins shows two inferior venae cavae (c), one on each side of the aorta (Ao). The right-side cava is slightly larger than its counterpart on the left. **B:** At the level of the renal veins, the right renal vein (*arrowhead*) drains into the right-side cava. The left renal vein (*arrow*) drains into the left-side cava, which then crosses anterior to the aorta to join its counterpart on the right; (*open arrow*) inferior right crus. **C:** Above the level of the renal veins, there is only one inferior vena cava (c), which lies on the right side; (K) kidney.

A,B

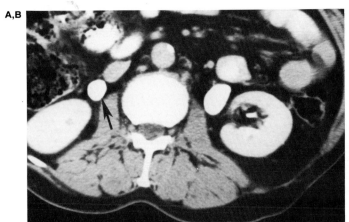 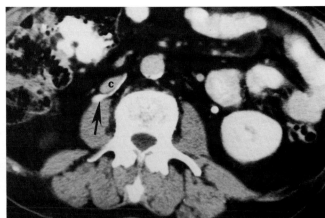

C

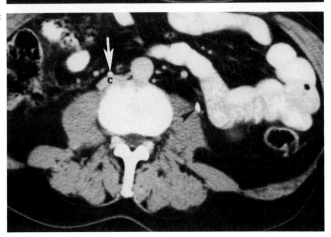

FIG. 33. Circumcaval ureter. **A:** Postcontrast CT image demonstrates a dilated proximal right ureter (*arrow*). **B:** One centimeter caudal to **A,** the right ureter (*arrow*) passes behind the inferior vena cava (c). **C:** One centimeter caudal to **B,** the right ureter (*arrow*) lies anterior to the inferior vena cava (c). This is in contrast to the normal left ureter (*arrowhead*), which lies along the anterolateral aspect of the psoas muscle.

Pathologic Conditions

Venous Thrombosis

CT

Tumoral and nontumoral thrombosis of the inferior vena cava can be identified but not differentiated from each other on CT images unless hypervascularity is shown in the tumoral thrombus by bolus dynamic CT (102,134,144,150). Thrombosis of the renal and gonadal veins has been similarly documented (61,131). In cases of septic thrombosis, inflammatory changes often can be observed surrounding the occluded vein (Fig. 34) (131). Because the right renal vein is shorter and more obliquely oriented than the longer, more horizontal left renal vein, direct demonstration of thrombus is achieved less frequently on the right than on the left. The involved segment of the vein can be either normal in caliber or substantially enlarged. Enlargement of the cava (or the renal vein) secondary to a thrombus can be strongly suggested on noncontrast-enhanced images alone because dilatation often is more focal in cases of thrombosis than in the more generalized dilatation seen secondary to increased blood flow or increased vascular resistance at the level of the diaphragm/right atrium. In cases of complete caval obstruction, extensive venous collaterals may also be identified by CT (113). These include the paravertebral venous system and its communications with the ascending lumbar veins and the azygos/hemiazygos system; gonadal, peri-ureteric, and other retroperitoneal veins; abdominal-wall veins; hemorrhoidal venous plexus; and the portal venous system.

Definitive diagnosis of venous thrombosis by CT depends on demonstration of an intraluminal thrombus (Fig. 35). Whereas a fresh thrombus has a density similar to that of circulating blood, an old thrombus is of lower density than the surrounding blood on noncontrast images. When the occlusion is complete, the involved segment remains unenhanced on postcontrast images. In the case of chronic occlusion, the inferior vena cava may become atrophic and calcified (Fig. 36). In cases where the venous occlusion is partial, the thrombus appears as a low-density filling defect surrounded by iodine-containing blood. However, caution must be taken not to confuse true intraluminal defects from those caused by a laminar-flow phenomenon, with the slower-flowing enhanced blood staying closest to the wall, and unopacified blood flowing centrally suggesting a luminal thrombus (9,60). This "defect" is commonly seen in the inferior vena cava at the end of a bolus injection when a foot vein is used. At present, there probably are few, if any, indications for administering contrast material via a foot vein injection. Bolus injection of contrast material through an arm vein, followed by serial dynamic images, is the preferred method for examining the patency of the venous system.

A "pseudothrombus" artifact also may occur in the suprarenal vena cava with a bolus injection or rapid infusion even when an arm vein is used (146). This defect is most pronounced just at and cephalad to the renal vein origins, although it can be seen as high as the intrahepatic vena cava (Fig. 37). It is caused by the poor mixing between the densely opacified renal venous effluent and the less densely opacified infrarenal caval blood. This artifact can be differentiated from a true thrombus by its unsharp border and higher attenuation, and by the use of delayed images.

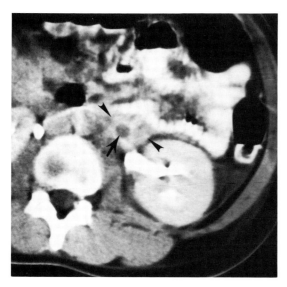 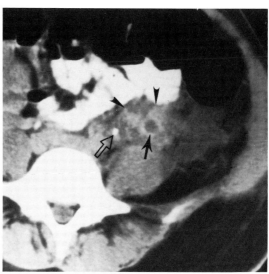

A,B

FIG. 34. Postpartum septic thrombosis of the left ovarian vein. Sequential postcontrast CT images demonstrate a thrombosed left ovarian vein (*arrow*) and its surrounding inflammatory changes (*arrowheads*); (*open arrow*) left ureter.

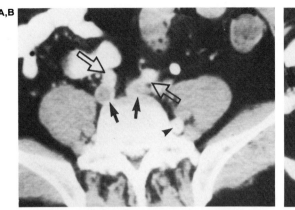

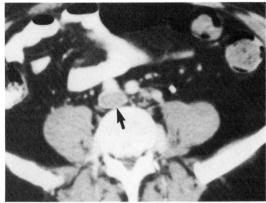

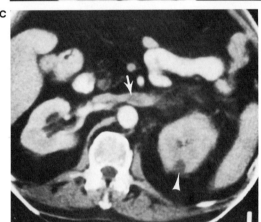

FIG. 35. Thrombosis of the inferior vena cava and its tributaries. **A:** Postcontrast CT image demonstrates nonenhancing thrombi within both common iliac veins (*arrows*). A large paravertebral collateral vein (*arrowhead*) is seen on the left side; (*open arrows*) common iliac arteries. **B:** Three centimeters cephalad to **A,** thrombus is seen in the inferior vena cava (*arrow*) as well. **C:** Postcontrast CT image from another patient shows a thrombus (*arrow*) within a nondilated left renal vein. The patient also has a small left renal cyst (*arrowhead*).

FIG. 36. Chronic vena caval thrombosis. Postcontrast CT image demonstrates a calcified, atrophic inferior vena cava (*arrow*). Note multiple enhancing collateral vessels in the retroperitoneum (*arrowheads*).

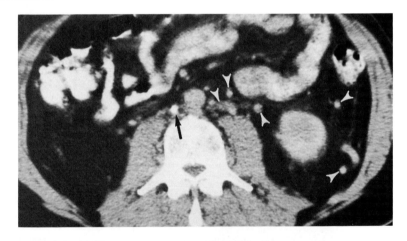

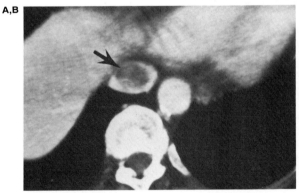

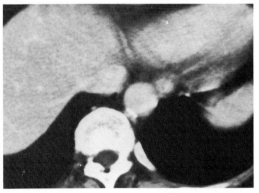

FIG. 37. Pseudothrombus in the inferior vena cava. **A:** CT image at the level of the diaphragm obtained 1 min after a bolus intravenous injection of contrast material into an arm vein shows a central, hypodense defect within the inferior vena cava (*arrow*). **B:** Repeat image at the same level several minutes later demonstrates uniform enhancement of the inferior vena cava, without evidence of a thrombus.

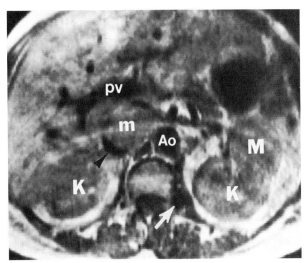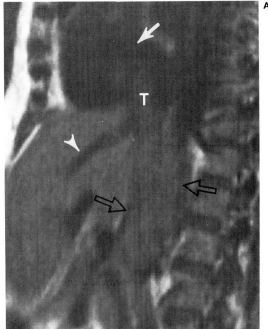

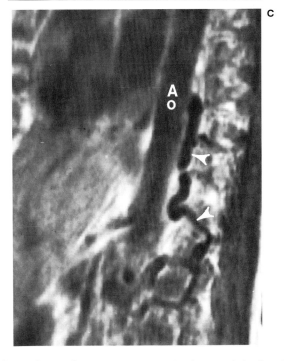

FIG. 38. Left renal cell carcinoma invading the inferior vena cava and right atrium. **A:** Transverse MR image (TR = 2,100 msec, TE = 35 msec) shows a 4-cm left renal mass (M). A mass (m) with a signal intensity similar to that of renal cell carcinoma is present within the inferior vena cava. The posterolateral portion of the inferior vena cava (*arrowhead*) is still patent; (pv) portal vein; (Ao) aorta; (K) kidney; (*arrow*) enlarged paravertebral collateral vein. **B:** Sagittal MR image (TR = 500 msec, TE = 35 msec) shows the tumor thrombus (T) extending into the right atrium (*arrow*). Tumor extension into the right atrium was not appreciated on a prior CT study; (*arrowhead*) middle hepatic vein; (*open arrows*) inferior vena cava. **C:** Sagittal MR image through the aorta (Ao) demonstrates a large paravertebral collateral vein (*arrowheads*).

MRI

Venous thrombus produces intraluminal signal (Fig. 38) and can be differentiated from slow flow by comparing the signal intensities on the first and second echoes or by using a phase-sensitive imaging sequence (46,51,75,76). Additional MRI manifestations of caval thrombosis include focal dilatation of the vena cava and the presence of venous collateral vessels that appear as tubular structures emitting little or no signal. MRI may distinguish tumor thrombus from bland thrombus on the basis of their signal characteristics. The MRI features of tumor thrombus include isointensity with the primary neoplasms and loss of definition of the vena caval wall. High signal

intensity on first- and second-echo images is indicative of a bland thrombus. Thrombi of intermediate signal intensity can be seen in both entities. In one study, bland thrombus could be differentiated from tumor thrombus in 11 of 16 cases (75). However, the reliability of MRI in making such a distinction needs to be determined in a larger group of patients.

Transverse views are often sufficient for the diagnosis of caval thrombosis; sagittal and coronal sections more directly display the cephalocaudal extent of the thrombus. The latter information is particularly important for the planning of resection of tumor thrombus (Figs. 38 and 39).

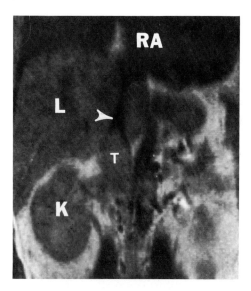

FIG. 39. Renal cell carcinoma extending into the inferior vena cava. The cephalic extent of caval invasion could not be accurately determined on a prior contrast-enhanced CT study. Coronal MR image (TR = 500 msec, TE = 70 msec) clearly shows the cephalic extent of tumor thrombus (T). Most of the intrahepatic portion of the inferior vena cava (*arrowhead*) is uninvolved; (K) kidney; (L) liver; (RA) right atrium.

Clinical Application

Although there are no data comparing the accuracy of CT and venography in detecting nontumoral thrombosis of the inferior vena cava and its major branches, CT is reported to have a similar overall accuracy in the detection of inferior vena cava and main renal vein invasion by

renal cell carcinoma. In one study (150), the overall accuracy of CT was 93% in detecting inferior vena caval invasion and 82% in detecting main renal vein invasion. It is often harder to be certain of tumor thrombus in the right renal vein, which is shorter than its counterpart on the left. CT is not able to detect tumor thrombus in intrarenal venous branches; however, this is of limited clinical significance because the presence of only intrarenal vein invasion by tumor does not alter surgical management (150).

Because of its high degree of accuracy, CT has largely replaced inferior vena cavography in detecting invasion of the main renal veins and inferior vena cava in patients with renal cell carcinoma. Likewise, because of its ease of performance and because of its ability to examine the entire retroperitoneum simultaneously, CT has become the procedure of choice for evaluating patients suspected of having nontumoral venous thrombosis.

MRI is as accurate as contrast-enhanced CT in demonstrating vena caval thrombus (51,75). The ability to evaluate the inferior vena cava without iodinated contrast material represents a major advantage of MRI. At present, MRI is reserved for either patients who have a contraindication to iodinated contrast material or patients in whom the prior CT findings are equivocal (Figs. 38 and 39).

Ultrasound is another well-established technique for detecting thrombus in the inferior vena cava (115,130). Ultrasound can evaluate the inferior vena cava from the level of the renal veins to the right atrium in most patients. However, the inability of ultrasound to clearly demonstrate the rest of the vena cava because of overlying bowel gas has limited its use.

A,B

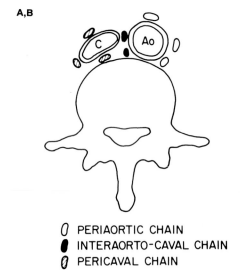

(*) PERIAORTIC CHAIN
(●) INTERAORTO-CAVAL CHAIN
(*) PERICAVAL CHAIN

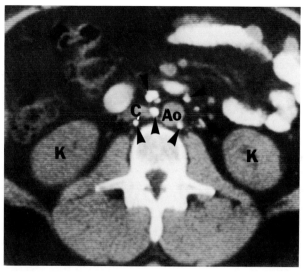

FIG. 40. A: Schematic drawing denoting distribution of periaortic and pericaval lymph nodes. **B:** CT image in a patient following lymphangiography showing normal distribution of retroperitoneal lymph nodes (*arrowheads*); (Ao) aorta; (C) inferior vena cava; (K) kidney.

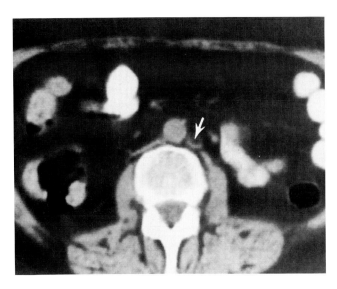

FIG. 41. Fibrolipomatous changes in a paraaortic lymph node. Note that the central portion (*arrow*) of this lymph node has an attenuation value similar to that of retroperitoneal fat.

LYMPH NODES

Normal Anatomy

Normal unopacified lymph nodes are routinely seen on CT images. They appear as small soft-tissue densities, ranging from 3 to 10 mm in size. In the retroperitoneum, lymph nodes can be found adjacent to the anterior, posterior, medial, and lateral walls of the inferior vena cava and aorta (Fig. 40). Lymph nodes also can be seen as nonenhancing soft-tissue densities in the root of the mesentery and along the course of the major venous structures draining to the inferior vena cava and portal vein (132). In the pelvis, lymph nodes can be identified in close proximity with the iliac vessels. Although the internal architecture of a lymph node generally is not discernible on CT, benign fibrolipomatous changes have been shown on CT images on rare occasions (Fig. 41).

Normal abdominal and pelvic lymph nodes can likewise be seen on MRI (35,154). However, because of their small size and the poorer spatial resolution of MRI, normal nodes are seen less frequently on MRI studies than on CT images. As with CT, the internal architecture of a normal lymph node generally cannot be evaluated with MRI. The signal intensity of normal nodes usually is similar to that of pathologically enlarged lymph nodes.

Pathologic Conditions

CT

The diagnosis of retroperitoneal lymphadenopathy by CT is based on recognition of nodal enlargement, sometimes concomitant with displacement or obscuration of normal structures in far-advanced disease (2,11,17,84,87,119,128). Except in unusually lean or cachectic patients, enlarged lymph nodes generally are well profiled by surrounding fat. In the abdomen and pelvis, lymph nodes are considered unequivocally abnormal if they exceed 1.5 cm in cross-sectional diameter. Lymph nodes in the retrocrural space are considered to be pathologic if they exceed 6 mm in size (20). An isolated abdominal or pelvic lymph node between 1 and 1.5 cm is regarded as a suspicious finding; clustering of nodes of this size should increase the index of suspicion. A CT-guided percutaneous needle biopsy or a follow-up study may be indicated in such problem cases.

The CT presentation of malignant lymphadenopathy may vary from (a) one or several discrete enlarged lymph nodes to (b) a more conglomerate group of contiguous enlarged nodes similar in size to the aorta or inferior vena cava to (c) a large homogenous mass in which individual nodes are no longer recognizable, obscuring the contours of normal surrounding structures (Fig. 42). Massive enlargement of retroaortic and retrocaval nodes may cause anterior displacement of these vessels.

Because intranodal architecture is not discernible on CT, lymph nodes that are normal in size but infiltrated with neoplastic cells cannot be distinguished as abnormal by CT. Furthermore, CT usually cannot differentiate between benign and malignant causes of lymph node enlargement. Diffuse lymph node enlargement secondary to viral or granulomatous disease cannot be differentiated from lymphoma or metastases based on CT findings alone (93), although the massive type of conglomeration described almost never is seen with the benign conditions. The inability of CT to distinguish benign from malignant causes of lymphadenopathy is particularly troublesome for patients with AIDS-related disease, because benign nodal hyperplasia, lymphoma, and metastases from Kaposi's sarcoma occur with equal frequency in these patients (109) (Fig. 43). Percutaneous needle biopsy of the enlarged nodes under CT guidance often is needed to establish a histologic diagnosis.

A definitive CT diagnosis may be possible in Whipple's disease. In this disease, the attenuation value of the enlarged lymph nodes often is quite low, ranging from +10 HU to +30 HU (96) (Fig. 44). This relatively low density most likely is caused by the deposition of fat and fatty acids in the lymph nodes. Enlarged, low-density lymph nodes also may be seen in patients with tuberculosis, testicular neoplasms, particularly teratocarcinoma (Fig. 45), and epidermoid carcinoma of the genitourinary tract, and rarely in patients with lymphoma. Usually this is the result of necrosis or liquefaction within the neoplasm.

Other entities, such as retroperitoneal fibrosis (Fig. 46), perianeurysmal fibrosis, and false aortic aneurysm (Fig. 11), also may exhibit findings on CT resembling those of malignant lymphadenopathy (1,18,137). However, the soft-tissue mass seen in idiopathic retroperitoneal fibrosis

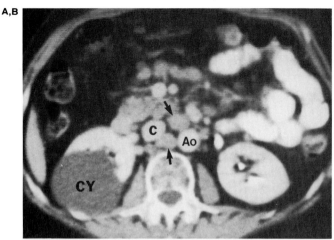

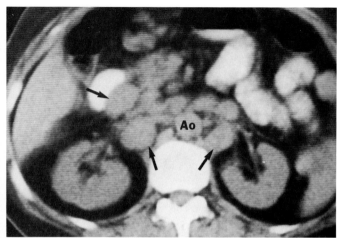

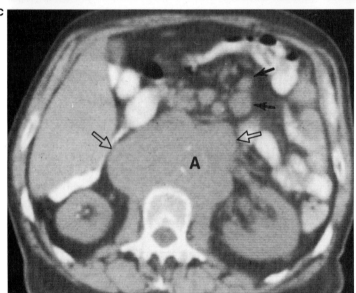

FIG. 42. Retroperitoneal lymphadenopathy in three different patients with lymphoma. **A:** Mild lymph node enlargement. Postcontrast CT image shows that individual lymph nodes (*arrows*) are enlarged, but their discrete outlines have been maintained; (Ao) aorta; (C) inferior vena cava; (CY) renal cyst. **B:** Moderate lymph node enlargement. Enlarged lymph nodes have coalesced to form soft-tissue masses (*arrows*), each of which is slightly larger than the adjacent aorta (Ao). **C:** Massive lymph node enlargement is seen as a large, homogeneous soft-tissue mass (*open arrows*), resulting in obscuration of retroperitoneal vascular structure. Note that the location of aorta (A) is identified by virtue of its mural calcification; (*arrows*) enlarged mesenteric nodes.

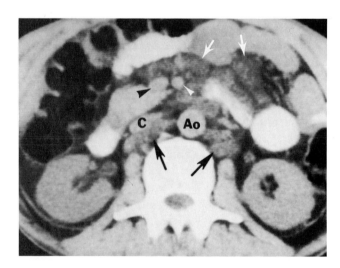

FIG. 44. Whipple disease. Enlarged retroperitoneal and mesenteric lymph nodes (*white arrows*) are present. Note that the attenuation value of the lymph nodes is lower than that of adjacent vascular structures and psoas muscles; (Ao) aorta; (C) inferior vena cava; (*black arrowhead*) superior mesenteric vein; (*white arrowhead*) superior mesenteric artery.

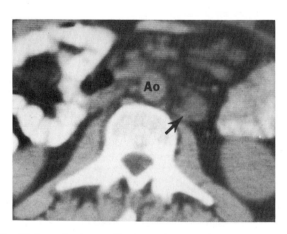

FIG. 43. Lymphadenopathy (*arrow*) secondary to *Mycobacterium intracellularis* in a patient with AIDS; (Ao) aorta.

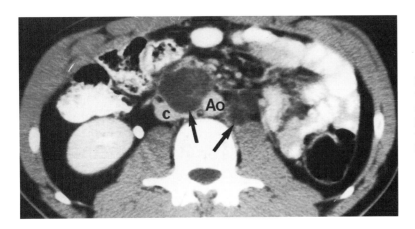

FIG. 45. Low-density nodal metastases due to testicular teratocarcinoma. Postcontrast CT image demonstrates enlarged paraaortic and precaval lymph nodes (*arrows*). Note that the attenuation value of these lymph nodes is lower than that of back muscles; (Ao) aorta; (c) inferior vena cava.

or perianeurysmal fibrosis usually has a more regular border than that seen with malignant lymphadenopathy (Fig. 47). False aortic aneurysms usually can be distinguished from lymphadenopathy on postcontrast images. Although the inferior extent of the right crus of the diaphragm or vascular abnormalities and anomalies—such as an enlarged gonadal vein (Fig. 24), a duplicated inferior vena cava, or a dilated azygos or hemiazygos vein—conceivably could be confused with an enlarged lymph node, careful examination of multiple contiguous images and perhaps concomitant use of intravenous iodinated contrast material can distinguish these entities from lymphadenopathy.

MRI

Abnormal retroperitoneal lymph nodes are identified on the basis of nodal enlargement rather than by any characteristic signal intensity (89). Although *in vitro* study has shown that lymph nodes containing metastases have a significantly longer T2 than normal and hyperplastic nodes (148), *in vivo* tissue characterization based on relaxation times or signal intensities is not yet possible (36,89). Enlarged lymph nodes due to malignant disease cannot be distinguished from those due to benign processes. Furthermore, lymph nodes that are of normal size but are partially or totally replaced with a neoplasm will not be identified as abnormal by MRI.

Abnormal lymph nodes usually have a homogeneous MRI appearance, but may appear inhomogeneous as a result of calcification or necrosis (Fig. 48). On T1-weighted images, the signal intensity of lymph nodes is slightly higher than that of iliopsoas muscle and diaphragmatic crura and is much lower than the signal intensity of fat (Fig. 49). On images obtained with longer repetition times and/or longer echo-delay times, the contrast between lymph nodes and muscle increases, and that between nodes and fat decreases (Fig. 49). Thus, on T2-weighted images, lymph nodes are easily distinguished from muscle and diaphragmatic crura, but may be difficult to differentiate from surrounding retroperitoneal fat because of their similar signal intensities (35,89). In general, abnor-

FIG. 46. Retroperitoneal fibrosis. A large soft-tissue mass is present in the retroperitoneum, resulting in total obscuration of the aorta and inferior vena cava. Also note the presence of mild hydronephrosis bilaterally. Streaky soft-tissue densities posterior to both kidneys may be due to collateral vessels or previous renal inflammatory disease. This CT appearance is indistinguishable from that of malignant lymphadenopathy. Surgical biopsy yielded fibrosis.

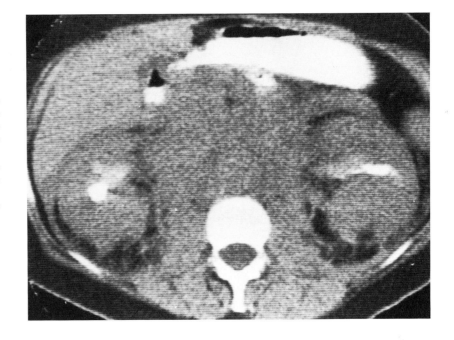

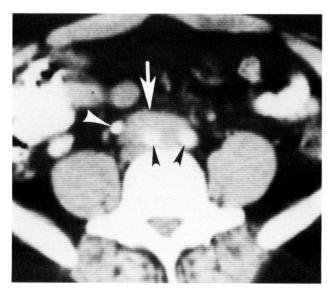

FIG. 47. Idiopathic retroperitoneal fibrosis. Postcontrast CT image demonstrates a mantle of soft-tissue density (*arrow*) encasing both iliac arteries (*black arrowheads*). Note that the mass has well-defined borders. Although not pathognomonic, this CT appearance is more characteristic of retroperitoneal fibrosis than malignant lymphadenopathy; (*white arrowhead*) mildly dilated right ureter.

mal lymph nodes are better demonstrated on T1-weighted images. The multiplanar capability of MRI has not facilitated the detection of lymphadenopathy. Images obtained in the sagittal or coronal planes do not contribute additional clinically useful information.

Lymph nodes are well distinguished from blood vessels because of the signal void usually demonstrated by vascular structures. As a result, displacement or encasement of blood vessels by lymphadenopathy is well demonstrated by MRI (Fig. 50). In patients with sparse retroperitoneal fat, MRI may not be able to differentiate between loops of bowel and lymph nodes. This will continue to be a potential problem until an efficacious and convenient oral contrast agent is developed.

Clinical Application

Lymphoma

The accuracy of CT in detecting intraabdominal and pelvic lymphadenopathy in patients with lymphoma has been studied by several groups of investigators. Results from these studies are generally influenced by the types of CT scanners used, expertise of the interpreters, and types of patients selected. The reported accuracy has ranged from 68 to 100%, with a false-positive rate varying from zero to 25% (2,11,12,17,21,40,93,103,119,152). False-positive cases are largely due to confusion with unopacified bowel loops or normal vascular structures, a problem that is easily resolved by rigorous attention to technique. False-positive diagnoses also can be due to misinterpretation of lymphadenopathy secondary to benign inflammatory disease as malignant. False-negative interpretations almost always are secondary to inability to recognize replaced but normal-size or minimally enlarged lymph nodes as abnormal. Even with increasing experience in image interpretation, coupled with meticulous scanning techniques, this limitation remains a problem for CT and accounts for most of the false-negative interpretations.

Bipedal lymphangiography has been the technique employed in the past to investigate possible retroperitoneal lymph node abnormalities. However, the method is time-consuming, occasionally difficult to perform, and uncomfortable for the patient. In patients with severe cardiopulmonary disease, lymphangiography may be medically contraindicated. The introduction of CT has provided a method for easy assessment of the retroperitoneal lymph nodes and for simultaneous evaluation of lymph nodes and organs elsewhere in the abdomen. Efforts have been made by several investigators to compare the clinical efficacy of lymphangiography with that of CT. Although most investigators, including ourselves, found CT to have an accuracy comparable to that of lymphan-

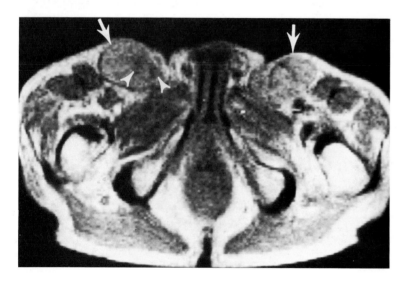

FIG. 48. Bilateral inguinal lymphadenopathy (*arrows*) due to non-Hodgkin lymphoma (TR = 900 msec, TE = 30 msec). The lymph nodes are inhomogeneous, with areas of lower intensity (*arrowheads*), corresponding to lower attenuation values on CT images, believed to represent necrosis. (From ref. 89.)

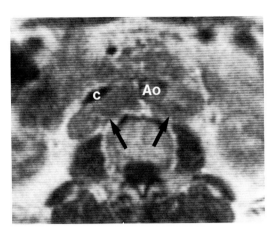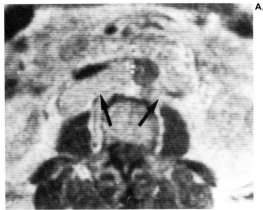

FIG. 49. Retroperitoneal lymphadenopathy due to non-Hodgkin lymphoma. **A:** MR image (TR = 500 msec, TE = 30 msec). The intensity of enlarged retrocaval and paraaortic nodes (*arrows*) is slightly higher than that of the psoas muscle and much lower than that of fat on this relatively T1-weighted image; (Ao) aorta; (c) inferior vena cava. **B:** MR image (TR = 1,500 msec, TE = 60 msec). The contrast between enlarged lymph nodes (*arrows*) and adjacent fat is decreased on this relatively T2-weighted image.

giography in detecting retroperitoneal and pelvic lymph node involvement by lymphoma (11,12,40,42,152), others (21) showed lymphangiography to be a slightly more accurate test in evaluating patients in the clinically early stages of Hodgkin disease. However, all groups found CT capable of detecting lymph nodes in areas where the lymphographic contrast material does not reach, i.e., nodes around the celiac axis, retrocrural space, renal hilus, and splenic and hepatic hila, as well as in the mesentery (Fig. 51). Lymphomatous infiltration of various intraabdominal organs, such as the liver, the spleen, the kidneys, and the gastrointestinal tract, also can be seen on CT images (Figs. 52–54), although the sensitivity of CT in detecting early or minimal parenchymal lymphoma is low (2,21,107). Such nodal and extranodal areas frequently are involved at presentation with non-Hodgkin lymphomas. Demonstration of lymphomatous involvement of iliopsoas muscle, adrenal glands, gynecologic organs, and pancreas by CT also has been reported (63). CT also may be superior to lymphangiography in delineating the exact extent of intraabdominal nodal involvement, because lymph nodes totally replaced by lymphoma are not opacified at all by lymphography.

There is nearly unanimous agreement (22,30,87,111) that CT should assume the primary radiologic role in staging patients with non-Hodgkin lymphomas because of the tendency of these diseases to exhibit bulky lymphadenopathy in multiple sites and because of their high incidence of mesenteric lymph node involvement (>50%). Lymphangiography is rarely needed in this group of patients. Other radiologic studies such as upper gastrointestinal series and barium enema are necessary only when specific symptoms in a patient suggest involvement of these organs.

Controversy regarding whether CT or lymphangiography should be used for the initial staging of Hodgkin

disease has become less heated in recent years. Although some centers continue to use lymphangiography as a primary imaging method and use CT only as a complementary tool in a few selected cases, others, including ourselves, have replaced lymphangiography with CT as the primary imaging method. A positive CT study eliminates the need for a lymphangiogram. A negative CT study can exclude nodal disease with a high degree of confidence. Lymphangiography certainly is valuable when the CT images are equivocal and, following a negative CT study, can be reassuring and on rare occasion may detect replaced but normal-size lymph nodes. Staging laparotomy is still required for many patients at the time of initial presentation because of the inability of CT to detect microscopic disease in both lymph nodes and the spleen.

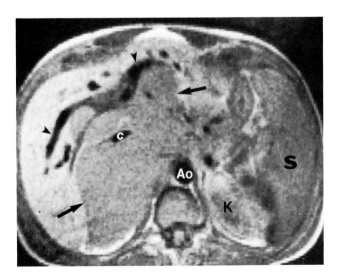

FIG. 50. Non-Hodgkin lymphoma: MR image (TR = 500 msec, TE = 35 msec). A large nodal mass (*arrows*) can be easily distinguished from adjacent vessels; (Ao) aorta; (c) inferior vena cava; (*arrowheads*) portal vein branches; (S) spleen; (K) kidney.

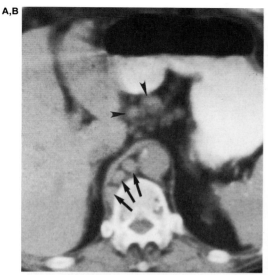

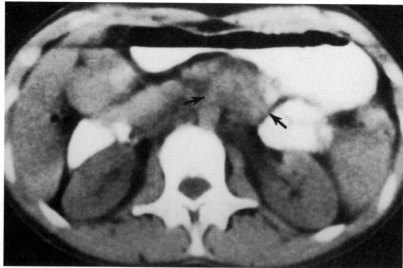

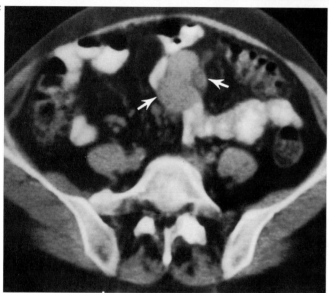

FIG. 51. Lymphoma involving nodes (*arrows*) in areas where lymphographic contrast material does not reach. **A:** Retrocrural (*arrows*) and left gastric (*arrowheads*). **B:** Celiac. **C:** Mesenteric.

In addition to being used as an initial staging procedure, CT also has been used to follow responses to various methods of treatment (Fig. 55). It should be emphasized that in patients with massive lymphadenopathy seen on the initial study, the findings on follow-up images may not always revert to normal even when patients are in complete clinical remission. Fibrotic changes secondary to prior radiation or chemotherapy may appear either as discrete, albeit smaller, soft-tissue masses or as a thin sheath causing obscuration of the discrete outlines of the aorta and inferior vena cava (Fig. 56). Unfortunately, CT is incapable of differentiating between viable residual neoplasm and such fibrotic changes caused by chemotherapy or radiotherapy. Additional follow-up studies or surgical/percutaneous biopsy often are necessary for such a differentiation. Despite this limitation, CT provides a more accurate delineation of progression or regression of the disease process than any other radiologic procedure (90).

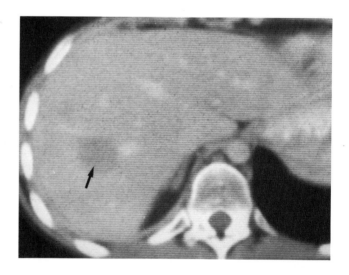

FIG. 52. Hepatic lymphoma. A single hypodense lesion (*arrow*) representing lymphoma is present in the right lobe of the liver.

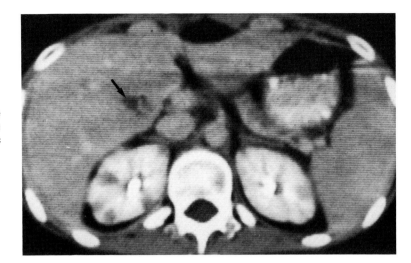

FIG. 53. Renal lymphoma. Postcontrast CT image demonstrates multiple low-density lesions in both kidneys. The spleen is also enlarged; (*arrow*) hepatic lymphoma.

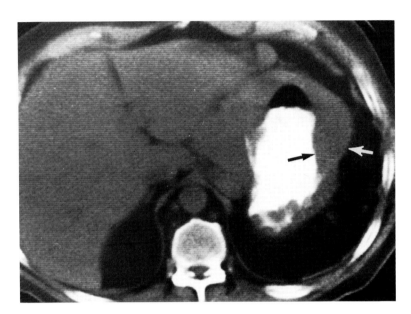

FIG. 54. Gastric lymphoma. Marked thickening of the gastric wall (*arrows*) is caused by non-Hodgkin lymphoma.

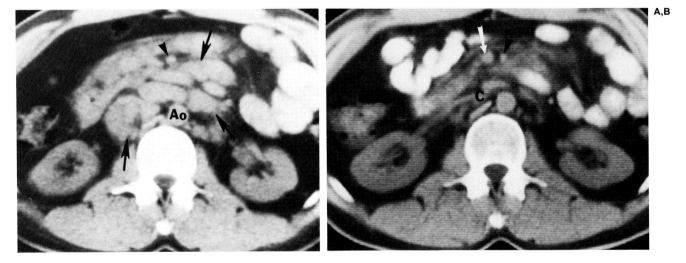

FIG. 55. A: Initial CT image in patient with poorly differentiated lymphocytic lymphoma showed retroperitoneal and mesenteric adenopathy (*arrows*). **B:** A follow-up CT study after six courses of chemotherapy demonstrated nearly complete resolution of intraabdominal lymphadenopathy. Note that the inferior vena cava (C) and superior mesenteric vein (*white arrow*) can be much better appreciated on this examination; (Ao) aorta; (*black arrowhead*) superior mesenteric artery.

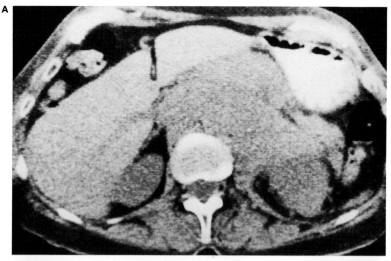

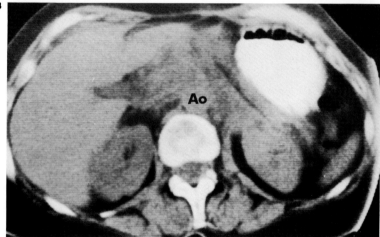

FIG. 56. Residual fibrosis following chemotherapy. **A:** Initial image in this patient with Hodgkin disease shows massive retroperitoneal lymphadenopathy obscuring the aorta and inferior vena cava. Patient was started on chemotherapy, and serial CT images documented gradual improvement. **B:** A follow-up study 2 years after **A** demonstrates persistent residual soft-tissue density partially obscuring the aorta (Ao). Surgical biopsy of this area showed only residual fibrosis.

Testicular Tumors

Testicular neoplasms are the most common solid cancers in male patients 15 to 34 years old, accounting for a significant percentage of all cancer deaths in this group. Histologically, the germ cell testicular tumors are composed of different cell types. For therapeutic purposes, they are classified into seminomatous and nonseminomatous categories. Although most seminomas are treated by radiation therapy, most nonseminomatous tumors (and some seminomatous) are treated by retroperitoneal lymphadenectomy or chemotherapy (23). Accurate preoperative determination of tumor extent helps in the design of radiation ports for seminomas and in the choice of initial mode of treatment (surgery versus chemotherapy) in the nonseminomatous group. Testicular tumors tend to metastasize via the lymphatic system. A thorough understanding of the distribution and pattern of lymphatic spread by testicular cancer will be helpful in interpretation of CT findings. In general, the testicular lymphatics, which follow the course of the testicular arteries/veins, drain directly into the lymph nodes in or near the renal hilum (Fig.

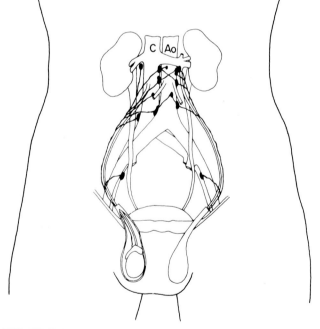

FIG. 57. Schematic diagram showing lymphatic drainage from the testis and epididymis. The testis primarily drains into lymph nodes at or below the level of the renal hilum, whereas the epididymis drains into the distal aortic or proximal iliac nodal group.

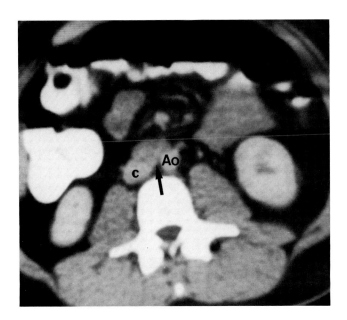

FIG. 58. Nodal metastases from right testicular seminoma. CT image through the lower poles of both kidneys shows a single 2.5-cm interaortocaval lymph node (*arrow*). Metastases from the right testis have a predilection for this nodal chain; (Ao) aorta; (c) inferior vena cava.

57). These lymph nodes (sentinel nodes) lie lateral to the lumbar nodes and usually are not opacified by bipedal lymphangiography (24). After involvement of these sentinel nodes, the lumbar paraaortic nodes will become involved (unilaterally or bilaterally), followed by spread to the mediastinal and supraclavicular nodes or hematogenous dissemination to the lungs, liver, and brain.

Data from a large surgical series showed that nodal metastases from the right testis tend to be midline, with primary zones of involvement being the interaortocaval, precaval, and preaortic lymph node groups (34) (Fig. 58). Although previous studies showed that the lymphatic drainage from the right testis not infrequently "crosses over" to the left side without involving the ipsilateral side, involvement of contralateral left paraaortic node(s) without concomitant involvement of interaortocaval nodes in patients with right-side testicular tumor was not found. If lymph nodes in the right renal hilar region are normal in size, then lymph nodes in the right suprahilar area are always uninvolved.

Nodal metastases from the left testis show a predilection for left paraaortic nodes, followed by preaortic and interaortocaval nodal groups (Fig. 59). In contradistinction to

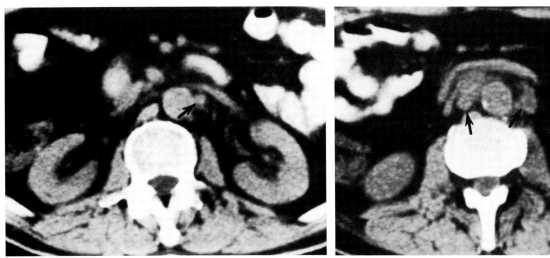
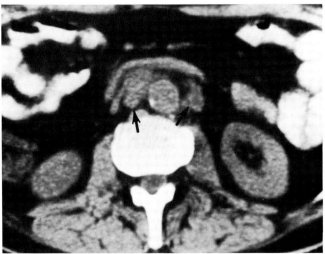

A,B

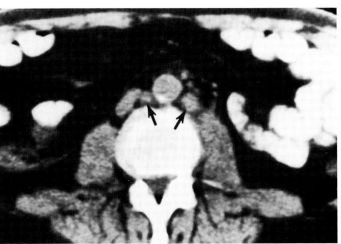

C

FIG. 59. Nodal metastases from embryonal cell carcinoma of left testis. Enlarged lymph nodes (*arrows*) are noted in the left paraaortic and interaortocaval chains at several levels. **A:** CT image through renal hilus. **B:** CT image through lower poles of both kidneys. **C:** CT image below both kidneys.

A,B

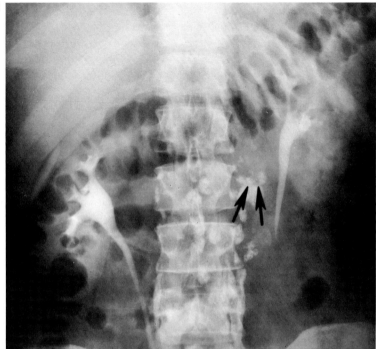

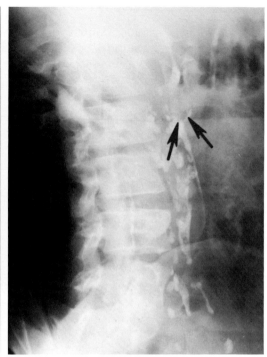

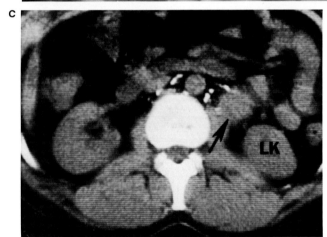

FIG. 60. Metastatic retroperitoneal lymphadenopathy in a patient with left testicular seminoma. Anteroposterior (**A**) and left posterior oblique (**B**) views of the abdomen from a bipedal lymphangiogram show a well-defined peripheral filling defect involving at least one left paraaortic lymph node (*arrows*) at the level of the second lumbar vertebra, compatible with nodal metastases. **C:** CT image demonstrates a large metastatic mass (*arrow*) not appreciated on the preceding lymphangiogram; (LK) left kidney.

right-side testicular drainage, left suprahilar nodes have been found to be involved even when renal hilar nodal groups are grossly normal. However, contralateral hilar nodes are always free of disease if the ipsilateral lymph nodes are not involved.

Although both testes have lymphatic channels to the ipsilateral external iliac nodes, isolated involvement of the external iliac, inguinal, and femoral nodes is most common when the primary drainage routes have been altered by previous inguinal surgery. Also, if the tumor locally involves the epididymis, it may spread via lymphatic routes to the distal aortic or proximal common iliac group.

The overall accuracy achieved by CT examinations performed on early model scanners (scanning times of 10–18 sec) compares very favorably with that for lymphangiography (19,39,42,92,98,125,140). The reported

accuracy of CT is in the range of 70 to 90%. With routine use of sub-5-sec scanners, which have better spatial resolution and increased contrast sensitivity, coupled with increasing experience in image interpretation, the results from CT should be even better, although no such study has yet been reported. Furthermore, because testicular tumors first metastasize to lymph nodes at the renal hilar level, a nodal group not normally opacified with bipedal lymphangiography, CT has a definite advantage in detecting early metastases to these lymph nodes. Similarly, CT is superior to lymphangiography in delineating the exact extent of the tumor mass, knowledge important in the planning of radiation therapy (Fig. 60). CT also can be used to detect metastases to extralymphatic organs such as the liver and the lung. Lymphangiography has a theoretical advantage over CT in detecting neoplastic replacement in normal-size lymph nodes.

CT is the preferred method in staging patients with known testicular neoplasms. Lymphangiography should be reserved for cases where the CT findings are equivocal or negative. Because more than 90% of nonseminomatous testicular tumors produce alpha-fetoprotein (AFP) or the beta subunit of human chorionic gonadotropin (β-HCG), serial determinations of serum levels of these tumor markers provide an extremely accurate method to follow therapeutic responses and to detect possible recurrence (78,85). CT can be used to confirm the lesion anatomically when such markers become positive. Because the great majority of pure seminomas do not produce either HCG or AFP, CT has become the procedure of choice in following responses to chemotherapy and radiation therapy in this group of patients (78,92). As described previously, with substantial lymphomatous lymph node involvement, fibrotic changes secondary to prior radiation or chemotherapy cannot be differentiated from viable residual neoplasm (133). Additional follow-up studies or biopsy often are necessary for such a differentiation.

Other Metastatic Diseases

Nodal metastases from other primary tumors likewise can be detected on CT images when the involved lymph nodes are enlarged. Because of its ability to evaluate the liver, adrenals, and abdominal lymph nodes simultaneously, CT has been used as part of an abdominal oncologic survey in patients with known malignant neoplasms with a propensity for metastases to these areas, such as melanoma and colon carcinoma. CT is also used to document suspected recurrence or to follow responses to various treatments in these patients.

In contradistinction to lymphoma, nodal metastases from primary epithelial cancer of the genitourinary tract frequently cause replacement without enlarging the lymph node, a condition not discernible on CT images (94). Furthermore, metastases to the pelvic lymph nodes usually antedate involvement of retroperitoneal lymph nodes in these cases. The role of CT in primary epithelial carcinoma of the genitourinary tract will be covered in the chapter on the pelvis.

Roles of Other Noninvasive Imaging Methods

Besides lymphangiography and CT, other noninvasive diagnostic tests (i.e., ultrasound and gallium scintigraphy) have been reported to be of some value in the detection of abdominal lymphadenopathy. Ultrasound has been quite accurate in detecting retroperitoneal adenopathy (15,19); however, it is often difficult to obtain adequate images of the lower abdomen because of bowel gas. In obese patients, examination of the retroperitoneal area by ultrasound also is difficult because of marked attenuation of the sound beam by the abundant subcutaneous and mesenteric fat. The use of gallium-67 imaging in detecting intraabdominal nodal involvement by malignant lymphoma has been generally disappointing. In a large cooperative study (80), the true-positive rate for detecting intraabdominal disease was 48%.

In recent years, MRI has been shown to be comparable to CT in the detection of retroperitoneal lymphadenopathy (35,45,89). There are several advantages of MRI with respect to CT. One advantage is its ability to distinguish vascular structures from soft-tissue structures without the use of iodinated contrast material (Fig. 61). In particular, mildly enlarged pelvic lymph nodes may be difficult to detect by CT because of the great variability in location, diameter, and orientation of the pelvic arteries and veins. Even with intravenous administration of contrast mate-

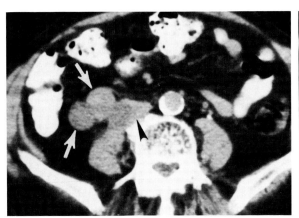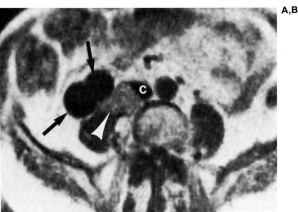

A,B

FIG. 61. Nodal metastases from primary bladder carcinoma. **A:** Postcontrast CT image at the level of the iliac crest shows dilated ureters on the right side (*arrows*) in this patient with a duplicated collecting system. Retrocaval adenopathy (*arrowhead*) was mistaken for an enlarged inferior vena cava. **B:** MR image (TR = 900 msec, TE = 30 msec) at a similar level as **A** shows a normal-size inferior vena cava (c) displaced by retrocaval adenopathy (*arrowhead*); (*arrows*) dilated ureters.

A,B

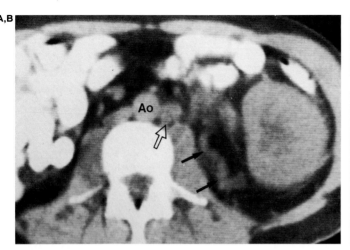

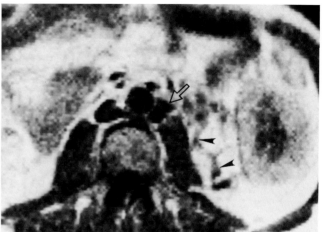

FIG. 62. Differentiation between collateral vessels and adenopathy in a 50-year-old man with left renal cell carcinoma. **A:** Postcontrast CT image at a level lower than the tumor demonstrates a tortuous collateral vessel (*arrows*). A round soft-tissue density (*open arrow*) is seen anterior to the left psoas muscle, suspicious for an enlarged lymph node. **B:** MR image (TR = 900 msec, TE = 30 msec) at the same level as **A.** The suspected lymphadenopathy (*open arrow*) appears as an area of signal void, indicating that it is a vessel rather than a lymph node. A tortuous collateral vessel (*arrowheads*) is also seen. (From ref. 89.)

rial, adequate opacification of both the arteries and veins is not always achieved. In these patients, pelvic lymphadenopathy is more easily demonstrated by MRI. Venous anomalies, prominent gonadal veins, and collateral vessels all may mimic retroperitoneal lymphadenopathy on non-contrast-enhanced CT studies, but are easily shown to be vascular structures by MRI (Fig. 62).

Another advantage of MRI is in the evaluation of some postsurgical patients. On CT images, metallic clips and prostheses produce streak artifacts that can obscure significant regions of interest. In contradistinction, the surgical clips most commonly used at our institutions for

abdominal surgical procedures are made of tantalum or other material that causes minimal artifacts and does not degrade the MR images (36,45,105). Large metallic objects, such as hip prostheses, produce a focal loss of signal, but otherwise do not interfere with MRI of the pelvis.

MRI does have several limitations as compared with CT. With optimal opacification of the bowel loops, CT can more easily detect lymphadenopathy in patients who have little retroperitoneal fat and patients in whom the retroperitoneal tissue planes have been altered by surgery. Because of the poorer spatial resolution of MRI, a cluster of normal-size lymph nodes could appear as a single en-

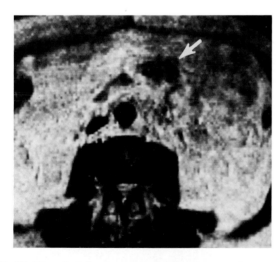

FIG. 63. Fibrosis following successful treatment of non-Hodgkin lymphoma. T2-weighted MR image (TR = 2,100 msec, TE = 90 msec) shows a low-intensity mass (*arrow*) in the mesentery, representing residual fibrosis. Lymphadenopathy would have a signal intensity similar to that of fat on this sequence.

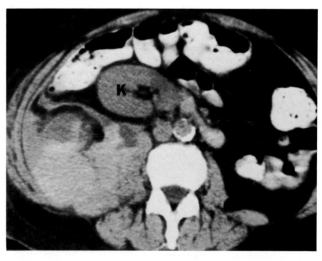

FIG. 64. Spontaneous retroperitoneal hemorrhage in a patient on anticoagulant therapy. Non-contrast-enhanced CT image shows a mixed-attenuation mass involving right perirenal and posterior pararenal spaces. Some areas of this mass have relatively high attenuation values, compatible with acute hemorrhage. Note anteromedial displacement of the right kidney (K).

larged node on an MRI study. Finally, MRI is unable to detect small calcifications in lymph nodes, a limitation that is of greater significance for evaluation of the mediastinum than for the retroperitoneum and pelvis.

At present, a thorough MRI examination of the abdomen and pelvis takes more time than a comparable CT study. Therefore, CT remains the imaging procedure of choice for screening the retroperitoneum for evidence of lymphadenopathy. If the CT findings are equivocal, an MRI study should be performed. MRI should be considered as the primary imaging technique in those patients whose exposure to ionizing radiation should be limited. This includes pediatric patients, especially if multiple follow-up examinations are anticipated, and pregnant patients in the second and third trimesters.

A potential application of MRI is in the evaluation of a patient who has undergone radiation therapy or chemotherapy and has a residual retroperitoneal mass. As mentioned previously, CT frequently is unable to distinguish residual fibrotic changes from viable neoplasm (95,97). The initial experience suggests that MRI may be able to distinguish radiation fibrosis from recurrent tumor in some patients (64). Demonstration of low signal intensity (similar to that of muscle) on T1- and T2-weighted images suggests that the soft-tissue mass represents fibrosis (Fig. 63). However, regions of intermediate to high signal intensity on T2-weighted images may represent not only viable tumor but also benign processes such as necrosis or inflammation. Determination of the clinical utility of MRI in differentiating residual tumor from fibrosis will require the evaluation of a larger population of post-therapy patients.

RETROPERITONEAL HEMORRHAGE

Retroperitoneal hemorrhage occurs most commonly in patients on anticoagulant therapy, following trauma, or as a complication of an aortic aneurysm or a retroperitoneal tumor. Bleeding into the retroperitoneal space has been reported to occur in a high percentage of patients following translumbar aortography (10,25) and percutaneous renal biopsy (121). It can also occur in patients with bleeding diatheses or vasculitis (126).

Although acute onset of abdominal pain and development of an abdominal mass in association with a decreasing hematocrit are suggestive of retroperitoneal hemorrhage, clinical signs and symptoms may be ambiguous, delayed, or misleading. The diagnosis of retroperitoneal hemorrhage by plain abdominal radiographs lacks both sensitivity and specificity.

CT

CT is an accurate noninvasive imaging method for detecting retroperitoneal hemorrhage (38,50,126). On CT images, it appears as an abnormal soft-tissue density, either well localized or diffusely enlarging the retroperitoneal space (126) (Fig. 64). Its location and attenuation characteristics depend on the source and duration of the hemorrhage.

Hemorrhage following renal biopsy is centered around the traumatized kidney, whereas that associated with a leaking abdominal aortic aneurysm (Fig. 9) or translumbar aortography will surround the aorta before extending into the surrounding retroperitoneum. An acute hematoma (+70 to +90 HU) has a higher attenuation value than circulating blood because clot formation and retraction cause greater concentration of red blood cells (139,151). A subacute hematoma often has a lucent halo and a soft-tissue-density center. A chronic hematoma appears as a low-density mass (+20 to +40 HU) with a thick, dense rim (112,139). Peripheral calcification also may be present. Although hyperdensity is quite specific for acute hematoma, the appearance of retroperitoneal hemorrhage on CT is by no means pathognomonic. A subacute hematoma can be confused with a retroperitoneal tumor; a chronic hematoma may have an appearance similar to that of an abscess, lymphocele, cyst, or urinoma. Differentiation among these entities often requires correlation with the patient's clinical history. The use of serial scanning showing decreasing attenuation values for the retroperitoneal mass provides a reassuring sign that a diagnosis of hematoma is correct in cases where the clinical features are equivocal (28).

MRI

The MRI appearance of retroperitoneal hemorrhage depends not only on the age of the hematoma but also on the magnetic-field strength. The signal intensity of an acute hematoma imaged with a low magnetic field (0.15–0.5 T) is less than that of muscle on T1-weighted images and slightly higher than that of muscle on T2-weighted images (138). This is in contradistinction to the findings of acute hematomas having a signal intensity similar to that of the muscle on T1-weighted images and marked hypointensity on T2-weighted images when examined at high magnetic field (1.5 T) (66,153). A fluid-fluid level with greater signal in the dependent layer on T1-weighted images also has been described in large, acute hematomas (70).

As the hematoma ages, it assumes a more characteristic MRI appearance. On T1-weighted images, a subacute hematoma often has three distinct layers of signal: a low-intensity rim, a high-intensity (similar to fat) peripheral zone, and a medium-intensity central core (slightly greater than muscle) (70,124,143) (Fig. 65). On T2-weighted images, the signal intensity of the central core increases relative to the peripheral zone, whereas the rim remains low in intensity. With further maturation of the hematoma, the central core, which represents the retracted clot, con-

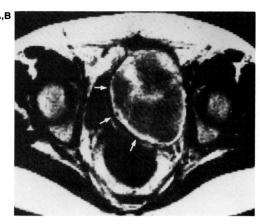 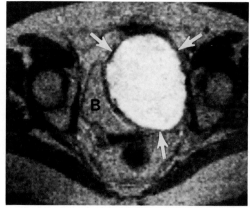

FIG. 65. Pelvic hematoma 2 weeks after hysterectomy. **A:** T1-weighted MR image (TR = 500 msec, TE = 30 msec) shows a large pelvic mass with three zones of signal intensities: a low-intensity rim (*arrows*), a peripheral zone of high signal intensity, and a central core of medium signal intensity. **B:** T2-weighted MR image (TR = 2,100 msec, TE = 90 msec) demonstrates the entire hematoma to be of homogeneously high signal intensity, surrounded by a low-intensity rim (*arrows*); (B) urinary bladder. (From ref. 143.)

tinues to diminish in size, and the entire hematoma eventually becomes a homogeneous high-intensity mass surrounded by a low-intensity rim on both T1- and T2-weighted images. Progressive increase in signal intensity of a hematoma parallels the formation of methemoglobin (13).

Although hematomas may have a characteristic MRI appearance, the specificity of this appearance is still unknown. Hemorrhage into a tumor may be indistinguishable from a bland hematoma, and fluid-fluid levels due to settling of debris within an abscess may simulate the appearance of sedimented blood. Because of the limited availability of MR imagers and because of the ease with which the diagnosis of acute hematoma can be made with CT, CT will remain the procedure of choice for imaging patients suspected of having acute retroperitoneal hemorrhage (<2 weeks duration). However, MRI may provide a more specific diagnosis than CT in less acute cases in which CT findings are nonspecific.

RETROPERITONEAL FIBROSIS

Retroperitoneal fibrosis, a disease process often insidious in its clinical presentation, is characterized pathologically by fibrous-tissue proliferation along the posterior aspect of the retroperitoneal cavity, causing encasement of blood vessels and ureters. The histologic features range from an active inflammatory process to a more acellular, hyalinized reaction (49). Although most of the reported cases have been idiopathic, certain drugs (such as methysergide), primary or metastatic tumors, aneurysms, and aneurysm surgery have all been associated with similar pathologic alterations in the retroperitoneum (1,106,145). In cases where retroperitoneal fibrosis is associated with an aortic aneurysm, a heterogeneous population of leukocytes, i.e., polymorphonuclear leukocytes, lymphocytes,

and plasma cells, can be found within the perianeurysmal tissues. Therefore, it has been suggested that perianeurysmal fibrosis may be the end result of an exaggerated inflammatory response to luminal thrombi or their breakdown products permeating the aortic wall (1). The lack of any hemosiderin-laden macrophages in the periaortic tissue negates the possibility of prior dissection or rupture (106).

The CT appearance of retroperitoneal fibrosis is quite variable. Although some have no detectable abnormality, others may present as a well-marginated sheath of soft-tissue density, with obscuration of the aorta and inferior vena cava (18,49) (Fig. 47). On rare occasion, retroperitoneal fibrosis may even present as single or multiple soft-tissue masses with irregular borders. The latter appearance is quite similar to that of primary retroperitoneal tumor or malignant lymphadenopathy, although marked anterior displacement of the great vessels is not seen in idiopathic retroperitoneal fibrosis and may serve as a useful sign in differentiating these entities (32).

On non-contrast-enhanced CT images, retroperitoneal fibrosis usually has an attenuation value similar to that of muscle, although focal or uniform hyperdensity also has been reported (123). On postcontrast images, it may exhibit exuberant enhancement (1,123,145). Whereas the precontrast hyperdensity of retroperitoneal fibrosis has been attributed to the high physical density of collagen within these tissues, contrast enhancement is said to be in part due to the abundant capillary network (123).

In view of the spectrum of histologic findings, a variable MRI appearance for retroperitoneal fibrosis would be expected. At present, there has been limited experience with the MRI appearance of retroperitoneal fibrosis. Although some have reported it to have a signal intensity intermediate between that of psoas muscle and fat (77,91) (Fig. 66), we also have seen cases in which the signal intensity was similar to that of psoas muscle on both T1- and T2-

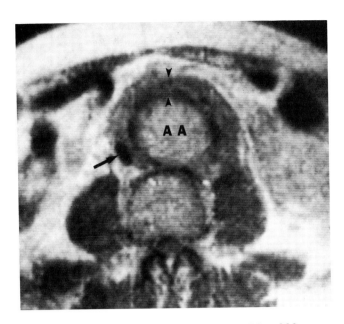

FIG. 66. Perianeurysmal fibrosis. MR image (TR = 900 msec, TE = 30 msec) shows a rind of tissue (*arrowheads*) surrounding an aortic aneurysm (AA). This tissue has a signal intensity intermediate between those of fat and muscle; (*arrow*) inferior vena cava.

weighted sequences. The latter appearance may reflect a more quiescent stage of the disease.

PRIMARY RETROPERITONEAL TUMORS

Retroperitoneal tumors tend to be quite large when first suspected clinically, because only when they reach such size are adjacent structures affected that produce symptoms (Fig. 67). Diagnosis of tumors arising from the retroperitoneal tissues is readily accomplished with CT even

when they are relatively small (135,136). Such neoplasms, usually sarcomas, appear on CT generally as soft-tissue-density masses that displace, compress, or obscure the normal retroperitoneal structures. Provided that some perivisceral fat is present, CT can accurately define the size, extent, and composition of such a tumor as well as its effects on neighboring structures. Adjacent organs may be invaded, but clear planes of separation cannot always be seen. Predictions as to definite invasion of normal structures, with implications toward surgical resectability, should be offered with caution.

Although most solid retroperitoneal tumors have attenuation values similar to that of muscle tissue, a specific histologic diagnosis occasionally can be suggested based on unique CT findings. Lipomas appear as sharply marginated, homogeneous masses with CT densities equal to that of normal fat. A lymphangioma with high lipid content can simulate a lipoma on CT images (55).

With the exception of an exceedingly rare, very well differentiated liposarcoma that is difficult to distinguish from a lipoma even at surgery and on pathologic examination, most malignant liposarcomas can be distinguished from benign lipoma by CT (55,147). Liposarcomas usually are inhomogeneous and poorly marginated or infiltrative and have CT numbers greater than that for the patient's normal fat (Fig. 68). They also may exhibit contrast enhancement. Three distinct CT patterns have been described that reflect the amount and distribution of fat within the liposarcoma (55). The solid pattern has CT numbers greater than +20 HU; the mixed pattern has discrete fatty areas less than −20 HU and other areas greater than +20 HU; a pseudocystic pattern has a homogeneous density between +20 HU and −20 HU. The well-differentiated liposarcoma with abundant mature fat generally still has a mixed pattern; poorly differentiated

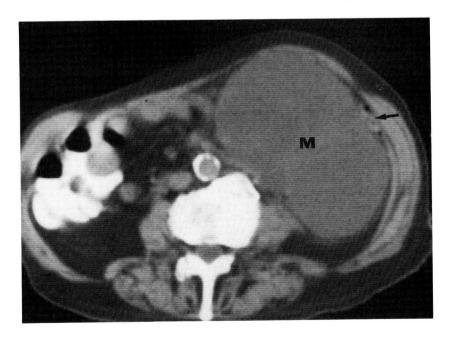

FIG. 67. Primary retroperitoneal liposarcoma. CT image shows a large mass (M) compressing the descending colon (*arrow*) and causing an anterior bulge of the abdominal wall. The mass has a near-soft-tissue density.

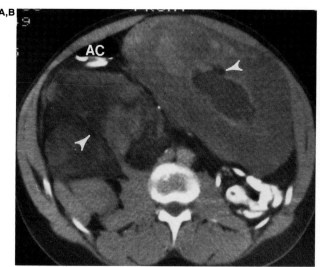 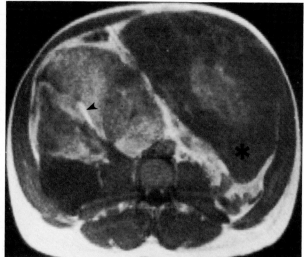

FIG. 68. Retroperitoneal liposarcoma. A: CT image demonstrates a large mixed-density mass nearly occupying the entire abdomen. The mass has only a few foci of fat density (*arrowheads*); (AC) ascending colon. B: T1-weighted MR image (TR = 500 msec, TE = 15 msec) at a similar level as A. Note that the tumor has heterogeneous signal intensities. While some areas are isointense to muscle (*), other areas are isointense to fat (*arrowhead*).

tumors with little fat are seen as solid patterns and are indistinguishable on CT images from other soft-tissue-density neoplasms. The pseudocystic pattern results from averaging of a homogeneous mixture of fat and solid connective tissue and may simulate a cystic lymphangioma (127).

Tissue necrosis and cystic degeneration with areas of tumor approaching water in attenuation value are particularly common in leiomyosarcomas (104). Although a malignant hemangiopericytoma may have a similar CT appearance, it frequently contains speckled calcifications (3).

As with CT, MRI cannot provide a specific histologic diagnosis in most cases. The only tumors that can be diagnosed on the basis of their MRI appearance are lipomas

and possibly liposarcomas (37). Unlike lipomas, which are homogeneous and have the same signal intensity as fat on all pulse sequences, liposarcomas usually are inhomogeneous and may not have any areas of fat-like signal intensity (Fig. 68B). As with CT, the MRI features of a liposarcoma depend on the relative amounts of intracellular lipid and mucin and the degree of cellularity (147).

CT should be the procedure of choice in screening patients suspected of having retroperitoneal tumors because of abnormal findings on physical examination or other radiologic studies; its accuracy is exceedingly high, quite comparable to that in patients with retroperitoneal lymphoma or metastatic testicular cancer. In patients with known primary retroperitoneal tumors, CT can be used to assess responses to treatment and to document possible recurrence.

PSOAS MUSCLE

Normal Anatomy

CT

The psoas major, psoas minor, and iliacus muscles compose a group of muscles that function as flexors of the thigh and trunk. The psoas major muscle originates from fibers arising from the transverse processes of the 12th thoracic vertebra as well as all lumbar vertebrae. The muscle fibers fuse and pass inferiorly in a paraspinal location. As it exits from the pelvis, the psoas major assumes a more anterior location, merging with the iliacus to become the iliopsoas muscle. The iliopsoas passes beneath the inguinal ligament to insert on the lesser trochanter of the femur. At its superior attachment, the psoas muscle

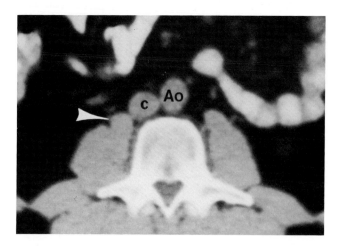

FIG. 69. The psoas minor muscle (*arrowhead*), prominent in some muscular individuals on CT, should not be confused with an enlarged lymph node; (Ao) aorta; (c) inferior vena cava.

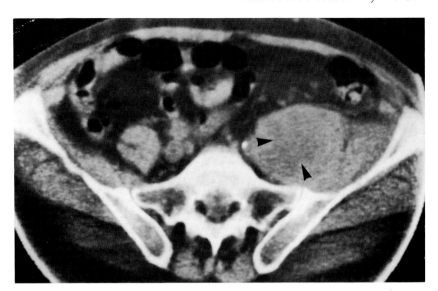

FIG. 70. Non-Hodgkin lymphoma involving the left psoas muscle. CT image from a patient with left back pain and fever demonstrates a markedly enlarged left psoas muscle, with areas of lower attenuation value (*arrowheads*). The CT findings are nonspecific and can be confused with hemorrhage or infection involving the psoas muscle. A definitive diagnosis was made by surgical biopsy.

passes beneath the arcuate ligament of the diaphragm. The psoas muscle is in a fascial plane that directly extends from the mediastinum to the thigh.

The psoas minor is a long, slender muscle, located immediately anterior to the psoas major. When present, it arises from the sides of the body of the 12th thoracic and 1st lumbar vertebrae and from the fibrocartilage between them. It ends in the long flat tendon that inserts on the iliopectineal eminence of the innominate bone.

On CT images, the normal psoas major muscles are delineated clearly in almost every patient as paired paraspinal structures. The proximal portion of the psoas muscle is triangular in shape, whereas the distal end has a more rounded appearance. The size of the psoas major muscle increases in a cephalocaudad direction. When visible, especially in young, muscular individuals, the psoas minor appears as a small, rounded, soft-tissue mass anterior to the psoas major (Fig. 69). Caution must be taken not to confuse this muscle with an enlarged lymph node. The sympathetic trunk as well as the lumbar veins and arteries are sometimes seen as small soft-tissue densities located just medial to the psoas muscles and lateral to the lumbar spine. However, differentiation between an artery, a vein, and a nerve in this location is not possible on non-contrast-enhanced images.

MRI

The psoas muscle has a low signal intensity on both T1- and T2-weighted images. A T1-weighted pulse sequence provides the best contrast between the muscle and adjacent retroperitoneal fat; a T2-weighted sequence best differentiates normal and abnormal psoas (88,149). To evaluate the psoas muscle, images in the transaxial plane should be obtained. If an abnormality is noted in the muscle, additional coronal or sagittal views may help delineate the extent of disease and determine if there is involvement of the spine (149).

Pathologic Conditions

Neoplasms

Neoplastic disease can involve the psoas muscle by one of three mechanisms: total replacement, medial displacement, or lateral displacement (88). In the case of lateral displacement, a paraspinal mass that often represents enlargement of lymph nodes is present between the spine and psoas muscle.

On CT, lymphomas and other malignant retroperitoneal neoplasms can result in enlargement or obscuration of the psoas muscle regardless of the underlying mechanism. The involved muscle most often has an attenuation value similar to that for the normal muscle, although areas of low attenuation also may be present (Fig. 70).

On MRI, the abnormal muscle has a signal intensity higher than that of normal psoas on both T1- and T2-weighted images. On T1-weighted images, the signal intensity of the diseased muscle is less than that for fat unless hemorrhage has occurred, in which case high-intensity signal may be observed in the abnormal region. Because of its superior contrast sensitivity, MRI is superior to CT in separating normal and abnormal psoas muscle. We have encountered cases in which the CT study showed apparent enlargement of the psoas muscle and subsequent MRI examination demonstrated that the psoas muscle was compressed and displaced laterally by a mass (Fig. 71). However, neither examination can reliably differentiate between mere contiguity and actual invasion.

Inflammatory Lesions

Infection within the psoas muscle is commonly due to direct extension from contiguous structures such as the spine, kidney, bowel loops, and pancreas. With the decreasing incidence in tuberculous involvement of the

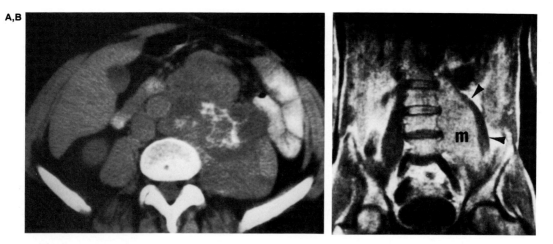

FIG. 71. Apparent psoas enlargement due to metastatic colon carcinoma. **A:** CT image demonstrates a large retroperitoneal mass, with amorphous calcifications obscuring the contour of the left psoas muscle. **B:** Coronal MR image (TR = 900 msec, TE = 30 msec) shows a large, medium-intensity paraspinal mass (m) displacing a relatively normal left psoas (*arrowheads*) laterally. The paraspinal mass most likely represents nodal metastases. Calcification is not seen on this MR image. (From ref. 88.)

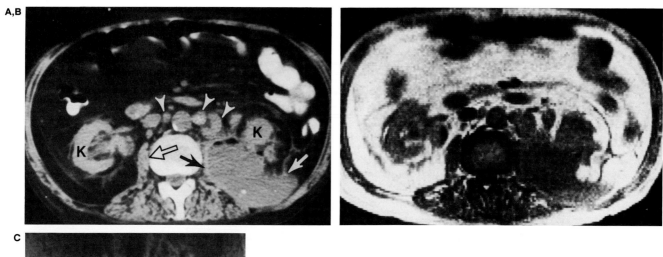

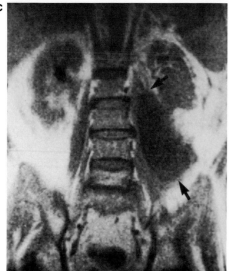

FIG. 72. Psoas abscess in a patient with transitional cell carcinoma of the left ureter. **A:** Non-contrast-enhanced CT image shows an air-containing fluid collection (*arrows*) involving the left psoas muscle and extending into left perirenal and posterior pararenal spaces; (K) kidney; (*arrowheads*) metastatic lymphadenopathy; (*open arrow*) normal right psoas. **B:** Transverse MR image (TR = 500 msec, TE = 30 msec) at the same level as **A** shows similar findings as CT. However, gas bubbles are not visible on this MR image. **C:** Coronal MR image (TR = 500 msec, TE = 30 msec) better delineates the cephalocaudal extent of this abscess (*arrows*).

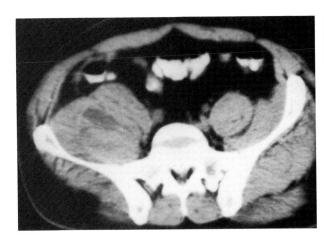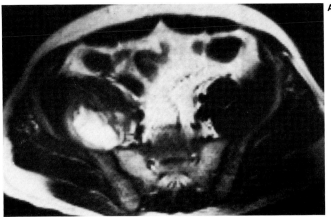

FIG. 73. Psoas hematoma in a patient on anticoagulant therapy. **A:** Non-contrast-enhanced CT image demonstrates marked enlargement of right iliopsoas muscle compared with the normal left side. An area of lower attenuation value is noted centrally. Due to lack of hyperdensity, this CT appearance is nonspecific and also can be seen with abscess or neoplasm. **B:** Transverse MR image (TR = 500 msec, TE = 30 msec) shows that a portion of the lesion has an extremely high signal intensity compatible with a subacute hematoma.

spine, the majority of psoas abscesses now encountered are of pyogenic origin. On CT images, the involved psoas muscle often is diffusely enlarged, usually with central areas of lower density (0–30 HU) (52,79,108,118). The size and extent of the abscess usually can easily be delineated; visualization of the abscess frequently can be improved on the images by intravenous administration of iodinated contrast material. Although uniform enlargement of a psoas muscle with areas of lower density is not specific for an inflammatory process, demonstration of gas bubbles within the psoas muscle is virtually pathognomonic of an abscess (Fig. 72). In cases in which the CT findings are nonspecific, CT can be used to guide percutaneous needle aspiration of the observed abnormality to obtain tissue for histologic examination and bacteriologic culture. In cases in which the diagnosis of psoas abscess is certain, CT can be used to guide percutaneous drainage (110).

Psoas abscess can likewise be detected by MRI. Abscesses have a signal intensity equal to or greater than that of normal muscle on T1-weighted images and a high signal intensity on T2-weighted images (88,149). Because of the similarity in signal characteristics, psoas inflammation or abscess cannot be differentiated by MRI from psoas involvement by neoplastic disease. A major limitation of MRI is its inability to consistently detect small collections of air that may be present within the abscess (Fig. 72B). If detected, a collection of air would appear as a focal region of signal void on both T1- and T2-weighted images. However, a focal calcification in the muscle could also have a similar appearance.

Other Conditions

Although the psoas muscle may be involved in spontaneous hemorrhage, a hematoma in this muscle also can result from a leaking aortic aneurysm. As mentioned pre-

viously, the CT attenuation value of a hematoma varies from about +20 to +90 HU, depending on its age. Hematoma, abscess, and neoplasm, with or without central necrosis, all can have identical CT appearances (Fig. 73A).

The MRI appearance of intramuscular hemorrhage also depends on the age of the hematoma (143). As stated previously, acute hematoma may have a nonspecific MRI appearance, whereas subacute and chronic hematomas often contain more characteristic features (Fig. 73B).

Atrophy of the psoas muscle secondary to neuromuscular disorders similarly can be shown. A uniform decrease in the size of the muscle bulk on the involved side is seen (Fig. 74). On occasion, it also has a low density on CT because of partial fatty replacement of the muscle.

Clinical Application

The plain radiograph is neither sensitive nor specific in assessment of disease processes involving the psoas muscle. Both psoas margins may be poorly visualized or not visualized in a substantial number of normal subjects (43). Furthermore, pathologic conditions involving the medial aspect of the psoas muscle cannot be initially identified on plain radiographs. Although ultrasound is also capable of demonstrating the normal and abnormal psoas muscle, this examination often can be difficult or impossible to complete because of overlying bowel gas. In addition, sonography may be difficult to perform successfully in obese patients.

Although MRI can clearly depict psoas disease and provide better contrast between normal and abnormal psoas than can CT, it presently does not appear to offer any advantages over CT in terms of either sensitivity or specificity. Furthermore, most patients with abnormalities of the psoas muscle may not present with specific signs and symptoms that would enable the clinician to limit diagnosis of the lesion to the psoas compartment. In most

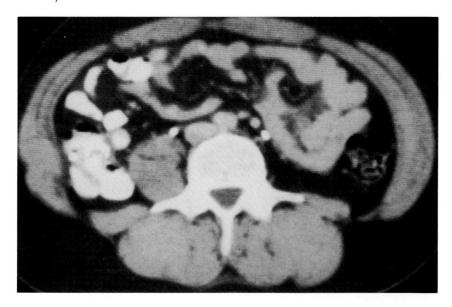

FIG. 74. Psoas atrophy. Note absence of left psoas muscle in this patient with a history of polio. The right psoas is normal.

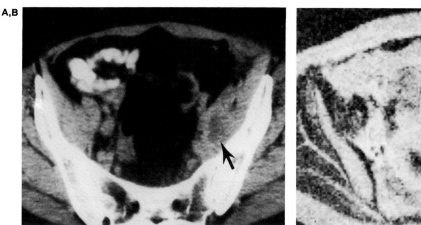

FIG. 75. Psoas metastases: value of MRI. A 60-year-old woman previously treated for cervical carcinoma presented with left-lower-extremity edema. **A:** CT image demonstrates slight enlargement of iliopsoas muscle. An ill-defined area of lower density (*arrow*) is noted posteriorly. **B:** Transverse MR image (TR = 2,100 msec, TE = 90 msec) more clearly separates the normal anterior portion (*arrowhead*) from the involved posterior portion (*arrow*) of left iliopsoas muscle. The MRI finding facilitates placement of the biopsy needle. (From ref. 88.)

instances, the psoas is mentioned only as one of many possible areas affected. At present, CT is still a better screening procedure in these situations, because it requires a shorter imaging time and is more readily available (88). An MRI study should be performed if the CT findings are equivocal. In these instances, MRI may help facilitate the planning of any additional diagnostic or therapeutic procedures (Fig. 75).

REFERENCES

1. Aiello MR, Cohen WM. Inflammatory aneurysms of the abdominal aorta. *J Comput Assist Tomogr* 1980;4:265–267.
2. Alcorn FS, Mategrano VC, Petasnick JP, Clark JW. Contributions of computed tomography in the staging and management of malignant lymphoma. *Radiology* 1977;125:717–723.
3. Alpern MB, Thorsen MK, Kellman GM, Pojunas K, Lawson TL. CT appearance of hemangiopericytoma. *J Comput Assist Tomogr* 1986;10:264–267.
4. Amparo EG, Higgins CB, Hricak H, Sollitto R. Aortic dissection: magnetic resonance imaging. *Radiology* 1985;155:399–406.
5. Amparo EG, Hoddick WK, Hricak H, et al. Comparison of magnetic resonance imaging and ultrasonography in the evaluation of abdominal aortic aneurysms. *Radiology* 1985;154:451–456.
6. Andersen PE Jr, Lorentzen JE. Comparison of computed tomography and aortography in abdominal aortic aneurysms. *J Comput Assist Tomogr* 1983;7:670–673.
7. Atlas SW, Vogelzang RL, Bressler EL, Gore RM, Bergan JJ. CT diagnosis of a mycotic aneurysm of the thoracoabdominal aorta. *J Comput Assist Tomogr* 1984;8:1211–1212.
8. Axelbaum SP, Schellinger D, Gomes NM, Ferris RA, Hakkal HG. Computed tomographic evaluation of aortic aneurysms. *AJR* 1976;125:75–78.
9. Barnes PA, Bernardino ME, Thomas JL. Flow phenomenon mimicking thrombus: a possible pitfall of the pedal infusion technique. *J Comput Assist Tomogr* 1982;6:304–306.
10. Bergman AB, Neiman HL. Computed tomography in the detection of retroperitoneal hemorrhage after translumbar aortography. *AJR* 1978;131:831–833.
11. Best JJK, Blackledge G, Forbes WSC, et al. Computed tomography of abdomen in staging and clinical management of lymphoma. *Br Med J* 1978;2:1675–1677.

12. Blackledge G, Best JJK, Crowther D, Isherwood I. Computed tomography in the staging of patients with Hodgkin's disease: a report on 136 patients. *Clin Radiol* 1980;31:143–148.

13. Bradley WG Jr, Schmidt PG. Effect of methemoglobin formation on the MR appearance of subarachnoid hemorrhage. *Radiology* 1985;156:99–103.

14. Bradley WG Jr, Waluch V. Blood flow: magnetic resonance imaging. *Radiology* 1985;154:443–450.

15. Brascho DJ, Durant JR, Green LE. The accuracy of retroperitoneal ultrasonography in Hodgkin's disease and non-Hodgkin's lymphoma. *Radiology* 1977;125:485–487.

16. Breckenridge JW, Kinlaw WB. Azygos continuation of inferior vena cava: CT appearance. *J Comput Assist Tomogr* 1980;4:392–397.

17. Breiman RS, Castellino RA, Harell GS, Marshall WH, Glatstein E, Kaplan HS. CT-pathologic correlations in Hodgkin's disease and non-Hodgkin's lymphoma. *Radiology* 1978;126:159–166.

18. Brun B, Laursen K, Sorensen IN, Lorentzen JE, Kristensen JK. CT in retroperitoneal fibrosis. *AJR* 1981;137:535–538.

19. Burney BT, Klatte EC. Ultrasound and computed tomography of the abdomen in the staging and management of testicular carcinoma. *Radiology* 1979;132:415–419.

20. Callen PW, Korobkin M, Isherwood I. Computed tomographic evaluation of the retrocrural prevertebral space. *AJR* 1977;129:907–910.

21. Castellino RA, Hoppe RT, Blank N, et al. Computed tomography, lymphography, and staging laparotomy: correlations in initial staging of Hodgkin disease. *AJR* 1984;143:37–41.

22. Castellino RA, Marglin S, Blank N. Hodgkin disease, the non-Hodgkin lymphomas, and the leukemias in the retroperitoneum. *Semin Roentgenol* 1980;15:288–301.

23. Catalona WJ. Current management of testicular tumors. *Surg Clin North Am* 1982;62:1119–1127.

24. Chiappa S, Uslenghi C, Bonadonna G, et al. Combined testicular and foot lymphangiography in testicular carcinomas. *Surg Gynecol Obstet* 1966;123:10–14.

25. Chuang VP, Fried AM, Chen CQ. Computed tomographic evaluation of para-aortic hematoma following translumbar aortography. *Radiology* 1979;130:711–712.

26. Chuang VP, Mera CE, Hoskins PA. Congenital anomalies of the inferior vena cava. Review of embryogenesis and presentation of a simplified classification. *Br J Radiol* 1974;47:206–213.

27. Churchill RJ, Wesby G III, Marsan RE, Moncada R, Reynes CJ, Love L. Computed tomographic demonstration of anomalous inferior vena cava with azygous continuation. *J Comput Assist Tomogr* 1980;4:398–402.

28. Cisternino SJ, Neiman HL, Malave SR Jr. Diagnosis of retroperitoneal hemorrhage by serial computed tomography. *J Comput Assist Tomogr* 1979;3:686–688.

29. Cory DA, Ellis JH, Bies JR, Olson EW. Retroaortic left renal vein demonstrated by nuclear magnetic resonance imaging. *J Comput Assist Tomogr* 1984;8:339–340.

30. Crowther D, Blackledge G, Best JJK. The role of computed tomography of the abdomen in the diagnosis and staging of patients with lymphoma. *Clin Hematol* 1979;83:567–591.

31. Davis JH. Complications of surgery of the abdominal aorta. *Am J Surg* 1975;130:523–527.

32. Degesys GE, Dunnick NR, Silverman PM, Cohan RH, Illescas FF, Castagno A. Retroperitoneal fibrosis: use of CT in distinguishing among possible causes. *AJR* 1986;146:57–60.

33. Dinsmore RE, Wedeen VJ, Miller SW, et al. MRI of dissection of the aorta: recognition of the intimal tear and differential flow velocities. *AJR* 1986;146:1286–1288.

34. Donohue JP, Zachary JM, Maynard B. Distribution of nodal metastases in non-seminomatous testis cancer. *J Urol* 1982;128:315–320.

35. Dooms GC, Hricak H, Crooks LE, Higgins CB. Magnetic resonance imaging of the lymph nodes: comparison with CT. *Radiology* 1984;153:719–728.

36. Dooms GC, Hricak H, Moseley ME, Bottles K, Fisher M, Higgins CB. Characterization of lymphadenopathy by magnetic resonance relaxation times: preliminary results. *Radiology* 1985;155:691–697.

37. Dooms GC, Hricak H, Sollitto RA, Higgins CB. Lipomatous tumors and tumors with fatty component: MR imaging potential and comparison of MR and CT results. *Radiology* 1985;157:479–483.

38. Druy ME, Rubin BE. Computed tomography in the evaluation of abdominal trauma. *J Comput Assist Tomogr* 1979;3:40–44.

39. Dunnick NR, Javadpour N. Value of CT and lymphography: distinguishing retroperitoneal metastases from non-seminomatous testicular tumors. *AJR* 1981;136:1093–1099.

40. Earl HM, Sutcliffe SBJ, Fry IK, et al. Computerised tomography (CT) abdominal scanning in Hodgkin's disease. *Clin Radiol* 1980;31:149–153.

41. Egan TJ, Neiman HL, Herman RJ, Malave SR, Sanders JH. Computed tomography in the diagnosis of aortic aneurysm dissection or traumatic injury. *Radiology* 1980;136:141–146.

42. Ehrlichman RJ, Kaufman SL, Siegelman SS, Trump DL, Walsh PC. Computerized tomography and lymphangiography in staging testis tumors. *J Urol* 1980;126:179–181.

43. Elkin M, Cohen G. Diagnostic value of the psoas shadow. *Clin Radiol* 1962;13:210–217.

44. Ellert J, Kreel L. The role of computed tomography in the initial staging and subsequent management of the lymphomas. *J Comput Assist Tomogr* 1980;4:368–391.

45. Ellis JH, Bies JR, Kopecky KK, Klatte EC, Rowland RG, Donohue JP. Comparison of NMR and CT imaging in the evaluation of metastatic retroperitoneal lymphadenopathy from testicular carcinoma. *J Comput Assist Tomogr* 1984;8:709–719.

46. Erdman WA, Weinreb JC, Cohen JM, Buja LM, Chaney C, Peshock RM. Venous thrombosis: clinical and experimental MR imaging. *Radiology* 1986;161:233–238.

47. Evancho AM, Osbakken M, Weidner W. Comparison of NMR imaging and aortography for preoperative evaluation of abdominal aortic aneurysm. *Mag Res Med* 1985;2:41–55.

48. Faer MJ, Lynch RD, Evans HO, Chin FK. Inferior vena cava duplication: demonstration by computed tomography. *Radiology* 1979;130:707–709.

49. Fagan CJ, Larrieu AJ, Amparo EG. Retroperitoneal fibrosis: ultrasound and CT features. *AJR* 1979;133:239–243.

50. Federle MP, Goldberg HI, Kaiser JA, Moss AA, Jeffrey RB, Mall JC. Evaluation of abdominal trauma by computed tomography. *Radiology* 1981;138:637–644.

51. Fein AB, Lee JKT, Balfe DM, et al. Diagnosis and staging of renal cell carcinoma: a comparison of MR imaging and CT. *AJR* 1987;148:749–753.

52. Feldberg MAM, Koehler PR, van Waes PFGM. Psoas compartment disease studied by computed tomography. *Radiology* 1983;148:505–512.

53. Fisher MR, Hricak H, Higgins CB. Magnetic resonance imaging of developmental venous anomalies. *AJR* 1985;145:705–709.

54. Flak B, Li DKB, Ho BYB, et al. Magnetic resonance imaging of aneurysms of the abdominal aorta. *AJR* 1985;144:991–996.

55. Friedman AC, Hartman DS, Sherman J, Lautin EM, Goldman M. Computed tomography of abdominal fatty masses. *Radiology* 1981;139:415–429.

56. Gale ME, Johnson WC, Gerzof SG, Robbins AH. Problems in CT diagnosis of ruptured abdominal aortic aneurysms. *J Comput Assist Tomogr* 1986;10:637–641.

57. Gefter WB, Arger PH, Mulhern CB, Pollack HM, Wein AJ. Computed tomography of circumcaval ureter. *AJR* 1978;131:1086–1087.

58. Geisinger MA, Risius B, O'Donnell JA, et al. Thoracic aortic dissection: magnetic resonance imaging. *Radiology* 1985;155:407–412.

59. Ginaldi S, Chuang VP, Wallace S. Absence of hepatic segment of the inferior vena cava with azygous continuation. *J Comput Assist Tomogr* 1980;4:112–114.

60. Glazer GM, Callen PW, Parker JJ. CT diagnosis of tumor thrombus in the inferior vena cava: avoiding the false-positive diagnosis. *AJR* 1981;137:1265–1267.

61. Glazer GM, Francis IR, Gross BH, Amendola MA. Computed tomography of renal vein thrombosis. *J Comput Assist Tomogr* 1984;8:288–293.

62. Glazer HS, Gutierrez F, Levitt RG, Lee JKT, Murphy WA. The thoracic aorta studied by MR imaging. *Radiology* 1985;157:149–156.

63. Glazer HS, Lee JKT, Balfe DM, Mauro M, Griffith RC, Sagel SS.

Unusual CT manifestations of non-Hodgkin's lymphoma. *Radiology* 1983;149:211–217.

64. Glazer HS, Lee JKT, Levitt RG, et al. Radiation fibrosis: differentiation from recurrent tumor by MR imaging. *Radiology* 1985;156:721–726.

65. Gomes NM, Hufnagel CA. CT scanning: a new method for the diagnosis of abdominal aortic aneurysms. *J Cardiovasc Surg* 1979;20:511–515.

66. Gomori JM, Grossman RI, Goldberg HI, Zimmerman RA, Bilaniuk LT. Intracranial hematomas: imaging by high-field MR. *Radiology* 1985;157:87–93.

67. Goodwin JD, Herfkens RL, Skioldebrand CG, Federle MP, Lipton MJ. Evaluation of dissections and aneurysms of the thoracic aorta by conventional and dynamic CT scanning. *Radiology* 1980;136:125–133.

68. Gross SC, Barr I, Eyler WR, Khaja F, Goldstein S. Computed tomography in dissection of the thoracic aorta. *Radiology* 1980;136:135–139.

69. Haaga JR, Baldwin N, Reich NE, et al. CT detection of infected synthetic grafts: preliminary report of a new sign. *AJR* 1978;131:317–320.

70. Hahn PF, Saini S, Stark DD, Papanicolaou N, Ferrucci JT Jr. Intraabdominal hematoma: the concentric-ring sign in MR imaging. *AJR* 1987;148:115–119.

71. Heiberg E, Wolverson MK, Sundaram M, Shields JB. CT characteristics of aortic atherosclerotic aneurysm versus aortic dissection. *J Comput Assist Tomogr* 1985;9:78–83.

72. Herfkens RJ, Higgins CB, Hricak H, et al. Nuclear magnetic resonance imaging of atherosclerotic disease. *Radiology* 1983;148:161–166.

73. Higgins CB, Goldberg H, Hricak H, Crooks LE, Kaufman L, Brasch R. Nuclear magnetic resonance imaging of vasculature of abdominal viscera: normal and pathologic features. *AJR* 1983;140:1217–1225.

74. Hilton S, Megibow AJ, Naidich DP, Bosniak MA. Computed tomography of the postoperative abdominal aorta. *Radiology* 1982;145:403–407.

75. Hricak H, Amparo E, Fisher MR, Crooks L, Higgins CB. Abdominal venous system: assessment using MR. *Radiology* 1985;156:415–422.

76. Hricak H, Demas BE, Williams RD, et al. Magnetic resonance imaging in the diagnosis and staging of renal and perirenal neoplasms. *Radiology* 1985;154:709–715.

77. Hricak H, Higgins CB, Williams RD. Nuclear magnetic resonance imaging in retroperitoneal fibrosis. *AJR* 1983;141:35–38.

78. Javadpour N, Doppman JL, Bergman SM, Anderson T. Correlation of computed tomography and serum tumor markers in metastatic retroperitoneal testicular tumor. *J Comput Assist Tomogr* 1978;2:176–180.

79. Jeffrey RB, Callen PW, Federle MP. Computed tomography of psoas abscesses. *J Comput Assist Tomogr* 1980;4:639–641.

80. Johnston GS, Go MF, Benna RS, Larson SM, Andrews GA, Hubner KF. Gallium-67 citrate imaging in Hodgkin's disease: final report of cooperative group. *J Nucl Med* 1977;18:692–698.

81. Justich E, Amparo EG, Hricak H, Higgins CB. Infected aortoiliofemoral grafts: magnetic resonance imaging. *Radiology* 1985;154:133–136.

82. Kam J, Patel S, Ward RE. Computed tomography of aortic and aortoiliofemoral grafts. *J Comput Assist Tomogr* 1982;6:298–303.

83. Korobkin M, Callen PW, Fisch AE. Computed tomography of the pelvis and retroperitoneum. *Radiol Clin North Am* 1979;17:301–318.

84. Kreel L. The EMI whole body scanner in the demonstration of lymph node enlargement. *Clin Radiol* 1976;27:421–429.

85. Lange PH, Fraley EE. Serum alpha-fetoprotein and human chorionic gonadotropin in the treatment of patients with testicular tumors. *Urol Clin North Am* 1977;4:383–406.

86. Larde D, Belloir C, Vasile N, Frija J, Ferrane J. Computed tomography of aortic dissection. *Radiology* 1980;136:147–151.

87. Lee JKT, Balfe DM. Computed tomographic evaluation of lymphoma patients. *CRC Crit Rev Diagn Imaging* 1981;18:1–28.

88. Lee JKT, Glazer HS. Psoas muscle disorders: MR imaging. *Radiology* 1986;160:683–687.

89. Lee JKT, Heiken JP, Ling D, et al. Magnetic resonance imaging of abdominal and pelvic lymphadenopathy. *Radiology* 1984;153:181–188.

90. Lee JKT, Levitt RG, Stanley RJ, Sagel SS. Utility of body computed tomography in the clinical follow-up of abdominal masses. *J Comput Assist Tomogr* 1978;2:607–611.

91. Lee JKT, Ling D, Heiken JP, et al. Magnetic resonance imaging of abdominal aortic aneurysms. *AJR* 1984;143:1197–1202.

92. Lee JKT, McClennan BL, Stanley RJ, Sagel SS. Computed tomography in the staging of testicular neoplasms. *Radiology* 1978;130:387–390.

93. Lee JKT, Stanley RJ, Sagel SS, Levitt RG. Accuracy of computed tomography in detecting intraabdominal and pelvic adenopathy in lymphoma. *AJR* 1978;131:311–315.

94. Lee JKT, Stanley RJ, Sagel SS, McClennan BL. Accuracy of CT in detecting intraabdominal and pelvic lymph node metastases from pelvic cancers. *AJR* 1978;131:675–679.

95. Lewis E, Bernardino ME, Salvador PG, Cabanillas FF, Barnes PA, Thomas JL. Post-therapy CT-detected mass in lymphoma patients: is it viable tissue? *J Comput Assist Tomogr* 1982;6:792–795.

96. Li DKB, Rennie CS. Abdominal computed tomography in Whipple's disease. *J Comput Assist Tomogr* 1981;5:249–252.

97. Libshitz HI, Jing BS, Wallace S, Logothetis CJ. Sterilized metastases: a diagnostic and therapeutic dilemma. *AJR* 1983;140:15–19.

98. Lien HH, Kolbenstvedt A, Talle K, Fossa SD, Klepp O, Ous S. Comparison of computed tomography, lymphography, and phlebography in 200 consecutive patients with regard to retroperitoneal metastases from testicular tumor. *Radiology* 1983;146:129–132.

99. Machida K, Tasaka A. CT patterns of mural thrombus in aortic aneurysms. *J Comput Assist Tomogr* 1980;4:840–842.

100. Mark AS, McCarthy SM, Moss AA, Price D. Detection of abdominal aortic graft infection: comparison of CT and In-labeled white blood cell scans. *AJR* 1985;144:315–318.

101. Mark AS, Moss AA, Lusby R, Kaiser JA. CT evaluation of complications of abdominal aortic surgery. *Radiology* 1982;145:409–414.

102. Marks WM, Korobkin M, Callen PW, Kaiser JA. CT diagnosis of tumor thrombosis in the renal vein and inferior vena cava. *AJR* 1978;131:843–846.

103. Marshall WH, Breiman RS, Harell GS, Glatstein E, Kaplan HS. Computed tomography of abdominal paraaortic lymph node disease: preliminary observations with a 6 second scanner. *AJR* 1977;128:759–764.

104. McLeod AJ, Zornoza J, Shirkhoda A. Leiomyosarcoma: computed tomographic findings. *Radiology* 1984;152:133–136.

105. Mechlin M, Thickman D, Kressel HY, Gefter W, Joseph P. Magnetic resonance imaging of postoperative patients with metallic implants. *AJR* 1984;143:1281–1284.

106. Megibow AJ, Ambos MA, Bosniak MA. Computed tomographic diagnosis of ureteral obstruction secondary to aneurysmal disease. *Urol Radiol* 1980;1:211–215.

107. Megibow AJ, Balthazar EJ, Nadich DP, Bosniak MA. Computed tomography of gastrointestinal lymphoma. *AJR* 1983;141:541–547.

108. Mendez G, Isikoff MB, Hill MC. Retroperitoneal processes involving the psoas demonstrated by computed tomography. *J Comput Assist Tomogr* 1980;4:78–82.

109. Moon KL, Federle MP, Abrams DI, Volberding P, Lewis BJ. Kaposi sarcoma and lymphadenopathy syndrome: limitations of abdominal CT in acquired immunodeficiency syndrome. *Radiology* 1984;150:479–483.

110. Mueller PR, Ferrucci JT Jr, Wittenberg J, Simeone JF, Butch RJ. Iliopsoas abscess: treatment by CT-guided percutaneous catheter drainage. *AJR* 1984;142:359–362.

111. Neumann CH, Robert NJ, Canellos G, Rosenthal D. Computed tomography of the abdomen and pelvis in non-Hodgkin lymphoma. *J Comput Assist Tomogr* 1983;7:846–850.

112. New PFJ, Aronow S. Attenuation measurements of whole blood and blood fractions in computed tomography. *Radiology* 1976;121:635–640.

113. Pagani JJ, Thomas JL, Bernardino ME. Computed tomographic manifestations of abdominal and pelvic venous collaterals. *Radiology* 1982;142:415–419.

114. Papanicolaou N, Wittenberg J, Ferrucci JT Jr, et al. Preoperative evaluation of abdominal aortic aneurysms by computed tomography. *AJR* 1986;146:711–715.

115. Park JH, Lee JB, Han MC, et al. Sonographic evaluation of inferior vena caval obstruction: correlative study with vena cavography. *AJR* 1985;145:757–762.

116. Perrett LV, Sage MR. Computed tomography of abdominal aortic aneurysms. *J Surg* 1978;48:275–277.

117. Pripstein S, Cavoto FV, Gerritsen RW. Spontaneous mycotic aneurysm of the abdominal aorta. *J Comput Assist Tomogr* 1979;3: 681–683.

118. Ralls PW, Boswell W, Henderson R, Rogers W, Boger D, Halls J. CT of inflammatory disease of the psoas muscle. *AJR* 1980;134: 767–770.

119. Redman HC, Glatstein E, Castellino RA, Federal WA. Computed tomography as an adjunct in the staging of Hodgkin's disease and non-Hodgkin's lymphomas. *Radiology* 1977;124:381–385.

120. Rosen A, Korobkin M, Silverman PM, Moore AV Jr, Dunnick NR. CT diagnosis of ruptured abdominal aortic aneurysm. *AJR* 1984;143:265–268.

121. Rosenbaum R, Hoffsten PE, Stanley RJ, Klahr S. Use of computerized tomography to diagnose complications of percutaneous renal biopsy. *Kidney Int* 1978;14:87–92.

122. Royal SA, Callen PW. CT evaluation of anomalies of the inferior vena cava and left renal vein. *AJR* 1979;132:759–763.

123. Rubenstein WA, Gray G, Auh YH, et al. CT of fibrous tissues and tumors with sonographic correlation. *AJR* 1986;147:1067–1074.

124. Rubin JI, Gomori JM, Grossman RI, Gefter WB, Kressel HY. High-field MR imaging of extracranial hematomas. *AJR* 1987;148: 813–817.

125. Safer ML, Green JP, Crews QE Jr, Hill DR. Lymphangiographic accuracy in the staging of testicular tumors. *Cancer* 1975;35:1603–1605.

126. Sagel SS, Siegel MJ, Stanley RJ, Jost RG. Detection of retroperitoneal hemorrhage by computed tomography. *AJR* 1977;129:403–407.

127. Sarno RC, Carter BL, Bankoff MS. Cystic lymphangiomas: CT diagnosis and thin needle aspiration. *Br J Radiol* 1984;57:424–426.

128. Schaner EG, Head GL, Doppman JL, Young RC. Computed tomography in the diagnosis, staging, and management of abdominal lymphoma. *J Comput Assist Tomogr* 1977;1:176–180.

129. Schultz CL, Morrison S, Bryan PJ. Azygous continuation of the inferior vena cava: demonstration by NMR imaging. *J Comput Assist Tomogr* 1984;8:774–776.

130. Schwerk WB, Schwerk WN, Rodeck G. Venous renal tumor extension: a prospective US evaluation. *Radiology* 1985;156:491–495.

131. Shaffer PB, Johnson JC, Bryan D, Fabri PJ. Diagnosis of ovarian vein thrombophlebitis by computed tomography. *J Comput Assist Tomogr* 1981;5:436–439.

132. Silverman PM, Kelvin FM, Korobkin M, Dunnick NR. Computed tomography of the normal mesentery. *AJR* 1984;143:953–957.

133. Soo CS, Bernardino ME, Chuang VP, Ordonez N. Pitfalls of CT findings in post-therapy testicular carcinoma. *J Comput Assist Tomogr* 1981;5:39–41.

134. Steele JR, Sones PJ, Heffner LT Jr. The detection of inferior vena cava thrombosis with computed tomography. *Radiology* 1978;128: 385–386.

135. Stephens DH, Sheedy PF, Hattery RR, Williams B. Diagnosis and evaluation of retroperitoneal tumors by computed tomography. *AJR* 1977;129:395–402.

136. Stephens DH, Williamson B Jr, Sheedy PF II, Hattery RR, Miller WE. Computed tomography of the retroperitoneal space. *Radiol Clin North Am* 1977;15:377–390.

137. Sterzer SK, Herr HW, Mintz I. Idiopathic retroperitoneal fibrosis misinterpreted as lymphoma by computed tomography. *J Urol* 1979;122:405–406.

138. Swensen SJ, Keller PL, Berquist TH, McLeod RA, Stephens DH. Magnetic resonance imaging of hemorrhage. *AJR* 1985;145:921–927.

139. Swensen SJ, McLeod RA, Stephens DH. CT of extracranial hemorrhage and hematomas. *AJR* 1984;143:907–912.

140. Thomas JL, Bernardino ME, Bracken RB. Staging of testicular carcinoma: comparison of CT and lymphangiography. *AJR* 1981;137:991–996.

141. Thorsen MK, San Dretto MA, Lawson TL, Foley WD, Smith DF, Berland LL. Dissecting aortic aneurysms: accuracy of computed tomographic diagnosis. *Radiology* 1983;148:773–777.

142. Turner RJ, Young SW, Castellino RA. Dynamic continuous computed tomography: study of retroaortic left renal vein. *J Comput Assist Tomogr* 1980;4:109–111.

143. Unger EC, Glazer HS, Lee JKT, Ling D. MRI of extracranial hematomas: preliminary observations. *AJR* 1986;146:403–407.

144. VanBreda A, Rubin BE, Druy EM. Detection of inferior vena cava abnormalities by computed tomography. *J Comput Assist Tomogr* 1979;3:164–169.

145. Vint VC, Usselman JA, Warmath MA, Dilley RB. Aortic perianeurysmal fibrosis: CT density enhancement and ureteral obstruction. *AJR* 1980;134:577–580.

146. Vogelzang RL, Gore RM, Neiman HL, Smith SJ, Deschler TW, Vrla RF. Inferior vena cava CT pseudothrombus produced by rapid arm-vein contrast infusion. *AJR* 1985;144:843–846.

147. Waligore MP, Stephens DH, Soule EH, McLeod RA. Lipomatous tumors of the abdominal cavity: CT appearance and pathologic conditions. *AJR* 1981;137:539–545.

148. Weiner JI, Chako AC, Merten CW, Gross S, Coffey EL, Stein HL. Breast and axillary tissue MR imaging: correlation of signal intensities and relaxation times with pathologic findings. *Radiology* 1986;160:299–305.

149. Weinreb JC, Cohen JM, Maravilla KR. Iliopsoas muscles: MR study of normal anatomy and disease. *Radiology* 1985;156:435–440.

150. Weyman PJ, McClennan BL, Stanley RJ, Levitt RG, Sagel SS. Comparison of computed tomography and angiography in the evaluation of renal cell carcinoma. *Radiology* 1980;137:417–424.

151. Wolverson MK, Crepps LF, Sundaram M, Heiberg E, Vas WG, Shields JB. Hyperdensity of recent hemorrhage at body computed tomography: incidence and morphologic variation. *Radiology* 1983;148:779–784.

152. Zelch MG, Haaga JR. Clinical comparison of computed tomography and lymphangiography for detection of retroperitoneal lymphadenopathy. *Radiol Clin North Am* 1979;17:157–168.

153. Zimmerman RD, Deck MDI. Intracranial hematomas: imaging by high-field MR. *Radiology* 1986;159:565–566.

154. Zirinsky K, Auh YH, Rubenstein WA, Kneeland JB, Whalen JP, Kazam E. The portacaval space: CT with MR correlation. *Radiology* 1985;156:453–460.

CHAPTER 18

Kidney

Bruce L. McClennan and David N. Rabin

Computed tomography (CT) has been used to image the complete spectrum of renal and ureteral diseases. The impact of CT on diagnostic uroradiology has been substantial, with a clear role for CT in the diagnosis, management, and follow-up of patients with urologic disease (138,139,182,184). The superb contrast sensitivity of CT is a clear advantage over conventional radiography and allows resolution of tissues with only minor differences in their attenuation values. Modern CT scanners with sub-5-sec imaging times make CT of the kidney an imaging study that is rapid and easy to perform and one that is free from operator dependence, but nevertheless requires careful attention to technique. It is a nearly noninvasive technique with little or no risk to the patient or operator, except that related to the use of intravenous radiopaque contrast material and ionizing radiation confined mainly to the slice that is imaged. The use of low osmolality ionic and nonionic contrast material may further reduce the side effects of contrast-assisted CT imaging (136).

The cross-sectional anatomic display made possible with CT has made visible areas previously considered "blind" to most imaging techniques, particularly the perirenal and pararenal fascial compartments (115,157,168). For optimal renal CT, transaxial images usually suffice, but direct coronal or sagittal imaging is possible on some systems. Reformatted or reconstructed images can occasionally be useful for evaluating the spread of renal or ureteral diseases.

The indications for CT for evaluation of patients known to have or suspected of having urinary tract disease are continuously evolving (139) (Table 1). Contrast-enhanced CT usually can permit differentiation between a benign renal cyst and a solid renal neoplasm (146). Therefore, renal CT has been accepted as the preferred method for evaluation of most renal masses (Fig. 1). The "nonvisualized" kidney at urography is no longer as enigmatic a problem, because CT is able to demonstrate the site, cause, and extent of most cases of obstructive hydrone-

phrosis. Azotemia is no longer a stumbling block to adequate uroradiologic diagnosis, because CT can be performed in lieu of a urogram or with a smaller dose of low osmolality contrast material than would be necessary for conventional urography (134).

The direct multiplanar imaging capability of magnetic resonance imaging (MRI), along with its superior contrast resolution, has made it an extremely useful method for evaluation of the kidney (76,91,92). Renal and perirenal anatomy and abnormalities can be displayed without the need for ionizing radiation or intravenous radiopaque contrast material. MRI is useful for diagnosis of renal allograft rejection, differentiation between benign fluid-filled masses (cysts) and complex or malignant cystic lesions, staging renal cell carcinoma, especially large bulky tumors with vascular involvement, and identification of hemorrhage in simple cysts or in polycystic kidney disease (12,56,77,91-4,108,131,154,167,172). The use of a variety of compounds as contrast materials, such as gadolinium-DTPA (33), nitroxide stable free radicals (NSFR) (73), or ferromagnetic complexes (180), may allow improvement

TABLE 1. *Indications for renal CT*

1. Renal masses
    Cyst, tumor, infections (e.g., abscess), hematoma, cortical nodule (pseudotumor), calcification, AVM, AV fistula.
2. Renal failure
    Hydronephrosis (degree and cause), parenchymal diseases
3. Juxtarenal processes (perirenal, pararenal)
    Blood, pus, urine, lymph, effusion, tumor, fat, air
4. Oncologic management
    Tumor detection, staging, treatment planning, and follow-up
5. Miscellaneous
    Trauma, interventional CT, contrast-material sensitivity, congenital anomalies, allografts, renal vein thrombosis, renal ischemia or infarction

755

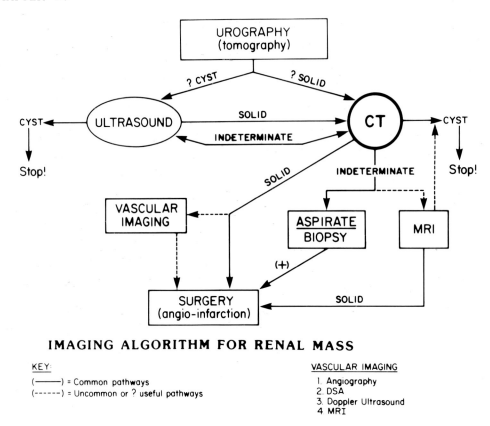

IMAGING ALGORITHM FOR RENAL MASS

KEY:
(———) = Common pathways
(------) = Uncommon or ? useful pathways

VASCULAR IMAGING
1. Angiography
2. DSA
3. Doppler Ultrasound
4. MRI

FIG. 1. Imaging algorithm for evaluation of a renal mass.

in the visualization of the urinary tract using MRI (53). However, the slower image-acquisition times, environmental restrictions, lack of optimal gastrointestinal tract contrast agents, and respiration-related artifacts in the abdomen have limited MRI as a primary renal imaging tool. Improved surface-coil technology and computer software, as well as magnetic resonance spectroscopy (MRS), may further increase the capability of MRI for evaluation of renal abnormalities, thereby expanding its role in uroradiologic diagnosis. This chapter will address the role of MRI and other imaging techniques relative to CT of the upper urinary tract.

NORMAL ANATOMY

CT

The cross-sectional anatomy of the normal kidney is clearly demonstrated using CT. The renal sinus and perinephric fat provide the tissue contrast necessary for definition of the renal contours and collecting system. Renal margins, particularly the anterior and posterior surfaces, are seen in their entirety with contiguous or overlapping transaxial slices. The renal capsule, which is tightly adherent to the parenchyma, is rarely, if ever, visualized,

but the perirenal fascia is commonly seen (Fig. 2A). The bridging reno-renal septae, which are identified as soft-tissue strands within the perirenal space, appear to provide linkage between the kidney and the anterior or posterior leaves of perirenal fascia (115). The posterior leaf of perinephric fascia (Gerota's) is not a single-layer structure but rather a laminated fascial structure that is capable of becoming thicker because of the spread of an inflammatory process between the lamina (168).

On noncontrast-enhanced CT images, the renal parenchyma appears homogeneous, with attenuation values measuring between 30 and 60 Hounsfield units (HU), depending on patient hydration and hematocrit. Segments of the urine-filled collecting system have near-water attenuation values. Occasionally, calices can be seen on noncontrast images, but they are best studied after intravenous administration of radiopaque contrast material. The renal vascular pedicle is easily imaged, with the larger renal vein lying anterior to the renal artery (Fig. 2A).

MRI

The MRI appearance of renal parenchyma varies depending on the imaging technique and pulsing parameters used. On T1-weighted images, the renal cortex has a me-

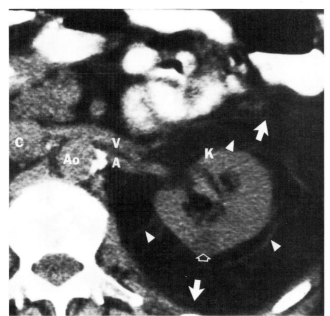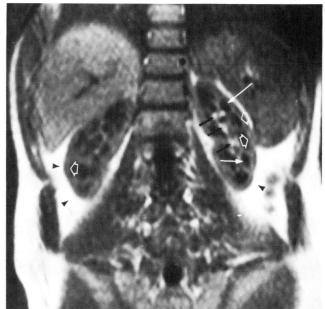

FIG. 2. Normal renal anatomy. **A:** The kidney (K) is surrounded by abundant perinephric fat. The renal hilum generally contains fat and can be differentiated from the adjacent parenchyma. The renal vein (V) lies anterior to the renal artery (A); (Ao) aorta; (C) inferior vena cava; (*arrowheads*) bridging reno-renal septae; (*arrows*) perirenal fascia; (*open arrow*) cyst with volume averaging. **B:** Coronal MRI (TR = 1,650 msec, TE = 400 msec) demonstrates normal pyramids (*white arrows*), corticomedullary junction or pyramid/cortex junction (*white open arrows*), sinus fat (*black arrows*), and perinephric fat (*black arrowheads*).

dium signal intensity, whereas the renal medulla has a low signal intensity (Fig. 2B). Renal sinus fat and perinephric fat both have a high signal intensity. The renal pelvis may occasionally be seen as a low-intensity structure, and the normal intrarenal calices are almost never seen. Both the renal artery and vein usually are seen as areas of signal void. On T2-weighted images, the signal intensity of the renal medulla increases relative to the renal cortex, making their differentiation difficult. Likewise, the renal fascia is better seen on T1-weighted than on T2-weighted images, although neither sequence is as good as high-resolution contrast-enhanced CT.

NORMAL VARIANTS AND CONGENITAL ANOMALIES

As with urography, knowledge of the myriad CT/MRI appearances of congenital renal anomalies and minor anatomic variants is essential to correct interpretation. The diagnosis of renal abnormalities depends on knowing variations of renal anatomy such as the dromedary (splenic) hump that can mimic a mass. Duplex kidneys, with hydronephrosis of either the upper- or lower-pole moieties, can be a difficult differential diagnostic problem. Large extrarenal pelves may simulate hydronephrosis when stressed by diuresis. Suspected mass lesions indicated by urography occasionally are found to be merely prom-

inent persistent fetal lobations when imaged by CT or MRI. Parenchymal (cortical) nodules will be enhanced after administration of contrast material like normal renal tissue, with clear corticomedullary distinction (Fig. 3). When centrally placed, a column of Bertin that simply represents a prominent, centrally placed cortical septation may be mistaken for a pathologic finding (Fig. 4). Compensatory hypertrophy of the kidney may be a focal process that requires dynamic contrast-enhanced CT to distinguish it from neoplastic renal enlargement.

Common congenital anomalies of the fusion variety, such as horseshoe kidney, crossed fused ectopy, and duplex kidneys, as well as ectopic, malrotated, or hypoplastic kidneys, have characteristic CT appearances (3,96) (Figs. 5–7). Small, unilaterally hypoplastic kidneys usually are caused by trauma, infection, or some ischemic or obstructive insult during the growth phase. True congenital hypoplasia is distinctly rare or very difficult to document. Renal agenesis will result in a contralateral solitary kidney that may, on rare occasion, be ectopic. Attention should be paid to the genital system in these patients because of the common coexistence of müllerian duct abnormalities. A kidney that is merely ptotic or a truly ectopic kidney may simulate an intraabdominal or pelvic neoplasm. Enlargement of the spleen and particularly the liver will displace the corresponding kidney medially or caudad, rotating it about its horizontal axis, causing a spuriously enlarged appearance (Fig. 8). When a kidney is congenitally absent or has been removed, the splenic flexure and

Text continues on page 763.

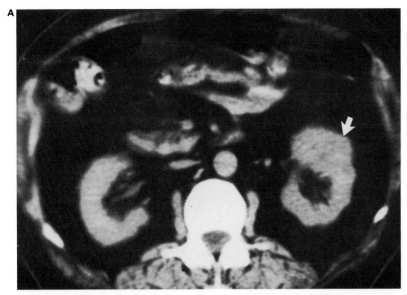

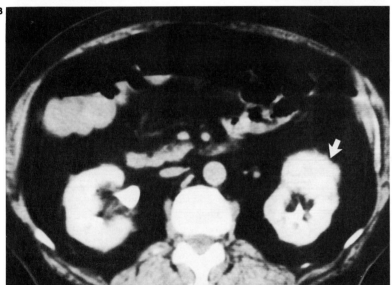

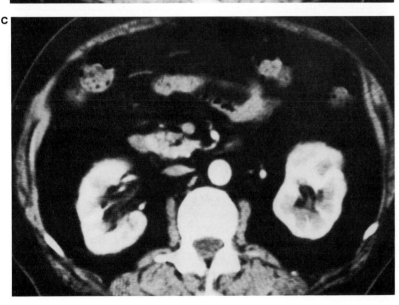

FIG. 3. Cortical nodules. A prominence (*arrow*) is seen to the contour of the anterior portion of the left kidney on noncontrast CT (**A**), and equilibrium-phase contrast-enhanced CT of the kidney (**B**) suggested an enhancing mass (*arrow*). **C:** After a repeat bolus of contrast material, the area of mass effect is seen to enhance as normal renal parenchyma. A sharp corticomedullary junction exists in the area that had previously been suspicious for a mass.

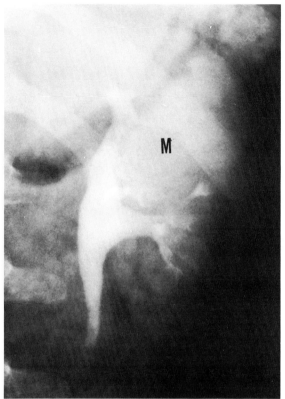

A

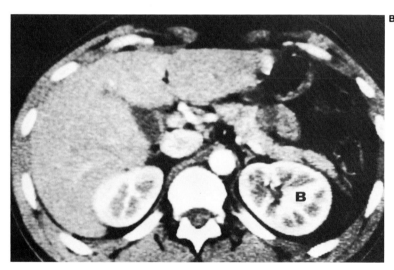

B

FIG. 4. Column of Bertin. **A:** An apparent mass (M) separates the superior and middle infundibula of the left kidney on an excretory urogram. **B:** CT following bolus injection of contrast material shows that the column of Bertin (B) (area of mass effect) enhances as normal renal parenchyma. **C:** An image obtained a few seconds later at a slightly more caudad level shows that the density difference between the column of Bertin and the medulla has decreased to the same extent as the contrast difference between the remainder of the cortex and the medulla. The ''mass'' is a column of Bertin that is normal invaginated renal cortex. (Courtesy of Dr. Gaston Morillo.)

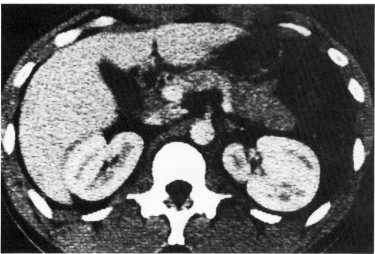

C

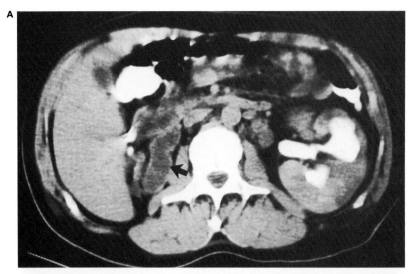

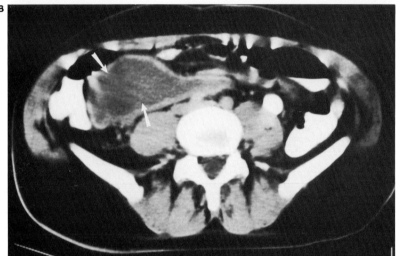

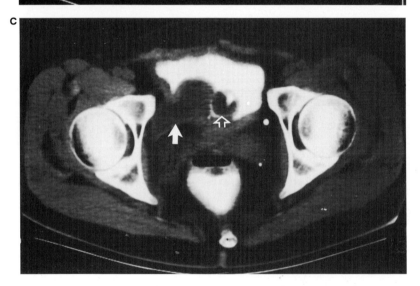

FIG. 5. End-stage duplex right kidney, with obstruction of the upper-pole moiety. **A:** A dilated obstructed right-upper-pole moiety (*arrow*) is seen after contrast enhancement. **B:** A more caudad image shows further dilatation of the upper moiety (*arrows*). **C:** An image obtained at the level of the bladder shows the presence of a (common insertion) ureterocele (*arrow*); (*open arrow*) Foley catheter. (Courtesy of Dr. Gaston Morillo.)

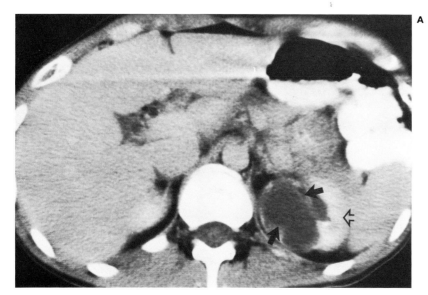

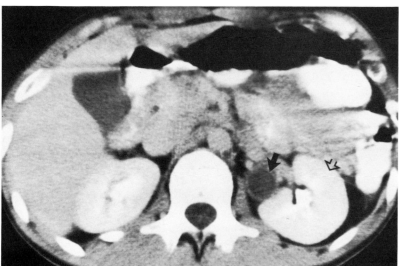

FIG. 6. Obstructed upper-pole duplication. A: A dilated obstructed upper-pole moiety (*arrows*) is seen with adjacent normal cortex (*open arrow*). B: A more caudal image shows the dilated upper-pole ureter (*arrow*) adjacent to the normal lower-pole moiety (*open arrow*). C: T1-weighted coronal MR image (TR = 300 msec, TE = 15 msec) shows the dilated upper-pole moiety (*arrow*) and ureter (*arrowhead*) and adjacent normal lower-pole moiety (*open arrow*).

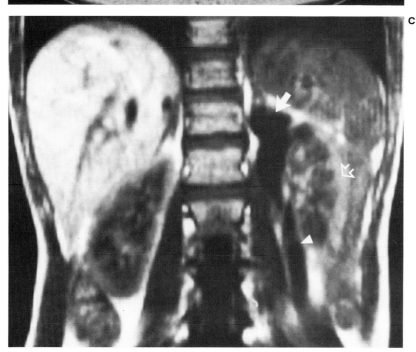

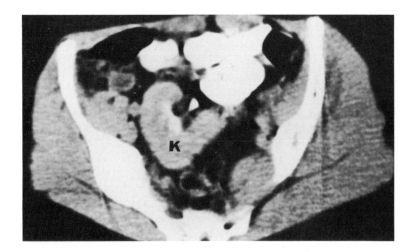

FIG. 7. Pelvic kidney. The right kidney (K) is located in the pelvis.

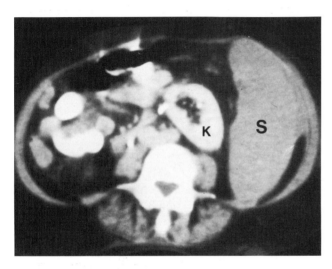

FIG. 8. Caudal displacement of the left kidney (K) by a markedly enlarged spleen (S) in a patient with non-Hodgkin lymphoma. The anteroposterior diameter of the kidney is increased because of rotation about its horizontal axis.

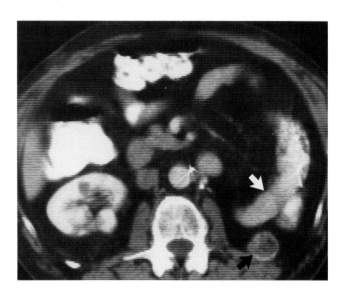

FIG. 9. Normal postnephrectomy changes. Left kidney has been removed for renal cell carcinoma. Contrast-filled loops of small bowel (*white arrow*) and colon (*black arrow*) are seen in the left renal bed.

A,B

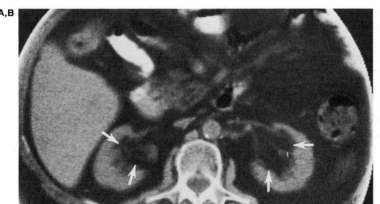

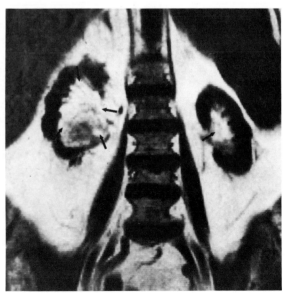

FIG. 10. Renal sinus lipomatosis. **A:** There is an increased amount of renal sinus fat (*arrows*) bilaterally, causing compression of the renal hilar vessels and pyelocaliceal system. **B:** Coronal MRI (TR = 300 msec, TE = 15 msec) shows bilateral enlargement of the high-intensity renal sinus fat (*arrows*) in a different patient.

pancreatic tail may fill the renal fossa on the left (13) (Fig. 9). On the right, the duodenum, proximal small bowel, and/or hepatic flexure may fill the corresponding space. Intravenous contrast material and oral contrast material are mandatory in these instances for proper identification of these structures.

Renal sinus lipomatosis, seen in 0.6% to 1.25% of the adult population, can cause diagnostic problems, particularly if there are coincident peripelvic cysts (75). Hydronephrosis may be mimicked by renal sinus lipomatosis on noncontrast CT images. Renal sinus lipomatosis may have a near-water density if only a small amount of fat is present because of partial-volume effects or if the fat and fibrous tissue are equally mixed (Fig. 10). This is not a problem on MRI, because fat has a high signal intensity on T1-weighted images, whereas the dilated pyelocaliceal system is of very low signal intensity. Most space-occupying processes in the renal sinus are not clinically significant, i.e., peripelvic cysts and sinus lipomatosis, but occasional infiltration of or encroachment on the renal sinus by inflammatory processes, neoplasms (lymphoma, cavernous hemangioma), hemorrhage, or urine leakage may occur. Renal sinus lipomatosis may be associated with abundant accumulation of retroperitoneal fat. Retroperitoneal fat accumulations may cause renal axis shift, especially on the right side in adult females. The rotation of the kidney usually is about its longitudinal or vertical axis, with resultant shift of the lower pole of the right kidney laterally over time.

CONTRAST MATERIAL IN CT

Intravenous radiopaque contrast material is essential for optimal CT examination of the kidneys. It improves both the detection and definition of disease. After intravascular administration of the contrast agent, there is rapid diffusion into the extracellular space and extravascular compartments. Immediately following this, plasma reentry occurs, and renal excretion ensues. Contrast-assisted renal CT involving dynamic imaging techniques uses these physiologic properties of contrast material to provide information on the enhancement characteristics of normal and pathologic tissues (31,53,98) (Fig. 11). A crude functional assessment of the kidney can be achieved relying on the phenomena of vascular opacification and contrast-material excretion. Dynamic renal CT is related to the same urographic principles that account for the appearance of the urographic nephrogram and pyelogram. Such functional and morphological information helps determine the status of the vascular supply to an ischemic or traumatized kidney, or the salvagability of an obstructed system, by revealing the amount of residual functional parenchyma (25-7,30,31,66,84,98). Precontrast renal CT images may be necessary for organ or lesion localization and for identification of hemorrhage or calcification (53).

The methods for delivery of contrast material for renal CT are typically intravenous bolus or infusion methods or some combination of both, utilizing a peripheral vein. Manual or mechanical-injector methods yield suitable opacification if a large peripheral vein is the injection site. Central venous injection, intraarterial injection, or foot vein infusions are rarely required. Rapid bolus injections (less than 30 sec) of 20 to 40 g of iodine usually suffice. High-speed injections will lead to more rapid peak plasma concentrations, and, ideally, a square-wave form to the plasma concentration curve is desirable (30). In practice, this is difficult to achieve, and on occasion additional injections may be required. Mechanical injectors can accomplish this task with programmed injection rates. Increasing the speed of injection from 4 ml to 8 ml per second will enhance opacification, but rates above this level are rarely needed (37). The time of the peak plasma level is directly proportional to the quantity of contrast material given and inversely proportional to the patient's blood volume (30). It is also dependent on cardiac output and on the type (osmolality) of contrast material used (30). Time–density curves and serial densitometric measurements can be calculated using existing software programs (228,229); however, they are rarely, if ever, used in clinical practice.

Infusion techniques usually are reserved for opacification of major vascular structures, such as the inferior vena cava, which may be opacified via a foot vein or femoral vein when staging large, bulky renal cell carcinomas, but such methods are rarely needed with sub-5-sec CT scanners. If study of a large area is desired, infusion techniques can be of value. Large doses of contrast material may be given by either bolus or infusion techniques, which, though rarely needed, may provide suitable opacification for up to an hour after delivery (83). Total doses between 20 and 40 g of iodine per patient are common for renal CT. Small intravenous bolus injections of 10 to 40 cc of a 32% to 66% solution of contrast material usually are sufficient for assessment of mass enhancement, differentiation of juxtarenal and intrarenal lesions, and assessment of renal vascular integrity. Evaluation of small transitional cell carcinomas of the kidney requires smaller doses of contrast material, because dense caliceal opacification will mask subtle tumoral invasion of renal parenchyma, calices, sinus, or hilar fat.

To date, there is no dominant influence of any of the physiochemical or molecular structural features of contrast material that significantly affects the choice of one agent over another for renal CT. Factors relating to patient tolerance, safety, and cost should dictate the choice of a contrast agent for CT (197,198).

With contrast-enhanced renal CT, there is a linear relationship between iodine concentration and CT number (HU) (25,26). Therefore, an increase in the plasma concentration of contrast material will increase the CT number of the renal parenchyma. A higher peak plasma level,

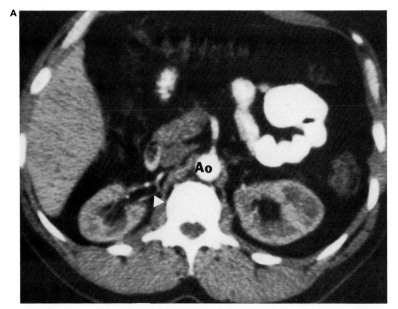

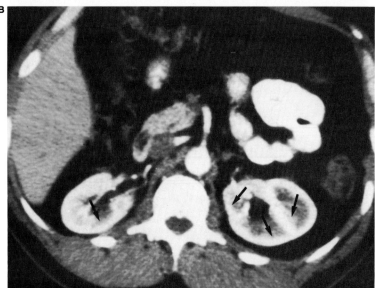

FIG. 11. Dynamic intravenous-contrast CT sequence. Normal CT nephrogram following a bolus injection. **A:** Vascular phase. Note that the aorta (Ao) and arterial branches (*arrowhead*) are opacified. **B:** Vascular nephrogram. The markedly enhanced renal cortex can be clearly differentiated from lower-density medulla on this image; (*arrows*) corticomedullary junction. **C:** Medullary phase. The corticomedullary distinction is fading as contrast material is now in both the cortex and medulla. The medulla is now more opacified than the cortex. Parts **D** and **E** on *facing page.*

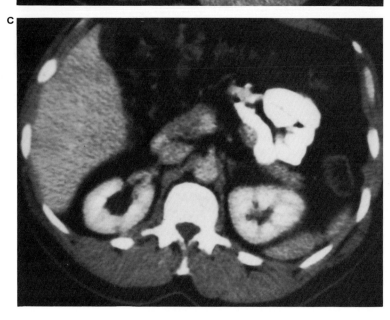

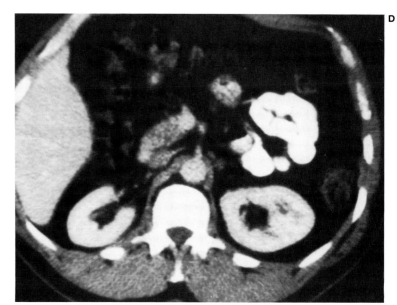

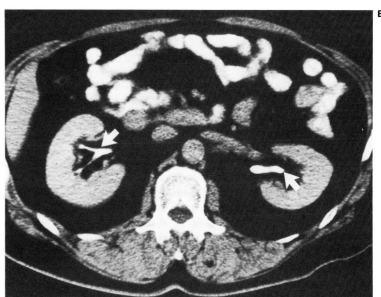

FIG. 11. (*Continued.*) Parts **A–C** on *facing* page. **D:** Nephrogram phase. The medulla and cortex now have similar degrees of opacification (tubular nephrogram). **E:** Pyelogram phase in a different patient. The pyelocaliceal system is opacified (*arrows*) by contrast material; nephrogram is less pronounced.

and therefore higher cortical CT number, is achieved after a bolus injection of contrast—on the average at least 80 HU. The peak plasma concentration and renal cortical CT number achieved after infusion techniques are lower than with bolus injections, but the peak may be maintained longer (31).

With serial dynamic CT imaging, the handling of contrast material can be observed to be triphasic: (a) major vascular opacification (arteries and veins), (b) nephrogram phase, and (c) pyelogram phase (caliceal filling). Some authors refer to these phases as the bolus effect and the nonequilibrium and equilibrium phases, respectively (30,31,47,171) (Fig. 11).

With serial dynamic imaging after an intravenous bolus of contrast material, the aorta, the main renal arteries, and the renal vein are first opacified, followed immediately

by an intense vascular nephrogram defining the corticomedullary junction. Interstitial diffusion is not as important a consideration as it may be in other organ systems because of the excretory nature of the kidney (47,113). A time–density curve (TDC) for each renal artery should parallel the aorta in the absence of significant renal artery stenosis or increased intrarenal vascular resistance (98,104,164,165,226,228,229). The attenuation value of the normal renal parenchyma will increase to 80 to 120 HU after contrast-material injection. The appearance time for the corticomedullary junction and the degree of opacity will depend on the patient's renal function, cardiac output, and the method of contrast delivery (98,113,164,165). The arteriovenous difference measured during this second (nonequilibrium) phase is less than initially observed, in the range of 10 to 30 HU. As contrast

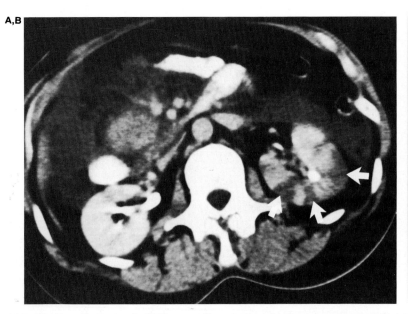 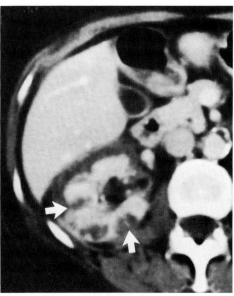

FIG. 12. Renal infarcts. A: CT image after a bolus injection of contrast material demonstrates multiple wedge-shaped peripheral-based cortical defects (*white arrows*) in the left kidney. Normal enhancement is seen in the right kidney. B: CT image on another patient after a bolus injection of contrast material shows multiple peripheral areas of nonenhancement (infarction) in the right kidney (*arrows*). The kidney is enlarged.

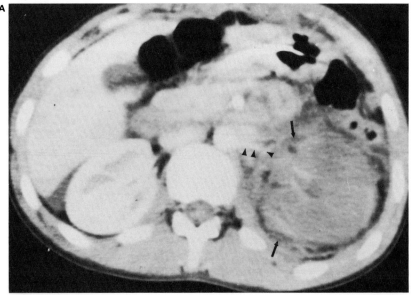

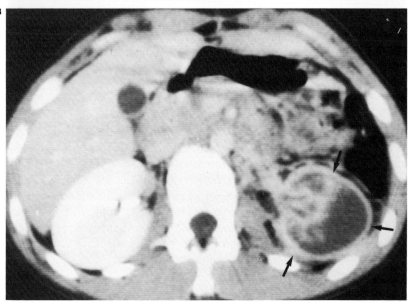

FIG. 13. Global infarction due to trauma. A: CT image obtained after a motor vehicle accident shows an enlarged left kidney, with perirenal (*arrows*) fluid (hematoma) and very minimal enhancement in the vascular phase of a dynamic CT image. Left renal artery (*arrowheads*) appears disrupted. B: CT image obtained 1 month later shows that there is only peripheral cortical (*arrows*) enhancement of the left kidney following global infarction and trauma to the left renal vascular pedicle. Note that the perirenal soft-tissue densities have decreased since the previous image.

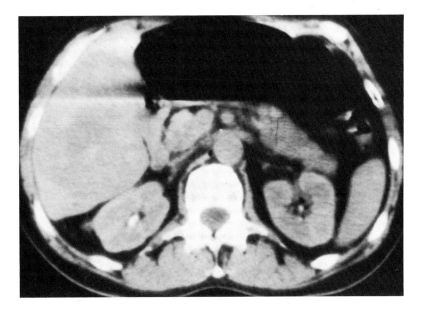

FIG. 14. Prolonged dense nephrogram. The corticomedullary junction is still seen 24 hr after intravenous injection of contrast material. This can be seen in patients with or without obstruction, or in cases of subclinical acute tubular necrosis.

material reaches the renal tubules, medullary opacification occurs, typically between 1 and 3 min. During this time, the medulla may even appear denser than cortex. The third phase (equilibrium) occurs at approximately 2 min post injection and progresses rapidly within 3 to 4 min to the pyelographic phase of observed caliceal and pelvic filling. The degree of distension is proportional to the dose and type of contrast material used.

The improved spatial resolution of CT compared with radionuclide imaging may allow assessment of renal perfusion in cases of real or suspected renal ischemia after trauma or percutaneous transluminal angioplasty (164,165,206). The attenuation value of the ischemic kidney actually increases, in the range of 10 HU, over the control value prior to administration of contrast material (158,164,165). Prolonged ischemia or frank infarction tends to lower CT numbers both before and after contrast-material administration. The segmental nature of renal infarcts makes their detection relatively straightforward in most cases (66,158,159) (Figs. 12 and 13). However, persistent wedge-shaped cortical defects (patchy nephrogram pattern) have been described in a number of conditions, including ischemia (3,24,66,69,100,101,159).

Prolonged or diffusely dense CT nephrograms may occur in patients with glomerulonephritis, acute tubular necrosis, leukemia, urate nephropathy, myoglobinuria, and obstruction (69,139,148,158,161) (Fig. 14). Delayed enhancement in the areas of initial lower attenuation, wedge-shaped defects, can be seen in patients with bacterial nephritis (7,69,100,101). The cause of these nephrographic patterns may relate to intrarenal vasoconstriction, secondary either to some degree of acute tubular necrosis or to intrarenal obstruction, with diminution in excretion (glomerular filtration) (24,69).

Renal vein thrombosis or renal artery aneurysms can be demonstrated using contrast-assisted CT, often obviating arteriographic studies (67,130) (Fig. 15).

PATHOLOGIC CONDITIONS

Renal Masses

One of the greatest impacts of CT imaging has been in the diagnosis of renal mass lesions (6,44,121,139,184). Intravenous excretory urography, with tomography, remains the major screening test for detection of renal masses. However, once detected, further definition and diagnosis can be achieved by CT imaging (Fig. 1). The diagnostic accuracy of properly performed contrast-assisted renal CT for distinguishing cyst and neoplasm is extremely high, well over 90% in our experience (146).

Ultrasound is also highly accurate in differentiating between a cystic lesion and a solid renal neoplasm. Often it is the first procedure performed to characterize a mass lesion detected on excretory urography. Likewise, ultrasound frequently is used to guide percutaneous needle aspiration. However, we prefer to use CT for staging renal neoplasms because it provides a better topographic display of perirenal spaces than does ultrasound (126). Although MRI can often distinguish a cystic lesion and a solid lesion, it is rarely used for such a purpose (108,131). At present, MRI is reserved for staging patients with proven renal neoplasms in whom the CT findings are equivocal or for evaluation of CT-indeterminate renal masses.

Cysts

The most common renal mass in the adult is a cyst. Most cysts are cortical in location and round in shape (46,146). They may be solitary or multiple, and they often occur on the anterior or posterior surface of the kidney. Masses in these locations often are very difficult to detect by excretory urography, even with linear tomography (Fig.

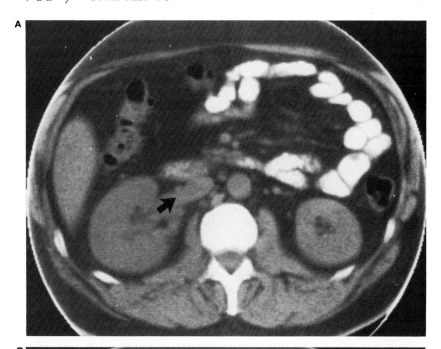

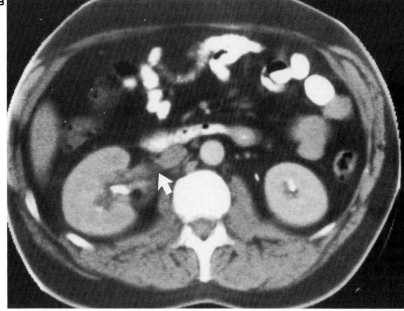

FIG. 15. Renal vein thrombosis. **A:** Noncontrast CT image shows widening of the right renal vein as it joins the inferior vena cava (*arrow*). **B:** An image obtained after intravenous administration of contrast material shows a filling defect in the right renal vein (*arrow*).

16). Cortical cysts increase in number with age, and nearly 50% of patients over the age of 50 years have one or more renal cysts at autopsy (146). Cysts tend to increase in number more frequently than they increase in size (46). The requisite CT or MRI features for a benign (simple) renal cyst are as follows: (a) homogeneous, of near-water density (0–20 HU) on CT, low signal intensity on T1-weighted images, and high signal intensity on T2-weighted images; (b) no detectable wall when cyst projects beyond the renal outline; (c) no enhancement with intravenous contrast material; (d) smooth parenchymal interface (146). When these criteria are strictly met, CT or MRI diagnosis of a renal cyst is virtually certain. It is current policy not to aspirate all renal cysts routinely, because CT reveals a large number of incidental renal cysts daily. In patients without symptoms or signs, i.e., hematuria, if the CT criteria for renal cysts are met, no further imaging studies are required. Renal angiography, ultrasound-guided mass aspiration, MRI, and surgery are reserved for those cyst-like masses that cannot be categorized confidently as simple cysts.

Renal cysts often are small, less than 1 cm, but they can be detected down to 5 mm in diameter using current-generation CT imaging (20). Masses smaller than the image slice (collimation) thickness may be volume-averaged, leading to spurious attenuation measurements both before

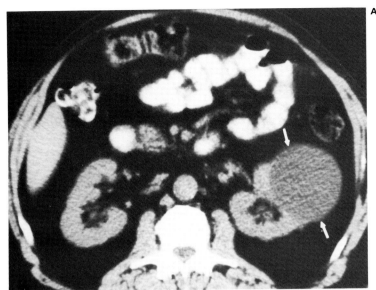

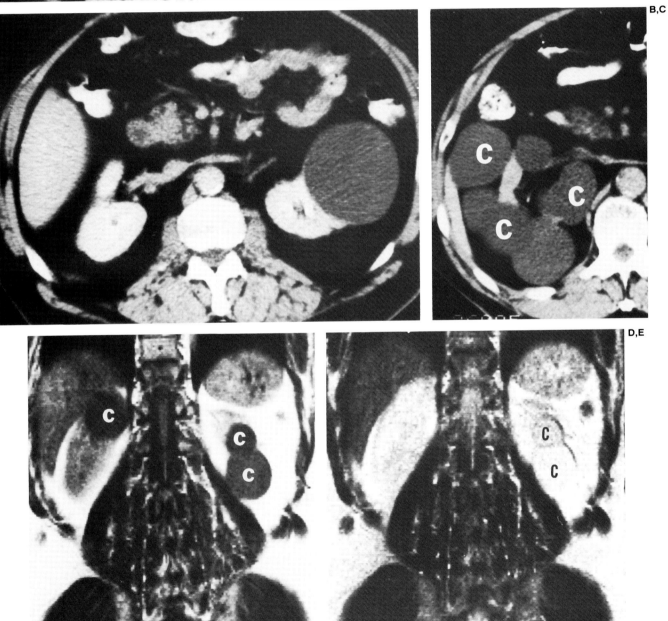

FIG. 16. Simple renal cyst. **A:** Precontrast CT image demonstrates a well-marginated mass (*arrows*) arising from the lateral aspect of the left kidney. The attenuation value of this mass was +4 HU. **B:** Postcontrast image demonstrates no enhancement within the mass. The interface between the kidney and the mass is sharp and smooth. These CT features are characteristic of a benign renal cyst. **C:** Another patient demonstrates multiple near-water-density renal cysts (C). **D:** Coronal MR image in another patient (TR = 2,100 msec, TE = 35 msec) shows low-intensity (T1 image) homogeneous round lesions with smooth surfaces in both kidneys. These are cysts (C). **E:** Coronal MR image (TR = 2,100 msec, TE = 90 msec) of the same patient shows that the cysts have increased in signal intensity (T2 image). It is now difficult to see the right-upper-pole cyst.

A

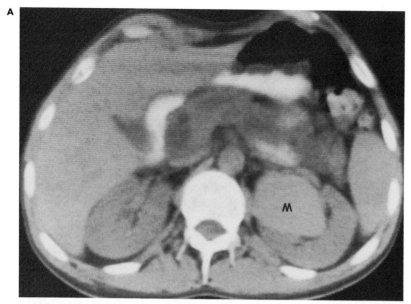

B

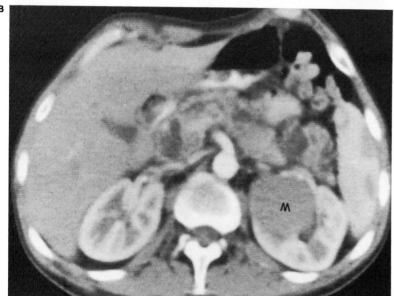

FIG. 17. Hyperdense renal cyst. **A:** Precontrast CT image shows a mass arising from the hilum of the left kidney. The mass has a higher attenuation value than adjacent renal parenchyma. **B:** Dynamic bolus CT shows no enhancement of the mass (M). **C:** Postcontrast image demonstrates a sharp interface between the nonenhanced mass and enhanced renal parenchyma. Ultrasound confirmed a cyst (see Fig. 35 for an example of a hyperdense renal cancer).

C

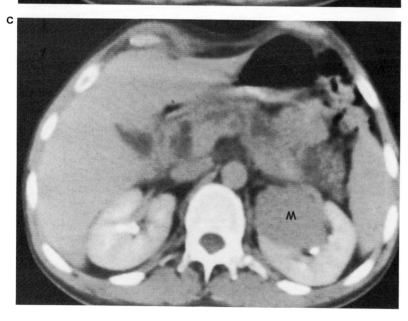

and after contrast enhancement. Accumulated experience has made it clear that CT numbers (HU) cannot be considered as absolute values. A wide range of CT numbers has been observed for a given tissue, depending on various factors such as kv or kilovoltage, location within the imaging ring, and adjacent structures, i.e., bone. Often it is valuable to compare the attenuation value of a renal mass with the density of a known standard such as paraspinal muscle, gallbladder bile, the contralateral renal pelvis, or the urinary bladder. Furthermore, the range of acceptable attenuation values for benign cyst fluid must be determined for each individual scanner and calculated to a water standard. Overreliance on precise attenuation measurements, particularly at the high end of the scale, near 20 HU, can lead to diagnostic errors. Recalibration and water-phantom measurements may be required when equivocal measurements are obtained. Simple cysts almost never measure greater than 20 HU. Similar precautions must be exercised with the degree of contrast enhancement for small lesions lest false-positive enhancement readings due to volume averaging lead to the erroneous diagnosis of neoplasm.

Uncommonly, a simple renal cyst may appear to be of higher attenuation, or "hyperdense," compared with normal renal parenchyma on non-contrast-enhanced CT sections (39,40,42,44,170,190,204,233) (Fig. 17). High-attenuation, hyperdense cysts usually are solitary, but may be multiple, and can be seen in cases of adult polycystic kidney disease (123). These masses demonstrate all the typical CT features of a benign renal cyst, except for their uniformly high attenuation values. Ultrasound confirmation is required if they are 1 cm or larger, because solid neoplasms may give an appearance similar to that for hyperdense cysts (50). Pathologically, some hyperdense cysts contain thick, dark, crankcase-oil-type contents or inspissated milky white material (e.g., milk of calcium or calcium carbonate), whereas others will have amber, clear fluid with high protein content (59,123,133,204,205). The etiology of hyperdense cysts is still uncertain.

Because renal cyst fluid is in limited equilibrium with urine, the theory that intravenous contrast material may account for some high central-attenuation measurements has been suggested (133,170,190). One study performed with early CT scanners showed that iodine did enter the renal cyst, remaining there for up to 96 hr. However, the iodine levels in the cyst fluid were insufficient to cause measurable attenuation increases and the appearance of a hyperdense cyst. In another study performed with a modern sub-5-sec scanner, in only a single case was a renal cyst found to fill with contrast material after a high-dose urogram (170). In the remaining cases, there were no increases in the attenuation values of renal cysts on delayed CT images performed 1 to 3 days after large doses of contrast material (170).

Hemorrhagic cysts can appear hyperdense. Clot retraction may increase attenuation values, causing the hyper-

dense appearance on CT because of concentration of the protein components of blood (39). Hemorrhagic cysts can be distinguished from simple cysts by MRI because the former have a higher signal intensity on T1-weighted images (90) (Fig. 18). However, hemorrhagic renal cancers may also appear hyperintense on T1-weighted images and simulate hemorrhagic cysts (167). Therefore, ultrasound evaluation is still of critical value in these cases.

If a renal cyst is cortical in location and of sufficient size to project beyond the renal margin, the wall of the cyst should be imperceptible on CT. A parenchymal spur or beak may occasionally be seen, similar to the beak of compressed renal parenchyma seen on nephrotomography in renal cysts. If the cyst is polar (upper or lower), transaxial CT images through the base may show the beak-like deformity simulating a true cyst wall (189). This appearance of an apparent thick wall in the portion of the cyst still surrounded by renal parenchyma can simulate a cystic, thick-walled neoplasm and may lead to inappropriate additional studies or unnecessary surgery. Care must be exercised so that the full complement of slices includes images of the cyst outside the confines of the normal kidney. Direct coronal or sagittal images, though rarely necessary in most cases, may be of use because reconstructed multiplanar images may not provide suitable resolution. MRI has proven useful in the coronal or sagittal plane when evaluating complex cystic lesions at either renal pole. The wall of a simple cyst should not be calcified (43) (Fig. 19). Focal or diffuse wall thickening may occur in cystic neoplasms or with tumor at the base of a renal cyst or, more rarely, in the wall of a benign cystic mass (44) (Fig. 20). Totally intrarenal cysts do occur, making evaluation of any wall impossible. In patients with hematuria, other imaging tests, such as magnification pharmacodynamic renal angiography, may be required on occasion to evaluate small cystic lesions suspected of occult renal neoplasia.

Another potential source for confusion in the evaluation of the simple renal cyst is the presence of a single, thin intracystic septation (9,20,79,81,128,177) (Fig. 21). Solitary or multiple thin septations by themselves probably are of no clinical significance if all other CT features of a renal cyst are present. The septation should not have any solid elements or calcifications, but may partially or completely traverse the cyst in question. Although a minimal amount of calcification in one or more internal septations has been encountered in benign cystic lesions, further follow-up or needle aspiration may be required for satisfactory clinical confirmation, because confusion with a multilocular cystic nephroma or adult Wilms tumor may occur (9,128) (Figs. 29 and 30).

Peripelvic or Parapelvic Cysts

Peripelvic cysts or parapelvic uriniferous pseudocysts are thought to be acquired lesions secondary to prior ob-

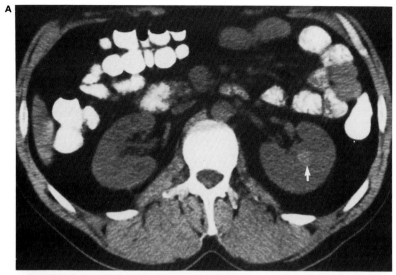

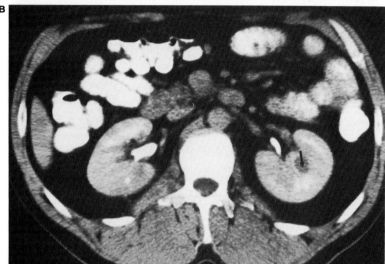

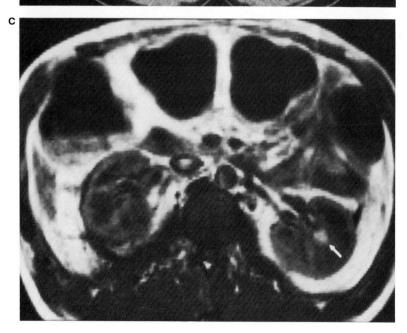

FIG. 18. Hemorrhagic cyst. **A:** Noncontrast CT image shows a high-attenuation area within the left kidney (*arrow*). **B:** Following intravenous administration of contrast material, the area of previous high attenuation (cursor in center) is now an area of relatively low attenuation due to nonenhancement (*arrow*). **C:** Axial MRI (TR = 500 msec, TE = 17 msec) shows the lesion (*arrow*) seen on CT to have a high signal intensity on this T1-weighted sequence. Part **D** continued on *facing page*.

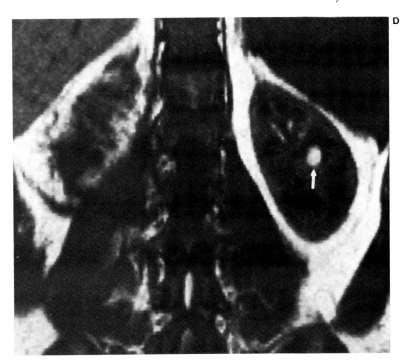

FIG. 18. *(Continued.)* Parts **A–C** on *facing page.* **D:** Coronal MRI (TR = 300 msec, TE = 15 msec) localizes the lesion *(arrow)* more precisely.

struction, with subsequent urine extravasation (85,145) (Fig. 22). Those found in the renal hilar area may be lymphatic in origin. Parapelvic cysts are distinctly rare in children, but they display the same CT features as cortical renal cysts. They have near-water attenuation values and are not enhanced after contrast-material administration. They may be single, multiple, or even multilocular. Commonly, displacement or replacement of the renal sinus or hilar fat is seen as the parapelvic cyst insinuates itself among the infundibulae and intrarenal blood vessels

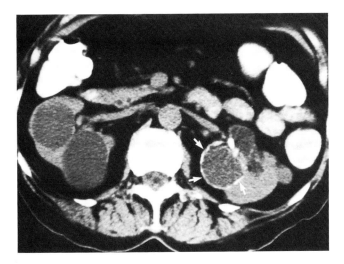

FIG. 19. Calcified cyst. There is a water-density multiloculated mass with a calcified rim involving the medial aspect of the left kidney *(arrows)*. This does not fulfill the CT criteria for a simple cyst, but proved to be a benign cyst. Additional cysts involving the left kidney are present. The right kidney also had several cysts.

within the renal sinus. Areas of compressed renal tissue, hilar vessels, or contiguous calices may simulate thick cyst walls. Parapelvic cysts may be bilateral and on occasion may communicate with the collecting system. On noncontrast CT images, parapelvic cysts may mimic hydronephrosis or a large extrarenal pelvis. After intravenous administration of contrast material, the cyst can be seen separate and distinct from the nonobstructed but frequently attenuated central portions of the collecting system. Parapelvic cysts may increase in attenuation after retrograde administration of pyelographic contrast material, which is thought to be due to extravasation and communication during the study (133).

Adult Polycystic Kidney Disease

Adult polycystic kidney disease (APCKD) usually is a bilateral process, although unilateral involvement has been described (118,119). Patients often present with hypertension or an abdominal mass, or after trauma. Frequently there is no evidence of renal failure at the time of diagnosis. The disease tends to involve other organs, namely, the liver, spleen, and pancreas (Fig. 23). When patients with the disease are examined with CT, the search often is for focal neoplastic change, abscess, or hemorrhage, particularly in the symptomatic patient. Kidneys may vary in size from normal to massively enlarged. The cysts vary in number, but usually are multiple, unequal in size, and scattered throughout the parenchyma—peripherally and

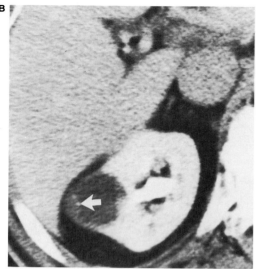 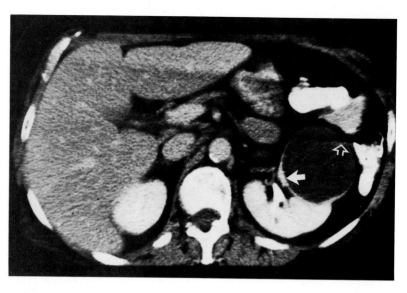

FIG. 20. Abnormal cyst walls in different patients. **A:** Renal cell carcinoma in a cyst. There is an enhancing cancer nodule (*arrow*) in the wall of this near-water-density right renal mass. **B:** This cyst has a thick wall (*arrow*) and does not fulfill the criteria for a simple cyst. Note that streak artifacts can simulate septae (*open arrow*). Cyst aspiration was performed. Diagnosis: simple cyst.

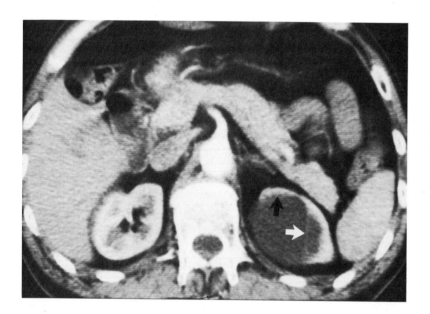

FIG. 21. Septated cyst. CT image obtained after intravenous administration of contrast material shows irregular parenchymal margin (*black arrow*) and a single septation (*white arrow*) within the water-density left renal mass. This is an indeterminate mass because it does not fulfill the CT criteria for a simple cyst.

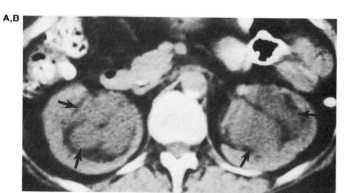 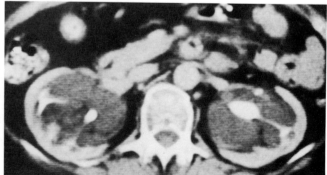

FIG. 22. Peripelvic/parapelvic cyst. **A:** Multiple near-water-density masses (*arrows*) are present in the renal sinus bilaterally. **B:** Postcontrast image accentuates the density difference between enhanced renal parenchyma and nonenhanced parapelvic cysts. Note compression of pelvocaliceal system and renal sinus fat by these cysts.

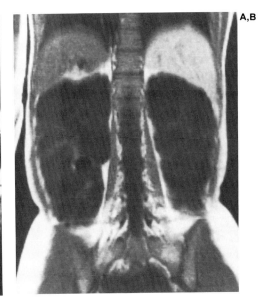

FIG. 23. Adult polycystic kidney disease, advanced stage. **A:** Both kidneys are markedly enlarged and contain numerous cysts of varying sizes. Only islands of functioning renal parenchyma (*arrowheads*) are left. Multiple cysts are also present in the liver (*arrows*). **B:** Coronal MRI (TR = 300 msec, TE = 15 msec) shows bilateral large kidneys, with almost total replacement of the parenchyma by cysts.

centrally. The cysts may calcify (Fig. 24). Asymmetrical involvement of the two kidneys may occur. Although most of the cysts are of near-water density, they may have higher attenuation values because of the presence of blood products or mucoid material (Fig. 25). The occurrence of hemorrhagic cysts demonstrated by MRI (90), or hyperdense cysts on CT (123), or, rarely, renal cell carcinoma should prompt a most careful evaluation of the symptomatic patient with APCKD. On rare occasion, simple, multiple cortical renal cysts may be confused with APCKD, as may a severe form of medullary sponge kidney. Medullary (uremic) cystic disease or juvenile nephronopthesis typically affects younger or teenage patients. CT study usually is not required, because the diagnosis in these normal-size kidneys is made by ultrasound or urography and by clinical and biochemical features.

Acquired Cystic Disease of Dialysis

Cystic replacement of kidneys in patients on chronic intermittent hemodialysis occurs in a large percentage of patients: 46% to 49% in some series (34,97,124). The incidence increases with the years on dialysis, particularly after the third year (Fig. 26). Cystic disease of dialysis may reverse or regress after renal transplantation, and, on rare occasion, patients with chronic renal failure may develop this disease without ever having received dialysis (34,97,124). The etiology is uncertain but is thought to be secondary to ischemia, fibrosis, and unknown metabolites. Men outnumber women with this process, and the cysts vary in size from a few millimeters to several centimeters. Most of the involved kidneys are reduced in size at the time of diagnosis, but the renal contour is preserved because most cysts are intrarenal. Complications include

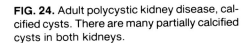

FIG. 24. Adult polycystic kidney disease, calcified cysts. There are many partially calcified cysts in both kidneys.

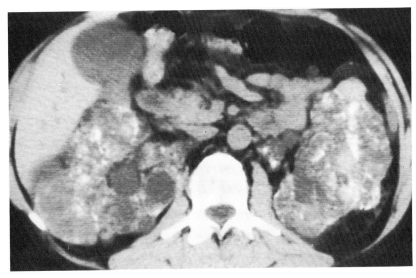

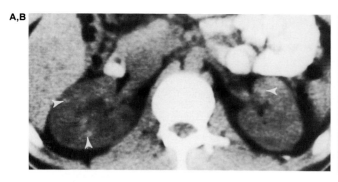
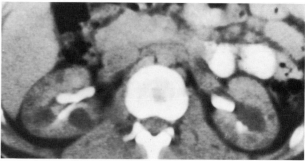

FIG. 25. Adult polycystic kidney disease, early stage. **A:** Multiple small to medium-size cysts are present bilaterally in a young man with a family history of polycystic disease. Areas of high attenuation (*arrowheads*) believed to represent inspissated mucoid material or calcified walls can be seen in several cysts. **B:** Postcontrast image shows renal cysts more clearly.

hemorrhage within the cyst and subcapsular or perinephric hematoma formation. The incidence of neoplasms, both adenomas and carcinomas, is definitely increased, up to seven times over the normal population (34,97,124). Renal cell carcinomas with metastases have been found in patients with acquired cystic disease of dialysis, particularly in patients on dialysis for 3 years or more. Bleeding into existing cysts may cause increased attenuation measurements, irregular cyst walls, calibration, and other CT features of malignancy. Aspiration

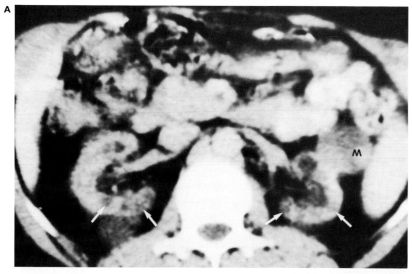

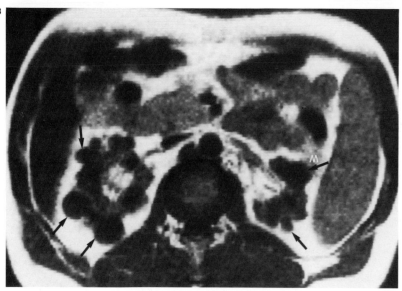

FIG. 26. Acquired cystic disease of dialysis. **A:** CT image shows numerous low-attenuation cystic masses (*arrows*). A renal cell carcinoma (M) is noted on left. **B:** MRI (TR = 500 msec, TE = 30 msec). Note that both kidneys have decreased in overall mass and volume. There are many small cortical cysts (*arrows*). MR image is slightly more caudad. Renal cell carcinoma (M) is only partially in the image plane.

and angiography are rarely useful, and nephrectomy should be considered in these cases. Careful follow-up of these patients with ultrasound and/or CT is required. Most of the time, CT without contrast-material administration is more useful than ultrasound, because the smaller, diffusely involved kidneys are difficult to image adequately, even with state-of-the-art ultrasound equipment.

Tuberous Sclerosis

Involvement of the kidneys in patients with tuberous sclerosis usually takes the form of multiple hamartomas (angiomyolipomas) (22,74,179) (Fig. 27). Cystic renal involvement is a part of the spectrum of this disease, but the cysts typically are small (143,208). Hemorrhage within

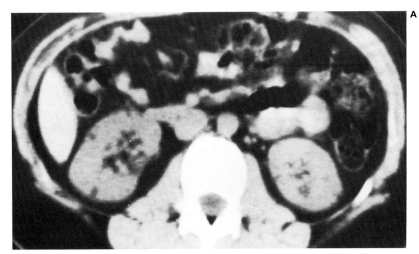

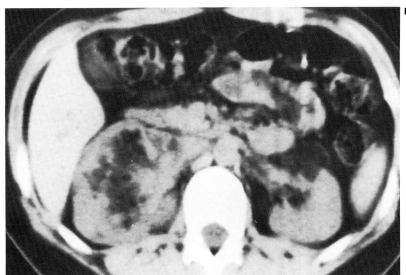

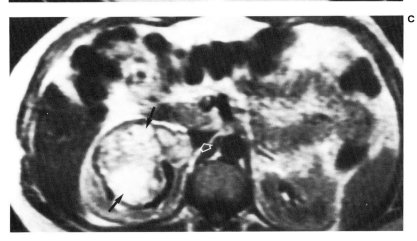

FIG. 27. Tuberous sclerosis. **A:** There are numerous small fat-density masses within the kidneys. **B:** There is a larger angiomyolipoma in the right kidney. **C:** Transaxial T1-weighted MR image demonstrates a large mixed-intensity mass (*arrows*) representing the larger angiomyolipoma seen in (**B**). The IVC (*open white arrow*) is compressed but patent. (Courtesy of Dr. John Fries.)

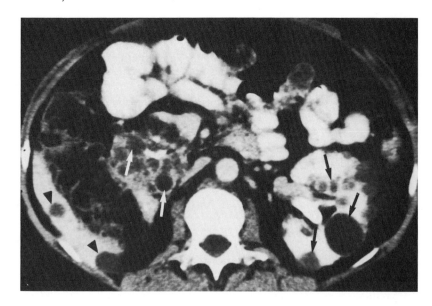

FIG. 28. Von Hippel-Lindau disease. Post-contrast CT image shows that the left kidney is enlarged, with numerous cystic masses (*black arrows*). Cystic masses are also present within the head of the pancreas (*white arrows*) and the liver (*arrowheads*).

the larger angiomyolipomatous masses can create confusing CT images (65). Differentiation between the cysts and small fatty tumors by CT may require thin collimation for accurate measurement of attenuation values. However, the distinction between small cysts and small angiomyolipomas is in essence an academic endeavor when renal involvement is diffuse. The renal failure associated with this syndrome may be severe and is thought to be due to cystic involvement, with compression of normal renal parenchyma. Confusion with APCKD or lymphangiomatosis may sometimes occur, but the cysts in tuberous sclerosis rarely exceed 3 cm in size even when the kidneys are markedly enlarged (179).

von Hipple-Lindau Disease

In patients with von Hipple-Lindau disease (VHL), cystic renal involvement, renal carcinoma, and renal adenoma often are seen (122,125) (Fig. 28). Involvement may be unilateral or bilateral and often is multicentric. Compression of normal renal parenchyma causes a confusing CT appearance when cystic involvement is extensive. Cysts may occur in the pancreas, and a picture mimicking that of APCKD may be seen. Periodic screening of patients and their relatives is best performed with CT, although ultrasound and MRI may provide similar information (122,125). The renal carcinomas can be small, less than 2 cm in size, and can occur within the cysts themselves; therefore, early detection is difficult. Magnification renal angiography may be required, because renal-sparing surgery is the current preferred management option for these patients (209).

Other Cystic Diseases

Considerable semantic confusion exists concerning the nomenclature of multilocular cysts in adults (132). Most

cases are reported in children, but adults also develop the condition (155,156). The etiology remains uncertain. Pathologically, multilocular cystic nephroma (MLCN) is a localized cystic disease of the kidney, with a female predilection in adults (132). The cyst-like mass has thick walls or septations that may be enhanced after contrast-material administration. Calcifications may be seen in the septations or may appear as a stellate conglomerate. These le-

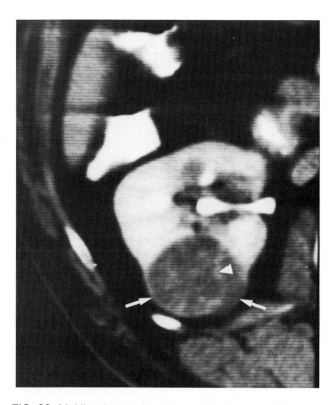

FIG. 29. Multilocular cystic nephroma in a man. A CT image obtained after a bolus injection of contrast material shows a low-density mass (*arrows*) arising from the posterior aspect of the right kidney. Linear internal septations are visible (*arrowhead*).

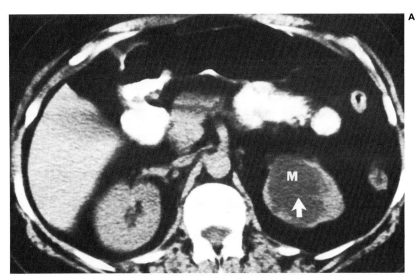

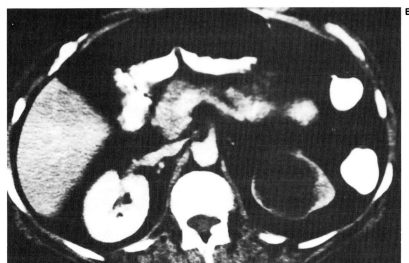

FIG. 30. Multilocular cystic nephroma in a woman. **A:** Noncontrast CT shows a low-density mass (M) with a single septum (*arrow*). **B:** Contrast-material administration shows rim enhancement without central enhancement. **C:** A more caudal image shows an enhancing wall (*arrow*) and a slightly irregular parenchymal interface (*arrowhead*), as well as an incidental right renal cyst (*open arrow*).

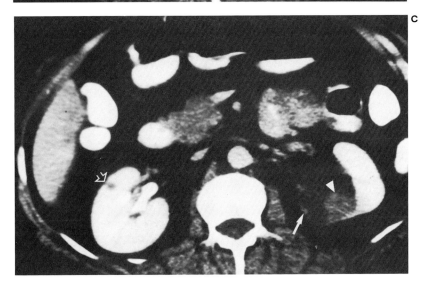

sions range in size from a few centimeters to over 10 cm, but the patients often are asymptomatic, with the mass being discovered incidentally (Figs. 29 and 30). Blastomatous elements in the lining of MLCN have led most observers to consider them premalignant. Therefore, the treatment usually is renal-sparing surgery. However, cystic renal cell carcinomas can closely mimic MLCN (57,79–81,155,156,223). Cyst or mass aspiration usually is not useful, because the walls frequently are irregular or calcified, and aspirated fluid turbid or hemorrhagic.

Multicystic dysplastic kidney usually is encountered as an abdominal mass in a child. The CT appearance is fairly characteristic, with peripheral or central calcification within a small or large single-chamber or multiloculated cystic mass replacing most recognizable parenchyma (Fig. 31). The contralateral kidney usually is enlarged, often with an element of ureteropelvic junction obstruction, suggesting that this is a congenital anomaly. Usually, no functional renal parenchyma is seen, but there may be vascular enhancement on early CT images because of the total body effect of contrast material (36,207).

Other processes, either extrinsic, like pancreatic pseudocysts, or intrinsic, such as hydatid disease, may simulate renal cysts on CT (89,107). Pancreatic pseudocysts frequently insinuate themselves within the anterior pararenal fascia or enter the perinephric space (see Fig. 81). When present, they may be bound by the bridging reno-renal septae and appear subcapsular in location (168).

Echinococcal (hydatid) cysts of the kidney may be solitary or multiple (89,102,107). They typically have en-hancing thick walls with numerous central septations, some having calcifications. They may communicate with the collecting system when they rupture. The presence of daughter cysts (scolices) within the dominant cystic mass is pathognomonic. Cyst aspiration is discouraged because of the risk of seeding and anaphylaxis.

RENAL NEOPLASMS

Renal Cell Carcinoma

Malignant tumors of the kidney account for 2% to 3% of all neoplasms, with renal cell carcinoma accounting for over 85% of all renal neoplasms (135,137). One-third of patients have metastases at the time of initial diagnosis, and these metastatic deposits often involve a single organ site (135,137). CT imaging is the preferred imaging method for patients known to have or suspected of having renal neoplasia (232). For detection and delineation of

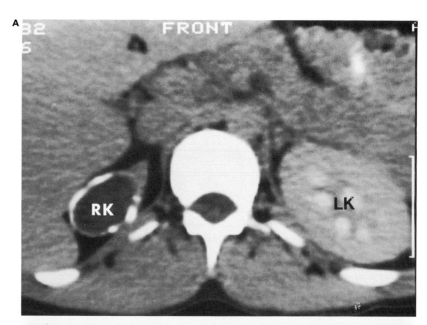

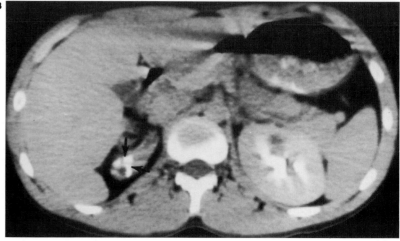

FIG. 31. Adult multicystic dysplastic kidney. **A:** Postcontrast CT image shows enlarged left kidney (LK) and the calcified cystic remnant of the right kidney (RK). **B:** One centimeter cephalad, clumps of calcification (*arrows*) are noted within the posterior aspect of the dysplastic right kidney.

TABLE 2. *Indications for CT for renal neoplasms*

1. Urograms suspicious for renal neoplasms
2. Normal findings on urograms but suspicious signs/ symptoms, e.g., hematuria
3. Paraneoplastic syndromes
4. Unknown primary tumors
5. Syndromes associated with renal neoplasia, e.g., von Hippel-Lindau disease, acquired renal cystic disease of dialysis
6. Previous therapy for renal cancer
7. Renal scarring, focal hypertrophy, xanthogranulomatous pyelonephritis, ectopia and fusion anomalies

the renal and extrarenal extent (TNM stage) of neoplasms, CT is the most reliable cross-sectional imaging study. As a complementary imaging test, MRI can give similar information about the local stage (T stage), as well as involvement of major vessels and lymph nodes (N stage), when the lymph nodes are enlarged (105,135,137). The indications for CT in patients with real or suspected renal neoplasms are listed in Table 2.

The diagnosis of a renal cell carcinoma by CT or MRI depends on distortions of the renal parenchyma and contour, the collecting system, or the sinus fat. Diagnostic criteria include the following: (a) a mass with heterogeneous or homogeneous appearance and attenuation normally less than that of normal renal parenchyma; less commonly, tumors appear isodense or hyperdense to renal parenchyma on precontrast CT images; (b) variable signal intensities on MRI, with the majority having a lower signal intensity than normal renal cortex on T1-weighted images, but an equal or higher signal intensity than normal renal cortex on T2-weighted images; (c) contrast enhancement, but usually less than that of surrounding parenchyma, although transient increased enhancement (tumor staining) may be seen during the early arterial phase of dynamic CT imaging when rapid bolus techniques are used; (d) unsharp parenchymal interface, but encapsulation (pseudocapsule) may exist; (e) when present, the wall or rim of the neoplasm is perceptibly thick and usually irregular; (f) secondary characteristics, such as renal vein or inferior vena cava (IVC) enlargement or invasion, renal artery enlargement, collateral circulation, nodular areas of soft-tissue attenuation in the perinephric space, enlarged lymph nodes, tumor calcification, and metastases (Fig. 32). On the basis of these criteria, CT is extremely accurate in the diagnosis of renal cell carcinoma, with CT being correct in 59 of 62 cases in one study (220). The positive predictive value of contrast-assisted CT for renal neoplasms reaches over 96% (43). MRI is less accurate than CT in diagnosing small renal cell carcinomas. A CT diagnosis of papillary-type renal cell carcinoma can be suggested if the neoplasm displays calcification, diminished

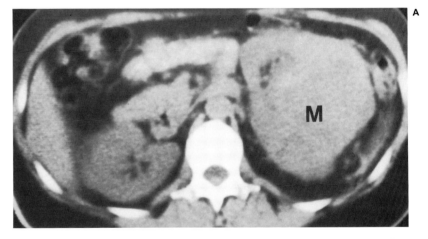

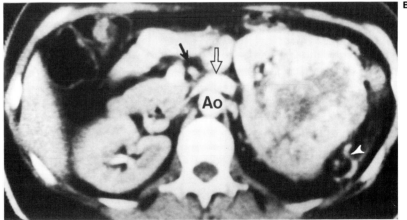

FIG. 32. Renal cell carcinoma. **A:** Precontrast CT image shows a large mass (M) arising from the posterior lateral surface of the left kidney. The kidney is displaced anteromedially. The mass is essentially isodense with normal renal parenchyma and effaces the renal collecting system. **B:** Postcontrast image following a bolus injection demonstrates nonuniform enhancement of the tumor. The central low-density area consists of necrotic, avascular tissue. In spite of its large size, the tumor remains confined within Gerota's fascia. The *open arrow* points to a normal-appearing main left renal vein. Note the compression ("nutcracker effect") of the left renal vein between the aorta (Ao) and superior mesenteric artery (*black arrow*); (*arrowhead*) large capsular vessel supplying the tumor.

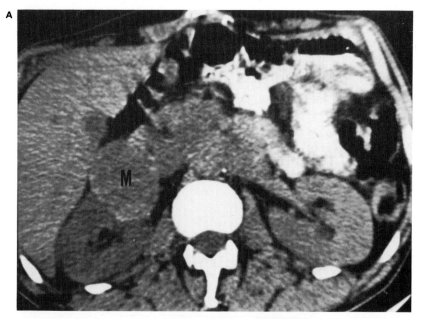

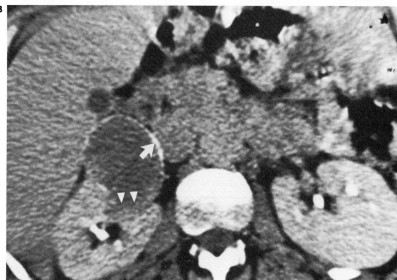

FIG. 33. Papillary renal cell cancer. **A:** There is a mass (M) arising from the anterior aspect of the right kidney, with higher attenuation than the normal renal parenchyma. The periphery of the mass appears to be calcified. Attenuation measurements indicated a solid process. **B:** Following contrast-material administration, the mass is enhanced to a lesser degree than the normal renal parenchyma. The calcified rim (*arrow*) is better shown on this image. Note that the border with the normal parenchyma is not sharply defined (*arrowheads*). (From ref. 219.)

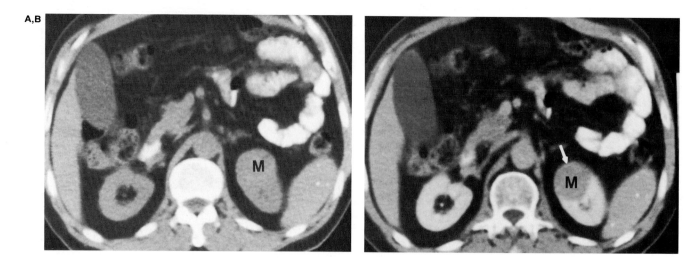

FIG. 34. Stage I renal cell carcinoma. **A:** Focal mass (M) in left upper pole has attenuation similar to that for renal parenchyma. **B:** After dynamic CT with contrast material, central enhancement and a perceptible rim (*white arrow*) were noted.

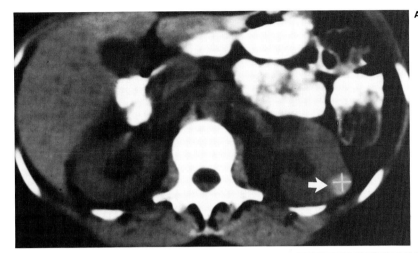

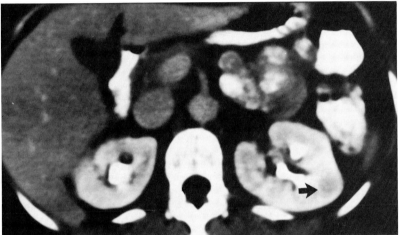

FIG. 35. Hyperdense renal cell carcinoma. **A:** A round mass (*arrow*) with higher density than normal renal parenchyma is seen involving the lateral aspect of the left kidney. **B:** After bolus intravenous injection of contrast material, the lesion is lower in attenuation than the renal cortex and similar in attenuation to the renal medulla. This proved to be a renal cell carcinoma. (From ref. 50.)

enhancement (vascularity), and low stage (I or II) on initial evaluation (163) (Fig. 33). Low-stage disease often connotes small size, but renal cell carcinoma, papillary or nonpapillary varieties, may present with concurrent metastases even when masses are less than 3 cm in size (44,227) (Figs. 34 and 35). Cyst and carcinoma may coexist along with synchronous adenomas or even, rarely, other neoplasms such as hamartoma (angiomyolipoma) or transitional cell carcinoma (68,74,208). Extensive retroperitoneal, adrenal, or renal capsular tumors involving the kidney may cause confusing CT appearances. Angiography or MRI may be useful for determining organ of origin and tumor type and extent (87). Diffuse involvement by a rare variant of renal cell carcinoma—carcinosarcoma—may cause a confusing picture mimicking metastatic disease to the kidney from another primary or invasion by contiguous adrenal or retroperitoneal tumors. Renal cell carcinomas with oncocytic features (central scar) may mimic the more benign tumor—oncocytoma (8,38,103) (Fig. 36). Other entities such as lymphoma, metastases, and xanthogranulomatous pyelonephritis may exhibit CT features similar to those of renal cell carcinomas.

Knowledge of Robson's classification, as well as the TNM system, for staging renal cell carcinoma is important for understanding the many CT and MRI appearances and for decisions concerning resectability and patient prognosis (135,175) (Table 3). Tumor extension through the capsule into the perinephric space is recognized as an indistinct tumor margin, with strands (webs) of thickened

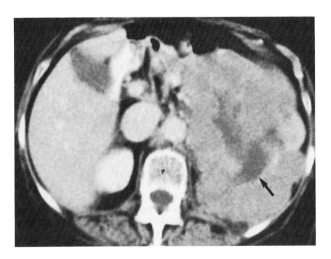

FIG. 36. Renal cell carcinoma with central scar. An irregular mass replaces the left kidney. The tumor's central necrosis (*arrow*) mimics an oncocytoma's central scar. (From ref. 135.)

TABLE 3. *Staging renal cell carcinoma: Robson's classification versus TNM*

Robson	Disease extent	TNM
I	Tumor confined to kidney (small, intrarenal)	T1
	Tumor confined to kidney (large)	T2
II	Tumor spread to perinephric fat, but within Gerota's fascia	T3a
IIIA	Tumor spread to renal vein or cava	T3b
IIIB	Tumor spread to local lymph nodes (LN)	N1–N3
IIIC	Tumor spread to local vessels and LN	T3b, N1–N3
IVA	Tumor spread to adjacent organs (excluding ipsilateral adrenal)	T4
IVB	Distant metastasis	M1a–d, N4

connective-tissue septa extending radially into the perinephric fat (Fig. 37). These strands are of soft-tissue density on CT images and of low or medium signal intensity on MR images. This feature is seen posteriorly and laterally, where the perinephric fat is most abundant. Direct anterior tumor spread is limited by the anterior pararenal fascia. Such regular streaky densities may be seen in the perinephric space in the absence of true tumor spread and may merely represent thickened or coalescent normal connective-tissue septae. These septae, the so-called bridging reno-renal septae, often become more prominent as a result of edema, vascular collaterals, inflammation, hemorrhage, and previous or concurrent disease. Large tumors may expand the perinephric space, displacing or compressing the fat without microscopic perinephric invasion. Gross tumor extension to or through Gerota's fascia obliterates normal tissue boundaries, with invasion of contiguous organs, bowel, or flank muscles. Because Gerota's fascia can be readily visualized in a significant number of individuals using current CT and MR imagers, caution must be used when interpreting "thickening" of Gerota's fascia as an indicator of tumor invasion. Local or diffuse thickening of Gerota's fascia is a nonspecific sign, particularly in the absence of gross tumor invasion of adjacent structures. There is the same lack of correlation between tumor size and extracapsular extension with CT imaging as existed in previous angiographic renal tumor staging (23,220). Areas where the assessment of perinephric extension are difficult are posteromedially where the kidney abuts the psoas muscle, anteriorly where the perinephric fat is thin or not well developed, and on the right where the duodenum may be in direct contiguity with the kidney. Some pathologists consider perirenal, hilar, or sinus fat invasion (because they are contiguous areas) in the same category as perinephric extension. Assessment of the hilum or renal sinus is very difficult with large bulky tumors that compress or invade the hilum.

Hilar or sinus fat may appear hazy or "dirty," reflecting edema or microscopic tumor invasion. This finding often is a harbinger of local lymph node spread (Fig. 38).

The presence of lymph node metastases confers a poor prognosis on the patient with renal cell carcinoma (135,139). There is a high association between local tumor recurrence and lymph node involvement (persistent tumor in local lymph nodes). Complete excision of the tumor and local lymph nodes (radical nephrectomy) is thought to improve survival, although simple nephrectomy without extensive lymph node dissection is considered by some to be equally effective (139). Lymph nodes less than 1 cm in size can be seen using CT or MRI, but they are considered normal. Lymph nodes in the 1- to 2-cm-diameter range, especially if numerous and located in the hilar, periaortic, or paracaval areas, should be regarded with suspicion and considered indeterminate by size criteria alone. Nodes greater than 2 cm are almost always enlarged by tumor. Enlarged lymph nodes due to reactive hyperplasia or granulomatous disease and normal-size nodes containing microscopic foci of tumor are rare causes of false-positive and false-negative CT/MRI interpretations, respectively. Both CT and MRI are capable of assessing lymph nodes in the upper abdomen and retrocrural spaces. Attention should also be paid to the mediastinum and pulmonary hila, because renal lymphatic drainage can be directly to the thorax. Care must be taken not to confuse lymph nodes with enlarged venous collaterals. Serial imaging after contrast-material injection on CT or MRI (with or without contrast) may be required for definitive evaluation in such cases. Local lymph nodes may actually be an ineffectual barrier to tumor spread, because the incidence of distant metastases is 50% higher in patients who have positive local lymph nodes (135).

Intrarenal venous invasion by tumor is not resolvable (visible), but major renal vein and IVC involvement can be detected (130,135,231). Major surgical decisions depend on the extent of renal vein and IVC invasion. IVC involvement does not preclude surgical resection. The right renal vein and left renal vein can be identified when normal or enlarged by thrombus, unless the veins are compressed, displaced, or engulfed by extensive local tumor (Fig. 39). The right renal vein may be difficult to see because it is short, vertically oriented, and usually solitary. It is easier to see the left renal vein because it is longer and horizontally oriented (32). The tendency for the left renal vein to be compressed between the aorta and superior mesenteric artery, the so-called nutcracker phenomenon, must be recognized as a normal variation, because it can cause some proximal venous enlargement (Fig. 32). Retroaortic left renal veins and large gonadal veins are important to describe so as to avoid inadvertent surgical resection.

The diagnosis of venous thrombosis by CT/MRI depends on the demonstration of focal enlargement of the involved vein or, more definitively, an intraluminal

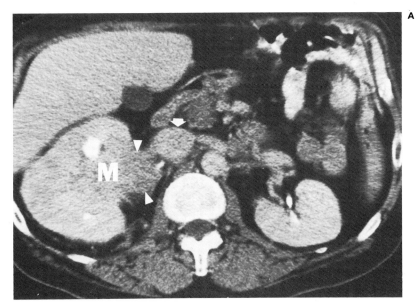

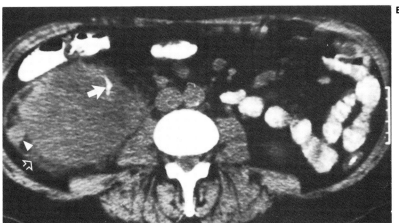

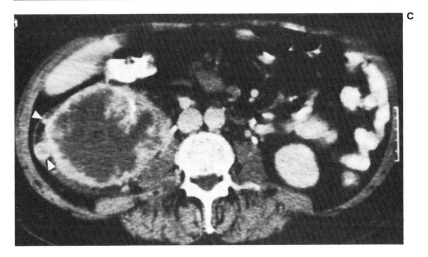

FIG. 37. Renal cell carcinoma, with perinephric extension and renal vein involvement. **A:** A large mass (M) is present in the right kidney. There is a dilated right renal vein filled with tumor thrombus (*arrowheads*). The inferior vena cava appears dilated (*arrow*). **B:** A more caudal image shows that the mass is necrotic, with low-attenuation regions, and has an area of calcification (*arrow*). A tumor nodule is also seen in the perinephric space (*arrowhead*); (*open arrow*) thickened Gerota's fascia. **C:** After a repeat bolus intravenous injection of contrast material, the necrotic nature of the mass and the perinephric extension is more clearly seen (*arrowheads*).

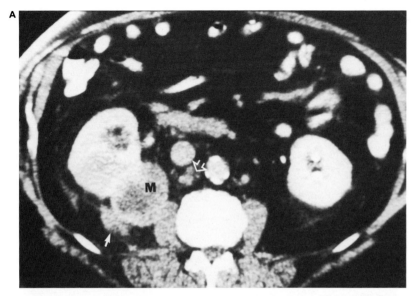

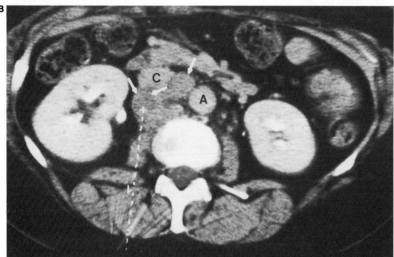

FIG. 38. Renal cell cancer, with local nodal spread. **A:** There is a large mass (M) growing off the inferior surface of the right kidney, with perinephric extension (*arrow*). An enlarged lymph node is present between the IVC and the aorta (*open arrow*). **B:** Confluent lymphadenopathy in a different patient. There is retrocaval and inter-aortocaval adenopathy (*arrows*). The primary cancer is not seen on this image. The IVC (C) is displaced anteriorly; (A) aorta. *Dotted line* shows biopsy route that confirmed metastatic renal cell cancer. **C:** Extensive retroperitoneal lymphadenopathy in a third patient. The left-side renal cell cancer obliterates the sinus fat and collecting system. There is bulky retroperitoneal adenopathy (*arrows*).

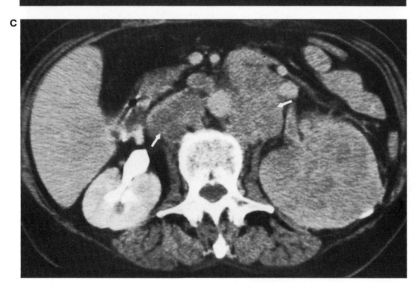

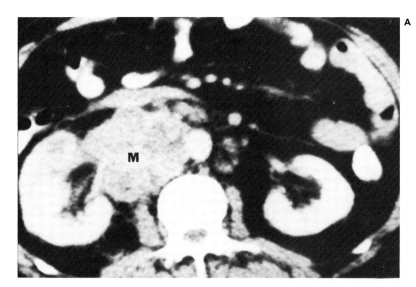

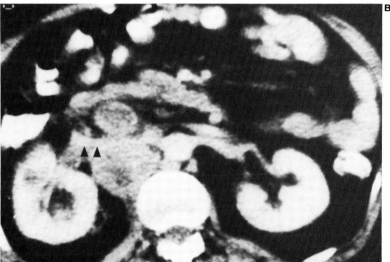

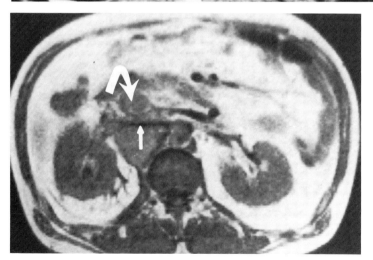

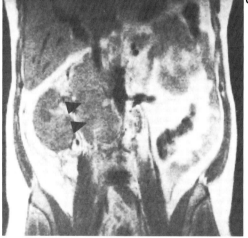

FIG. 39. Renal cell carcinoma, with invasion of the IVC. **A:** Postcontrast CT shows a large perihilar lymph node mass (M) in this patient with a right-lower-pole carcinoma. **B:** More caudal image shows compression of the renal artery by the mass (*arrowheads*). The status of the IVC is uncertain. **C:** MRI (TR = 500 msec, TE = 30 msec) at same level as (**B**) reveals an encased right renal artery (*arrow*), and the IVC lacks flow-void artifact because it is filled with tumor thrombus (*curved arrow*). **D:** Coronal MRI (TR = 500 msec, TE = 30 msec) shows the cephalocaudad extent of the adenopathy (*arrowheads*).

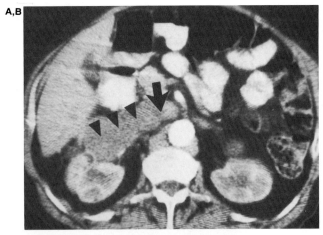

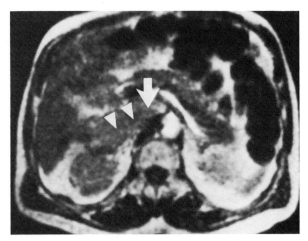

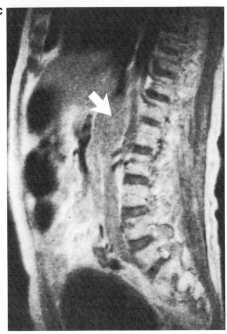

FIG. 40. Renal cell cancer, with invasion of the renal vein and IVC. **A:** CT image after intravenous administration of contrast material shows a dilated right renal vein, with tumor thrombus (*arrowheads*) and extension into the IVC (*arrow*). **B:** Transaxial MR image (TR = 500 msec, TE = 30 msec) at the same level as (**A**) shows similar findings. **C:** A sagittal MR image (TR = 500 msec, TE = 30 msec) shows tumor thrombus within the inferior vena cava (*white arrow*).

thrombus (199) (Figs. 39–41). When venous occlusion is complete, the involved segment remains unenhanced, and paravertebral collaterals may be identified on postcontrast CT images (58). In cases in which the venous occlusion is partial, the thrombus appears as a low-density filling defect surrounded by iodine-containing blood on CT, and it shows variable signal intensities on MRI. On CT, caution must be taken not to confuse true intraluminal defects from those caused by (a) influx of unopacified blood from large adjacent venous branches and (b) laminar flow phenomena that often are encountered with lower-extremity injections (199). As the contrast material layers against the periphery of the IVC, the faster-moving central column of blood may cause a "doughnut-like" appearance due to nonenhanced flowing blood representing the hole in the doughnut. Likewise, intraluminal signals related to slow flow should not be confused with a thrombus on MRI (see Chapter 4).

Tumoral thrombus and nontumoral thrombus usually cannot be differentiated from each other on CT images

unless hypervascularity is shown in the tumoral thrombus. However, bland thrombi occasionally may be distinguished from tumor thrombi on MRI. Enhancement of the caval wall suggests wall adherence of a tumor thrombus or frank wall invasion on CT. Although the cephalic extent of the tumor thrombus in the IVC can be estimated by examining consecutive transaxial CT images, sagittal or coronal MRI provides a more direct display of the cephalocaudal dimension of the thrombus and its relationship to the adjacent hepatic veins (195). Doppler ultrasound and venography may provide similar information, but rarely are they needed.

Other Organ Involvement

Local spread of renal cell carcinoma depends on individual tumoral characteristics: grade, size, degrees of necrosis and hemorrhage, as well as tumor vascularity (135,139). Tumors with extensive necrosis have a limited

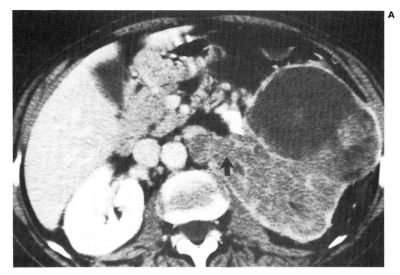

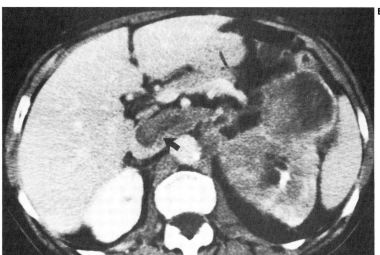

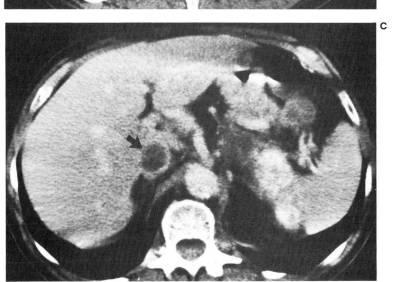

FIG. 41. Renal cell carcinoma, with left-renal-vein and IVC invasion. **A:** There is a huge left renal cancer extending into the left renal vein (*arrow*). **B:** The tumor thrombus extends into the IVC (*arrow*). **C:** A more cephalad image at the level of the liver shows tumor thrombus (*arrow*) extending up the IVC.

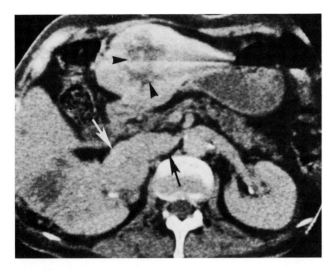

FIG. 42. Renal cell carcinoma, with hepatic metastases. A large mass arises from the lateral surface of the right kidney and invades the liver. There is an irregular low-density metastasis (*black arrowheads*) in the left lobe of the liver. The right renal vein (*white arrow*) and IVC (*black arrow*) are markedly enlarged because of tumor invasion.

ability to generate a good blood supply, and they rarely metastasize. As a general rule, the extent and number of metastases relate to tumor size and vascularity; so tumors over 10 cm in size frequently (80%) have metastases, whereas tumors less than 5 cm in diameter usually do not have metastases at the time of initial diagnosis (135). On rare occasions, renal cell carcinoma, papillary or non-papillary varieties, may present with concurrent metastases even when the primary is less than 3 cm in size (43,44,227). The lung, mediastinum, axial skeleton, brain, and liver are the most common sites (Fig. 42). Direct involvement of the liver and spleen is more common than metastatic spread. Additionally, the pancreas, psoas muscles, and ipsilateral adrenal gland are common targets for direct tumor invasion. Because bilateral synchronous and asynchronous renal cell carcinomas do occur, careful analysis of the contralateral kidney in a patient with renal neoplasm is mandatory (135,139). Although the prognosis is dismal in these patients, renal-sparing surgery is the treatment of choice.

Angiography

The role of angiography for diagnosis, staging, and detection of extrarenal extension of renal cell carcinoma has changed drastically since the advent of CT and MRI. Both CT and MRI are more accurate and more sensitive than angiography for detection of perinephric extension and lymph node involvement, and they are equally as accurate for renal venous and IVC invasion (56,91,132,220). Renal venography is reserved for cases in which CT and/or MRI findings are equivocal. Renal arteriography is performed

for patients with solitary kidneys, renal anomalies, multifocal or bilateral tumor involvement, and any other situation in which renal-sparing surgery is contemplated. In some instances, digital techniques have replaced the conventional film–screen combination (62).

Follow-up

In addition to the initial diagnosis and staging of renal cell carcinoma, CT and MRI play an important role in the follow-up of patients treated with surgery, angioinfarction, or chemotherapy (1,10,14). Those patients who are at the highest risk for postoperative recurrence include those with large bulky tumors, incomplete resection, and lymph node or adrenal involvement (135). Because most late metastases develop intraabdominally, the liver, mesentery, remaining kidney, adrenals, and paraaortic or paracaval areas require close scrutiny. The features that suggest tumor recurrence are a soft-tissue mass in the renal fossa (distinct from bowel loops filled with oral contrast material), asymmetric or ipsilateral psoas muscle enlargement, and local organ abnormalities (Figs. 43 and 44). In addition to bowel loops, the tail of the pancreas, liver, and spleen may partially fill the vacated renal bed postoperatively and should not be confused with a recurrent neoplasm. Abscesses, seromas, or lymphoceles can also mimic a recurrent cancer. MRI may be useful in distinguishing between tumor recurrence and scar tissue or fibrosis.

Renal cell carcinoma treated by angioinfarction (e.g., absolute alcohol) has a characteristic CT appearance (224). Within the first 48 hr following the procedure, persistent or trapped contrast material may be seen, along with branching peripheral gas collections. Later, 5 to 7 days after the procedure, air collections become more central, depending on the extent of infarction and necrosis (14) (Fig. 45). Eventually, the kidney size will decrease or stay the same. If the size increases, regenerated tumor must be suspected.

Transitional Cell Carcinoma

Transitional cell carcinoma of the ureter, pelvis, and collecting system accounts for 5% to 10% of all renal tumors (11,139). They expand or compress surrounding urothelial structures, obliterating or invading renal sinus fat, peripelvic or periureteric fat, and tissue planes. Intraparenchymal invasion may occur focally, or tumor spread may be suburothelial, causing a urographic picture of caliceal, pelvic, or ureteric stricture. These strictures may have a relatively smooth appearance on urography or retrograde pyelography. The kidney usually retains its reniform shape, even though some transitional cell carcinomas can be quite large.

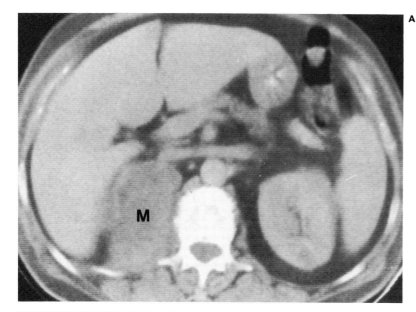

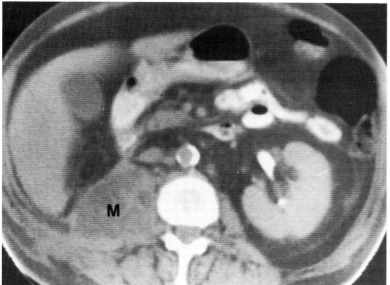

FIG. 43. Recurrent renal cell carcinoma. **A:** A large mass (M) fills the renal fossa on the right in this patient who had had prior radical right nephrectomy for carcinoma. Compensatory hypertrophy of the left kidney is present. **B:** Two centimeters caudal, the tumor mass (M) is noted to invade the right psoas. Percutaneous biopsy confirmed recurrence.

CT frequently is used to evaluate patients known to have or suspected of having transitional cell carcinoma of the ureter or pelvis. The role of CT is twofold (11,35,110,160). First, CT is used to determine the cause of a radiolucent filling defect seen on a urogram. Although CT is not histospecific, differentiation between soft-tissue masses and fresh blood clots or stones is straightforward (Fig. 46). Relatively radiolucent stones like struvite or urate calculi can be detected with CT because they have a higher attenuation value than urine or renal parenchyma (Fig. 47). Second, CT is often used to delineate actual tumor extent after its detection by urography, retrograde pyelography, or ureterorenoscopy. Because conservative surgery, i.e., local resection, is occasionally an option for ureteral tumors, CT plays an important preoperative role for staging and surgical planning.

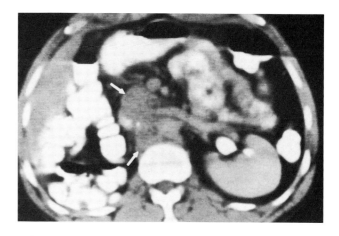

FIG. 44. Recurrent renal cell cancer. Retrocrural and paracaval lymph nodes (*arrows*) were involved with renal cell cancer. Right kidney had been removed 1 year earlier.

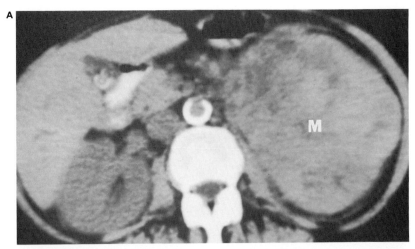

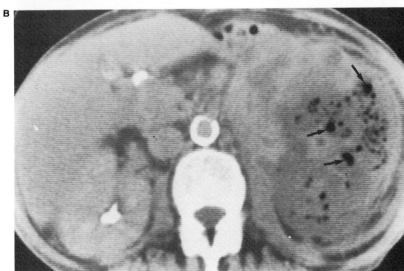

FIG. 45. Gas collection in an angioinfarcted kidney. **A:** Preinfarction: There is a large mass (M), with perinephric extension and thickening of Gerota's fascia on the left. **B:** Postinfarction: The mass contains gas (*arrows*), is not enhanced, and is lower in attenuation than the normal kidney.

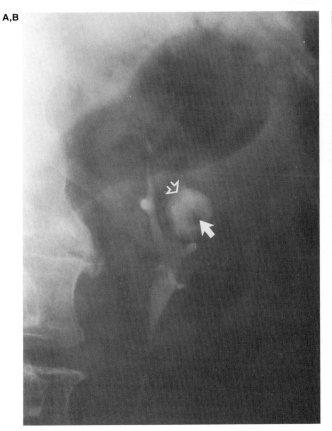

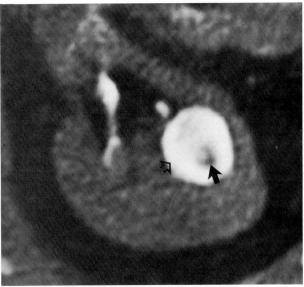

FIG. 46. Organized hematoma in a hydrocalix mimicking transitional cell carcinoma. **A:** Film from intravenous urography (IVU) shows a filling defect (*arrow*) in a hydrocalix (*open arrow*). This could represent a transitional cell carcinoma. **B:** CT image shows the same filling defect (*arrow*) in the hydrocalix (*open arrow*). This proved to be an organizing hematoma that mimicked a transitional cell carcinoma. (Courtesy of Dr. Melvin Conrad.)

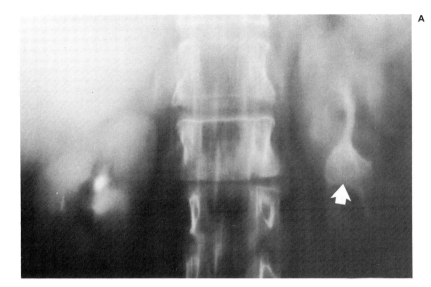

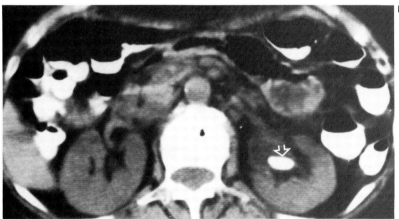

FIG. 47. Urate stone. A: IVU tomogram shows a radiolucent filling defect in the left renal pelvis (*arrow*). B: CT image without intravenous contrast material shows a high-density calculus (*open arrow*) present in the left renal pelvis. This corresponds to the radiolucent filling defect seen on the IVU.

When CT is performed to assess known or suspected transitional cell carcinoma, precontrast images are obtained only for localization and slice selection prior to contrast enhancement. Single or serial bolus injection of 10 to 25 cc of a 32% to 60% solution is routinely used, because opacification that is too dense may mask subtle degrees of tumor invasion or the tumorous filling defect itself.

Transitional cell carcinoma may be solitary or multiple, with CT attenuation values approaching those of soft tissue on noncontrast images, but usually greater than those of urine and similar to or slightly less than those for renal parenchyma (8–70 HU) (11) on postcontrast studies. Rarely, speckles of calcification may be present on the surfaces of some tumors, resulting in their higher attenuation values (Fig. 48). Intratumoral calcification suggests squamoid elements within the transitional cell carcinoma (24). Adherent blood can increase measured values as well. The surface of the tumor may appear smooth or irregular, depending on tumor architecture and degree of hemorrhage. Although characteristically hypovascular or avascular at angiography, contrast-enhanced CT may show subtle transient enhancement of a transitional cell carcinoma (8–55 HU ± S.D. after contrast injection) (11) (Fig. 49).

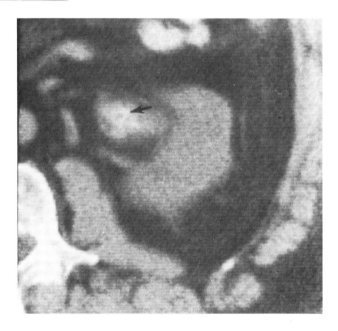

FIG. 48. Calcified transitional cell carcinoma. A soft-tissue mass with amorphous calcification (*arrow*) is present in the left renal pelvis. Although most transitional cell carcinomas have attenuation values approaching those for soft tissue (40–70 HU), calcification may rarely be seen. (From ref. 11.)

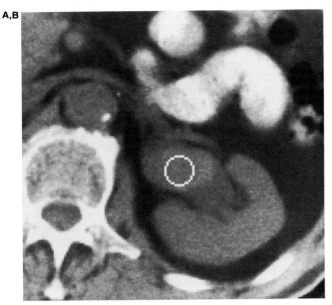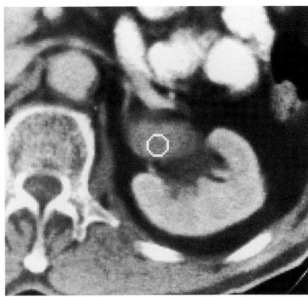

FIG. 49. Transitional cell carcinoma: contrast enhancement. **A:** Precontrast CT image shows a soft-tissue mass (cursor) with attenuation value of +49 HU in the left renal pelvis. **B:** Following a 25-cc bolus injection of iodinated contrast material, the attenuation value of the tumor under cursor increased to +78 HU. (From ref. 11.)

At least three CT patterns have been described with transitional cell carcinoma involving the ureter or collecting system (11). Most commonly, tumors appear as sessile intraluminal masses (Fig. 50). Other patterns include concentric or eccentric ureteral or pelvic-wall thickening (Figs. 51 and 52). When large infiltrating masses are present, they may locally invade the renal pelvis, causing a hazy appearance to the surrounding fat or obliteration of the intrarenal pericaliceal sinus fat. Parenchymal expansion may occur, with obliteration of any normal landmarks, in which case invasive transitional cell carcinoma may mimic invasive renal cell carcinoma, lymphoma, or metastases (Figs. 53 and 54). On occasion, an obstructive nephrogram proximal to the tumor may be

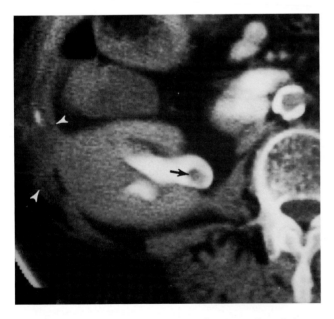

FIG. 50. Transitional cell carcinoma. A fixed, sessile soft-tissue mass (*arrow*) is seen in the right renal pelvis. This has been the most common CT pattern of transitional cell tumor. Soft-tissue changes in right-flank musculature (*arrowheads*) are secondary to previous ureterotomies for transitional cell carcinoma.

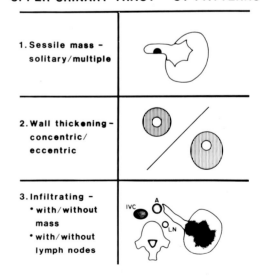

TRANSITIONAL CELL CARCINOMA OF UPPER URINARY TRACT - CT PATTERNS

1. Sessile mass - solitary/multiple

2. Wall thickening - concentric/eccentric

3. Infiltrating -
   • with/without mass
   • with/without lymph nodes

FIG. 51. CT patterns of transitional cell carcinoma of the pelvis and ureter.

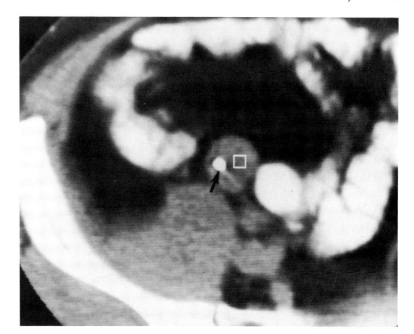

FIG. 52. Transitional cell carcinoma of the right ureter: semilunar pattern. The cursor is placed over an eccentric portion of the thickened ureteral wall. The *arrow* points to the eccentrically situated ureteral stent. (From ref. 11.)

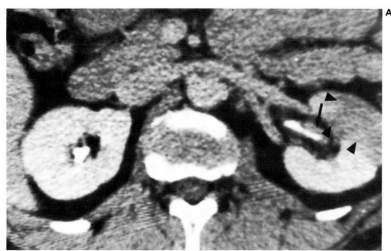

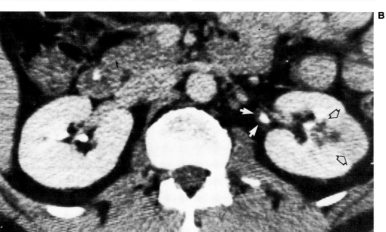

FIG. 53. Invasive transitional cell carcinoma. **A:** Postcontrast CT image shows a soft-tissue-density lesion in the renal pelvis (*arrow*) representing the primary transitional cell carcinoma. Note that the anterior half of the kidney (*arrowheads*) is invaded by the neoplasm. **B:** More caudal image shows thickening of the proximal ureter (*white arrows*). The lateral portion of the kidney is also infiltrated by the neoplasm (*open arrows*). (Courtesy of Dr. Gaston Morillo.)

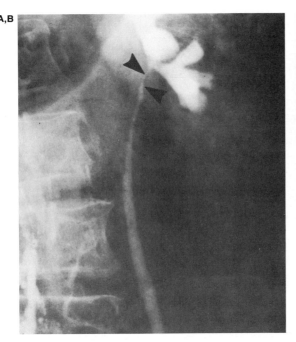 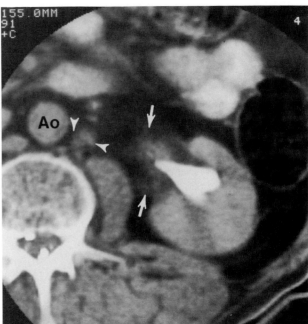

FIG. 54. Stage IV transitional cell carcinoma. **A:** Retrograde pyelogram shows irregular constriction of the ureteral-pelvic junction (*arrowheads*), causing dilatation of intrarenal collecting system. The exact tumor extent cannot be appreciated on this study. **B:** Postcontrast CT image through left renal pelvis demonstrates an extraureteral soft-tissue mass, with spiculations extending out into the perirenal fat (*arrows*). A cluster of minimally enlarged lymph nodes (*arrowheads*) is noted lateral to the aorta (Ao). (From ref. 11.)

seen, causing a localized patchy nephrographic appearance (24). Contrast may pool around the intracaliceal tumor mass, causing a rim or crescent-shaped collection outlining the neoplasm.

CT can offer valuable staging information in patients with transitional cell carcinoma, but it cannot differentiate between tumors limited to the urothelial mucosa (stage I) and muscle-wall invasion (stage II) (Table 4). However, the treatment is not significantly different for stage I and stage II tumors of transitional cell origin. Stage III, with focal or diffuse parenchymal invasion, still is treated by nephroureterectomy. Extrarenal spread usually is central, extending out through the renal hilum, with or without local lymph node enlargement. This pattern usually is easily discernible by CT imaging. Extensive local invasion, lymph node involvement, or distant metastases preclude curative surgery, and more conservative treatment methods usually are employed (11).

Other tumors may involve the kidney or urothelial surfaces. Squamous cell carcinoma (215,225), cholesteatoma,

metastases to the urothelium, and mucinous adenocarcinoma of the urothelium may all have CT appearances similar to those of multiple transitional cell carcinomas (5,11) (Fig. 55). Cytology, ureterorenoscopy, or surgery is necessary for definite diagnosis in these cases.

LYMPHOMA

Renal involvement by lymphoma is considered a late manifestation of the disease. Widespread use of CT imaging for staging of patients known to have or suspected of having lymphoma has shown renal changes in at least 5% of patients (86). The incidence is higher in autopsy series (33%–52%), confirming the fact that renal involvement usually is late. Appreciation of the many CT patterns of renal lymphoma will improve early detection rates (78,86).

Various patterns have been encountered with renal lymphoma: enlargement, with maintenance of the normal renal contour (most commonly); multiple soft-tissue nodules unilaterally or bilaterally (in more than 50% of renal lymphoma cases); direct invasion from contiguous disease in the lymph nodes or retroperitoneal spaces (approximately 25%); a solitary renal mass (5%–10%); diffuse infiltration (confluence of multifocal disease) in up to 10% of cases; perinephric involvement, compressing or displacing the kidney with fascial thickening and/or obliteration of perinephric spaces (74,86) (Figs. 56 and 57).

TABLE 4. *Staging classification of transitional cell carcinoma*

I	Limited to uroepithelial mucosa and lamina propria
II	Invasion to but not beyond the pelvic and ureteric muscularis
III	Invasion beyond the muscularis to adventitial fat or parenchyma
IV	Distant metastases

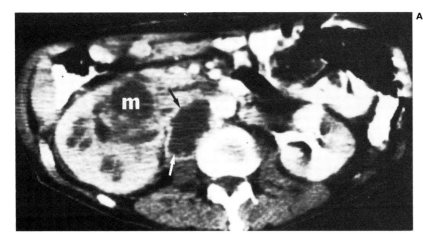

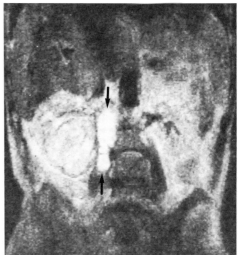

FIG. 55. Squamous carcinoma of the kidney. **A, B:** CT and axial MR (TR = 500 msec, TE = 30 msec) images at the same level show a large necrotic right renal mass (m), with extension into the psoas (*arrows*). **C:** Coronal T2-weighted MR image (TR = 2,100 msec, TE = 90 msec) shows full extent of the psoas involvement (*arrows*).

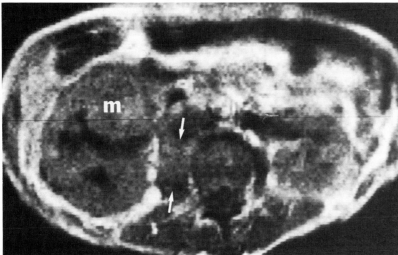

Secondary renal manifestations of lymphoma include urinary tract obstruction, with hydronephrosis, urate or hypercalcemic nephropathy, and retroperitoneal fibrosis in treated lymphoma patients.

Because the kidney is devoid of lymphoid tissue, primary renal lymphoma is considered very rare or merely occult secondary involvement. Renal lymphoma almost always results from hematogenous dissemination or direct contiguous invasion. Lymphomatous renal masses generally appear homogeneous, with attenuation values (density) similar to those for normal renal parenchyma on precontrast CT images. A heterogeneous appearance due to necrosis and hemorrhage may be seen post treatment. Uncommonly, renal lymphoma may appear lower

FIG. 56. Enlarged kidneys due to lymphoma. There is bilateral obliteration of the renal sinus, with compression of sinus fat (left > right) and perihilar and periaortic lymphadenopathy on the left.

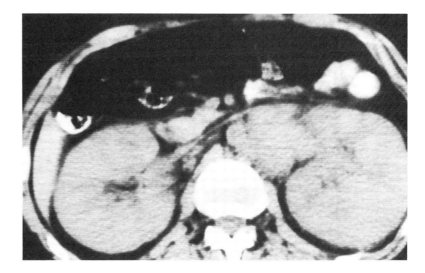

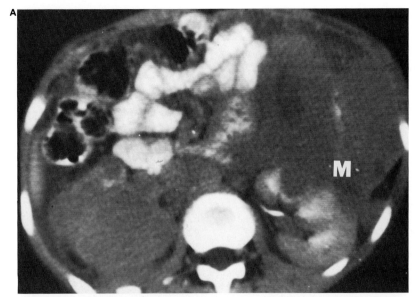

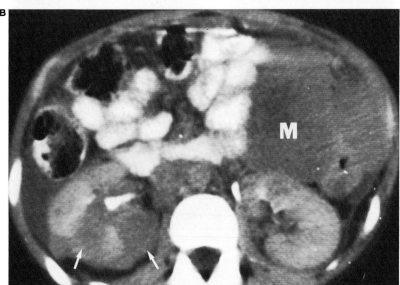

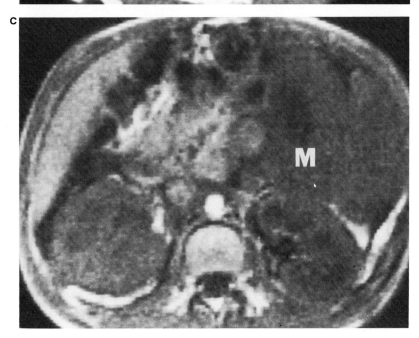

FIG. 57. Lymphoma. **A:** There is a large mass (M) extending out of the left kidney. The right kidney is almost entirely replaced by lymphoma. **B:** More caudal image again shows lymphomatous infiltration of the right kidney (*arrows*). Normal residual parenchyma is noted anteriorly. **C:** Transaxial MR image (SE, TR = 2,100 msec, TE = 35 msec) shows the left renal mass (M) and the abnormal right kidney.

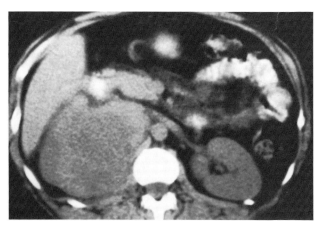
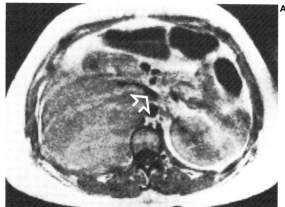

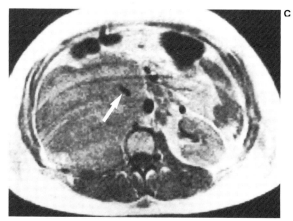

FIG. 58. Renal lymphoma. **A:** CT image demonstrates massive enlargement of the right kidney and extrarenal extension of the lymphomatous mass. The IVC cannot be clearly identified. **B:** Transaxial MR image (SE, TR = 500 msec, TE = 30 msec) demonstrates the IVC (*open arrow*) more readily than noncontrast CT. **C:** Transaxial MRI (SE, TR = 500 msec, TE = 30 msec). The IVC (*arrow*) is engulfed by the lymphomatous mass.

or higher in density than normal kidneys. After contrast-material administration, lymphomatous tissue increases in attenuation only slightly (10–30 HU), whereas normal tissue is enhanced to a greater extent (60–120 HU) (78,86). The enhancement may be patchy or wedge-shaped. The MRI appearance is commonly one of mixed or inter-mediate-signal-intensity masses distorting the renal or perirenal anatomy, with occasional displacement of adjacent structures (78). Encased vascular structures can be displayed with MRI (Fig. 58), and the multiplanar-im-

aging features allow more precise determination of true tumor volume and extent. A differential diagnosis of renal lymphoma usually is not a clinical problem, but the presence or persistence of renal involvement is important as regards treatment options, e.g., radiation and/or chemotherapy. The pattern of renal and perirenal lymphomatous involvement may be mimicked by primary neoplasms, metastatic carcinoma to the kidney, multiple angiomyolipomas, infections, leukemia, or sinus histiocytosis (Figs. 59 and 60).

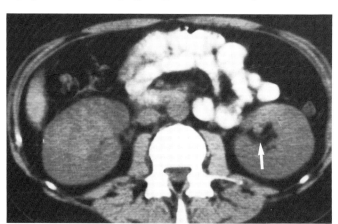
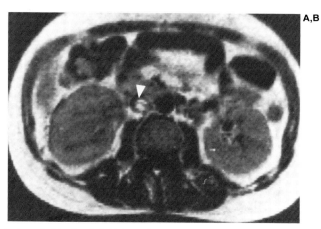

FIG. 59. Renal metastasis. **A:** CT image demonstrates normal renal sinus fat in the left kidney (*arrow*), but not in the right. The latter has a swollen "faceless" appearance due to the presence of infiltrative metastatic disease. **B:** Transaxial MR image (SE, TR = 500 msec, TE = 30 msec) shows findings noted in (**A**). High signal in the IVC (*arrowhead*) is due to slow flow rather than invasion of the IVC.

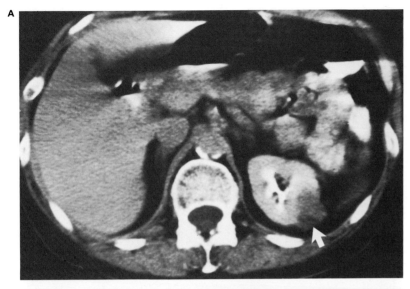

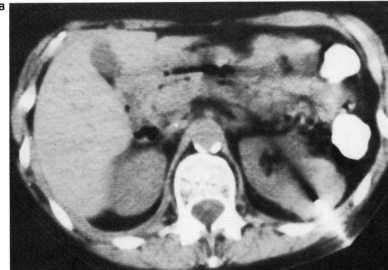

FIG. 60. Renal metastasis. **A:** Postcontrast CT image demonstrates an inhomogeneous, poorly enhancing mass (*arrow*) protruding from the lateral border of the left kidney. **B:** Biopsy revealed metastatic oat cell carcinoma.

BENIGN RENAL TUMORS

Adenoma

It remains controversial whether a renal adenoma is a benign neoplasm or in fact a precursor of renal cell carcinoma. The criteria of a well-encapsulated, solid neoplasm less than 3 cm in diameter, without necrosis, hemorrhage, cellular mitosis, or atypia, confined to the renal cortex, in a patient with no metastases, have been widely considered to define an adenoma. Currently, the diagnosis of an adenoma is made only when the lesion is less than 2 cm in size (135,166). However, solid renal cell carcinomas in the range of 2 to 3 cm in size have been detected with CT and MRI (44) (Fig. 34). The CT and MRI appearances of a renal adenoma of any size may be similar to those for renal cell carcinoma. Calcification has been encountered, but is of no significant differential diagnostic importance. Adenomas may be solitary, multiple, or bilateral and may coexist with renal cell carcinoma in a single kidney or a single patient.

Some adenomas will have so-called oncocytic features (large polysomal cells with eosinophilic cytoplasm) and thus be designated oncocytomas (8,38,117,166). A helpful, although not pathognomonic, CT feature of an oncocytoma is a central stellate, nonenhancing "scar" (8) (Figs. 61 and 62). Angiographically, these tumors have a spoke-and-wheel palisading peripheral vascular pattern, with central stellate avascular areas. Oncocytomas are rare, accounting for only 0.9% to 1.4% of all renal parenchymal neoplasms. The so-called central scar histologically is composed of white fibrous tissue. These tumors rarely metastasize, but renal cell carcinomas may have oncocytic features histologically and radiographically (Fig. 36). Therefore, the treatment remains biopsy or surgery, with consideration given to renal-sparing surgery (109).

On CT and MRI, papillary renal cell carcinomas may appear identical with renal adenomas or oncocytomas

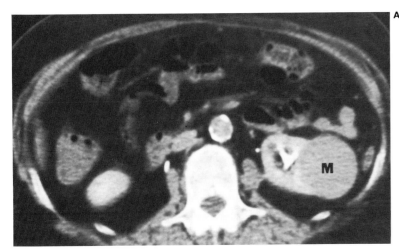

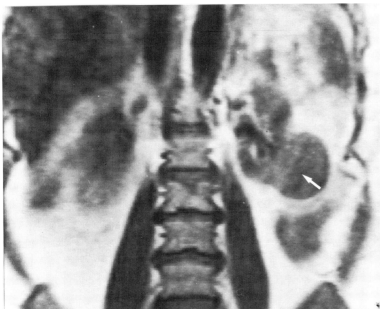

FIG. 61. Oncocytoma. **A:** CT image shows a mass (M) extending from the lateral aspect of the left kidney. The mass has an attenuation value slightly lower than that of paraspinal muscles. **B:** Coronal MR image demonstrates the mass and a subtle suggestion of a central scar (*arrow*). Diagnosis: oncocytoma. (Courtesy of Dr. Suresh Patel.)

without central scars, making categorical CT/MRI diagnosis of adenoma or oncocytoma impossible (163). Other benign renal neoplasms, such as fibroma, leiomyoma, plasmacytoma, intrarenal pheochromocytoma, hamartoma, extramedullary hematopoiesis, and fibrous histiocytoma, do not have specific CT or MRI features to allow a specific histologic diagnosis (179) (Fig. 63). On occasion, a solitary metastasis of lymphoma (lymphomatous deposit or mass) may also appear as a "benign" solitary renal mass. Some benign neoplasms may degenerate or differentiate into malignant neoplasms, i.e., malignant fibrous histiocytoma and malignant leiomyosarcoma, with CT and MRI appearances consistent with their typical aggressive local behavior.

Hemangiomas (capillary or cavernous) may have CT features that suggest their identification. Bleeding within the neoplasm or into the collecting system may be clinically evident. Capillary hemangiomas may be too small to image with CT, and hemangiomas may occur in the wall of a benign renal cyst. Cavernous hemangiomas, typically seen as avascular space-occupying processes on angiography, may present as masses within the renal sinus and renal medulla (15) (Fig. 64). Associated hemorrhage may be evident on CT.

Angiomyolipoma

Angiomyolipomas occur as isolated lesions in middle-aged females or as the renal manifestation of tuberous sclerosis (19,82,212). Frequently they are small, less than 1 cm in size, multiple or bilateral (19,28,185,212) (Fig. 65). Histologically, angiomyolipomas are composed mainly of three elements: (a) blood vessels, (b) smooth muscle, and (c) fat in varying proportions. They are considered benign mesenchymal tumors, but occasionally are found to have cellular pleomorphism and mitoses and even regional lymph node involvement. Rarely, if ever,

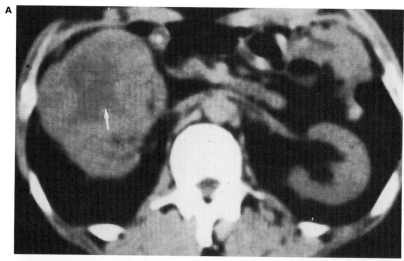

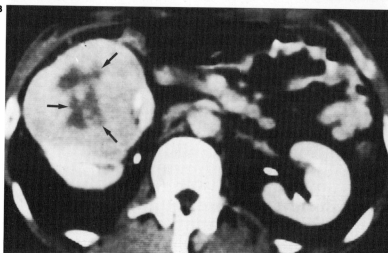

FIG. 62. Oncocytoma. **A:** Noncontrast CT image shows a large mass involving the right kidney, with a central scar (*arrow*). **B:** After intravenous administration of contrast material, the central scar is much more prominent (*arrows*). (Courtesy of Dr. Robert Boltuch.)

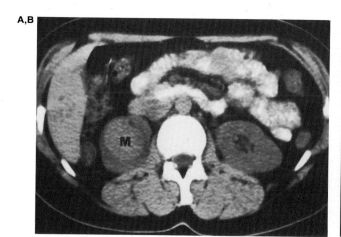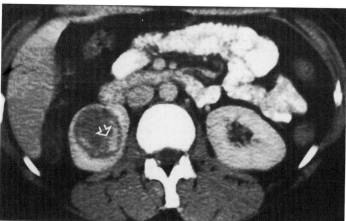

FIG. 63. Renal fibroma. **A:** Precontrast CT image shows a well-circumscribed mass (M) arising from the central portion of the right kidney. The mass is slightly higher in attenuation than the normal renal parenchyma. **B:** Following intravenous administration of contrast material, the mass has heterogeneous contrast enhancement (*open arrow*), but the majority of the mass is lower in attenuation than the normal renal parenchyma. (Courtesy of Dr. Mark Schwimmer.)

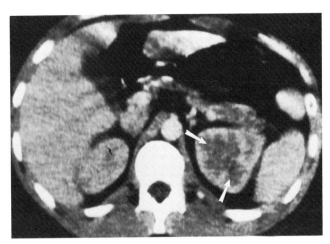 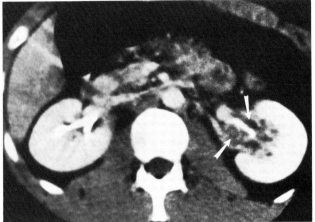

A,B

FIG. 64. Cavernous hemangioma. **A:** Expanded left upper pole shows irregular peripheral enhancement (*arrows*). **B:** Mass that proved to be cavernous hemangioma expands the renal sinus and insinuates itself (*arrows*) between the vessels and the renal pelvis. (Courtesy of Dr. Arthur Bishop.)

do they metastasize, but some may be locally aggressive, displacing contiguous structures and parasitizing local vasculature (82,212). When enough fatty tissue is present within the tumor, the CT and MRI appearances are virtually pathognomonic, that is, a well-circumscribed fat-density mass or masses either partially or totally within the renal substance. However, intramural hemorrhage and predominant muscle or vascular components may make differential diagnosis difficult. Almost all cases will display some low-density, fat-like components suggesting the diagnosis. Very narrow collimation may be necessary in tiny lesions. In cases in which the tumor is predominantly extrarenal in location, distinction between angiomyolipoma and primary retroperitoneal lipoma or liposarcoma

invading the kidney may be difficult (Fig. 66). Very small lesions may be confused with renal cysts because of volume averaging, and in children, Wilms's tumors may contain small amounts of fat. Rarely, angiomyolipomas can coexist with renal cell carcinoma in a given kidney or patient, prompting further evaluation with more invasive studies like angiography or biopsy. Currently, conservative surgical therapy is used for patients with angiomyolipomas, whether solitary or multiple or in patients with tuberous sclerosis (152). Tumors that are less than 4 cm in size and asymptomatic can be followed up at leisure (152). Larger angiomyolipomas should be monitored closely with CT, MRI, or ultrasound. Symptomatic patients should be carefully evaluated, with consideration

FIG. 65. Small angiomyolipoma. A fat-density (−40 HU) mass is present in the posterior aspect of the right kidney (*arrowhead*). Two, more subtle, low-density lesions in the right kidney represent volume averaging with other small angiomyolipomas (*arrows*).

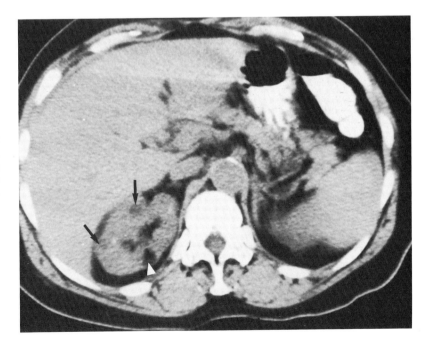

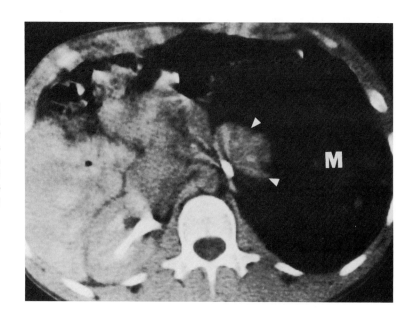

FIG. 66. Angiomyolipoma, with a large extrarenal component. Postcontrast CT image demonstrates a predominantly fatty mass (M) displacing the kidney (*arrowheads*) anteriorly and medially. When the tumor has a large extrarenal component, as in this case, differentiation between angiomyolipoma and a primary retroperitoneal liposarcoma invading the kidney may be difficult. (Courtesy of Dr. Gaston Morillo.)

A
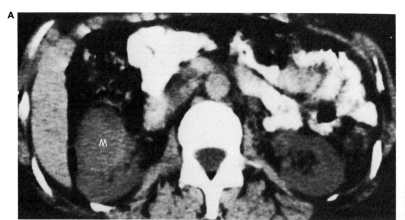

B,C
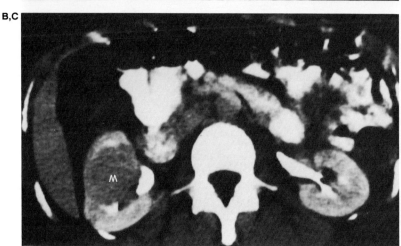

FIG. 67. Arteriovenous malformation (AVM). **A:** CT image (from another hospital) without intravenous contrast material shows a mass (M) with higher attenuation than the normal renal parenchyma in the right kidney. **B:** A delayed, nondynamic, postcontrast CT image shows that the mass (M) is now lower in attenuation than the renal parenchyma. **C:** Coronal MR image (SE, TR = 1,500 msec, TE = 35 msec) demonstrates a large vein (*arrow*) draining from the malformation (V) into the IVC. Parts **D** and **E** on *facing page*.

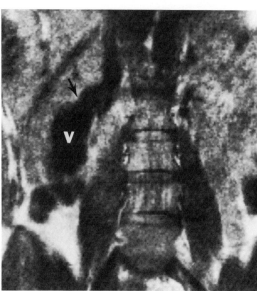

given to angioinfarction and segmental surgery if the tumors are less than 4 to 5 cm in size (152). Conservative surgery may not be possible with larger lesions.

Arteriovenous Malformation

Large arteriovenous malformations (AVM) or large arteriovenous fistulas (AVF) may or may not be clinically evident, depending on the presence or absence of a hemodynamically significant shunt, audible bruit, hematuria, or subjective symptoms. Whether suspected on clinical grounds or encountered incidentally on a CT examination, AVMs and AVFs should be distinguishable from true neoplasms by their degree of contrast enhancement, large feeding and draining vessels, and occasional curvilinear calcifications in their walls. The precontrast density of the fast-flowing blood within the AVM will be similar to that in the aorta and IVC, but rapid bolus injections of contrast material coupled with serial dynamic CT imaging are necessary for optimal opacification and correct diagnosis. Contrast-assisted CT performed with a slow or low-volume drip infusion may mask the true nature of the AVM, demonstrating only minimal "total-body enhancement" of the lesion in question when compared with normal renal parenchyma. Unless the malformations are thrombosed, MRI easily identifies their vascular nature, because rapidly flowing blood appears as an area of signal void (Fig. 67).

Indeterminate Masses

Some masses do not fit satisfactorily into the CT categories of cyst, tumor, or abscess, even with optimal contrast-assisted CT and correlation with pertinent history and physical examination. Such renal masses are therefore considered indeterminate by CT criteria (6). Masses that display indeterminate CT features in patients with obvious urinary tract infections or sepsis most likely are focal bacterial nephritis or abscess and will be discussed later in this chapter. One study of 815 patients referred for CT evaluation of one or more renal masses revealed that 8% of masses were CT-indeterminate (6). The numbers of indeterminate masses will vary, but have remained near or slightly less than this percentage in our current practice. Causes for an indeterminate diagnosis relate most frequently to confusing features such as wall thickening, calcification, variable attenuation, hemorrhage, and variable enhancement or to other reasons placing the mass in the "gray" zone between cyst and neoplasm (6,43). Broad categories of CT-indeterminate masses include the following categories: (I) technically indeterminate CT images; (II) "cyst-like" masses; and (III) "tumor-like" (solid) masses with complex features.

Technically indeterminate CT images of renal masses result mainly from respiratory artifacts or volume-averaging effects on small masses, polar lesions, or intracaliceal defects. Other technical causes include data-poor or photopenic images in very large patients, slower scanners,

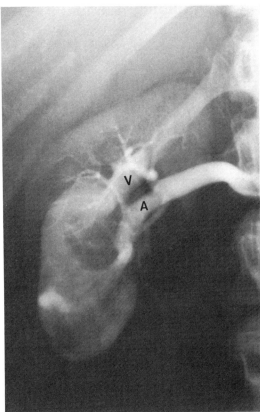

D,E

FIG. 67. (Continued.) Parts **A–C** on facing page. **D:** Transaxial MR image (SE, TR = 1,500 msec, TE = 35 msec) shows a large "signal-void" (V) area in the right renal hilum compatible with a vascular malformation. **E:** Angiogram demonstrates that there is a large AVM. The draining vein (V) and feeding artery (A) are well seen.

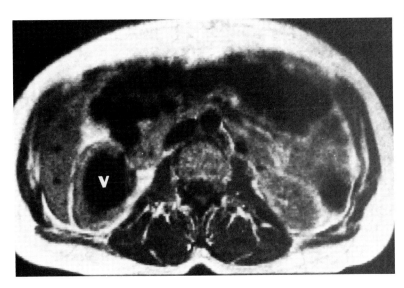

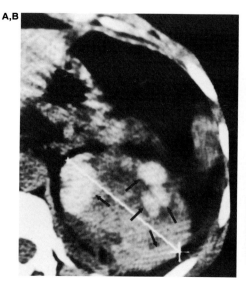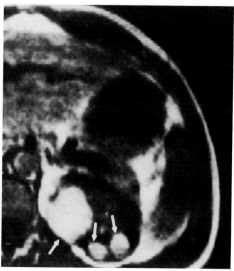

FIG. 68. Indeterminate masses due to hemorrhage into renal cysts. **A:** Noncontrast CT image shows an enlarged left kidney, with multiple round, high-attenuation lesions (*arrows*). **B:** MRI (TR = 500 msec, TE = 17 msec) at a slightly different level shows multiple round, high-intensity lesions (*arrows*). A T2-weighted MR image also demonstrated these lesions to have extremely high signal intensity, compatible with hemorrhagic fluid.

incorrect ring size, lack of or inappropriate use of intra-venous contrast material (i.e., nonbolus infusion), and artifactual density measurements. Most masses for which technically indeterminate CT images prevent a definitive diagnosis will be renal cysts, resolvable by repeat CT, ultrasound with aspiration, or MRI. Those considered truly indeterminate or possibly solid after other imaging tests must be considered surgical lesions.

On technically adequate, contrast-enhanced CT images, cyst-like renal masses may still be considered indeterminate by CT criteria alone. Causes include (a) a uniformly thick wall, (b) calcification involving the septae, the entire thickened wall, or portions of it, where the contents of the "cystic mass" consist of homogeneous, low-density, presumably fluid material, (c) numerous strands or septations inside the cysts, (d) high attenuation of the cyst contents (20–60 HU or more), (e) irregular contour, parenchymal interface, or delineation from adjacent structures, and (f) variable or poor contrast enhancement (154) (see Figs. 20, 21, 29, 30, 68, and 69).

The presence of one or more noncystic features increases the likelihood of malignancy; therefore, confirmatory or complementary imaging procedures may be required. Thick walls, high attenuation, and indistinct interfaces are common features resulting in an indeterminate CT diagnosis in this group (category II) of lesions (6). Although lesions in this group may not be enhanced after administration of contrast material, they may be better defined; so contrast enhancement is essential to their evaluation. Some of the indeterminate masses in this group will be abscesses, but a large proportion will be benign or malignant cystic neoplasms or complicated (hemorrhagic) cysts (see Fig. 18). Angiography usually is

not contributory in this group of lesions, but ultrasound with aspiration or biopsy has been most helpful in our experience. On rare occasions, MRI may provide confirmatory evidence that the indeterminate mass is predominantly fluid-filled (131).

The last category of CT indeterminacy, category III, involves masses that closely resemble neoplasms and are likely solid, but exhibit confusing CT features. These may be large, complex renal masses with ill-defined contours, sometimes extending beyond the expected renal confines or diffusely infiltrating and enlarging the kidney. Often the extent of involvement, hemorrhagic or otherwise, of the perinephric spaces is out of proportion to the size of the suspected intrarenal tumor. Irregular postcontrast enhancement or inhomogeneous precontrast attenuation measurements are common findings. Secondary features such as renal vein invasion and lymph node involvement may be absent. Adrenal enlargement may be present on the ipsilateral or contralateral side, raising the possibility of coincidental adrenal adenoma or metastases. Large percentages of such lesions in our experience have been xanthogranulomatous pyelonephritis, renal cell carcinoma, or transitional cell carcinoma complicated by extensive perinephric hemorrhage or urinoma formation (6). Lesions in this category require surgical intervention or percutaneous biopsy. Angiography may be necessary for diagnosis of a small intrarenal primary neoplasm that has bled, or for "road-mapping" if renal-sparing surgery is considered. Routinely, however, angiography is rarely contributory to the preoperative diagnosis, and ultrasound may be indeterminate as well (43,132). MRI may be useful in differentiating between hemorrhagic collections and a neoplastic process, or for determining the organ of origin

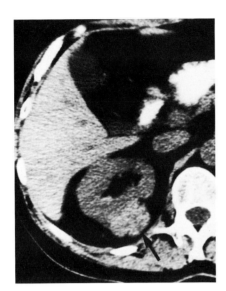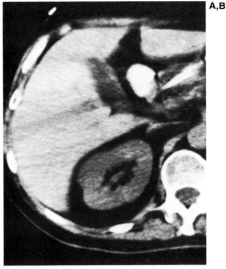

A,B

FIG. 69. Indeterminate renal mass (renal hematoma). **A:** There is a mass (*arrow*) protruding from the posterior surface of the right kidney. The mass has higher attenuation (hyperdense) than the normal renal parenchyma. **B:** A CT image at the same level done 3 months later demonstrates disappearance of the mass. Diagnosis: renal hematoma.

of a neoplasm. Biopsy or follow-up CT images may be useful to confirm the diagnosis and plan the surgical approach when a large amount of intrarenal or perinephric blood is present.

The diagnostic strategy for evaluating indeterminate renal masses is shown in Fig. 1 and is designed to provide information sufficient for the decision on nonoperative versus operative (radical versus conservative) management. The optimal approach will include the following: (a) repeat CT with and without contrast enhancement if technical problems exist, as well as consideration of ultrasound, MRI, or biopsy; (b) for a mass that is cyst-like, with only one or two of the dissonant features previously described, i.e., thick wall, one should consider ultrasound or needle-aspiration biopsy; (c) apparently solid, tumor-like masses with complex features deserve consideration for surgery. MRI, angiography, or biopsy may be considered if it will alter the surgical management toward a more conservative option. In Curry's series, if three or more noncystic criteria were present, even when lesions were not obviously solid, the predictive value for malignancy approached 96% (43). Renal infarcts or occult focal inflammatory disease (hemorrhagic acute focal bacterial nephritis) may account for false-positive diagnoses in this last group. MRI may be useful if specific features are seen as fluid–iron levels in hemorrhagic cysts, thus distinguishing these indeterminate masses from true carcinomas (90). However, in most instances, renal masses that are indeterminate on CT remain indeterminate after MRI. The same is true for angiography; in fact, its decreased use for CT-indeterminate renal masses is reflected in the marked decrease cost for evaluation of all renal masses because of the infrequent use of angiography and nephrotomography documented at the Mayo Clinic (232).

Calcified Renal Masses

Calcifications in a renal mass may occur in both benign and malignant conditions (127,219). Because CT has the ability to localize calcifications more accurately than other imaging techniques and to determine the cystic or solid nature of a renal mass, a distinction between benign and malignant categories of calcified renal masses is often possible (Fig. 70). Thus, not all calcified masses are indeterminate by CT criteria. Calcified renal masses fall mainly into three groups, based on CT features: (a) soft-tissue tumors, (b) cyst-like lesions with focal, mural, or septal calcification, and (c) indeterminate masses (6,43,219). The distinguishing feature of masses in the tumor group is calcification that is not truly peripheral in location (Fig. 71). There is almost always a soft-tissue component to the mass outside the confines of the calcium. Although the calcification may appear peripheral on conventional radiographs, it does not always truly define the perimeter of the mass on CT. Calcifications that are curvilinear, amorphous, punctate, or some combination thereof have been encountered. Although the diagnosis of calcified renal tumor often can be entertained on the basis of intravenous urography, CT confirms the diagnosis and provides further valuable staging information. Renal neoplasms that are calcified have a better prognosis than noncalcified lesions; so both the presence and the distribution of calcium are important for diagnosis and prognosis (111,216,219).

The major distinguishing features of cyst-like lesions include the absence of any soft-tissue mass and the presence of thick walls (focal or uniform) and a homogeneous, near-water-density center (fluid). The calcifications are largely curvilinear or punctate and focal, but they truly

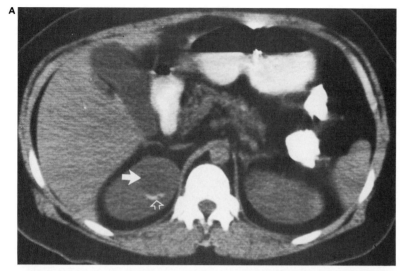

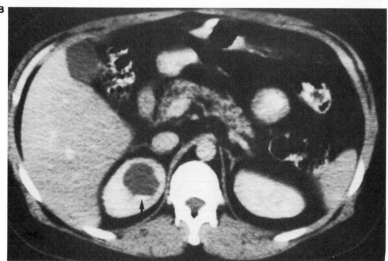

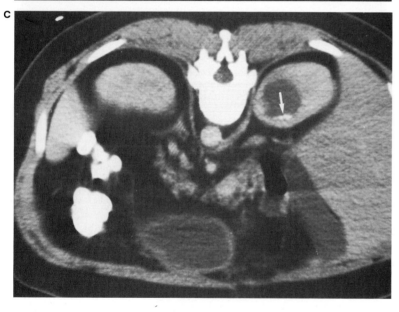

FIG. 70. Indeterminate renal mass, with a mobile calcification that simulated a calcified cyst wall. **A:** Precontrast CT image shows a low-attenuation lesion in the right kidney (*arrow*), with a calcification (*open arrow*) at the posterior rim of this lesion, suggesting calcification in the wall. **B:** CT image following intravenous administration of contrast material shows that the low-attenuation lesion has a slightly irregular wall, and the calcification appears to be in the posterior wall (*arrow*). **C:** Turning the patient prone resulted in shifting the calcification (*arrow*) to the anterior surface of this cyst.

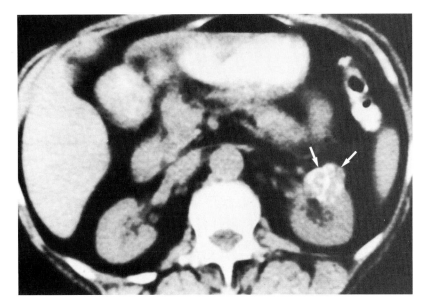

FIG. 71. Calcified papillary renal cell carcinoma. There is an irregular soft-tissue mass (*arrows*) with multiple central and peripheral calcifications arising from the anterolateral aspect of the left kidney.

are peripheral in the mass (219) (see Fig. 19). These lesions are typically benign. Although MRI is insensitive in detecting calcification, it has been helpful in confirming the "fluid" nature of these lesions in troublesome cases (131).

Hydatid cystic involvement of the kidney may give a CT appearance strikingly similar to that for the cyst-like calcified renal masses (group 2) (147). Echinococcosis is rare in the United States, but endemic in many parts of the world. CT accurately displays either the solitary or diffuse form of this disease, with daughter cysts (brood capsules) seen within larger cysts (89,107). The calcifications occur in the walls of the cysts, and the appearance usually is pathognomonic. Cyst walls may be thin or thick in this entity, and enhancement of the walls may be seen on CT. Attenuation values may be 10 to 20 HU higher than for typical benign cyst fluid (161).

Indeterminate calcified renal masses are those masses in which the calcification is but one indeterminate CT feature present. Occasionally the calcification is peripheral, but central attenuation values are higher than those for water density and more in the range of those for soft tissue.

Contrast enhancement may be minimal or nondetectable. This group of lesions comprises a wide spectrum of pathologic conditions, ranging from adenoma (oncocytoma) to papillary adenocarcinoma to hemorrhagic cysts (153). Other neoplasms that may calcify include adult Wilms's tumor (80), transitional cell carcinoma, squamous cell carcinoma, and metastases (4,114,188) (Fig. 72). Although aneurysms, AVMs and AVFs, or even angiomyolipomas may calcify and have CT appearances confusingly similar to those for calcified renal masses described herein, proper contrast-assisted CT usually allows a precise diagnosis of these conditions.

INFECTION

Acute Infection

When a patient presents with fever, chills, flank pain, and a focal mass or diffusely enlarged kidney as revealed by excretory urography, inflammatory disease must be

FIG. 72. Metastatic osteosarcoma. Precontrast CT image shows a round lesion involving the lateral aspect of the right kidney (*arrow*). The attenuation value of the lesion is similar to that of osseous structure.

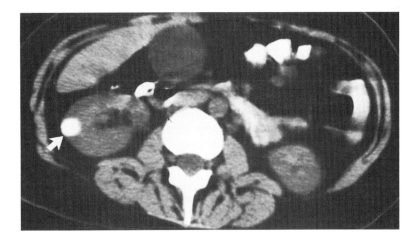

A

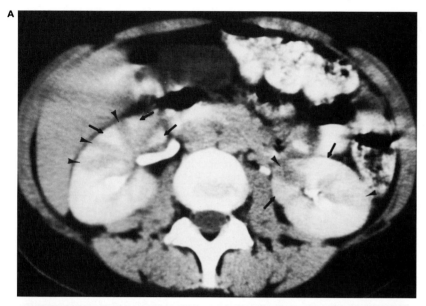

B

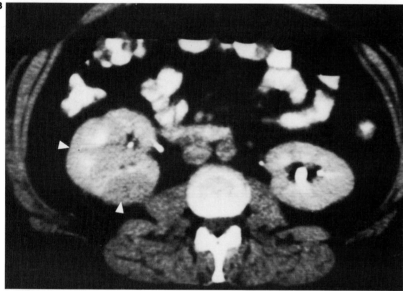

FIG. 73. Acute focal bacterial nephritis. **A:** Postcontrast CT image shows "patchy" enhancement (*arrows*) in both kidneys. Wedge-shaped areas of parenchyma that do not enhance (*arrowheads*) are involved by inflammation. **B:** Globular nature of some wedge-shaped areas (*arrowheads*) is noted in another patient.

strongly considered. Various terms have been used to describe this clinical entity, including pyelonephritis (acute, focal, or suppurative), acute bacterial nephritis (focal or diffuse), and acute lobar nephronia (7,120,218,230). The renal pathophysiology is due to interstitial edema and intense vasoconstriction that may be "patchy" in a lobar distribution (69,174) (Fig. 73). Although most patients with acute pyelonephritis do not require any radiographic examination, they may be referred for a CT study to exclude the possibility of renal or perirenal abscess.

On CT, the kidneys may be diffusely enlarged. The involved kidney usually is of normal attenuation value on noncontrast CT studies; it may contain areas of lower density due to edema. Gas may be seen in the collecting system or the interstitium or both in cases of emphysematous pyelonephritis (95,151,214) (Fig. 74). After intravenous administration of contrast material, one or more wedge-shaped, poorly enhancing or nonenhancing areas

may be seen initially. These nonenhanced areas may slowly fill with contrast material, resulting in persistent hyperdensity on delayed CT images, occasionally up to 24 hr. Additional CT findings include loss of corticomedullary junction definition, obliteration of renal sinus fat, and caliceal distortion.

Although acute pyelonephritis usually causes enlargement of the entire kidney, it may, on occasion, result in a focal mass or masses. Acute focal bacterial nephritis (AFBN) best describes the early, more edematous or solid phase of focal renal infection caused most commonly by a Gram-negative organism. The CT appearance of AFBN is similar to that of acute pyelonephritis, except that the abnormality is more focal in the former.

The CT features of an uncommon form of AFBN, hemorrhagic AFBN, may include focal wedge-shaped areas of increased attenuation on noncontrast images. These areas are thought to be due to different stages of

A,B

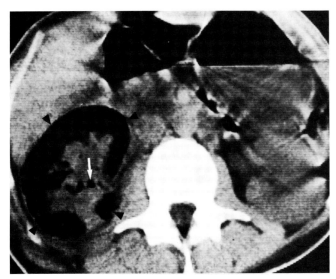 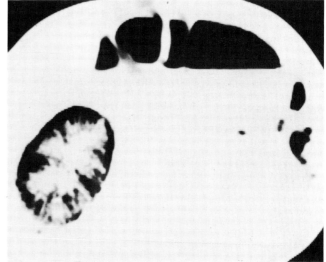

FIG. 74. Emphysematous pyelonephritis. **A:** CT image shows intrarenal (*arrow*) and subcapsular (*arrowheads*) gas. **B:** The same image as in (**A**), but at lung windows, redemonstrates diffuse gaseous involvement of right kidney. (Courtesy of Dr. Gaston Morillo.)

hemorrhage caused by infection and venous congestion (18,22).

MRI remains an adjunctive imaging procedure for evaluation of focal or diffuse inflammatory renal disease, largely because of its limited spatial resolution and only limited experience with renal contrast enhancement, e.g. gadolinium.

Abscess

Whereas acute pyelonephritis can be adequately treated with antibiotics alone, resulting in complete resolution in most instances, it may, on rare occasion, progress into an abscess cavity, and these frequently require percutaneous or surgical drainage. An abscess can also develop from infection of a preexisting renal cyst (18,22). Renal abscesses may project beyond the normal contour of the kidney or be totally intrarenal in location (22) (Figs. 75 and 76). The CT picture of a renal abscess typically is a well-defined mass of lower density than normal renal-parenchyma, having a thick, slightly irregular, and occasionally enhancing wall. No central contrast enhancement is seen. CT demonstration of gas, present in only a small percentage of patients, virtually assures the diagnosis of an abscess (Fig. 77). In the absence of gas bubbles, an abscess may mimic a necrotic renal neoplasm. Other inflammatory processes that may present with focal CT findings or an abscess-like appearance include tuberculosis, fungal infection (candidiasis), actinomycosis, and brucellosis (45,48,60,70,106,162,186).

Renal tuberculosis, which is infrequently seen in the United States, may have a variety of CT appearances, depending on the severity of the disease. Kidney size may be normal, or large if hydronephrosis is present, or small

with or without focal calcification. Enhancement after contrast-material administration, which is a gross reflection of renal function, may be poor depending on the degree of parenchymal destruction. Rim enhancement of hydronephrotic segments may be a transient finding. Caliceal, pelvic, or ureteric narrowing (strictures) may cause secondary dilatation. Low-density areas have been described representing hydrocalices containing caseous material or representing focal parenchymal caseous necrosis (45,162). Milk of calcium may exist within the obstructed portions of the kidney (205). Ureteric calcification not visible on intravenous urography may be noted on CT. Renal scarring and perinephric extension may be observed, and these findings often are only unilateral. The

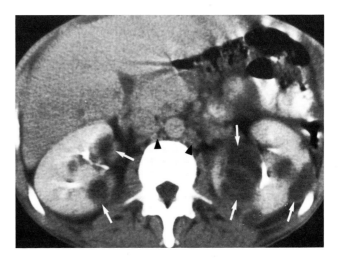

FIG. 75. Renal abscesses due to *Nocardia*. Postcontrast CT image shows multiple nonenhancing round areas (*arrows*) in both kidneys. These represent focal nocardial abscesses. Also noted is paraaortic adenopathy (*arrowheads*). (Courtesy of Dr. Gaston Morillo.)

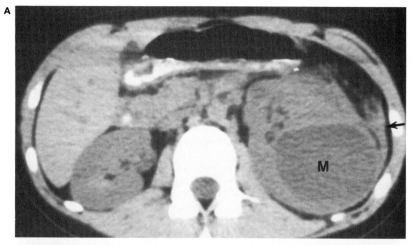

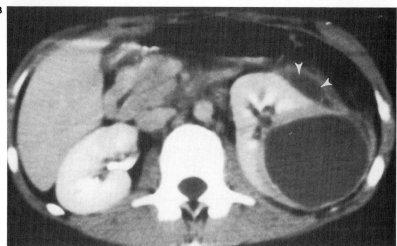

FIG. 76. Renal abscess with perirenal extension. **A:** Noncontrast-enhanced CT image shows a large, low-density mass (M) in the left kidney. Thickening of renal fascia (*arrow*) anterolaterally is present. **B:** After intravenous administration of contrast material, a slightly enhanced thick wall is seen. The center of the mass remains unenhanced. Perinephric collection is seen anterior to kidney (*arrowheads*). **C:** Two centimeters caudal to (**B**), a perirenal collection (*arrowheads*) and the thickening of renal fascia (*arrow*) are again noted.

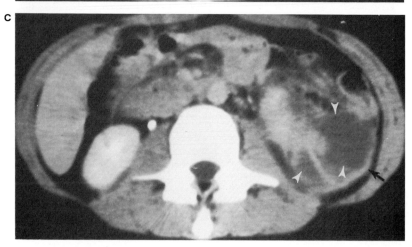

CT manifestations of tuberculosis are protean and frequently are observed late, but their appearance may be helpful in supporting a urographic diagnosis when persistent pyuria exists (Fig. 78).

Chronic Infection

The characteristic changes of chronic pyelonephritis seen with urography are also readily identified using CT imaging (Fig. 77). The focal parenchymal scars with underlying caliceal distortion or more global shrinkage with irregular contours are hallmarks of chronic inflammation (168).

Xanthogranulomatous pyelonephritis (XGPN) is an interesting pathologic condition that results from chronic infection in an obstructed kidney (71). Focal involvement, so-called tumefactive XGPN, and renal pelvic involvement may occur (88,213). The usual CT appearance of XGPN includes the following: (a) a large central calculus

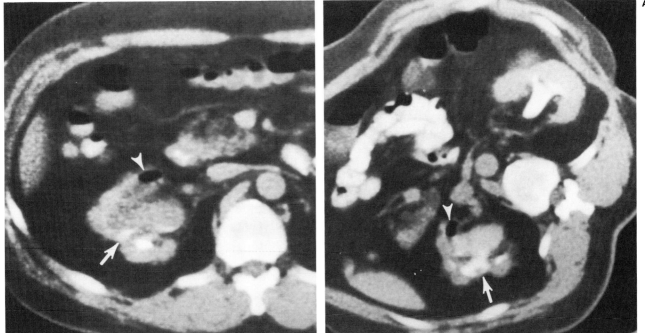

FIG. 77. Chronic atrophic pyelonephritis, with acute exacerbation. **A:** Precontrast supine CT image shows a small and irregular right kidney, with deep cortical scar (*arrow*) posterolaterally, compatible with chronic atrophic pyelonephritis. In addition, a gas bubble (*arrowhead*) is seen within the dilated pyelocaliceal system, indicative of an acute infectious process caused by gas-forming organisms. **B:** Image obtained with patient in right lateral decubitus position confirms the gas bubble (*arrowhead*) to be within a dilated calix. *Arrow* points to the deep cortical scar and blunted calix.

(staghorn) occupying most of the renal pelvis and collecting system; (b) poor or no excretion of contrast material (global or focal); (c) multiple nonenhancing round areas within the renal contour, with attenuation values higher than that for urine, and arranged radially, corresponding to dilated calices; (d) discrete solid masses, representing enlarged coalescent inflammatory infiltrates (granulomatous masses); (e) frequent perinephric involvement (71,88,213) (Fig. 79). XGPN can be locally aggressive and may present with gas-containing intrarenal abscesses. This is not to be confused with emphysematous pyelonephritis, which presents a different CT picture, including gas within the collecting system and in the surrounding perirenal spaces (178) (Fig. 74). Pyohydronephrosis may mimic XGPN, and only pathologic evaluation will reveal the typical inflammatory changes and lipid-laden macrophages of XGPN. Although XGPN has not been shown to be a predisposing factor, concomitant XGPN and renal cell carcinoma have been reported (187).

Because XGPN may be focal, renal-sparing surgery can be performed if the disease is suitably staged. A staging system has been suggested similar to the staging criteria

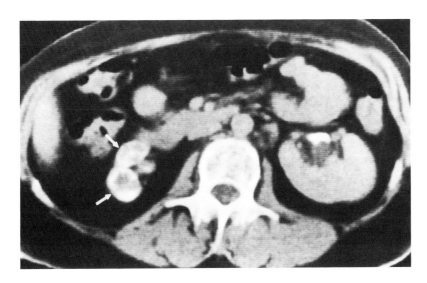

FIG. 78. End-stage renal tuberculosis. Postcontrast CT image shows a small nonfunctioning right kidney with rim calcifications (*arrows*). Diagnosis: autonephrectomy (putty kidney).

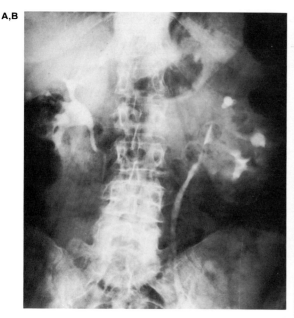

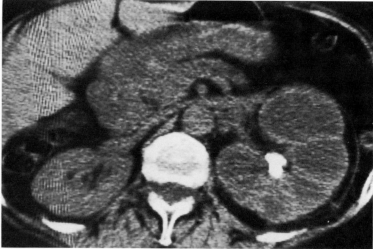

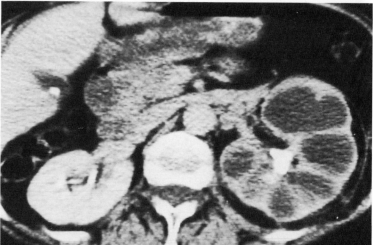

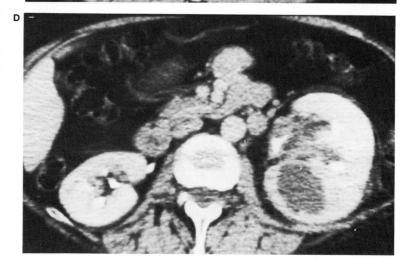

FIG. 79. Focal xanthogranulomatous pyelonephritis. **A:** IVU shows an enlarged left kidney, with distorted renal collecting system and absence of the upper-pole collecting system. **B:** Noncontrast CT image shows a central calculus within a hydronephrotic-appearing left kidney. **C:** Postcontrast CT image shows the hydronephrosis more clearly. **D:** A more caudal image shows the junction of the hydronephrotic upper pole with the more normal lower pole of the left kidney.

for renal cell carcinoma. CT can precisely define the full extent of XGPN and assist in the planning of surgical therapy.

Excessive proliferation of fat, both within the renal sinus and around the kidney, may be observed on CT and may be due to a chronic inflammatory stimulus (75,202,211).

Total renal replacement by fatty tissue, with some fibrous components, has been described in patients with staghorn or branched calculi. Frequently this is seen in conjunction with XGPN, and CT optimally displays the calculus and surrounding fat (Fig. 80).

Other chronic renal infections include malacoplakia,

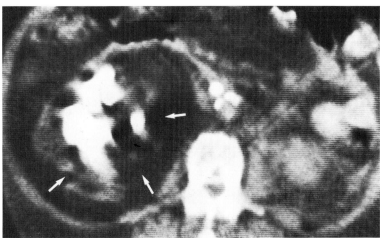

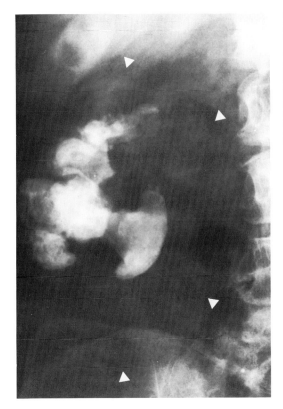

A,B

FIG. 80. Fatty replacement of the kidney. **A:** Plain radiograph shows a staghorn calculus within a surrounding envelope of fat (*arrowheads*). **B:** CT image shows parenchymal replacement by fat. The staghorn calculus is in an enlarged (fatty-replaced) kidney (*arrows*). The perinephric fat has also proliferated.

megalocytic interstitial nephritis, brucellosis, and fungal diseases, but CT reports of these entities are rare. Chronic hydatid infections have already been mentioned.

Juxtarenal Processes

Many of the disease processes that involve the juxtarenal areas begin as primary renal processes, and CT often can reveal the origin and nature of these processes (126). The various fascial boundaries to the kidney are illustrated in Chapter 11, and they divide the retroperitoneal area at the renal level into three separate compartments: an anterior pararenal space, a perirenal space, and a posterior pararenal space. The perirenal and posterior pararenal spaces typically are filled with fat, whereas the anterior pararenal space is only a potential space. The bridging reno-renal septae, described in the section under normal anatomy, may serve to limit the spread of diseases. Processes that frequently affect the extraperitoneal pararenal spaces are hemorrhage, infection, urine or lymph extravasation (lymphocele), fat deposition, pancreatic effusions (pseudocysts) (Fig. 81), and primary tumors (tumors of mesenchymal origin) and metastases (e.g., cervix and melanoma) (64,72,190–2,194,196).

Hemorrhage

Hemorrhage into the perirenal or posterior pararenal spaces may be extensive without showing any significant

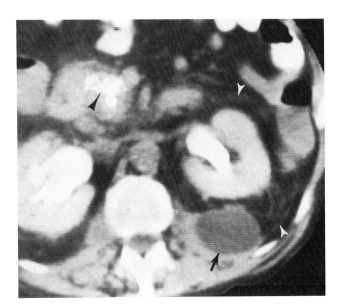

FIG. 81. Pancreatic pseudocyst involving posterior pararenal space. A low-density mass (*arrow*) abuts the left psoas and quadratus lumborum muscles and displaces the left kidney anteriorly. This mass was traced to be contiguous with the pancreas on more cephalic images. Also note a cluster of calcifications (*black arrowhead*) within the pancreatic head and thickening of the renal fascia (*white arrowheads*). (Courtesy of Dr. George Wilson.)

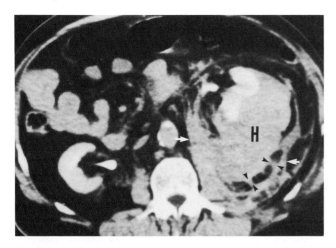

FIG. 82. Perinephric hemorrhage. CT image with intravenous contrast material shows subcapsular mass due to hemorrhage (H), with extension into the perinephric space (*arrows*). There is thickening of the bridging renal septae (*arrowheads*).

change on plain abdominal radiographs or intravenous urography (181,196). Acute hemorrhage typically measures 60 to 80 HU, whereas more chronic or subacute hematomas may measure 10 to 40 HU. Whereas hematomas less than 24 hr of age have a low signal intensity on T1-weighted MR images, subacute and chronic hematomas have a high signal intensity. A more detailed discussion of MRI features of hematoma can be found in Chapter 16. A hematoma may be only subcapsular, perinephric, or paranephric, but usually a combination occurs (Fig. 82). The extent is determined by the perinephric fascial investments (Gerota's fascia) and by the presence or extent of the bridging reno-renal septae. Correct identification of the location of the blood, e.g., subcapsular or perinephric, may well be determined by the degree to which the bridging septa and/or the renal capsule become effective barriers to bleeding or boundary-forming structures.

Trauma, either blunt or penetrating, is the most common cause of hemorrhage into the juxtarenal spaces. Penetrating injuries, including renal biopsy and percutaneous nephrolithotomy, result in hematoma formation in the perinephric space and posterior pararenal space overlying the puncture site (176). Subcapsular collections are less frequently seen with penetrating trauma. Other causes of perirenal hemorrhage include arteritis, interstitial nephritis (lupus), acquired cystic disease of dialysis, anticoagulation, small renal tumors, and extracorporeal shock-wave lithotripsy.

Although most abdominal aortic aneurysms rupture into the perirenal spaces or psoas compartments, blood under pressure may dissect into the anterior pararenal space or within the anterior pararenal fascia (2,183). Extravasated blood mixed with urine or extravasated contrast material may result in a confusing CT appearance, thus obscuring the underlying cause of hemorrhage, i.e., renal neoplasm.

Urinoma

Urine extravasation into the perirenal spaces can occur spontaneously, secondary to urinary tract obstruction, after renal trauma, after ureterorenoscopic or percutaneous manipulation, and after extracorporeal shock-wave lithotripsy (144). CT is superior to intravenous urography or ultrasound for defining size, location, and cause of urinoma formation (51,144). Urinomas usually are of low density, with attenuation values ranging from −10 to +20 HU. They are of low signal intensity on T1-weighted images and high signal intensity on T2-weighted images. Long-standing urinomas may have well-defined walls, some with calcification, and their CT appearance may mimic that of a chronic hematoma or seroma, abscess, retroperitoneal cyst, or lymphocele.

Abscess

A number of conditions predispose to perinephric inflammatory disease, most of which are extensions of underlying renal disease (146,191) (Fig. 83). Although usually confined within Gerota's fascia, aggressive infections may break down existing fascial barriers and involve contiguous spaces and organs. Patients with diabetes mellitus, stone disease, renal obstruction, congenital anomalies, and polycystic kidney disease are prone to perinephric abscess formation, but perinephric abscesses most frequently occur when there is a concomitant renal abscess. Other local inflammatory conditions, such as diverticulitis or appendicitis, may spread to the perinephric space, and hematogenous cause for perinephric abscess may also be found, but is rare today. Pancreatic abscesses, pseudocyst formation, and even thoracic inflammatory processes may likewise present or extend into the perinephric space (10,194) (Fig. 81). Gram-negative enteric organisms are common etiologic agents, but amebic and fungal infections may also occur (191). Perinephric abscesses are most common on the right side, and CT is regarded as the best imaging test for displaying the complete extent of a perinephric inflammatory process.

The CT and MRI appearances of a perinephric abscess are similar to those for abscesses elsewhere. It usually has a low density on CT and a mixed signal intensity on MRI. The abscess often insinuates itself throughout the perinephric spaces, often with thick, irregular walls. The walls may be enhanced, but unless gas is present within the abscess itself, it cannot always be differentiated from a hematoma, a urinoma, or a necrotic neoplasm (Fig. 84). In addition to a dominant mass, often there is thickening of Gerota's fascia, as well as strands or webs of soft-tissue density within the perinephric space. CT has made the previously difficult diagnosis of perinephric abscess a more common event, and CT is used to direct management, which most often is percutaneous catheter drainage. Small

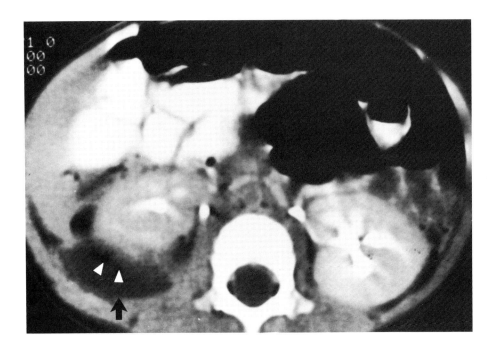

FIG. 83. Perinephric abscess. There is a low-attenuation fluid collection (*arrow*) with gas (*arrowheads*) in the perinephric space. (Courtesy of Dr. Gaston Morillo.)

perinephric extensions of largely intrarenal abscesses often may be effectively treated with intravenous antibiotics alone.

Neoplasms

Tumors arising in the perinephric spaces (renal capsular neoplasms) often present diagnostic difficulties, because their CT appearance may resemble that of aggressive renal cell carcinoma, carcinosarcomas, primary extrarenal lymphoma, or local metastases (e.g., adrenal) (49,222). The posterior perinephric and pararenal spaces may contain a large amount of fat; therefore, liposarcoma is the most common capsular or perinephric neoplasm of mesenchymal origin (49,72,222) (Fig. 84). Some authors have defined the renal capsule in general terms as the renal fascial investments and the fat contained therein. More

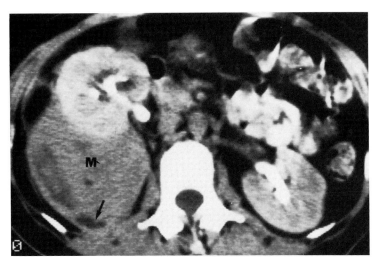

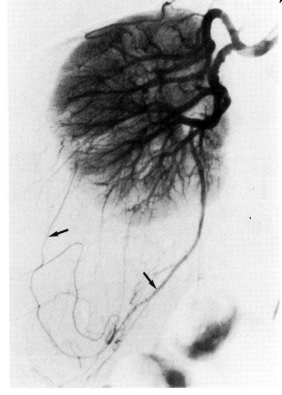

A,B

FIG. 84. Primary liposarcoma of the perinephric space. **A:** CT image shows a large mass (M) growing off the posterior surface of the right kidney. It is not distorting the collecting system. The mass has fat-density material within it (*arrow*). **B:** Subtraction angiogram shows feeding capsular arteries (*arrows*). (Courtesy of Dr. George Leopold.)

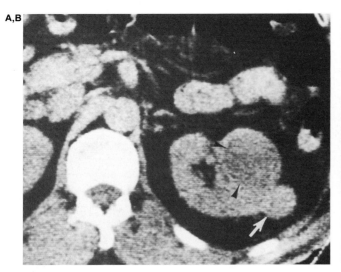
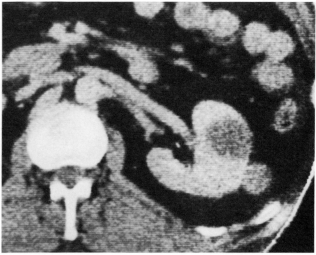

FIG. 85. Renal capsular fibroma. **A:** Precontrast CT image shows a well-circumscribed 2-cm mass (*arrow*) arising from the posterolateral surface of the left kidney. The mass has the same attenuation value as the normal renal parenchyma. In addition, an intrarenal cyst (*arrowheads*) is present in the lateral aspect of the kidney, which is partial-volume-averaged. **B:** Postcontrast image demonstrates the cyst to a better degree. The cyst was not enhanced; the fibroma was enhanced to a lesser extent than normal renal parenchyma.

specifically, the renal capsule is a densely adherent, fibrous covering to the renal parenchyma. Although malignant tumors (mesenchymal sarcomas) tend to dominate the list of so-called capsular neoplasms, benign tumors such as fibromas do occur (Fig. 85).

Typical CT features of juxtarenal mesenchymal sarcomas may include (a) inward displacement of renal parenchyma, with smooth interfaces (although the tumor–parenchyma interface may be indistinct on transaxial CT slices), (b) enlarged capsular collateral vessels, (c) little or no contrast enhancement, and (d) large tumors that displace rather than invade local structures. The CT appearance of a liposarcoma correlates with the gross and histologic features of the tumor (222). Liposarcomas that are well differentiated may look like benign lipomas.

Myxoid liposarcomas contain a fibrous stroma and may have mixed or soft-tissue attenuation values on CT. Similar CT patterns may exist for other primary perinephric neoplasms, such as fibrous histiocytoma, leiomyosarcoma, angiosarcoma, neuroblastoma, and lymphoma (72). CT often suggests a primary extrarenal origin for the tumor, and MRI may play a valuable adjunctive imaging role for determining the organ or site of origin when a large, bulky tumor is present, showing it clearly in coronal and sagittal planes (222).

Renal Failure

Renal evaluation using CT to determine size, shape, location, number, and calcification of kidneys in azotemic

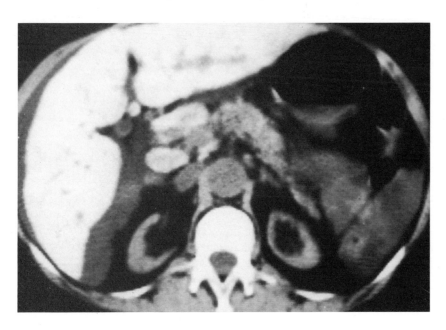

FIG. 86. End-stage renal disease, with secondary hemochromatosis. Bilateral shrunken kidneys are noted in this adult with severe renal failure and hemochromatosis. The increased attenuation of the liver is due to hemochromatosis. The marked diminution of kidney size implies irreversibility and chronicity. Ascites is present.

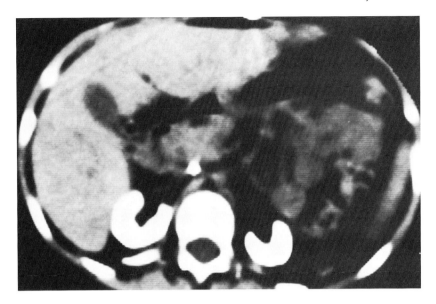

FIG. 87. Oxalosis. Both kidneys are small and densely calcified because of oxalosis.

patients is feasible in virtually all patients (Fig. 86). However, high-resolution real-time ultrasound is the procedure of choice for differentiating between obstructive uropathy and intrinsic renal parenchymal disease (134,217). CT usually is reserved for cases in which ultrasound is technically unsuccessful because of extreme obesity or in which ultrasound cannot define the level and cause of the urinary tract obstruction (61). CT diagnosis of hydronephrosis can be made without the use of intravenous contrast material, although it is easier with contrast-enhanced CT images (21,134). A small dose (10–20 cc) of a low osmolality agent may be all that is required to distinguish parenchyma from dilated calices. Extra-renal pelves, dilated calices secondary to postobstructive atrophy, and parapelvic cysts may account for a false-positive diagnosis of hydronephrosis. On non-contrast-enhanced images, the dilated urine-filled calices appear as low-attenuation fluid-density structures within the normal or enlarged renal silhouette. High-density urine in obstructed systems may be nearly isodense with parenchyma. This is commonly encountered in pyonephrosis. A "reverse-layering" effect may occur that is due to high-density (attenuation) urine laden with products of infection that rise to the top of a dilated calix or ureter, causing the appearance of a fluid–fluid level, but with a high-attenuation substance on the top and regular urine on the bottom. Typically, enhanced urine containing contrast material layers posteriorly on supine CT images.

In cases of obstruction, a faint nephrogram and pyelogram may be more apparent on contrast-enhanced CT than with conventional urography. The obstructive nephrogram may persist for several hours if delayed CT images are performed. Persistent nephrograms may also be seen in patients with acute renal failure from a variety of nonobstructive causes, including acute glomerulonephritis, leukemia, acute tubular necrosis (ATN), infection, and trauma (129). Parenchymal thickness can be assessed, thus providing valuable information on potential salvageability

and appropriate intervention, i.e., CT-guided drainage. Although MRI can similarly reveal the site and cause of obstructive uropathy, it is rarely needed for such a purpose.

In addition to hydronephrosis, various renal parenchymal diseases that result in impaired renal function or end-stage renal disease have been evaluated with CT. Chronic pyelonephritis results in an irregular renal contour, with cortical scarring and caliceal distortion, whereas renal ischemia may lead to small, smooth kidneys. Chronic glomerulonephritis, advanced tuberculosis, and acquired cystic disease with or without dialysis will lead to small, sometimes calcified, kidneys. Calcification may be focal, diffuse, medullary, or cortical in cases of oxalosis, AIDS with superinfection, e.g., *Mycobacterium avium,* and acute cortical necrosis (16,116,193) (Fig. 87). Nephrocalcinosis may mimic acute cortical necrosis on CT images, but variations in window setting and image collimation should allow correct diagnosis (169,193,203).

Acute intrarenal hemorrhage and hypercalciuric states may cause confusing high-attenuation appearances on non-contrast-enhanced CT images of the kidney (42). Serial CT images or MRI to rule out bleeding may be necessary. The CT finding of small end-stage kidneys implies irreversibility and often terminates the imaging evaluation of an azotemic patient (Fig. 88).

Renal Transplants

Evaluation of renal allografts for known or suspected complications has relied on radionuclide imaging for determination of flow and function. Doppler ultrasound is the preferred adjunctive imaging study to radionuclide evaluation for the diagnosis of rejection (201). CT has been reserved for cases in which ultrasound has been unsuccessful in evaluating peritransplant collections and hydronephrosis or in which an open wound or bowel gas

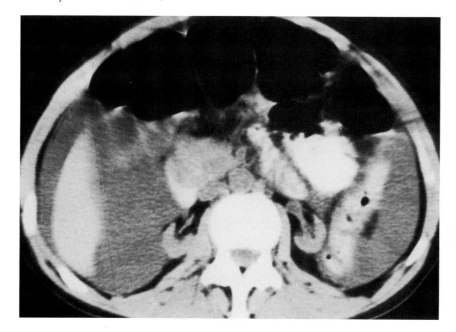

FIG. 88. End-stage renal disease. Bilateral shrunken kidneys are noted in this patient with severe renal failure. The marked diminution of kidney size implies irreversibility and chronicity. Marked ascites is present.

has precluded an adequate ultrasound examination (41,63,112). CT is able to distinguish acute hematoma, urinoma, lymphocele, or abscess, but gas in an abscess must be differentiated from residual postoperative gas (15,141,150) (Fig. 89).

MRI can be used to evaluate ATN, cyclosporin toxicity, and acute rejection. Although the corticomedullary differentiation is well preserved on T1-weighted images in cases of ATN and cyclosporin toxicity, it is often obscured or absent in cases of acute rejection (12,93,94,172) (Fig. 90). A decrease in the number of cortical vessels seen on MRI is another indication of acute rejection (12). However, neither of these two MRI features is absolutely sensitive or specific (12,77,93,94,210). Furthermore, these MRI changes may persist even after the patient has clin-

ically returned to normal. Although the accuracy of MRI in differentiating between ATN and acute rejection is still being determined, the expense and limited availability of MRI have made it unsuitable for use as a screening procedure. Doppler ultrasound and radionuclide studies provide equivalent, more economical, and more readily available information regarding the renal allografts.

Renal Trauma

Trauma to the kidney as an isolated event, or more frequently as a concomitant injury in patients with blunt abdominal trauma, is a daily occurrence. Motor vehicle accidents account for a large number of cases, and patients

A,B

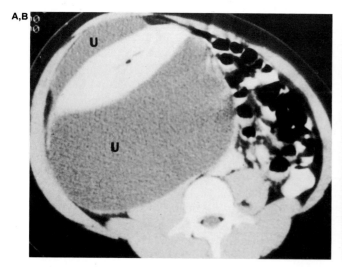
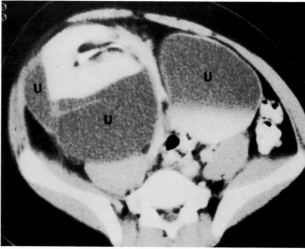

FIG. 89. Renal transplant complication. A transplant kidney is being displaced anteriorly and compressed by several urinomas (U). (Courtesy of Dr. Joel Sigeti.)

A,B

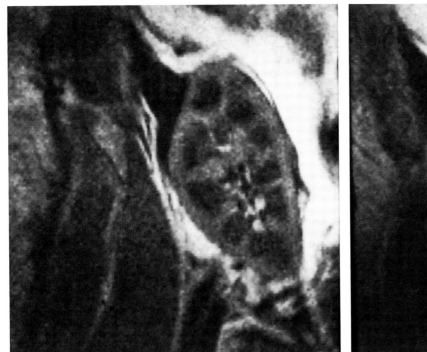
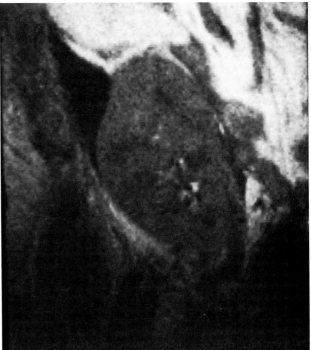

FIG. 90. Acute rejection of renal transplant: MRI demonstration. **A:** Coronal MRI performed on 9/25/87 (TR = 300 msec, TE = 15 msec) shows normal corticomedullary differentiation. **B:** A repeat study on 10/2/87 (TR = 500 msec, TE – 15 msec) shows loss of the corticomedullary differentiation. Histologic examination of the biopsy specimen revealed acute rejection.

in the young age groups are frequently the victims. Although most renal trauma is blunt, resulting in renal contusion, penetrating abdominal injuries occur that require accurate radiologic evaluation and prompt management (Fig. 91). Whereas unstable patients with penetrating abdominal or retroperitoneal injuries often require immediate surgical intervention, with a minimal radiologic evaluation, accurate assessment of the type and extent of renal injury is recommended in stable patients (29,54,55,149,173) (Fig. 92). In patients who suffer only minor trauma and are clinically stable, excretory urography with tomography may be all that is required for satisfactory patient management. However, in patients with unsatisfactory findings on urogram or labile clinical conditions, i.e., persistent hematuria or declining hematocrit, a CT examination should be the next imaging study considered. Overall, CT is more sensitive, specific, and accurate than urography for evaluating renal trauma (149,200). Extravasation of urine may be detected with CT when not visible on conventional urography. Preexisting renal tumors that may be masked on urography by extensive renal/perirenal hemorrhage after blunt trauma may be seen on CT. With dynamic contrast-enhanced CT, renal pedicle injuries can be imaged (84,200). Likewise, parenchymal contusion, which often appears as an area of diminished enhancement, and perirenal and intrarenal hematuria all can be detected by CT. Other associated abdominal injuries, particularly hepatic, splenic, and retroperitoneal, often are optimally displayed as well.

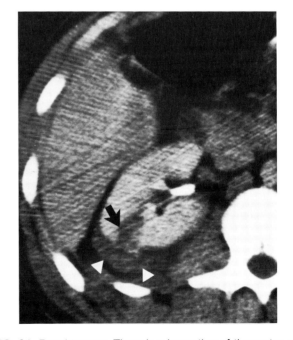

FIG. 91. Renal trauma. There is a laceration of the cortex of the right kidney (*arrow*) following a stab wound. Perinephric hematoma is also present (*arrowheads*).

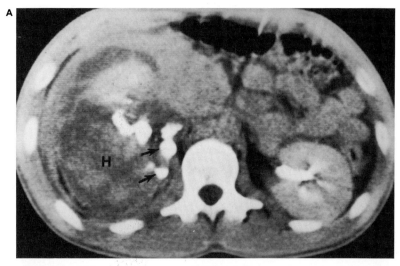

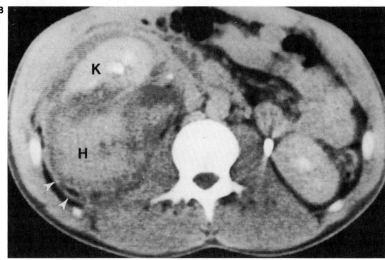

FIG. 92. Renal trauma. **A:** Postcontrast CT image demonstrates a large hematourinoma (H) from fracture through midpole of the right kidney. Extravasation of contrast material (*arrows*) is seen. The patient was in stable condition and was treated conservatively. **B:** Two centimeters caudal, a large hematoma (H) is noted, with thickening of the renal fascia (*arrowheads*). The remaining normal right kidney (K) is displaced anteriorly by the hematoma.

Other imaging studies also have been used to evaluate patients with renal trauma. Although Doppler ultrasound is capable of revealing the integrity of renal vessels and detecting renal/perirenal hematoma, it is inferior to CT in depicting extension into other retroperitoneal spaces. The restrictive environment of many MRI units precludes a significant role for MRI in the seriously injured patient.

REFERENCES

1. Alter AJ, Uchling DT, Zwiebel WJ. Computed tomography of the retroperitoneum following nephrectomy. *Radiology* 1979;133:663–668.
2. Amendola MA, Tisnado J, Fields WR, et al. Evaluation of retroperitoneal hemorrhage by computed tomography before and after translumbar aortography. *Radiology* 1979;133:401–404.
3. Andersen BL, Lauver JW, Ross P, Fitzgerald RH. Demonstration of radiation nephritis by computed tomography. *Comput Radiol* 1982;6:187–191.
4. Ayers R, Curry NS, Gordon L, Bradford BF. Renal metastases from osteogenic sarcoma. *Urol Radiol* 1985;7:39–41.
5. Balfe DM, McClennan BL, AufderHeide J. Multimodal imaging in evaluation of two cases of adenocarcinoma of the renal pelvis. *Urol Radiol* 1981;3:19–23.
6. Balfe DM, McClennan BL, Stanley RJ, Weyman PJ, Sagel SS. Evaluation of renal masses considered indeterminate on computed tomography. *Radiology* 1982;142:421–428.
7. Balfe DM, Stanley RJ, McClennan BL. The CT spectrum of renal inflammatory disease. In: Siegelman S, Gatewood O, Goldman S, eds. *Computed tomography of the kidney and adrenals.* New York: Churchill-Livingstone, 1984;167–188.
8. Ball DS, Friedman AC, Hartman DS, Radecki PD, Caroline DF. Scar sign of renal oncocytoma: magnetic resonance imaging appearance and lack of specificity. *Urol Radiol* 1986;8:46–48.
9. Banner MP, Pollack HM, Chatten J, Witzleben C. Multilocular renal cysts: radiologic-pathologic correlation. *AJR* 1981;136:239–247.
10. Barlaza GS, Kuhns LR, Siegel RS, Rapp R. The posterior pararenal space: an escape route for retrocrural masses. *J Comput Assist Tomogr* 1979;3:470–473.
11. Baron RL, McClennan BL, Lee JKT, Lawson T. Transitional cell carcinoma of the pelvis and ureter—CT evaluation. *Radiology* 1982;144:125–130.
12. Baumgartner BR, Nelson RC, Ball TI, et al. MR imaging of renal transplants. *AJR* 1986;147:949–953.
13. Bernardino ME, Chuang VP, Wallace S, Thomas JL, Soo CS. Therapeutically infarcted tumors: CT findings. *AJR* 1981;136:527–530.
14. Bernardino ME, deSantos LA, Johnson DE, Bracken RB. Computed tomography in the evaluation of post-nephrectomy patients. *Radiology* 1979;130:183–187.
15. Bia MJ, Baggish D, Katz L, Gonzalez R, Kliger AS, Rosenfield AT. Computed tomography in the diagnosis of pelvic abscesses in renal transplant patients. *JAMA* 1981;246:1435–1437.
16. Billimoria PE, Fabian TM, Schulz EE, Chase DR. Acquired renal oxalosis. *J Comput Assist Tomogr* 1983;7:158–160.
17. Bishop AF, Stanley RJ, Kissane JM, McClennan BL. Spontaneous hematuria and left renal enlargement in a young man. *Urol Radiol* 1982;4:52–56.

18. Borrero GO, Jafri SZ, Vazquez PM, Hollowell ML, Kling GA. Computed tomography of acute renal abscess due to *Salmonella*. *Comput Radiol* 1986;10:41–44.
19. Bosniak MA. Angiomyolipoma (hamartoma) of the kidney: a preoperative diagnosis is possible in virtually every case. *Urol Radiol* 1981;3:135–142.
20. Bosniak MA. The current radiological approach to renal cysts. *Radiology* 1986;158:1–10.
21. Bosniak MA, Megibow AJ, Ambos MA, Mitnick JS, Lefleur RS, Gordon R. Computed tomography and ureteral obstruction. *AJR* 1982;138:1107–1114.
22. Bova JG, Potter JL, Arevalos E, Hopens T, Goldstein HM, Radwin HM. Renal and perirenal infection: the role of computerized tomography. *J Urol* 1985;133:375–378.
23. Bracken B, Jonsson K. How accurate is angiographic staging of renal carcinoma? *Urology* 1979;14:96–99.
24. Breatnach ES, Stanley RJ, Lloyd K. Focal obstructive nephrogram: an unusual CT appearance of a transitional cell carcinoma. *J Comput Assist Tomogr* 1984;8:1019–1022.
25. Brennan RE, Curtis JA, Pollack HM, Weinberg I. Sequential changes in the CT numbers of the normal canine kidney following intravenous contrast administration. I. The renal cortex. *Invest Radiol* 1979;14:141–148.
26. Brennan RE, Curtis JA, Pollack HM, Weinberg I. Sequential II. The renal medulla. *Invest Radiol* 1979;14:239–245.
27. Brennan RE, Rapoport S, Weinberg I, Pollack HM, Curtis JA. CT-determined canine kidney and urine iodine concentrations following intravenous administration of sodium diatrizoate, metrizamide, iopamidol, and sodium ioxaglate. *Invest Radiol* 1982;17:95–100.
28. Bret PM, Bretagnolle M, Gaillard D, et al. Small, asymptomatic angiomyolipomas of the kidney. *Radiology* 1985;154:7–10.
29. Bretan PN, McAninch JW, Federle MP, Jeffrey RB. Computerized tomographic staging of renal trauma: 85 consecutive cases. *J Urol* 1986;136:561–565.
30. Burbank FH. Determinants of contrast enhancement for intravenous digital subtraction angiography. *Invest Radiol* 1983;18:308–316.
31. Burgener FA, Hamlin DJ. Contrast enhancement in abdominal CT: bolus vs. infusion. *AJR* 1981;137:351–358.
32. Buschi AJ, Harrison RB, Brenbridge ANAG, Williamson BRJ, Gentry RR, Cole R. Distended left renal vein: CT/sonographic normal variant. *AJR* 1980;135:339–342.
33. Carr DH, Brown J, Bydder GM, et al. Gadolinium-DTPA as a contrast agent in MRI: initial clinical experience in 20 patients. *AJR* 1984;143:215–224.
34. Cho C, Friedland GW, Swenson RS. Acquired renal cystic disease and renal neoplasms in hemodialysis patients. *Urol Radiol* 1984;6:153–157.
35. Cholankeril JV, Freundlich R, Ketyer S, Spirito AL, Napolitano J. Computed tomography in urothelial tumors of renal pelvis and related filling defects. *J Comput Assist Tomogr* 1986;10:263–272.
36. Christianson PJ, Clark MA, Meek J, Sharer W, Anclair PL, O'Connell KJ. Unusual case of dysgenetic renal cyst. *Urology* 1982;19:447–449.
37. Claussen CD, Banzer D, Pfretzschner C, Kalender WA, Schorner W. Bolus geometry and dynamics after intravenous contrast medium injection. *Radiology* 1984;153:365–368.
38. Cohan RH, Dunnick NR, Degesys GE, Korobkin M. Computed tomography of renal oncocytoma. *J Comput Assist Tomogr* 1984;8:284–287.
39. Coleman BG, Arger PH, Mintz MC, Pollack HM, Banner MP. Hyperdense renal masses. A computed tomographic dilemma. *AJR* 1983;143:291–294.
40. Curry NS, Brock JG, Metcalf JS, Sens MA. Hyperdense renal mass: unusual CT appearance of a benign renal cyst. *Urol Radiol* 1982;4:33–36.
41. Curry NS, Frangos DN, Tague DF. Computed tomography of end-stage renal transplant rejection. *J Comput Assist Tomogr* 1986;10:51–53.
42. Curry NS, Gordon L, Gobien RP, Lott M. Renal medullary "rings": a possible CT manifestation of hypercalcemia. *Urol Radiol* 1984;6:48–50.
43. Curry NS, Reinig J, Schabel SI, Ross P, Vujic I, Gobien RP. An evaluation of the effectiveness of CT vs. other imaging modalities in the diagnosis of atypical renal masses. *Invest Radiol* 1984;19:447–452.
44. Curry NS, Schabel SI, Bettsill WL. Small renal neoplasms: diagnostic imaging, pathologic features, and clinical course. *Radiology* 1986;158:113–117.
45. Dahlene DH, Stanley RJ, Koehler RE, Shin MS, Tishler JM. Abdominal tuberculosis: CT findings. *J Comput Assist Tomogr* 1984;8:443–445.
46. Dalton D, Neiman H, Grayhack JT. The natural history of simple renal cysts: a preliminary study. *J Urol* 1986;135:905–908.
47. Dean PB, Kivisaari L, Kormano M. Contrast enhancement pharmacokinetics of six ionic and nonionic contrast media. *Invest Radiol* 1983;18:368–374.
48. Denton AE. Computed tomographic findings in thoracic and renal actinomycosis: case report and review of literature. *J Am Osteopath Assoc* 1985;85:57–60.
49. Dooms GC, Hricak H, Sollitto RA, Higgins CB. Lipomatous tumors and tumors with fatty component: MR imaging potential and comparison of MR and CT results. *Radiology* 1985;157:479–483.
50. Dunnick NR, Korobkin M, Clark WM. CT demonstration of hyperdense renal carcinoma. *J Comput Assist Tomogr* 1984;8:1023–1024.
51. Dunnick NR, Long JA, Javadpour N. Perirenal extravasation of urographic contrast medium demonstrated by computed tomography. *J Comput Assist Tomogr* 1980;4:538–539.
52. Engelstad BL. Most promising MR contrast agents affect signal by enhancing relaxation. *Diagnostic Imaging* 1987;145–156.
53. Engelstad B, McClennan BL, Levitt RG. The role of precontrast images in CT of the kidney. *Radiology* 1980;136:153–155.
54. Erturk E, Sheinfeld J, DiMarco PL, Cockett ATK. Renal trauma: evaluation by computerized tomography. *J Urol* 1985;133:946–949.
55. Federle MP, Goldberg HI, Kaiser JA, Moss AA, Jeffrey RB, Mall JC. Evaluation of abdominal trauma by computed tomography. *Radiology* 1981;138:637–644.
56. Fein AB, Lee JKT, Balfe DM, et al. Diagnosis and staging of renal cell carcinoma: a comparison of MR and CT. *AJR* 1987;148:749–754.
57. Feldberg MAM, vanWaes PFGM. Multilocular cystic renal cell carcinoma. *AJR* 1982;138:953–955.
58. Ferris RA, Kirschner LP, Mero JH, McCabe DJ, Moss ML. Computed tomography in the evaluation of inferior vena caval obstruction. *Radiology* 1979;130:7–10.
59. Fishman MC, Pollack HM, Arger PH, Banner MD. High protein content: uncommon cause of CT hyperdense benign renal cysts. *J Comput Assist Tomogr* 1983;7:1103–1106.
60. Flechner SM, McAninch JW. Aspergillosis of the urinary tract: ascending route of infection and evolving patterns of disease. *J Urol* 1981;125:598–601.
61. Forbes WSC, Isherwood I, Fawcitt RA. Computed tomography in the evaluation of the solitary or unilateral nonfunctioning kidney. *J Comput Assist Tomogr* 1987;2:389–394.
62. Ford KK, Braun SD, Miller GA, Newman GE, Dunnick NR. Intravenous digital subtraction angiography in the preoperative evaluation of renal masses. *AJR* 1985;145:323–326.
63. Fuld IL, Matalon TA, Vogelzang RL, et al. Dynamic CT in the evaluation of physiologic status of renal transplants. *AJR* 1984;142:1157–1160.
64. Gebel M, Kuhn K, Dohring W, Freise J. Ultrasonography and computed axial tomography in the detection and monitoring of renal hematomas following ultrasonically guided percutaneous renal biopsy. *Radiology* 1985;28:25–27.
65. Gentry LR, Gould HR, Alter AJ, Wegenke JD, Atwell DT. Hemorrhagic angiomyolipoma: demonstration by computed tomography. *J Comput Assist Tomogr* 1981;5:861–865.
66. Glazer GM, Francis IR, Brady TM, Teng SS. Computed tomography of renal infarction: clinical and experimental observations. *AJR* 1983;140:721–727.
67. Glazer GM, Francis IR, Gross BH, Amendola MA. Computed tomography of renal vein thrombosis. *J Comput Assist Tomogr* 1984;8:288–293.
68. Godec CJ, Murrah VA. Simultaneous occurrence of transitional cell carcinoma and urothelial adenocarcinoma associated with xanthogranulomatous pyelonephritis. *Urology* 1985;26:412–415.
69. Gold RP, McClennan BL, Rottenberg RR. CT appearance of acute inflammatory disease of the renal interstitium. *AJR* 1983;141:343–349.
70. Goldman SM, Fishman EK, Hartman DS, Kim YC, Siegelman

SS. Computed tomography of renal tuberculosis and its pathological correlates. *J Comput Assist Tomogr* 1985;9:771–776.

71. Goldman SM, Hartman DS, Fishman EK, Finizio JP, Gatewood OM, Siegelman SS. CT of xanthogranulomatous pyelonephritis: radiologic-pathologic correlation. *AJR* 1984;142:963–969.

72. Goldman SM, Hartman DS, Weiss SW. The varied radiographic manifestation of retroperitoneal malignant fibrous histiocytoma revealed through 27 cases. *J Urol* 1986;135:33–38.

73. Griffeth LK, Rosen GM, Rauckman EJ, Drayer BP. Pharmacokinetics of nitroxide NMR contrast agents. *Invest Radiol* 1984;19:553–562.

74. Gutierrez OH, Burgener FA, Schwartz S. Coincident renal cell carcinoma and renal angiomyolipoma in tuberous sclerosis. *AJR* 1979;132:848–850.

75. Hadar H, Meiraz D. Renal sinus lipomatosis. Differentiation from space-occupying lesion with aid of computed tomography. *Urology* 1980;15:86–90.

76. Haggar AM, Kressel HY. Magnetic resonance imaging of the genitourinary tract. *Urol Clin North Am* 1985;12:725–736.

77. Halasz NA. Differential diagnosis of renal transplant rejection: is MR imaging the answer? *AJR* 1986;147:954–955.

78. Hartman DS, Davis CJ Jr, Goldman SM, Friedman AC, Fritzsche P. Renal lymphoma: radiologic-pathologic correlation of 21 cases. *Radiology* 1982;144:759–766.

79. Hartman DS, Davis CJ, Johns T, Goldman SM. Cystic renal cell carcinoma. *Urology* 1986;28:145–153.

80. Hartman DS, Davis CJ Jr, Madewell JE, Friedman AC. Primary malignant renal tumors in the second decade of life: Wilms tumor versus renal cell carcinoma. *J Urol* 1982;127:888–891.

81. Hartman DS, Davis CJ, Sanders RC, Johns TT, Smirniotopoulos J, Goldman SM. The multiloculated renal mass: considerations and differential features. *RadioGraphics* 1987;7:29–52.

82. Hartman DS, Goldman SM, Friedman AC, David CJ, Madewell JE, Sherman JL. Angiomyolipoma: ultrasonic-pathologic correlation. *Radiology* 1981;139:451–458.

83. Hayman LA, Evans RA, Fahr LM, Hinck VC. Renal consequences of rapid high dose contrast CT. *AJR* 1980;134:553–555.

84. Haynes JW, Walsh JW, Brewer WH, Vick CW, Allen HA. Traumatic renal artery occlusion: CT diagnosis with angiographic correlation. *J Comput Assist Tomogr* 1984;8:731–733.

85. Healy ME, Teng SS, Moss AA. Uriniferous pseudocyst: computed tomographic findings. *Radiology* 1984;153:757–762.

86. Heiken JP, McClennan BL, Gold RP. Renal lymphoma. *Semin Ultrasound, CT, MR* 1986;7:58–66.

87. Herman SD, Friedman AC, Siegelbaum M, Ramchandani P, Radecki PD. Magnetic resonance imaging of papillary renal cell carcinoma. *Urol Radiol* 1985;7:168–171.

88. Hertle L, Becht E, Klose K, Rumpelt HJ. Computed tomography in xanthogranulomatous pyelonephritis. *Eur Urol* 1984;10:385–386.

89. Hertz M, Zissin R, Dresnik Z, Morag B, Itzchak Y, Jonas P. Echinococcus of the urinary tract: radiologic findings. *Urol Radiol* 1984;6:175–181.

90. Hilpert PL, Friedman AC, Radecki PD, et al. MRI of hemorrhagic renal cysts in polycystic kidney disease. *AJR* 1986;146:1167–1172.

91. Hricak H, Demas BE, Williams RD, et al. Magnetic resonance imaging in the diagnosis and staging of renal and perirenal neoplasms. *Radiology* 1985;154:709–715.

92. Hricak H, Fisher MR. Magnetic resonance imaging of the genitourinary tract. *Postgrad Radiol* 1986;6:173–190.

93. Hricak H, Terrier F, Demas BE. Renal allografts: evaluation by MR imaging. *Radiology* 1986;159:435–441.

94. Hricak H, Terrier F, Marotti M, et al. Post-transplant renal rejection: comparison of quantitative scintigraphy, US and MR imaging. *Radiology* 1987;162:685–688.

95. Hudson MA, Weyman PJ, van der Vliet AH, Catalona WJ. Emphysematous pyelonephritis: successful management by percutaneous drainage. *J Urol* 1986;136:884–886.

96. Hulnick DH, Bosniak MA. "Faceless kidney": CT sign of renal duplicity. *J Comput Assist Tomogr* 1986;10:771–772.

97. Ishikawa I. Uremic acquired cystic disease of kidney. *Urology* 1985;26:101–107.

98. Ishikawa I, Onouchi Z, Saito Y, et al. Renal cortex visualization and analysis of dynamic CT curves of the kidney. *J Comput Assist Tomogr* 1981;5:695–701.

99. Ishikawa I, Saito Y, Onouchi Z, et al. Delayed contrast enhancement in acute focal bacterial nephritis: CT features. *J Comput Assist Tomogr* 1985;9:894–897.

100. Ishikawa I, Saito Y, Shinoda A, Onouchi Z. Evidence for patchy renal vasoconstriction in man: observation by CT scan. *Nephron* 1981;27:31–34.

101. Ishikawa I, Tateishi K, Onouchi Z, et al. Persistent wedge-shaped contrast enhancement of the kidney. *Urol Radiol* 1985;7:45–47.

102. Ismail MA, Al-Dabagh MA, Al-Janabi A, et al. The use of computerised axial tomography (CAT) in the diagnosis of hydatid cysts. *Clin Radiol* 1980;31:287–290.

103. Jasinski RW, Amendola MA, Glazer GM, Bree RL, Gikas PW. Computed tomography of renal oncocytoma. *Comput Radiol* 1985;9:307–314.

104. Jensen LI, Dean PB, Nyman U, Goldman K. Contrast media for CT. An analysis of the early pharmacokinetics. *Invest Radiol* 1985;20:867–870.

105. Johnson CD, Dunnick NR, Cohan RH, Illescas FF. Renal adenocarcinoma: CT staging of 100 tumors. *AJR* 1987;148:59–64.

106. Jorulf H, Lindstedt E. Urogenital schistosomiasis. *Radiology* 1985;157:745.

107. Kalovidouris A, Pissiotis C, Pontifex G, Gouliamos A, Pentea S, Papavassiliou C. CT characterization of multivesicular hydatid cysts. *J Comput Assist Tomogr* 1986;10:428–431.

108. Karstaedt N, McCullough DL, Wolfman NT, Dyer RB. Magnetic resonance imaging of the renal mass. *J Urol* 1986;136:566–570.

109. Kavoussi LR, Torrence RJ, Catalona WJ. Renal oncocytoma with synchronous contralateral renal cell carcinoma. *J Urol* 1985;134:1193–1196.

110. Kenney PJ, Stanley RJ. Computed tomography of ureteral tumors. *J Comput Assist Tomogr* 1987;11:102–107.

111. Kim WS, Goldman SM, Gatewood OMB, et al. Computed tomography in calcified renal masses. *J Comput Assist Tomogr* 1981;5:855–860.

112. Kittredge RD, Brensilver J, Pierce JC. Computed tomography in renal transplant problems. *Radiology* 1978;127:165–169.

113. Kormano M, Partaren K, Soimakallio S, Kivimaki T. Dynamic contrast enhancement of the upper abdomen and effect of contrast medium and body weight. *Invest Radiol* 1983;18:364–367.

114. Kumar R, Amparo EG, David R, Fagan CJ, Morettin LB. Adult Wilms' tumor: clinical and radiographic features. *Urol Radiol* 1984;6:164–169.

115. Kunin M. Bridging septa of the perinephric space: anatomic, pathologic and diagnostic consideration. *Radiology* 1986;158:361–365.

116. Laupacis A, Vlan RA, Rankin RN, Stiller CR, Keown PA. Acute cortical necrosis: CT findings in post-partum renal cortical necrosis. *J Can Assoc Radiol* 1983;34:53–55.

117. Lautin EM, Gordon PM, Friedman AC, et al. Radionuclide imaging and computed tomography in renal oncocytoma. *Radiology* 1981;138:185–190.

118. Lawson TL, McClennan BL, Shirkhoda A. Adult polycystic kidney disease: ultrasonographic and computed tomographic appearance. *J Clin Ultrasound* 1981;6:295–302.

119. Lee JKT, McClennan BL, Kissane JM. Unilateral polycystic kidney disease. *AJR* 1978;130:1165–1167.

120. Lee JKT, McClennan BL, Melson GL, Stanley RJ. Acute focal bacterial nephritis: emphasis on gray scale sonography and computed tomography. *AJR* 1980;135:87–92.

121. Levine E. CRC diagnosis: computed tomography of renal masses. *Crit Rev Diagn Imag* 1985;24:91–200.

122. Levine E, Collins DL, Horton WA, Schmenke RN. CT screening of the abdomen in von Hippel-Lindau disease. *AJR* 1982;139:505–510.

123. Levine E, Grantham JJ. High density renal cysts in autosomal dominant polycystic kidney disease demonstrated by CT. *Radiology* 1985;154:477–482.

124. Levine E, Grantham JJ, Slucher SL, Greathouse JL, Krohn BP. CT of acquired cystic kidney disease and renal tumors in long-term dialysis patients. *AJR* 1984;142:125–131.

125. Levine E, Lee KR, Weigel JW, Farber B. Computed tomography in the diagnosis of renal carcinoma complicating Hippel-Lindau syndrome. *Radiology* 1979;130:703–706.

126. Love L, Meyers MA, Churchill RJ, Reynes CJ, Moncada R, Gibson D. Computed tomography of extraperitoneal spaces. *AJR* 1981;136:781–789.

127. Love L, Yedicka J. Computed tomography of internally calcified renal cysts. *AJR* 1985;145:1225–1227.
128. Madewell JE, Goldman SM, Davis CJ, Hartman DS, Feigin DS, Lichtenstein JE. Multilocular cystic nephroma. A radiologic-pathologic correlation in 58 patients. *Radiology* 1983;146:309–321.
129. Mangano FA, Zaontz M, Pahira JJ, et al. Computed tomography of acute renal failure secondary to rhabdomyolysis. *J Comput Assist Tomogr* 1985;9:777–779.
130. Marks WM, Korobkin M, Callen PW, Kaiser JA. CT diagnosis of tumor thrombosis of the renal vein and inferior vena cava. *AJR* 1978;131:843–846.
131. Marotti M, Hricak H, Fitzsche P, Crooks LE, Hedgcock MW, Tanagho EA. Complex and simple renal cysts: comparative evaluation by magnetic resonance imaging. *Radiology* 1987;162:679–684.
132. Mauro MA, Wadsworth DE, Stanley RJ, McClennan BL. Renal cell carcinoma: angiography in the CT era. *AJR* 1982;139:1135–1138.
133. Mayer DP, Baron RL, Pollack HM. Increase in CT attenuation values of parapelvic renal cysts after retrograde pyelography. *AJR* 1982;139:991–993.
134. McClennan BL. Current approaches to the azotemic patient. *Radiol Clin North Am* 1979;17:197–211.
135. McClennan BL. Computed tomography in the diagnosis and staging of renal cell carcinoma. *Semin Urol* 1985;3:111–131.
136. McClennan BL. Low osmolality contrast media: premises and promises. *Radiology* 1987;162:1–8.
137. McClennan BL, Balfe DM. Oncologic imaging: kidney and ureter. *Int J Radiat Oncol Biol Phys* 1983;9:1683–1704.
138. McClennan BL, Fair WR. CT scanning in urology. *Urol Clin North Am* 1979;6:343–373.
139. McClennan BL, Lee JKT. Kidney. In: Lee JKT, Sagel SS, Stanley RJ, eds. *Computed body tomography.* New York: Raven Press, 1983.
140. McClennan BL, Stanley RJ, Melson GL, Levitt RJ, Sagel SS. Computed tomography of the renal cyst—is cyst aspiration necessary? *AJR* 1979;133:671–675.
141. McDonald JE, Lee JKT, McClennan BL, et al. Natural history of extraperitoneal gas after renal transplantation: CT demonstration. *J Comput Assist Tomogr* 1982;6:507–510.
142. McMillin KI, Gross BH. CT demonstration of peripelvic and periureteral non-Hodgkin lymphoma. *AJR* 1985;144:945–946.
143. Mitnick JS, Bosniak MA, Mitton S, Raghavendra BN, Subramanyam BR, Genieser NB. Cystic renal disease in tuberous sclerosis. *Radiology* 1983;147:85–87.
144. Mitty HA. CT for diagnosis and management of urinary extravasation. *AJR* 1980;134:497–501.
145. Morag B, Rubenstein ZJ, Hertz M, Solomon A. Computed tomography in the diagnosis of renal parapelvic cysts. *J Comput Assist Tomogr* 1983;7:833–836.
146. Morgan WR, Nyberg LM Jr. Perinephric and intrarenal abscesses. *Urology* 1985;26:529–536.
147. Morris DL, Buckley J, Gregson R, Worthington BS. Magnetic resonance imaging in hydatid disease. *Clin Radiol* 1987;38:141–144.
148. Mukherji SK, Siegel MJ. Rhabdomyolysis and renal failure in child abuse. *AJR* 1987;148:1203–1204.
149. Nicolaisen GS, McAninch JW, Marshall GA, Bluth RF, Carroll PR. Renal trauma: re-evaluation of the indications for radiographic assessment. *J Urol* 1985;133:183–187.
150. Novick AC, Irish C, Steinmuller D, Buonocore E, Cohen C. The role of computerized tomography in renal transplant patients. *J Urol* 1981;125:15–18.
151. Olazabal A, Velasco M, Martinez A, Villavicencio H, Codina M. Emphysematous pyelonephritis. *Urology* 1987;29:95–98.
152. Osterling JE, Fishman EK, Goldman SM, Marshall FF. The management of renal angiomyolipoma. *J Urol* 1986;135:1121–1124.
153. Paling MR, Williamson BJR. The renal parenchymal stone: a benign calcified renal mass. *Urol Radiol* 1984;6:170–174.
154. Papanicolaou N, Hahn PF, Edeman RR, et al. Magnetic resonance imaging of the kidney. *Urol Radiol* 1986;8:139–150.
155. Parienty RA, Pradel J, Imbert MC, Picard JD, Savant P. Computed tomography of multilocular cystic nephroma. *Radiology* 1981;140:135–139.
156. Parienty RA, Pradel J, Parienty I. Cystic renal cancer: CT characteristics. *Radiology* 1985;157:741–744.
157. Parienty RA, Pradel J, Picard JD, Ducellier R, Lubrano JM, Smolarski N. Visibility and thickening of the renal fascia on computed tomograms. *Radiology* 1981;139:119–124.
158. Parker MD. Acute segmental renal infarction: difficulty in diagnosis despite multimodality approach. *Urology* 1981;18:523–526.
159. Pazmino P, Pyatt R, Williams E, Bohan L. Computed tomography in renal ischemia. *J Comput Assist Tomogr* 1983;7:102–105.
160. Pollack HM, Arger PH, Banner MP, Mulhern CB, Coleman BG. Computed tomography of renal pelvic filling defects. *Radiology* 1981;138:645–651.
161. Pope TL, Buschi AJ, Moore TS, Williamson BRJ, Brenbridge ANAG. CT features of renal polyarteritis nodosa. *AJR* 1981;136:986–987.
162. Premkumar A, Lattimer J, Newhouse JH. CT and sonography of advanced urinary tract tuberculosis. *AJR* 1987;148:65–69.
163. Press GA, McClennan BL, Melson GL, Weyman PJ, Mauro MA, Lee JKT. Papillary renal cell carcinoma: CT and sonographic evaluation. *AJR* 1984;143:1005–1010.
164. Probst P, Link L, Futterlieb A, Wehrli HP. Experimental acute renal artery stenosis: dynamic CT and renal perfusion. *Invest Radiol* 1984;19:87–95.
165. Probst P, Mahler F, Roesler H, Fuchs WA. Renal artery stenosis and evaluation of the effect of endoluminal dilatation: comparison of dynamic CT scanning and I-131-OIHA renogram. *Invest Radiol* 1983;18:264–271.
166. Quinn MJ, Hartman DS, Friedman AC, et al. Renal oncocytoma: new observations. *Radiology* 1984;153:49–53.
167. Ramchandani P, Soulen RL, Schnall RI, et al. Impact of magnetic resonance on staging of renal carcinoma. *Urology* 1986;27:564–568.
168. Raptopoulous V, Kleinman PK, Marks S, Snyder M, Silverman PM. Renal fascial pathway: posterior extension of pancreatic effusions within the anterior pararenal space. *Radiology* 1986;158:367–374.
169. Rausch HP, Hanefeld F, Kaufman HJ. Medullary nephrocalcinosis and pancreatic calcifications demonstrated by ultrasound and CT in infants after treatment with ACTH. *Radiology* 1984;153:105–107.
170. Rawas M, Tao H. Intravenous contrast medium and renal cyst. *J Can Assoc Radiol* 1985;36:301–303.
171. Reiser UJ. Study of bolus geometry after intravenous contrast medium injection: dynamic and quantitative measurement (chronogram) using an x-ray CT device. *J Comput Assist Tomogr* 1984;8:251–262.
172. Rholl KS, Lee JKT, Ling D, Sicard GA, Griffith RC, Freeman M. Acute renal rejection versus acute tubular necrosis in a canine model: MR evaluation. *Radiology* 1986;160:113–117.
173. Rhyner P, Federle MP, Jeffrey RB. CT of trauma to the abnormal kidney. *AJR* 1984;142:747–750.
174. Rigsby CM, Rosenfield AT, Glickman MG, Hodson J. Hemorrhagic focal bacterial nephritis: findings on gray-scale sonography and CT. *AJR* 1986;146:1173–1177.
175. Robson CJ. The results of radical nephrectomy for renal cell carcinoma. *J Urol* 1969;101:297–301.
176. Rosenbaum R, Hoffsten PE, Stanley RJ, Klahr S. Use of computerized tomography to diagnose complications of percutaneous renal biopsy. *Kidney Int* 1978;14:87–92.
177. Rosenberg ER, Korobkin M, Foster W, Silverman PM, Bowie JD, Dunnick NR. The significance of septations in a renal cyst. *AJR* 1985;144:593–595.
178. Rosi P, Selli C, Carini M, Rosi MF, Mottola A. Xanthogranulomatous pyelonephritis: clinical experience with 62 cases. *Eur Urol* 1986;12:96–100.
179. Rumancik WM, Bosniak MA, Rosen RJ, Hulnich D. Atypical renal and pararenal hamartoma associated with lymphangiomatosis. *AJR* 1984;142:971–972.
180. Runge VM, Clanton JA, Foster MA, et al. Paramagnetic NMR contrast agents. Development and evaluation. *Invest Radiol* 1984;19:408–415.
181. Sagel SS, Siegel MJ, Stanley RJ, Jost RG. Detection of retroperitoneal hemorrhage by computed tomography. *AJR* 1977;129:403–407.
182. Sagel SS, Stanley RJ, Levitt RJ, Geisse G. Computed tomography of the kidney. *Radiology* 1977;124:359–370.
183. Sandler CM, Jackson H, Kaminsky RI. Right perirenal hematoma secondary to a leaking abdominal aortic aneurysm. *J Comput Assist Tomogr* 1981;5:264–266.

184. Sandler CM, Raval B, David CR. Computed tomography of the kidney. *Urol Clin North Am* 1985;12:657–665.

185. Sant GR, Ucci AA Jr, Meres EM Jr. Multicentric angiomyolipoma: renal and lymph node involvement. *Urology* 1986;28:111–113.

186. Schaffer RM, Schwart GE, Becker JA, et al. Renal ultrasound in acquired immunodeficiency syndrome (AIDS). *Radiology* 1984;153:511–513.

187. Schoborg TW, Saffos RO, Urdaneta L, Lewis CW. Xanthogranulomatous pyelonephritis associated with renal cell carcinoma. *J Urol* 1980;124:125–127.

188. Scully RE, Mark EJ, McNeely BU. Case records of the Massachusetts General Hospital. Case 32-1981. *N Engl J Med* 1981;305:331–336.

189. Segal AJ, Spitzer RM. Pseudo thick-walled renal cyst by CT. *AJR* 1979;132:827–828.

190. Shanser JD, Hedgcock MW, Korobkin M. Transit of contrast material into renal cyst following urography or arteriography. Presented at the Society of Uroradiology meeting, New York, 1978.

191. Sheinfeld J, Erturk E, Spataro RF, Cockett ATK. Perinephric abscess: current concepts. *J Urol* 1987;137:191–194.

192. Shirkhoda A. Computed tomography of perirenal metastases. *J Comput Assist Tomogr* 1986;10:435–438.

193. Shuman WP, Mack LA, Rogers JV. Diffuse nephrocalcinosis: hyperechoic sonographic appearance. *AJR* 1981;136:830–832.

194. Siegelman SS, Copeland BE, Saba GP, Cameron JL, Sanders RC, Zerhouni EA. CT of fluid collections associated with pancreatitis. *AJR* 1980;134:1121–1132.

195. Smith WP, Levine E. Sagittal and coronal CT image reconstruction: application in assessing the inferior vena cava in renal cancer. *J Comput Assist Tomogr* 1980;4:531–535.

196. Somogyi J, Cohen WN, Omar MM, Makhuli Z. Communication of right and left perirenal spaces demonstrated by computed tomography. *J Comput Assist Tomogr* 1979;3:270–273.

197. Spataro RF, Fischer HW, Boylan L. Urography with low osmolality contrast media: comparative urinary excretion of iopamidol, Hexabrix and diatrizoate. *Invest Radiol* 1982;17:494–500.

198. Spataro RF, Katzberg RW, Fischer HW, McMannis MJ. High-dose clinical urography with the low-osmolality contrast agent Hexabrix: comparison with a conventional contrast agent. *Radiology* 1987;162:9–14.

199. Steele JR, Sones PJ, Heffner LT. The detection of inferior vena caval thrombosis with computed tomography. *Radiology* 1978;128:385–386.

200. Steinberg DL, Jeffrey RB, Federle MP, McAninch JW. The computerized tomography appearance of renal pedicle injury. *J Urol* 1984;132:1163–1164.

201. Steinberg HV, Nelson RC, Murphy FB, et al. Renal allograft rejection: evaluation by Doppler US and MR imaging. *Radiology* 1987;162:237–242.

202. Subramanyam BR, Bosniak MA, Horii SC, Megibow AJ, Balthazar EJ. Replacement lipomatosis of the kidney: diagnosis by computed tomography and sonography. *Radiology* 1983;148:791–792.

203. Sumner RE, Volberg FM, Karstaedt N, Ward CF, Lorentz WB. Hypophosphatasia and nephrocalcinosis demonstrated by ultrasound and CT. *Clin Nephrol* 1984;22:317–319.

204. Sussman S, Cochran ST, Pagani JJ, et al. Hyperdense renal masses: a CT manifestation of hemorrhagic renal cysts. *Radiology* 1984;150:207–211.

205. Sussman SK, Goldberg RP, Griscom HT. Milk of calcium hydronephrosis in patients with paraplegia and urinary-enteric diversion: CT demonstration. *J Comput Assist Tomogr* 1986;10:257–259.

206. Takahashi M, Tamakawa Y, Shibata A, Fukushima Y. Computed tomography of "page" kidney. *J Comput Assist Tomogr* 1977;1:344–348.

207. Takao R, Amamoto Y, Matsunaga N, et al. Computed tomography of multicystic kidney. *J Comput Assist Tomogr* 1980;4:548–549.

208. Takeyama M, Arima M, Sagawa S, Sonoda T. Preoperative diagnosis of coincident renal cell carcinoma and renal angiomyolipoma in nontuberous sclerosis. *J Urol* 1982;128:579–581.

209. Tarr RW, Carter MR, Shaff MI, Tishler JMA, Page DL, Kulkarni MV. Hypertension in a patient with multiple renal and adrenal masses. *Invest Radiol* 1985;20:455–459.

210. Terrier F, Hricak H, Revel D, et al. Magnetic resonance imaging in the diagnosis of acute renal allograft rejection and its differentiation from acute tubular necrosis. Experimental study in the dog. *Invest Radiol* 1985;20:617–625.

211. Thierman D, Haaga JR, Anton P, LiPuma JP. Renal replacement lipomatosis. *J Comput Assist Tomogr* 1983;7:341–343.

212. Totty WG, McClennan BL, Melson GL, Patel R. Relative value of computed tomography and ultrasonography in the assessment of renal angiomyolipoma. *J Comput Assist Tomogr* 1981;5:173–177.

213. Varma DG, Rojo JR, Thomas R, Walker PD. Computed tomography of xanthogranulomatous pyelonephritis. *J Comput Assist Tomogr* 1985;9:241–247.

214. Vas W, Carlin B, Salimi Z, Tang-Barton P, Tucker D. CT diagnosis of emphysematous pyelonephritis. *Comput Radiol* 1985;9:37–39.

215. Vas W, Salimi Z, Tang-Barton P, Vargas F, Sidarthan AS. Computed tomography and ultrasound demonstration of squamous cell carcinoma. *Comput Tomogr* 1985;9:87–89.

216. Wasserman NF, Ewing SL. Calcified renal oncocytoma. *AJR* 1983;141:747–749.

217. Webb JAW, Reznek RH, White FE, Cattell WR, Fry IK, Baker LRI. Can ultrasound and computed tomography replace high-dose urography in patients with impaired renal function. *Q J Med [New Series 53]* 1984;211:411–425.

218. Wegenke JD, Malek GH, Alter AJ, Olson JG. Acute lobular nephronia. *J Urol* 1986;135:343–345.

219. Weyman PJ, McClennan BL, Lee JKT, Stanley RJ. CT of calcified renal masses. *AJR* 1982;138:1095–1099.

220. Weyman PJ, McClennan BL, Stanley RJ, Levitt RG, Sagel SS. Comparison of computed tomography and angiography in the evaluation of renal cell carcinoma. *Radiology* 1980;137:417–424.

221. Whittemore DM, Wendel RG. Bilateral involvement of renal hamartoma in two cases without tuberous sclerosis. *J Urol* 1981;125:99–101.

222. Wilgore M, Stephens D, Soule E, McLeod R. Lipomatous tumors of the abdominal cavity: CT appearance and pathologic correlation. *AJR* 1981;137:539–545.

223. Wills JS. Cystic adenocarcinoma of the kidney mimicking multilocular renal cyst. *Urol Radiol* 1983;5:51–53.

224. Wilms G, Baert AL, Marchal G, Bruneel M. CT demonstration of gas formation after renal tumor embolization. *J Comput Assist Tomogr* 1979;3:838–839.

225. Wimbish JK, Sanders MM, Samuels BI, Francis IR. Squamous cell carcinoma of the renal pelvis: case report. *Urol Radiol* 1983;5:267–269.

226. Wong WS, Moss AA, Federle MP, Cochran ST, London SS. Renal infarction: CT diagnosis and correlation between CT findings and etiologies. *Radiology* 1984;150:201–205.

227. Yashiro N, Yuoshida H, Arai S, Ohtomok, Itai Y, Lio M. Incidentally discovered small renal carcinoma: CT and angiography. *Radiat Med* 1985;3:42–46.

228. Young SW, Noon MA, Marincek B. Dynamic computed tomographic time-density study of normal human tissue after intravenous contrast administration. *Invest Radiol* 1980;16:36–39.

229. Young SW, Turner RJ, Castellino RA. A strategy for the contrast enhancement of malignant tumors using dynamic computed tomography and intravascular pharmacokinetics. *Radiology* 1980;137:137–141.

230. Zaontz MR, Pahira JJ, Wolfman M, Gargurevich AJ, Zeman RK. Acute focal bacterial nephritis: a systematic approach to diagnosis and treatment. *J Urol* 1985;133:752–757.

231. Zeman RK, Cronan JJ, Rosenfield AT, Lynch JH, Jaffe MH, Clark LR. Renal cell carcinoma: dynamic thin-section CT assessment of vascular invasion and tumor vascularity. *Radiology* 1988;167:393–396.

232. Zimmer WD, Williamson B Jr, Hartman GW, Hattery RR, O'Brien PC. Changing patterns in the evaluation of renal masses: economic implications. *AJR* 1984;143:285–289.

233. Zirinsky K, Auh YH, Rubenstein WA, Williams JJ, Pasmantier MW, Kazam E. CT of hyperdense renal cyst: sonographic correlation. *AJR* 1984;143:151–156.

CHAPTER 19

The Adrenals

David Ling and Joseph K. T. Lee

Computed tomography (CT) is the primary radiologic technique for imaging the adrenals, and both the normal adrenal glands and adrenal masses can be accurately demonstrated by CT (1,46,96). Using optimal scanning technique, both adrenal glands can be clearly identified in nearly 100% of patients. Occasionally, an adrenal gland may be difficult to delineate if there is a paucity of surrounding retroperitoneal fat or if the image quality is degraded by patient motion or excessive artifacts from nearby surgical clips.

Most adrenal masses will be detected if the adrenals are evaluated with contiguous 8- to 10-mm-collimated images. If the initial examination is equivocal or if small adrenal masses are suspected, 4- to 5-mm-collimated images at 4- to 5-mm intervals should be obtained. Orally administered contrast material should be given routinely to help differentiate the adrenals from adjacent gastrointestinal structures. Most patients can be evaluated without intravenous iodinated contrast material. However, especially in thin patients, intravenous contrast material can be useful not only in delineating the normal adrenal gland but also to distinguish an adrenal mass from the kidney, liver, or pancreas. In particular, rapid sequential imaging of the adrenals following a bolus intravenous injection of contrast material helps differentiate a small adrenal mass from adjacent vascular structures (Fig. 1).

Normal and abnormal adrenal glands also can be imaged with magnetic resonance imaging (MRI). An MRI study of the adrenals should include a T1-weighted sequence to determine if an adrenal mass is present and a T2-weighted sequence for additional characterization of any detected mass. When 7- to 10-mm-thick slices are obtained, the normal right adrenal can be seen in about 90% of patients, and the normal left adrenal gland can be identified in nearly every patient (11,61). The most common cause for nonvisualization of the normal right adrenal is lack of surrounding fat. Because of its multiplanar imaging capability, MRI is particularly useful in displaying the relationships between a large adrenal mass and adjacent structures. It is also useful in differentiating a metastasis from a nonhyperfunctioning adenoma (11,30,76).

NORMAL ANATOMY

The adrenal glands are small retroperitoneal structures enclosed within the perinephric fascia, and are usually surrounded by a sufficient amount of fat for CT identification (Figs. 2–4). The right adrenal gland is commonly seen on images beginning 1 to 2 cm above the upper pole of the right kidney. The right adrenal lies immediately posterior to the inferior vena cava and between the right crus of the diaphragm medially and the right lobe of the liver laterally. The caudal aspect of the right adrenal gland often is seen anterior and medial to the upper pole of the right kidney. Differentiation of the right adrenal gland from the adjacent liver and crus of the diaphragm can be difficult if there is a paucity of retroperitoneal fat. The left adrenal gland is seen at the same level or just caudal to the level of the right adrenal gland. It lies lateral to the aorta and left crus of the diaphragm and anteromedial to the upper pole of the left kidney. A portion of the left adrenal gland often is seen just posterior to the pancreas and/or splenic vessels. The adrenals normally extend 2 to 4 cm in the craniocaudal direction. As a result, a sufficient number of images must be obtained to ensure that the entire gland is imaged, because a small adrenal mass may be shown on one section, with the rest of the images showing a normal-appearing gland (Fig. 5).

The normal adrenals display a variety of shapes, depending on the orientation of the gland and the level of the image. The right adrenal most commonly has an oblique linear configuration that parallels the crus of the diaphragm. It may also have an inverted V, Y, or L con-

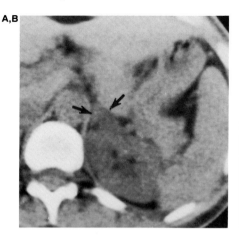 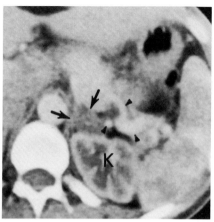

FIG. 1. A 33-year-old woman with primary aldosteronism. **A:** Precontrast CT image suggests enlargement of the left adrenal gland (*arrows*), but it is difficult to distinguish surrounding organs and vessels from the adrenal gland. **B:** CT image following 35-ml intravenous bolus injection of iodinated contrast material more clearly distinguishes the left adrenal from the left kidney (K) and splenic vessels (*arrowheads*). Histologic examination of the surgical specimen revealed an adenoma.

figuration (Fig. 2). Triangular, K, and H shapes are also encountered (Fig. 3). The left adrenal often has an inverted V, Y, or T shape. It also may assume a triangular shape (Figs. 2C, 3, and 4). The caudal aspects of both adrenal glands often have a horizontal linear configuration (Fig. 4B). The lengths of the limbs of the adrenal glands on any cross section are highly variable, and the limbs may measure up to 4 cm in length. Except at the apex of the gland, where the limbs converge, the limbs of the adrenal glands have a uniform thickness, with straight or concave margins. On any cross section, the normal thickness of these limbs perpendicular to their long axes usually is 5 to 7

mm, and any measurement greater than 10 mm is suggestive of adrenal disease (46,60).

In patients with congenital renal anomalies, such as agenesis or inferior ectopy, the ipsilateral adrenal is disk-shaped, with a paraspinal orientation that produces a linear configuration on CT images (48). In patients with acquired renal atrophy or patients who have had prior simple nephrectomy, the adrenals have a normal appearance (48), but may be difficult to see secondary to alteration of the normal anatomy. The right adrenal may be obscured by medial movement of the right lobe of the liver and posterior displacement of bowel loops. Similarly, the left ad-

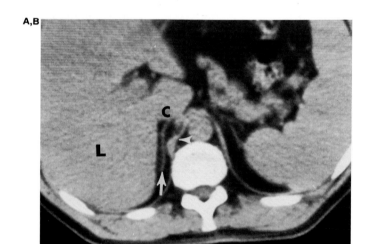 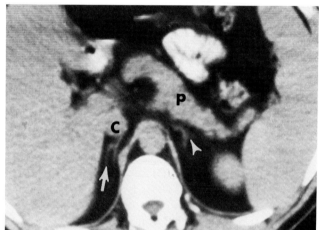

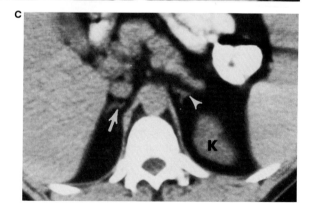

FIG. 2. Normal adrenal glands. **A:** The long vertical limb of the right adrenal (*arrow*) is seen posterior to the inferior vena cava (C) between the crus of the right hemidiaphragm (*arrowhead*) and right lobe of the liver (L). Part of the left adrenal gland is also seen at this level. **B:** One centimeter caudal, both limbs of the right adrenal gland are seen and have the appearance of an inverted Y (*arrow*). The left adrenal (*arrowhead*) is seen posterior to the pancreas (p). **C:** One centimeter more caudal, the left adrenal gland is still seen as an inverted Y, whereas only the lateral limb of the right adrenal gland (*arrow*) is visible; (K) kidney.

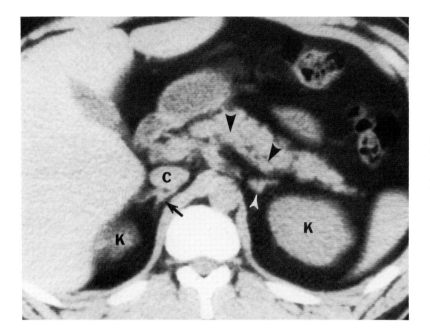

FIG. 3. Normal adrenal glands. The right adrenal gland (*arrow*) is shaped like the letter H, and the left adrenal has a triangular shape (*white arrowhead*); (*black arrowheads*) splenic vein; (C) inferior vena cava; (K) kidney.

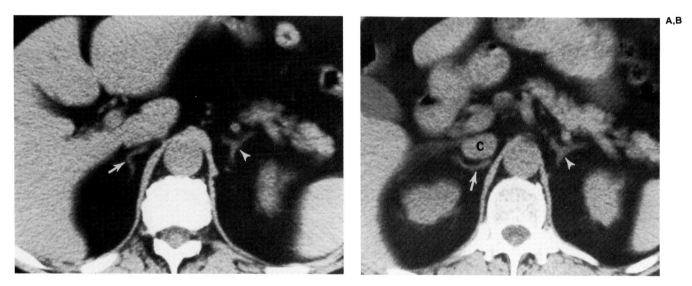

FIG. 4. Normal adrenal glands. A: The right adrenal gland has an inverted L shape (*arrow*); the left adrenal looks like an inverted T (*arrowhead*). B: One centimeter caudal, only the horizontal portion of the right adrenal (*arrow*) is imaged parallel to the posterior wall of the inferior vena cava (C). The appearance of the left adrenal (*arrowhead*) is similar to that in (A).

FIG. 5. Incidental nonhyperfunctioning adenoma. CT image was obtained to evaluate abnormal findings on liver function tests. There was no clinical or biochemical evidence of adrenal disease. A: A 1-cm low-density mass (*arrow*) is seen projecting from the medial limb of the right adrenal. Follow-up CT image 5 months later showed no change in the size of the mass. B: A normal right adrenal (*arrow*) is seen 2 cm inferiorly. (From ref. 32.)

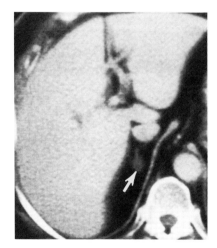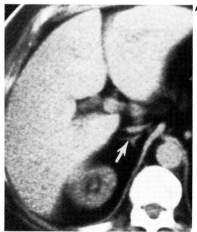

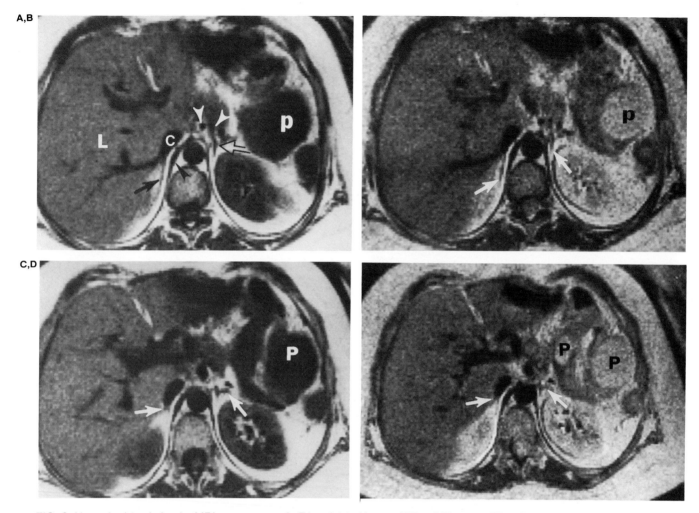

FIG. 6. Normal adrenal glands: MRI appearance. **A:** T1-weighted image (TR = 500 msec, TE = 35 msec). The medial limb of the right adrenal gland (*arrow*) is seen between the crus of the right hemidiaphragm (*black arrowhead*) and the posterior right lobe of the liver (L). The signal intensity of the right adrenal gland is similar to that of the liver, but higher than that of the crus. The left adrenal gland (*open arrow*), which has an inverted V shape, is seen behind the splenic vein (*white arrowheads*). **B:** T2-weighted image (TR = 1,500 msec, TE = 90 msec) at the same level as (**A**). Although both the right and left adrenals (*arrows*) are still visible, the signal-intensity difference between the adrenals and the surrounding fat is less with this sequence, thereby making their identification more difficult. **C:** T1-weighted image (TR = 500 msec, TE = 35 msec). One centimeter caudal to (**A**), both adrenals (*arrows*) appear as an inverted V; (P) pancreatic pseudocyst. **D:** T2-weighted image (TR = 1,500 msec, TE = 90 msec) obtained at the same level as (**C**) shows similar findings.

renal gland may be difficult to see because of posterior movement of the tail of the pancreas, splenic vessels, or small-bowel loops or medial movement by the spleen (38).

The normal adrenals usually have a homogeneous MRI appearance (11,61). Sometimes the adrenal cortex can be differentiated from the medulla because the latter has a lower signal intensity (61,81). On all pulse sequences, the adrenals have a signal intensity greater than that of the diaphragmatic crura and less than that of fat (11,14) (Figs. 6 and 7). The signal-intensity difference between the adrenal gland and surrounding fat is greater on T1-weighted images than on T2-weighted images. Therefore, the normal adrenal gland is most easily seen on T1-weighted images. The adrenal glands are easily distinguished from the inferior vena cava and splenic vessels because of the lack of signal from the flowing blood.

PSEUDOTUMORS

Occasionally, an adjacent vascular or gastrointestinal structure may mimic an adrenal mass. In these situations, intravenous administration of contrast material or additional oral contrast material helps distinguish these "pseudotumors" from true adrenal masses. On the left, a prominent medial lobulation of the spleen or accessory spleen may produce a rounded density resembling an adrenal mass. In most cases, a splenic lobulation can be shown to be contiguous with the spleen, with the normal adrenal identified at a different level. If the findings are still equivocal, intravenous administration of contrast material will demonstrate equal enhancement of the splenic pseudotumor and the remainder of the spleen. Both left renal and pancreatic masses may also mimic a

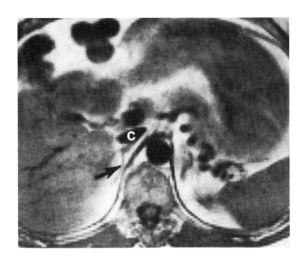

FIG. 7. Normal right adrenal gland: MRI appearance. T1-weighted image (TR = 500 msec, TE = 35 msec). The right adrenal gland (*arrow*) lies posterior to the inferior vena cava (c) and appears as an inverted L.

configuration on contiguous images. A definitive diagnosis can be established by obtaining rapid serial images after bolus intravenous administration of contrast material. Adjacent small bowel, a gastric diverticulum (83), or a redundant posteriorly folded gastric fundus may mimic an adrenal mass, and additional oral contrast material is useful in distinguishing these structures (Fig. 8).

Pseudotumors are less common on the right, but in some cases tortuous renal vessels or masses arising from the liver or the right kidney can cause confusion. The use of narrow collimation and intravenous contrast material helps delineate the normal right adrenal gland. If post-contrast images are confusing or if there is a contraindication to intravenous administration of iodinated contrast material, the possibility of a vascular structure simulating an adrenal mass can be further evaluated by MRI. The absence of signal within the structure will confirm its vascular nature.

left adrenal mass. In some individuals, the close proximity of a tortuous splenic artery to the lateral limb of the left adrenal can produce the appearance of a small adrenal mass. In addition, a left adrenal mass may be simulated by portal-systemic periadrenal venous collaterals that are dilated in the presence of portal hypertension (7,59). In particular, the left inferior phrenic vein passes immediately anterior to the left adrenal gland and may dilate as a collateral pathway from the splenic vein to the left renal vein (7). The vascular nature of these pseudotumors often can be suspected as a result of their elongated and tubular

PATHOLOGY

In patients with biochemical evidence of adrenal hyperfunction, a CT examination is valuable not only because of its ability to detect adrenal masses but also because CT generally is able to exclude such lesions by demonstration of normal adrenal glands. If an adrenal mass is detected, despite the nonspecific CT appearance of most adrenal masses, a specific histologic diagnosis often can be suggested when CT findings are combined with the biochemical information. Even if there is no bio-

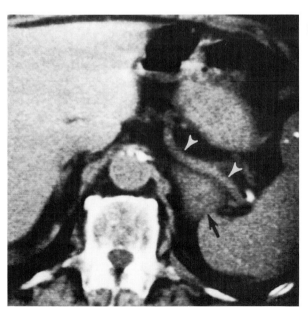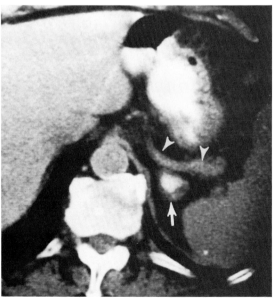

FIG. 8. Adrenal pseudotumor. A: CT image shows a triangular-shaped soft-tissue mass (*arrow*) posterior to the splenic artery (*arrowheads*) in the region of the left adrenal gland. B: A repeat image after administration of additional oral contrast material demonstrates the previously noted soft-tissue mass to contain contrast material (*arrow*), thus representing a portion of gastric fundus; (*arrowheads*) splenic artery.

A,B

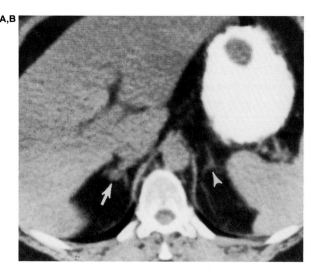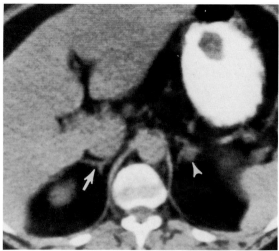

FIG. 9. Bilateral nonhyperfunctioning adrenal adenomas discovered incidentally on a CT examination performed for vague abdominal pain. **A:** An 8-mm soft-tissue nodule located between the two limbs of right adrenal gland causes minimal distortion to its normal appearance. The left adrenal (*arrowhead*) is normal at this level. **B:** One centimeter caudad, a similar nodule is noted in the left adrenal gland (*arrowhead*); (arrow) normal-appearing right adrenal.

chemical evidence of adrenal hyperfunction, the clinical history and the appearance of the detected adrenal mass often are sufficient to suggest a pathologic diagnosis. Otherwise, additional imaging studies or biopsy may be necessary to further characterize the adrenal mass.

The accuracy of CT in diagnosing adrenal masses exceeds 90% (1,20,51). Adrenal masses as small as 5 mm in diameter can be detected by CT. A small adrenal mass may have an attenuation value identical with that of normal adrenal parenchyma (Fig. 9). In such cases, the only sign of an adrenal neoplasm is focal enlargement of a portion of the adrenal gland that produces a convex configuration of the normally concave or straight margin of

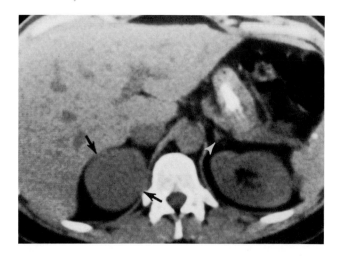

FIG. 10. Cushing syndrome due to a cortical adenoma. The normal right adrenal tissue is obscured by this 5-cm round mass (*arrows*); (*arrowhead*) normal left adrenal gland.

the gland. Therefore, focal enlargement is more significant in the detection of small adrenal masses than any absolute measurement of adrenal size. Larger masses appear as rounded or oval densities, often replacing or obliterating the normal adrenal tissue (Fig. 10). With very large masses, the primary site of origin can be difficult to determine by CT. Large renal, hepatic, or primary retroperitoneal tumors may be indistinguishable from huge adrenal lesions because of obscuration of the usual organ boundaries on the CT images. An adrenal origin may be established by biochemical testing if the lesion is a hormonally active adrenal tumor. In some cases, the vectors of displacement of adjacent structures and the location of the epicenter of the mass are helpful clues. For example, anterior displacement of the inferior vena cava is more often caused by a retroperitoneal mass than by a hepatic lesion (Fig. 11).

In contradistinction to focal mass lesions, hyperplastic adrenal glands may demonstrate thickening of the limbs, but they usually maintain a normal adrenal configuration (Fig. 12). Also, with hyperplasia, both adrenals are enlarged, whereas primary adrenal masses usually are unilateral, with a normal-appearing or atrophic contralateral adrenal. However, in as many as 50% of patients with clinical and biochemical evidence of adrenal hyperplasia, the adrenal glands have a normal CT appearance (20,51). Because the normal thickness of the adrenal cortex is only 2 mm, a large increase in cortical thickness is necessary before hyperplasia causes sufficient adrenal enlargement to be detected by CT.

Hyperplastic adrenal glands may contain microscopic or macroscopic nodules. Although usually less than 5 mm in diameter, nodules can be as large as 2 cm (84) and can be detected by CT (51), especially if narrowly collimated

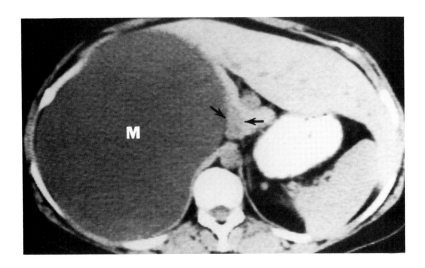

FIG. 11. Adrenal cyst. A large, near-water-density mass (M) displaces the inferior vena cava (*arrows*) anteriorly and medially. Anteromedial displacement of the inferior vena cava usually is caused by an adrenal mass rather than by a hepatic or a renal mass.

sections are obtained. Nodularity concomitant with bilateral adrenal enlargement suggests adrenal hyperplasia rather than primary adrenal tumors, because in the presence of a functioning tumor, the contralateral adrenal gland usually appears normal or atrophic on CT. However, a single hyperplastic nodule with otherwise normal-appearing adrenal glands cannot reliably be distinguished from an adenoma by CT.

Occasionally, mild to moderate enlargement of the adrenal glands is noted on CT in patients without clinical suspicion of adrenal abnormality and without accompanying biochemical abnormalities. These findings are almost never of clinical significance. Nonspecific hyperplasia of the adrenal glands may occur in patients with acromegaly (nearly 100%), hyperthyroidism (40%), hypertension with arteriosclerosis (16%), diabetes mellitus (3%), and a variety of malignant diseases (84).

On MR images, adrenal lesions may produce an abnormal signal intensity, as well as alteration of the normal adrenal morphology. Enlargement of the adrenal gland is most easily appreciated using T1-weighted pulse sequences. With rare exception, such as in the presence of hemorrhage, adrenal tumors exhibit a low signal intensity on T1-weighted images. As a result, adrenal tumors are easily distinguished from surrounding fat. As TR and TE are increased, adrenal lesions often show increasing signal intensity such that on T2-weighted pulse sequences, differentiation between the lesion and fat may be difficult (Fig. 13). MRI has been shown to be comparable to CT in the detection of adrenal masses (76,81).

CUSHING SYNDROME

Cushing syndrome most often is due to adrenal cortical hyperplasia (70%) secondary to excessive production of ACTH by a pituitary microadenoma (Cushing disease) or less commonly by an ectopic source. The rest of the patients with hypercortisolism have either adrenal adenomas (20%) or adrenal cortical carcinomas (10%) (84). CT has been highly accurate in localizing adrenal adenomas (18,20). Most cortisol-producing hyperfunctioning adenomas are at least 2 cm in diameter and are readily detected by CT, particularly in the Cushingoid patient, who has abundant retroperitoneal fat. Adenomas are well-defined masses that usually have a homogeneous appearance. These lesions may be of soft-tissue density, but because of their high lipid content, adenomas often have attenuation values less than that of soft tissue and near that of water (80) (Fig. 14). A low-density adenoma can be distinguished from an adrenal cyst if there is slight inhomogeneity of the adenoma; however, if these two possibilities cannot be differentiated, an ultrasound ex-

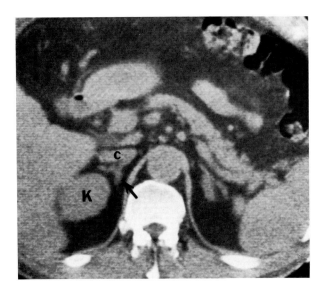

FIG. 12. Conn syndrome due to adrenal hyperplasia. Mild enlargement of both adrenals (*arrow*) is seen. Note that the normal adrenal configuration is maintained; (K) kidney; (c) inferior vena cava.

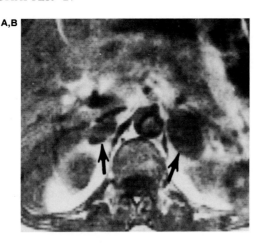 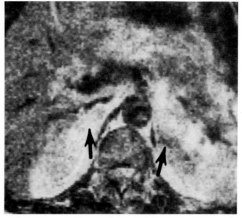

FIG. 13. Bilateral adrenal metastases from primary bronchogenic carcinoma. **A:** T1-weighted image (TR = 500 msec, TE = 35 msec) shows two well-defined adrenal masses (*arrows*) with signal intensities much lower than that of surrounding fat. **B:** T2-weighted image (TR = 2,100 msec, TE = 90 msec) at the same level as (**A**). Adrenal masses (*arrows*) are much more difficult to see because their signal intensities are similar to those of adjacent fat in this sequence.

amination should confirm the solid nature of the adrenal mass. Occasionally, calcification may be present in an adrenal adenoma.

Normal results on CT examination in patients with biochemical evidence of Cushing syndrome usually indicate adrenal hyperplasia and exclude an adrenal tumor as the cause. The accuracy of CT in diagnosing an adrenal neoplasm as the cause of hypercortisolism approaches 100%, and if a unilateral mass is demonstrated by CT, no further localization studies are indicated. With ACTH-dependent hypercortisolism, the adrenals may be enlarged as a result of macronodular hyperplasia (Fig. 15) or may

be normal in size. Although usually bilateral, the adrenal enlargement may be unilateral (72). A dexamethasone suppression test can help differentiate between pituitary and ectopic ACTH production. If the Cushing syndrome is due to ectopic ACTH production, urinary cortisol excretion is not suppressed by high-dose dexamethasone administration (12).

On MRI, both the cortisol-producing adenomas and adrenal hyperplasia may exhibit a signal intensity similar to that of the normal adrenals (21,76). Hemorrhage into an adenoma, a rare occurrence, may produce a high signal intensity on a T2-weighted sequence (2).

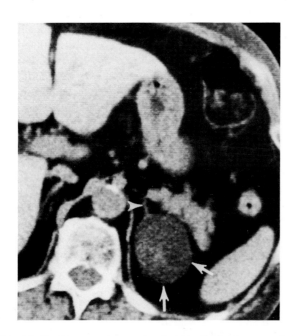

FIG. 14. Cushing syndrome due to a cortical adenoma. A 4-cm low-density (−4 HU) inhomogeneous mass (*arrows*) can be seen originating from the left adrenal (*arrowhead*).

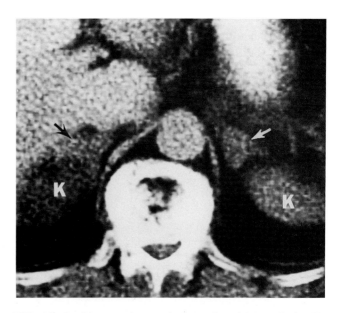

FIG. 15. Cushing syndrome due to adrenal hyperplasia. Although the adrenal glands are enlarged (*arrows*), their normal configuration is maintained; (K) kidneys.

THE ADRENALS / 835

PRIMARY ALDOSTERONISM

Primary aldosteronism (Conn syndrome) is a rare cause of hypertension and is characterized by hypokalemia, decreased plasma renin activity, and increased plasma aldosterone following sodium loading (12). Hyperaldosteronism is most commonly due to an adrenal cortical adenoma (75%), with hyperplasia (25%) and, very rarely, adrenal carcinoma as other causes (42). The distinction between an adenoma and hyperplasia is critical to patient management, because adenomas are treated surgically, whereas hyperplasia is best managed medically. In the majority of patients with hyperaldosteronism secondary to adrenal hyperplasia, partial or total adrenalectomy fails to correct the hypertension (33).

Aldosteronomas are indistinguishable from other adenomas on CT and MRI examinations. They usually are homogeneous and may have a low attenuation value, near that of water on CT (Figs. 1 and 16). Compared with the normal adrenals, aldosteronomas may be slightly hypointense on T1-weighted images and slightly hyperintense on T2-weighted images (21,30,76). Unlike cortisol-secreting tumors, aldosteronomas can be quite small (5 mm or less) and usually are less than 3 cm in diameter (29). CT has been shown to detect 70% of aldosteronomas (29). Despite optimal imaging techniques, such as utilizing 4- to 5-mm sections, small aldosteronomas occasionally may not be detected. As in Cushing syndrome, hyperplastic glands may appear enlarged; however, most patients with primary aldosteronism due to adrenal hyperplasia have normal findings on CT examinations.

In a patient with biochemical evidence of hyperaldosteronism, CT should be the initial imaging procedure. MRI offers no advantage over CT. If the CT findings are negative, adrenal venous sampling should be considered. Selective adrenal venous sampling for aldosterone levels appears to be more sensitive (>96%) than CT for detecting aldosteronomas; however, this procedure is invasive and at times is technically difficult to perform (29). Bilateral adenomas rarely occur (92) and may be indistinguishable from bilateral focal hyperplasia (77).

ADRENAL CARCINOMA

Adrenal carcinomas are rapidly growing tumors that may remain clinically silent until symptoms are produced secondary to metastatic disease, mass effect, or hormonal hyperfunction. Approximately 50% of adrenal carcinomas present as functioning tumors, and patients may develop Cushing syndrome, virilization, feminization, or, rarely, hyperaldosteronism (84). Functioning carcinomas are more common among female patients, whereas nonfunctioning tumors are more common among male patients (41). Functioning tumors may not be detected any earlier than nonfunctioning carcinomas, because the malignant cells inefficiently synthesize steroids (usually 17-ketosteroids) and require a large mass in order to produce elevated levels of steroids (54). As a result, adrenal carcinomas usually are large masses at the time of presentation, at least 4 cm and often more than 10 cm in diameter (4,19,41), and are readily detectable by CT or MRI (Figs. 17 and 18). These neoplasms often contain low-density areas on CT, representing necrosis. Irregular contrast enhancement and calcifications sometimes occur. On T1-weighted MR images, adrenal carcinomas may have a heterogeneous appearance; on T2-weighted images, the tumors may have a signal intensity greater than that of fat (11,21,76). Because the tumor often is locally extensive or even metastatic at its time of initial diagnosis, the CT or MRI study should be carefully scrutinized for evidence of hepatic metastases and retroperitoneal lymphadenopathy, as well as renal vein and inferior vena cava tumor extension, prior to any attempt at resection of the primary lesion (17,62).

PHEOCHROMOCYTOMA

Pheochromocytomas are catecholamine-secreting tumors that may cause sustained or paroxysmal hypertension. In nearly every patient with a symptomatic pheochromocytoma, urinary catecholamine, vanillylmandelic acid (VMA), and metanephrine levels are elevated (13). Patients with multiple endocrine adenomatosis type II (MEA-II) have an increased incidence of pheochromocytomas and may be asymptomatic, with normal laboratory values (86). There is also an increased incidence of pheochromocytomas among patients with neurofibromatosis, von Hippel–Lindau disease, and multiple cuta-

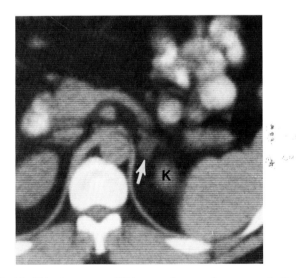

FIG. 16. Aldosteronoma. CT image shows a 1-cm mass in the medial limb of the left adrenal (*arrow*). The mass has an attenuation value slightly lower than that of adjacent normal adrenal tissue.

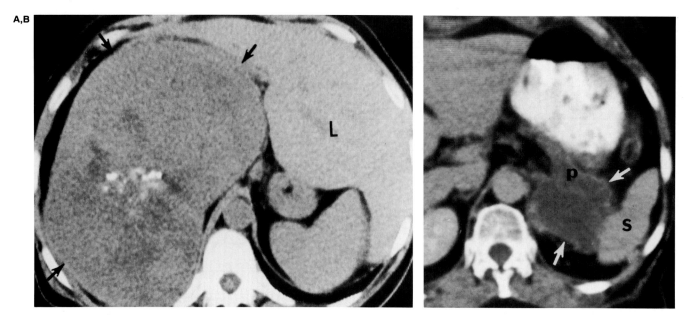

FIG. 17. Adrenal carcinomas. **A:** A large right-upper-quadrant mass (*arrows*) is demonstrated displacing the liver (L) toward the left. Coarse central calcifications as well as low-density areas of necrosis are seen within the mass. (Courtesy of Dr. Larry Anderson, Everett, Washington.) **B:** In another patient, postcontrast CT image demonstrates an irregular mass, with mixed attenuation values in the left adrenal gland (*arrows*). The mass abuts the spleen (S) and invades the pancreatic tail (p).

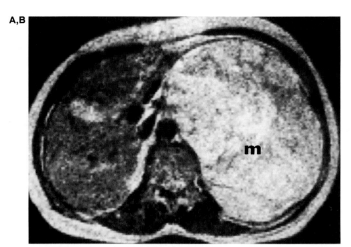

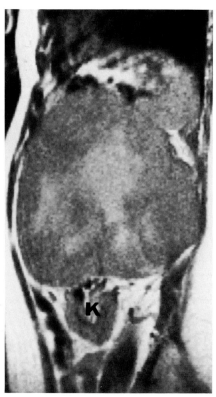

FIG. 18. Adrenal carcinoma: MRI appearance. **A:** Transaxial T2-weighted image (TR = 2,100 msec, TE = 90 msec) shows a large inhomogeneous adrenal mass (m) occupying the entire left upper quadrant. The center of the mass has a signal intensity higher than that of fat, indicating necrosis. **B:** Sagittal T1-weighted image (TR = 500 msec, TE = 35 msec) better delineates the cephalocaudal extent of the mass. The left kidney (K) is displaced inferiorly. Portions of the mass have a higher signal intensity representing areas of hemorrhage.

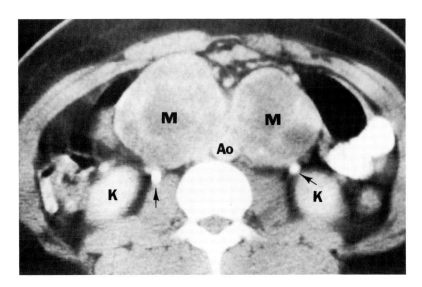

FIG. 19. Pheochromocytomas involving the organ of Zuckerkandl. Postcontrast CT image shows two large, mixed-density masses (M) surrounding the distal abdominal aorta (Ao); (*arrow*) contrast-filled ureters; (K) kidneys.

neous neuromas (84). Pheochromocytomas are bilateral in approximately 10% of cases (44).

Pheochromocytomas arise from the chromaffin cells of the sympathetic nervous system. Although most pheochromocytomas arise in the adrenal medulla, as many as 10% of the tumors occur in extraadrenal locations, most frequently in the paracaval or paraaortic regions along the course of the sympathetic ganglia (7%) or near the organ of Zuckerkandl (Fig. 19). These tumors also occur in the mediastinum (1%) and in the wall of the urinary bladder (1%) (28) (Fig. 20). Extraadrenal pheochromocytomas may occur singly or as multicentric lesions (38). Unlike most pheochromocytomas, which are unilateral, those associated with MEA-II syndrome are more often bilateral (75%) (Fig. 21) and are rarely extraadrenal (86). Pheo-

chromocytomas are malignant in 6% to 10% of cases (44). However, approximately 40% of extraadrenal pheochromocytomas are malignant. The diagnosis of a malignant pheochromocytoma may depend on detection of metastatic disease, because histologic differentiation between benign and malignant tumors can be difficult (38).

Most pheochromocytomas are larger than 3 cm at the time of clinical presentation (87). On CT images, the tumors may appear as homogeneous masses of soft-tissue density (Figs. 21 and 22). With the larger tumors, necrosis frequently is present, producing central regions of low density. Rarely, extensive central necrosis results in a cystic appearance that may resemble an adrenal cyst on CT (8). Calcifications may occur within the tumors (Fig. 21). Following intravenous administration of contrast material, there is enhancement of the tumors, and any inhomogeneity of the tumors is more easily visualized.

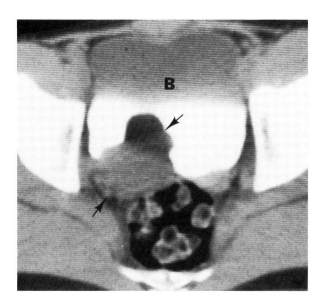

FIG. 20. Pheochromocytoma originating from the wall of the urinary bladder in a 16-year-old boy presenting with severe hypertension and postmicturition syncope. Postcontrast CT image shows an irregular mass (*arrows*) indenting the posterior bladder wall; (B) urinary bladder.

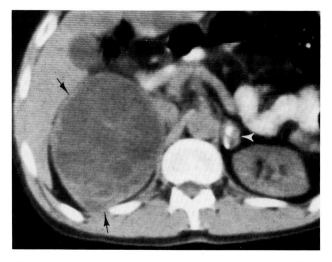

FIG. 21. Bilateral pheochromocytomas in a patient with MEA-II syndrome. Noncontrast CT image demonstrates a large, low-attenuation mass with a thick, soft-tissue-density rim and multiple internal septae in the region of the right adrenal gland (*arrows*). A 1.5-cm, partially calcified mass (*arrowhead*) is seen in the left adrenal gland.

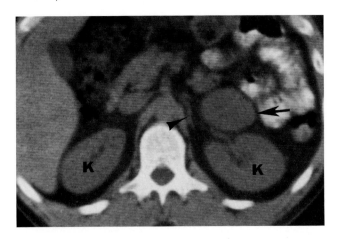

FIG. 22. Pheochromocytoma. A 4-cm mass (*arrow*) with an attenuation value similar to that of paraspinal muscle originates from the caudal portion of the lateral limb of the left adrenal. The normal medial limb (*arrowhead*) is also seen; (K) kidney.

CT has been able to detect approximately 90% of pheochromocytomas (94); false-negative examinations most commonly occur as a result of difficulty in detecting small tumors in patients with little retroperitoneal fat or in those cases in which the tumor is located outside the area surveyed by the CT examination. Pheochromocytomas originating in the mediastinum, especially those that are intrapericardial in location, can be difficult to detect because they are similar in density to the surrounding mediastinal structures on noncontrast images. In addition, the tumor and mediastinal vascular structures may appear isodense even on postcontrast images unless serial dynamic images are obtained during a bolus injection of contrast material (27).

Except for patients who have a predisposition for developing pheochromocytomas, a CT examination to search for a pheochromocytoma probably is not indicated in any hypertensive patient who has normal urinary catecholamines and VMA. If a patient with hypertension, but without documented biochemical evidence of pheochromocytoma, is referred for a CT examination, the study may be restricted to the adrenal glands. However, in patients with biochemical evidence suggestive of a pheochromocytoma, the entire retroperitoneum and pelvis should be surveyed if the adrenal glands are found to be normal. If still no tumor is found, a CT study of the chest should be considered. Most pheochromocytomas can be detected without intravenous injection of contrast material. Administration of contrast material may help detect extraadrenal pheochromocytomas, but it also exposes the patient to possible contrast-material-induced hypertensive crisis. Unpredictable and occasionally significant elevations in plasma norepinephrine have been reported following intravenous administration of contrast material. As a result, it has been suggested that a patient suspected of having a pheochromocytoma may benefit from α-adrenergic blockade if contrast material is to be given during the CT examination (74). CT is less successful (73%) in detecting recurrent disease, primarily because of either the small size of the recurrent tumor or artifacts secondary to surgical clips (94). Possible sites of recurrence include the contralateral adrenal, the bed of the resected gland, lung, bone, and liver (94).

Pheochromocytomas as small as 1.1 cm have been detected by MRI (76). As with CT, small pheochromocytomas often have a homogeneous appearance, whereas the larger tumors appear inhomogeneous. Malignant and benign pheochromocytomas may have similar signal intensities (76). On T1-weighted images, they are similar to the liver, kidney, and muscle in signal intensity and are easily distinguished from surrounding fat (21,76). Using a T2-weighted pulse sequence, pheochromocytomas demonstrate a high signal intensity that is markedly greater than that of the liver and muscle (30,76) and may be greater than that of fat (21) (Fig. 23). If a large tumor is present, coronal or sagittal views may help delineate the extent of the lesion, as well as define interfaces between the pheochromocytoma and adjacent organs such as the liver. In addition, coronal views may be helpful for screening the sympathetic chain (25).

NONHYPERFUNCTIONING TUMORS

Most patients with nonhyperfunctioning adrenal tumors do not have any symptoms referable to the adrenal lesion unless there is hemorrhage within the tumor or the tumor is large enough to cause symptoms on the basis of size alone. As a result, nonhyperfunctioning adrenal tu-

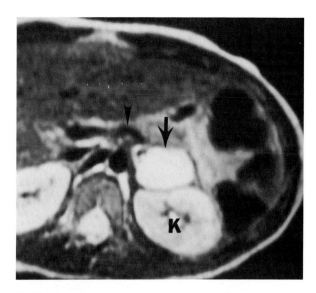

FIG. 23. Pheochromocytoma in an 8-year-old boy with severe hypertension. T2-weighted image (TR = 2,000 msec, TE = 70 msec) obtained from a 1.5-T imager shows a well-defined, markedly hyperintense left adrenal mass (*arrow*); (K) kidney; (*arrowhead*) splenic vein. (Courtesy of Dr. Arthur Bishop, Peoria, Illinois.)

mors often are discovered incidentally on CT examinations performed for other indications.

Nonhyperfunctioning Adenomas

Not infrequently, adrenal adenomas are detected by CT in patients with no clinical or biochemical evidence of adrenal hyperfunction. Small incidental adenomas have been found in 2% to 8% of autopsies and are most common in elderly, obese diabetics (30%), elderly women (29%), and hypertensives (20%) (84). Nonhyperfunctioning adenomas also occur at increased incidence in association with malignant tumors of the bladder, kidney, and endometrium. In these patients, differentiation between an incidental adenoma and a metastasis by CT may not be possible.

The CT appearance of nonhyperfunctioning adenomas may be indistinguishable from those of other adenomas. They usually are well defined, have a smooth contour, and have no perceptible wall. These adenomas usually are homogeneous in appearance and often have an attenuation value that is less than that of muscle and may be near that of water, depending on the amount of lipid within the tumor (11,32) (Figs. 24 and 25). Calcifications may be present, and there may be mild enhancement after intravenous administration of contrast material (58). Nonhyperfunctioning adenomas range from 1 to 6 cm in diameter, with the majority of lesions less than 3 cm in diameter (4,32,66), and can be bilateral.

On MRI, nonhyperfunctioning adenomas usually have a homogeneous appearance, with a signal intensity less than that of fat but greater than that of muscle on all pulse sequences (11). The signal intensity of a nonhyperfunc-

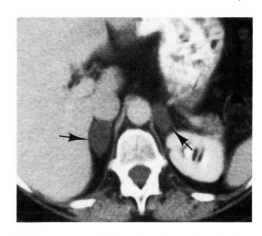

FIG. 25. Biopsy-proved bilateral nonhyperfunctioning adenomas in a patient with bronchogenic carcinoma. Postcontrast CT image demonstrates bilateral adrenal masses (*arrows*), each measuring 1.5 cm in diameter. Both masses have homogeneous near-water attenuation values. This CT appearance is fairly characteristic of a nonhyperfunctioning adenoma.

tioning adenoma is similar to that of the liver and normal adrenal on both T1-weighted and T2-weighted images (11,21,30,76) (Fig. 26).

Metastatic Disease

The adrenals are frequent sites of metastatic disease. The most common primary tumors that metastasize to the adrenal gland are lung and breast malignancies. In addition, metastatic disease from thyroid, renal, gastric, colon, pancreatic, and esophageal carcinomas, as well as melanoma, occur not infrequently. Adrenal metastases have been detected by CT in up to 15% of patients with carcinoma of the lung (90). It is not unusual for the adrenals to be the only demonstrable sites of metastatic disease in patients with bronchogenic carcinoma (68,78). Preoperative CT evaluation of the adrenal glands has been recommended in patients with non-small-cell carcinoma of the lung (63,78). If an adrenal metastasis is identified, chemotherapy or radiation therapy becomes the primary therapeutic option, rather than thoracotomy and surgical resection. Therefore, any patient who has a CT study of the chest for suspected lung carcinoma should also have the adrenal glands evaluated at the same time. Examination of the adrenal glands also has been advocated in patients with small-cell carcinoma of the lung, because accurate staging of the extent of disease may help determine the prognosis for the patient (90).

As demonstrated by CT, adrenal metastases vary considerably in size, frequently are bilateral, and most commonly have a round or ovoid shape (Fig. 27). When metastases are large and bilateral, they may lead to adrenal insufficiency. Adrenal metastases may have well-defined smooth contours or may have irregular, lobulated margins. Occasionally, metastatic disease can result in a small

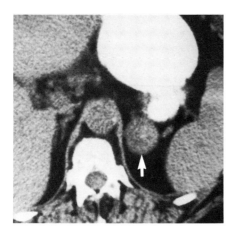

FIG. 24. Incidentally discovered nonhyperfunctioning adenoma. CT image performed because of low-back pain demonstrates a 2.5-cm, slightly inhomogeneous left adrenal mass (*arrow*) with near-soft-tissue density. Biochemical evaluation of adrenal function was normal. Follow-up image 6 months later demonstrated no interval change.

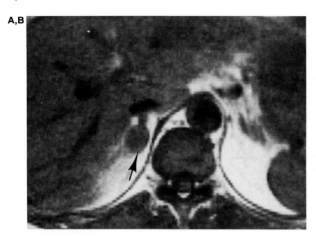 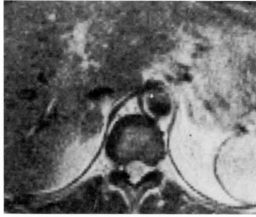

FIG. 26. Nonhyperfunctioning adenoma: MRI appearance. **A:** T1-weighted image (TR = 500 msec, TE = 35 msec) shows a 1.5-cm right adrenal mass (*arrow*). The mass has a signal intensity similar to that of the liver, but much lower than that of fat. **B:** T2-weighted image (TR = 2,100 msec, TE = 90 msec). The adrenal mass has a signal intensity similar to that of the liver, but much lower than that of fat.

adrenal mass that appears to retain the normal adrenal shape, but careful evaluation of the enlarged gland usually will show abnormal focal convexity of the contour of the adrenal lesion. Most often, an adrenal metastasis is of soft-tissue density; however, the larger masses frequently appear inhomogeneous as a result of focal areas of necrosis or hemorrhage (Fig. 28). On rare occasion, adrenal metastases may even calcify (Fig. 29). Although CT can accurately detect metastatic disease that has produced gross morphologic enlargement of the adrenals, adrenal glands that have a normal appearance on CT may still contain microscopic foci of metastatic disease (10,68,69).

When evaluated by MRI, adrenal metastases frequently appear inhomogeneous on T2-weighted images and sometimes on T1-weighted images as well (11) (Figs. 30 and 31). With a T1-weighted pulse sequence, adrenal me-

tastases appear either hypointense or isointense to the liver (11,21,30,76). On T2-weighted images, all adrenal metastases appear hyperintense as compared with the liver (11,76) and frequently have a signal intensity equal to or greater than that of fat (11,21,76). If hemorrhage has occurred within the tumor, the metastasis may have areas of high signal intensity on both T1- and T2-weighted images.

Although adrenal metastases may simulate nonhyperfunctioning adrenal adenomas on T1-weighted images, these usually can be differentiated from one another on T2-weighted sequences (11,30,75) (Fig. 30). With few exceptions (2), nonhyperfunctioning adenomas usually appear hypointense to fat, whereas metastases frequently

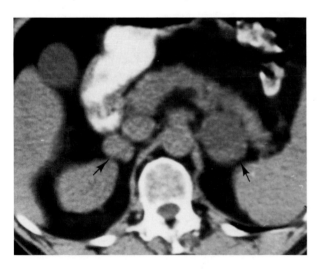

FIG. 27. Bilateral adrenal metastases from primary bronchogenic carcinoma. Noncontrast CT image shows bilateral adrenal masses (*arrows*), the left having an attenuation value slightly lower than that of the right.

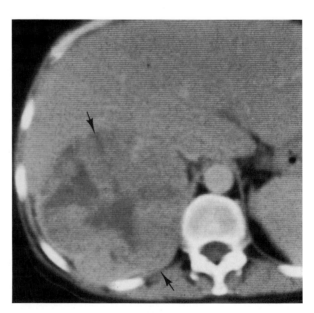

FIG. 28. Metastatic melanoma to the right adrenal gland. Postcontrast CT image shows a large, inhomogeneous mass (*arrows*) with central necrosis.

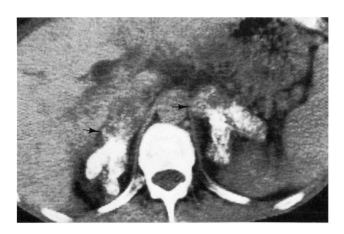

FIG. 29. Calcified adrenal metastasis in a patient with carcinoma of the colon. Noncontrast CT image demonstrates diffuse calcifications in two markedly enlarged adrenal glands. Although both adrenal glands maintain their overall configuration, focal bulges (*arrows*) are nevertheless present. (Courtesy of Dr. David DiSantis, Norfolk, Virginia.)

are isointense to fat on T2-weighted images. The distinction between these two entities also can be achieved by calculating the intensity ratio between the adrenal mass and fat or between the adrenal mass and the liver. In one study using images obtained with a 0.5-T imager using a

TR of 2,100 msec and TE of 90 msec, none of the metastases had an intensity ratio (adrenal mass vs. fat) less than 0.6, and none of the nonhyperfunctioning adenomas had a ratio greater than 0.8. However, in one-third of the cases, the ratio was between 0.6 and 0.8, making distinction between these two entities impossible (11).

Because an adrenal metastasis may be indistinguishable from an adrenal adenoma on CT, an MRI study should be performed to further characterize a solitary adrenal mass discovered in any patient with carcinoma who has no other evidence of metastatic disease. If the MRI findings are equivocal, a biopsy of the adrenal mass should then follow. This can be achieved percutaneously utilizing CT or ultrasound guidance.

Myelolipoma

Myelolipomas are rare benign tumors, with an autopsy incidence of 0.2% to 0.4% (67). These tumors probably arise from reticulum-cell metaplasia (71) and are composed of myeloid and erythroid elements as well as fatty tissue. Myelolipomas usually are unilateral and asymptomatic. However, they may enlarge to 10 to 12 cm in diameter, and patients rarely may develop flank or ab-

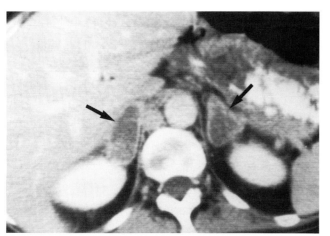

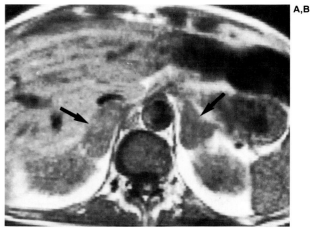

A,B

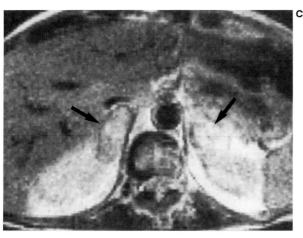

C

FIG. 30. Bilateral adrenal metastases. **A:** Postcontrast CT image demonstrates slightly inhomogeneous, but predominantly low-density, masses with enhanced walls in both adrenal glands (*arrows*). **B:** T1-weighted image (TR = 500 msec, TE = 35 msec) at a similar level as (**A**) confirms the presence of bilateral adrenal masses (*arrows*). The MRI appearance of these masses is indistinguishable from that of nonhyperfunctioning adenomas on this sequence. **C:** T2-weighted image (TR = 2,100 msec, TE = 90 msec) shows the masses (*arrows*) to have inhomogeneous signals. The intensity in the central portions of both masses is similar to that of perirenal fat, compatible with metastases.

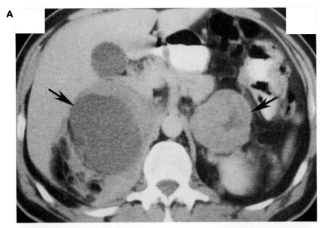

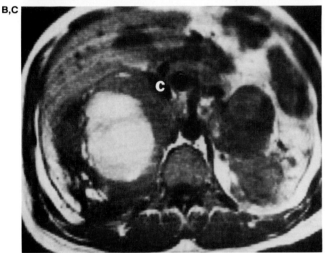

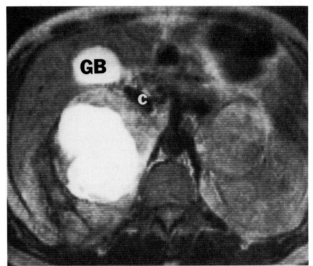

FIG. 31. Hemorrhagic adrenal metastases due to melanoma. **A:** Postcontrast CT image demonstrates bilateral, inhomogeneous adrenal masses (*arrows*), the right being more irregular than the left. **B:** T1-weighted image (TR = 500 msec, TE = 35 msec) shows basically the same findings as CT. The extremely high signal intensity seen in the right adrenal mass is due to subacute hemorrhage. **C:** T2-weighted image (TR = 2,100 msec, TE = 90 msec). With the exception of hemorrhage, both adrenal masses have signal intensities similar to that of fat; (c) inferior vena cava; (GB) gallbladder.

dominal pain secondary to hemorrhage or necrosis within the mass (24).

On CT images, myelolipomas are well-defined masses. The appearance of the mass depends on the relative amount of fatty tissue within the lesion. As a result, these tumors vary in appearance from a predominantly fatty mass with a surrounding thin rim of soft tissue to a lesion that is predominantly of soft-tissue density but contains small regions of fat density (Fig. 32). The fatty component of the tumor may be isodense with subcutaneous and retroperitoneal fat or may have an attenuation value between those of subcutaneous fat and water. High-density areas

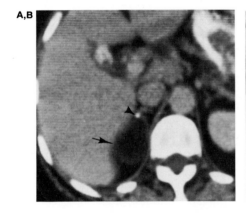

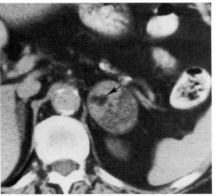

FIG. 32. Myelolipoma. **A:** Postcontrast CT image demonstrates a predominantly fatty mass originating from the right adrenal gland (*arrow*). A speckle of calcification is noted anteriorly (*arrowhead*). **B:** In another patient, a noncontrast CT image shows a 4-cm inhomogeneous mass replacing the left adrenal gland. Only a small portion of the mass is of fat density (*arrow*), whereas the remaining portion has mixed attenuation values.

A,B

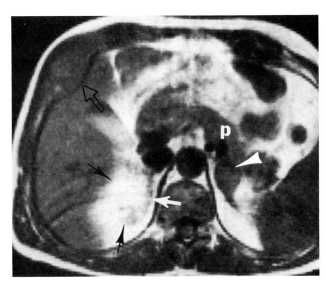 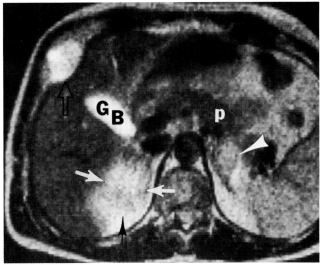

FIG. 33. Myelolipoma: MRI appearance. **A:** T1-weighted image (TR = 500 msec, TE = 30 msec) shows a large right adrenal mass (*arrows*) composed predominantly of fat. Also noted is a metastasis to a right rib (*open arrow*) and the left adrenal gland (*arrowhead*) from a primary bronchogenic carcinoma. **B:** T2-weighted image (TR = 2,100 msec, TE = 90 msec). Both the adrenal metastases (*arrowhead*) and myelolipoma (*arrows*) have a signal intensity similar to that of fat on this sequence; (*open arrow*) rib metastasis; (GB) gallbladder; (p) pancreas.

occasionally are observed within a myelolipoma that probably are secondary to prior hemorrhage (88). Calcifications may be present, and occasionally the tumor may appear to extend into the perinephric space (91). Although functioning adrenal tissue may be found within a myelolipoma, it almost never leads to hyperfunction (5). However, a hyperfunctioning adrenal adenoma and a myelolipoma may coexist within the same adrenal gland (93,95). In most cases, the characteristic CT appearance of a myelolipoma allows the diagnosis to be made without additional studies, and in an asymptomatic patient surgical intervention is not indicated. In one case, a metastasis to the adrenal gland from adenocarcinoma of the lung had an appearance similar to that of a myelolipoma and was believed to be secondary to the malignancy invading and engulfing a portion of surrounding fat (35). If confirmation of the diagnosis of a myelolipoma is indicated, percutaneous needle aspiration or biopsy may be performed. The histologic diagnosis of myelolipoma requires the presence of myeloid and erythroid elements as well as mature fat cells. In particular, the most important cytologic feature is the presence of megakaryocytes (15). If the specimen is composed primarily of hematopoietic tissue, the lesion may not be distinguishable from other adrenal neoplasms (15). Extramedullary hematopoiesis rarely involves the adrenal gland and will also demonstrate erythroid and myeloid precursors by needle aspiration; however, fat cells will not be seen (49).

As in the case of CT, the MRI appearance of myelolipomas varies with the amount of fat contained in the tumor (30,81) (Fig. 33). Myelolipomas containing little or no fat cannot be distinguished from other types of adrenal neoplasms.

Other Neoplasms

The adrenals occasionally are involved by lymphoma, with diffuse non-Hodgkin lymphoma the most frequent cell type (31,45,70). On CT images there is enlargement of one or both adrenal glands, usually concomitant with retroperitoneal lymphadenopathy (31,45) (Fig. 34), although lymphoma limited to the adrenal glands can occur (23). The MRI appearance of adrenal lymphoma is nonspecific and is indistinguishable from that of metastatic disease to the adrenals (11,30) (Fig. 35).

Adult neuroblastoma is a rare tumor that is different from childhood neuroblastoma in that extraadrenal sites frequently are involved, and calcification of the neoplasm is rare. In one series of 27 cases (85), the mediastinum was the most common primary site, followed by the adrenal gland, retroperitoneum, and pelvis. Also, at the time of presentation, there often are multiple sites of involvement (22,85). The most common sites of metastatic disease include the skeletal system, lungs, liver, and lymph nodes. The presentation of adult neuroblastoma typically is nonspecific, with symptoms usually due to compression of adjacent organs or nerves. On CT, the tumor may simulate an adrenal carcinoma or even a renal-cell carcinoma, including extension into the renal vein (89) (Fig. 36A). The MRI signal intensities of neuroblastomas are nonspecific and vary from slightly to markedly hyperintense relative to the liver on T2-weighted images (21,30) (Fig. 36B,C).

The CT appearance of an adrenal cavernous hemangioma is that of a low-density mass with central and peripheral calcifications, some of which may have a phlebolith-like appearance on plain radiographs (52).

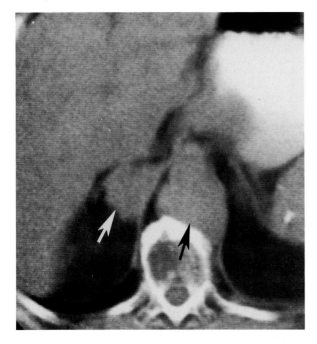

FIG. 34. Adrenal lymphoma. CT image shows a large, irregular right adrenal gland (*white arrow*). Retrocrural lymphadenopathy (*black arrow*) is also present.

CYSTS

Cystic lesions of the adrenal are extremely rare. The most common adrenal cysts are endothelial cysts (45% of all adrenal cysts), which are predominantly lymphangiomatous cysts (47). These cysts usually are small (1–15 mm) and asymptomatic. Pseudocysts (39% of all adrenal cysts) are the most common clinically detected cysts and result from hemorrhage into normal adrenal glands or into adrenal neoplasms (26,47). Pseudocysts may become very large and produce lumbar or flank pain due to compression of adjacent structures or rupture. Rare cystic lesions of the adrenals include parasitic cysts (7%), which usually are echinococcal, and true epithelial cysts (9%).

Benign adrenal cysts typically are well-defined, near-water-density masses (Fig. 11). The wall of an adrenal pseudocyst may contain calcification and may be enhanced after administration of contrast material (101). A pseudocyst may contain multiple septations. Differentiation between a cyst and a low-density adenoma can be difficult with CT; if clinically indicated, either ultrasound or MRI can be used to distinguish the two.

INFLAMMATORY DISEASE

Active granulomatous disease of the adrenals usually causes diffuse enlargement of both adrenal glands (16,39,57,98). Low-density areas within the adrenals represent regions of caseous necrosis (98). Bilaterally enlarged adrenal glands in a patient with a reactive tuberculin skin test are suggestive of active tuberculosis, even though characteristic lung lesions may not be present and pulmonary cultures may be negative (79). The adrenals also may be involved by disseminated histoplasmosis, in which the enlarged adrenals frequently maintain their normal shape (98) (Fig. 37). Infiltration of adrenal glands by North American blastomycosis also has been reported (37). Documentation of an infectious process may require percutaneous aspiration of the adrenals (16,37,98). The adrenals may develop calcifications as a result of the inflam-

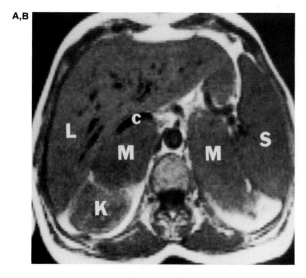
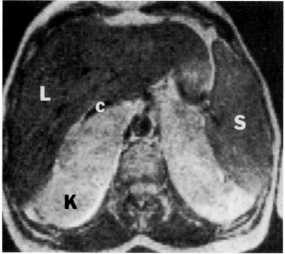

FIG. 35. Primary adrenal lymphoma: MRI appearance. **A:** T1-weighted image (TR = 500 msec, TE = 35 msec) shows two oblong-shaped adrenal masses (M). **B:** T2-weighted image (TR = 2,100 msec, TE = 90 msec). The masses are slightly inhomogeneous and have a signal intensity similar to that of fat. Based on MRI signal characteristics, adrenal lymphoma cannot be distinguished from metastases; (K) kidney; (c) inferior vena cava; (L) liver; (S) spleen.

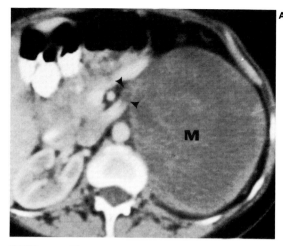

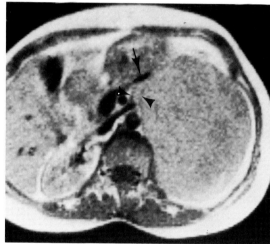

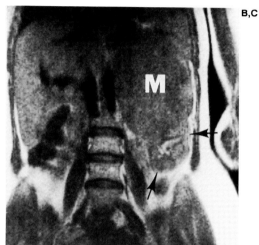

FIG. 36. Adrenal neuroblastoma in a 50-year-old woman. **A:** Postcontrast CT image demonstrates a large, inhomogeneous left adrenal mass (M) invading the proximal left renal vein (*arrowheads*). **B:** Transaxial MR image (TR = 1,500 msec, TE = 35 msec) at a similar level demonstrates essentially the same findings. Again note the extension of the tumor into the proximal left renal vein (*arrowheads*); (*arrow*) splenic vein. **C:** Coronal MR image (TR = 500 msec, TE = 35 msec) shows inferior displacement of the left kidney (*arrows*) by the mass (M). The high-intensity structures in the kidney represent renal sinus fat surrounding the pyelocalyceal system.

matory process. The calcifications may be quite dense, and at times no noncalcified glandular tissue can be seen. The absence of an associated soft-tissue mass helps differentiate postinflammatory adrenal calcifications from calcifications arising within an adrenal tumor. Rarely, an

abscess may develop in the adrenal gland as a result of bacterial infection (64).

On MRI, adrenal masses due to tuberculosis may have a high signal intensity, similar to that of fat on T2-weighted images (2).

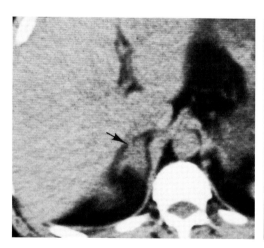

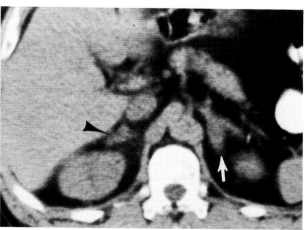

FIG. 37. Bilateral adrenal enlargement secondary to disseminated histoplasmosis. **A:** Enlarged right adrenal gland (*arrow*). **B:** One centimeter caudad, an enlarged left adrenal gland is seen (*arrow*). Only the lateral limb of the right adrenal (*arrowhead*) is seen at this level.

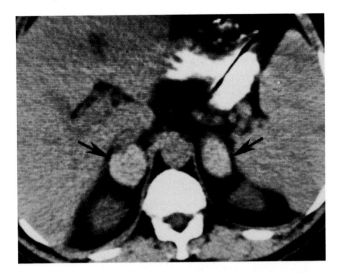

FIG. 38. Acute adrenal hemorrhage. Noncontrast CT image demonstrates bilateral adrenal masses (*arrows*), each measuring 3.5 cm in diameter. The attenuation value of both masses is uniformly higher than that of paraspinal muscle.

Adrenal Hemorrhage

Bilateral adrenal hemorrhage is an uncommon condition that usually occurs in association with a bleeding diathesis or severe stress to the patient, such as major surgery or sepsis. In particular, anticoagulant therapy is a predisposing factor with most anticoagulant-related adrenal hemorrhages occurring during the initial 3 weeks of treatment (65,100). Potentially fatal acute adrenal insufficiency may develop as a result of the adrenal hemorrhage. Because the clinical manifestations of adrenal insufficiency often are nonspecific, the diagnosis may be first suggested or confirmed by CT (53,99). Failure of the adrenal glands to respond to an ACTH stimulation test confirms the diagnosis of adrenal insufficiency.

Typically, spontaneous bilateral adrenal hemorrhage presents as adrenal masses up to 3 cm in diameter (53,99) (Fig. 38) that may appear hyperdense or may be of soft-tissue density. When they have an attenuation value of soft tissue, hemorrhage-related adrenal masses may be indistinguishable from adrenal metastases, although adrenal insufficiency secondary to metastatic disease is uncommon (6). Follow-up CT studies will show progressive decreases in size and density of the adrenal masses (53,99), and calcification of the gland may develop as a late sequela (Fig. 39).

Posttraumatic adrenal hemorrhage usually (85% of cases) involves the right adrenal gland (82). It is believed that elevation of the inferior vena cava pressure as a result of blunt trauma may be more directly transmitted to the right adrenal gland as compared with the left adrenal. Characteristically, CT demonstrates a hyperdense right adrenal mass, streaky infiltration of the periadrenal tissue,

and enlargement of the right diaphragmatic crus (97). The CT appearance may resemble bleeding into an adrenal tumor.

As with CT, the signal intensity of adrenal hemorrhage on MR images will depend on the age of the hematoma. Subacute adrenal hemorrhage may have a high signal intensity on T1- and T2-weighted images (50).

Addison Disease

The CT appearance of the adrenals in patients with Addison disease may help determine the cause of the adrenal hypofunction and as a result may occasionally help in the management of the patient. Adrenal atrophy on the basis of either autoimmune disease or a deficiency of ACTH production by the pituitary gland results in bilateral small glands, without adrenal calcification (16,43). Bilateral adrenal enlargement in the clinical setting of adrenal insufficiency may be secondary to adrenal hemorrhage (53), to an infectious process such as tuberculosis or histoplasmosis (57,98), or, less likely, to metastatic disease (6). Small adrenals that are partially or completely calcified suggest a prior inflammatory process, whereas dense bilateral adrenal calcifications in a patient with normal adrenal function are more likely to be posthemorrhagic in origin. In addition, patients with secondary hemochromatosis may have mild adrenal insufficiency associated with normal-size or small adrenal glands that are slightly hyperdense (16).

CT AND OTHER IMAGING TECHNIQUES

As compared with CT, ultrasound has a higher false-positive rate and lower specificity (1). Also, evaluation of

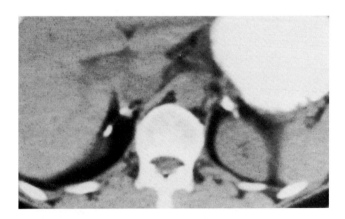

FIG. 39. Bilateral adrenal calcifications incidentally discovered on a CT study performed for another reason. Patient had a history of adrenal hemorrhage, but had no clinical evidence of adrenal insufficiency.

the adrenals, especially the left adrenal, often is limited by the size of the patient or by overlying bowel gas. Therefore, except in the pediatric population, ultrasound is not used as the primary test, but rather in selected cases to further characterize adrenal masses demonstrated by CT. Occasionally, with large upper abdominal masses, the ability to use ultrasound to image in any plane helps determine the organ of origin. Also, ultrasound can be used to determine whether a low-density adrenal mass is cystic or solid.

Although adrenal angiography and venography have been replaced by CT, adrenal venous sampling is still performed if a patient is suspected of having a hyperfunctioning tumor, but has normal or equivocal findings on CT study. Although venous sampling is an invasive, technically difficult procedure with potential complications of adrenal infarction and hemorrhage (3,29), it is more sensitive than CT in detecting aldosteronomas (29).

In the evaluation of adrenocortical disease, adrenal scintigraphy with ^{131}I-labeled iodocholesterol preparations offers no significant advantage over CT. Although the overall accuracies of the two techniques are similar (36), adrenal scintigraphy has several disadvantages. Compared with CT, radionuclide scintigraphy is more expensive, requires several days for completion of the study, and exposes the patient to a greater radiation dose. In addition, there is limited availability of the radiopharmaceutical (36). Similar disadvantages limit the use of adrenergic tissue-localizing radiopharmaceuticals, such as ^{131}I-labeled metaiodobenzylguanidine (MIBG), that have been reported to be comparable to CT for evaluation of adrenal pheochromocytomas (73). One advantage of ^{131}I-MIBG is that the entire body can be imaged in a patient suspected of having primary extraadrenal or metastatic pheochromocytomas. Use of ^{123}I-MIBG may increase the sensitivity of the test, because a higher dose of radiopharmaceutical can be administered; however, there is greater uptake by the normal adrenal medulla as compared with ^{131}I-MIBG, and differentiation between abnormal and normal tracer uptake may be difficult (55).

Although MRI is able to demonstrate both normal and abnormal adrenal glands accurately, it is presently limited by its longer examination time, greater cost, and more stringent patient requirements as compared with CT. However, MRI is extremely useful in selected cases. As stated previously, MRI can differentiate between a nonfunctioning adrenal adenoma and a metastasis (11,30,75). In addition, in patients with large upper abdominal masses, MRI may be more accurate in demonstrating the adrenal as the organ of origin and the extent of the mass. Also, MRI can better delineate recurrent disease in postoperative patients, in whom the prior tumor bed often is obscured on CT images by surgical-clip-related artifacts (76). Lastly, pregnant patients suspected of having adrenal disease can be more safely studied with MRI (34).

CLINICAL APPLICATION

Because of its high accuracy and ease of performance, CT remains the procedure of choice for imaging the adrenal gland. A CT examination should be performed whenever an adrenal mass is suggested either by the clinical history or by another radiologic study such as excretory urography or ultrasound. If an adrenal mass is detected, the patient should be evaluated for evidence of hyperfunction. Of the nonhyperfunctioning adrenal masses, those larger than 3 cm most likely represent either an adenoma or a metastasis, and differentiation of the two by CT may not be possible. In one study of patients without any known primary extraadrenal malignancy, only 39% of the incidental adrenal masses detected by CT represented malignant tumors (4). In another series of patients with non-small-cell bronchogenic carcinoma, 68% of patients with isolated adrenal masses demonstrated on preoperative CT studies had benign adenomas (66). Therefore, in any patient with a resectable primary malignancy that has a high propensity to metastasize to the adrenal gland, an MRI study should be performed to distinguish a metastasis from a nonhyperfunctioning adenoma, especially in cases in which there is no other evidence of possible metastatic disease. If the MRI findings are equivocal, the lesion should then be biopsied. Percutaneous needle biopsy of the adrenal gland under CT or ultrasound guidance is a safe and accurate procedure (40,68). Prior to biopsy of any adrenal mass, the possibility of a pheochromocytoma should be excluded by clinical history or by a urine screening test, because needle biopsy of a pheochromocytoma may precipitate a potentially fatal catecholamine crisis (9,56).

Any small adrenal mass that has a smooth contour, has an attenuation value less than that of soft tissue, and appears homogeneous is highly suggestive of a benign adenoma. If the patient has no known primary extraadrenal malignancy, such a mass may be managed conservatively, with a follow-up CT study in 3 to 6 months. If there is no interval growth of the mass, the diagnosis of a benign adenoma is confirmed. Alternatively, an MRI study can be used to corroborate its benign nature. In rare cases in which a suspected adenoma is biopsied percutaneously, localization of the needle tip within the mass must be verified. Because an adenoma cannot be differentiated cytologically from normal adrenal parenchyma cells, a false-negative result may be obtained if the normal parenchyma is sampled instead of the mass (40).

REFERENCES

1. Abrams HI, Siegelman SS, Adams DF, et al. Computed tomography versus ultrasound of the adrenal gland: a prospective study. *Radiology* 1982;143:121–128.

2. Baker ME, Spritzer C, Blinder R, Herfkens RJ, Leight GS, Dunnick NR. Benign adrenal lesions mimicking malignancy on MR imaging: report of two cases. *Radiology* 1987;163:669–671.

3. Bayliss RI, Edwards OM, Starer F. Complications of adrenal venography. *Br J Radiol* 1970;43:531–533.

4. Belldegrun A, Hussain S, Seltzer SE, Loughlin KR, Gittes RF, Richie JP. Incidentally discovered mass of the adrenal gland. *Surg Gynecol Obstet* 1986;163:203–208.

5. Bennett BD, McKenna TJ, Hough AJ, Dean R, Page DL. Adrenal myelolipoma associated with Cushing's disease. *Am J Clin Pathol* 1980;73:443–447.

6. Black RM, Daniels GH, Coggins CH, Mueller PR, Data RE, Lichtenstein N. Adrenal insufficiency from metastatic colonic carcinoma masquerading as isolated aldosterone deficiency. Report of a case and review of the literature. *Acta Endocrinol* 1981;98:586–591.

7. Brady TM, Gross BH, Glazer GM, Williams DM. Adrenal pseudomasses due to varices: angiographic–CT–MRI–pathologic correlations. *AJR* 1985;145:301–304.

8. Bush WH, Elder JS, Crane RE, Wales LR. Cystic pheochromocytoma. *Urology* 1985;25:332–334.

9. Casola G, Nicolet V, van Sonnenberg E, et al. Unsuspected pheochromocytoma: risk of blood-pressure alterations during percutaneous adrenal biopsy. *Radiology* 1986;159:733–735.

10. Cedermark BJ, Ohlsen H. Computed tomography in the diagnosis of metastases of the adrenal glands. *Surg Gynecol Obstet* 1981;152: 13–16.

11. Chang A, Glazer HS, Lee JKT, Ling D, Heiken JP. Adrenal gland: MR imaging. *Radiology* 1987;163:123–128.

12. Cryer PE. The adrenal cortex. In: Cryer PE, ed. *Diagnostic endocrinology.* 2nd ed. New York: Oxford University Press, 1979:55–94.

13. Cryer PE. The adrenergic nervous system. In: Cryer PE, ed. *Diagnostic endocrinology.* 2nd ed. New York: Oxford University Press, 1979:117–134.

14. Davis PL, Hricak H, Bradley WG Jr. Magnetic resonance imaging of the adrenal glands. *Radiol Clin North Am* 1984;22:891–895.

15. DeBlois GG, DeMay RM. Adrenal myelolipoma diagnosis by computed-tomography-guided fine-needle aspiration. *Cancer* 1985;55:848–850.

16. Doppman JL, Gill JR Jr, Nienhuis AW, Earll JM, Long JA Jr. CT findings in Addison's disease. *J Comput Assist Tomogr* 1982;6: 757–761.

17. Dunnick NR, Doppman JL, Geelhoed GW. Intravenous extension of endocrine tumors. *AJR* 1980;135:471–476.

18. Dunnick NR, Doppman JL, Gill JR, Strott CA, Keiser HR, Brennan MF. Localization of functional adrenal tumors by computed tomography and venous sampling. *Radiology* 1982;142:429–433.

19. Dunnick NR, Heaston D, Halvorsen R, Moore AV, Korobkin M. CT appearance of adrenal cortical carcinoma. *J Comput Assist Tomogr* 1982;6:978–982.

20. Eghrari M, McLoughlin MJ, Rosen IE, et al. The role of computed tomography in assessment of tumoral pathology of the adrenal glands. *J Comput Assist Tomogr* 1980;4:71–77.

21. Falke TH, te-Strake L, Shaff MI, et al. MR imaging of the adrenals: correlation with computed tomography. *J Comput Assist Tomogr* 1986;10:242–253.

22. Feinstein RS, Gatewood OMB, Fishman EK, Goldman SM, Siegelman SS. Computed tomography of adult neuroblastoma. *J Comput Assist Tomogr* 1984;8:720–726.

23. Feldberg MAM, Hendriks MJ, Klinkhamer AC. Massive bilateral non-Hodgkin's lymphomas of the adrenals. *Urol Radiol* 1986;8: 85–88.

24. Fink DW, Wurtzebach LR. Symptomatic myelolipoma of the adrenal. *Radiology* 1980;134:451–452.

25. Rink IJ, Reinig JW, Dwyer AJ, Doppman JL, Linehan WM, Keiser HR. MR imaging of pheochromocytomas. *J Comput Assist Tomogr* 1985;9:454–458.

26. Foster DG. Adrenal cysts. *Arch Surg* 1966;92:131–143.

27. Francis IR, Glazer GM, Shapiro B, Sisson JC, Gross BH. Complementary roles of CT and ^{131}I-MIBG scintigraphy in diagnosing pheochromocytoma. *AJR* 1983;141:719–725.

28. Fries JG, Chamberlin JA. Extra-adrenal pheochromocytoma: literature review and report of a cervical pheochromocytoma. *Surgery* 1968;63:268–279.

29. Geisinger MA, Zelch MG, Bravo EL, Risius BF, O'Donovan PB, Borkowski GP. Primary hyperaldosteronism: comparison of CT, adrenal venography, and venous sampling. *AJR* 1983;141:299–302.

30. Glazer GM, Woolsey EJ, Borrello J, et al. Adrenal tissue characterization using MR imaging. *Radiology* 1986;158:73–79.

31. Glazer HS, Lee JKT, Balfe DM, Mauro MA, Griffeth R, Sagel SS. Non-Hodgkin lymphoma: computed tomographic demonstration of unusual extranodal involvement. *Radiology* 1983;149:211–217.

32. Glazer HS, Weyman PJ, Sagel SS, Levitt RG, McClennan BL. Nonfunctioning adrenal masses: incidental discovery on computed tomography. *AJR* 1982;139:81–85.

33. Grant CS, Carpenter P, Van Heerden JA, Hamberger B. Primary aldosteronism. Clinical management. *Arch Surg* 1984;119:585–590.

34. Greenberg M, Moawad AH, Wienties BM, et al. Extraadrenal pheochromocytoma: detection during pregnancy using MR imaging. *Radiology* 1986;161:475–476.

35. Greene KM, Brantly PN, Thompson WR. Adenocarcinoma metastatic to the adrenal gland simulating myelolipoma: CT evaluation. *J Comput Assist Tomogr* 1985;9:820–821.

36. Guerin CK, Wahner HW, Gorman CA, Carpenter PC, Sheedy PF. Computed tomographic scanning versus radioisotope imaging in adrenocortical diagnosis. *Am J Med* 1983;75:653–657.

37. Halvorsen RA Jr, Heaston DK, Johnston WW, Ashton PR, Burton GM. Case report. CT guided thin needle aspiration of adrenal blastomycosis. *J Comput Assist Tomogr* 1982;6:389–391.

38. Hattery RR, Sheedy PF II, Stephens DH, Van Heerden JA. Computed tomography of the adrenal gland. *Semin Roentgenol* 1981;16: 290–300.

39. Hauser H, Gurret JP. Miliary tuberculosis associated with adrenal enlargement: CT appearance. *J Comput Assist Tomogr* 1986;10: 254–256.

40. Heaston DK, Handel DB, Ashton PR, Korobkin M. Narrow gauge needle aspiration of solid adrenal masses. *AJR* 1982;138:1143–1148.

41. Henley DJ, Van Heerden JA, Grant CS, Carney JA, Carpenter PC. Adrenal cortical carcinoma—a continuing challenge. *Surgery* 1983;94:926–931.

42. Horton R, Finck E. Diagnosis and localization in primary aldosteronism. *Ann Intern Med* 1972;76:885–890.

43. Huebener KH, Treugut H. Adrenal cortex dysfunction: CT findings. *Radiology* 1984;150:195–199.

44. Hume DM. Pheochromocytoma in the adult and in the child. *Am J Surg* 1960;99:458–496.

45. Jafri SZ, Francis IR, Glazer GM, Bree RL, Amendola MA. CT detection of adrenal lymphoma. *J Comput Assist Tomogr* 1983;7: 254–256.

46. Karstaedt N, Sagel SS, Stanley RJ, Melson GL, Levitt RG. Computed tomography of the adrenal gland. *Radiology* 1978;129:723–730.

47. Kearny GP, Mahoney EM, Maher E, Harrison JH. Functioning and nonfunctioning cysts of the adrenal cortex and medulla. *Am J Surg* 1977;134:363–368.

48. Kenney PJ, Robbins GL, Ellis DA, Spirt BA. Adrenal glands in patients with congenital renal anomalies: CT appearance. *Radiology* 1985;155:181–182.

49. King BF, Kopecky KK, Baker MK, Clark SA. Extramedullary hematopoiesis in the adrenal glands: CT characteristics. *J Comput Assist Tomogr* 1987;11:342–343.

50. Koch KJ, Cory DA. Simultaneous renal vein thrombosis and bilateral adrenal hemorrhage: MR demonstration. *J Comput Assist Tomogr* 1986;10:681–683.

51. Korobkin M, White EA, Kressel HY, Moss AA, Montagne JP. Computed tomography in the diagnosis of adrenal disease. *AJR* 1979;132:231–238.

52. Lee WJ, Weinreb J, Kumari S, Phillips G, Pochaczevsky R, Pillari G. Adrenal hemangioma. *J Comput Assist Tomogr* 1982;6:392–394.

53. Ling D, Korobkin M, Silverman PM, Dunnick NR. CT demonstration of bilateral adrenal hemorrhage. *AJR* 1983;141:307–308.

54. Lipsell MB, Hertz R, Ross GT. Clinical and pathophysiologic aspects of adrenocortical carcinoma. *Am J Med* 1963;35:374–383.

55. Lynn MD, Shapiro B, Sisson JC, et al. Pheochromocytoma and

the normal adrenal medulla: improved visualization with I-123 MIBG scintigraphy. *Radiology* 1987;156:789–792.

56. McCorkell SJ, Niles NL. Fine-needle aspiration of catecholamine-producing adrenal masses: a possibly fatal mistake. *AJR* 1985;145:113–114.

57. McMurry JF Jr, Long D, McClure R, Kotchen TA. Addison's disease with adrenal enlargement on computed tomographic scanning. Report on two cases of tuberculosis and review of the literature. *Am J Med* 1984;77:365–368.

58. Mitnick JS, Bosniak MA, Megibow AJ, Naidich DP. Non-functioning adrenal adenomas discovered incidentally on computed tomography. *Radiology* 1983;148:495–499.

59. Mitty HA, Cohen BA, Sprayregen S, Schwartz K. Adrenal pseudotumors on CT due to dilated portosystemic veins. *AJR* 1983;141:727–730.

60. Montagne JP, Kressel HY, Korobkin M, Moss AA. Computed tomography of the normal adrenal glands. *AJR* 1978;130:963–966.

61. Moon KL, Hricak H, Crooks LE, et al. Nuclear magnetic resonance imaging of the adrenal gland: a preliminary report. *Radiology* 1983;147:155–160.

62. Nader S, Hickey RC, Sellin RV, Samaan NA. Adrenal cortical carcinoma: a study of 77 cases. *Cancer* 1983;52:707–711.

63. Nielsen ME Jr, Heaston DK, Dunnick NR, Korobkin M. Preoperative CT evaluation of adrenal glands in non-small-cell bronchogenic carcinoma. *AJR* 1982;139:317–320.

64. O'Brien WM, Choyke PL, Copeland J, Klappenbach RS, Lyunch JH. Computed tomography of adrenal abscess. *J Comput Assist Tomogr* 1987;11:550–551.

65. O'Connel TX, Aston SJ. Acute adrenal hemorrhage complicating anticoagulant therapy. *Surg Gynecol Obstet* 1974;139:355–357.

66. Oliver TW, Bernardino ME, Miller JI, Mansour K, Greene D, Davis WA. Isolated adrenal masses in non-small-cell bronchogenic carcinoma. *Radiology* 1984;153:217–218.

67. Olsson CA, Krane RJ, Klugo RC, Selikowitz SM. Adrenal myelolipoma. *Surgery* 1973;73:665–670.

68. Pagani JJ. Non-small-cell lung carcinoma adrenal metastases. Computed tomography and percutaneous needle biopsy in their diagnosis. *Cancer* 1984;53:1058–1060.

69. Pagani JJ. Normal adrenal glands in small cell lung carcinoma: CT-guided biopsy. *AJR* 1983;140:949–951.

70. Paling MR, Williamson BRJ. Adrenal involvement in non-Hodgkin lymphoma. *AJR* 1983;141:303–305.

71. Plaut A. Myelolipoma in the adrenal cortex. *Am J Pathol* 1958;34:487–515.

72. Pojunas KW, Daniels DL, Williams AL, Thorsen MK, Haughton VM. Pituitary and adrenal CT of Cushing syndrome. *AJR* 1986;146:1235–1238.

73. Quint LE, Glazer GM, Francis IR, Shapiro B, Chenevert TL. Pheochromocytoma and paraganglioma: comparison of MR imaging with CT and I-131 MIBG scintigraphy. *Radiology* 1987;165:89–93.

74. Raisanen J, Shapiro B, Glazer GM, Desai S, Sisson JC. Plasma catecholamines in pheochromocytoma: effect of urographic contrast media. *AJR* 1984;143:43–46.

75. Reinig JW, Doppman JL, Dwyer AJ, Frank J. MRI of indeterminate adrenal masses. *AJR* 1986;147:493–496.

76. Reinig JW, Doppman JL, Dwyer AJ, Johnson AR, Knop RH. Adrenal masses differentiated by MR. *Radiology* 1986;158:81–84.

77. Roberts L Jr, Dunnick NR, Thompson WM, et al. Primary aldosteronism due to bilateral nodular hyperplasia: CT demonstration. *J Comput Assist Tomogr* 1985;9:1125–1127.

78. Sandler MA, Pearlberg JL, Madrazo BL, Gitschlag KF, Gross SC. Computed tomographic evaluation of the adrenal gland in the preoperative assessment of bronchogenic carcinoma. *Radiology* 1982;145:733–736.

79. Sawczuk IS, Reitelman C, Libby C, Grant D, Vita J, White RD. CT findings in Addison's disease caused by tuberculosis. *Urol Radiol* 1986;8:44–45.

80. Schaner EG, Dunnick NR, Doppman JL, Strott CA, Gill JR, Javadpour N. Adrenal cortical tumors with low attenuation coefficients: a pitfall in computed tomography diagnosis. *J Comput Assist Tomogr* 1978;2:11–15.

81. Schultz CL, Haaga JR, Fletcher BD, Alfidi RJ, Schultz MA. Magnetic resonance imaging of the adrenal glands: a comparison with computed tomography. *AJR* 1984;143:1235–1240.

82. Scully RE, Mark EJ, McNeeley BU. Case 28, case records of the Massachusetts General Hospital: weekly clinicopathological exercises. *N Engl J Med* 1984;311:783–790.

83. Silverman PM. Gastric diverticulum mimicking adrenal mass: CT demonstration. *J Comput Assist Tomogr* 1986;10:709–710.

84. Sommers SC. Adrenal glands. In: Anderson WAD, Kissane JM, eds. *Pathology.* vol 2. St Louis: Mosby, 1977:1658–1679.

85. Tang CK, Hajdu SI. Neuroblastoma in adolescence and adulthood. *NY State J Med* 1975;75:1434–1438.

86. Thomas JL, Bernardino ME. Pheochromocytoma in multiple endocrine adenomatosis. Efficacy of computed tomography. *JAMA* 1981;245:1467–1469.

87. Tisnado J, Amendola MA, Konerding KF, Shirazi KK, Beachley MC. Computed tomography versus angiography in the localization of pheochromocytoma. *J Comput Assist Tomogr* 1980;4:853–859.

88. Tsukaguchi I, Sato K, Ohara S, Kadowaki T, Shin T, Kotoh K. Adrenal myelolipoma: report of a case with CT and angiographic evaluation. *Urol Radiol* 1983;5:47–49.

89. van der Vliet AH, Ling D. Renal and scapular masses in a 57-year-old woman. *Urol Radiol* 1986;8:56–59.

90. Vas W, Zylak CJ, Mather D, Figueredo A. The value of abdominal computed tomography in the pre-treatment assessment of small cell carcinoma of the lung. *Radiology* 1981;138:417–418.

91. Vick CW, Zeman RK, Mannes E, Cronan JJ, Walsh JW. Adrenal myelolipoma: CT and ultrasound findings. *Urol Radiol* 1984;6:7–13.

92. Weinberger MH, Grim CE, Hollifoeld JW, et al. Primary aldosteronism. Diagnosis, localization and treatment. *Ann Intern Med* 1979;90:386–395.

93. Weiner SN, Bernstein RG, Lowy S, Karp H. Combined adrenal adenoma and myelolipoma. *J Comput Assist Tomogr* 1981;5:440–442.

94. Welch TJ, Sheedy PJ, van Heerden JA, Sheps SG, Hattery RR, Stephens DH. Pheochromocytoma: value of computed tomography. *Radiology* 1983;148:501–503.

95. Whaley D, Becker S, Presbrey T, Shaff M. Adrenal myelolipoma associated with Conn syndrome: CT evaluation. *J Comput Assist Tomogr* 1985;9:959–960.

96. Wilms G, Baert A, Marchal G, Goddeeris P. Computed tomography of the normal adrenal glands: correlative study with autopsy specimens. *J Comput Assist Tomogr* 1979;3:467–469.

97. Wilms G, Marchal G, Baert A, Adisoejoso B, Mangkuwerdojo S. CT and ultrasound features of post-traumatic adrenal hemorrhage. *J Comput Assist Tomogr* 1987;11:112–115.

98. Wilson DA, Muchmore HG, Tisdal RG, Fahmy A, Pitha JV. Histoplasmosis of the adrenal glands studied by CT. *Radiology* 1984;150:779–783.

99. Wolverson MK, Kannegiesser H. CT of bilateral adrenal hemorrhage with acute adrenal insufficiency in the adult. *AJR* 1984;142:311–314.

100. Xarli VP, Steele AA, Davis PJ, Buescher ES, Rios CN, Garcia-Bunuel R. Adrenal hemorrhage in the adult. *Medicine* 1978;57:211–221.

101. Yamakita N, Yasuda K, Goshima E, et al. Comparative assessment of ultrasonography and computed tomography in adrenal disorders. *Ultrasound Med Biol* 1986;12:23–29.

CHAPTER 20

Pelvis

Joseph K. T. Lee and Mary Victoria Marx

Radiologic evaluation of pelvic diseases has undergone a remarkable transition and evolution during the past decade. In recent years, computed tomography (CT) has become an essential imaging tool for evaluating patients suspected of having pelvic disease because it provides excellent cross-sectional display of bony and soft-tissue pelvic structures regardless of body habitus. The development of magnetic resonance imaging (MRI) has further expanded our capability to examine the pelvis. Although the clinical utility of MRI in pelvic imaging is still being explored, MRI has several unique features that make it an ideal method for imaging the pelvis. First, the ability of MRI to produce images in multiple planes without the degradation that results from CT reconstruction is especially helpful with complex pelvic anatomy. Second, MRI has superior contrast sensitivity, causes no known biologic effects, and can distinguish vascular from non-vascular structures without the use of intravenous contrast material. Finally, respiratory motion, which often degrades the quality of upper abdominal and thoracic MR images, is virtually absent in the pelvis.

TECHNIQUES

CT

A successful CT examination of the pelvis depends on careful patient preparation. Because multiple small-bowel loops reside in the pelvis, complete opacification of the alimentary tract is essential lest they be misinterpreted as mass lesions. This can be achieved by giving the patient 600 to 1,000 ml of dilute oral contrast material at least 1 hr before the examination. Although the rectosigmoid colon usually can be recognized by its location and its fecal content, opacification of this segment of the bowel may be desirable in selected patients. Rectosigmoid opacifi-

cation frequently is achieved via the oral route if contrast material is administered 6 to 12 hr before the study; a contrast-material enema (200 ml) occasionally may be necessary to expedite opacification of this region.

Imaging when the urinary bladder is distended is often helpful, because small-bowel loops can be displaced out of the pelvis, thus making identification of other pelvic structures easier. As dense contrast material in the bladder sometimes results in imaging artifacts and obscures adjacent structures, it is generally best to obtain images when the bladder is filled with unopacified urine. However, when staging patients with bladder neoplasms or other genitourinary neoplasms, it is often necessary to opacify the urinary bladder and distal ureters. Optimal opacification of these structures can be achieved by intravenous administration of 25 to 30 ml of 60% iodinated contrast material approximately 15 min before the study.

A vaginal tampon may be useful in female patients to facilitate identification of the vaginal canal (25).

Although intravenous contrast material is routinely used in some institutions, we reserve it for cases where there are uncertainties about soft-tissue densities on pre-contrast images. When used, we prefer to give 30 to 50 ml of 67% iodinated compound as a bolus, followed by dynamic imaging at a single level. In spite of the great variability in location and diameter of the pelvic arteries and veins, intravenous contrast material, when used properly, allows easy differentiation between a lymph node and a blood vessel (Fig. 1).

Transaxial CT images are used as the routine imaging format. Although direct coronal imaging with the patient sitting on the specially designed support device provides a clear display of the pelvic floor and its adjacent structure (145), it has not gained widespread acceptance because of the additional time required to assemble such a device and because of the ease with which such images can be obtained with MRI.

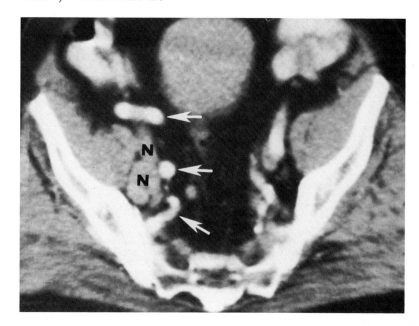

FIG. 1. Enlarged iliac nodes (N) due to metastatic prostate cancer are easily distinguished from enhancing iliac vessels (*arrows*) on this image obtained after a bolus intravenous injection of contrast material.

MRI

Patients scheduled for MRI of the pelvis require no special preparation. They are usually examined supine during shallow respiration, with the urinary bladder at least half full before the study is begun.

Both T1-weighted (TR = 300–500 msec, TE = 15–35 msec) and T2-weighted (TR = 1,500–2,100 msec, TE = 90–120 msec) spin-echo sequences are necessary for complete examination of the pelvis. Whereas T1-weighted images are best for detecting lymphadenopathy and extension of pelvic neoplasms into adjacent fat, T2-weighted images provide clear delineation of the bladder wall, as well as the internal morphology of the prostate gland and the uterus.

Transaxial images are obtained in every case; additional views are performed in either the coronal or sagittal plane. Coronal images are useful for evaluating the seminal vesicles and bladder neoplasms that involve the lateral wall. Sagittal views are best for defining the uterine body, cervix, and vaginal canal. Sagittal images are also necessary in cases in which a bladder neoplasm is located along the anterior or posterior wall.

NORMAL ANATOMY

The pelvis is a complex structure that is composed of an osseous ring formed by the innominate bones and sacrum, with numerous attached muscles for support and ambulation. Within this musculo-osseous skeleton reside various internal organs and major blood vessels, lymphatics, and nerves. Most of these structures are either midline or bilaterally symmetrical within this skeletal framework. This section will cover the essential CT and MRI features of the internal pelvic organs. Information

concerning the relationship between the peritoneal and extraperitoneal spaces of the pelvis can be found in Chapter 11.

CT

The pelvic muscles (psoas, iliacus, obturator internus, pyriformis, and levator ani) are well delineated on CT images and are symmetrical in the normal individual (see Figs. 43D, 57B, and 57D in Chapter 11). Pelvic lymph nodes can be found in close proximity to the pelvic blood vessels. Although lymph nodes less than 1 cm in size cannot be confidently identified as such in the pelvis, lymph nodes that are enlarged or calcified or that contain fibro-lipomatous changes are readily recognized on CT. Small-bowel loops are easily identified if they contain oral contrast material; unopacified bowel loops may simulate a mass lesion. The rectum and the ascending, descending, and sigmoid colon can be recognized even if they are not opacified by oral contrast material because of their relatively fixed locations. Furthermore, they often contain various amounts of air and/or feces, thereby allowing distinction from other structures.

The urinary bladder is a homogeneous midline structure whose size and configuration vary greatly depending on the amount of urine it contains. Whereas urine is of near-water density, the bladder wall has a soft-tissue density.

In the male pelvis, the seminal vesicles are seen posterior to the bladder, cephalad to the prostate gland and anterior to the rectum (Fig. 2A). They are oval or tear-shaped structures. A small amount of fat usually is present between the seminal vesicles and the posterior wall of the bladder. This relationship may be distorted by a distended rectum or when the patient is prone (129,130). The prostate gland has a homogeneous soft-tissue density and is

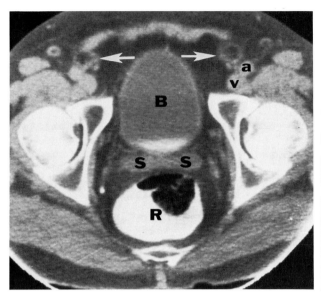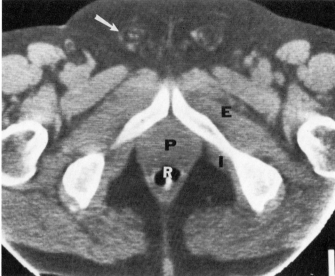

FIG. 2. Normal male pelvis. **A:** The seminal vesicles (S) lie between the bladder (B) and rectum (R) and have a "bow-tie" configuration centered in the midsagittal plane. Fat separates the seminal vesicles from adjacent structures; (a) femoral artery; (v) femoral vein. **B:** Four centimeters caudad, the prostate gland (P) lies posterior to the pubic symphysis. The spermatic cord (*arrow*) contains fat, vessels, and the vas deferens; (R) rectum; (I) obturator internus; (E) obturator externus.

located just posterior to the pubic symphysis and anterior to the rectum (Fig. 2B). The spermatic cords are seen anterolateral to the pubic symphysis and medial to the femoral vein. They may appear either as small oval soft-tissue structures or as thin-walled, ring-like elements, containing several soft-tissue densities representing the vas deferens and the spermatic vessels. The spermatic cord can be traced to the scrotum. The testes and the epididymis are of soft-tissue density; they cannot be separated from each other.

In the female pelvis, the uterus is seen as an oval or triangular soft-tissue mass located posterior to the urinary bladder (Fig. 3). A central area of lower attenuation, which probably represents secretions within the endometrial cavity, sometimes can be seen on non-contrast images. After intravenous administration of contrast material, the myometrium exhibits intense contrast enhancement, and the endometrial cavity is better delineated (4). Although demarcations between the vagina, cervix, and uterus are not clearly shown by CT images, they can nevertheless be separated from one another by their configurations. The uterine body usually is triangular in shape, whereas the cervix has a more rounded appearance. At the level of the fornix, the vagina is seen as a flat rectangle. CT identification of the rest of the vaginal canal is facilitated if a tampon is used. The normal adult premenopausal ovaries may be seen. Although highly variable, they are most often found slightly posterolateral to the body of the uterus. They usually are of uniform soft-tissue density; small cystic areas representing normal follicles occasionally can be seen (Fig. 3). The broad ligaments can sometimes be seen as a band of soft tissue extending laterally

from the uterus to the pelvic side wall. The cardinal ligaments (lateral cervical ligaments) cause widening of the base of the broad ligament and can occasionally be seen on CT as triangular densities extending from the cervix and upper vagina laterally. On rare occasion, uterosacral ligaments are visible on CT images as arc-like structures extending from the cervix to the sacrum.

MRI

Normal pelvic anatomy similarly can be depicted with MRI. With the exception of differences in gray scale, the pelvic anatomy as displayed on T1-weighted or proton-density MR images is quite similar to that obtained with CT. The cortical bone has an extremely low intensity due to the lack of mobile protons; fat, whether inside or outside the marrow, has a high signal intensity. Pelvic musculature and visceral organs have low-to-medium signal intensities. Because rapidly flowing blood emits no signal, pelvic vessels usually are seen as areas of "signal void" (12). Vessels containing more sluggish blood flow are identified as structures with high signal intensity on a second-echo image.

The urinary bladder appears as a homogeneous low-intensity structure, and the bladder wall cannot be differentiated from urine on T1-weighted sequences (15,36) (Fig. 4A). The signal intensity of urine compared with adjacent perivesical structures increases with prolongation of TR and TE. Therefore, on a T2-weighted sequence, urine, which has a high signal intensity, can be easily distinguished from the low-intensity bladder wall (Fig. 4B).

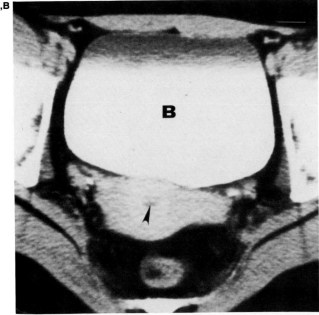

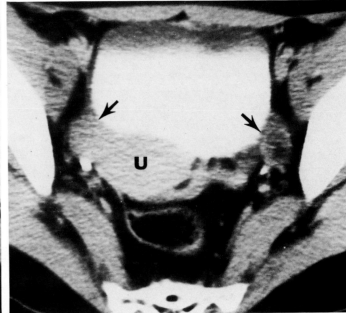

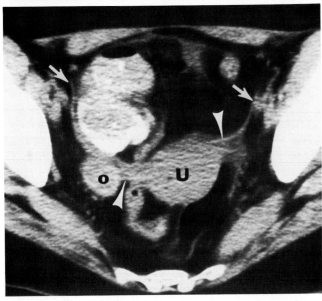

FIG. 3. Normal female pelvis. **A:** CT image at the level of acetabula demonstrates a normal uterus located behind the opacified urinary bladder (B). The central lower-attenuation area (*arrowhead*) represents the endometrial cavity. **B:** CT image at the level of iliac wings in another patient shows the uterine fundus (U) and both ovaries (*arrows*). Note that the left ovary has areas of lower attenuation value representing ovarian follicles. **C:** CT image in a third patient shows the round ligament (*arrow*) emanating from the broad ligament (*arrowhead*). Also of note is a soft-tissue-density right ovary (o); (U) uterus.

The low-intensity bladder wall may be obscured by the chemical-shift artifact that results from the difference in resonance frequency between fat and water protons. The chemical-shift artifact occurs at the water–fat interface (bladder–perivesical fat) in the direction of the readout (frequency) gradient, which is different for different imaging planes (i.e., with some imagers, the chemical-shift artifact will affect lateral walls on transaxial views; it will affect the superior and inferior bladder walls on sagittal sections) (7). The chemical-shift artifact can be recognized on a transverse image as a dark band along the lateral wall on one side and a bright band along the lateral wall on the opposite side. If the pixel bandwidth stays the same, this artifact is more pronounced with increasing field strength. In extreme cases, the chemical-shift artifact may lead to apparent thickening of the bladder wall on one side and apparent absence of the bladder wall on a contralateral side (Fig. 5).

The prostate gland has a homogeneous low signal intensity, similar to that of skeletal muscle, on T1-weighted images. With thinner slice collimation and better imaging equipment, the central and transitional zones can be differentiated from the peripheral zone because the latter has a higher signal intensity on T2-weighted sequences (62,112,132) (Fig. 6). The higher signal intensity of the peripheral zone has been attributed to its more abundant glandular components and its more loosely interwoven muscle bundles. The distinction between peripheral and central zones is consistently made in men younger than 35 years of age, but it can be made in only 35% of men older than 40 years of age (62). In older men, the peripheral zone shows variation in size and signal intensity.

A,B

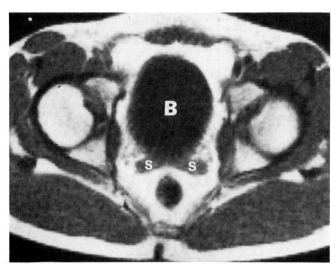

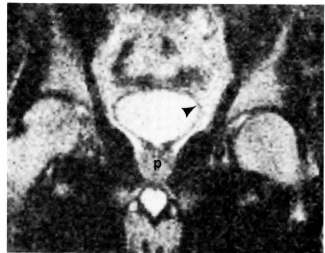

FIG. 4. Normal urinary bladder. **A:** Transaxial T1-weighted MR image (TR = 500 msec, TE = 30 msec) shows a low-intensity urinary bladder (B). The bladder wall cannot be distinguished from urine with this sequence; (s) seminal vesicles. **B:** Coronal T2-weighted MR image (TR = 2,100 msec, TE = 90 msec). The bladder wall, which has a low signal intensity (*arrowhead*), can be easily differentiated from the high-intensity urine; (p) prostate.

Although the prostatic capsule is not usually visible, the prostate gland can be distinguished from adjacent structures because of interposed fatty tissue. The Denonvilliers fascia sometimes can be seen as a low-intensity band separating the rectum from the prostate gland. Periprostatic venous plexus are seen as curvilinear, high-intensity structures on the second echo of a T2-weighted sequence (Fig. 6). They are most abundant anterior and lateral to the prostate gland (117).

The seminal vesicles have a medium-to-low signal intensity on T1-weighted sequences and appear brighter than fat on T2-weighted images (Fig. 7).

Normal scrotal contents can be seen when imaged with a surface coil (9,125,131). The signal intensity of the testes is similar to that of thigh muscle on T1-weighted images and greater than that of subcutaneous fat on T2-weighted images (Fig. 8). The tunica albuginea has a low signal intensity on both T1- and T2-weighted images; the epididymis has an intensity similar to that of the testis on T1-weighted images, but much less than that of the testis

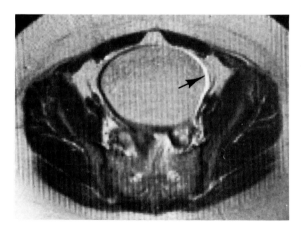

FIG. 5. Chemical-shift artifact obscuring normal urinary bladder wall. Transaxial T2-weighted MR image (TR = 2,100 msec, TE = 90 msec) obtained with a 1.5-T imager shows a bright line (*arrow*) replacing the normally low-intensity bladder wall. Note the apparent thickening of the right lateral wall.

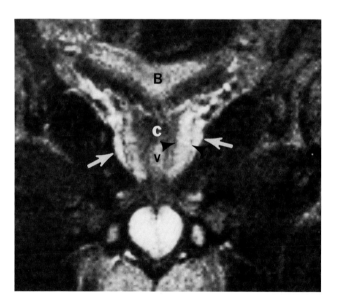

FIG. 6. Normal prostate gland in a 25-year-old man. Coronal T2-weighted MR image (TR = 2,100 msec, TE = 90 msec) obtained with 5-mm slice thickness and a Helmholtz-type surface coil shows clear differentiation between the peripheral zone (*arrowheads*) and the central/transition zone (c). The verumontanum (v) is also depicted; (B) urinary bladder; (*arrows*) periprostatic venous plexus.

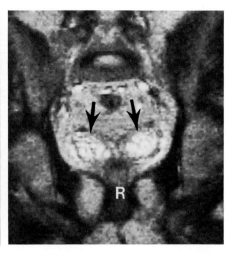

FIG. 7. Normal seminal vesicles. **A:** Coronal T1-weighted MR image (TR = 500 msec, TE = 30 msec). The seminal vesicles (*arrows*) have relatively low signal intensity. **B:** Coronal T2-weighted MR image (TR = 2,100 msec, TE = 90 msec). The signal intensity of the seminal vesicles (*arrows*) is higher than that of fat; (R) rectum.

on T2-weighted images. The pampiniform plexus often can be seen as a convoluted structure located cephalad to the epididymal head. The wall of the plexus has a low signal intensity on both T1- and T2-weighted images, whereas the internal structure contains both medium- and high-signal areas, the latter undoubtedly related to slow blood flow. The skin, the dartos muscle, and different scrotal fascia cannot be separated from one another and are imaged as a band of medium-to-low intensity.

Although the uterus has a homogeneous low-to-medium signal intensity on a T1-weighted sequence, it exhibits three different signal intensities on a T2-weighted sequence (59,82) (Fig. 9). With the latter sequence, the central portion of the uterus (endometrium) has a signal intensity higher than that of subcutaneous fat, whereas the peripheral myometrium has a signal intensity higher than that of striated muscle. Between these two layers is a narrow band that corresponds to the inner myometrium. It has a signal intensity similar to that of striated muscle.

The MRI appearance of normal uterus is influenced by hormonal changes (27,56,101). In women of reproductive age, the central high-intensity zone is thin immediately following menstruation and achieves its maximal thickness at the midcycle (27,56,101). Likewise, the signal intensity of the myometrium and uterine volume reaches a maximal value during the secretory phase. In women taking oral contraceptive pills, the endometrium is atrophic, and the zonal anatomy is indistinct. Such an appearance is also seen in premenarchal and postmenopausal uteri.

Similar to the uterus, the cervix has a homogeneous low-to-medium signal intensity on T1-weighted images.

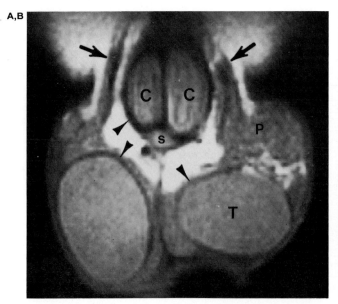
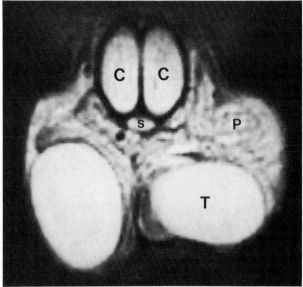

FIG. 8. Normal scrotum. **A:** Coronal T1-weighted MR image (TR = 500 msec, TE = 15 msec). The testis (T) has a lower signal intensity than subcutaneous fat; (*arrow*), spermatic cord; (P) pampiniform plexus; (*arrowhead*) tunica covering the testis and penis; (C) corpus cavernosum, (s) corpus spongiosum. **B:** Coronal T2-weighted MR image (TR = 2,100 msec, TE = 90 msec) obtained at a slightly more posterior level than (**A**). Note that the signal intensity of the testis is higher than that for fat.

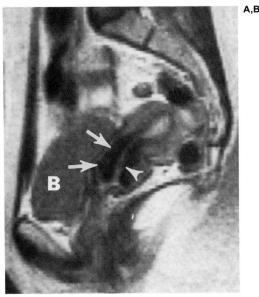

A,B

FIG. 9. Normal uterine anatomy. A: Sagittal MR image (TR = 1,500 msec, TE = 70 msec) shows a retroverted uterus with three zones of different signal intensities. Note the low-intensity junctional band (*arrowheads*) extending from the uterine body to the cervix. B: Sagittal MR image (TR = 2,100 msec, TE = 70 msec) of a different patient shows nearly the entire cervical lip (*arrows*) to be of low signal intensity. The endocervix (*arrowhead*) has a high signal intensity similar to that of endometrium; (B) urinary bladder.

On T2-weighted images, the central zone in the cervix has a high signal intensity similar to that of the central uterine signal. This is believed to represent the cervical epithelium and mucus (59,82). The peripheral cervical zone in some patients has a homogeneous low signal intensity similar to the junctional low-intensity band of the uterine body (Fig. 9B). In other patients, two distinct signal intensities can be seen in this peripheral zone: an inner low-intensity band and an outer medium-intensity layer (82,162) (Fig. 9A).

The vagina can be identified distinct from the surrounding structures on a T2-weighted image. It has a high-intensity center representing the vaginal epithelium and mucus, surrounded by a low-intensity wall (Fig. 10). The normal ovaries are more difficult to demonstrate on MRI. When seen, they have a low-to-medium signal intensity on T1-weighted images and an intensity similar to or higher than that of fat on T2-weighted images (30) (Fig. 11).

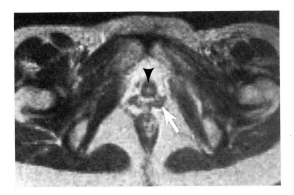

FIG. 10. Normal vagina. Transaxial MR image (TR = 2,100 msec, TE = 90 msec). The vaginal wall (*arrow*) has a low signal intensity, whereas the center has a high signal intensity due to its mucus content; (*arrowhead*) urethra.

Because the parametrium is composed mainly of fat, it has a high signal intensity on T1-weighted images. However, the parauterine ligaments and vessels have a low signal intensity. Because of slow blood flow, parauterine vessels are imaged as structures of extremely high intensity on second-echo images.

The rectosigmoid colon, which often is surrounded by abundant, high-signal pelvic fat, has a medium signal intensity on a T2-weighted sequence. It may be either collapsed or distended with air, which appears as an area of extremely low signal intensity.

STAGING OF PELVIC NEOPLASMS

Urinary Bladder

Most neoplasms of the urinary bladder are of uroepithelial origin, with transitional cell carcinoma much more common than the squamous cell variety. Although the prognosis depends on the extent of the tumor involvement at presentation, the degree of cellular differentiation affects the rate of bladder-wall invasion. There is a higher tendency for the poorly differentiated tumors to infiltrate the bladder wall than for the well-differentiated types (1,44).

Because cystoscopy is very sensitive in detecting small bladder neoplasms, and biopsy of these lesions at cystoscopy often can define the depth of tumor extension into the submucosa and muscular layers, these methods remain the primary diagnostic procedures in patients suspected of having bladder carcinomas. The role of any imaging method in bladder cancer is therefore to determine the presence or absence of invasion into the surrounding perivesical fat, adjacent viscera, and pelvic lymph nodes. Accurate determination of the extent of a bladder tumor is important because it dictates the treatment and prognosis for such a patient (44,76). One of the more com-

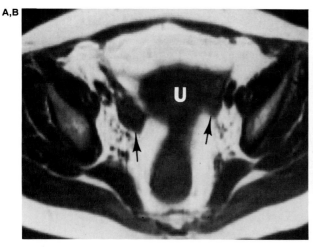
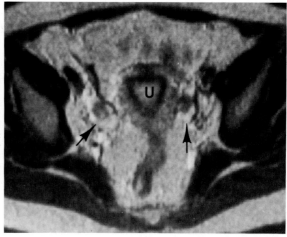

FIG. 11. Normal ovaries. **A:** Transaxial MR image (TR = 500 msec, TE = 35 msec). The signal intensity of both ovaries (*arrows*) is similar to that of the uterus (U), but much lower than that of fat. **B:** On a T2-weighted image (TR = 2,100 msec, TE = 90 msec), the peripheral portion of the ovary (*arrows*) is isointense with fat, whereas the central portion is of lower signal intensity.

monly used staging systems for bladder carcinomas is listed in Table 1. In general, stage A lesions can be treated adequately with fulguration or transurethral resection; low-grade stage B_1 lesions may be treated with segmental cystectomy. Radical cystectomy is the procedure of choice for stage B_2 or stage C lesions, whereas palliative radiation therapy with an ileal loop is the common management for stage D disease (32).

CT

On CT images, a bladder neoplasm appears as a sessile or pedunculated soft-tissue mass projecting into the bladder lumen (58,69,108,129,130) (Fig. 12). It can also present as a focal or diffuse thickening of the bladder wall (Fig. 13). When a neoplasm causes diffuse thickening of the bladder wall, it can be confused with cystitis, although the thickening usually is more uniform in the latter entity (Fig. 14). The density of a bladder neoplasm is similar to that of normal bladder wall; calcification within the tumor may be seen on rare occasions.

Extravesical extension of the tumor is recognized on CT images as blurring or obscuration of the perivesical fat planes (Fig. 15). In more advanced cases, a soft-tissue mass can be seen extending from the bladder into adjacent viscera (Fig. 16) or muscles (e.g., obturator internus). However, it is often difficult to determine whether actual tumor invasion is present or the tumor is merely contiguous with the pelvic-wall muscle. When invasion of the pelvic bone is present, the diagnosis can be readily made by CT. Invasion of the seminal vesicles can be predicted when the normal angle between the seminal vesicle and the posterior wall of the bladder is obliterated (129,130). Caution must be taken not to overuse this sign, as the normal seminal vesicle angle can be distorted by a dis-

TABLE 1. *Staging of bladder tumors according to the Marshall system[a]*

0	Epithelial	
A	Lamina propria	
B_1	Superficial muscle	
B_2	Deep muscle	
C	Perivesical fat	
D_1	Adjacent organs, lymph nodes	
D_2	Distant metastases	

[a] From Marshall (97), with permission.

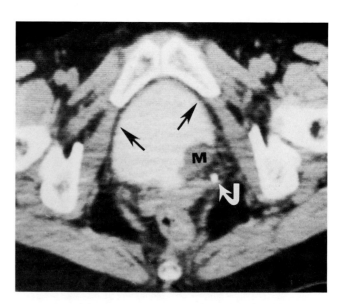

FIG. 12. Bladder carcinoma. A pedunculated mass (M) projects into the bladder lumen in the region of the left ureteral orifice, causing mild hydroureter (*curved white arrow*). In other areas, the bladder wall is uniformly thin and almost nondetectable (*black arrows*).

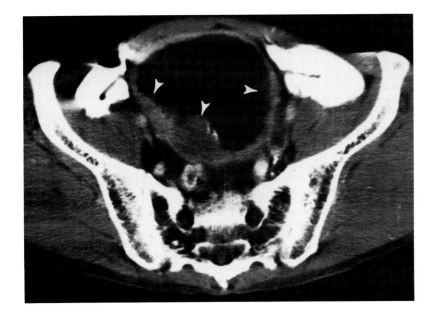

FIG. 13. Bladder carcinoma. Extensive involvement is indicated by diffuse nodular thickening of the bladder wall (*arrowheads*). The left anterolateral wall is spared.

tended rectum or when the patient is prone (129,130). Because no distinct fat plane is present between the urinary bladder and the vagina or prostate in normal subjects, a confident CT diagnosis of early invasion into the neighboring structures is difficult. Metastases into the pelvic lymph nodes can be diagnosed only when the involved nodes are enlarged (89,150). Although there are no well-established size criteria to distinguish normal and abnormal pelvic lymph nodes on CT, we consider nodes greater than 1.5 cm to be pathologic. Nodes smaller than 1 cm in size are considered to be normal, and nodes between 1 and 1.5 cm are viewed with high suspicion, especially if they are within the expected course of lymphatic spread. In these cases, CT-guided needle aspiration of the suspicious area is often performed and the aspirate sent for

cytologic examination. In the lymphatic spread from bladder cancer, the medial (obturator) and the middle groups of the external iliac nodes are often affected first (Fig. 17), followed by the internal iliac and the common iliac nodes (1). Obturator nodal metastases are best seen on slices obtained 1 to 3 cm superior to the acetabulum.

CT is capable of differentiating between bladder neoplasms with extravesical extension and those confined to the wall, but is incapable of distinguishing tumors within

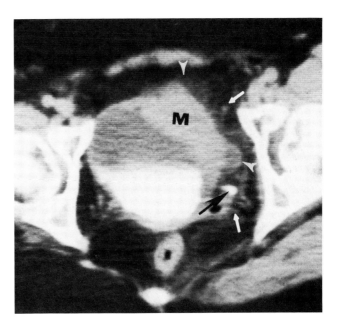

FIG. 15. Bladder carcinoma, with extension into perivesical fat. A large mass (M) arises from the bladder wall and is associated with left hydroureter (*black arrow*). The mass projects beyond the expected boundary of the bladder anteriorly and to the left (*white arrowheads*). Wispy streaks of soft tissue (*white arrows*) infiltrate the left perivesical fat.

FIG. 14. Cytoxan-induced cystitis, producing diffuse thickening of the bladder wall.

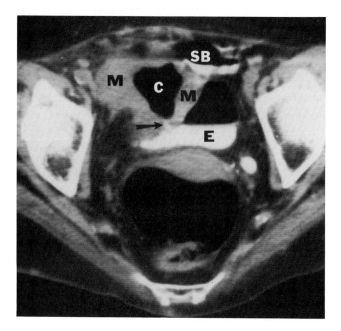

FIG. 16. Bladder carcinoma with bowel invasion. A large right anterior bladder mass (M) has eroded into small bowel (SB) and has cavitated (C). Enteric contrast material (E) has entered the bladder via a neoplastic enterovesical fistula (*arrow*); intravenous contrast material was not given.

the latter group (stages 0, A, B$_1$, and B$_2$) from each other (41,58,69,108,129,130). The overall accuracy of CT in detecting perivesical and seminal vesicular involvement is in the range of 65% to 85% (41,58,126); the accuracy in detecting lymph node metastases ranges from 70% to 90%, with a false-negative rate of 25% to 40% (58,89,108,150). The major limitation of CT in staging bladder cancer lies in its inability to detect microscopic invasion of the perivesical fat and to recognize normal-

size but neoplastically involved lymph nodes as abnormal. False-positive cases are mostly due to confusion produced by normal contiguous extravesical structures mimicking tumor spread or asymmetrical perivesical fat planes caused by inflammation or fibrosis.

MRI

Tumors of the bladder, whether infiltrative, sessile, or pedunculated, can be detected if they exceed 1 to 2 cm (37). The signal intensity of a bladder neoplasm is higher than that for urine, but lower than that for fat, on both T1-weighted and proton-density images; the signal of a bladder neoplasm is similar to or slightly lower than that of urine on T2-weighted images. Thus, a bladder neoplasm is best seen on a spin-echo sequence with a short TE (37,87) (Fig. 18).

Neoplastic infiltration of bladder wall can be differentiated from bladder-wall hypertrophy secondary to bladder outlet obstruction because the former has a signal intensity higher than that of normal wall, whereas the latter has a signal intensity similar to that of normal wall (36). However, both mucosal edema and inflammation of the bladder wall have high signal intensities on T2-weighted images that overlap that for bladder neoplasms (37).

MRI cannot distinguish stage A from stage B$_1$ tumors (2,16,37,124). However, MRI can identify deep muscular invasion (stage B$_2$). On a T2-weighted sequence, gross tumor involvement of a deep muscular layer often leads to disruption of the low-intensity bladder wall; a low-intensity line usually is preserved in neoplasms with either no muscle involvement or superficial muscle invasion (37,124) (Fig. 19).

A,B

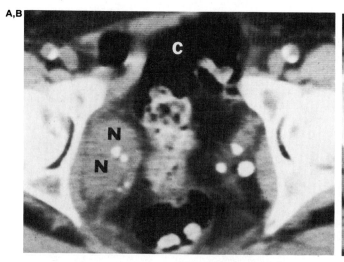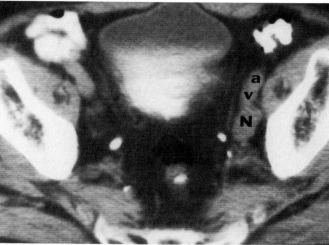

FIG. 17. Lymph node metastases of bladder carcinoma. **A:** Enlarged right obturator lymph nodes (N) represent recurrent bladder carcinoma in this patient who had had prior cystectomy. Sigmoid colon (C) fills the space previously occupied by bladder. Note calcified phleboliths. **B:** In another patient with bladder carcinoma, postcontrast CT image shows an enlarged middle external iliac lymph node (N) just posterior to the external iliac artery (a) and vein (v). The primary bladder carcinoma was seen on a more caudal image.

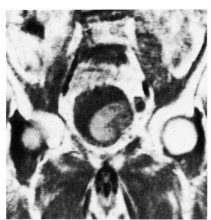
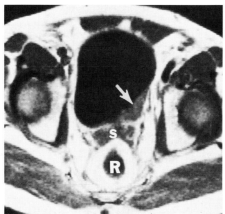

A,B

FIG. 18. Carcinoma of the urinary bladder. **A:** Coronal MR image (TR = 2,100 msec, TE = 35 msec) shows a large polypoid mass in the bladder. The mass has a signal intensity intermediate between those of urine and fat. **B:** Transaxial MR image (TR = 500 msec, TE = 35 msec) in another patient shows a plaque-like lesion (*arrow*) along the left posterolateral wall of the bladder; (s) seminal vesicle; (R) rectum.

Tumor extension into the perivesical fat (stage C) also can be detected and is seen as an area of diminished signal relative to the pelvic fat on a T1-weighted image. It often has a wipsy appearance, but occasionally may be more confluent. It is best appreciated on T1-weighted images because of sharp contrast between fat and tumor (Fig. 20). Tumor invasion into adjacent organs, such as the seminal vesicles and the rectum, can similarly be detected (Fig. 21). The diagnosis of seminal vesicular involvement can be made by noting not only changes in its size or morphology but also its signal intensity. Normal seminal vesicles have a high signal intensity on T2-weighted images; invasion of the seminal vesicles by carcinomas may lead to a lower signal intensity. Other conditions, such as atrophy and fibrosis, may cause a similar decrease in signal intensity.

Lymph node metastases can be seen if the involved nodes are enlarged. Lymphadenopathy is best appreciated on T1-weighted images. Unfortunately, tissue characterization based on MR signals is not possible. Lymphadenopathy from benign causes cannot be distinguished from malignant disease. Likewise, a normal-size lymph node replaced with tumor cannot be recognized as abnormal by MRI (29,84).

Preliminary data show that MRI has an accuracy of 75% to 85% in staging bladder neoplasms (2,16,37,124). MRI is slightly more sensitive than CT in detecting invasion of perivesical fat, the prostate, and the seminal

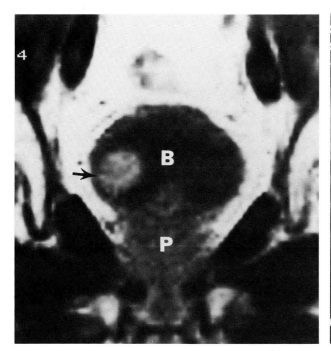
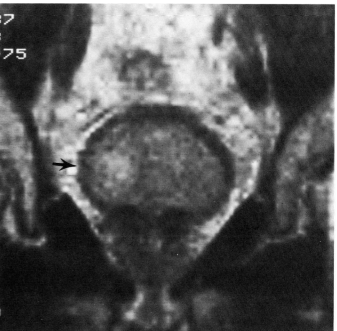

A,B

FIG. 19. Carcinoma of the urinary bladder. **A:** Coronal T1-weighted image (TR = 500 msec, TE = 35 msec) shows a medium-intensity polypoid mass (*arrow*) along the right lateral wall of the bladder (B); (P) prostate. **B:** Coronal T2-weighted image (TR = 2,100 msec, TE = 90 msec) shows the neoplasm to be nearly isointense with urine. The bladder wall (*arrow*) underlying the tumor is well preserved. Histologic examination of the resected specimen revealed no muscle invasion.

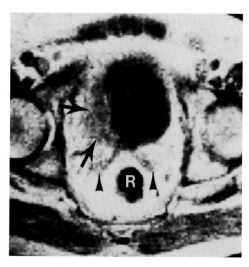

FIG. 20. Bladder carcinoma invading perivesical fat. Transaxial MR image (TR = 500 msec, TE = 30 msec) shows medium-intensity tumor (*arrows*) extending into high-intensity fat; (*arrowhead*) seminal vesicles; (R) rectum. (From ref. 87.)

vesicles. It is also superior to CT in distinguishing between an enlarged lymph node and a small blood vessel (84). However, like CT, MRI is not able to detect microscopic invasion of the perivesical fat or lymph nodes. Furthermore, asymmetrical perivesical fat planes caused by inflammation may lead to false-positive MRI interpretations. MRI is more time-consuming than CT. Because of lack of optimal oral contrast agents, small-bowel loops may be mistaken for lymphadenopathy on MR images.

Clinical Application

Arteriography, triple-contrast cystography, and lymphangiography have all been used in the past in the pre-

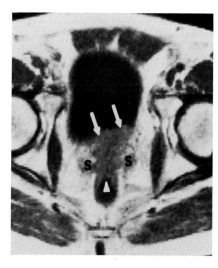

FIG. 21. Bladder carcinoma invading the rectum. Transaxial MR image (TR = 500 msec, TE = 30 msec) shows invasion of the anterior wall of the rectum (*arrowhead*) by a posterior bladder carcinoma (*arrows*); (s) seminal vesicles.

operative staging of bladder neoplasms (74,80,148). The first two procedures are invasive and have produced variable results (74,80); lymphangiography evaluates the status of only the pelvic and retroperitoneal lymph nodes, not the visceral organs (148). None of these procedures has been routinely applied. CT provides a noninvasive method of differentiating between early and advanced stages of bladder neoplasms and therefore helps avoid needless radical surgery in advanced cancers. In spite of its limitations, CT is now routinely used in the preoperative evaluation of patients with biopsy-proven bladder neoplasms. Although MRI is slightly more accurate than CT in staging bladder neoplasms, the disadvantages of MRI, including higher cost, longer examination time, and more stringent patient requirements, have limited its use. Other than being used to clarify equivocal CT findings (Fig. 22), the role of MRI in bladder neoplasms remains to be defined.

Prostate

Prostatic carcinoma is an exceedingly common tumor and is the third leading cause of death among American men (133). Adenocarcinomas account for more than 95% of malignant prostatic neoplasms, with the rest being transitional or squamous cell carcinoma or sarcomas (21). Approximately 65% of newly diagnosed cases will present as advanced disease. The prognosis and treatment depend on the stage of the disease when first seen. A commonly used staging classification for prostatic carcinoma is shown in Table 2 (70). In general, stage A_1 lesions are managed by repeated examinations or prostatic biopsies at 6-month intervals; stage A_2 lesions are treated by either radical prostatectomy or external and/or internal radiation in the form of ^{125}I seeds. Stage B lesions are treated by pelvic lymphadenectomy to exclude micrometastases to lymph nodes, followed by radical prostatectomy. Stage C tumors are generally treated by external-beam radiation to the involved regions; stage D tumors are treated with palliative hormonal therapy such as diethylstilbestrol (DES), orchiectomy, or antiandrogens (111).

Clinical staging based on bimanual rectal examination, serum acid phosphatase determination, and radionuclide

TABLE 2. *Clinical staging classification for prostatic carcinoma*[a]

A	Occult cancer
B	Cancer nodule confined within prostatic capsule
C	Cancer with extracapsular extension into surrounding structures or confined within capsule with elevation of serum alkaline phosphatase; pelvic nodes may be involved
D	Bone or extrapelvic involvement

[a] From Jewett (70).

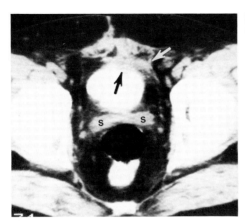
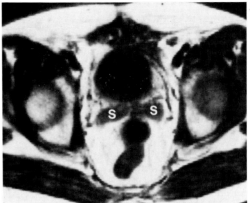
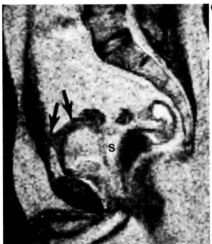

C

FIG. 22. Postoperative scar simulating extravesical tumor invasion: use of MRI. **A:** Contrast-enhanced CT image. A plaque-like tumor (*black arrow*) is noted in the anterior portion of the urinary bladder. A band of soft-tissue density (*white arrow*) is seen between the tumor and abdominal wall, findings suggestive of extravesical tumor extension. **B:** Transaxial T1-weighted image (TR = 500 msec, TE = 35 msec) shows findings similar to those of CT. **C:** Sagittal T2-weighted image (TR = 2,100 msec, TE = 90 msec). The extravesical soft tissue (*arrows*) noted superior and anterior to the bladder has a signal intensity similar to that of the anterior abdominal wall; this finding is compatible with fibrosis rather than tumor extension. Note that the bladder neoplasm is invisible on this image because it has a signal intensity similar to that of urine; (s) seminal vesicles. (From ref. 124.)

bone scintigraphy may underestimate the extent of disease in 40% to 50% of cases (34). The purpose of preoperative diagnostic imaging evaluation is to increase the accuracy of the assigned clinical stage, usually by elevating it to stage C or D, thereby eliminating unnecessary surgical procedures.

CT

CT is not used as a screening procedure for the detection of prostatic carcinoma because of its inability to differentiate among normal, hyperplastic, and cancerous glands (121,137,144). Nevertheless, CT does provide useful information as to the extent of the tumor once a histologic diagnosis is established. CT is capable of differentiating patients with stage A and B diseases from those with stage C and D diseases (Figs. 23–25). The criteria used to diagnose extracapsular extension from prostatic carcinomas are essentially the same as those used in the staging of bladder carcinomas, namely, lack of symmetry of peripelvic fat planes and obliteration of the seminal vesicle angles. Metastases to pelvic lymph nodes can also be detected if they cause nodal enlargement (Fig. 26). The size criterion used to differentiate a normal and an abnormal pelvic lymph node in prostatic carcinoma is similar to

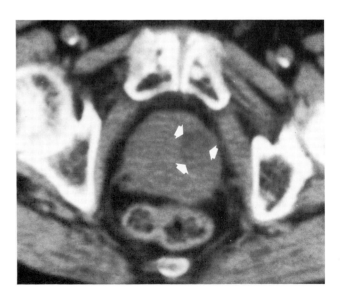

FIG. 23. Prostatic carcinoma, stage B. The irregular low-attenuation nodule (*arrows*) in this mildly enlarged prostate gland is a biopsy-proven carcinoma. Periprostatic fat planes are intact, and there are no distant metastases.

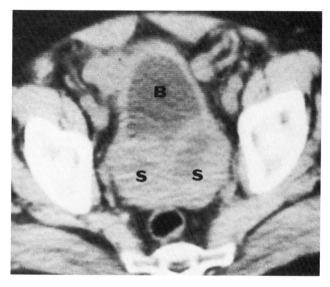

FIG. 24. Prostatic carcinoma, stage C. The seminal vesicles (S) are markedly enlarged because of direct invasion by an adjacent prostatic carcinoma; (B) bladder.

that used in bladder carcinoma. Percutaneous CT-guided biopsy of any suspicious lymph node often is helpful in establishing a histologic diagnosis and improves its overall accuracy (39). As with urinary bladder neoplasms, lymphatic drainage of the prostate is mainly into external and internal iliac nodal groups. Similarly, understaging by CT occurs in cases where there is microscopic invasion into periprostatic fat or involved but normal-size pelvic lymph nodes. The overall accuracy of CT in detecting pelvic lymph node metastases from prostatic cancer is in the range of 70% to 80%, with a sensitivity as low as 50% (39,48,90,108,155). Although the sensitivity in detecting extracapsular extension is low, the specificity is high, with no false-positive CT interpretations reported in some series

(34,48). Because of its low sensitivity in detecting extracapsular extension of the prostatic carcinoma, especially in early clinical stages, it seems reasonable to reserve CT for cases in which there is a high clinical suspicion of advanced disease (stages C and D). In patients who are scheduled to receive radiation therapy for prostatic carcinoma, CT can also be used to help design radiation ports because of its high accuracy in assessing the size and precise location of the prostate gland (28,115). CT is also valuable for evaluation of patients suspected of having recurrent disease.

MRI

There have been conflicting reports on the ability of MRI to differentiate between prostatic carcinoma and benign hyperplasia. Although studies performed with low-field-strength units (0.04–0.15 T) have shown that prostatic carcinoma can be differentiated from benign hyperplasia because of its longer T1 and T2 (81,136), the results based on medium-field (0.3–0.6 T) superconducting-magnet imagers have been less encouraging. With the exception of one report (65), most investigators have found it difficult to distinguish these two entities (17,93,113,117). Although prostatic carcinoma often creates an area of high signal intensity on T2-weighted images, this appearance is not specific for carcinoma. Benign prostatic hyperplasia may also appear as hyperintense nodules (93). Benign hyperplasia has a variable appearance (high or low signal intensity), a reflection of its heterogeneous composition. Some nodules are cellular, whereas others are fibrous. Other benign conditions, such as acute and chronic prostatitis, are also of heterogeneous intensity on MRI, with areas of high signal intensity indistinguishable from carcinoma (18).

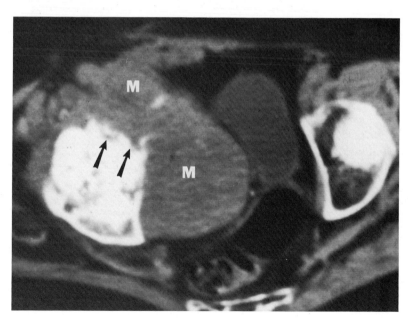

FIG. 25. Prostatic carcinoma, stage D. The large soft-tissue mass (M) involving the right pelvic side wall and inguinal area is due to metastatic prostate cancer and is associated with sclerosis and cortical destruction (*arrows*) of the acetabulum.

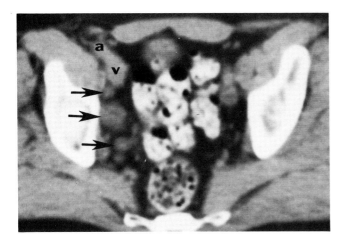

FIG. 26. Prostatic carcinoma, stage C. Right external iliac lymphadenopathy (*arrows*) demonstrated by CT changed the clinical stage of this tumor from B to C; (a) external iliac artery; (v) external iliac vein.

Although differentiation between benign prostatic hyperplasia and carcinoma is not possible, MRI has value in staging prostatic carcinoma. Because the prostatic capsule is not reliably visualized with MRI, the diagnosis of extracapsular extension depends on identification of signal alteration in periprostatic fat. Tumor extension into periprostatic fat is best detected on T1-weighted images and appears as wispy or confluent areas of low signal intensity surrounded by high-intensity fat (Fig. 27). Extracapsular tumor extension can also be predicted when there is disruption of periprostatic venous plexus, which appears on the anterior and the lateral aspects of the prostate as a high-signal-intensity rim on a second-echo image (11,117) (Fig. 28). Involvement of seminal vesicles can likewise be detected. As mentioned previously, seminal vesicular invasion can be suggested if there is asymmetrical enlarge-

ment of the seminal vesicle, obliteration of one of the seminal vesicle angles, or abnormally low signal intensity on T2-weighted images. Whereas normal seminal vesicles have a high signal intensity (higher than that for fat) on T2-weighted images, invasion of the seminal vesicles by carcinomas may lead to a lower signal intensity. Recognition of changes in the signal intensity of seminal vesicles may sometimes be a more sensitive indicator of tumor invasion than are changes in their size (Fig. 29).

Extension of prostatic carcinoma into adjacent pelvic organs can be detected by MRI. Because of the Denonvilliers fascia, tumor often grows around the rectum to occupy the presacral space, rather than invading the rectum directly (Fig. 30). As in the case of bladder neoplasm, metastases to lymph nodes can be seen on MRI if the involved nodes are enlarged. Because of the ease with which small blood vessels can be identified on MRI, it is superior to CT in differentiating between small pelvic vessels and lymphadenopathy (Fig. 31). The experience in using MRI for staging prostatic carcinoma is limited, with accuracies of 83% and 89% reported in two relatively small series (11,61). Understaging (false-negative interpretations) usually results from the inability of MRI to detect microscopic or early extracapsular invasion; overstaging (false-positive interpretations) is often due to misinterpreting inflammatory changes as tumor infiltration.

Clinical Application

Although neither CT nor MRI is capable of detecting minimal or microscopic involvement of the periprostatic fat and seminal vesicles, such involvement does not change therapy in most centers. The value of preoperative CT is its ability to detect unsuspected gross local disease

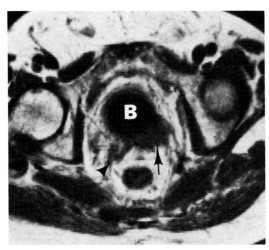
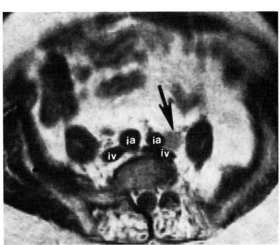

A,B

FIG. 27. Prostatic carcinoma, with extracapsular invasion and lymph node metastases. **A:** Transaxial MR image (TR = 500 msec, TE = 35 msec) shows tumor infiltration into left periprostatic fat (*arrow*). The left seminal vesicle is also obscured; (B) urinary bladder; (*arrowhead*) right seminal vesicle. **B:** Six centimeters cephalad, a 1.5-cm left common iliac nodal metastasis (*arrow*) is seen; (ia) common iliac arteries; (iv) common iliac vein.

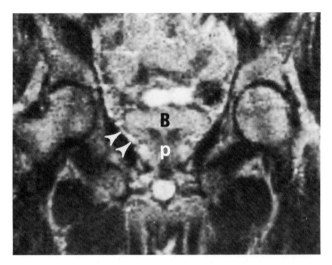

FIG. 28. Prostatic carcinoma extending into left periprostatic tissue: T2-weighted coronal image (TR = 2,100 msec, TE = 90 msec). A high-intensity structure representing periprostatic venous plexus (*arrowheads*) is noted along right supralateral aspect of the prostate. No such structure is present on the left side. Histologic examination of the resected specimen showed that left periprostatic tissue was infiltrated by prostatic carcinoma; (B) urinary bladder; (p) prostate. (From ref. 11.)

and nodal metastases in patients with clinical stage B lesions who are scheduled to undergo radical prostatectomy. CT is also used to confirm the extent of tumor in patients clinically suspected of having advanced disease and to provide additional information useful for radiotherapy planning. Although one study suggests that neither CT nor MRI can significantly improve on the information obtained by digital rectal examination (109), other studies have shown that CT can upstage 10% to 15% of patients clinically thought to have stage B disease (28,34,43).

Although MRI is more accurate than CT for detecting local extension of prostatic carcinoma (61), a complete staging examination by MRI is more time-consuming than with CT (1 hr for MRI vs. 15 min for CT). In addition, an MRI examination is more expensive than a CT study. It still needs to be determined if it is cost-effective

to replace CT with MRI for routine preoperative staging of prostatic carcinoma.

Transrectal ultrasound is another method that has been used for local staging (118). Although tumor detection by transrectal ultrasound appears promising, operator dependence and the limited field of view present obstacles to tumor staging.

Cervix

Carcinoma of the cervix is the fifth most common form of cancer in American women, after breast, colorectum, lung, and endometrium. The incidence rises after the age of 20 years, reaching its maximum for the group between 45 and 55 years of age. The overwhelming majority of carcinomas of the cervix are epidermoid. In general, grading (degree of histological differentiation) of epidermoid carcinoma is of little prognostic value (1). After the histological diagnosis of cervical carcinoma is established, assessment of actual extent of the disease will dictate the method of treatment. Whereas radical hysterectomy with lymph node sampling or radiation therapy are treatment options in stages I to IIA (Table 3), radiation therapy is the treatment of choice in stages IIB to IVB. Clinical staging procedures involve bimanual pelvic examination and conventional radiologic methods, such as excretory urography, barium enema, and lymphangiography. Cystoscopy and proctoscopy are also used in cases where there is a clinical suspicion of direct invasion to the urinary bladder and the rectum.

CT

Carcinoma of the cervix may be recognized on noncontrast CT images as a large cervix with regular or irregular borders. On postcontrast CT images, the tumor may appear as a soft-tissue mass enlarging the cervix, with

A,B

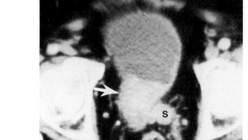
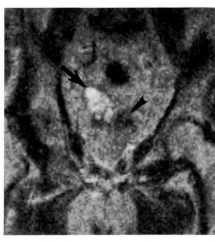

FIG. 29. Prostatic carcinoma extending into left seminal vesicle. **A:** CT image shows a soft-tissue mass (*arrow*) obscuring the right seminal vesicle, changes suggestive of tumor invasion; (s) normal left seminal vesicle. **B:** Coronal MR image (TR = 2,100 msec, TE = 90 msec) shows a large but normal-intensity seminal vesicle on the right (*arrow*). The left seminal vesicle is smaller and has an abnormally low signal intensity (*arrowhead*). Pathologic examination of the resected specimen showed total replacement of the left seminal vesicle with prostatic carcinoma. The right side was normal. (From ref. 87.)

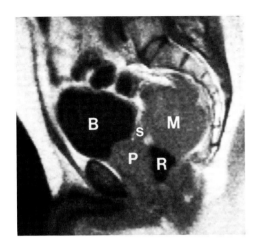

FIG. 30. Prostatic carcinoma, with rectal invasion: sagittal MR image (TR = 500 msec, TE = 30 msec). A large mass (M) representing contiguous spread of prostatic carcinoma lies posterior to the rectum (R); (s) seminal vesicles; (B) urinary bladder; (P) prostate. (From ref. 87.)

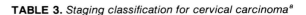

TABLE 3. *Staging classification for cervical carcinoma*[a]

0	Carcinoma in situ
I	Carcinoma strictly confined to the cervix
	Ia Microinvasive carcinoma
	Ib All other cases of stage I
II	Carcinoma extends beyond the cervix
	IIa No obvious parametrial involvement
	IIb Obvious parametrial involvement
III	Carcinoma involves the lower third of the vagina
	IIIa No extension to the pelvic wall
	IIIb Extension to the pelvic wall and/or hydronephrosis or nonfunctioning kidney
IV	Carcinoma has extended beyond the true pelvis or has involved the mucosa of the bladder or rectum
	IVa Spread to adjacent organs
	IVb Spread to distant organs

[a] From Kottmeier (79).

hypodense areas in the tumor due to necrosis, ulceration, and diminished intravenous contrast enhancement compared with normal cervical tissue (Fig. 32). Fluid collections in the endometrial cavity and uterine enlargement are frequently seen because of tumor obstruction of the endocervical canal (Fig. 33C). CT is capable of differentiating between tumor confined to the cervix and tumor that has invaded the parametrium (78,140,151,160) (Figs. 33 and 34).

CT criteria for parametrial tumor invasion are (a) irregularity or poor definition of the lateral cervix margins,

(b) prominent parametrial soft-tissue strands or an eccentric soft-tissue mass, and (c) obliteration of the periureteral fat plane (146) (Fig. 33). A parametrial soft-tissue mass and loss of the periureteral fat plane are essential for a definitive CT diagnosis of parametrial tumor extension. Caution must be taken not to overinterpret loss of the cervical border and minimal soft-tissue infiltration of the paracervical fat as parametrial tumor invasion, because parametritis secondary to prior instrumentation may result in similar CT findings (Fig. 35). Furthermore, normal broad, round, cardinal, and uterosacral ligaments should not be mistaken for lateral tumor extension.

Pelvic side-wall tumor extension (stage IIIB) is characterized by confluent, irregular, linear parametrial soft-tissue strands extending to and/or enlarging the obturator

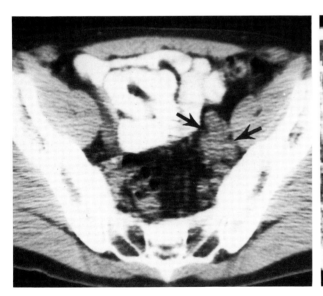
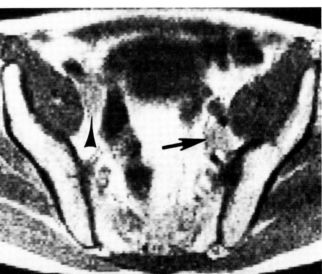

A,B

FIG. 31. Pelvic lymphadenopathy secondary to prostatic carcinoma. **A:** Noncontrast CT image shows increased soft-tissue densities around left iliac vessels (*arrows*), indicating possible lymphadenopathy. **B:** Transaxial MR image (TR = 900 msec, TE = 30 msec) confirms the presence of enlarged left external iliac node (*arrow*). Enlarged right iliac lymph node (*arrowhead*), not suspected on previous CT study, is also seen. Lymphadenopathy can be easily distinguished from adjacent low-intensity iliac vessels. (From ref. 87.)

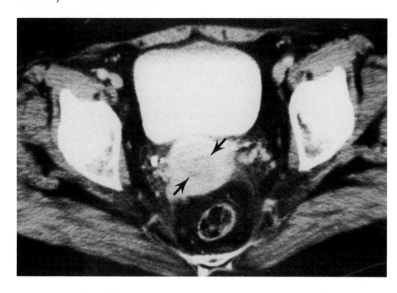

FIG. 32. Cervical carcinoma. A central low-attenuation area in the cervix (*arrows*) following contrast enhancement corresponds to clinically known tumor.

A,B

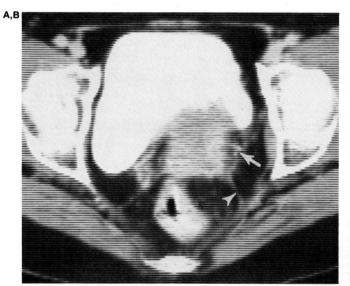 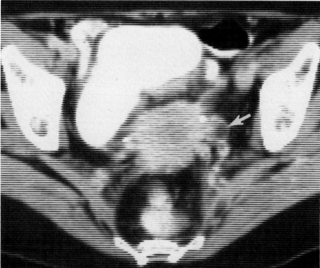

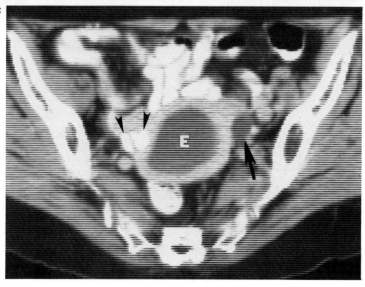

C

FIG. 33. Cervical carcinoma causing left hydronephrosis and obstructed uterus. **A:** Postcontrast CT image demonstrates a large cervix with an irregular left lateral border, indicating left parametrial invasion (*arrow*). There is also thickening of the left uterosacral ligament (*arrowhead*). **B:** Two centimeters cephalad, a dilated left distal ureter (*arrow*) is seen. The presence of hydroureter makes this stage IIIb disease. **C:** Two centimeters more cephalad, an enlarged fluid-filled endometrial cavity (E) is noted; (*arrow*) dilated left ureter; (*arrowheads*) calcified leiomyomata.

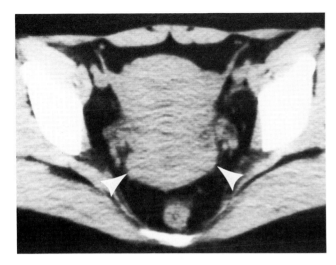

FIG. 34. Cervical carcinoma confined to the cervix. The cervix is enlarged (*arrowheads*), but its border is smooth, and there is no abnormal parametrial soft tissue. The adnexal structures are symmetric, and the pelvic fat appears "clean."

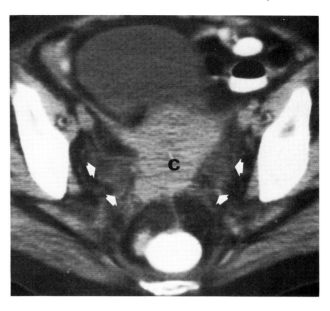

FIG. 35. Cervical carcinoma: pitfall in CT staging. In this case, wispy, soft-tissue infiltration in the parametrial fat (*arrows*) was due to inflammation. The tumor was confined to the cervix (C).

internus and pyriformis muscle (151). When a parametrial mass is within 2 to 3 mm of the pelvic side wall, even though there is a small intervening fat plane, the tumor should be staged as IIIB. In these cases, the gynecologist usually cannot interpose his or her examining fingers between the bulky tumor and the pelvic side wall and stages the tumor as IIIB. CT demonstration of hydronephrosis due to distal ureteral obstruction, with or without pelvic side-wall extension, indicates a stage IIIB tumor (Fig. 33B). Tumor extension into the urinary bladder and/or rectum (stage IVA) can be suggested if there is focal loss of the perivesical/perirectal fat plane accompanied by asymmetric wall thickening. Additional features include nodular indentation or serrations along the bladder/rectal wall and intraluminal tumor mass (Fig. 36).

Besides local invasion, carcinoma of the cervix metastasizes primarily by the lymphatic system. Initial metastases are found in the external and internal iliac lymph nodes. With more extensive primary neoplasms, metastases to the periaortic nodes, in addition to the pelvic nodes, frequently will be present at the time of initial evaluation. Although the clinical staging classification does not recognize pelvic lymph node metastases, demonstration of such lymph node metastases by CT precludes surgical salvage.

CT is slightly more accurate than pelvic examination and other radiologic studies (e.g., excretory urography, barium enema) in detecting tumor extension into the parametrium and the pelvic side wall. The reported accuracy for CT ranges from 58% to 88% (50,78,151,160), whereas the accuracy of clinical staging is generally cited as 60% to 70% (73). Both false-positive and false-negative CT interpretations may occur. False-positive CT diagnoses are often due to misinterpreting normal or inflammatory parametrial soft-tissue strands as tumor invasion; false-

negative diagnoses are usually due to its inability to detect microscopic or early disease. In addition, CT may not be able to determine if invasion of a structure has occurred or if the tumor is only contiguous, especially in the rectal area.

The overall accuracy for CT in detecting pelvic nodal metastases from cervical carcinoma is in the range of 70% to 80% (42,78,147,151). As with other pelvic malignant neoplasms, false-negative cases are mostly due to microscopic disease or metastases less than 1 cm in size; false-

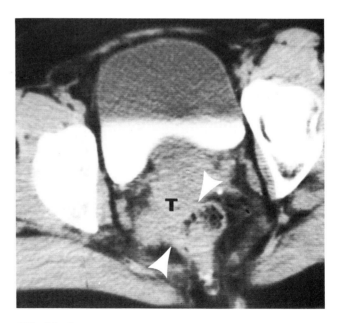

FIG. 36. Cervical carcinoma: stage IV. Parametrial tumor extends almost to the right pelvic side wall and invades the rectum (*arrowheads*).

A,B

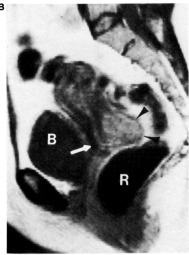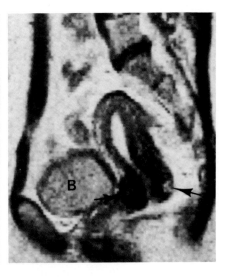

FIG. 37. Cervical carcinoma. **A:** Sagittal MR image (TR = 1,500 msec, TE = 35 msec) shows a mass (*arrowheads*) projecting from the posterior cervical lip. The anterior cervical lip (*arrow*) is normal. **B:** Sagittal MR image (TR = 1,500 msec, TE = 70 msec) in another patient demonstrates two small nodules (*arrows*), one in each cervical lip; (B) urinary bladder.

positive cases are largely secondary to misinterpretation of hyperplastic lymph nodes as metastatic disease. Because metastases from cervical carcinoma often replace a portion of a lymph node without enlarging it, the reported false-negative rate for CT exceeds 20% (147). Because lymphangiography is capable of delineating intranodal architecture, and hyperplastic changes usually can be differentiated from metastatic disease, lymphangiography is more accurate than CT in diagnosing lymph node involvement from cervical carcinoma (42).

MRI

Cervical carcinoma can be detected by MRI (14,-20,82,114,141,162). On T2-weighted images, cervical carcinoma most often appears as a mass of high signal intensity (Fig. 37). In some instances, no discrete mass is

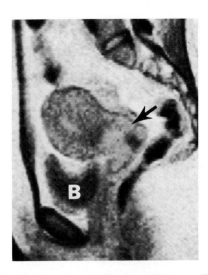

FIG. 38. Cervical carcinoma. Sagittal MR image (TR = 1,500 msec, TE = 70 msec) shows that the cervix (*arrow*) has an abnormally high signal intensity without a well-defined mass; (B) urinary bladder.

seen; however, the tumor may still be identified in these cases because of the disruption of part or all of the normally low-intensity cervical lips (Fig. 38).

When the cervical carcinoma is large (>4 cm), additional MRI findings may be noted (Fig. 39). These include blurring and widening of the uterine junctional low-intensity band, as well as broadening of the central uterine high-intensity zone. The latter finding is caused by uterine secretions retained within an enlarged uterine cavity—the so-called obstructed uterus (162). When the retained uterine secretions are not bloody, problems can arise in differentiating between uterine secretions in an obstructed uterus and merely thickened endometrium. This difficulty arises because both entities have low signal intensities on T1-weighted images and high signal intensities on T2-weighted images. However, if the retained uterine secretions are bloody, they will have a high signal intensity on both T1- and T2-weighted images. This allows one to differentiate between sequestered bloody uterine secretions and thickened endometrium.

Besides being able to image the primary cervical carcinoma, MRI is also able to detect extension of the tumor into the parametria and pelvic side walls. Because fat has a short T1 and cervical carcinoma has a long T1, tumor extension into the parametria is best evaluated on T1-weighted images. Parametrial extension is diagnosed either by an asymmetric appearance of the parametria or by abnormal tumor intensity extending into the parametrial ligaments, coupled with local disruption of the normal low-intensity cervix (141) (Fig. 40A). Invasion of the vagina is better seen on T2-weighted images (Fig. 40B). Infiltration of adjacent organs, such as the urinary bladder and the rectum, can similarly be detected. It is not certain, however, whether or not MRI is superior to CT in differentiating between mere contiguity and frank invasion. Metastases to lymph nodes can also be detected by MRI. As stated previously, the diagnosis of malignant lymphadenopathy by MRI is similar to that of CT and is based on recognition of enlargement of the involved node.

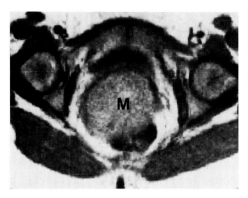
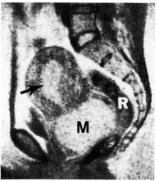

FIG. 39. Obstructed uterus secondary to a large cervical carcinoma. A: Transaxial MR image (TR = 1,500 msec, TE = 30 msec). A large cervical mass (M) is seen. B: Sagittal MR image (TR = 1,500 msec, TE = 60 msec) shows an enlarged uterine cavity filled with secretions (*arrow*). The cervical mass (M) is again noted; (R) rectum.

In one study of 19 patients with cervical carcinoma, the MRI diagnosis was correct in 14 patients with no parametrial disease and 3 patients with parametrial invasion (141). The MRI interpretation was falsely positive in 2 patients.

Clinical Application

CT is not indicated in patients with carcinoma *in situ.* In addition, CT is not routinely used in clinical stage IB to IIA tumors because clinical staging by experienced gynecologists has a higher accuracy than CT staging in evaluating these tumors (50,147). Although some use CT to evaluate the pelvis and the retroperitoneum in all patients having more than microinvasive disease (78), others, including ourselves, continue to use conventional radiologic procedures (barium enema, excretory urography, and lymphangiography) to stage patients with clinical evidence of low-stage disease (42,47,95).

CT should be used as the initial staging procedure in patients suspected of having clinical stage IIIB to IVB tumors (42,47,95,147). It is also used to confirm clinical stage IIB tumors by showing tumor invading the parametria. Not only is CT more accurate than other available imaging methods in detecting pelvic side-wall invasion, it also provides direct delineation of the tumor mass, thereby assisting in the design of radiation ports. Cystos-

copy and sigmoidoscopy should be reserved for patients with hematuria or guaiac-positive stool. In patients with documented advanced disease, CT can be used to monitor tumor response to treatment. CT is also the procedure of choice in patients suspected of having recurrence (149,151). Although MRI often can delineate the primary tumor more clearly than CT, it is as yet undetermined whether MRI or CT is more accurate in the staging of cervical carcinoma. At present, CT is still being used for staging cervical carcinoma because of its superior spatial resolution and the ease with which the entire abdomen and pelvis can be examined. However, at our institution, MRI is being used with increasing frequency to delineate tumor volume for planning of radiation therapy.

Uterus

The predominant neoplasm of the uterine body is adenocarcinoma of the endometrium. The prognosis for this neoplasm, which usually affects women in the fifth decade, depends on the histology, the grade (degree of cellular differentiation), and the stage (anatomical extent) of the tumor. Whereas well-differentiated adenocarcinomas of the endometrium often are localized on initial presentation, poorly differentiated adenocarcinomas and endometrial sarcomas tend to metastasize widely. In addition, the incidence of distant metastases increases with increas-

FIG. 40. Advanced-stage cervical carcinoma. A: Transaxial T1-weighted image (TR = 500 msec, TE = 35 msec) shows a large cervix (c), with thickening of the left uterosacral ligament (*arrowheads*) representing pelvic side-wall invasion. An enlarged left external iliac lymph node (*arrow*) is also seen. B: Sagittal T2-weighted MR image (TR = 1,500 msec, TE = 70 msec) demonstrates invasion of cervical carcinoma into the vagina (*arrow*) as well as the posterior bladder wall (*arrowhead*); (R) rectum. (From ref. 114.)

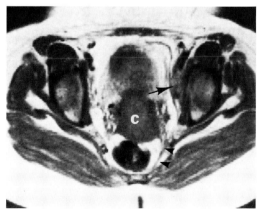
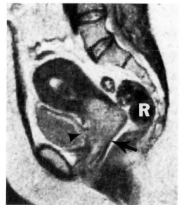

ing depth of myometrial invasion. In lymphatic spread from neoplasms of the uterine body, the paraaortic and paracaval groups are most frequently involved, followed by external iliac and inguinal nodes (1). Local spread to the broad ligament and adnexal structures, as well as metastases to the omentum and peritoneum, also may occur.

The clinical management of patients with endometrial cancer varies from institution to institution. At our institution, the treatment of stage I (Table 4) disease depends on the degree of cellular differentiation: low-grade tumors are managed by hysterectomy; high-grade tumors receive staging laparotomy after brief intracavitary radiation. In addition to hysterectomy, random sampling of pelvic lymph nodes and peritoneal washing are also performed. The subsequent therapy depends on the operatively determined tumor extent. Treatment of stage II disease depends on the extent of cervical involvement; patients with macroscopic tumors undergo a staging laparotomy as described for high-grade stage I patients. In patients with stage III and IV tumors, palliative radiation or surgery often is the only treatment rendered.

CT

On noncontrast CT images, focal or diffuse enlargement of the uterine body can be seen. After administration of contrast material, an endometrial neoplasm appears as a mass that is enhanced to a lesser degree than normal myometrium, but to a greater degree than nonenhancing uterine secretions (51,55,128,152) (Fig. 41). In some cases the primary tumor may occlude the internal cervical os, resulting in hydrometra, hematometra, or pyometra. When this occurs, CT demonstrates a symmetrically en-

TABLE 4. *Staging classification for endometrial carcinoma*[a]

I	Tumor confined to the corpus
	A Uterine cavity less than 8 cm
	B Uterine cavity greater than 8 cm
II	Tumor involving corpus and cervix
III	Involvement of parametria, adnexae, pelvic side wall, or pelvic nodes
IV	A Bladder or rectal involvement
	B Metastases outside the true pelvis

[a] From International Federation of Gynecology and Obstetrics (67).

larged uterus containing a central low-attenuation mass surrounded by a large amount of fluid (128). Such an appearance may be confused with that of a cystic ovarian cancer. Occlusion of the internal os also may be due to senile contraction, primary or recurrent carcinoma of the cervix, radiation therapy, or postsurgical scarring (Fig. 42). The depth of myometrial invasion can be determined from postcontrast images (31,51,55) (Fig. 43). Endometrial tumor involvement of the cervix by CT is characterized by cervical enlargement and hypodense areas within the fibromuscular stroma of the cervix (10,55). CT findings of parametrial and pelvic side-wall extension from endometrial carcinoma are similar to those seen in cervical carcinoma.

The reported accuracy for CT in staging patients with endometrial cancer ranges from 84% to 88% (10,152). CT often upstages clinical stage I and II tumors by detecting occult metastases to pelvic and paraaortic lymph nodes or the omentum (Fig. 41). Most of the staging errors by CT are due to its failure to identify microscopic tumor spread to the parametria, lymph nodes, or other pelvic viscera.

A,B

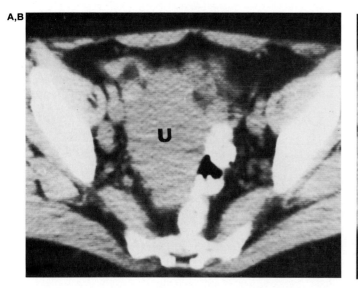 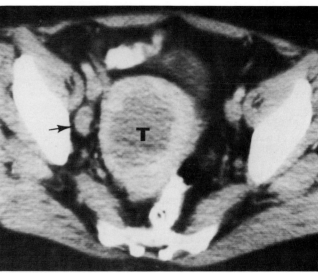

FIG. 41. Endometrial carcinoma. **A:** Without intravenous contrast material, the endometrial tumor is isodense with normal myometrium; (U) uterus. **B:** After intravenous administration of contrast material, the tumor (T) is lower in attenuation than the enhancing myometrium surrounding it; (*arrow*) enlarged external iliac node.

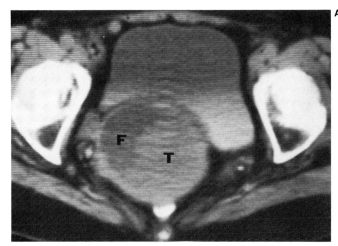

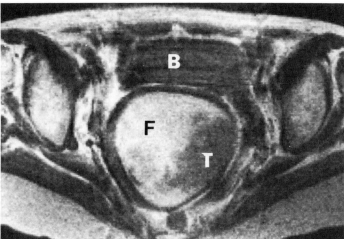

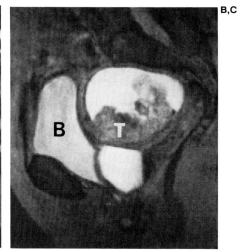

FIG. 42. Endometrial carcinoma. **A:** Postcontrast CT image shows an irregular endometrial tumor (T) outlined by fluid (F). The uterus was obstructed because of postsurgical cervical fibrosis. **B:** Transaxial MR image (TR = 500 msec, TE = 70 msec) at a slightly higher level than (**A**) shows similar findings. The high intensity of the fluid (F) is due to hemorrhage; (T) tumor. **C:** Sagittal MR image (TR = 1,500 msec, TE = 90 msec) better delineates the cephalocaudal extent of the tumor (T); (B) urinary bladder.

MRI

Endometrial carcinoma has a variable MRI appearance. In some patients, low-to-medium-intensity tumor nodules, ranging from a few millimeters to a few centimeters in size, can be identified within the uterine cavity on T2-weighted images (63,82,162) (Figs. 42B, 42C, and 44). However, in other patients, MRI will show only expansion of the central high-intensity area of the uterus, without discrete nodules. Although the expanded central high-intensity area corresponds to the tumor mass and thickened endometrium in most cases, it correlates with increased uterine secretion in some patients. As stated previously, it is not yet possible to differentiate between nonbloody uterine secretions and the underlying endometrium because of their similar signal intensities on both T1- and T2-weighted images. Because endometrial carcinoma occurs predominantly in postmenopausal women, and because normal postmenopausal uteri have a very thin central high-intensity zone (often less than 5 mm in width), expansion of the central high-intensity zone in this age group should raise the suspicion of uterine abnormality.

In contradistinction to endometrial carcinoma, a uter-

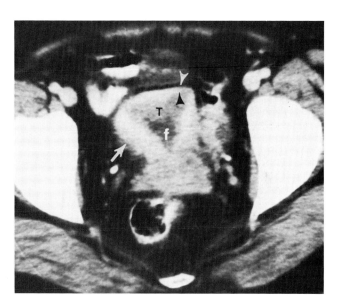

FIG. 43. Endometrial carcinoma, with deep myometrial invasion. Postcontrast CT image demonstrates that the tumor (T) is enhanced to a lesser degree than normal myometrium (*arrow*), but more than endometrial fluid (f). Marked thinning of the anterior myometrium (*arrowheads*) is due to tumor invasion.

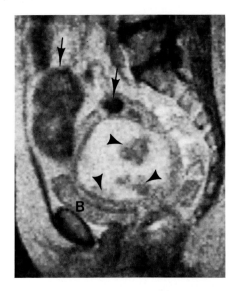

FIG. 44. Endometrial carcinoma. Sagittal MR image (TR = 1,500 msec, TE = 60 msec) shows a large uterine cavity containing several medium-to-low-intensity nodules (*arrowheads*) representing adenocarcinomas of the endometrium. Incidentally noted are two leiomyomas (*arrows*); (B) urinary bladder.

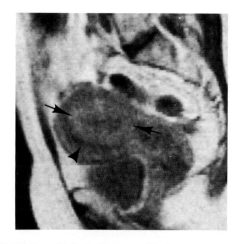

FIG. 46. Endometrial carcinoma, with deep myometrial invasion. Sagittal MR image (TR = 1,500 msec, TE = 70 msec) shows a large endometrial carcinoma (*arrows*) replacing most of the posterior myometrium. Note the preservation of low-intensity junctional band anteriorly (*arrowhead*), but not posteriorly.

interpret this finding, because the entire junctional zone may not be visible in some healthy postmenopausal women (27). Although MRI also can detect tumor extension into the cervix (Fig. 47), it is less accurate in detecting metastases to the adnexa, the peritoneum, and the lymph nodes (63).

ine sarcoma generally appears as a large mass of inhomogeneous signal intensity, totally obscuring the uterine contour (82,162) (Fig. 45).

Preliminary data have shown that MRI is useful in assessing the depth of myometrial invasion by endometrial cancer (63,120,162). On T2-weighted images, preservation of the junctional low-intensity band usually implies absence of myometrial invasion; focal disruption or total obliteration of this band suggests myometrial involvement (Fig. 46). However, caution must be taken not to over-

Clinical Application

Because the initial symptom is postmenopausal bleeding, most patients with endometrial cancer seek medical care when the disease is at an early stage. The diagnosis is established by fractional dilatation and curettage. Clin-

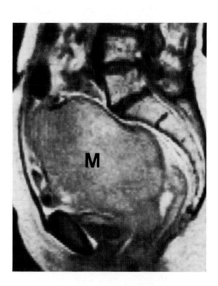

FIG. 45. Endometrial sarcoma. Sagittal MR image (TR = 1,500 msec, TE = 35 msec) shows a lobulated mass (M) obliterating the normal uterine anatomy.

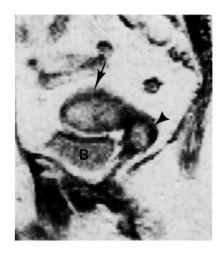

FIG. 47. Endometrial carcinoma invading the cervix. Sagittal MR image (TR = 1,500 msec, TE = 60 msec) shows expansion of the uterine body (*arrow*) and endocervix (*arrowhead*). Ill-defined medium-intensity nodules can be seen within these two regions; (B) urinary bladder. (From ref. 162.)

ical staging is based on bimanual pelvic examination, sonographic determination of the depth of the uterine cavity, and conventional roentgenographic studies, including chest radiographs and excretory urography. Cystoscopy and sigmoidoscopy are used in selected cases.

CT is not routinely performed in patients with well-differentiated stage I adenocarcinoma of the endometrium. However, CT is extremely useful in detecting clinically unsuspected extrauterine metastases in patients with sarcomas and high-grade endometrial carcinomas. Furthermore, CT is also useful in determining the depth of myometrial invasion in these patients. Preoperative radiation is often given to patients in whom CT shows deep myometrial invasion. CT is also valuable in patients suspected of having neoplastic recurrence and in following the response to chemotherapy or radiation treatment.

Although MRI can more clearly demonstrate the primary neoplasm and determine the depth of myometrial invasion than CT, it has not replaced CT for staging of endometrial carcinoma because MRI is less sensitive to extrauterine metastases, is more expensive, and requires longer examination time.

Ovary

Ovarian cancer is the most lethal of all gynecologic malignancies. The peak incidence is in women between 40 and 65 years of age. The prognosis depends on the clinical stage, the degree of cellular differentiation, and the histological type of ovarian cancer. Because of a paucity of symptoms in early stages, most patients present with advanced disease. Approximately 85% of ovarian cancers are epithelial in origin, with the remaining 15% derived from germ or stroma cells (1). In patients with epithelial ovarian carcinomas, the great majority (90%) have either serous or mucinous cystadenocarcinoma, with the rest being endometrial or solid carcinomas. Stage for stage (Table 5), the prognosis for patients with solid carcinomas is worse than that for either serous or mucinous tumors.

TABLE 5. *Staging classification for ovarian carcinoma[a]*

I	Growth limited to the ovaries
	IA One ovary; no ascites
	IB Both ovaries; no ascites
	IC One or both ovaries; ascites present, with malignant cells in the fluid
II	Growth involving one or both ovaries, with pelvic extension
	IIA Extension and/or metastases to the uterus and/or tubes only
	IIB Extension to other pelvic tissues
III	Growth involving one or both ovaries, with widespread intraperitoneal metastases (the omentum, the small intestine, and its mesentery), limited to the abdomen
IV	Growth involving one or both ovaries, with distant metastases outside the peritoneal cavity

[a] From International Federation of Gynecology and Obstetrics (67).

Ovarian carcinomas usually spread by implanting widely on the omental and peritoneal surfaces. Although not pathognomonic, demonstration of an "omental cake" is highly suggestive of an ovarian malignancy (91) (Fig. 48). An "omental cake" appears as an irregular sheet of nodular soft-tissue densities beneath the anterior abdominal wall on CT and masses of medium signal intensities on MRI. Peritoneal tumor implants are recognized as soft-tissue or medium-signal-intensity nodules/plaques along the lateral peritoneal surfaces of the abdomen (68). Subdiaphragmatic peritoneal nodules are most easily detected between the abdominal wall and the liver in the presence of ascites (68) (Fig. 49). Rarely, peritoneal and omental metastases may calcify (104) (Fig. 50). Although intraperitoneal seeding is the almost exclusive metastatic mode in mucinous carcinomas, lymphatic metastases to the paraaortic lymph nodes and occasionally to the inguinal nodes do occur in serous and other types of ovarian carcinomas.

In most centers, neither CT nor MRI plays a primary role in the initial evaluation of ovarian carcinoma. When the diagnosis of an ovarian carcinoma is suspected, based on physical examination or sonographic findings, exploratory laparotomy usually follows. Because the sensitivity of CT and MRI in detecting small intraperitoneal implants (<1 cm) is low, surgical exploration is necessary to document the exact stage of the disease in all cases (3,24,72). Surgical debulking of the neoplasm is particularly helpful in patients with stage III or IV ovarian cancer (49). Cytoreductive surgery not only allows for greater drug exposure and penetration but also may favorably affect tumor cell kinetics, allowing for greater cell kill with

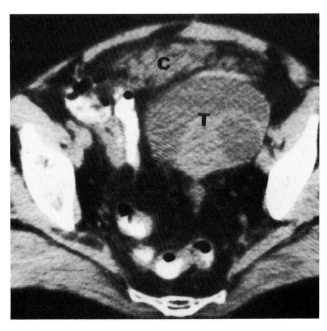

FIG. 48. Ovarian carcinoma: stage IV. The primary tumor (T) is a complex mass with solid and cystic components. Peritoneal spread is indicated by an omental cake (C).

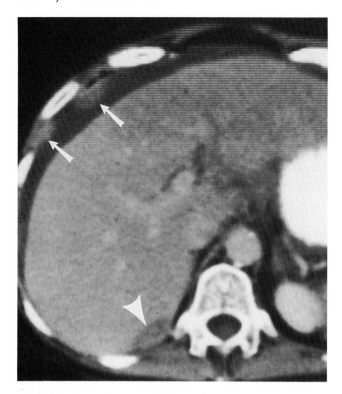

FIG. 49. Ovarian carcinoma: stage IV. Tumor implants in the parietal peritoneum (*arrows*) are outlined by ascites. A subdiaphragmatic lesion is also present (*arrowhead*).

chemotherapeutic agents (49). Although CT is valuable in following treatment responses in patients with ovarian malignancy (3), it cannot replace a second-look laparotomy for accurate assessment of disease status because of its low accuracy in detecting small peritoneal metastases (13,24).

CLARIFICATION OF KNOWN AND SUSPECTED PELVIC ABNORMALITY

Evaluation of Urinary Bladder Deformity

When the lateral aspect of the urinary bladder is noted to be compressed on an excretory urogram, either uni-

laterally or on both sides, the differential diagnosis usually includes pelvic lipomatosis, pelvic lymph node enlargement, hypertrophic iliopsoas muscles (22), lymphocele, urinoma, hematoma, or pelvic venous thrombosis. Documentation of a urinoma/hematoma or pelvic lymphadenopathy can be accomplished quickly with sonography (106). Pelvic lipomatosis is often suspected from apparent increased lucency on the plain radiograph. A diagnosis of venous thrombosis and pelvic collateral venous congestion causing bladder deformity usually requires prior venography. Because of the superior contrast sensitivity of CT and MRI, both are capable of differentiating among fat, water, and soft tissues (Fig. 51). Because neutral fat has a characteristic CT and MRI appearance, a definitive diagnosis of pelvic lipomatosis can be made by either method, and surgical exploration or percutaneous biopsy obviated (23,54,138,159). The true nature of venous collaterals can be established on CT images by administering contrast material intravenously. Such a diagnosis can also be made by MRI without the use of intravenous contrast material. In cases where the bladder deformity is due to compression by enlarged pelvic lymph nodes, either CT or MRI can be used to assess the status of the retroperitoneal and mesenteric lymph nodes as well.

Characterization of Presacral Masses

Ultrasonography is not as accurate in detecting presacral masses as in diagnosing gynecologic masses. Sonographic studies are often suboptimal in obese patients because of marked attenuation of the sound beam by abundant subcutaneous fat. Furthermore, ultrasound is incapable of evaluating bony abnormalities, which are often associated with presacral masses. Both CT and MRI are useful in these circumstances in confirming the presence of a pelvic mass when one is suspected either by physical examination or by other radiologic tests (e.g., barium enema) (92). In general, CT is superior to MRI in evaluating the integrity of cortical bone and in demonstrating gas bubbles and

A,B

FIG. 50. Calcified peritoneal metastases due to recurrent ovarian carcinoma. **A:** Noncontrast CT image shows two specks of calcification (*arrows*) near the surface of the liver. **B:** Postcontrast CT study obtained 6 months later demonstrates interval increase in the size of the calcification. Percutaneous biopsy confirmed ovarian metastases.

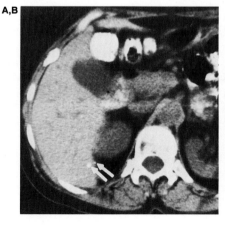
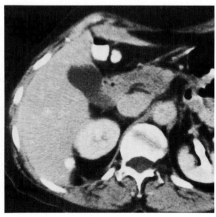

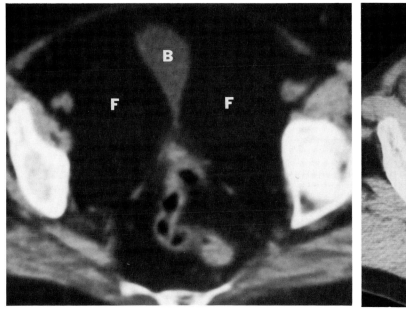

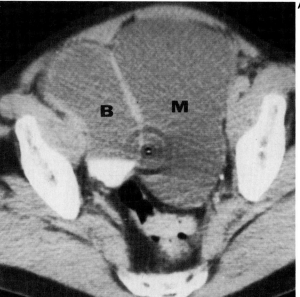

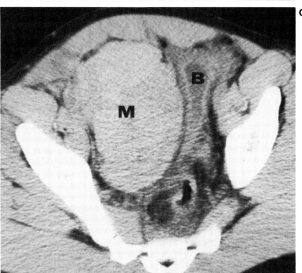

FIG. 51. Bladder deformity. **A:** Pelvic lipomatosis. The midline bladder (B) is elevated and narrowed by an excessive amount of pelvic fat (F), easily differentiated from higher-attenuation soft tissue. **B:** Bladder diverticulum. The contrast-containing bladder (B) is displaced to the right by a thin-walled water-density mass (M), which on delayed images was also filled with contrast material. **C:** Hematoma. A large mass (M) with an attenuation value slightly higher than that of gluteal muscle displaces the bladder (B) to the left. The high density is characteristic of an acute hematoma.

calcifications. In contradistinction, MRI is more sensitive than CT in detecting marrow alteration and provides a better topographic display of a presacral mass because of its direct multiplanar imaging capability. When a mass is detected, either CT or MRI can characterize many lesions and give an accurate assessment of possible bony involvement. Air, fat, fluid, and soft tissue are easily differentiated. An air-containing mass suggests an abscess cavity (6), whereas a mass with the density of fat is compatible with a benign lipoma. Masses with near-water density or signal intensity include seroma, urinoma, and cystic teratoma, although the latter often contains areas of fatty and calcific elements and usually has a thick wall. When the mass is composed of soft tissue, definitive histologic diagnosis by CT or MRI is not possible. Although both CT and MRI are capable of delineating the size and shape of the mass,

as well as its effects on neighboring viscera, differentiation between a benign tumor and a malignant tumor may be difficult unless secondary findings such as lymph node metastases or bony destruction are also present. The attenuation values of an abscess, a hematoma, and a necrotic tumor also may overlap, and distinction among these entities often depends on the clinical history and physical findings. Likewise, the signal intensity of an abscess overlaps that of a necrotic tumor.

Evaluation of Gynecologic Masses

Because it does not involve ionizing radiation and because of the ease in obtaining longitudinal and transverse images, ultrasonography is used as the primary imaging

A–C

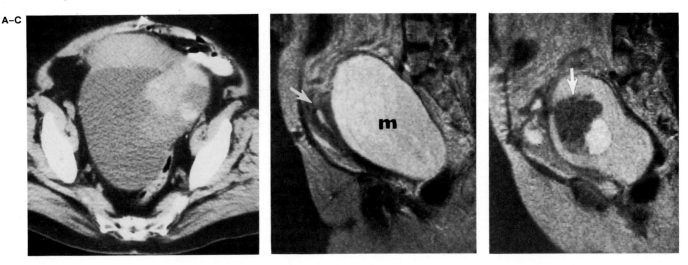

FIG. 52. Ovarian cystadenocarcinoma. **A:** Postcontrast CT image demonstrates a large, complex pelvic mass with both cystic and solid components. The exact location of the uterus is difficult to determine. **B:** Sagittal T2-weighted MR image (TR = 1,500 msec, TE = 90 msec) shows the uterus (*arrows*), with its characteristic high-intensity endometrium, to be displaced anteriorly by the mass (m). This portion of the mass is filled with fluid. **C:** Sagittal T2-weighted MR image (TR = 1,500 msec, TE = 90 msec) 2 cm lateral to (**B**) shows solid components (*arrow*) of the mass, convincingly demonstrating that the mass is extrauterine in origin.

method in the evaluation of patients suspected of having gynecologic abnormalities. Ultrasonography can accurately differentiate cystic and solid lesions and uterine and ovarian masses (153). Also, ultrasonography is superior to CT in detecting internal septations within a cystic mass (35). However, CT can be helpful when ultrasonography is suboptimal either because of abundant intestinal gas

or because of marked obesity. Because a successful pelvic sonographic study is dependent on the presence of a distended urinary bladder, CT also can be beneficial in patients with a small irritable bladder and in patients who have had prior cystectomy. Although MRI is more time-consuming and more costly than ultrasonography or CT, it has nevertheless added a new dimension to the evalu-

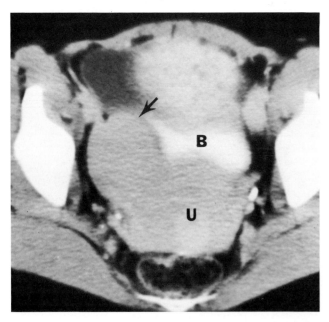

FIG. 53. Noncalcified uterine leiomyoma. Postcontrast CT image demonstrates a round, soft-tissue mass (*arrow*) representing a leiomyoma. The mass is inseparable from the uterine body (U); (B) urinary bladder.

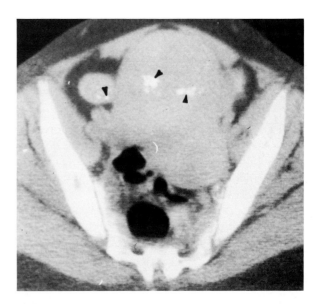

FIG. 54. Calcified uterine leiomyomata. The uterus is markedly enlarged and lobulated. Clusters of calcification (*arrowheads*) are noted in several areas.

ation of gynecologic masses. It is most useful in determining the organ of origin in large pelvic masses (Fig. 52).

Leiomyomas

CT

Leiomyomas usually are of soft-tissue density similar to that of normal uterus (Fig. 53). Necrosis or degeneration may result in a low-attenuation mass, sometimes simulating adnexal abnormality. Although contour deformity was the most common CT finding in one series, calcification was a more specific CT sign (139) (Fig. 54). It has been reported that a leiomyoma may be distinguished from an endometrial carcinoma because the former tends to exhibit contrast enhancement similar to normal myometrium, whereas the latter is enhanced to a lesser degree and appears as a hypodense mass (55). However, the reliability of this potentially distinctive CT feature is unknown. In our experience, a noncalcified uterine myoma cannot be distinguished from a malignant uterine neoplasm based on CT density alone (Fig. 55).

MRI

The signal intensity of uterine leiomyoma is variable (20,53,64,82). On T2-weighted images, it may have a signal intensity similar to that of endometrium, myometrium, or the junctional band (Figs. 44 and 56). This variable appearance is related to the degree of cellularity of the tumor. The lesions with low signal intensity generally have low cellularity, hyaline degeneration, and/or calcification. The medium- and high-intensity lesions generally have normal cellularity (82). However, other investigators have shown that leiomyomas without degeneration have a homogeneous low-intensity appearance, whereas degenerative leiomyomas have an inhomogeneous MRI appearance, with areas of both high and low signal intensities (64). Pathologically, these high-intensity areas correlate with areas of fatty and cystic degeneration. Although the explanations for why different leiomyomas have varying signal intensities differ, all agree that there is no reliable MRI feature for detecting malignant degeneration within a benign leiomyoma.

MRI may be able to differentiate between an adenomyoma (focal adenomyosis) and a leiomyoma (96). Whereas an adenomyoma often appears as a poorly marginated low-intensity mass, a leiomyoma usually is well defined and has a variable signal intensity. However, if a leiomyoma has a homogeneous low intensity and indistinct margins, it cannot be distinguished from an adenomyoma by MRI.

Ovarian Masses

CT

Both benign and malignant ovarian tumors have been diagnosed by CT. A benign ovarian cyst appears as a well-circumscribed, round, near-water-density structure with an almost imperceptible wall (Fig. 57). It is not enhanced after intravenous administration of water-soluble iodinated contrast material. The CT appearance of an ovarian cyst is quite similar to those for cysts in other organs (e.g., renal cysts, hepatic cysts). A follicular cyst cannot be differentiated from a corpus luteum cyst based on CT ap-

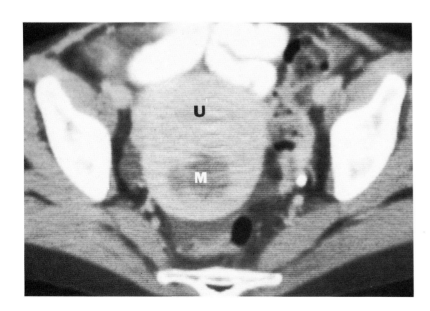

FIG. 55. Uterine leiomyoma. An irregular mass (M) with central low attenuation enlarges the posterior uterine fundus (U) in this contrast-enhanced image. By CT criteria, this leiomyoma is indistinguishable from uterine malignancy.

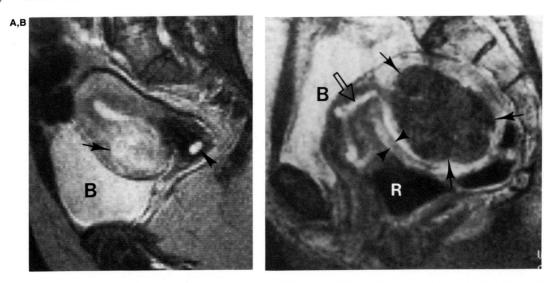

FIG. 56. Uterine leiomyomata. A: Sagittal MR image (TR = 2,000 msec, TE = 70 msec) shows a mixed-intensity leiomyoma (*arrow*) originating from the anterior wall of the lower uterine segment; (B) urinary bladder; (*arrowhead*) nabothian cyst. **B:** In another patient, sagittal MR image (TR = 2,500 msec, TE = 70 msec) shows a large leiomyoma (*arrows*) in the fundus of a retroverted uterus. Note that the signal intensity of the leiomyoma is lower than that of adjacent myometrium (*arrowheads*); (*open arrow*) endometrium; (B) urinary bladder; (R) rectum.

pearance alone. In patients with the Stein-Leventhal syndrome, both ovaries are enlarged and contain numerous cysts. The diagnosis usually can be made by CT. On occasion, the cysts are too small to be discernible by CT, and the ovaries may simply appear as two enlarged soft-tissue masses (Fig. 58). Under these circumstances, polycystic ovarian disease cannot be differentiated from other solid ovarian neoplasms.

Dermoid cysts (cystic teratomas) occur in young women and are bilateral in 25% of patients. They are composed of ectodermal, mesodermal, and endodermal elements. When calcific (or osseous) and fatty elements are present within the tumor, its diagnosis by CT is quite easy (Fig. 59).

Endometriosis is a disease affecting a significant portion of the menstruating population. Symptoms have classi-

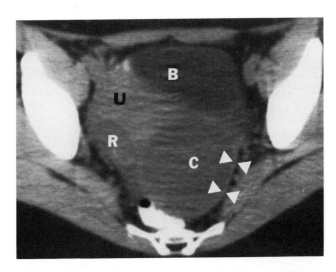

FIG. 57. Simple ovarian cyst. A left ovarian cyst (C) displaces the uterus (U) to the right and effaces the rectum. The cyst is of near-water density and is well defined, with a thin wall (*arrowheads*). A smaller right ovarian cyst (R) appears slightly higher in attenuation because of partial-volume averaging with the uterus; (B) bladder.

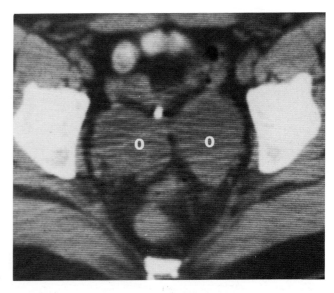

FIG. 58. Polycystic ovaries. The ovaries (O) are symmetrically enlarged. Although they are inhomogeneous in attenuation, no well-defined cyst is seen. Bilateral solid ovarian neoplasm cannot be excluded on the basis of this appearance.

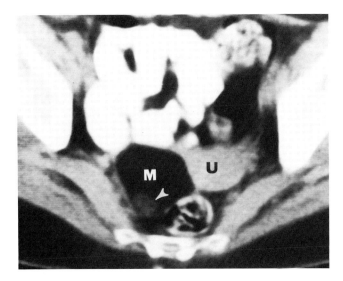

FIG. 59. Ovarian dermoid. A well-defined mass (M), with attenuation value equal to that of subcutaneous fat, lies to the right of the uterus (U). A small nodule of soft-tissue density is present within the mass (*arrowhead*). Despite the absence of calcification, the fatty component is adequate to identify this mass as a dermoid.

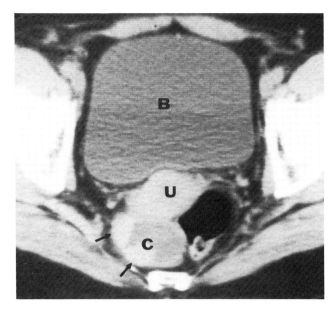

FIG. 61. Ovarian cystadenoma. The cystadenoma (C) is a complex mass lying posterior to the uterus (U). Two soft-tissue nodules (*arrows*) lie in the wall. The attenuation value of the fluid component is between that of soft tissue and water; (B) urinary bladder.

cally been characterized as the triad of dysmenorrhea, dyspareunia, and infertility. On CT, it may have a soft-tissue density, a near-water density, or a mixture of the two (38) (Fig. 60).

Ovarian cystadenomas often are quite large when they first present. They appear as well-defined low-density masses, with thick, irregular walls and multiple internal septae (153) (Fig. 61). Papillary projections of soft-tissue density may be seen within the tumor. Whereas serous cystadenoma has a central CT density approaching that

of water, mucinous cystadenoma has a density slightly less than that of soft tissue. Amorphous, coarse calcifications sometimes can be seen in the wall or within the soft-tissue component of a serous cystadenoma. Malignant ovarian cystadenocarcinomas cannot be reliably distinguished from benign cystadenomas unless metastases are present (Fig. 62).

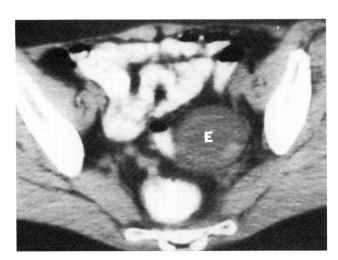

FIG. 60. Endometrioma. This well-defined mass, with attenuation value slightly less than that of gluteal muscle, proved to be an endometrioma (E) or "chocolate cyst." A specific histologic diagnosis cannot be provided based on CT findings alone.

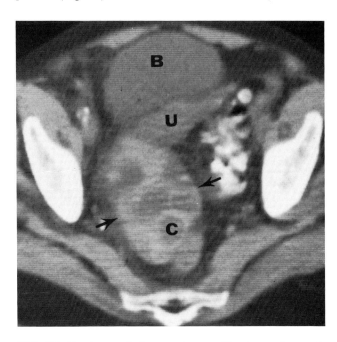

FIG. 62. Ovarian cystadenocarcinoma. The tumor (*arrows*), which contains several thick-walled cysts (C), cannot be diagnosed definitively as malignant by CT criteria because there is no evidence of extraovarian disease; (U) uterus; (B) bladder.

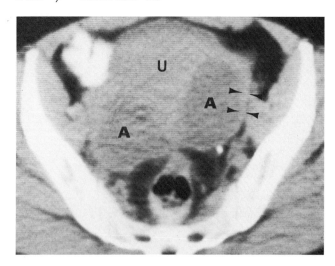

FIG. 63. Tubo-ovarian abscess. Bilateral abscesses (A) are present. Thick, nonuniform walls (*arrowheads*) surround the low-density masses. Correlation of the CT findings with clinical history is necessary to distinguish abscess from other ovarian lesions; (U) uterus.

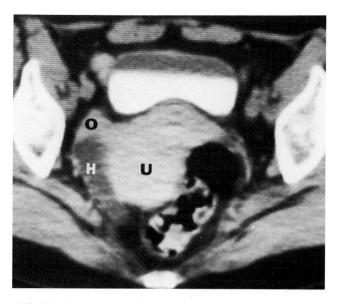

FIG. 64. Hydrosalpinx. The right fallopian tube (H) appears as a tubular near-water-density mass adjacent to the retroverted uterine fundus (U) and behind the right ovary (O).

The CT appearances of primary solid ovarian carcinomas are similar to those of their benign counterparts. Concomitant metastases to the lymph nodes, other organs, and omentum may be detected.

The CT appearance of a tubo-ovarian abscess is similar to those for abscesses occurring in other parts of the body. It appears as a soft-tissue mass, with central areas of lower density and a thick irregular wall (Fig. 63). An associated hydrosalpinx sometimes also may be seen (Fig. 64). If the abscess contains air, a precise diagnosis can be provided. In the absence of gas bubbles, a tubo-ovarian abscess cannot be differentiated from a necrotic tumor or a hematoma based on the CT findings alone. Pelvic inflammatory disease that does not present as a discrete abscess also has a nonspecific CT appearance. The normal pelvic structures are poorly defined because of obliteration of fat planes by the inflammatory process.

MRI

The MRI appearance of an uncomplicated ovarian cyst is similar to that of cyst elsewhere in the body (30,52,105). An ovarian cyst usually has an extremely low signal intensity on T1-weighted images and a very high signal intensity on T2-weighted images (Fig. 65). Hemorrhage into an ovarian cyst may result in higher signal intensity on T1-weighted images (Fig. 66). In patients with polycystic ovary disease, T2-weighted images often show multiple

A,B

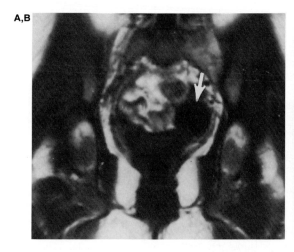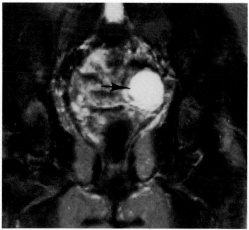

FIG. 65. Ovarian cyst. **A:** Coronal MR image (TR = 500 msec, TE = 17 msec) shows a 2.5-cm round, low-intensity mass (*arrow*) in the left adnexa. **B:** On T2-weighted image (TR = 3,000 msec, TE = 90 msec), the mass has a uniformly high signal intensity (*arrow*).

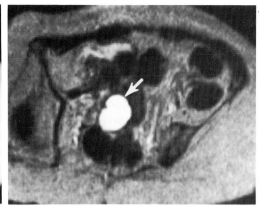

FIG. 66. Hemorrhagic ovarian cyst. **A:** Transaxial T1-weighted image (TR = 500 msec, TE = 17 msec) shows a relatively high-signal-intensity mass (*arrow*) in the right ovary. The pelvis is deformed in this patient with a congenital neuromuscular disorder. **B:** On T2-weighted image (TR = 2,100 msec, TE = 90 msec), the mass (*arrow*) has a higher signal intensity than fat.

small peripheral cysts of high signal intensity surrounding abundant low-intensity central stroma (103).

Dermoid cysts (cystic teratomas) vary in signal intensity depending on their tissue composition (20,59,105,143) (Fig. 67). The majority of cystic teratomas have appeared as masses with high signal intensity due to their large fat content. However, calcifications, bone, hair, and fibrous tissue, all of which are frequently found in teratomas, will appear as low-intensity foci. A unique chemical-shift artifact that is the exact reverse of what can be seen around the urinary bladder may be seen in some cases of cystic teratomas (143).

An endometrioma may appear as a unilocular or multilocular cystic mass (20,52,59,110). On T1-weighted images, the signal intensity of an endometrioma may be similar to that of urine or fat, depending on the amount of hemorrhage within the lesion (52). A distinct low-intensity capsule has been seen in some cases (110).

Ovarian cystadenomas often appear as large pelvic masses (52,105). The signal characteristics of these masses

differ depending on the chemical composition of the cyst fluid and the amount of solid components contained within the tumor (Fig. 68). As with CT, malignant ovarian cystadenocarcinomas cannot be reliably distinguished from benign cystadenomas unless metastases are present.

Congenital Uterine Anomalies

Congenital uterine anomalies, such as bicornuate uterus and hydrometrocolpos, may also be diagnosed on CT images (Fig. 69), but ultrasonography usually suffices as the diagnostic technique.

Because the normal zonal anatomy of the uterus is clearly shown on T2-weighted images, MRI also has been used to evaluate patients suspected of having congenital uterine anomalies (Fig. 70). MRI can differentiate a bicornuate uterus and a septate uterus (102). MRI is also helpful in assessing the status of the uterus in patients with vaginal agenesis (142).

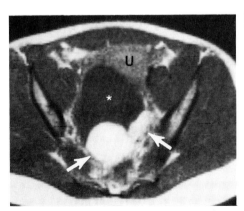

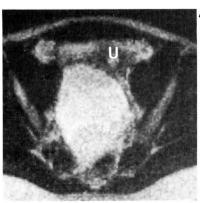

FIG. 67. Dermoid. **A:** Transaxial T1-weighted image (TR = 500 msec, TE = 30 msec). A large mass is noted in the right adnexa. The anterior portion of the mass (*) has a low signal intensity, whereas the posterior portion has a high signal intensity similar to that of fat (*arrows*). **B:** On T2-weighted image (TR = 1,500 msec, TE = 90 msec), the signal intensity of the anterior portion of the mass is higher than that of fat, whereas the posterior portion is again similar to subcutaneous fat; (U) uterus.

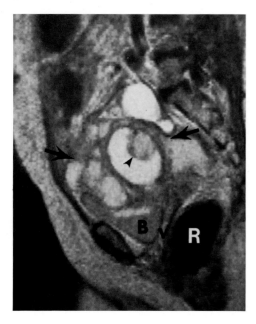

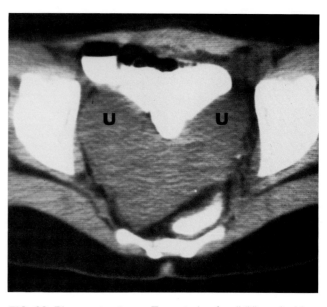

FIG. 68. Ovarian cystadenocarcinoma. Sagittal MR image (TR = 1,500 msec, TE = 90 msec) shows a complex mass (*arrows*) in the pelvis in this posthysterectomy patient. The high-intensity areas contain fluid, and the medium-intensity area (*arrowhead*) represents solid tumor nodule; (B) urinary bladder; (v) vagina; (R) rectum.

FIG. 69. Bicornuate uterus. Two uterine fundi (U) are incidentally identified on this CT image obtained for other reasons. The typical V shape of the bicornuate uterus is demonstrated.

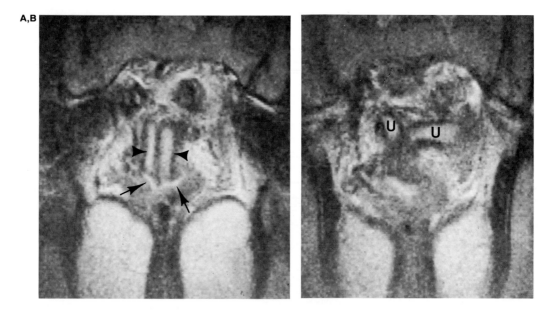

FIG. 70. Complete duplication of the uterus and vagina. **A:** Coronal MR image (TR = 2,100 msec, TE = 90 msec) shows two vaginal canals (*arrows*) and two cervices (*arrowheads*). **B:** One centimeter posterior to (**A**), two separate uterine bodies (U) are noted.

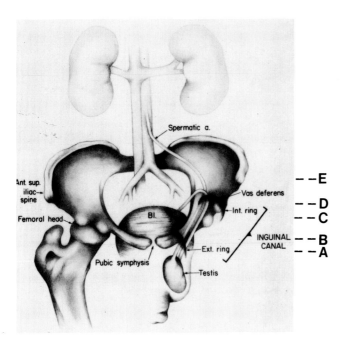

FIG. 71. Schematic drawing showing the relationships among the inguinal canal, the spermatic cord (containing spermatic vessels and vas deferens), and adjacent bony landmarks. The inguinal canal is a superficial structure that runs parallel to the iliac wing. The internal inguinal ring is located halfway between the pubic symphysis and anterior superior iliac spine, i.e., approximately 5 to 6 cm caudad to the anterior superior iliac spine. The external inguinal ring is just cephalad to the pubic ramus. Letters A–E correspond to planes of imaging in Fig. 72. (From ref. 86.)

LOCALIZATION OF UNDESCENDED TESTES

Gray-scale sonography is the procedure of choice in the evaluation of a patient suspected of having testicular abnormalities when the testis lies within the scrotal sac. However, CT can almost always accurately depict the presence and location of the testis when it is not palpable on physical examination.

The testis develops from the elongated embryonic gonad lying ventral to the mesonephric ridge. It migrates from its intraabdominal position to the scrotal sac during the latter third of gestation (5). Interruption of this normal migratory process results in ectopic positioning of the testis. Because malignant neoplasms occur 12 to 40 times more commonly in the undescended (intraabdominal) testis than in the descended testis, it is widely agreed that orchiopexy be performed in patients younger than 10 years of age and orchiectomy be performed in patients who are seen after puberty (116). Preoperative localization of a nonpalpable testis by radiologic methods often helps in planning the surgical approach and shortens the anesthesia time.

Detection of an undescended testis by CT is based on recognition of a mass, which is of soft-tissue density and oval in shape, along the expected course of testicular descent (83,86,161) (Figs. 71–73). When the undescended testis is unusually large, this may be due to either malignant transformation or epididymitis (Fig. 74). In general, it is easier to detect an undescended testis in the inguinal canal or in the lower pelvis, where structures usually are bilaterally symmetrical. Undescended testes as small as 1 cm have been accurately located in these areas. Detection of such an atrophic testis and differentiation from adjacent structures are more difficult in the upper pelvis and lower abdomen because bowel loops, vascular structures, and lymph nodes are more abundant. Despite these limitations, CT has proved accurate in localization of nonpalpable testes (83).

Other radiologic methods that have been used to localize undescended testes include testicular arteriography, venography, gray-scale ultrasound, and, recently, MRI (40,46,77,94). Testicular arteriography is not only technically difficult but also painful. Although testicular venography is less traumatic than arteriography, it is also associated with a high radiation dose and some morbidity, although the false-negative rate is relatively low. Selective catheterization of the right testicular vein is technically difficult; selective venography of either testicular vein can be unsuccessful because of the presence of venous valves. Although ultrasound is useful in localizing an undescended testis within the inguinal canal, usually it is not reliable in the pelvis or abdomen (94). MRI may have a problem similar to that of ultrasonography in detecting intraabdominal testis (40). On MRI, undescended testes, which often are atrophic, may have a lower signal intensity than their contralateral normal testes.

Because of its ease of performance and noninvasive nature, we believe CT is the procedure of choice for preoperative localization of a nonpalpable testis. In cases where CT cannot resolve the problem, testicular venography or arteriography can still be employed for further evaluation.

EVALUATION OF SCROTAL ABNORMALITIES

CT is not used for primary evaluation of scrotal abnormalities because testicular lesions are poorly defined on CT images. However, in some studies obtained for other indications, CT may reveal herniation of fat into the scrotum or a hydrocele.

In contradistinction, MRI is capable of differentiating intratesticular and extratesticular lesions (8,125,131) (Figs.

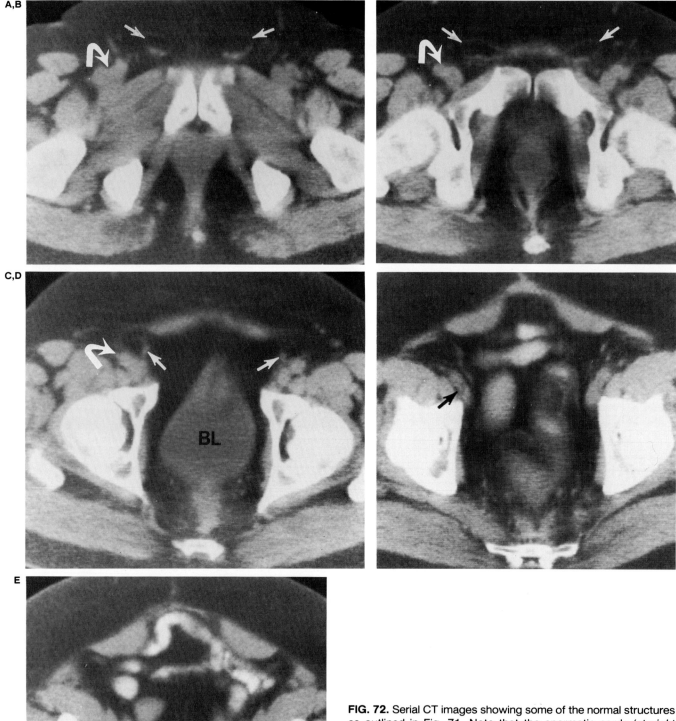

FIG. 72. Serial CT images showing some of the normal structures as outlined in Fig. 71. Note that the spermatic cords (*straight white arrows*) move laterally as they ascend along the inguinal canal; (BL) bladder; (*curved white arrows*) femoral vessels; (*black arrows*) iliac vessels.

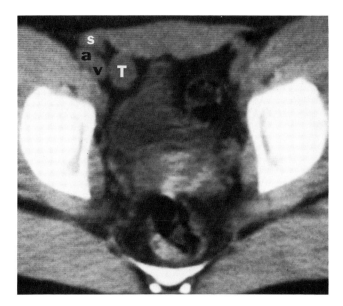

FIG. 73. Intraabdominal testis. The slightly atrophic right testis (T) lies medial to the right iliac artery (a) and vein (v). This is a common site for an intraabdominal testicle. The spermatic cord (s) is anterior to the vessels.

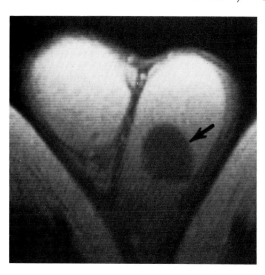

FIG. 75. Testicular cyst. Transaxial MR image (TR = 1,500 msec, TE = 35 msec) shows a well-defined, low-intensity mass (*arrow*) in the left testis. The increased signal intensity in the anterior portions of both testes is due to nonuniform response of a single-loop surface coil.

75 and 76). Except for an old hematoma, all intratesticular disease processes appear less intense than normal testicular tissue, especially on T2-weighted images. Based on the MR signal intensity, a cystic lesion can be differentiated from a solid neoplasm, and a simple fluid collection (e.g., spermatocele, hydrocele) can be distinguished from one complicated by infection or hemorrhage (Figs. 76–79).

At present, MRI provides information similar to that obtained with sonography in most cases. Therefore, ultrasonography remains the procedure of choice for evaluating scrotal abnormalities because of its ease of performance and lower cost. However, MRI is helpful in patients with painful scrotal lesions. Whereas sonographic examination requires good contact with the scrotal surface, MRI can be performed with a minimum of patient discomfort. The ability of MRI to clearly delineate the tunica albuginea is also helpful in the evaluation of scrotal trauma, because surgical intervention often is needed in cases in which the tunica is disrupted.

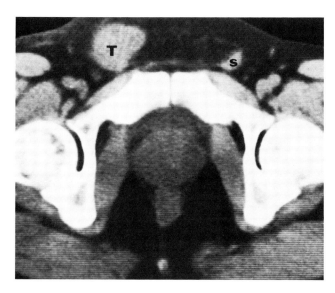

FIG. 74. Intracanalicular testis. The enlarged undescended right testis (T) is in the inguinal canal. The enlargement in this case was due to epididymitis rather than malignancy. The left spermatic cord (s) is normal.

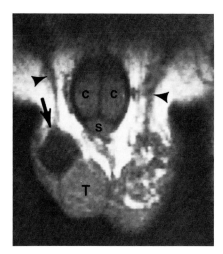

FIG. 76. Simple spermatocele. Coronal MR image (TR = 500 msec, TE = 35 msec) shows a round, low-intensity mass (*arrow*) superior and lateral to the right testis (T); (*arrowheads*) spermatic cords; (c) corpora cavernosum; (s) corpus spongiosum.

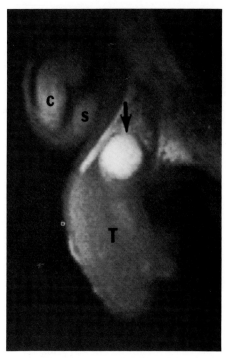

FIG. 77. Hemorrhagic epididymal cyst. Sagittal MR image (TR = 500 msec, TE = 35 msec) shows a high-intensity lesion (*arrow*) in the region of left epididymal head; (T) testis; (c) corpora cavernosum; (s) corpus spongiosum.

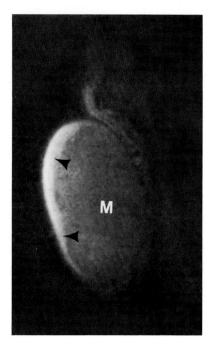

FIG. 79. Testicular seminoma. Sagittal T2-weighted MR image (TR = 2,100 msec, TE = 90 msec) shows a large hypointense mass (M) almost completely replacing the right testis. A crescentic layer of normal parenchyma is seen anteriorly (*arrowheads*).

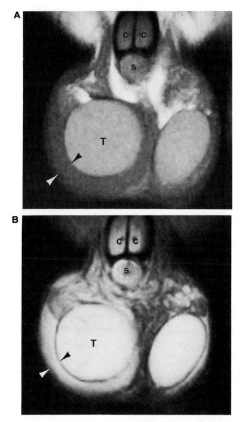

FIG. 78. Simple hydrocele. A: Coronal MR image (TR = 1,500 msec, TE = 35 msec) shows a crescentic collection with homogeneous signal intensity (*arrowheads*) in the right hemiscrotum; (T) testis; (c) corpora cavernosum; (s) corpus spongiosum. B: Coronal T2-weighted MR image (TR = 2,100 msec, TE = 90 msec) shows that the collection (arrowheads) has a signal intensity similar to that of the testis, thereby confirming its fluid nature.

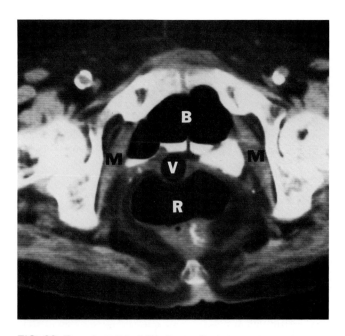

FIG. 80. Female pelvis following radical cystectomy. Air- and contrast-filled bowel loops (B) lie anterior to the vagina, which is marked by a tampon (V). The obturator internus muscles (M) are bilaterally symmetrical and normal. No recurrent disease is present; (R) rectum.

ASSESSMENT OF THE POSTOPERATIVE PELVIS

Post Cystectomy

The detection of possible surgical complications and local neoplastic recurrences has been difficult by conventional radiologic methods in patients with prior cystectomy for bladder cancers. Barium gastrointestinal studies are insensitive in detecting masses not closely related to the bowel; gallium radionuclide imaging is of little help in the immediate postoperative period. Because the ability to detect pelvic abnormalities by sonography is highly dependent on the presence of a distended urinary bladder, sonography also is of limited use in postcystectomy patients. Furthermore, the presence of surgical wounds, with or without drains, further constrains its usefulness.

CT is well suited for evaluation of such patients (85). Normal surrounding anatomy and pathologic alterations can be delineated in patients who have had prior cystectomy. In male patients after radical cystectomy, the bladder, the prostate, and the seminal vesicles are absent. In female patients, the uterus, both fallopian tubes, and the urinary bladder are absent. Small-bowel loops and, rarely, a loop of sigmoid colon fill in the space previously occupied by these structures (Fig. 80). Although the perivesical fat plane often is disrupted in postcystectomy patients, the muscle groups lining the pelvic side wall, namely, the obturator internus in the lower pelvis and the iliopsoas in the upper pelvis, remain symmetrical. Recognition of alterations in the symmetry of the remaining structures enables diagnosis of pathologic conditions at a much earlier stage than formerly possible (Fig. 17A). Local recurrences, surgical complications (e.g., urinomas, lymphoceles, abscesses), and distant metastases all can be recognized on postoperative CT examinations (Fig. 81). A recurrent tumor often appears as a mass of soft-tissue density, separate from bowel, with or without central necrosis. Although unopacified bowel loops and other normal pelvic structures may masquerade as recurrent disease, routine use of oral and intravenous contrast material has largely eliminated this potential problem. An abscess cavity can be confidently diagnosed if an extraalimentary tract mass containing gas is shown on CT images (6). However, in the absence of gas bubbles, an abscess cavity may be confused with a necrotic tumor based on the CT findings alone. Correlation with clinical history and physical examination, or biopsy of the lesion directly at surgery or via a percutaneous needle, often is required. A urinoma is seen as a low-density mass with an imperceptible wall located outside the genitourinary tract. Although the density of a urinoma is close to that of water in most cases, it varies with the specific gravity of the urine (134); enhancement may occur after intravenous administration of contrast material. A urinoma could be confused with a seroma, lymphocele, or even an

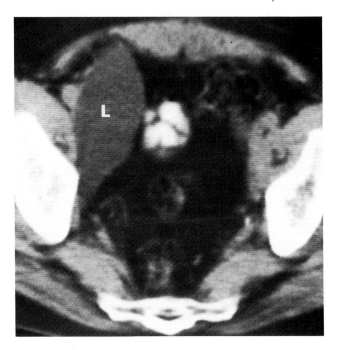

FIG. 81. Lymphocele following radical cystectomy. The ellipsoid, well-defined, water-density lymphocele (L) is in the extraperitoneal space along the right pelvic side wall. The diagnosis was established by chemical analysis of the aspirated fluid.

abscess on CT. Again, correlation with clinical information and sometimes chemical analysis of the aspirated fluid is needed for such a differentiation.

Post Abdominoperineal Resection

Abdominoperineal (AP) resection of the rectum and distal sigmoid colon is the standard surgical procedure in treating patients with middle-to-distal rectal carcinoma. The incidence of tumor recurrence following AP resection is high in patients initially presenting with advanced-stage disease. In one study (154), more than half of the patients with Duke's B and C rectal carcinoma (Table 6) developed recurrent disease within 5 years. Approximately 50% of the patients with recurrence manifested only distant metastases; the rest had local recurrence either alone or in conjunction with distant metastases.

Because conventional radiologic methods, including contrast gastrointestinal studies, are insensitive in detecting pelvic recurrence, the ability to detect local recurrence has relied largely on the presence of a palpable mass on physical examination or the development of severe pelvic

TABLE 6. *Dukes classification of colon cancer[a]*

A	Confined to the bowel wall
B	Tumor invasion through the muscularis into the serosa or into the mesenteric fat
C	Tumor distant from the bowel

[a] From Dukes (33).

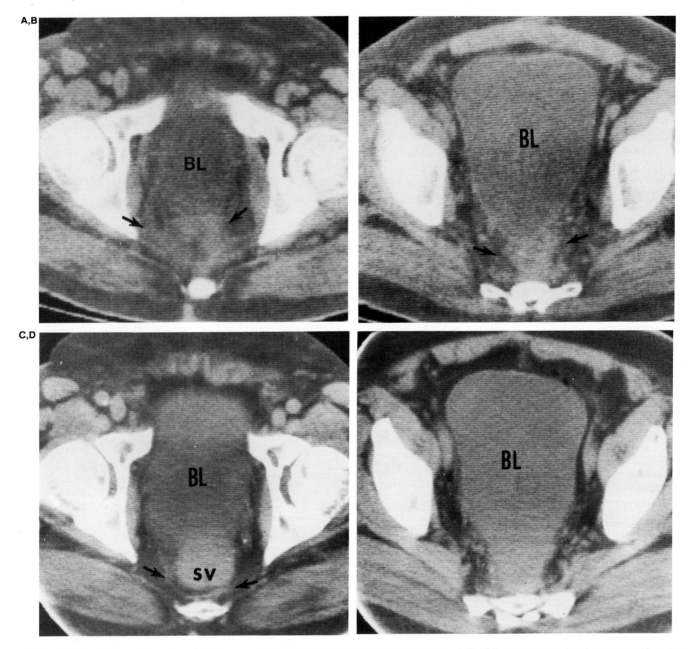

FIG. 82. Resolution of postsurgical changes following AP resection of the rectum. **A,B:** CT images obtained 1 month after AP resection show amorphous soft-tissue densities (*arrows*) obliterating normal fascial planes in the operative bed. **C,D:** Follow-up images obtained 8 months after surgery demonstrate much clearer delineation of the seminal vesicles (SV), with only minimal streaky densities (*arrows*) in the postsurgical space in front of the coccyx; (BL) urinary bladder. (From ref. 88.)

pain. Knowledge of the size of the recurrent tumor is essential in designing radiation ports so that a maximal dose can be given to the tumor, with sparing of adjacent normal structures.

Because of its ability to provide detailed cross-sectional images of the pelvic anatomy easily, CT has become the imaging method of choice in following these patients for possible recurrence. In the immediate postoperative period, amorphous soft-tissue densities, believed to represent edema or hemorrhage, can be seen in the surgical bed

(Fig. 82). The normal fascial planes and contour of the remaining pelvic organs often are obscured. Although the duration of the postoperative changes varies from patient to patient, such changes resolve within several months in most cases. In some instances, postoperative changes may persist and appear as mass-like lesions in the presacral area (66,75,123).

Several months after AP resection, the urinary bladder can be seen on CT images to occupy a presacral (precoccygeal) location. Although the prostate gland remains fixed

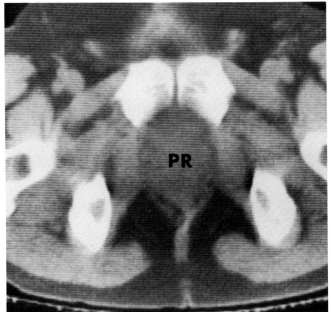

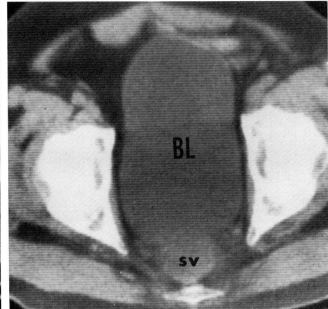

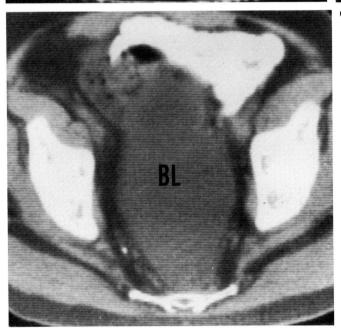

FIG. 83. A–C: Normal male pelvic anatomy following AP resection of the rectum. The prostate gland (PR) remains fixed in its anterior position; the seminal vesicles (sv) and the posterior wall of the bladder both fall posteriorly to occupy the empty rectal fossa. Other than these relocated pelvic structures, the operative bed contains no soft-tissue masses; (BL) urinary bladder.

in its preoperative position, the seminal vesicles in men (Fig. 83) and the uterus in women move with the bladder and can be seen in a presacral location (88) (Fig. 84). In addition, loops of small bowel also may be seen in the previous rectal fossa if the surgical procedure does not include restoration of the peritoneal floor or if the surgical sutures are disrupted.

On CT images, recurrent tumor appears as an irregular soft-tissue mass with or without central necrosis. When the recurrence is large or is associated with metastases to other organs such as lymph nodes, the bones, and the liver, the diagnosis can be confidently made. When the local recurrent tumor is small, difficulty in differentiation between recurrent tumor and postoperative fibrosis has been reported (66,75,123). However, our own studies

showed that pelvic CT images in patients without local recurrence usually contained no detectable abnormality or minimal streaky densities located anterior to the sacrococcygeal bone (88). Thus, postoperative changes usually are quite distinct and can be confidently distinguished from a local recurrent tumor, which often appears as a mass-like lesion (Fig. 85). Because our patients had uncomplicated postoperative courses, it is conceivable that surgical complications, including prolonged wound infection, may lead to extensive scar formation and therefore result in a mass-like lesion on CT images. Because postoperative changes theoretically could simulate recurrent neoplasm, a base-line CT study several months following the AP resection may be beneficial. Changes detected on subsequent CT evaluations will then be more readily

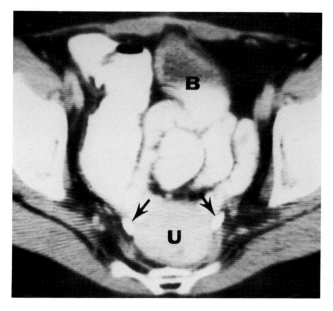

FIG. 84. Normal female pelvis following AP resection. The uterus (U) lies in a presacral position, and small bowel fills the area previously occupied by the uterus. The ureters (*arrows*) are displaced medially and posteriorly; (B) bladder.

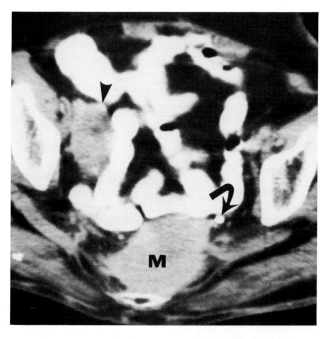

FIG. 85. Recurrent rectal cancer following abdominoperineal resection. A bulky presacral mass (M) displaces bowel anteriorly and is associated with left hydronephrosis (*arrow*). Note that the fat surrounding the mass is infiltrated; (*arrowhead*) external iliac lymphadenopathy.

identified as recurrent tumor or as evolving postoperative tissue alterations. Percutaneous biopsy of any visible mass lesion in the operative bed is valuable to confirm recurrent neoplasms (19). Alternatively, MRI can be used to differentiate between recurrent neoplasm and postoperative fibrosis. Whereas recurrent neoplasm usually has a medium-to-high signal intensity on T2-weighted images, fibrosis has a very low signal intensity similar to that skeletal muscle (45) (Fig. 86).

OBSTETRICAL APPLICATION

General

Ultrasonography is the procedure of choice in imaging the gravid uterus because it does not involve ionizing radiation, and it features high accuracy, lower cost, flexi-

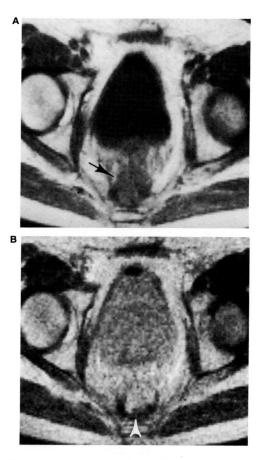

FIG. 86. Local recurrence after abdominoperineal resection for rectal carcinoma. **A:** Transaxial T1-weighted image (TR = 500 msec, TE = 35 msec) shows a medium-intensity mass (*arrow*) in the rectal fossa. **B:** Transaxial T2-weighted MR image (TR = 2,100 msec, TE = 90 msec) shows that the mass is isointense with fat, compatible with recurrent neoplasm. The low-intensity rim posterior to the mass (*arrowhead*) represents postsurgical scar.

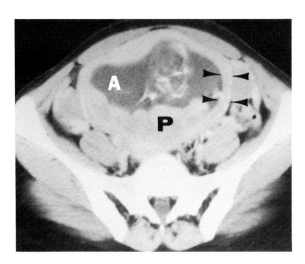

FIG. 87. Intrauterine pregnancy. The enlarged endometrial cavity contains the fetus, floating in amniotic fluid (A), and the posteriorly placed placenta (P). The myometrium is thin (*arrowheads*).

bility, and real-time capability. Ideally, the gravid uterus should never be examined using CT. However, when the gravid uterus is scanned inadvertently, intrauterine pregnancies can be demonstrated by CT (Fig. 87). On rare occasion, CT is used to confirm an equivocal sonographic finding of fetal anomaly.

Although there are yet no known hazards associated with MRI, women in their first trimester of pregnancy are not imaged for fear of inducing fetal anomalies. Furthermore, fetal anatomy is less well delineated at this stage of pregnancy because of rapid fetal motion (71,157). Fetal anatomy is better demonstrated during the last part of the first trimester and in patients with severe oligohydramnios due to restricted fetal motion. The heart and major vessels are seen as areas of signal void; the fluid-filled lungs are seen as high-intensity structures on T2-weighted images. The brain and some of the major abdominal organs also can be seen (99,157,158). Intracranial and extracranial fetal anomalies can likewise be demonstrated by MRI (98,158). Preliminary data suggest that assessment of fetal subcutaneous fat by MRI is a better indicator for detecting intrauterine growth retardation than is sonographic measurement of fetal growth parameters (135). MRI is most useful in delineating the relationship of the placenta and fetal presenting part to the internal cervical os (100,119,158) (Fig. 88) and in demonstrating maternal pelvic masses (156).

Although ultrasound will remain as the primary obstetric imaging method, MRI can provide important data about fetal anomalies and growth and development when sonographic evaluation is limited by oligohydramnios or maternal obesity. It can also be used to confirm fetal abnormalities when ultrasonography is equivocal and to demonstrate maternal pelvic structures when ultrasonography is unsuccessful because of underlying bowel gas or obesity.

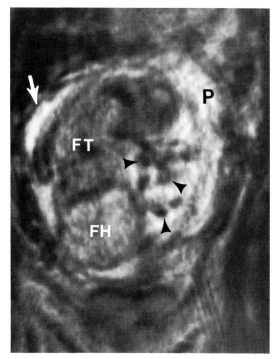

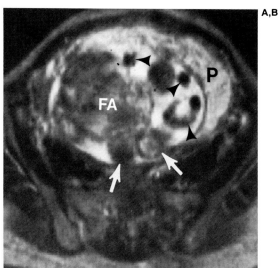

FIG. 88. Gravid uterus. A: Coronal MR image (TR = 2,100 msec, TE = 90 msec) shows a single fetus in vertex presentation; (P) placenta; (FH) fetal head; (FT) fetal trunk; (*arrow*) amniotic fluid; (*arrowheads*) umbilical vessels. B: Transaxial MR image (TR = 2,100 msec, TE = 90 msec) through the midportion of fetal abdomen (FA). Fetal extremities (*arrows*), umbilical vessels (*arrowheads*), and placenta (P) are seen.

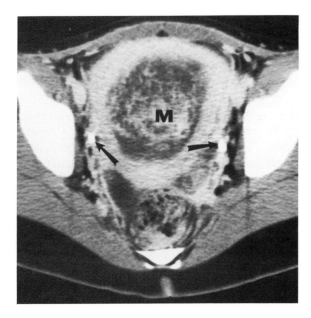

FIG. 89. Gestational trophoblastic disease. A large hydatidiform mole (M) occupies the uterine cavity. The mole is enhanced inhomogeneously with intravenous contrast material and contains numerous small cystic spaces. The ureters (*arrows*) are dilated because of extrinsic compression. Vascular engorgement accounts for soft-tissue strands in the parametrial fat.

Gestational Trophoblastic Disease

Gestational trophoblastic disease represents a spectrum of gynecologic abnormalities, from benign hydatidiform mole to choriocarcinoma (57). Ultrasonography is effective in the initial diagnosis of molar disease, but is not as useful in staging patients with invasive molar disease or choriocarcinoma (sometimes referred to as gestational trophoblastic neoplasia, GTN) (122). Both CT and MRI have been used to evaluate this group of patients (26,60,107,127).

Although uteri in patients with GTN often are diffusely enlarged, they may also be normal in size or focally enlarged. Although the size of the uterus does not correlate with the serum level of human chorionic gonadotropin (HCG), a patient with an enlarged uterus is more likely to have distant metastases and to require hysterectomy for successful treatment. On CT, the uterus often exhibits inhomogeneous contrast enhancement, with multiple areas of lower density (Fig. 89). Myometrial tumor nodules appear as hypodense areas on postcontrast CT images. The ovaries often are enlarged and contain numerous thecalutein cysts. Local invasion as well as distant metastases to the liver and lung can be seen on CT images. On MRI, the gestational trophoblastic neoplasms appear as masses of heterogeneous signal intensities obliterating normal uterine zonal anatomy. Numerous tortuous, dilated vessels appearing as areas of signal void often are seen within the tumor.

REFERENCES

1. Ackerman LV, del Regato JA. *Cancer, diagnosis, treatment and prognosis.* 4th ed. St Louis: Mosby, 1970.
2. Amendola MA, Glazer GM, Grossman HB, Aisen AM, Francis R. Staging of bladder carcinoma: MRI-CT-surgical correlation. *AJR* 1986;146:1179–1183.
3. Amendola MC, Walsh JW, Amendola BE, Tisnado J, Hall DJ, Goplerud DR. Computed tomography in the evaluation of carcinoma of the ovary. *J Comput Assist Tomogr* 1981;5:179–186.
4. Ammann AM, Walsh JW. Normal anatomy and technique of examination. In: Walsh JW, ed. *Computed tomography of the pelvis.* New York: Churchill Livingstone, 1985:1–28.
5. Arey LB. *Developmental anatomy.* 7th ed. Philadelphia: Saunders, 1965:315–341.
6. Aronberg DJ, Stanley RJ, Levitt RG, Sagel SS. Evaluation of abdominal abscess with computed tomography. *J Comput Assist Tomogr* 1978;2:384–387.
7. Babcock EE, Brateman L, Weinreb JL, Horner SD, Nunnally RL. Edge artifacts in MR images: chemical shift effect. *J Comput Assist Tomogr* 1985;9:252–257.
8. Baker LL, Hajek PC, Burkhard TK, et al. MR imaging of the scrotum: pathologic conditions. *Radiology* 1987;163:93–98.
9. Baker LL, Hajek PC, Burkhard TK, et al. MR imaging of the scrotum: normal anatomy. *Radiology* 1987;163:89–92.
10. Balfe DM, van Dyke J, Lee JKT, Weyman PJ, McClennan BL. Computed tomography in malignant endometrial neoplasms. *J Comput Assist Tomogr* 1983;7:677–681.
11. Biondetti PR, Lee JKT, Ling D, Catalona WJ. Clinical stage B prostate carcinoma: staging with MR imaging. *Radiology* 1987;162:325–329.
12. Bradley WG, Waluch V. Blood flow: magnetic resonance imaging. *Radiology* 1985;154:443–450.
13. Brenner DE, Shaff MI, Jones HW, Grosh WW, Greco FA, Burnett LS. Abdominopelvic computed tomography: evaluation in patients undergoing second-look laparotomy for ovarian carcinoma. *Obstet Gynecol* 1985;65:715–719.
14. Bries JR, Ellis JH, Kopecky KK, et al. Assessment of primary gynecologic malignancies: comparison of 0.15T resistive MRI with CT. *AJR* 1984;143:1249–1257.
15. Bryan PJ, Butler HE, LiPuma JP, et al. NMR scanning of the pelvis: initial experience with a 0.3T system. *AJR* 1983;141:1111–1118.
16. Bryan PJ, Butler HE, LiPuma JP, Resnick MI, Kursh ED. CT and MR imaging in staging bladder neoplasms. *J Comput Assist Tomogr* 1987;11:96–101.
17. Bryan PJ, Butler HE, Nelson AD, et al. Magnetic resonance imaging of the prostate. *AJR* 1986;146:543–548.
18. Buonocore E, Hesemann C, Pavlicek W, Montie JE. Clinical and in vitro magnetic resonance imaging of prostatic carcinoma. *AJR* 1984;143:1267–1272.
19. Butch RJ, Wittenberg J, Mueller PR, Meyer JE, Ferrucci JT Jr. Presacral masses after abdominoperineal resection for colorectal carcinoma: the need for needle biopsy. *AJR* 1985;144:309–312.
20. Butler H, Bryan PJ, LiPuma JP, et al. Magnetic resonance imaging of the abnormal female pelvis. *AJR* 1984;143:1259–1266.
21. Catalona WJ, Scott WW. Carcinoma of the prostate: a review. *J Urol* 1978;119:1–8.
22. Chang SF. Pear-shaped bladder caused by large iliopsoas muscles. *Radiology* 1978;128:349–350.
23. Church PA, Kazam E. Computed tomography and ultrasound in diagnosis of pelvic lipomatosis. *Urology* 1979;14:631–633.
24. Clarke-Pearson DL, Bandy LC, Dudzinski M, Heaston D, Creasman WT. Computed tomography in evaluation of patients with ovarian carcinoma in complete clinical remission. Correlation with surgical-pathologic findings. *JAMA* 1986;255:627–630.
25. Cohen WN, Seidelmann FE, Bryan PJ. Use of a tampon to enhance vaginal localization in computed tomography. *AJR* 1977;128:1064–1065.
26. Davis WK, McCarthy S, Moss AA, Braga C. Computed tomography of gestational trophoblastic disease. *J Comput Assist Tomogr* 1984;8:1136–1139.
27. Demas BE, Hricak H, Jaffe RB. Uterine MR imaging: effects of hormonal stimulation. *Radiology* 1986;159:123–126.

28. Dobbs HJ, Husband JE. The role of CT in the staging and radiotherapy planning of prostatic tumours. *Br J Radiol* 1985;58:429–436.

29. Dooms GC, Hricak H, Moseley ME, Bottles K, Fisher M, Higgins CB. Characterization of lymphadenopathy by magnetic resonance imaging and tissue characterization. *Radiology* 1985;155:691–697.

30. Dooms GC, Hricak H, Tscholakoff D. Adnexal structures: MR imaging. *Radiology* 1986;158:639–646.

31. Dore R, Moro G, D'Andrea F, Fianza AL, Franchi M, Bolis PF. CT evaluation of myometrium invasion in endometrial carcinoma. *J Comput Assist Tomogr* 1987;11:282–289.

32. Droller MJ. Transitional cell cancer: upper tracts and bladder. In: Walsh PC, Gittes RF, Perlmutter AD, Stamey TA, eds. *Campbell's urology.* Philadelphia: Saunders, 1986:1343–1440.

33. Dukes CE. The classification of cancer of the rectum. *J Pathol Bacteriol* 1932;35:323–332.

34. Emory TH, Reinke DB, Hill AL, Lange PH. Use of CT to reduce understaging in prostatic cancer: comparison with conventional staging techniques. *AJR* 1983;141:351–354.

35. Federle MP, Filly RA, Moss AA. Cystic hepatic neoplasms: complementary roles of CT and sonography. *AJR* 1981;136:345–348.

36. Fisher MR, Hricak H, Crooks LE. Urinary bladder MR imaging: Part I. Normal and benign conditions. *Radiology* 1985;157:467–470.

37. Fisher MR, Hricak H, Tanagho EA. Urinary bladder MR imaging: Part II. Neoplasm. *Radiology* 1985;157:471–477.

38. Fishman EK, Scatarige JC, Saksouk FA, Rosenshein NB, Siegelman SS. Computed tomography of endometriosis. *J Comput Assist Tomogr* 1983;7:257–264.

39. Flanigan RC, Mohler JL, King CT, et al. Preoperative lymph node evaluation in prostatic cancer patients who are surgical candidates: the role of lymphangiography and computerized tomographic scanning with directed fine needle aspiration. *J Urol* 1985;134:84–87.

40. Fritzsche PJ, Hricak H, Kogan BA, Winkler ML, Tanagho EA. Undescended testis: value of MR imaging. *Radiology* 1987;164:169–173.

41. Frodin L, Hemmingsson A, Johansson A, Wicklund H. Computed tomography in staging of bladder carcinoma. *Acta Radiol* 1980;21:763–767.

42. Ginaldi S, Wallace S, Jing BS, Bernardino ME. Carcinoma of the cervix: lymphangiography and computed tomography. *AJR* 1981;136:1087–1091.

43. Giri PGS, Walsh JW, Hazra TA, Texter JH, Koontz WW. Role of computed tomography in the evaluation and management of carcinoma of the prostate. *Int J Radiat Oncol Biol Phys* 1982;8:283–287.

44. Gittes RF. Tumors of the bladder. In: Harrison JH, Gittes RF, Perlmutter AD, Stamey TA, Walsh PC, eds. *Urology.* Philadelphia: Saunders, 1970:1033–1070.

45. Glazer HS, Lee JKT, Levitt RG, et al. Radiation fibrosis: differentiation from recurrent tumor by MR imaging. *Radiology* 1985;156:721–726.

46. Glickman MG, Weiss RM, Itzchalk Y. Testicular venography for undescended testes. *AJR* 1977;129:71–75.

47. Goldman SM, Fishman EK, Rosenshein NB, Gatewood OMB, Siegelman SS. Excretory urography and computed tomography in the initial evaluation of patients with cervical cancer: are both examinations necessary? *AJR* 1984;143:991–996.

48. Golimbu M, Morales P, Al-Askari S, Shulman Y. CAT scanning in staging of prostatic cancer. *Urology* 1981;18:305–308.

49. Griffiths CT, Parker LM, Fuller AF Jr. Role of cytoreductive surgical treatment in the management of advanced ovarian carcinoma. *Cancer Treat Rep* 1979;63:235–240.

50. Grumbine FC, Rosenshein NB, Zerhouni EA, Siegelman SS. Abdominopelvic computed tomography in the preoperative evaluation of early cervical cancer. *Gynecol Oncol* 1981;12:286–290.

51. Hamlin DJ, Burgener FA, Beechman JB. CT of intramural endometrial carcinoma: contrast enhancement is essential. *AJR* 1981;137:551–554.

52. Hamlin DJ, Fitzsimmons JR, Pettersson H, Riggall RC, Morgan L, Wilkinson EJ. Magnetic resonance imaging of the pelvis: evaluation of ovarian masses at 0.15T. *AJR* 1985;145:585–590.

53. Hamlin DJ, Pettersson H, Fitzsimmons J, Morgan LS. MR imaging of uterine leiomyomas and their complications. *J Comput Assist Tomogr* 1985;9:902–907.

54. Harris RD, Bendon JA, Robinson CA, Seat SG, Herwig KR. Computed tomographic evaluation of pear-shaped bladder. *Urology* 1979;14:528–530.

55. Hasumi K, Matsuzawa M, Chen HF, Takahashi M, Sakura M. Computed tomography in the evaluation and treatment of endometrial carcinoma. *Cancer* 1982;50:904–908.

56. Haynor DR, Mack LA, Soules MR, Shuman WP, Montana MA, Moss AA. Changing appearance of the normal uterus during the menstrual cycle: MR studies. *Radiology* 1986;161:459–462.

57. Hilgers RD, Lewis JL. Gestational trophoblastic disease. In: Danforth DN, ed. *Obstetrics and gynecology.* New York: Harper & Row, 1982:393–406.

58. Hodson NJ, Husband JE, Macdonald JS. The role of computed tomography in the staging of bladder cancer. *Clin Radiol* 1979;30:389–395.

59. Hricak H, Alpers C, Crooks LE, Sheldon PE. Magnetic resonance imaging of the female pelvis: initial experience. *AJR* 1983;141:1119–1128.

60. Hricak H, Demas BE, Braga CA, Fisher MR, Winkler ML. Gestational trophoblastic neoplasm of the uterus: MR assessment. *Radiology* 1986;161:11–16.

61. Hricak H, Dooms GC, Jeffrey RB, et al. Prostatic carcinoma: staging by clinical assessment, CT, and MR imaging. *Radiology* 1987;162:331–336.

62. Hricak H, Dooms GC, McNeal JE, et al. MR imaging of the prostate gland: normal anatomy. *AJR* 1987;148:51–58.

63. Hricak H, Stern JL, Fisher MR, Shapeero LG, Winkler ML, Lacey CG. Endometrial carcinoma staging by MR imaging. *Radiology* 1987;162:297–305.

64. Hricak H, Tscholakoff D, Heinrichs L, et al. Uterine leiomyomas: correlation of MR, histopathologic findings and symptoms. *Radiology* 1986;158:385–391.

65. Hricak H, Williams RD, Spring DB, et al. Anatomy and pathology of the male pelvis by magnetic resonance imaging. *AJR* 1983;141:1101–1111.

66. Husband JE, Hodson NJ, Parsons CA. The use of computed tomography in recurrent rectal tumors. *Radiology* 1980;134:677–682.

67. International Federation of Gynecology and Obstetrics. Classification and staging of malignant tumors in the female pelvis. *J Int Fed Gynecol Obstet* 1965;3:204.

68. Jeffrey RB Jr. CT demonstration of peritoneal implants. *AJR* 1980;135:323–326.

69. Jeffrey RB, Palubinskas AJ, Federle MP. CT evaluation of invasive lesions of the bladder. *J Comput Assist Tomogr* 1981;5:22–26.

70. Jewett JH. The present status of radical prostatectomy for stages A and B prostatic cancer. *Urol Clin North Am* 1975;2:105–124.

71. Johnson IR, Symonds EM, Worthington BS, Pipkin FB, Hawkes RC, Gyngell M. Imaging of pregnant human uterus with nuclear magnetic resonance. *Am J Obstet Gynecol* 1984;148:1136–1139.

72. Johnson RJ, Blackledge G, Eddleston B, Crowther D. Abdominopelvic computed tomography in the management of ovarian carcinoma. *Radiology* 1983;146:447–452.

73. Kademian MT, Bosch A. Staging laparotomy and survival in carcinoma of the uterine cervix. *Acta Radiol* 1977;16:314–324.

74. Kafkas M. Study and diagnosis of bladder tumors by triple contrast cystography. *J Urol* 1973;109:32–34.

75. Kelvin FM, Korobkin M, Heaston DK, Grant JP, Akwari O. The pelvis after surgery for rectal carcinoma: serial CT observations with emphasis on nonneoplastic features. *AJR* 1983;141:959–964.

76. Kenny GM, Hardner GJ, Moore RM, Murphy GP. Current results from treatment of stages C and D bladder tumors at Roswell Park Memorial Institute. *J Urol* 1972;107:56–59.

77. Khademi M, Seebode JJ, Falla A. Selective spermatic arteriography for localization of impalpable undescended testis. *Radiology* 1980;136:627–634.

78. Kilcheski TS, Arger PH, Mulhern CB Jr, Coleman BG, Kressel HY, Mikuta JI. Role of computed tomography in the presurgical evaluation of carcinoma of the cervix. *J Comput Assist Tomogr* 1981;5:378–383.

79. Kottmeier HL. *Annual report on the results of treatment in carcinoma of the uterus, vagina, and ovary. Vol 16.* Stockholm: International Federation of Gynecology and Obstetrics. 1976.

80. Lang EK. The use of arteriography in the demonstration and staging of bladder tumors. *Radiology* 1963;80:62–68.
81. Larkin BT, Berquist TH, Utz DC. Evaluation of the prostate by magnetic resonance imaging. *Magn Reson Imaging* 1986;4:53–58.
82. Lee JKT, Gersell DJ, Balfe DM, Worthington JL, Picus D, Gapp G. The uterus: in vitro MR-anatomic correlation of normal and abnormal specimens. *Radiology* 1985;157:175–179.
83. Lee JKT, Glazer HG. CT in the localization of the nonpalpable testis. *Urol Clin North Am* 1982;9:397–404.
84. Lee JKT, Heiken JP, Ling D, et al. Magnetic resonance imaging of abdominal and pelvic lymphadenopathy. *Radiology* 1984;153:181–188.
85. Lee JKT, McClennan BL, Stanley RJ, Levitt RG, Sagel SS. Use of CT in evaluation of postcystectomy patients. *AJR* 1981;136:483–487.
86. Lee JKT, McClennan BL, Stanley RJ, Sagel SS. Utility of computed tomography in the localization of the undescended testis. *Radiology* 1980;135:121–125.
87. Lee JKT, Rholl KS. MRI of the bladder and prostate. *AJR* 1986;147:732–736.
88. Lee JKT, Stanley RJ, Sagel SS, Levitt RG, McClennan BL. CT appearance of the pelvis after abdominoperineal resection for rectal carcinoma. *Radiology* 1981;141:737–741.
89. Lee JKT, Stanley RJ, Sagel SS, McClennan BL. Accuracy of CT in detecting intraabdominal and pelvic lymph node metastases from pelvic cancers. *AJR* 1978;131:675–679.
90. Levine MS, Arger PH, Coleman BG, Mulhern CB, Pollack HM, Wein AJ. Detecting lymphatic metastases from prostatic carcinoma: superiority of CT. *AJR* 1981;137:207–211.
91. Levitt RG, Sagel SS, Stanley RJ. Detection of neoplastic involvement of the mesentery and omentum by computed tomography. *AJR* 1978;131:835–838.
92. Levitt RG, Sagel SS, Stanley RJ, Evens RG. Computed tomography of the pelvis. *Semin Roentgenol* 1978;13:193–200.
93. Ling D, Lee JKT, Heiken JP, Balfe DM, Glazer HS, McClennan BL. Prostatic carcinoma and benign prostatic hyperplasia: inability of MR imaging to distinguish between the two diseases. *Radiology* 1986;158:103–107.
94. Madrazo BL, Klugo RC, Parks JA, DiLoreto R. Ultrasonographic demonstration of undescended testis. *Radiology* 1979;133:181–183.
95. Marincek B, Devaud MC, Triller J, Fuchs WA. Value of computed tomography and lymphography in staging carcinoma of the uterine cervix. *Eur J Radiol* 1984;4:118–121.
96. Mark AS, Hricak H, Heinrichs LW, et al. Adenomyosis and leiomyoma: differential diagnosis with MR imaging. *Radiology* 1987;163:520–529.
97. Marshall VF. The relation of the preoperative estimate to the pathologic demonstration of the extent of vesical neoplasm. *J Urol* 1952;68:714–723.
98. McCarthy SM, Filly RA, Stark DD, Callen PW, Golbus MS, Hricak H. Magnetic resonance imaging of fetal anomalies in utero: early experience. *AJR* 1985;145:677–682.
99. McCarthy SM, Filly RA, Stark DD, et al. Obstetrical magnetic resonance imaging: fetal anatomy. *Radiology* 1985;154:427–432.
100. McCarthy S, Stark DD, Filly RA, Callen PW, Hricak H, Higgins CB. Obstetrical magnetic resonance imaging: maternal anatomy. *Radiology* 1985;154:421–425.
101. McCarthy S, Tauber C, Gore J. Female pelvic anatomy: MR assessment of variations during the menstrual cycle and with use of oral contraceptives. *Radiology* 1986;160:119–123.
102. Mintz MC, Thickman DI, Gussman D, Kressel HY. MR evaluation of uterine anomalies. *AJR* 1987;148:287–290.
103. Mitchell DG, Gefter WB, Spritzer CE, et al. Polycystic ovaries: MR imaging. *Radiology* 1986;160:425–429.
104. Mitchell DG, Hill MC, Hill S, Zaloudek C. Serous carcinoma of the ovary: CT identification of metastatic calcified implants. *Radiology* 1986;158:649–652.
105. Mitchell DG, Minta MC, Spritzer CE, et al. Adnexal masses: MR imaging observations at 1.5T, with US and CT correlation. *Radiology* 1987;162:319–324.
106. Mittelstaedt CA, Gosink BB, Leopold GR. Gray scale patterns of pelvic disease in the male. *Radiology* 1977;123:727–732.
107. Miyasaka Y, Hachiya J, Furuya Y, Seki T, Watanabe H. CT evaluation of invasive trophoblastic disease. *J Comput Assist Tomogr* 1985;9:459–462.
108. Morgan CL, Calkins RF, Cavalcanti EJ. Computed tomography in the evaluation, staging and therapy of carcinoma of the bladder and prostate. *Radiology* 1981;140:751–761.
109. Mukamel E, Hannah J, Barbaric Z, DeKernion JB. The value of computerized tomography scan and magnetic resonance imaging in staging prostatic carcinoma: comparison with the clinical and histological staging. *J Urol* 1986;136:1231–1233.
110. Nishimura K, Togashi K, Itoh K, et al. Endometrial cysts of the ovary: MR imaging. *Radiology* 1987;162:315–318.
111. Paulson DF, Perez CA, Anderson T. Genitourinary malignancies. In: DeVita VT, Hellman S, Rosenberg SA, eds. *Cancer principles and practice of oncology.* Philadelphia: Lippincott, 1982:758–768.
112. Phillips ME, Kressel HY, Spritzer CE, et al. Normal prostate and adjacent structures: MR imaging at 1.5T. *Radiology* 1987;164:381–385.
113. Phillips ME, Kressel HY, Spritzer CE, et al. Prostatic disorders: MR imaging at 1.5T. *Radiology* 1987;164:386–392.
114. Picus D, Lee JKT. Magnetic resonance imaging of the female pelvis. *Urol Radiol* 1986;8:166–174.
115. Pilepich MV, Perez CA, Prasad S. Computed tomography in definitive radiotherapy of prostatic carcinoma. *Int J Radiat Oncol Biol Phys* 1980;6:923–926.
116. Pinch L, Aceta T, Meyer-Hahlburg HFL. Cryptorchidism. A pediatric review. *Urol Clin North Am* 1974;1:573–592.
117. Poon PY, McCallum RW, Henkelman MM, et al. Magnetic resonance imaging of the prostate. *Radiology* 1985;154:143–149.
118. Pontes E, Eisenkraft S, Watanabe H, Ohe H, Saitoh M, Murphy GP. Preoperative evaluation of localized prostatic carcinoma by transrectal ultrasonography. *J Urol* 1985;134:289–291.
119. Powell MC, Buckley J, Price H, Worthington BS, Symonds EM. Magnetic resonance imaging and placenta previa. *Am J Obstet Gynecol* 1986;154:565–569.
120. Powell MC, Womack C, Buckley J, Worthington BS, Symonds EM. Pre-operative magnetic resonance imaging of stage I endometrial adenocarcinoma. *Br J Obstet Gynaecol* 1986;93:353–360.
121. Price JM, Davidson AJ. Computed tomography in the evaluation of the suspected carcinomatous prostate. *Urol Radiol* 1979;1:38–42.
122. Requard C, Mettler F. The use of ultrasound in the evaluation of trophoblastic disease and its response to therapy. *Radiology* 1980;135:419–422.
123. Reznek RH, White FE, Young JWR, Fry IK. The appearances on computed tomography after abdominoperineal resection for carcinoma of the rectum: a comparison between the normal appearances and those of recurrence. *Br J Radiol* 1983;56:237–240.
124. Rholl KS, Lee JKT, Heiken JP, Ling D, Glazer HS. Primary bladder carcinoma: evaluation with MR imaging. *Radiology* 1987;163:117–121.
125. Rholl KS, Lee JKT, Ling D, Heiken JP, Glazer HS. MR imaging of the scrotum with a high-resolution surface coil. *Radiology* 1987;163:99–103.
126. Sager EM, Talle K, Fossa S, Ous S, Stenwig AE. The role of CT in demonstrating perivesical tumor growth in the preoperative staging of carcinoma of the urinary bladder. *Radiology* 1983;146:443–446.
127. Sanders C, Rubin E. Malignant gestational trophoblastic disease: CT findings. *AJR* 1987;148:165–168.
128. Scott WW Jr, Rosenshein NB, Siegelman SS, Sanders RC. The obstructed uterus. *Radiology* 1981;141:767–770.
129. Seidelmann FE, Cohen WN, Bryan PJ. Computed tomographic staging of bladder neoplasms. *Radiol Clin North Am* 1977;15:419–440.
130. Seidenmann FE, Cohen WN, Bryan PJ, Temes SP, Kraus D, Schoenrock G. Accuracy of CT staging of bladder neoplasms using the gas-filled method: report of 21 patients with surgical confirmation. *AJR* 1978;130:735–739.
131. Seidenwurm D, Smathers RL, Lo RK, Carrol CL, Basset J, Hoffman AR. Testes and scrotum: MR imaging at 1.5T. *Radiology* 1987;164:393–398.
132. Sommer FG, McNeal JE, Carrol CL. MR depiction of zonal anatomy of the prostate at 1.5T. *J Comput Assist Tomogr* 1986;10:983–989.
133. Spirnak JP, Resnick MI. Carcinoma of the prostate. *Semin Urol* 1983;1:269–279.
134. Stanley RJ. Fluid characterization with computed tomography. In:

Moss AA, Goldberg HI, eds. *Computed tomography, ultrasound and X-ray: an integrated approach.* San Francisco: University of California, Department of Radiology, 1980:65–66.

135. Stark DD, McCarthy SM, Filly RA, Callen PW, Hricak H, Parer JT. Intrauterine growth retardation: evaluation by magnetic resonance. *Radiology* 1985;155:425–427.

136. Steyn JH, Smith FW. Nuclear magnetic resonance imaging of the prostate. *Br J Urol* 1982;54:726–728.

137. Sukov RJ, Scardino PT, Sample WF, Winter J, Confer DJ. Computed tomography and transabdominal ultrasound in the evaluation of the prostate. *J Comput Assist Tomogr* 1977;1:281–289.

138. Susmano DE, Dolin EH. Computed tomography in diagnosis of pelvic lipomatosis. *Urology* 1979;13:215–220.

139. Tada S, Tsukioka M, Ishii C, Tanaka H, Mizunuma K. Computed tomographic features of uterine myoma. *J Comput Assist Tomogr* 1981;5:866–869.

140. Tisnado J, Amendola MA, Walsh JW, Jordan RL, Turner MA, Krempa J. Computed tomography of the perineum. *AJR* 1981;136:475–481.

141. Togashi K, Nishimura K, Itoh K, et al. Uterine cervical cancer: assessment with high field MR imaging. *Radiology* 1986;160:431–435.

142. Togashi K, Nishimura K, Itoh K, et al. Vaginal agenesis: classification by MR imaging. *Radiology* 1987;162:675–677.

143. Togashi K, Nishimura K, Itoh K, et al. Ovarian cystic teratomas: MR imaging. *Radiology* 1987;162:669–673.

144. Van Engelshoven JMA, Kreel L. Computed tomography of the prostate. *J Comput Assist Tomogr* 1979;3:45–51.

145. Van Waes PFGM, Zonneveld FW. Direct coronal body computed tomography. *J Comput Assist Tomogr* 1982;6:58–66.

146. Vick CW, Walsh JW, Wheelock JB, Brewer WH. CT of the normal and abnormal parametria in cervical cancer. *AJR* 1984;143:597.

147. Villasanta U, Whitley NO, Haney PJ, Brenner D. Computed tomography in invasive carcinoma of the cervix: an appraisal. *Obstet Gynecol* 1983;62:218–224.

148. Wajsman Z, Baumgartner G, Murphy GP, Merrin C. Evaluation of lymphangiography for clinical staging of bladder tumors. *J Urol* 1975;114:714–724.

149. Walsh JW, Amendola MA, Hall DJ, Tisnado J, Goplerud DR. Recurrent carcinoma of the cervix: CT diagnosis. *AJR* 1981;136:117–122.

150. Walsh JW, Amendola MA, Konerding KF, Tisnado J, Hazra TA. Computed tomographic detection of pelvic and inguinal lymph node metastases from primary and recurrent pelvic malignant disease. *Radiology* 1980;137:157–166.

151. Walsh JW, Goplerud DR. Prospective comparison between clinical and CT staging in primary cervical carcinoma. *AJR* 1981;137:997–1003.

152. Walsh JW, Goplerud DR. Computed tomography of primary, persistent, and recurrent endometrial malignancy. *AJR* 1982;139:1149–1154.

153. Walsh JW, Rosenfield AT, Jaffe CC, et al. Prospective comparison of ultrasound and computed tomography in the evaluation of gynecologic pelvic masses. *AJR* 1978;131:955–960.

154. Walz BJ, Lindstrom FR, Butcher HR, Baglan RJ. Natural history of patients after abdominal-perineal resection: implications for radiation therapy. *Cancer* 1977;39:2437–2442.

155. Weinerman PM, Arger PH, Coleman BG, Pollack HM, Banner MP, Wein AJ. Pelvic adenopathy from bladder and prostate carcinoma: detection by rapid-sequence computed tomography. *AJR* 1983;140:95–99.

156. Weinreb JC, Brown CE, Lowe TW, Cohen JM, Erdman WA. Pelvic masses in pregnant patients: MR and US imaging. *Radiology* 1986;159:717–724.

157. Weinreb JC, Lowe T, Cohen JM, Kutler M. Human fetal anatomy: MR imaging. *Radiology* 1985;157:715–720.

158. Weinreb JC, Lowe TW, Santos-Ramos R, Cunningham FG, Parkey R. Magnetic resonance imaging in obstetric diagnosis. *Radiology* 1985;154:157–161.

159. Werboff LH, Korobkin M, Klein RS. Pelvic lipomatosis: diagnosis using computed tomography. *Urology* 1979;122:257–259.

160. Whitley NO, Brenner DE, Francis A, et al. Computed tomographic evaluation of carcinoma of the cervix. *Radiology* 1982;142:439–446.

161. Wolverson MK, Jagannadharao B, Sundaram M, Riaz A, Nalesnik WJ, Houttiun E. CT in localization of impalpable cryptorchid testes. *AJR* 1980;134:725–729.

162. Worthington JL, Balfe DM, Lee JKT, et al. Uterine neoplasms: MR imaging. *Radiology* 1986;159:725–730.

CHAPTER 21

Musculoskeletal System

William A. Murphy, William G. Totty, Judy M. Destouet, David C. Hardy, Barbara S. Monsees, William R. Reinus, and Louis A. Gilula

Computed tomography (CT) and magnetic resonance imaging (MRI) are major methods for evaluation of musculoskeletal anatomy and disease. Each has its own particular capabilities and effective applications, but the two are also complementary. The general aims of musculoskeletal imaging are to gain maximum information via the fewest studies, to achieve the highest possible diagnostic accuracy, and to do both at the lowest cost and lowest radiation dose to the patient. More than ever before, this requires sophisticated knowledge of the various imaging methods and their applications to a broad spectrum of anatomic regions and pathologic conditions. CT and MRI regularly make important contributions in this arena.

Each musculoskeletal imaging procedure contributes information in a unique manner and with a certain sensitivity and specificity dependent on the particular anatomic and clinical context. The job of the diagnostic radiologist is to apply each method wisely for the purposes of learning whether or not an abnormality exists, localizing a site of origin, estimating the seriousness or aggressiveness of the condition, defining local and distant relationships or extent, refining the data to yield a diagnosis, and, finally, providing a careful opinion to aid in treatment planning and determination of prognosis.

Initially, most musculoskeletal lesions are evaluated by conventional radiographs, which contribute a great deal of information concerning the presence of a skeletal lesion and assessment of its severity and cause. Conventional radiographs have intermediate sensitivity, but high specificity. Variations of conventional radiography (magnification, xeroradiography, conventional tomography) are sometimes employed to confirm a lesion, but they are only slightly more sensitive than radiography alone. If a skeletal lesion is suspected, but conventional studies are nonconfirmatory, or if lesion multiplicity is to be determined, radionuclide bone scintigraphy often is the second

study. It contributes greatly to confirming the presence of a skeletal lesion and establishing its local extent, distant spread, or multiplicity, and it does so with the highest sensitivity of any skeletal imaging examination, but at a low specificity. If a soft-tissue problem is to be studied, particularly in thin, lean extremities, ultrasonography may be a useful musculoskeletal imaging test.

CT has many advantages as a musculoskeletal imaging technique. Among these are its display of cross-sectional anatomy and spatial relationships, simultaneous display of bone and soft-tissue components, imaging of both sides of the body for comparison purposes, increased contrast sensitivity, and provision for image manipulation and reformation. These gains, which are beyond what is usually possible by conventional radiography, bone scanning, and ultrasonography, are accomplished at levels of sensitivity and specificity that are generally greater than those for any of the other imaging procedures. CT usually can confirm the presence of skeletal, articular, or soft-tissue disease and, once confirmed, can show its local extent and relationships to various structures.

At our institute, CT is used both as a primary imaging method and as a problem-solving examination following other imaging studies. CT is best when used to provide detailed information concerning bone or other mineralized tissue. It is well accepted as a primary method for imaging bone and soft-tissue tumors. It is complementary to plain radiography for evaluating multiple fractures in complex anatomic regions such as the pelvis. CT is also a commonly employed primary or secondary method for studying some joints, particularly when air and/or iodinated contrast agents have been previously injected into the joint.

MRI shares many of the advantages of CT as an imaging method, the most important of which is sectional display. Although MRI is inferior to CT for demonstration and assessment of small calcific deposits or detailed analysis

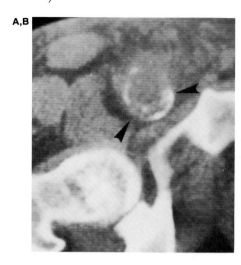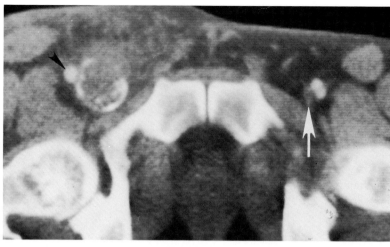

FIG. 1. Vascular enhancement on CT. **A:** Precontrast image shows a mass with shell-like peripheral calcification located in the region of the neurovascular bundle at the base of the femoral triangle (*arrowheads*). The mass displaces, but does not invade, adjacent muscles. **B:** CT after intravenous administration of contrast material shows the femoral artery (*arrowhead*) lateral to the mass. At surgery, the mass proved to be a tumor of the femoral vein. Compare the abnormal right femoral vein with the normal unopacified vein on the left side (*arrow*) just adjacent to the juxtaposed opacified superficial and deep femoral arteries.

of trabecular bone, MRI has superior contrast sensitivity and essentially equal spatial resolution. It is particularly effective for detection and delineation of bone marrow alterations, a function that no other method performs as well. The efficacy of MRI is enhanced by its multiplanar capability, its sensitivity to blood flow, and its ability to alter tissue contrast through pulse-sequence selection. Because MRI has no associated ionizing radiation, and because contrast agents are generally unnecessary, MRI is even more attractive for sectional imaging.

Compared with CT, MRI has equal or greater sensitivity for most soft-tissue applications, greater sensitivity for assessment of bone marrow changes, and lesser sensitivity for detection of small osseous alterations. Neither CT nor MRI can provide a specific histologic diagnosis under most circumstances.

Like CT, MRI is often a second imaging procedure following conventional radiographs or a radionuclide study. MRI is increasingly employed as a primary imaging test to evaluate soft-tissue masses and to confirm or exclude ischemic necrosis of the femoral head, and it probably will become a primary imaging test for internal derangements of most joints. It is commonly employed as a secondary test to verify bone marrow involvement in a large number of conditions.

Because the information gained by musculoskeletal CT and MRI is generally additive and is a refinement of that provided by the clinical circumstances and prior imaging tests, it is difficult to quantify the contribution of the additional information provided by these methods and its effect on clinical outcome (7,118,360). However, daily use of CT and MRI in the diagnosis of musculoskeletal conditions provides convincing clinical evidence of their efficacy. These methods are less invasive, they often im-

prove spatial appreciation of pathologic anatomy and better define the extent of disease, they can help determine the appropriate treatment, and they can simplify the monitoring of therapeutic responses.

TECHNIQUE

Because the musculoskeletal system is so variable from one region of the human anatomy to another, and because CT and MRI of musculoskeletal diseases are most commonly applied as problem-solving procedures, the technique for each patient or problem should be tailored to each clinical situation. The approach that follows is meant only as a guideline.

CT

Prior to CT imaging, a computed radiograph should be obtained. This is useful for visualization of osseous abnormalities, localization for the initial image, determination of the number and location of images needed, determination of angles for gantry position, selection of planes for image reconstruction, and verification of needle position during biopsy procedures.

Precise positioning of the patient or limb is important to ensure symmetric display of both sides. Many observations are facilitated if the opposite side is normal and is positioned exactly as the abnormal side; this is particularly true for the extremities. Usually, the plane of CT section should be perpendicular to the region of interest. This can be facilitated by use of bolsters, pillows, or sponges to elevate one portion of anatomy relative to another, or by gantry angulation. Variations of positioning may be required for specific anatomic regions and for various orthopedic measurements, such as femoral anteversion or tibial torsion.

Beam collimation can be varied according to the type and size of the lesion to be studied, as well as the need to reformat the data. For example, 0.8- to 1.0-cm slices are suitable for most soft-tissue and bone tumors; 0.4- to 0.5-cm slices may be necessary for small skeletal lesions, fractures, and confirmation of bone scan abnormalities and usually are required when reformation is anticipated; 0.2-cm slices may be necessary for certain regions (e.g., foot or wrist) when fine detail is needed.

Section sequencing must be tailored for the problem undergoing evaluation. Large soft-tissue and bone tumors can be evaluated with slices having a 100% interval or less between slices. Smaller lesions, joints, and fractures may require contiguous slices. A decision must be made each time whether to survey an area or to study it thoroughly.

Once the images are obtained and are available for review, they should always be displayed at two basic window settings. The usual soft-tissue window settings should be followed by skeletal window settings (high window level and wide window width). It may be necessary for the reviewer to select settings optimal for the individual case. Appropriate software programs can provide average attenuation values for regions of interest. For example, if long-bone medullary metastasis or infection is suspected, the attenuation values of diaphyseal medullary canals should be measured and compared with those for the opposite side. Multiplanar and three-dimensional reconstructions may have value, particularly in the evaluation of fractures (39,95,148,259,339,345,361).

Intravenous administration of contrast material should be considered according to the problem under evaluation. If it is necessary to evaluate the degree of vascularity of a tumor, appropriate CT sections may be obtained during rapid intravenous infusion of a contrast agent. Similar techniques are valuable in showing the relationships of major arteries or veins to musculoskeletal masses or for evaluation of enlargements of the vessels themselves (Fig. 1). Joints may also be studied following intraarticular instillation of air with or without iodinated contrast agents (323).

Candidates for musculoskeletal CT need not be excluded on the basis of plaster casts or orthopedic slings and traction devices. Plaster does not degrade a CT image. In fact, CT displays casted musculoskeletal anatomy better than does conventional radiography. If handled with care and approached with ingenuity, almost any patient in orthopedic traction can be imaged by CT.

MRI

In preparation for obtaining the imaging sequences, the region of interest should be localized. This may be accomplished by use of anatomic landmarks or by employing a short-duration pulse sequence in a plane perpendicular to the plane of choice for the imaging procedure in order to provide a scout view for determination of subsequent sections.

As with CT, precise positioning of the patient or limb is critical to ensure optimal imaging. The MRI plane should be parallel or perpendicular to the anatomic region or lesion of interest and as close to the center of the magnet as possible. When working within the three traditional orthogonal planes (transaxial, coronal, sagittal), it may be necessary to position the patient (particularly an extremity) to provide an image with the long axis of a bone or region in a single section. This can be made easier by liberal use of supporting sponges. On many occasions it is important to position the extremities similarly so that symmetrical anatomy will be displayed in individual sections.

Slice thickness should be varied according to the problem being evaluated. As with CT, 1.0-cm slices are adequate for survey of most bone and soft-tissue tumors. Thinner slices are necessary when greater detail is required, ranging to less than 0.1 cm for small joints such as the temporomandibular joint. With MRI, most studies are performed with contiguous slices. When this is not possible with a single pulse sequence, a second sequence is employed to image the remaining gaps.

As opposed to CT, MRI provides more choices and trade-offs for the radiologist to consider in order to achieve an optimal signal-to-noise ratio, resolution, and tissue contrast in the shortest possible time. These decisions are frequent and varied in musculoskeletal MRI because of the broad range of anatomic regions and pathologic conditions encountered. Thus, each examination must be tailored to the regional anatomy and the suspected condition. The appropriate coil, the correct plane, the proper slice thickness, the optimal pulse sequences, and the number of excitations averaged must each be selected.

The coil should be selected to complement the anatomy as closely as possible (182). This choice directly affects signal intensity, field of view, and resolution. A variety of coils (planar, solenoid, saddle, Helmholtz, etc.) should be available. For large parts (e.g., the pelvis), the body coil generally is employed, although a Helmholtz coil may be used when only a portion of the pelvis is of interest. For intermediate-size parts (e.g., thigh, knee, shoulder), small specialized coils are more appropriate. The resultant images are characterized by improved signal intensity and spatial resolution. Even smaller, more specialized coils are required to image distal appendicular anatomy (e.g., wrists or ankles) or small superficial parts (e.g., temporomandibular joint).

Once the coil has been selected to complement regional anatomy, the trade-offs involving slice thickness, field of view, number of excitations averaged, resultant signal-to-noise ratio, and resolution must be considered and bal-

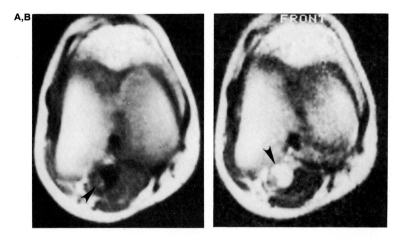

FIG. 2. Cystic degeneration of popliteal artery. **A:** MRI (TR = 500 msec, TE = 15 msec) shows popliteal artery (*arrowhead*) adjacent to low-signal-intensity mass. **B:** MRI (TR = 2,100 msec, TE = 90 msec) shows bright signal from cystic portion of popliteal artery (*arrowhead*).

anced. Generally, a choice of thinner slices and smaller field of view results in less available signal, but better in-plane resolution. Likewise, increasing the number of excitations averaged improves the signal-to-noise ratio, but increases the imaging time. Systems with higher field strengths provide improved signal and resolution characteristics.

Tissue contrast (and, to some degree, signal intensity) is controlled by pulse-sequence selection (247). On T1-weighted images of musculoskeletal tissues, subcutaneous fat and fatty bone marrow yield the brightest signal. Hyaline cartilage is less bright, and muscle is even less bright. Cyst fluid, joint effusion, ligaments, tendon, and mineralized bone produce little or no signal. On T2-weighted images, cyst fluid or joint effusion has the brightest signal, followed in decreasing order by subcutaneous fat, bone marrow, and muscle. Again, ligaments, tendons, and bone produce little or no signal intensity.

Blood is a special fluid that varies in signal intensity depending on at least the following factors: (a) the rate of flow; (b) the character of flow (laminar or turbulent); (c) the direction of flow in relation to the slice sequence of a multislice acquisition; (d) the higher signal of blood on even-numbered slices in a multislice sequence because of even-echo rephasing; (e) the pulse sequence selected; and (f) the chemical state of hemoglobin in areas of hemorrhage (56). Thus, careful consideration of these factors is necessary to understand the appearance of blood for each combination of anatomic site, pathologic condition, and pulse sequence (Fig. 2).

Because tissue contrast is a function of the combined effects of proton density, T1 relaxation, T2 relaxation, and pulse-sequence selection, adjacent normal and pathologic tissues can have identical intensities with certain pulse sequences. Therefore, the general advantage of contrast control by MRI is also a potential disadvantage.

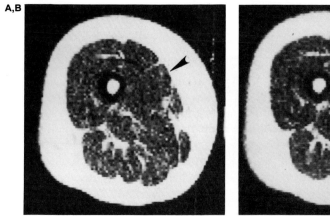

FIG. 3. Intramuscular myxoma. **A:** T1-weighted (TR = 300 msec, TE = 30 msec) MR image shows a very subtle mass effect (*arrowhead*) in the medial thigh, but no contrast difference between the mass and surrounding muscle. **B:** T2-weighted (TR = 900 msec, TE = 60 msec) MR image at same level shows distinct contrast between the mass and muscle, as well as clear definition of the interface between the two tissues. (From ref. 247.)

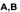

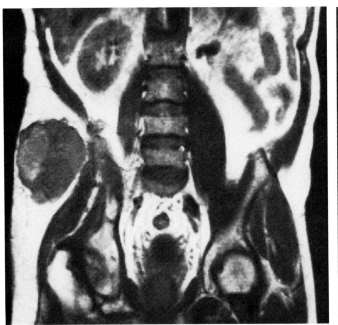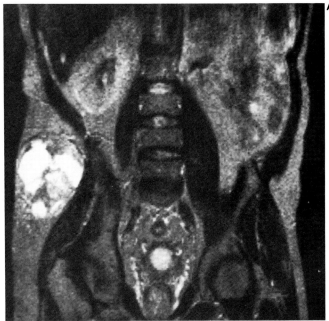

FIG. 4. Subcutaneous malignant fibrous histiocytoma. **A:** Coronal T1-weighted (TR = 600 msec, TE = 35 msec) MR image shows maximal contrast between tumor mass and surrounding subcutaneous fat. **B:** T2-weighted (TE = 1,500 msec, TR = 120 msec) MR image fails to show interface between mass and subcutaneous fat. Note that portions of the tumor show very high signal, presumably because of higher water content.

It is certainly possible to completely obscure a musculoskeletal lesion if only a single pulse sequence is employed (Fig. 3).

Guidelines for pulse-sequence selection are fairly simple. The initial sequence generally is chosen on the basis of the location and anticipated abnormality. When the abnormality is most likely in fatty tissue, such as subcutaneous fat or bone marrow, a T1-weighted sequence is employed to maximize contrast between the abnormality and surrounding fat (Fig. 4). Likewise, when the pathologic process is most likely located within muscle, the best sequence is T2-weighted to emphasize a contrast difference between the abnormality and surrounding muscle (Fig. 5). T2-weighted sequences are also used to emphasize the contrast provided by water or blood in tissues.

Metallic objects and artifacts

The presence of metal within a patient presents problems when imaging musculoskeletal tissues by CT or MRI (Fig. 6). With CT, metallic foreign bodies and orthopedic implants create major artifacts that often degrade the entire image. Although specialized computer programs have been developed to reduce these artifacts, they have not been totally successful. Nonetheless, the presence of metal within a patient is not a contraindication to CT, because sections adjacent to but not including metal are not affected, and even the affected sections often contain valuable anatomic details.

With MRI, the presence of metallic objects within a patient presents several potential problems, both within

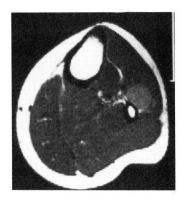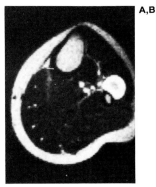

FIG. 5. Intramuscular lipomyxoma. **A:** Transverse T1-weighted (TR = 600 msec, TE = 35 msec) MR image shows little contrast between mass and surrounding muscle. **B:** T2-weighted (TR = 1,500 msec, TE = 90 msec) MR image shows maximal contrast between mass and muscle.

A,B

C,D

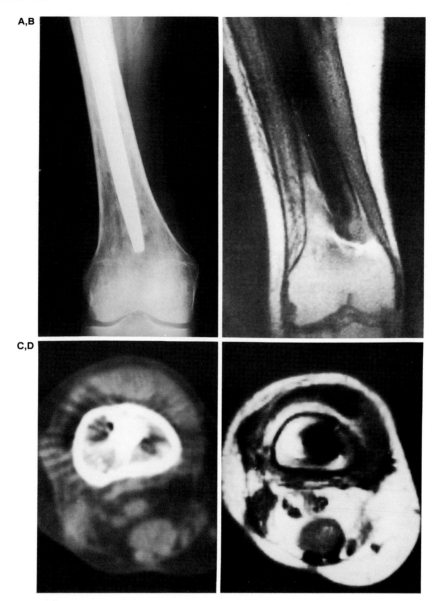

FIG. 6. Effects of metallic objects on CT and MR images. **A:** Anteroposterior (AP) radiograph of distal femur shows presence of an intramedullary (IM) rod. **B:** Coronal MR image (TR = 500 msec, TE = 30 msec) through IM rod shows loss of signal from medullary cavity, but preservation of signal from surrounding muscle and subcutaneous fat, as well as bone marrow distal to the tip of the rod. **C:** Transverse CT image through distal end of IM rod shows radial artifacts throughout most of the image. **D:** Transverse MR image (TR = 500 msec, TE = 30 msec) at same level as CT section shows that focal signal loss is restricted to the immediate vicinity of the IM rod, completely sparing the remainder of the section. (From ref. 247.)

the section and at a distance from it. Among these are (a) the possibility that the object might be moved by torque; (b) the possibility that an electronic device might malfunction; (c) the possibility that the metal might cause local tissue heating with certain pulse sequences; and (d) the likelihood that the metal will produce local image artifacts.

In musculoskeletal MRI, there are no known orthopedic devices that would be affected significantly by the torque within the magnetic field. The general contraindications for patients who have cerebral aneurysm clips or ocular metallic foreign bodies still apply. Although there are sev-

eral orthopedic stimulators being used to encourage fracture healing, it is not known how these respond to magnetic fields, and these patients are excluded from MRI examination, as are those with pacemakers.

For musculoskeletal MRI, focal loss of signal with or without regional distortion is the most important problem presented by metallic objects. Both ferromagnetic and nonferromagnetic metals cause focal signal loss as a result of local eddy currents associated with the devices. Metallic objects of any size create "holes" in the image, but ferromagnetic objects cause greater distortion. Even small ferromagnetic particles not detected on conventional ra-

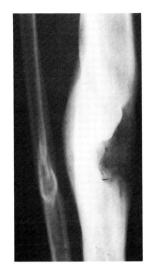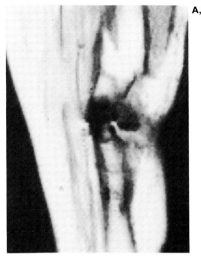

A,B

FIG. 7. Effect of ferromagnetic particle. **A:** Radiograph shows dense sclerosis of tibia resulting from prior fracture and osteomyelitis. No metallic fragments are identified. **B:** Coronal MRI section (TR = 500 msec, TE = 15 msec) shows focal signal deficiency and distortion caused by an embedded ferromagnetic particle resulting from prior surgery.

diographs can cause tiny holes in MR images (Fig. 7). The holes and distortions become greater as field strength increases.

Although various metallic objects cause focal image degradation, they seldom cause much difficulty in image interpretation. The closer to the metal, the greater the image degradation and any associated difficulty with interpretation. However, even when orthopedic devices are large, imaging of regional tissues is possible. Although both CT and MR images are degraded by metallic objects, there is more distortion on CT images than on MR images. Nonmetallic splints and casts cause no MRI artifacts and tend to be nearly invisible because they have few, if any, protons to produce a signal.

SOFT-TISSUE DISEASES AND MASSES

The basis of CT and MRI diagnosis of muscle disease and evaluation of soft-tissue masses is knowledge of normal anatomy. Because human body habitus and CT/MRI machinery configurations make positioning and study of the lean upper extremities technically difficult, and because the majority of soft-tissue diseases and masses involve the lower extremities, this analysis of normal anatomy will emphasize the lower extremities.

Normal Anatomy

Lower extremity

Figure 8 is a lower-extremity diagram that localizes sequential regions of soft-tissue anatomy that correspond to Fig. 9. The limbs are divided into flexor and extensor compartments. The chief hip flexors are the iliacus and

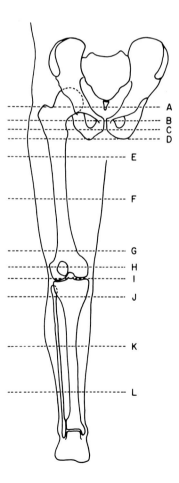

FIG. 8. Lower-extremity diagram. Each level indicated by a letter corresponds to a CT section displayed in Fig. 9.

A,B

C,D

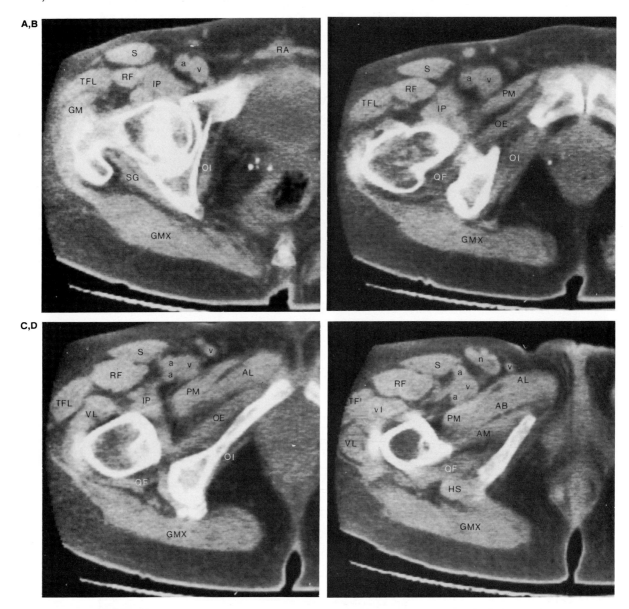

FIG. 9. Normal soft-tissue anatomy of the lower extremity. Each section is 1 cm thick and is identified according to the characteristic skeletal features: **A:** Midportion of hip. **B:** Femoral neck and symphysis pubis. **C:** Intertrochanteric femur and inferior pubic ramus. **D:** Lesser trochanter of femur and ischial tuberosity. Parts **E–L** on *facing page.* **E:** Proximal femoral shaft. **F:** Middle femoral shaft. **G:** Distal femoral metadiaphyseal junction. **H:** Distal femoral metaphysis and patella. **I:** Femoral condyles and patellar tendon. **J:** Proximal tibial metaphysis and tibiofibular joint. **K:** Junction of tibial proximal and middle thirds. **L:** Junction of tibial middle and distal thirds. The importance of discrete knowledge of soft-tissue anatomy is in the precision that it gives to confirmation, localization, and characterization of abnormal processes. All images are of the right side; (a) artery; (v) vein; (n) lymph node; (AB) adductor brevis muscle; (AL) adductor longus muscle; (AM) adductor magnus muscle; (BFT) biceps femoris muscles (tendon); (BLH) long head of biceps femoris muscle; (BSH) short head of biceps femoris muscle; (EDL) extensor digitorum longus muscle; (EHL) extensor hallucis longus muscle; (FDL) flexor digitorum longus muscle; (FHL) flexor hallucis longus muscle; (GT) gracilis muscle (tendon); (GM) gluteus medius muscle; (GML) gastrocnemius muscle lateral head; (GMM) gastrocnemius muscle medial head; (GMT) gastrocnemius tendon; (GMX) gluteus maximus muscle; (HS) hamstring muscles; (IP) iliopsoas muscle; (OE) obturator externus muscle; (OI) obturator internus muscle; (P) plantaris muscle; (PLB) peroneus longus and brevis muscles; (PM) pectineus muscle; (PO) popliteus muscle; (PT) patellar tendon; (QF) quadratus femoris muscle; (QT) quadriceps tendon; (RA) rectus abdominis muscle; (RF) rectus femoris muscle; (S) sartorius muscle; (SG) superior gemellus muscle; (SMT) semimembranosus muscle (tendon); (SO) soleus muscle; (STT) semitendinosus muscle (tendon); (TA) tibialis anterior muscle; (TFL) tensor fascia lata muscle; (TP) tibialis posterior muscle; (VI) vastus intermedius muscle; (VL) vastus lateralis muscle; (VM) vastus medialis muscle.

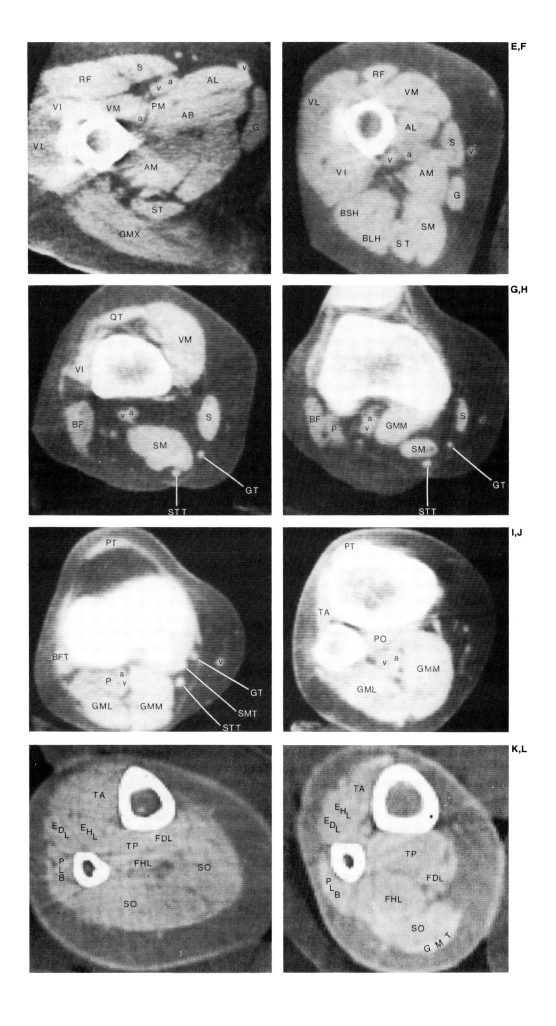

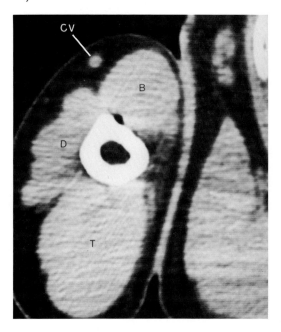

FIG. 10. Normal soft-tissue anatomy of the upper arm; (CV) cephalic vein; (B) biceps muscle; (D) deltoid muscle; (T) triceps muscle.

psoas major muscles, which, having crossed anterior to the hip joint, insert on the lesser trochanter via a common tendon (Fig. 9A–C). The rectus femoris muscle also crosses the hip joint, but it is a knee extensor and part of the quadriceps mechanism. The adductor group, the pectineus and sartorius, also contribute to hip flexion (Fig. 9B–E). The most powerful hip extensor is the gluteus maximus, but in normal gait, hip extension is achieved by the hamstring muscles. The hamstrings, which attach to the ischial tuberosity, include the semimembranosus, semitendinosus, long head of the biceps femoris, and a portion of adductor magnus muscles, to make up the muscle mass of the posterior thigh (Fig. 9E–I). With the exception of the adductor magnus, they insert distal to the knee and are also knee flexors. Hip adductors are the gluteus medius and gluteus minimus muscles. The adductor longus, brevis, and magnus muscles are the hip adductors (Fig. 9D–F). The lateral rotators of the hip include the piriformis, obturator internus, quadratus femoris, and obturator externus muscles (Fig. 9B–D).

The midportion of the thigh may be divided into three compartments: the extensor, adductor, and flexor (Fig. 9F). The extensor muscles (vastus group) almost surround the anterolateral aspect of the femur. The bulky adductors compose a medial compartment and insert into the femur distally. The knee flexor muscles (hamstrings) make up a posterior compartment. The adductor canal, a division between the flexor and adductor groups, spirals down the medial aspect of the thigh and is bordered medially by the sartorius muscle. Within the adductor canal descend the femoral vessels and saphenous nerve (Fig. 9F). The sciatic nerve is sandwiched between the hamstring and adductor magnus muscles.

The knee is a synovial joint that primarily functions as a hinge joint. The quadriceps tendon attaches to the patella superiorly (Fig. 9G). The patella then articulates with the femur, and at this point the knee joint is reinforced on each side of the patella by medial and lateral aponeurotic expansions known as patellar retinaculae (Fig. 9H–I). The patellar tendon arises from the inferior pole of the patella (Fig. 9I) and inserts at the tibial tubercle (Fig. 9J). In normal knees, the joint space, including the suprapatellar bursa, is not visualized because the potential intraarticular space is collapsed (Fig. 9G–I).

The thigh muscle, in addition to moving the hip, also moves the knee. The quadriceps muscles are its extensors, and the hamstrings its flexors. Leg muscles that attach to the femur assist in knee flexion. They include the gastrocnemius, popliteus, and plantaris muscles (Fig. 9H–I). The popliteal artery and vein are located centrally, just posterior to the distal femur.

The calf muscles that move the ankle and tarsus are divided into three compartments: anterior, posterior, and lateral (Fig. 9I–L). The anterior or extensor compartment contains the three dorsiflexors: the tibialis anterior, the extensor hallucis longus, and the extensor digitorum longus. In the posterior or plantar flexor compartment are the gastrocnemius, soleus, flexor hallucis longus, flexor digitorum longus, and tibialis posterior muscles. The peroneus longus and brevis muscles form the lateral or peroneal compartment and act to evert the foot. The principal inverter of the foot is the tibialis posterior, which is assisted by the tibialis anterior muscle.

Upper extremity

The upper arm is divided into ventral flexor and dorsal extensor compartments by the medial and lateral intermuscular septae (Fig. 10). The flexor compartment contains the biceps, brachialis, and part of the coracobrachialis muscles. It also transmits the brachial vessels and the median and ulnar nerves. The extensor compartment contains the triceps muscle, profunda artery, and radial nerve. A portion of the deltoid muscle is present in the proximal lateral aspect.

The forearm is similarly divided into ventral flexor and dorsal extensor compartments by the interosseous membrane (Fig. 11). The flexor group is subdivided into superficial and deep muscle groups. The superficial group consists of the pronator teres, flexor carpi radialis, palmaris longus, flexor carpi ulnaris, and flexor digitorum superficialis muscles. The deep group includes the flexor digitorum profundus, flexor pollicis longus, and pronator quadratus muscles.

The extensor muscles of the forearm are also divided into superficial and deep groups. From lateral to medial, the superficial muscle group includes the brachioradialis, extensor carpi radialis longus, extensor carpi radialis brevis, extensor digitorum, extensor digiti minimi, exten-

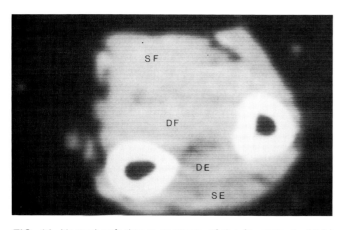
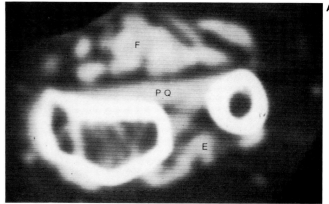

FIG. 11. Normal soft-tissue anatomy of the forearm. **A:** Middle forearm; (SF) superficial flexor muscle group; (DF) deep flexor muscle group; (DE) deep extensor muscle group; (SE) superficial extensor muscle group. **B:** Distal forearm; (F) flexor muscles and tendons; (PQ) pronator quadratus; (E) extensor muscles and tendons.

sor carpi ulnaris, and anconeus muscles. The deep group consists of the supinator, abductor pollicis longus, extensor pollicis brevis, extensor pollicis longus, and extensor indicis muscles.

It is sometimes difficult to distinguish the individual forearm muscle bundles by CT or MRI because of the paucity of fat in the forearm. However, MRI shows great promise for evaluation of tendons at the wrist in both coronal and cross-sectional planes (Fig. 12).

Muscle Diseases

Normal muscles are of soft-tissue density on CT, with muscle groups separated from one another by low-density fatty septae (36,119,334) (Fig. 9). On MRI, muscle is of intermediate signal intensity, bordered by fat planes of high signal intensity (94,248) (Fig. 13).

Minor variations of normal muscles depend on age, sex, and cerebral-dominance factors (36). Many muscle conditions, and muscular dystrophies in particular, typically are accompanied by some degree of muscle alteration, often with replacement of muscle fibers by fat cells and connective tissue. With the advent of CT and MRI, it is possible to make diagnoses prior to complete clinical presentation and to analyze muscle disorders both qualitatively and quantitatively (124,248).

Muscle diseases may be grouped into several categories, including metabolic myopathies, dystrophies, ischemias, neuropathies, systemic effects, and idiopathic. CT and MRI can characterize these conditions in terms of muscle size, the number and distribution of diseased mus-

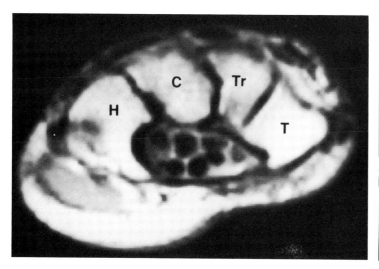
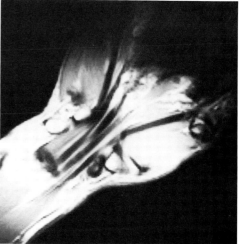

FIG. 12. MRI of the wrist. **A:** Transverse MRI (TR = 2,000 msec, TE = 25 msec) of the carpal tunnel; (T) trapezium; (Tr) trapezoid; (C) capitate; (H) hamate. Tendons in carpal tunnel are the flexor pollicis longus, the flexor digitorum superficialis group, and the flexor digitorum profundus group. **B:** Coronal MRI (TR = 2,100 msec, TE = 17 msec) of the carpal tunnel; tendons are the flexor pollicis longus and the flexor digitorum superficialis group.

A

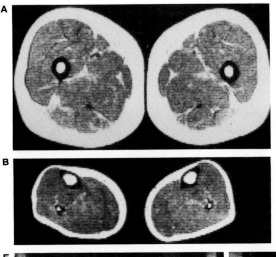

B

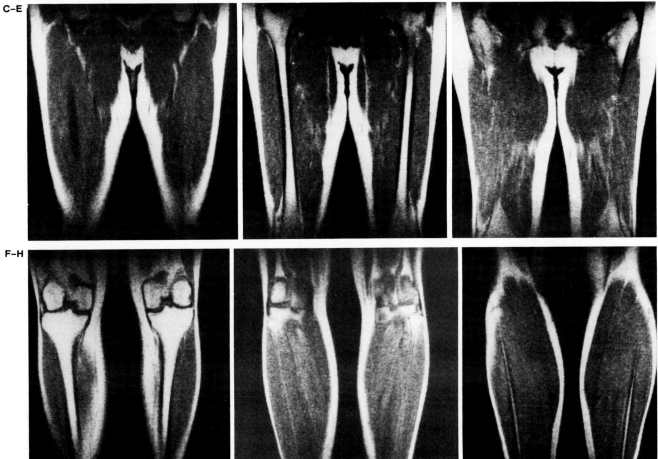

FIG. 13. Normal muscle in a 38-year-old man. **A:** Transverse MR image (TR = 1,500 msec, TE = 30 msec) through the middle thigh shows normal quadriceps, adductor, and hamstring muscle groups. **B:** Transverse MR image (TR = 500 msec, TE = 30 msec) through middle calf shows normal anterior, lateral, and posterior muscle groups. **C–E:** Coronal images through thigh show longitudinal anatomy of quadriceps, adductor, and hamstring muscle groups. **F–H:** Coronal MRI (TR = 500 msec, TE = 30 msec) through calf shows longitudinal anatomy of calf muscles. (From ref. 248.)

C–E

F–H

cles, and the pattern of fatty replacement (36,94, 119,248,252,334,364) (Figs. 14 and 15). The severity of involvement is not directly related to disease duration, but does parallel functional impairment. The distribution of muscle involvement and the pattern of replacement are not specific for a particular condition. Variable patterns are observed within diseases and even in individual patients. In the muscular dystrophies, the fatty replacement of muscle may be complete and homogeneous or incomplete and patchy. By surveying the muscular system

of the body, it is possible to show selective involvement and sparing of individual muscle groups. Thus, the localization, distribution, and extent of muscular involvement can be described.

MRI is the preferred study for detection and characterization of muscle diseases because of its superior contrast sensitivity, its multiplanar imaging capability, and its lack of ionizing radiation (248). The latter is especially important in imaging children or young adults who might require repeated examinations.

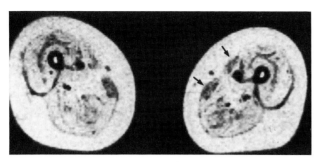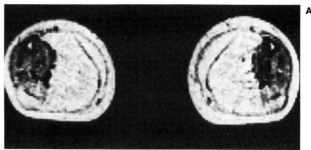

A,B

FIG. 14. Duchenne muscular dystrophy in 14-year-old boy. **A:** Transverse MRI (IR, TR = 1,600 msec, TI = 400 msec, TE = 300 msec) through middle thigh shows nearly complete fatty replacement of all muscle groups, with some sparing of sartorius and gracilis muscles (*arrows*). **B:** Transverse MRI (TR = 500 msec, TE = 30 msec) through middle calf shows complete replacement of gastrocnemius and soleus muscles, with apparent preservation of intermuscular fibrous septa. The large size of these muscles is MRI correlation for clinical "pseudohypertrophy." (From ref. 248.)

Soft-Tissue Masses

The evaluation of soft-tissue masses has been revolutionized—initially by the development of CT (140,294,349) and subsequently by MRI (57,247,338). The soft-tissue contrast resolution and sectional presentation of compartmental anatomy provided by CT and MRI make possible routine identification, characterization, and staging of soft-tissue masses.

CT is an effective method for study of soft-tissue masses of many causes. It usually permits distinction between one muscle and another, provides a cross-sectional image of limb compartments, is sensitive to anatomic distortion, localizes neurovascular bundles, and defines both the radial distribution of a mass and its local relationships. In select circumstances, these capabilities are improved by intravascular or intraarticular contrast enhancement (58).

CT has several disadvantages (19,67,85,109). In lean parts of the anatomy, there is insufficient fat to permit distinction between normal and pathologic anatomy, and a mass might not be detected because of isodensity with respect to surrounding muscle. There is also a risk that the size or extent of a mass might be overestimated because of adjacent edema or hemorrhage. Over-range artifacts caused by bone or metal in the imaging plane may obscure details of the margin or matrix of masses.

MRI is another effective method for detection, localization, and characterization of soft-tissue masses. Because of its high contrast sensitivity, MRI will demonstrate the boundaries of tumors with respect to fat, muscle, and bone. With the appropriate combination of imaging planes, distinction between the mass and adjacent structures usually can be achieved without difficulty.

MRI has certain disadvantages, the most important of which is insensitivity to small calcifications and collections of gas (338). These features often are diagnostically important, but must be detected by conventional radiography or CT. MR images are also degraded by metals in the section, but to a lesser degree than CT. As with CT,

there is a risk that the size or extent of a mass might be overestimated because of adjacent edema. However, appropriate selection of pulse sequences should resolve most questions (Fig. 16).

Comparative studies of CT and MRI show that MRI provides equal or greater information regarding lesion identification, characterization, and determination of extent (338,349). The greater inherent soft-tissue contrast resolution of MRI provides clearer definition of tumor margins than does CT.

Soft-tissue contrast

The contrast characteristics of soft-tissue masses depend on their compositions. For CT, density depends on the relative proportions of fat, water, and mineral. The MR signal intensity is a more complex phenomenon dependent on the balance of inherent tissue properties of hydrogen density and relaxation factors, blood flow, and pulse-sequence selection (247).

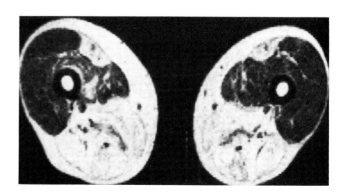

FIG. 15. Facioscapulohumeral dystrophy in 56-year-old man. Transverse MRI (TR = 300 msec, TE = 30 msec) through middle thigh shows symmetric fatty replacement of hamstring and rectus femoris muscles, but asymmetric involvement of vastus intermedius and adductor muscles.

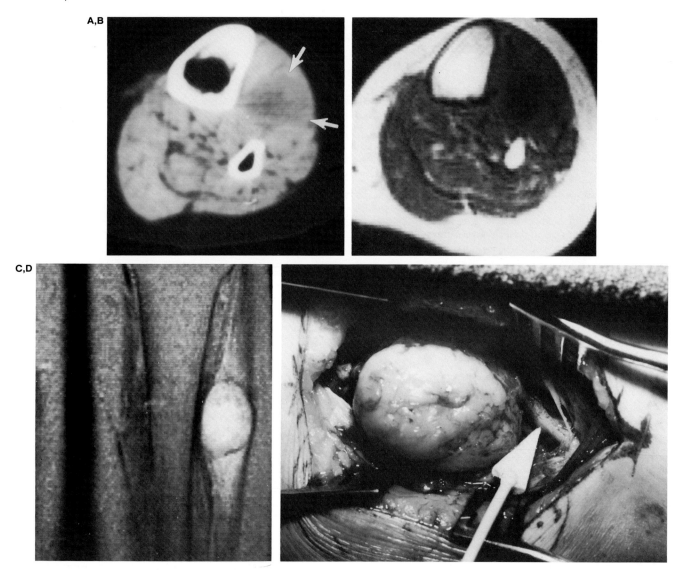

FIG. 16. Edema obscuring margins of mass (neurilemmoma). **A:** CT section shows ill-defined mass (*arrows*) localized to anterolateral calf, suggestive of an invasive tumor. **B:** T1-weighted (TR = 300 msec, TE = 15 msec) MR image at same level as CT section shows similar features, leading to the same conclusion. **C:** T2-weighted (TR = 3,000 msec, TE = 90 msec) MR image through the mass shows that it is sharply marginated, with no evidence of invasion; triangular regions of high signal intensity are seen proximal and distal to the mass, indicating edema around the tumor. **D:** Photograph at surgery confirms the encapsulated nature of the mass. *Arrow* points to the anterior tibial nerve from which the tumor arose. (Courtesy of Dr. T. Mustoe, St. Louis, Missouri.)

Cysts

Cystic masses usually are associated with a joint and arise from a synovial extension (195,196,310,328) (Fig. 17). These are sharply marginated, homogeneous masses with CT attenuation values or MR signal intensities similar to those for water. If hemorrhagic, their CT attenuation values or their T1-weighted signal intensities may increase. The largest synovial cysts tend to be found about the hip. Cysts show no CT enhancement after intravenous administration of contrast material, although this may make their margins more conspicuous because of enhancement of the surrounding tissues. Both CT and MRI

are effective methods for demonstration of the nature and origin of cysts. Neither is always effective for distinguishing between a pyogenic cystic collection and a sterile collection; cyst aspiration and fluid culture are necessary.

Abscesses

Soft-tissue abscesses infrequently present as masses. When they do, they generally are poorly defined, infiltrating lesions that distort normal muscle anatomy and fascial planes. Although abscesses may occur anywhere in the body, they are most commonly encountered in the paraspinal and pelvic muscles.

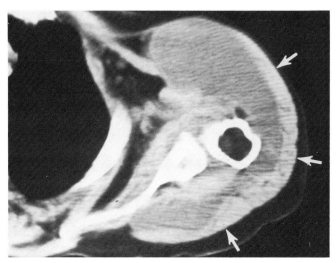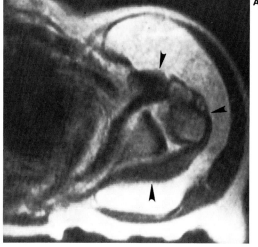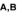

FIG. 17. Synovial cyst of shoulder joint. **A:** CT section shows near-water-density mass deep to deltoid muscle (*arrows*). **B:** MR image (TR = 3,000 msec, TE = 90 msec) at the same position obtained with a Helmholtz surface coil shows high-signal-intensity fluid-filled cyst interposed between deltoid muscle and rotator cuff muscles (*arrowheads*).

The CT or MRI appearance of an abscess is nonspecific and may be confused with that of hemorrhage or neoplasm unless soft-tissue gas is present. In the absence of percutaneous or open surgical intervention, the presence of soft-tissue gas is indicative of an inflammatory process (Fig. 18). CT is effective for definition of the extent of the abscess, guidance of percutaneous drainage procedures, and documentation of response to therapy. CT is generally preferred when intervention is contemplated. Otherwise, except for the detection of gas, MRI is as effective as CT for demonstration of the abscess (348) (Fig. 19).

Hemorrhage

Hemorrhages into soft tissue may have various causes, presentations, localizations, and appearances. Hemorrhage may occur spontaneously, following trauma, with bleeding diatheses, while a patient is receiving anticoagulants, with inflammatory diseases, into a tumor, and following surgery or percutaneous translumbar aortography. Because of the various causes and possible presentations, a physician may not always consider the diagnosis. If hemorrhage is suspected, confirmation and precise localization are difficult using conventional imaging tests.

CT or MRI nearly always shows the location and extent of soft-tissue hemorrhage, especially in anatomic regions that are difficult to examine physically. Intramuscular hemorrhage will cause an enlargement of the muscle that is easily recognized when the left and right sides are compared for symmetry (74). Whereas an acute hematoma is characteristically hyperdense, a subacute or chronic hematoma may not be readily differentiated from an abscess or a neoplasm on the basis of CT findings alone. Any of these may cause enlargement of a muscle with an isodense or low-density mass. With appropriate clinical history, a

diagnosis of hemorrhage may be suggested; in selected cases, CT can be used to guide a percutaneous needle aspiration for confirmation.

In addition to localization of soft-tissue hemorrhage, CT can characterize and display the various stages in the natural history of hemorrhage maturation (Fig. 20). Initially, the hematoma may be of homogeneous density, and then, as liquefaction begins, it may develop a patchy or heterogeneous appearance. When completely liquefied, the hematoma will have developed a pseudocapsule and homogeneous density lower than that of muscle. If the injury includes muscle necrosis, early mineralization may

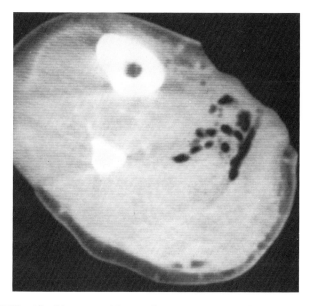

FIG. 18. Abscess with gas-forming organism. CT section shows a huge ulcer and a poorly defined infiltrating mass containing gas.

A,B

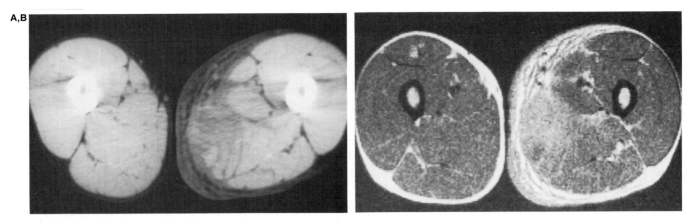

FIG. 19. Infected hematoma, comparison of CT and MRI. **A:** CT image through thigh shows mass in medial aspect, with associated edema of adjacent subcutaneous fat. **B:** MR image (TR = 500 msec, TE = 35 msec) at same anatomic level shows identical features.

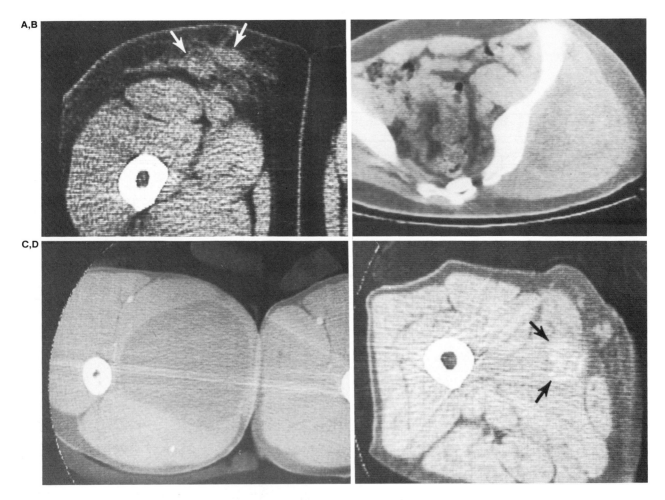

FIG. 20. Hematoma characterization. CT can demonstrate the degree of maturation when a hematoma is imaged. **A:** Early stage of subcutaneous hematoma, shortly after injury, when hematoma (*arrows*) is infiltrating the fat and remains similar to muscle in density. **B:** Intermediate stage of intramuscular hematoma maturation, when the gluteal hemorrhage is partially organized and partially liquefied and on CT is displayed as an inhomogeneous mass with regions that are less dense than muscle. **C:** Late stage of intramuscular hematoma, when the hemorrhage has liquefied and the CT shows a homogeneous mass of density less than muscle (contrast material is seen in vessels). **D:** Late stage of a small intramuscular hematoma or an early state of myositis ossificans, when the residual traumatized tissue begins to mineralize (*arrows*).

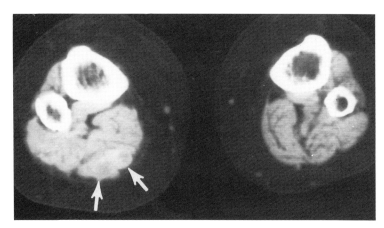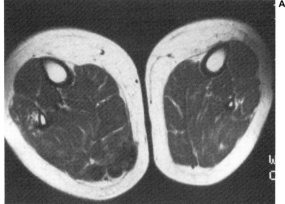

FIG. 21. Early myositis ossificans, comparison of CT and MRI. **A:** CT image through proximal calf shows early mineralization (*arrows*) of a muscle injury, indicative of myositis ossificans. **B:** Transverse MR image (TR = 600 msec, TE = 35 msec) distal to location of CT section shows low signal of involved muscle due to mineralization and fibrosis, but fails to specifically detect the calcium.

be detected by CT, indicating ossification of the hematoma or development of myositis ossificans (4). MRI will not identify the soft-tissue mineralization on which the specific diagnosis of myositis ossificans depends; it will only show a mass (Fig. 21).

The signal characteristics of soft-tissue hemorrhage on MRI change as the blood in the mass ages (299,331,341). Acute hemorrhage has a signal intensity close to that of muscle on T1-weighted images (Fig. 22) and a high signal intensity of T2-weighted images. After about 2 days, there is progressive shortening of the T1 relaxation value of the hematoma, and the signal intensity becomes much greater than that of muscle on T1-weighted images (Fig. 23). This

phenomenon is attributed to sequential changes that occur as the hemoglobin molecules are oxidized to methemoglobin. Within several days, and thereafter for many months, residual hematomas will have very strong signal intensities on both pulse sequences, permitting identification of blood.

Soft-tissue neoplasia

Benign and aggressive soft-tissue tumors can be evaluated by CT or MRI (67). The classic benign mass usually has a well-defined periphery or capsule and a homogeneous matrix. A typical aggressive mass has an ill-defined periphery and a heterogeneous or patchy matrix. On CT examination, tumors usually have an average attenuation value slightly lower than that for normal muscle. In general, on MRI examination, nonfatty tumors are of equal or lower signal intensity than skeletal muscle on T1-weighted sequences and of higher signal intensity than skeletal muscle on T2-weighted images. When compared

FIG. 22. Acute hematoma. Transverse T1-weighted (TR = 500 msec, TE = 15 msec) MR image of upper arm shows low signal intensity of acute biceps hematoma (*arrowheads*).

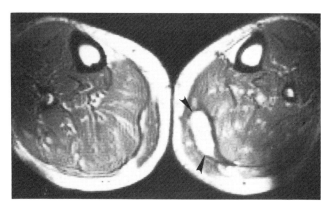

FIG. 23. Chronic hematoma. Transverse T1-weighted (TR = 700 msec, TE = 30 msec) MR image of lower leg shows bright signal intensity from old organized hematoma of calf (*arrowheads*).

A,B

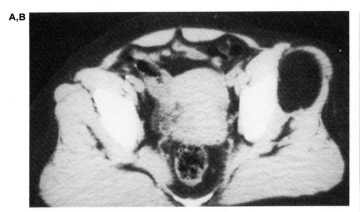
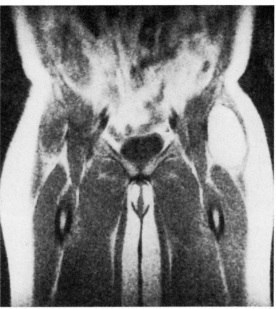

FIG. 24. Lipoma. **A:** CT image shows a homogeneous, fat-density, sharply marginated mass adjacent to the left acetabulum. **B:** Coronal MR image (TR = 500 msec, TE = 30 msec) shows a high-signal-intensity mass similar to subcutaneous fat. The cephalocaudad extent of the tumor is better displayed on this coronal image.

with fat, most lesions are lower in signal than fat on T1-weighted images and equal to or greater than fat on T2-weighted images. With MRI, lesions tend to be more inhomogeneous on T2-weighted images than on T1-weighted images.

Unfortunately, in most cases neither CT nor MRI can provide a specific histologic diagnosis. Both benign and malignant lesions may present morphologically as either well-defined or infiltrating masses. Relatively nonaggressive processes include cysts, lipomas, myositis ossificans,

and both benign and malignant neoplasms. Aggressive characteristics may be seen in acute hematomas, abscesses, some benign tumors, and many malignant neoplasms (166).

Benign tumors

Lipomas are common benign soft-tissue tumors. Most are subcutaneous and need no imaging evaluation. When deep or large or in an unusual location, both CT and MRI

A,B

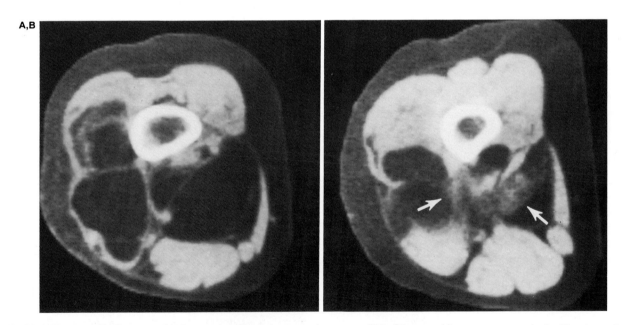

FIG. 25. Intramuscular lipoma, with focus of malignant mesenchymoma. This 61-year-old woman presented with a large lipoma of the thigh 12 years following resection. **A:** CT image through middle thigh shows adipose tissue replacing many muscles and displacing others. **B:** A more distal section shows an amorphous soft-tissue-density tumor infiltrating the lipoma, just posterior to the femur (*arrows*). This region of malignant mesenchymoma was very small in comparison with the bulky benign lipoma; histologically, it contained areas of osteosarcoma, chondrosarcoma, and liposarcoma.

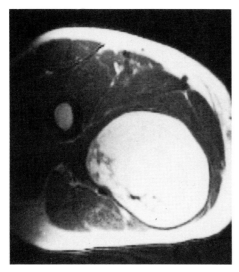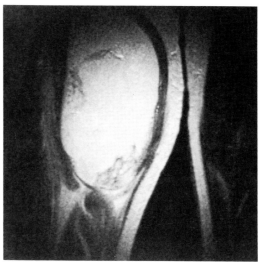

A,B

FIG. 26. Liposarcoma. **A:** Transverse MRI (TR = 300 msec, TE = 17 msec) using a Helmholtz surface coil shows large encapsulated fatty tumor, with a small area of streaky infiltration in the lateral portion of the tumor. **B:** Coronal MRI (TR = 3,000 msec, TE = 90 msec) confirms the fatty nature of this tumor and more directly displays its cephalocaudad extent.

can identify and localize the tumors as areas of fatty tissue distorting the surrounding tissues. Lipomas are composed almost exclusively of fatty tissue (−40 to −100 Hounsfield units, HU), although they may contain recognizable small, thin soft-tissue septae or vessels. In addition, they are well defined and homogeneous (167) (Fig. 24). When areas of soft-tissue density or intensity are present in the lesion, or when it invades the surrounding tissue, the possibility of a sarcoma must be considered, and a biopsy performed (Figs. 25 and 26). Larger, more infiltrating lipomatous lesions such as macrodystrophia lipomatosa and infiltrating angiolipomas are rare, but when present, CT or MRI can be used to map their extent and demonstrate where normal muscle is invaded or replaced (Figs. 27 and 28).

CT and MRI are effective for demonstration of hemangiomas and angiovenous dysplasias of the musculoskeletal system (54,173,205) (Fig. 29). These are best shown by MRI because the slowly flowing blood in the lesions has intense signal on T2-weighted images that facilitates their characterization and definition of extent (Fig. 30).

CT also has been used to evaluate a variety of other less common, benign masses, including benign mesenchymoma, intramuscular myxoma, endometriosis, and soft-tissue chondroma (367). The CT appearance in these lesions is not specific; however, CT does help identify, localize, and characterize each mass so that the surgical approach can be planned.

Malignant tumors

The value of CT and MRI in the evaluation and staging of soft-tissue sarcomas is now widely accepted (287). Cur-

rent therapy is based on accurate staging of the tumor, which in turn depends on accurate definition of the compartmental and longitudinal extent of the lesion. CT and MRI can provide this information as well as define the relationships of the tumor to adjacent vessels and nerves. Accurate preoperative characterization can facilitate the design and performance of limb surgery that will leave tumor-free surgical margins, preserve function, and lead to few tumor recurrences.

The most common malignant soft-tissue neoplasms are relatively indistinguishable by all imaging methods. Malignant fibrous histiocytomas, liposarcomas, and fibrosarcomas all present as inhomogeneous masses. They vary from fairly well encapsulated to very invasive. Both CT and MRI can define extent for most lesions on the basis of mass effect and associated distortion or infiltration of the surrounding normal tissues. MRI offers the advantages of increased contrast resolution and additional planes that may make the margins of lesions more conspicuous.

Malignant fibrous histiocytoma, the most common malignant soft-tissue neoplasm, generally is a lobulated inhomogeneous mass that often is invasive, but may be relatively well defined (93) (Fig. 31). Peripheral calcification may be present in some cases. On MRI, the tumor may consist of irregularly shaped regions of both high and low signal intensities, sometimes having areas of hemorrhage. Fibrosarcoma (332), another relatively common soft-tissue malignancy, is very difficult to distinguish from infection, hemorrhage, or other invasive neoplasm. It is often infiltrative and may replace muscles and invade bone. Its matrix is irregular and may be quite inhomogeneous.

Liposarcoma (66,67,76,167) usually is a bulky tumor with a pseudocapsule. Margins may be sharp or unsharp,

A,B

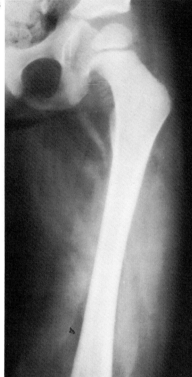

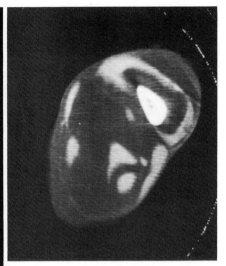

FIG. 27. Macrodystrophia lipomatosa. **A:** The left lower extremity is larger than the right, and normal muscle shadows have been replaced by bizarre fat planes. **B:** CT section through the distal thigh shows distortion of the femoral shape, as well as overly abundant adipose tissue that has replaced much of the muscle tissue. In this patient, CT localization of remaining musculature helped to plan a surgical debulking procedure.

and the matrix mixed or heterogeneous. The amount of fat is variable, with some poorly differentiated tumors containing almost no fat, whereas other tumors contain mostly fat (Fig. 25). If any solid or nonfatty component (other than small blood vessels) is present in a predominantly fatty tumor, the possibility of sarcomatous tissue must be considered. Neither CT nor MRI has any advantage in distinguishing benign and malignant fatty tumors (66,76).

Both CT and MRI are effective for identification, characterization, and staging of several less common malignant neoplasms, including extraosseous chondrosarcoma, neurofibrosarcoma, leiomyosarcoma, synovial sarcoma, and extraskeletal Ewing tumor. Most present as masses similar to the more common malignant lesions and vary in appearance from fairly well defined to infiltrating (Fig. 32). Metastases may also be detected.

Some soft-tissue tumors may present with a mineralized mass detected on plain films as the primary abnormality (83). In such cases, CT is the sectional imaging method of choice, because MRI is less effective for demonstration of the calcifications. On the basis of CT findings alone, it may not be possible to differentiate a benign mineralized lesion from a malignant lesion (Fig. 33). However, the CT study is helpful in determining precise location, radial spread of the tumor, and its local anatomic relationships.

In these cases, CT shows the tumor and its relationships to bone and extremity compartments better than do conventional radiographs.

Clinical Application

Soft-tissue masses sometimes are evaluated by a combination of conventional radiography, angiography, ra-

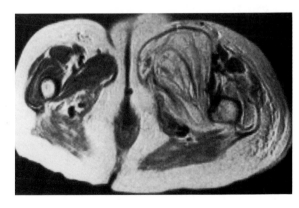

FIG. 28. Infiltrating lipoma. Transverse MR image (TR = 3,000 msec, TE = 35 msec) shows lipoma infiltrating and enlarging the adductor muscle group.

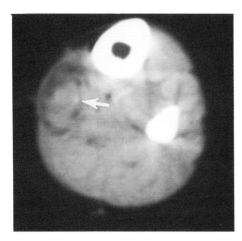
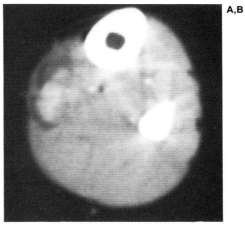

A,B

FIG. 29. Cavernous hemangioma in a 35-year-old woman. **A:** Noncontrast CT section through the calf shows a mass of the same density as muscle, but separated from muscle by a thin rim of fat. Note the single calcified phlebolith (*arrow*). **B:** Contrast-enhanced CT section at the same level shows the vascular nature of the mass. Note also the enhancement of several blood vessels.

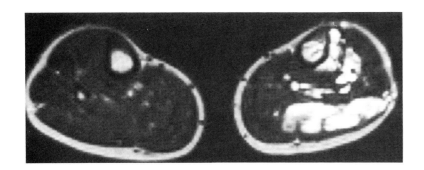

FIG. 30. Angiovenous dysplasia in an 18-year-old man. Transverse MR image (TR = 3,000 msec, TE = 90 msec) shows infiltrating nature of this large-vessel angiovenous dysplasia. Note muscular atrophy as compared with unaffected leg.

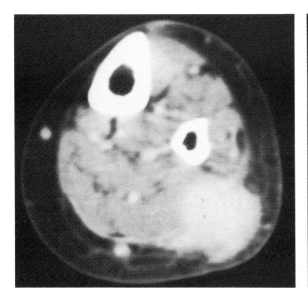
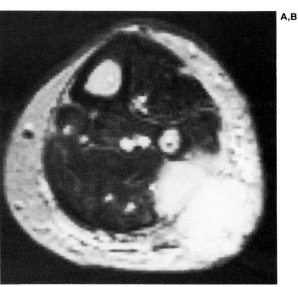

A,B

FIG. 31. Malignant fibrous histiocytoma. A 72-year-old woman presented with a hard, enlarging mass in the calf. **A:** Postcontrast CT image shows an enhancing mass involving both muscle and subcutaneous fat. The deep margins are poorly defined. **B:** Transverse MR image (TR = 3,000 msec, TE = 90 msec) at same level shows deep boundaries of the tumor better than CT because of greater contrast differences between tumor and muscle. Coronal and sagittal MR sections (not shown) established the craniocaudal extent of the tumor and better defined its local relationships.

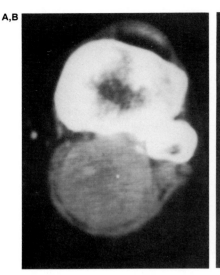
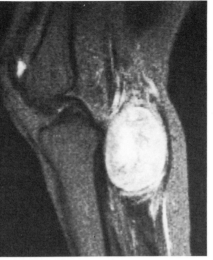

FIG. 32. Neurofibrosarcoma. A 53-year-old woman presented with a mass growing in the popliteal space. **A:** Contrast-enhanced cross-sectional CT image shows large, slightly inhomogeneous, encapsulated tumor in popliteal space. **B:** Parasagittal MR image (TR = 2,100 msec, TE = 120 msec) confirms features shown by CT and defines local relationships and craniocaudal extent.

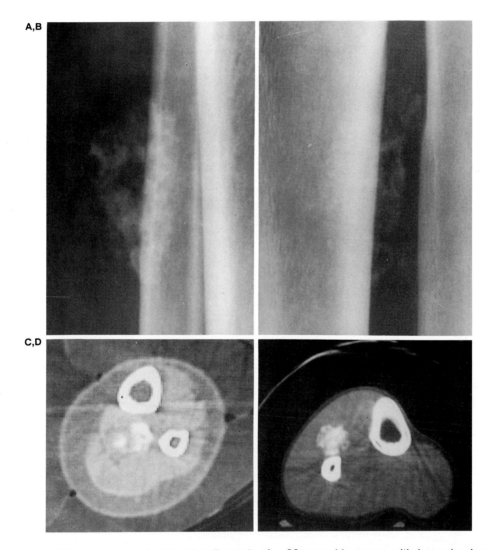

FIG. 33. Mineralized soft-tissue tumors. **A:** Lateral radiograph of a 26-year-old woman with leg pain shows a focal area of amorphous calcification posterior to the tibia. (From ref. 83.) **B:** CT section shows the mass located in the posterior (flexor) compartment of the leg. Whereas much of the mass is mineralized, the medial portion has an attenuation less than that of muscle. This mineralized tumor is an ossifying hemangioma. (From ref. 83.) **C:** Frontal radiograph of a 31-year-old man with leg pain shows a focus of amorphous calcification similar to that seen in part **A. D:** CT shows the mineralized mass located in the anterior (extensor) compartment. No soft-tissue component is apparent. This mineralized mass proved to be a mesenchymal chondrosarcoma.

dionuclide bone scintigraphy, ultrasonography (31,189), and sectional imaging (19,150,362). CT and MRI are far superior to conventional radiography for exclusion, confirmation, and characterization of soft-tissue masses. Both methods are superior to angiography and have essentially replaced it for lesion localization, definition of margins, determination of vascularity and vascular relationships, and aid in diagnosis (81). Angiography is reserved for those instances when sectional imaging fails to define vascular invasion adequately or when a preoperative vascular map is required. Sectional imaging is also superior to bone scintigraphy for determination of the anatomic relationship of a soft-tissue mass to a bone (85). However, bone scintigraphy is more effective for demonstration of a physiologic response of the bone to the adjacent mass (85,161). Radionuclide bone scintigraphy remains the best method to survey the skeleton for metastases. In most instances, CT and MRI are preferred to ultrasonography as the primary imaging tests for extremity masses.

We employ sectional imaging for preoperative characterization and staging of all soft-tissue neoplasia and prefer MRI as the initial or only method in most instances (263). The goal for therapy is complete excision of the tumor, with limb salvage (223) and preservation of function (61,84). Tumors that spare adjacent bone and major vessels and that are limited to a single soft-tissue compartment usually can be resected. When the entire tumor, its reactive rim, and a cuff of normal tissue are removed en bloc, local recurrences are few. If the tumor violates a second compartment, enters a joint, or invades major neurovascular structures, amputation may be required. We rely on sectional imaging to provide the necessary anatomic details. Whereas CT is more effective for analysis of soft-tissue calcification and bone mineral integrity, MRI is preferred for detailed evaluation of soft tissue and bone marrow.

Sectional imaging also is valuable for evaluation of regional soft-tissue anatomy following therapy. Both CT and MRI are effective for demonstration of tumor regression or recurrence. Neither will show microscopic residual or recurrent tumor (160).

BONE MARROW IMAGING

Normal bone marrow consists of three basic biological components (62). The first is the mineralized component that provides structural integrity. This is composed of the cancellous or trabecular bone, with its surrounding envelope of compact or cortical bone. The second component is the hematopoietic or cellular component, known as red marrow, that is responsible for replenishment of cellular components of the blood. The third basic component is fat, represented by numerous adipose cells throughout the medullary cavity in all bones. This com-

ponent is often termed "yellow marrow." All three components are important, and CT and MRI serve different purposes in their evaluation.

CT is an excellent sectional imaging method for analysis of the mineralized component of bone and bone marrow. In general, CT is employed to demonstrate alterations in the amount and condition of cortical and trabecular bone. It is much less effective for demonstration of alterations in the cellular or fatty elements, although it can be used for this purpose.

At birth, except for epiphyses and apophyses, which are fat or yellow marrow, bone marrow is entirely the hematopoietic or red component. Thereafter, bone marrow follows an orderly (though variable) conversion from red to yellow. This begins at the periphery of the appendicular skeleton and extends progressively centrally. The process results in a progressively smaller fraction of hematopoietic cells in marrow spaces (75). Larger fractions of hematopoietic cells persist longest at the proximal ends of the long bones and in the pelvis, vertebrae, and sternum. By adulthood, the appendicular skeleton has predominantly yellow marrow, and even those bones that have persistent red marrow contain roughly 50% yellow marrow.

MRI is the best imaging procedure for evaluation of the cellular marrow elements (267). Compared with other normal tissues, normal bone marrow yields relatively high signal intensity on all spin-echo sequences, because of the fat fraction. Marrow with greater fractions of hematopoietic cells (more water protons) shows lower signal intensity than that with greater fat fractions (more fat protons). This is particularly evident in children, where the epiphyses and apophyses (completely yellow marrow) are of much higher signal intensity than the metaphyses and diaphyses (higher fraction of red marrow) (Fig. 34). A relative difference between epiphyses and metaphyses may persist well into adult life. Overall, the trend is for marrow T1 relaxation times to become shorter with aging, as has been measured in the vertebral bodies of persons at various ages, indicating progressive fatty replacement.

Normal bone marrow appears uniform and homogeneous on MRI, except in specific anatomic locations where there is sufficient trabecular bone (load-bearing trabeculae in metaphyses), cartilage (physeal plate), or fibrosis (the physeal scar following epiphyseal closure) to cause focally decreased signal intensity or where there is focal fat deposition that causes increased signal intensity (126). Although the marrow signal intensity will vary somewhat from patient to patient, usually it is symmetric between sides in a given individual.

With physiologic stresses that require increased production of hematopoietic cells, the T1-weighted signal intensity falls as yellow marrow is converted to red marrow (Fig. 35).

Any process that replaces fat in the marrow will alter its signal characteristics (55,63,172,190,191,230,243,

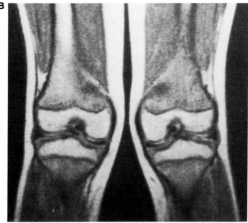
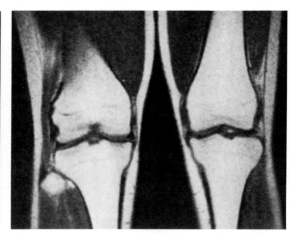

FIG. 34. Yellow and red marrow distribution. **A:** Coronal MR image (TR = 900 msec, TE = 30 msec) of knees of an 8-year-old girl shows high signal intensity from epiphyses (pure yellow marrow) and low signal intensity from metaphyses (primarily red marrow). **B:** Coronal MR image (TR = 300 msec, TE = 30 msec) of knees of a 25-year-old woman shows homogeneous high signal intensity from epiphyses and metaphyses, as all marrow is predominantly yellow.

253,278,297) (Fig. 36). Cellular, granulation, and fibrous tissues are common examples of tissues that may replace normal marrow elements. Because each of these has a longer T1 relaxation time than fat, T1-weighted images are effective to emphasize the contrast differences, to detect abnormal marrow conditions, and to characterize their extent. Although very sensitive, T1-weighted sequences are not specific. Likewise, T2-weighted sequences improve specificity only a small amount. The appropriate diagnosis of a bone marrow disorder is best determined by analysis of the patient's history and other clinical information and may require histologic sampling.

SKELETAL NEOPLASIA

Conventional radiography remains the first technique used for evaluation of skeletal tumors. In most cases, radiographs provide features resulting in the best differential diagnosis and the most probable histopathologic prediction. Occasionally radiographs will yield information clearly indicating that amputation is necessary. In these few cases, no further evaluation is needed. However, current therapeutic approaches emphasize combination chemotherapy and surgery to eradicate tumors and preserve

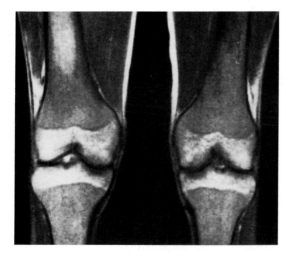

FIG. 35. Stimulation of red marrow production. Coronal MR image (TR = 500 msec, TE = 35 msec) of a 24-year-old man with sickle cell disease shows extensive red marrow distribution (even partially involving the epiphyses), out of proportion to what would normally be expected at this age. Red marrow production is stimulated to accommodate the increased requirement for hematologic cells due to the sickle cell anemia.

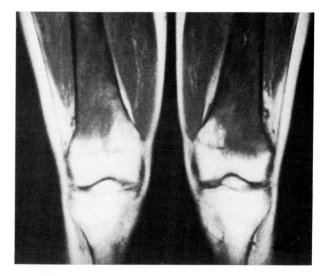

FIG. 36. Replacement of yellow marrow by tumor. Coronal MR image (TR = 300 msec, TE = 15 msec) of a 22-year-old woman with diffuse metastatic small-cell carcinoma shows extensive replacement of femoral diaphyseal and metaphyseal yellow marrow by low-signal-intensity tumor. The radiograph of the knee was normal.

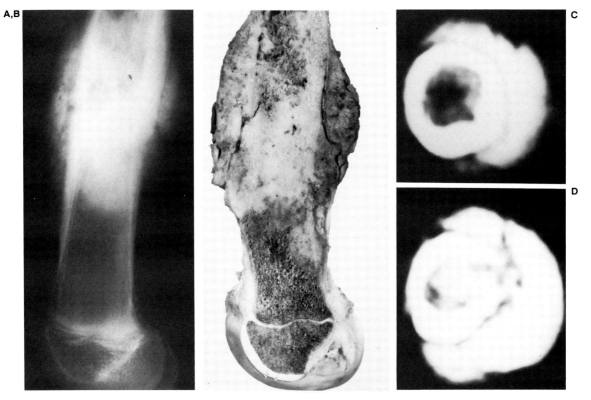

FIG. 37. Intraosseous and extraosseous tumor extent. **A:** Lateral radiograph shows central osteosarcoma of the femur, with mineralized tumor encircling the diaphysis. (From ref. 69.) **B:** Sagittally sectioned gross specimen shows close correlation with CT display of intraosseous and extraosseous tumor distribution. (Courtesy of Dr. Michael Kyriakos, St. Louis, Missouri.) **C:** CT section through the proximal portion of the tumor shows mineralized tumor within the medullary canal and surrounding the medial half. Soft-tissue window settings showed that the mineralized mass displaced normal muscles. (From ref. 69.) **D:** CT section through a distal portion of the tumor showed the sarcoma perforating the medial cortex, nearly filling the medullary canal and surrounding most of the shaft.

functional anatomy whenever possible (120,222). Thus, for most tumors, exact determination of the tumor extent is required (84). In such cases, CT and MRI can define the tumor extent and either confirm resectability or clearly show that amputation is necessary (57,330).

Both CT and MRI can fairly accurately show the location of the primary tumor within the bone, quantify the intramedullary component of the tumor, and define its extraosseous extent (247,365) (Figs. 37 and 38). CT is more sensitive to subtle cortical erosion and better for identification of small amounts of soft-tissue calcification than MRI. The ability of MRI to yield direct coronal and sagittal images and to display higher contrast between the tumor and surrounding normal tissues is a major advantage (12,22,26,286,365). MRI provides better tissue contrast, which allows easier definition of tumor margins. Exquisite sensitivity to marrow replacement allows detailed evaluation of tumor marrow extension. Using coronal or sagittal imaging, examiners can directly measure the craniocaudal tumor extent in marrow and identify "skip" lesions within the marrow cavity that do not erode the endosteal surface.

Both techniques may be used to identify compartmental anatomy, quantify the number of muscle layers involved by the tumor, and show three-dimensional spatial relationships in areas of complex skeletal and soft-tissue anatomy. Both accurately show tumor relationships to vital neural and vascular structures, as well as to adjacent articular surfaces, information that is especially important to the surgeon planning conservative, limb-sparing surgery. With both techniques, allowances must be made for the local effects of edema and postbiopsy hemorrhage, either of which may mimic tumor spread. For neither CT nor MRI have these tissue changes significantly decreased the accuracy of preoperative tumor staging.

Benign Neoplasms

Benign skeletal tumors usually are identified and easily characterized by conventional radiography. This information is generally sufficient for both probable diagnosis and appropriate treatment decisions. Sectional imaging, usually by CT, may be helpful when radiographs fail to

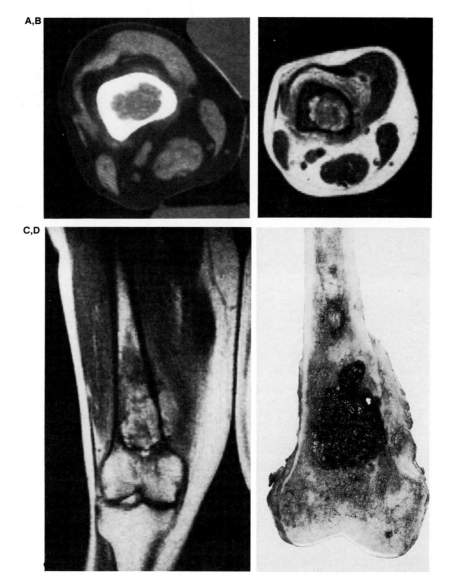

FIG. 38. Angiosarcoma: demonstration of tumor extent. **A:** CT section through distal thigh of a 35-year-old man shows tumor in medullary cavity and infiltration of fat around the femur. **B:** MR image (TR = 500 msec, TE = 30 msec) at similar level shows tumor in medullary cavity, penetration of posteromedial cortex, and more extensive infiltration of surrounding fat. **C:** Coronal MR image (TR = 500 msec, TE = 30 msec) shows proximal and distal extent of tumor, erosion of the medial femoral cortex, and direct extension of the medullary tumor into the medial soft tissues. **D:** Coronal section of amputated femur confirms the findings demonstrated on the coronal MR image. (Courtesy of Dr. Michael Kyriakos, St. Louis, Missouri.)

provide sufficient information about a tumor's characteristics to indicate whether or not a biopsy is necessary. Furthermore, sectional imaging may influence management by increasing diagnostic confidence or by better defining spatial relationships (e.g., in the pelvis, to help plan any contemplated operation).

Cartilaginous neoplasms

Among benign bone neoplasms, cartilaginous lesions are the most common tumors for which sectional imaging is helpful (158). They occur in most age groups, and at

times their radiologic appearances may not allow the radiologist to differentiate benign from malignant lesions. CT can show their mineralization pattern in cross section, an important advantage compared with radiography. Benign cartilaginous lesions have matrix calcification that is relatively evenly distributed, without sizable areas of uncalcified soft-tissue matrix. Occasionally the nature of calcification in a long-bone lesion may be difficult to classify on radiographs, and the differential diagnosis is between a chondrous lesion and a bone infarct. In these cases, bone infarcts can be recognized on CT by their peripherally marginated calcification, instead of the central, irregular calcification seen with chondrous tumors.

MRI often cannot detect small calcifications associated

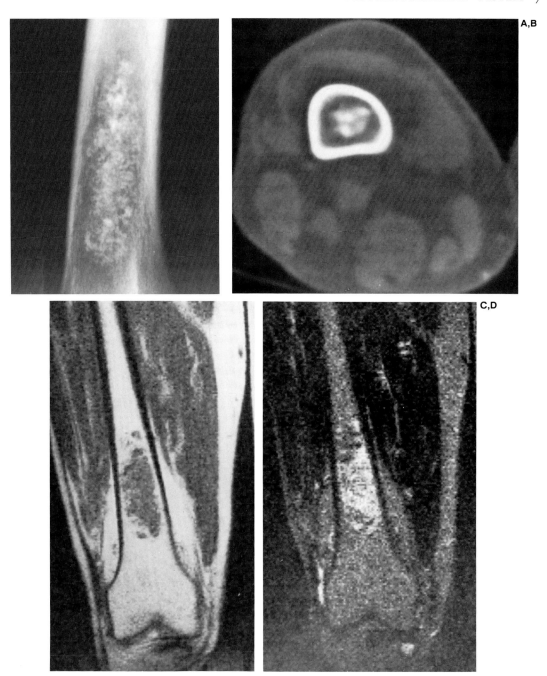

FIG. 39. Enchondroma in a 57-year-old man. **A:** Radiograph of distal femur shows numerous punctate calcifications within the medullary canal. The pattern suggests an enchondroma. **B:** CT section through the femoral metaphysis confirms the calcifications and shows that the endosteal bone surface is normal. **C:** T1-weighted (TR = 500 msec, TE = 35 msec) coronal MR image shows the intramedullary extent of the tumor, but fails to disclose the presence of calcification. **D:** T2-weighted (TR = 2,000 msec, TE = 120 msec) coronal MR image shows high signal intensity from the cartilaginous portion of the tumor, which has a higher fraction of water protons than does the adjacent unaffected marrow.

with a cartilaginous tumor, but it does show replacement of normal high-signal-intensity marrow with neoplastic tissue of low signal intensity on T1-weighted images and higher signal intensity than marrow on T2-weighted images (Fig. 39). In addition to showing any medullary calcifications, CT can be used to evaluate the endosteal sur-

face in cross section; benign lesions generally show no erosion of the endosteal surface. Subtle endosteal-surface erosions are more difficult to detect in cross section by MRI, primarily because of its inability to directly resolve the cortex itself. However, because MRI yields direct coronal and sagittal images, it can better define the longi-

A,B

C,D

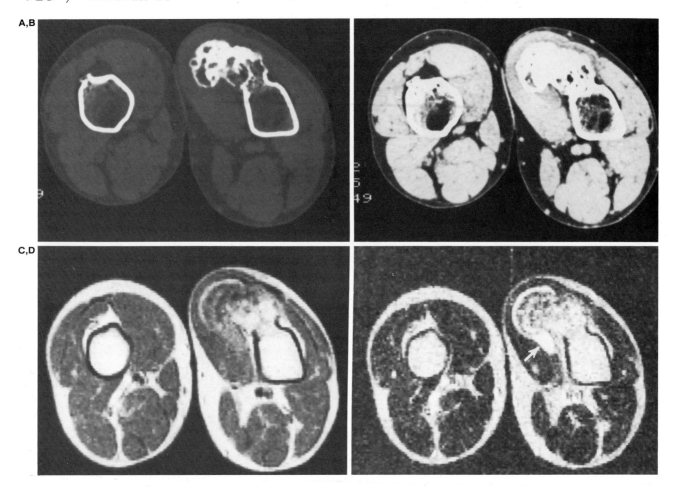

FIG. 40. Exostosis in young man with multiple hereditary exostoses in whom there was clinical concern that chondrosarcoma might be developing. CT sections through the pedunculated exostosis with (**A**) bone and (**B**) soft-tissue window settings show the usual anatomic features of an exostosis: continuity of the medullary cavity with the base of the exostosis, mixed mineralization of the tumor matrix, no soft-tissue mass, and a thin cartilage cap. MR images similar to CT section with (**C**) mixed T1/T2 weighting (TR = 1,500 msec, TE = 30 msec) and (**D**) more pronounced T2 weighting (TR = 1,500 msec, TE = 90 msec) show identical anatomic features. In addition, the MRI shows fluid (*arrow*) within the bursa adjacent to the periphery of the exostosis. This is best seen in the T2-weighted examination, but can also be identified on the CT examination. (From ref. 247.)

tudinal extent of intramedullary lesions than can radiography, scintigraphy, or CT.

Benign osteocartilaginous exostoses that have become symptomatic because of trauma or overlying inflammation may be difficult to distinguish from those in which a chondrosarcoma has developed. CT or MRI of exostoses characteristically shows a bony mass with a sharply defined periphery, an organized central matrix, a medullary cavity continuous with that of the bone from which it arose, and a thin cartilaginous cap (Fig. 40). When it is otherwise difficult to characterize, localize, and differentiate more sessile osteocartilaginous exostoses (such as those found in the spine or pelvis) from chondrosarcomas, cross-sectional imaging may be useful (176). The spatial and vascular relationships of pedunculated exostoses are easily demonstrated. Similarly, sectional imaging clearly demonstrates the cortical nature of juxtacortical (periosteal) chondromas (Fig. 41).

Other benign neoplasms

CT or MRI can be of value for evaluation of many of the less common benign bone lesions in much the same way as for the chondrous lesions. Bone cysts often can be identified on the basis of a thin osseous rim, a near-water-density/intensity central component, and lack of contrast enhancement. Aneurysmal bone cysts may show fluid–fluid levels and/or multiple compartments on either CT or MRI examination (18,155,157) (Fig. 42). Cortical margins may be so thinned that they cannot be appreciated radiographically, but the cyst extent may still be identified in sectional images (Fig. 43). Similar features, including high-attenuation components indicative of blood, may be seen in hemophilic pseudotumors (121,149). For each of these fluid- or blood-containing tumors, MRI typically shows bright signal intensity on T2-weighted sections.

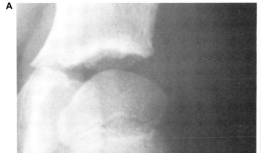

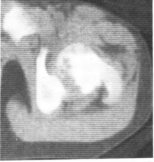

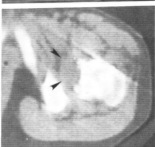

FIG. 41. Juxtacortical chondroma. **A:** Found incidentally in a 7-year-old girl during an excretory urogram, this lesion was radiologically characterized as a destructive process in the femoral neck. **B:** CT through the proximal margin of the lesion shows a productive bone reaction, with irregularity of the posteromedial aspect of the femoral neck. **C:** A section through the middle of the lesion shows an oval soft-tissue mass (*arrowheads*) next to the femoral neck medially, with reactive bone forming a rim around the mass anteriorly and posteriorly. CT correctly characterized the lesion as bone reaction to the adjacent soft-tissue mass, rather than a destructive lesion of the bone itself.

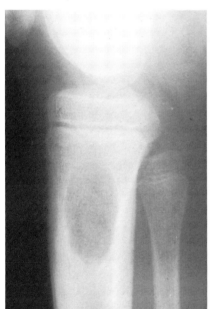

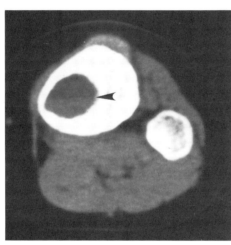

FIG. 42. Aneurysmal bone cyst with fluid layers. **A:** Lateral radiograph of leg of 10-year-old girl shows lytic lesion of proximal tibial metaphysis. **B:** CT image shows layering of fluid within the cyst (*arrowhead*). **C:** Parasagittal MR image (TR = 500 msec, TE = 30 msec) also shows layering of cyst fluid (*arrowhead*).

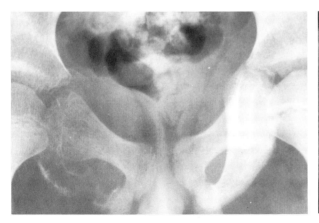

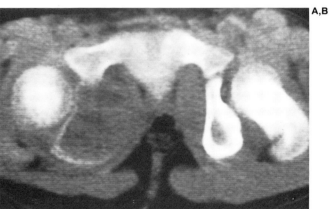

FIG. 43. Aneurysmal bone cyst. **A:** Frontal radiograph shows an expansile lesion of the right ischium, with destruction of the ischial teardrop and ischial portion of the acetabulum. A soft-tissue mass pushes into the pelvis. **B:** CT section through the ischial component of the acetabulum shows tumor expansion that impinges on the hip joint and displaces rather than invades pelvic soft tissue.

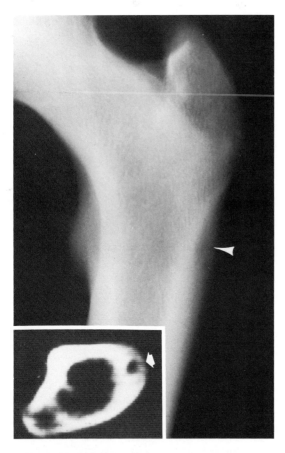

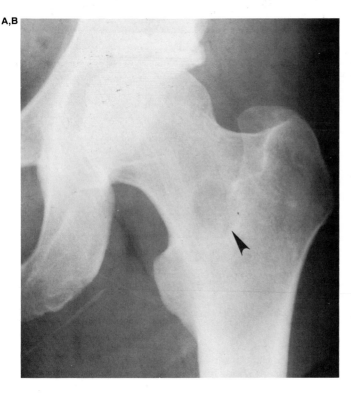

FIG. 44. Osteoid osteoma. Tomography of femur in a 13-year-old boy with hip pain suggested a lucent nidus (*arrowhead*) in the lateral cortex opposite the lesser trochanter. Inset: CT section through the lesser trochanter convincingly showed the nidus (*arrow*) and its location.

A,B

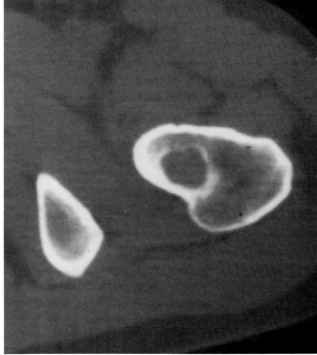

CT often is of particular value for evaluation of osteoid osteoma and osteoblastoma (136). In these lesions, proper identification of the nidus and/or the lesion extent is critical to complete surgical removal and avoidance of recurrence. An osteoid osteoma presents as a lucent focus within surrounding sclerosis (91) (Fig. 44). In some cases, a dense calcified center may be seen. The vascular nature of these lesions results in characteristic enhancement of the nidus following intravenous administration of contrast material (204). Because the nidus often is less than 1 cm in diameter, it may be obscured by surrounding trabecular bone or reactive sclerosis and thus not be identified by conventional radiographic methods. Thin, contiguous sections may be required in order to detect the nidus by CT (1). MRI also can demonstrate the tumor nidus (112).

Fibrous dysplasia characteristically has sharply defined, uninterrupted sclerotic margins on CT images (Fig. 45). A matrix of uniform density may be present, or thick, coarse dense bands may be seen (Fig. 46). MRI of fibrous dysplasia shows uniform or inhomogeneous low-signal marrow replacement on T1-weighted images and a mixed pattern with regions of high signal on T2-weighted sections (Fig. 47). Ossifying fibromas are seen as diffusely calcified cortical lesions on CT examination, a characteristic not seen in other benign lesions that involve the cortex.

CT is important in the evaluation of histologically benign but clinically aggressive lesions such as chondroblastoma and giant-cell tumor. It identifies subtle areas of cortical destruction, periosteal reaction, calcification, and soft-tissue extent not visible on plain radiographs, thereby helping to characterize either tumor. Chondro-

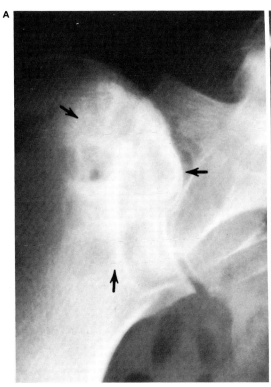

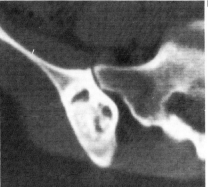

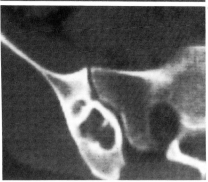

FIG. 46. Unconfirmed fibrous dysplasia. **A:** A mixed lytic and sclerotic lesion (*arrows*) was incidentally found in the right ilium of an 18-year-old girl with no musculoskeletal symptoms. The radiographs were insufficient for confident assignment of a diagnosis. **B, C:** CT sections through the lesion confirmed its mixed lytic and sclerotic nature, but also showed that the lesion was both confined to the ilium and circumscribed by a thick sclerotic rim. The summated features were sufficient for a presumptive diagnosis of fibrous dysplasia, and no surgery was performed.

blastomas are sharply defined lucent lesions in most cases (23,158,269) (Fig. 48). About one-third contain calcifications indicating their cartilage nature. CT may disclose certain complications, such as secondary aneurysmal bone cyst formation not identifiable on radiographs. CT of giant-cell tumors correlates well with the histologic features (68,162,202). CT is less effective for detection or exclusion of articular invasion than is arthrotomography. It helps to combine CT with intraarticular contrast (iodinated or air). MRI may even be more accurate.

Only limited descriptions of rare lesions such as osseous hydatid disease (echinococcosis) (28,30) and intraosseous lipoma (197,276) (Fig. 49) have been reported. Except for intraosseous lipoma, CT and MRI provide no histologically specific information about these lesions, but may be valuable in better characterizing the process.

Malignant Neoplasms

As with benign osseous neoplasms, malignant neoplasms of bone are almost always first identified and initially characterized by conventional radiography (53). In some cases, the radiographs show such extensive bone

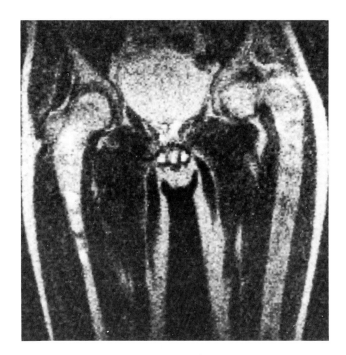

FIG. 47. Polyostotic fibrous dysplasia in a 13-year-old boy. T2-weighted (TR = 1,500 msec, TE = 90 msec) coronal MR image shows irregular replacement of marrow in both femora. Note the mixed signal pattern as well as the expansion and deformity of the left femur.

FIG. 45. Fibrous dysplasia in a 29-year-old man. **A:** AP radiograph of hip shows faint lytic area in intertrochanteric region (*arrowhead*). **B:** CT section through the lesion characterizes it as lucent, with a continuous thin sclerotic margin. The diagnosis was confirmed by percutaneous needle biopsy.

A,B

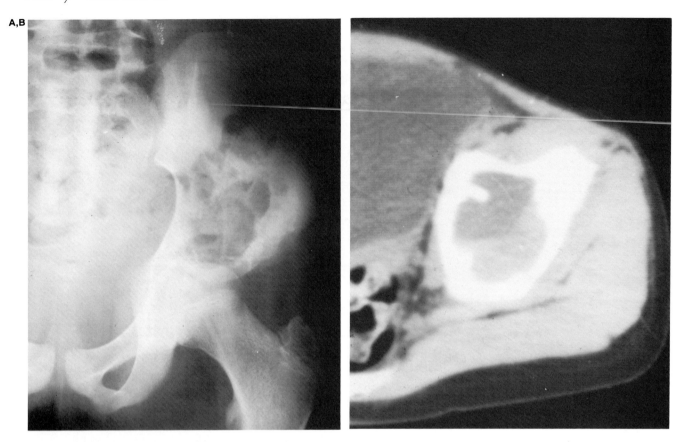

FIG. 48. Chondroblastoma in a 10-year-old girl. **A:** AP radiograph of left hemipelvis shows a destructive lesion of ilium. **B:** CT section shows that the lesion is better circumscribed than indicated by radiographic features. Note the fluid level within the tumor, indicating a cystic component.

and soft-tissue involvement that therapy can be chosen without further radiologic study. However, in most cases, precise definition of the longitudinal intraosseous and radial soft-tissue extent of the lesion is needed to plan adequate resection, while sparing the maximum amount of tissue and retaining as much function as possible (61).

Medullary osteosarcoma

Appropriate therapy depends on the extent of the tumor, and it is in the determination of tumor extent that CT and MRI are of most value (69,163). Osteosarcoma has a spectrum of sectional imaging characteristics that parallel its various descriptive clinical and pathologic subtypes. Lytic, sclerotic, and mixed lytic-sclerotic central (medullary) osteosarcomas are most common. Some osteosarcomas have considerable sclerosis because of production of new bone over large areas (Fig. 50). Other osteosarcomas produce little bone, presenting as primarily lytic lesions (65) (Fig. 51). Both cortical destruction and new bone production are easily demonstrated by CT (Figs. 52 and 53).

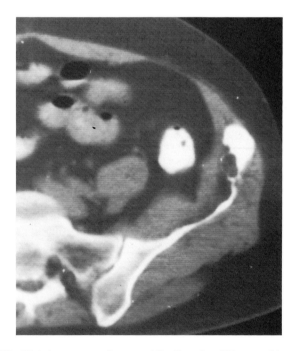

FIG. 49. Intraosseous lipoma of the ilium in a 57-year-old man is characterized by lipomatous replacement of the iliac wing.

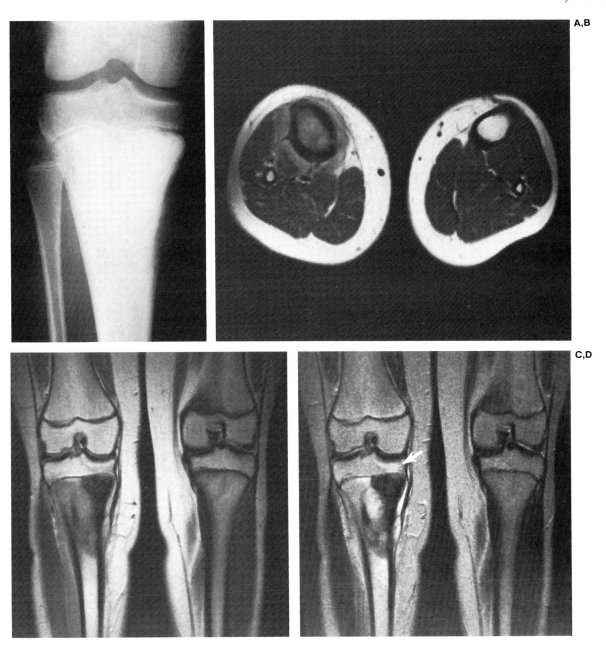

FIG. 50. Sclerotic osteosarcoma in the tibia of a 12-year-old boy. **A:** AP radiograph of the proximal leg shows sclerotic tumor throughout the metaphysis and diaphysis. Extraosseous tumor extent and integrity of the physeal plate cannot be determined. **B:** Transverse MR image (TR = 3,000 msec, TE = 35 msec) shows marrow replacement, cortical permeation, and radial spread around the tibia. **C:** T1-weighted (TR = 500 msec, TE = 17 msec) coronal MR image shows tumor involving the medial half of the physis and confirms extraosseous tumor extent. **D:** T2-weighted (TR = 3,000 msec, TE = 90 msec) coronal MR image shows high signal from epiphysis (*arrow*), indicating presence of tumor and emphasizing extraosseous extent of tumor.

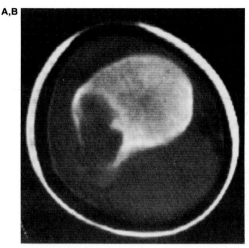

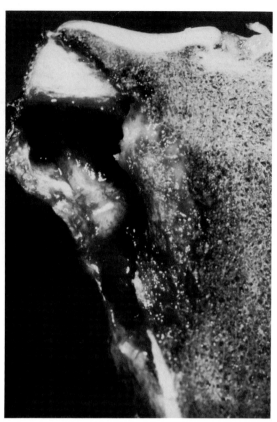

FIG. 51. Primary lytic osteosarcoma: character and extent unobscured by plaster cast. **A:** CT section through proximal tibial metaphysis shows a lytic, moderately well marginated lesion of the lateral tibial plateau. The tumor has perforated the posterolateral cortex and extended into the soft tissues. **B:** Correlation with the gross specimen of this telangiectatic osteosarcoma shows the blood-filled cavity and region of cortical destruction. (Courtesy of Dr. Michael Kyriakos, St. Louis, Missouri.)

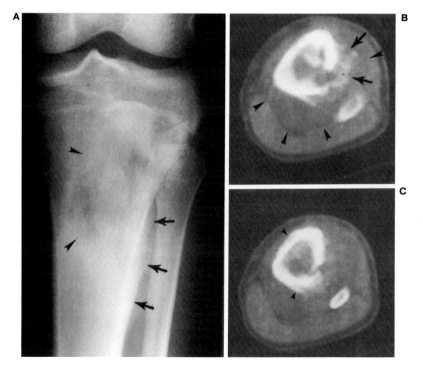

FIG. 52. Central osteosarcoma. **A:** Frontal radiograph shows a predominantly lytic lesion (*arrowheads*) in the lateral aspect of the proximal tibia. Periosteal reaction is present (*arrows*). (From ref. 69.) **B:** CT section through the metaphysis shows posterolateral cortical disruption, mineralizing tumor outside of bone (*arrows*), and a soft-tissue mass (tumor) surrounding the tibia (*arrowheads*). The fibular cortex adjacent to the soft-tissue mass is destroyed. (From ref. 69.) **C:** A section distally shows the periosteal reaction (*arrowheads*).

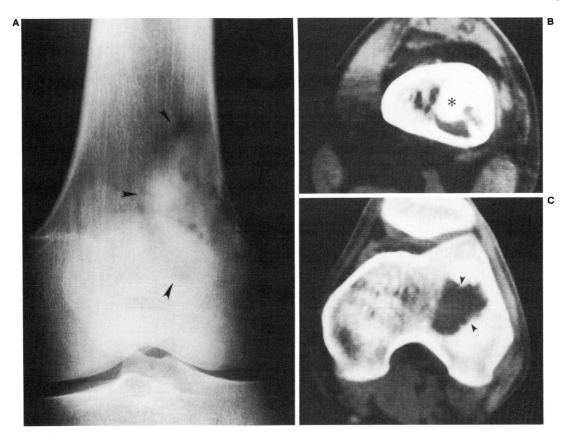

FIG. 53. Central osteosarcoma. **A:** Frontal radiograph shows an osteoblastic lesion in the lateral half of the distal femoral metaphysis (*arrowheads*). **B:** CT section through the proximal portion of the lesion shows its blastic component (*∗*). **C:** A section through the distal portion shows a more lytic zone in the lateral condyle (*arrowheads*). Contiguous CT sections showed that the osteosarcoma was confined to the medullary cavity, that no cortical disruption had occurred, and that the surrounding soft tissues were normal.

Neoplasm replaces the normal, low-attenuation marrow fat in the medullary canal with tumor cells of higher attenuation, allowing direct evaluation of intramedullary tumor extent by CT. Osteosarcoma typically permeates the cortex and extends into the surrounding muscles and fascial planes. The radial tumor extent is easily determined by CT when fat planes are prominent, but may be unclear when the patient is slender. Occasionally, osteosarcoma margins may be blurred by surrounding reactive edema, although generally this is not of clinical significance. More important problems are the edema and hemorrhage that follow biopsy; these alterations sometimes cannot be distinguished from tumor and may lead to an overestimate of tumor extent. Intravenous contrast enhancement can aid the determination of tumor spread, as it may make tumor margins more easily distinguishable and may facilitate demonstration of vascular relationships if the tumor is adjacent to the neurovascular bundle (308).

The possible presence of "skip" metastases is of vital importance in the staging of osteosarcoma; identifying or excluding such lesions in patients considered candidates for limb-sparing surgery is best accomplished with contiguous 1-cm imaging (308).

MRI is an effective sectional imaging method for staging osteosarcoma (329,366). The sensitivity of T1-weighted images to marrow fat replacement provides a stark outline of the low-signal tumor against the high-signal marrow fat (Figs. 50 and 54). Coronal or sagittal images along the long axis of the involved bone allow precise measurement of longitudinal extent, as well as identification of skip metastases in the marrow.

MRI takes advantage of intermuscular fat planes, but unlike CT, MRI is not fully dependent on them to distinguish between tumor and adjacent normal tissue. Osteosarcoma usually appears on a T2-weighted image as a high-signal mass that is clearly different from muscle (26,29,365,366) (Figs. 50 and 54). Lesions with a large amount of new bone will be of lower signal intensity on T2 images because of the absence of signal from the bone (22). An additional advantage of MRI is that vascular structures can be identified without injection of contrast material by the vascular flow-void phenomenon. MRI has

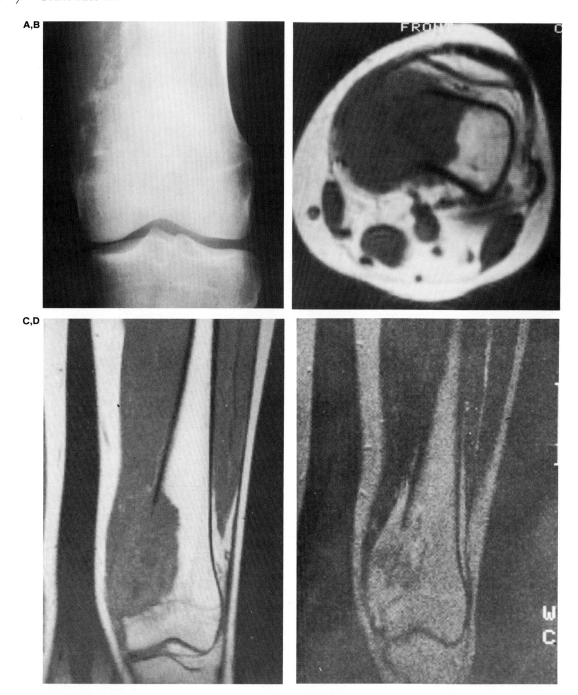

FIG. 54. Central osteosarcoma in the distal femur of an 18-year-old woman. **A:** AP radiograph of the distal left femur shows a destructive tumor that has broken out of the bone medially. **B:** Transverse T1-weighted (TR = 300 msec, TE = 17 msec) MR image shows sharp margins between tumor and marrow or adjacent fat. **C:** Coronal T1-weighted (TR = 500 msec, TE = 17 msec) MR image shows craniocaudal extent of tumor and invasion of the epiphysis. **D:** Coronal T2-weighted (TR = 3,000 msec, TE = 90 msec) MR image shows relationship of tumor to muscle.

been shown to be better than CT for delineating the marrow and soft-tissue extent of bone tumors in about one-third of cases and equal to CT in the other two-thirds (29).

Parosteal osteosarcoma

Parosteal osteosarcoma (343) is the second important subtype of osteosarcoma. Local resection, with tumor-free margins, is the accepted treatment because it leads to a less aggressive clinical course (40). Imaging with CT or MRI provides the same advantages for parosteal osteosarcoma as for medullary (central) osteosarcoma, including more precise definition of tumor spread along the cortex and into the medullary cavity (164,210) (Fig. 55). Radial growth into soft tissues and relationships to the neurovascular bundle are accurately depicted (Fig. 56).

Periosteal (127,342) and intracortical osteosarcomas are rare. Accurate definition of tumor extent is critical to surgical planning, as local recurrence is common if tumor-free margins are not achieved. CT is accurate for identification of these tumor types and mapping of their extent.

Beyond the initial evaluation of osteosarcomas, CT and

MRI have important roles in assessing a tumor's response to therapy and in detecting local and distant metastases. Base-line imaging studies of the surgical site after resection are necessary and provide a standard against which follow-up examinations can be compared. A response to chemotherapy is evidenced by a decrease in tumor size. Development of a new soft-tissue mass indicates recurrent tumor in most cases. Neither CT nor MRI is effective for demonstration of microscopic foci of residual or recurrent tumor.

Chondrosarcoma

Malignant chondrous tumors are clearly depicted by both CT and MRI (137,159,165,176,296). Malignant exostotic chondrosarcoma may show thickening of the cartilage cap, with development of a soft-tissue mass that invades surrounding normal tissues (Fig. 57). Irregular calcifications located within the cartilage cap, as shown by CT, suggest malignant transformation. Thin (less than 2.0 cm) cartilage caps may be more difficult to distinguish from overlying normal soft tissue on CT (165). Other

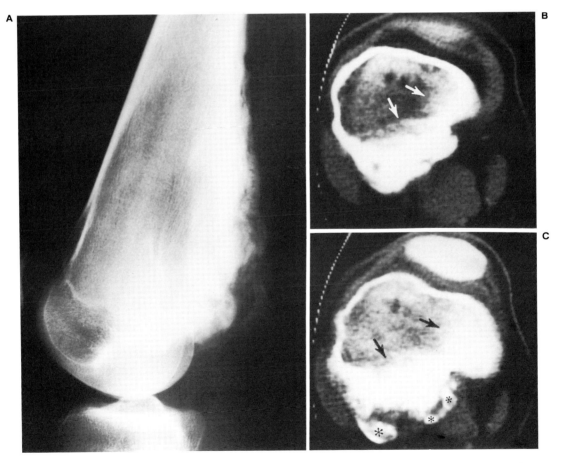

FIG. 55. Parosteal osteosarcoma. **A:** Lateral radiograph shows a long, dense knobby tumor along the posterior aspect of the femur. **B,C:** CT sections show the tumor arising from the posterior cortex and extending into the medullary trabecular bone (*arrows*). Other than small juxtaosseous mineralized nodules (∗), the tumor was confined to bone. On the basis of this information, a local resection was performed. (From ref. 69.)

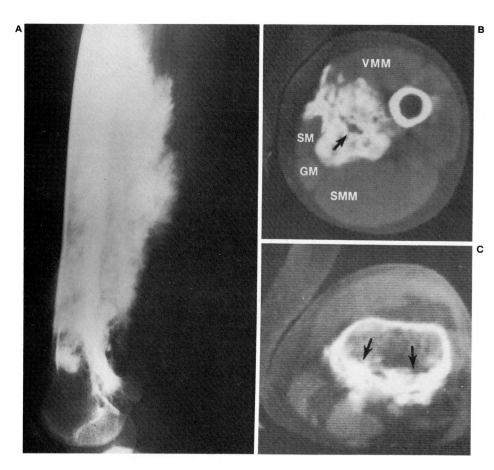

FIG. 56. Parosteal osteosarcoma. A: Lateral radiograph shows a huge mineralized mass in the thigh. B: CT of the proximal portion of the mass shows the tumor insinuated among the vastus medialis (VMM), sartorius (SM), gracilis (GM), and semimembranosus (SMM) muscles and extending from the bone surface to the subcutaneous fat. Furthermore, the mineralized mass encased the femoral artery, vein, and nerve (*arrow*). C: Distally, CT shows the tumor arising from the posterior femoral cortex and invading the medullary trabecular bone (*arrows*). On the basis of this information, a hip disarticulation was performed.

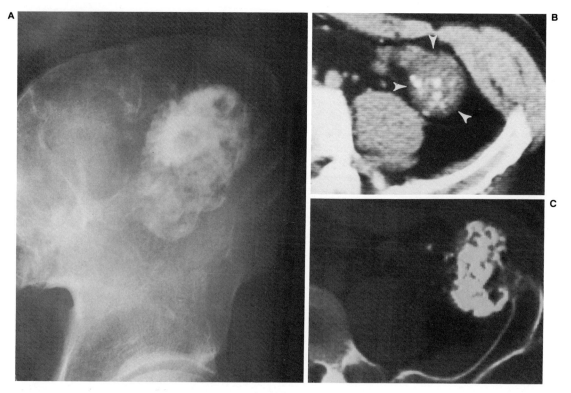

FIG. 57. Chondrosarcoma. A: In a 30-year-old man with multiple hereditary exostoses, a new calcified mass was discovered. (From ref. 176.) B: CT section at a soft-tissue window just cephalad to the densely mineralized mass shows a large, round soft-tissue mass (*arrowheads*), with a few small internal calcifications. This large cartilaginous component strongly suggested chondrosarcoma. C: A section at a bone window through the mineralized mass shows that it arises and projects medially from the anterior iliac crest.

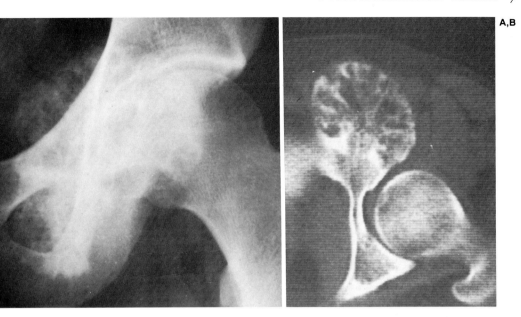

A,B

FIG. 58. Exostosis (osteochondroma). **A:** Frontal radiograph shows a large cartilaginous tumor superimposed on the left hip. Multiple special projections failed to adequately demonstrate its relationship to the pubis or to provide sufficient information to differentiate an exostosis from a chondrosarcoma. **B:** CT showed its origin from the superior pubic ramus, excluded any soft-tissue component, correctly indicated its benign nature, and provided anatomic information that helped in surgical planning. (From ref. 176.)

characteristics suggesting a malignant tumor include destruction of adjacent bone and the presence of large unmineralized areas within a partially calcified mass (296).

CT is the better sectional method for evaluation of the calcified or ossified portions of chondrous tumors and has been effective in distinguishing between benign cartilage tumors and chondrosarcomas (176) (Fig. 58). The increased sensitivity of MRI to soft-tissue differences may help distinguish between abnormal cartilage and normal tissue.

Central chondrosarcoma, a neoplasm located within the medullary cavity in long bones, sometimes contains irregular chondrous calcifications that are readily detected by CT, but may be missed with MRI (Fig. 59). The malignant nature of the lesion is suggested by destruction of the surrounding cortical bone ("pushing" margins), areas of necrosis within the tumor, and the presence of large noncalcified areas within the lesion (159).

The primary value of sectional imaging in evaluation of chondrosarcoma is the definition of tumor extent. CT provides an accurate depiction of tumor extent (137,159). MRI may better define both the intramedullary extent and soft-tissue extent of central chondrosarcoma in the same way that it does with osteosarcoma (Fig. 59). However, as with osteosarcoma, MRI will not identify small soft-tissue calcifications.

Other sarcomas of bone

CT also has been used to evaluate the less common primary malignant bone tumors, including chordomas

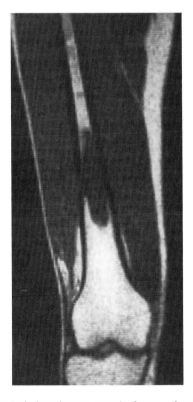

FIG. 59. Central chondrosarcoma in femur of a 30-year-old man. Coronal T1-weighted (TR = 300 msec, TE = 15 msec) MR image shows tumor extent, with replacement of fatty bone marrow.

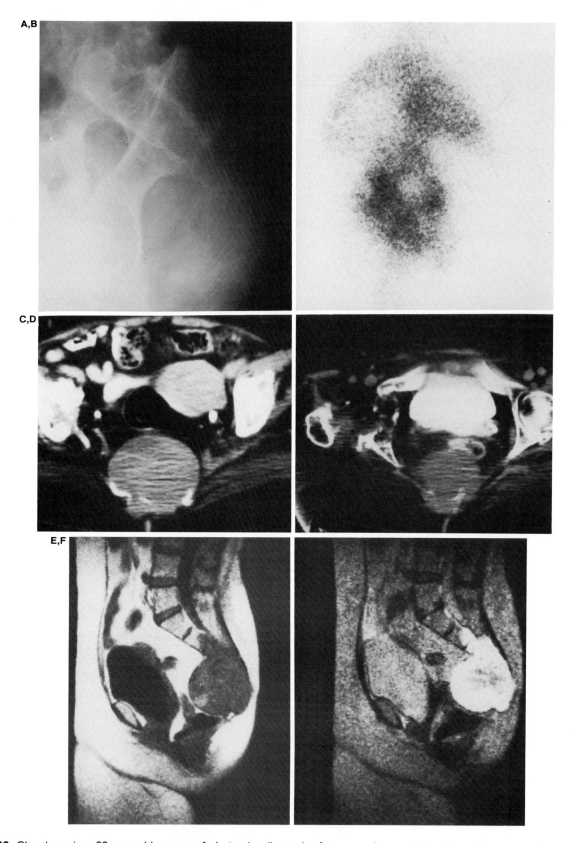

FIG. 60. Chordoma in a 60-year-old woman. **A:** Lateral radiograph of sacrum shows destruction of lower sacral segments and coccyx. There appears to be a soft-tissue mass. **B:** Lateral view from bone scan shows absence of radionuclide accumulation in the distal sacrum. Focal uptake anteriorly is due to hip osteoarthritis. Axial CT sections through middle of tumor (**C**) and caudal end of tumor (**D**) show relationships to sacrum and rectum. From the entire sequence of axial sections, it was still difficult to determine precisely the longitudinal extent and local relationships of the tumor. Note also the presence of osteoarthritis in the right hip. Parasagittal MR images with (**E**) T1-weighting (TR = 300 msec, TE = 30 msec) and (**F**) T2-weighting (TR = 1,500 msec, TE = 90 msec) show anteroposterior and craniocaudal extent and relationships to adjacent structures very well. Note the long T1 and T2 relaxation characteristics of the tumor. (From ref. 247.)

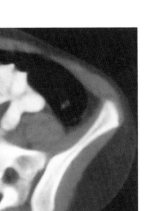

FIG. 61. Ewing sarcoma of right ilium in an 11-year-old girl. CT section shows permeative destruction of the right ilium, a large soft-tissue mass, and displacement of muscles and bowel.

(153,156,298) (Fig. 60), fibrosarcoma (332), malignant fibrous histiocytoma (77,332), and liposarcoma. In each case, the emphasis is on the ability of sectional studies to define tumor extent. MRI provides a better determination of marrow and soft-tissue extent, but a poorer evaluation of tumor calcification and bone mineral integrity, than does CT.

Small-cell neoplasms

CT and MRI have been shown to be of great value for recognition of abnormalities and for therapy planning. Several studies evaluating Ewing sarcoma (Fig. 61) have emphasized the ability to use CT and MRI to detect tumors in sites of complex anatomy, evaluate the radial extent of the tumor, plan radiation ports and surgery, and evaluate therapeutic responses (29,110,344) (Fig. 62).

In the evaluation of adult leukemia and lymphoma (Figs. 63 and 64), CT images display patterns of bone abnormality that parallel those seen on conventional radiographs. These patterns include skeletal permeation, destruction, and sclerosis. Soft tissue may be normal, displaced, or invaded by large or small masses. CT and MRI are particularly helpful in detecting, confirming, and defining the extent of abnormality, especially in areas of complex anatomy such as the chest wall. Such information may be essential in planning CT-guided biopsy. Both CT and MRI are useful in identifying recurrent disease.

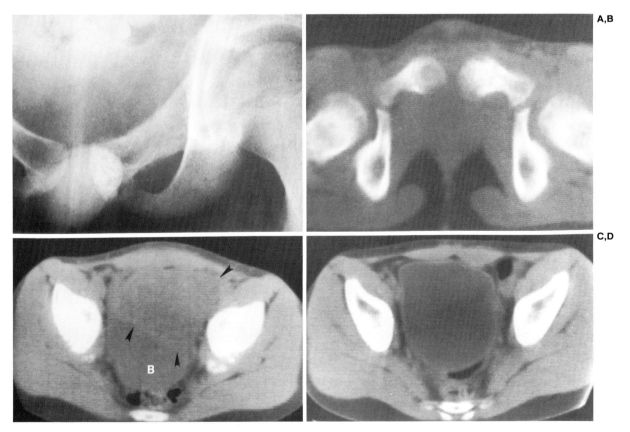

FIG. 62. Follow-up of Ewing sarcoma treated with chemotherapy. **A:** Frontal radiograph at initial presentation shows a motheaten, slightly sclerotic left superior pubic ramus. **B:** CT of the superior pubic ramus shows slight expansion and sclerosis of the bone. **C:** CT through the pelvis, just proximal to the hips, shows a large tumor mass (*arrowheads*) anterior to the bladder (B). **D:** Following chemotherapy, the mass has disappeared. The entire pelvis is now occupied by the fluid-filled bladder.

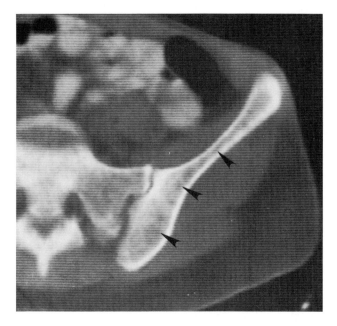

FIG. 63. Leukemia. CT of pelvis in 26-year-old woman with chronic myelogenous leukemia in blastic crisis shows numerous small foci of trabecular destruction (*arrowheads*).

Similar information may be provided in the evaluation of myeloma and solitary plasmacytoma (143,309) (Fig. 65). CT may also demonstrate lesions (initial or recurrent) when both radiography and bone scintigraphy findings are normal (Fig. 66).

Metastases

Most metastases to the skeleton are detected and confirmed by radiography or bone scintigraphy (128). Unsuspected bony metastases sometimes are recognized on CT images obtained for evaluation of another clinical problem. In some cases, metastases can be detected only by assessment of medullary marrow density (142).

CT patterns of metastases are similar to those seen with radiography (Fig. 67). However, in addition to confirmation of a lytic or sclerotic lesion, the radial extent of the metastasis is more easily appreciated. This may be important in planning radiation ports or biopsy sites. Occasionally, CT may be the only imaging procedure to detect and localize a metastasis convincingly, especially in areas of complex anatomy such as the spine (128). CT is particularly useful for detection and characterization of metastases that are suspected because of scintigraphic abnormalities, but not confirmed by standard radiography (128).

The high sensitivity of MRI for detection of marrow replacement makes it especially valuable for identifying

A,B

C,D

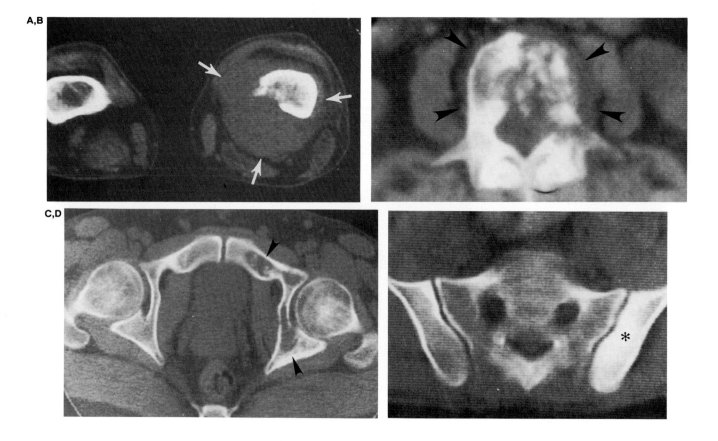

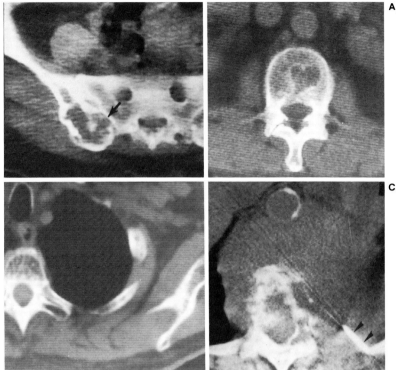

FIG. 65. Multiple myeloma. A: Plasmacytoma in a 45-year-old woman is characterized by an expansile lesion of the posterior iliac spine that has irregular margins, as well as focal cortical destruction adjacent to the sacroiliac joint (arrow). B: Plasmacytoma in a 71-year-old man incidentally found in L2 vertebral body is a sharply marginated, heart-shaped zone of trabecular lysis. C: Myelomatosis in a 65-year-old woman is manifested as many small holes in the vertebral body, ribs, and scapula. D: Myeloma with a large paravertebral soft-tissue mass, as well as vertebral-body dissolution, in an 81-year-old woman. Note the needle (arrowheads) in position for percutaneous biopsy of the paraspinal mass.

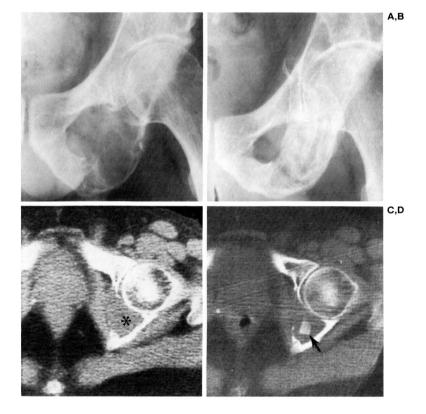

FIG. 66. Follow-up of plasmacytoma treated by curettage, bone graft, and radiation therapy. A: Frontal radiograph before treatment shows a lytic lesion of the ischium. B: A similar radiograph following therapy seems to show incorporation of the bone graft and healing. C: The pretherapy CT through the ischial contribution to the posterior acetabulum confirms the plasmacytoma (*). D: Following treatment, CT performed at the same time as the radiograph (B) shows the bone graft fragment (arrow) surrounded by a persistent soft-tissue mass.

FIG. 64. Lymphoma. A: Lymphocytic lymphoma of distal left femur fills the medullary cavity, destroys the posteromedial cortex, and surrounds the entire metaphysis (arrows). B: Histiocytic lymphoma has partially destroyed T11 vertebral body, but only a small paravertebral soft-tissue mass is present (arrowheads). C: Histiocytic lymphoma has completely replaced the marrow of the left superior pubic ramus and ischium (arrowheads). The involved marrow space has a lower attenuation value, except for several round calcifications. At no site was there cortical disruption or a soft-tissue mass. D: Histiocytic lymphoma has stimulated a diffuse sclerosis (*) of the left ilium. No bone destruction or soft-tissue mass was identified.

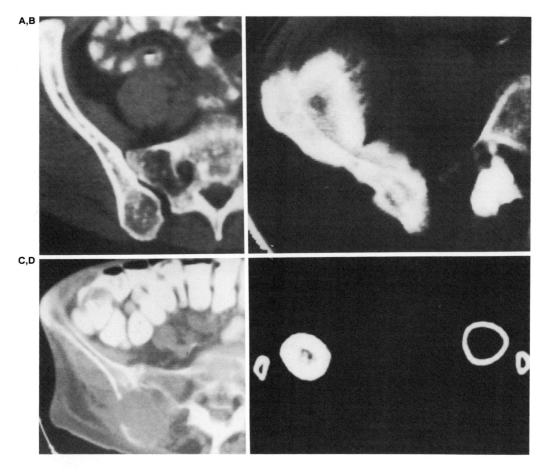

FIG. 67. Metastases. **A:** Multiple punctate, dense breast cancer metastases in the pelvis of a 52-year-old woman. **B:** Prostatic cancer metastasis completely permeates the ilium and pushes into the pelvis of this 70-year-old man. Note the "sunburst" orientation of the mineralized metastatic tumor as shown at this bone window. **C:** Metastatic carcinoma from an unknown primary tumor has replaced the entire posterior iliac spin of this 69-year-old woman. **D:** Breast cancer metastasis nearly fills the right tibial diaphysis of this 61-year-old woman.

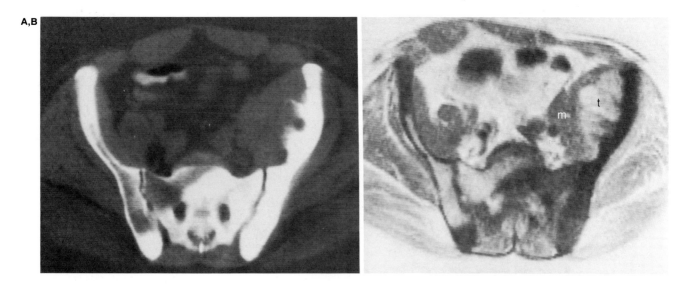

FIG. 68. Metastatic prostate carcinoma. **A:** Transverse CT section through pelvis shows blastic metastases in sacrum and both innominate bones. On the left side, there is extension of the blastic tumor medially associated with a soft-tissue mass. The tumor mass cannot be differentiated from the iliopsoas muscle. **B:** Transverse MR image (TR = 900 msec, TE = 30 msec) at same level as CT section shows identical distribution of marrow disease and clearly indicates the tumor extension from the left iliac wing. MRI is superior to CT for distinguishing tumor (t) and muscle (m). (From ref. 247.)

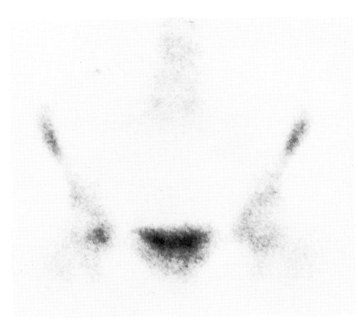
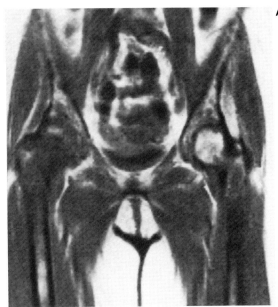

A,B

FIG. 69. Metastatic breast cancer to pelvis and femora of 63-year-old woman. **A:** Radionuclide bone scan shows faint radionuclide accumulation in right hip, but is otherwise unremarkable. **B:** Coronal T1-weighted (TR = 500 msec, TE = 30 msec) MR image shows diffuse marrow replacement by metastatic breast cancer. There are many round deposits in iliac bones, and almost total replacement of right femoral marrow.

tumor deposits in marrow (63) (Fig. 68). Detection of metastases by MRI in the presence of normal findings on bone scintigraphy is valuable (Fig. 69).

Skeletal pseudotumors

Hemophiliac patients develop intraosseous hemorrhages that may expand bone (121,149). As with a true neoplasm, CT can display the radial extent of such a lesion and define its spatial relationships with other important structures (Fig. 70). Such information can be important in their management, particularly if surgery becomes necessary. CT also can be used to differentiate between osseous dysplasia associated with neurofibromatosis and bony changes due to benign or malignant neural tumors (Fig. 71).

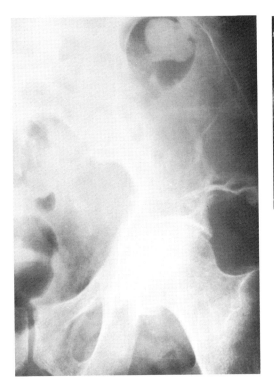
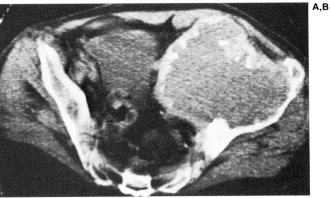

A,B

FIG. 70. Pseudotumor of hemophilia. **A:** Frontal radiograph shows a lytic, expansile lesion of the left ilium. Its true extent cannot be determined. **B:** CT section through midportion of the lesion shows its size, location, and homogeneous matrix.

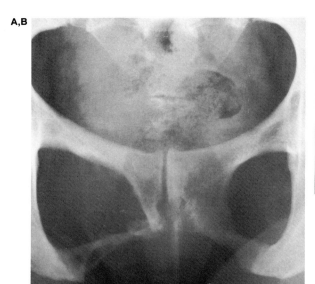

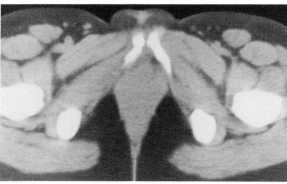

FIG. 71. Pseudotumor of neurofibromatosis. **A:** Frontal radiograph shows an enlarged right obturator foramen, as well as what appear to be pressure erosions of the pubic bones. **B:** CT section through the obturator foramina shows normal muscles and no tumor. Bone "erosions" were then attributed to the osseous dysplasia that sometimes accompanies neurofibromatosis.

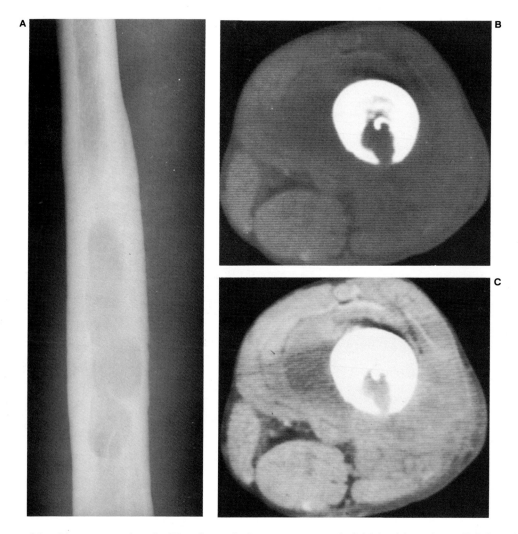

FIG. 72. Osteomyelitis with sequestration. **A:** AP radiograph demonstrates cortical thickening and a well-defined lucent lesion. **B:** CT with bone windows confirms cortical thickening and demonstrates an unsuspected posterior cortical defect. The study also demonstrates a dense crescentic bony fragment separate from the thickened cortex, consistent with a sequestrum not seen using conventional radiographs. **C:** Soft-tissue windowing at the same level demonstrates peripheral displacement of normal muscle groups by inhomogeneous regions representing soft-tissue inflammation.

Clinical Application

Conventional radiography is the imaging procedure of choice for initial evaluation of bone tumors. For benign neoplasms, this information usually is sufficient for both diagnosis and treatment. For malignant osseous neoplasms, staging the extent of the condition requires sectional imaging (2,67,203). Whereas CT is the preferred method for evaluation of trabecular and cortical integrity and characterization of tumor mineralization, MRI (T1-weighted sequences) is used for estimation of longitudinal intramedullary tumor spread. Both CT and MRI provide excellent estimates of radial spread of bone tumors into the surrounding soft tissues, but MRI (mixed or T2-weighted sequences) generally shows a more conspicuous interface between tumor and normal tissue (365,366). Likewise, both provide an estimate of major-vessel involvement by tumor, but MRI does so without the need for injection of a contrast agent and with better contrast conspicuity (200). Angiography is reserved for those rare occasions when a preoperative vascular map is required. Radionuclide scintigraphy provides information regarding axial spread, multiplicity of the primary tumor, and distant metastases.

Sectional imaging is also essential for evaluation of a tumor following therapy (141). If the tumor was not resected, the comparison should be with the study obtained just prior to institution of therapy and any subsequent studies. If the tumor was resected, the comparison should be with a study obtained soon after resection, as well as with any other subsequent examinations. It is advisable to use the same sectional method, CT or MRI, for monitoring therapeutic response, rather than alternating between the methods. This provides better continuity and an improved opportunity to detect an important anatomic change.

NONNEOPLASTIC MUSCULOSKELETAL CONDITIONS

Infection

CT and MRI are not generally necessary for initial documentation, localization, or diagnosis of infection because conventional radiographs usually are adequate (20). Radionuclide imaging remains the standard screening method for detection of subradiographic osteomyelitis. CT should be reserved for detailed delineation of bony cavities, sequestra, or cloacae (145,186,313,359) (Fig. 72), for demonstration of inflammatory bony changes in complex articulations or bones (151,213,240,244,271, 291,303), for demonstration of foreign bodies not visible by conventional radiography (359), and for guiding percutaneous aspiration biopsy or drainage procedures when indicated (151,271,313). These capabilities enable CT to play an important part in the treatment of selected cases of chronic osteomyelitis (151,313,359) (Fig. 73).

CT may detect specific signs of osteomyelitis, including

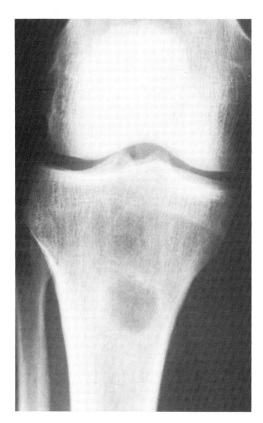
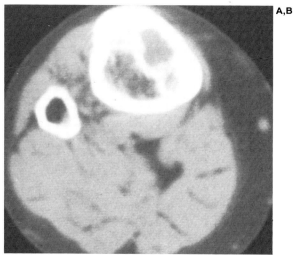

A,B

FIG. 73. Brodie's abscess. **A:** AP knee radiograph demonstrates a well-defined eccentric proximal tibial lucency, with sclerotic borders, in this 28-year-old woman with a 2-year history of a dull ache. **B:** CT demonstrates that the soft tissues about the tibia are normal. The lesion is localized to the anteromedial tibia and has a well-defined margin and a lobulated appearance.

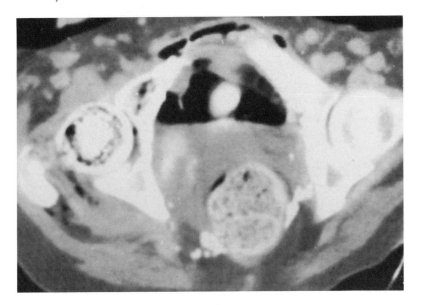

FIG. 74. Osteomyelitis with intraosseous gas. CT section at the level of the femoral heads demonstrates gas within the trabeculae of the right femoral head and superior pubic ramus, as well as in the soft tissues, in this 47-year-old woman with cervical carcinoma and multiple pelvic abscesses. The posterior pararectal densities are the result of prior parametrial injections of radioactive gold.

intraosseous gas (275,291) (Fig. 74), intracortical fissuring (290) (Fig. 75), and fat–fluid (pus) levels (217). The evaluation of osseous tuberculosis and hydatid disease (echinococcosis) of bone (28,30) has been aided by the use of CT (Fig. 76).

Osteomyelitis results in replacement of normal marrow with exudate, fibrosis, and hemorrhage. Fat necrosis and bony proliferation also may be present in varying proportions. CT analysis of the medullary content may detect the alterations in marrow composition that accompany osteomyelitis (186). However, the abnormal marrow of osteomyelitis is better imaged using MRI (20,247) (Fig. 77). T1-weighted sequences are used to maximize the

contrast between normal and infiltrated bone marrow (97). Normal marrow, with its homogeneous high signal, is replaced by tissues with longer T1 values (and hence decreased signal intensity on T1-weighted sequences). T2-weighted sequences usually will demonstrate increased signal intensity from the areas of marrow abnormality, reflecting prolonged T2 values (probably as a result of increased water and blood in the affected region). By taking advantage of the ability of MRI to image directly in the coronal and parasagittal planes along the long axis of an infected bone, peripheral interfaces of infection with normal marrow and adjacent soft tissues are more clearly demonstrated than with alternative methods (97,240,348).

A,B

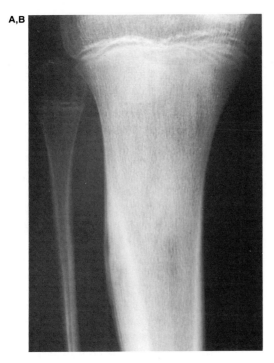

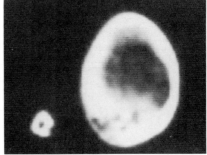

FIG. 75. Osteomyelitis with fissuring. A: This 11-year-old girl presented with mild right-leg pain of 2 years' duration. Radiographs showed cortical thickening and lamellar new bone formation of the posterolateral proximal tibial diaphysis. The characteristics were insufficient to distinguish between benign and malignant causes. B: CT confirmed the cortical thickening, but also showed intracortical tunnels (fissures), seen as holes in the sclerotic bone, and involvement of the medullary cavity. The lesion was removed surgically and proved to be chronic osteomyelitis.

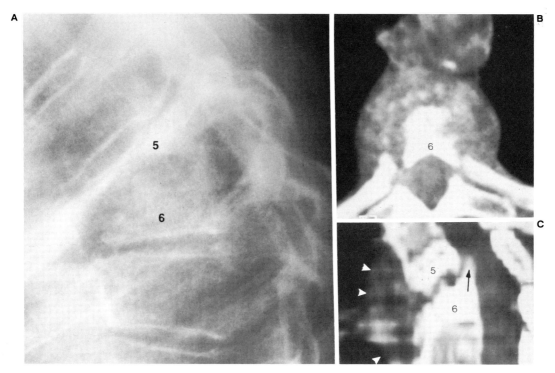

FIG. 76. Tuberculous discitis and spondylitis. **A:** This 93-year-old woman presented with a progressive paraplegia and a T6 localization of sensory deficit. Radiographs localized a disc-centered destructive lesion to the T5–T6 disc space, but did not further characterize the lesion. **B:** CT cross section through T6 shows the vertebral destruction, fragmentation, and paraspinal mass. **C:** CT section reformatted in a sagittal plane shows that T5 is largely destroyed and that a sharp posterosuperior spur of T6 encroaches on the canal (*arrow*), a condition aggravated by the gibbus deformity caused by disc and bone destruction. An anterior soft-tissue mass was also shown (*arrowheads*). Tuberculosis was proved by a percutaneous biopsy under fluoroscopic guidance.

An MRI examination of suspected osteomyelitis should be expected to confirm or exclude marrow abnormality, demonstrate cortical and soft-tissue involvement, and characterize the extent of marrow involvement (240,241). An MRI examination showing only normal marrow is a good indication that there is no infection. When conventional radiography and bone scintigraphy are nondiagnostic, MRI may detect or exclude an abnormality.

Both CT and MRI demonstrate soft-tissue changes notably better than conventional radiography (20,28,70, 97,186,240,247,271,348,359). They have been useful in evaluating primary soft-tissue abscesses, sinus tracts, joint effusions, swelling, edema, necrosis, sterile fluid collections, and infiltrative changes in fat adjacent to soft-tissue infections. Also, soft-tissue pressure ulcers and their complications have been successfully evaluated (92). Soft-tissue changes often are more conspicuous on MRI than on CT (20,247).

Arthritis

Conventional radiography remains the standard imaging method for evaluating joints in patients suspected of having arthritis. In most cases, a correct diagnosis can be established on the basis of the clinical history and physical examination, coupled with selected supplementary laboratory and plain roentgenographic tests. The de-

tailed display of cross-sectional anatomy provided by CT can be beneficial in demonstrating arthropathic processes in complex articulations and in bones difficult to evaluate fully by conventional radiography.

CT is especially useful in evaluating the sacroiliac joint in patients who may have sacroiliitis and spondyloarthropathy (27). The curved, angulated surfaces of the normal sacroiliac joint are easily displayed with CT (109,356). Although the advanced changes of sacroiliitis may be obvious on conventional radiographs, early evidence of inflammatory sacroiliitis can best be detected and differentiated from normal age-related degenerative changes by CT (27,47,48,88,185,194,300,347,357).

CT is superior to conventional radiography and tomography for assessing the sternoclavicular joint (70). It is particularly useful in evaluating patients suspected of having sternocostoclavicular hyperostosis, a disorder found most often in persons of Japanese descent (50,289,305).

In patients with rheumatoid arthritis, CT has been very useful for evaluating the region of the craniocervical junction, often more accurately demonstrating the extent of erosion, subluxation, soft-tissue changes, and atlantoaxial impaction (32,49,279).

MRI has no established role in the evaluation of arthritis involving the appendicular skeleton (187). It is capable of demonstrating articular cartilage and may be useful in

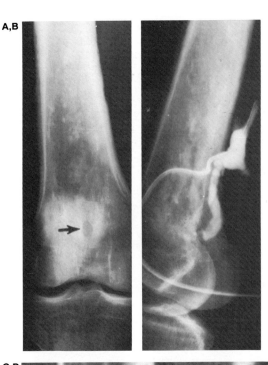

FIG. 77. Chronic osteomyelitis. **A:** AP radiograph of distal femur shows cortical thickening and cancellous sclerosis typical of chronic osteomyelitis. The extent of medullary involvement cannot be determined. An oval lucency (*arrow*) is observed that represents the cloaca, where the infection has perforated the cortex and periosteum to initiate a sinus tract to the skin. **B:** Lateral radiograph following filling of the sinus tract with an iodinated contrast agent shows the tract connecting with the femur at the level of the cloaca. **C:** Coronal MRI (TR = 300 msec, TE = 30 msec) through the distal femur shows the abscess as an irregularly marginated region of low signal (long T1) surrounded by higher-signal bone marrow. **D:** Coronal MRI (TR = 2,100 msec, TE = 30 msec) slightly more dorsal shows focal destruction of the metaphyseal cortex and a short segment of the soft-tissue sinus tract (*arrow*). The orifice of the cloaca is shown as a bright oval focus (*arrowhead*). **E:** Transverse MRI (TR = 300 msec, TE = 30 msec) through diametaphyseal junction shows the abscess cavity, cortical thickening, and focal thinning of the subcutaneous fat (*arrow*) near the opening of the sinus tract in the skin. **F:** T2-weighted transverse MR image (TR = 2,100 msec, TE = 120 msec) at same position shows abscess with bright signal, indicating the long T2 of inflammatory tissue. (From ref. 247.)

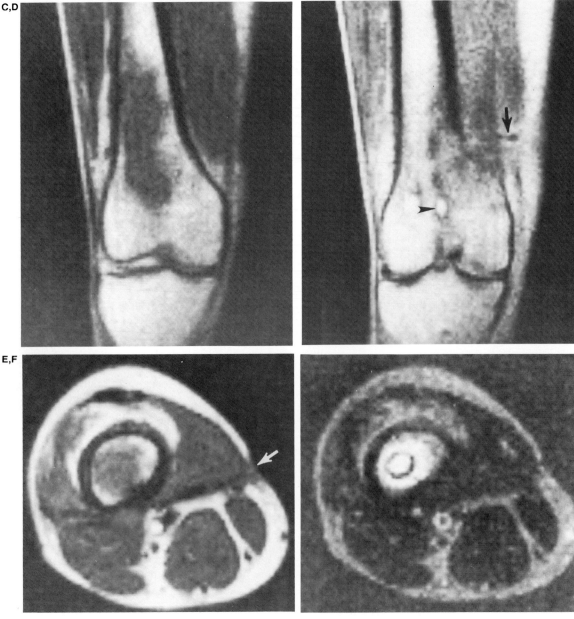

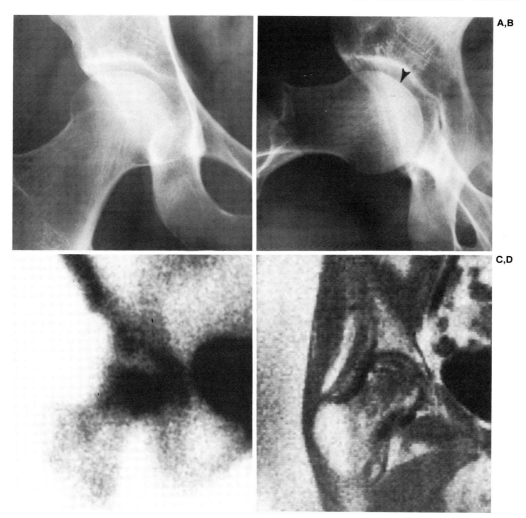

FIG. 78. Ischemic necrosis of femoral head: comparison of methods. **A:** AP radiographic findings in right hip are normal. **B:** Frog-leg lateral projection shows subtle infraction of subarticular cortex (*arrowhead*), indicating stage III ischemic necrosis. **C:** Radionuclide scintigraph shows intense tracer accumulation in femoral head, confirming the healing response to devascularization. **D:** Coronal MR image (TR = 500 msec, TE = 30 msec) shows focal decreased signal due to death of normal marrow cells and ingrowth of reparative tissues.

staging articular cartilage destruction (123). It is used extensively in the evaluation of cervical spine involvement by rheumatoid and degenerative conditions.

Ischemic necrosis and bone infarction

The processes of bone marrow devascularization are similar in all areas of the body and may result from a variety of insults, including fracture, dislocation, steroid therapy, sickle cell disease, hyperbaric pressure, and cellular infiltration. Although the causative events may vary, the pathophysiologic processes are similar. Ischemia causes cell death, followed by necrosis, granulation, and fibrosis. The repair process gradually replaces the dead trabecular bone and marrow. In some areas during the repair process, the bone may become so weak that local fracture results.

Although CT has been used for diagnosis of ischemic necrosis and bone infarction in various bones, MRI has now become the primary sectional imaging method for diagnosis. CT remains effective for detailed analysis of femoral-head ischemic necrosis when careful characterization is needed prior to an osteotomy for the purpose of rotating the affected segment of the femoral head. Multiplanar reformatted images (216) and three-dimensional images (339,345) are useful under these circumstances.

The primary anatomic site at which MRI has been used for detection of marrow devascularization has been the femoral head. In both children and adults, the signal derived from the normal femoral head is strong and homogeneous, except for certain anatomic features that are normally of lower signal intensity (physis, physeal scar, load-bearing trabeculae) or predictable variations in distribution of yellow and red marrow (212). The features of ischemic necrosis of the femoral head are similar in children (Legg-Calvé-Perthes disease) (336) and adults (108,247,337). Most necrotic areas appear as low-signal-intensity foci on T1-weighted images, bordered by the higher signal intensity of adjacent normal marrow (236,238) (Fig. 78). These abnormal areas remain of low signal intensity on all pulse sequences, except for areas of

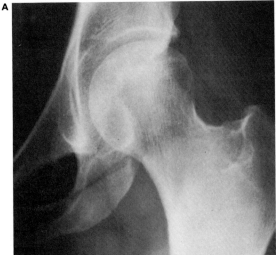

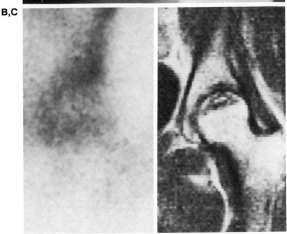

FIG. 79. Ischemic necrosis: sensitivity of MRI. **A:** AP radiograph shows normal findings. **B:** Radionuclide bone scan appears normal. **C:** MR examination shows focal abnormality of femoral head, consistent with devascularization.

revascularized granulation tissue, cyst formation, inflammation, or adjacent joint effusion that show increased signal intensities as TR and TE are lengthened.

In children, Legg-Calvé-Perthes disease is characterized by focally decreased signal intensity of the epiphyseal ossification center (24,336). In adults, four basic patterns of femoral-head devascularization (homogeneous, inhomogeneous, band, and ring) have been described (337), but without definition of prognostic or therapeutic significance.

Compared with conventional radiography, MRI is clearly more sensitive for detection of femoral-head devascularization (10,237,239,337). When radiographic findings are normal or indeterminate, MRI commonly confirms an abnormality. Compared with radionuclide imaging, MRI is also more sensitive for detection of femoral-head ischemic necrosis (226,237,239,337). In instances in which a bone scan shows focally decreased or focally increased radionuclide accumulation, MRI invariably confirms an abnormality. More important, when

findings on radionuclide studies are normal or indeterminate, MRI may demonstrate an abnormality (Fig. 79).

Devascularization of many other bone marrow sites likewise can be detected by MRI, including the humeral head, the knee, the talus, and the carpal bones (266,285,319,363). Here, too, MRI may be more sensitive than conventional radiography or radionuclide scanning for detection, characterization, and determination of the extent of the process.

Although MRI has high sensitivity, its specificity is more limited. It cannot distinguish among the various causes of marrow devascularization or replacement. However, when neoplastic replacement of the marrow or transient osteoporosis clinically mimics a devascularization pattern, MRI may be helpful. T2-weighted images may help distinguish between devascularized marrow and these other conditions. On these sequences, devascularized marrow remains of low signal intensity, whereas the other conditions, with greater water content, show increased signal intensity.

Paget disease of bone

Paget bone disease is best studied by radionuclide bone scintigraphy and conventional radiography (98). Most patients with Paget disease are asymptomatic. The condition may be discovered on CT studies obtained for other reasons (98). Recognition of its characteristic changes is important lest they be misinterpreted as malignant neoplasms (Fig. 80).

Paget disease is most commonly encountered during the later stages of its natural history. Usually it has involved a whole bone, increased the size of the bone, and replaced that bone with abnormal cortex and trabeculae. The cortex usually is thicker than normal and may have a very irregular surface. Increasing vertebral size and articular surface irregularity may result in spinal stenosis or Pagetic arthropathy.

The trabecular pattern may become globular or chaotic. The pattern seen on CT may be impossible to differentiate from metastasis without the aid of history, laboratory tests, and conventional radiographs. Paget disease also softens bone such that the bone is reshaped according to the mechanical forces on it. This may result in bowing or basilar invagination.

MRI is not commonly employed to study Paget disease. However, it does show the osseous expansion and disorganized mineralization of the condition. Because of the hypervascular marrow space and the cysts that occur in Pagetic bone, regions of high signal intensity are demonstrated on T2-weighted images.

Anywhere in its natural history, Paget disease may transform into a malignant neoplasm, commonly osteosarcoma (Fig. 81). When this happens, CT or MRI can be helpful in diagnosis, characterization, and treatment planning.

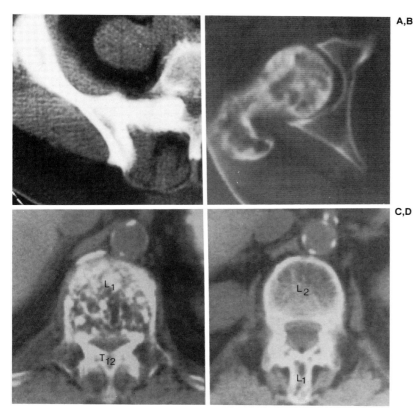

A,B

C,D

FIG. 80. Paget disease. **A:** Paget disease of the right ilium manifested as diffuse cortical thickening and mild focal unsharpness of the bone surface. **B:** Paget disease of the right femoral head and neck manifested as disorganized mineralization of the cancellous bone. Paget disease of L1: CT sections show involvement of the entire vertebra, including the body and pedicles (**C**), as well as the lamina and spinous process (**D**). Comparison of the latter two images shows the enlarged vertebra, with its disorganized trabeculae, as compared with the normal spinous process of T12 and body of L2.

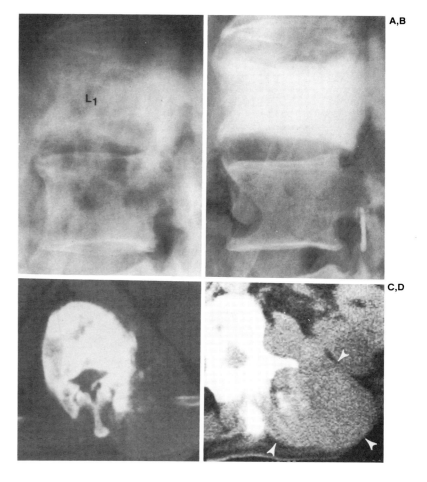

A,B

C,D

FIG. 81. Malignant transformation of Paget disease into osteosarcoma. **A:** This 68-year-old man had previously diagnosed Paget disease of L1 vertebra. **B:** Within a year, L1 became densely blastic. **C:** At bone window settings, CT section through L1 vertebral body shows the blastic lesion, with a large, left-side paraspinal mass containing radially oriented tumor mineralization. **D:** At soft-tissue window settings, CT section through L2 vertebral body and L1 inferior facets and spinous process shows tumor in the L1 spinous process. Caudal extension of the soft-tissue mass is also imaged (*arrowheads*).

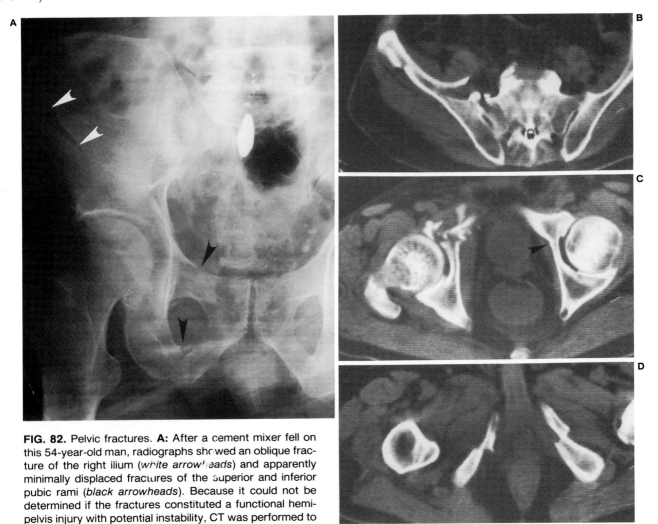

FIG. 82. Pelvic fractures. **A:** After a cement mixer fell on this 54-year-old man, radiographs showed an oblique fracture of the right ilium (*white arrowheads*) and apparently minimally displaced fractures of the superior and inferior pubic rami (*black arrowheads*). Because it could not be determined if the fractures constituted a functional hemipelvis injury with potential instability, CT was performed to provide information that would indicate whether or not the injury should be considered unstable. **B:** CT section through the ilia confirmed the oblique fracture and showed that the sacrum and sacroiliac joints were intact. **C:** CT section through the acetabulae showed an unsuspected shattered right superior pubic ramus and anterior acetabulum, as well as a nondisplaced buckle fracture of the left ischium (*arrowhead*). **D:** CT section through the distal ischiopubic junction showed bilateral fractures. On the basis of this information, the injury was judged potentially unstable, and the patient was carefully mobilized.

REGIONAL COMPLEX MUSCULOSKELETAL ANATOMY

CT and MRI excel in confirming, localizing, and characterizing soft-tissue masses, neoplastic bone disease, and other conditions in regions of complex musculoskeletal anatomy. Formerly, the pelvis, shoulder girdles, sternum, sternoclavicular joints, sacroiliac joints, accessory vertebral joints, and temporomandibular joints often were inadequately evaluated by various imaging techniques, either independently or in combination. The skeletal parts of these regions are curved, are of variable thickness, and are oriented at angles to the major axes of the whole body. The soft-tissue parts are small and are obscured by the bony parts, virtually invisible on images unless somehow enhanced by air or a contrast agent. Other parts of the

skeleton often are adjacent, a situation that may prevent obtaining an image of the desired bone or soft tissue without another bone superimposed.

Pelvis

The osseous anatomy of the pelvis is a complex union of the sacrum and two hemipelvic bones, each derived from three smaller bones: the ilium, ischium, and pubis. These bones are curved, are of variable thicknesses, and are spatially oriented at various angles with respect to each other and to the sagittal and coronal axes of the body. Because the pelvis is firmly fixed at the sacroiliac joints, it moves as a unit. This means that it is impossible to project some areas free of overlying osseous structures.

Thus, the deeper and more central structures such as the posterior iliac spines, the sacroiliac joints, and most of the sacrum are particularly difficult to image. Overlying fecal material and bowel gas further compromise conventional radiologic evaluation of the pelvis and sacrum (109).

Pelvic soft-tissue anatomy is as complex as pelvic skeletal anatomy (249). Muscles, lymph nodes, rectum, and genitourinary organs are present, in addition to nerves and vessels (207). Conventional radiography, urography, and barium studies may fail to show a soft-tissue abnormality or may show only limited secondary changes. CT and MRI can overcome these anatomic difficulties and graphically display both the anatomic location and intraosseous extent of lesions of the pelvis (109,201,207,254,356,357).

Trauma

CT provides more precise information about the presence, location, orientation, and number of pelvic fractures than does conventional radiography (242) (Fig. 82). CT also shows the soft-tissue relationships and provides a three-dimensional view of malalignments (Fig. 83). Plaster casts do not degrade CT or MR images. Another advantage is that the traumatized patient must be moved only minimally to obtain CT images; an ileus that obscures detail on conventional radiographs does not degrade CT information.

Neoplasia

CT and MRI have advantages over other procedures for evaluation of solid tumors of the pelvis (5). They more clearly define the extent of lesions and contribute information necessary for more precise treatment planning. Tumors of osseous or soft-tissue origin are easily localized to bone or soft tissue or both (109,121). Their intrapelvic or extrapelvic extent is readily defined.

Sacroiliac Joints

Each sacroiliac joint (SIJ) has two types of articulations: the anteroinferior third, which is synovial, and the pos-

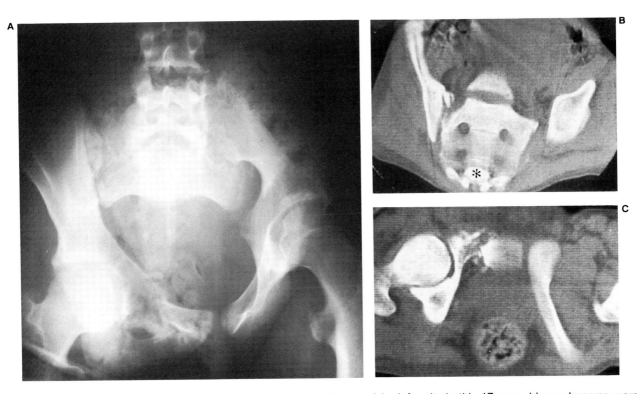

FIG. 83. Unstable pelvic fractures. **A:** Following a vehicular accident, pelvic deformity in this 17-year-old man became worse. Radiographs showed that the left hemipelvis was disassociated from the sacrum and displaced cranially. The junction of the right superior pubic ramus and ischium was shattered. **B:** CT section through the sacrum and sacroiliac joints showed disruption of both joints. A small fragment of the right first sacral ala remained attached to the subluxed ilium. The craniomedial dislocation of the left ilium was well shown. Whereas the first three sacral segments were imaged frontally, the last segments were viewed end-on (∗), indicating a transacral fracture between S3 and S4. **C:** A more caudal CT section graphically displayed the malalignment and severe deformity by imaging the left ischial tuberosity in the same plane as the right hip. On the basis of information provided by conventional radiographs and CT, a treatment plan was formulated to attempt reduction of this unstable pelvis.

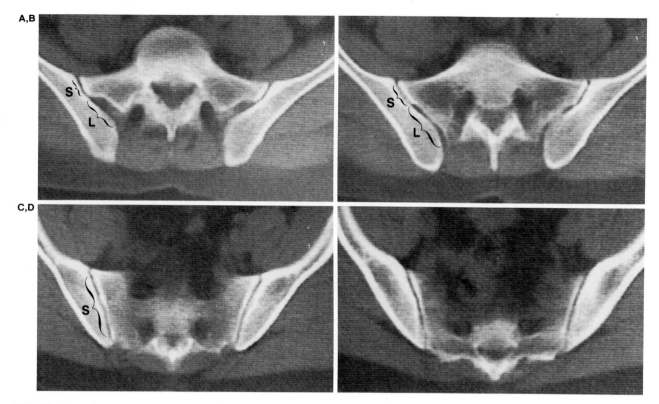

FIG. 84. Normal sacroiliac joints. Examined from cranial to caudal (**A–D**), CT shows both the synovial (S) and ligamentous (L) portions of the joints, as well as simultaneously demonstrating left and right joints in the same projection. The criteria of normalcy are that the joints be symmetric, with thin uniform cortices, and that the joint spaces be thin and of uniform width throughout. There should be no foci of sclerosis, erosion, or joint ankylosis. Focal unsharpness may occur as a result of partial-volume averaging of a curving cortex.

terior-superior two-thirds, which is ligamentous. The synovial portion has thinner articular cartilage than other synovial joints, has an undulating surface, and moves minimally. The ligamentous portion is V-shaped, narrowest adjacent to the synovial portion, and widens dorsally. It also undulates and has fairly deep concavities or pits for insertion of the interosseous ligaments. The criteria for normalcy of the synovial portions of the SIJs are that (a) the cartilage space be uniformly thick, (b) the cortices be uniformly thin and parallel to one another, (c) the left and right sides be symmetrical, and (d) no focal erosion, sclerosis, or fusion be present. The width of the normal synovial SIJ ranges from 2.5 to 4.0 mm. Less than 2 mm is considered joint-space narrowing (347). The criteria for normalcy of the ligamentous portions are that (a) the cortices be uniformly thin, (b) no erosion, sclerosis, or ligamentous mineralization be present, and (c) the sides be symmetrical (Fig. 84).

Trauma

The positions of sacral and pelvic fracture fragments sometimes are difficult to determine accurately on conventional radiographs. CT is very useful for evaluating fractures involving the sacroiliac joint and the remainder of the osseous pelvis (107,242) (Fig. 83). An important advantage is that adjacent soft-tissue structures can be

evaluated simultaneously. Furthermore, an overlying cast does not degrade the CT image.

More subtle injuries of the SIJ, particularly diastasis, may be particularly difficult to detect on conventional radiographs even if specialized views are obtained. A transaxial CT section makes comparison of the two SIJs relatively easy and thereby facilitates early diagnosis.

Infection

The majority of pyogenic sacroiliitis occurs in abusers of intravenous drugs; however, other predisposing causes of SIJ infection include trauma, pregnancy, and endocarditis, as well as adjacent skin, bone, and urinary tract infections.

Diagnosis of SIJ infection may be difficult because symptoms often are vague (9,291). Generally, SIJ tenderness is found on physical examination, but invariably the initial radiographic findings are normal. Technetium diphosphonate or gallium citrate images are more sensitive than conventional radiographs in confirming early sacroiliitis, but they are nonspecific. CT not only is useful for demonstrating early joint or bone changes but also may demonstrate soft-tissue abscess formation not evident on conventional radiographs and clinically unsuspected (244). Fluoroscopic or CT-guided arthrocentesis may be required for diagnosis of the specific pathogen.

Neoplasia

Because of the overlap of the sacrum and the ilium, occasionally it is difficult to ascertain if one or both bones are affected by a destructive neoplastic process (242). Although tumor of the SIJ itself is rare, direct extension into the joint from contiguous soft-tissue tumor or adjacent bone tumor is not uncommon (357). A neoplastic process in this region may present clinically as sacroiliitis. Findings on conventional radiographs may be normal, or the alterations that are seen may not adequately explain scintigraphic abnormalities. In these circumstances, the cross-sectional display of CT demonstrates the cortical margins and medullary region of the sacrum and the ilium and the surrounding soft tissues to best advantage (Fig. 85).

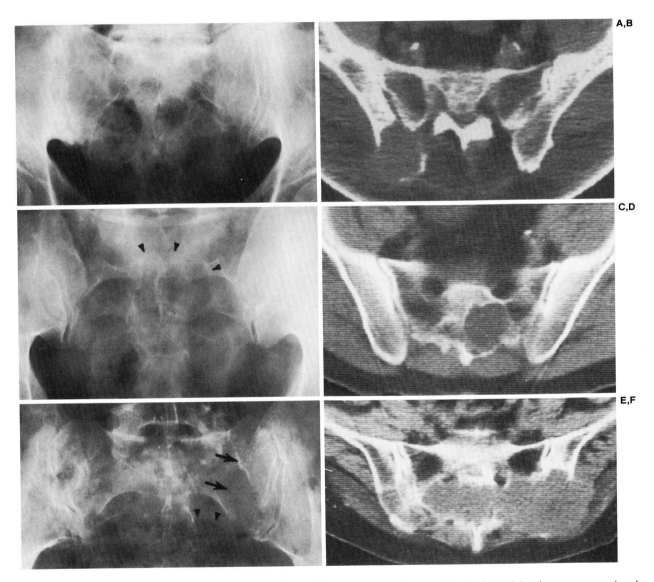

FIG. 85. Complex sacroiliac skeletal anatomy. CT readily confirms osseous abnormalities in the pelvis; they were previously interpreted as equivocal by conventional radiographic projections. **A,B:** A 55-year-old man 4 months following diagnosis of bronchogenic carcinoma developed right-hip pain and had a bone scan that was interpreted as showing an abnormal right sacroiliac joint. The radiograph (**A**) confirmed sacroiliac joint osteoarthritis. However, CT (**B**) showed that a metastasis had destroyed the right posterior iliac spine. **C,D:** A 55-year-old man presented with gait disturbance and low-back pain. A radiograph (**C**) showed a subtle curvilinear shadow over the sacrum (*arrowheads*) that could not be confirmed by other conventional studies. The CT image (**D**) clearly showed a well-defined lytic defect in the sacrum. Finally, films from 10 years previously were located, and they showed the same radiologic changes. **E,F:** A 55-year-old woman with parotid gland carcinoma presented with incontinence. The radiographs (**E**) showed destruction of the left posterior iliac spine (*arrows*) and subtle blurring of the second neural foraminal cortex (*arrowheads*). CT (**F**) showed a much more extensive metastasis than was apparent from the radiographs. The tumor extended from the right sacroiliac joint, across the sacrum and left sacroiliac joint, through the left ilium, and into the gluteal muscles. (From ref. 109.)

A,B

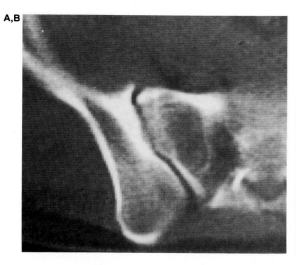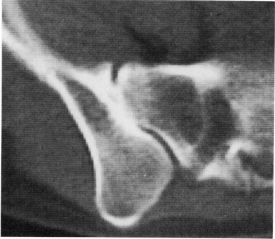

FIG. 86. Ankylosing spondylitis. A: CT shows focal iliac sclerosis adjacent to focal sacral erosion. The joint space and its apposing cortical surfaces are irregular. B: CT shows focal ankylosis of the sacroiliac joint.

MRI is also an effective method for demonstration of bone and soft-tissue neoplasia in this region.

Arthropathy

By far, the spondyloarthropathy most frequently associated with bilateral sacroiliitis is ankylosing spondylitis. However, rheumatoid arthritis, connective-tissue disorders, psoriasis, Reiter's syndrome, inflammatory bowel disease, and other disorders may be associated with either unilateral or bilateral sacroiliitis. The earliest changes of sacroiliitis, widening of the joint space, accompanied by loss of the sharp cortical margins of the articulating surfaces, may be impossible to detect on conventional radiographs. Cortical erosions and subchondral sclerosis are later findings. Intraarticular bony spurs or transarticular bony bridges typically are present before ankylosis of the

entire joint occurs. Frequently these changes are seen only with conventional tomography or CT. Ankylosis of the joint space can be readily appreciated on conventional radiographs, but by that time the clinical diagnosis is obvious.

Almost all patients with ankylosing spondylitis show their first radiologically detectable manifestation in the SIJ. Because of the major limitations of conventional radiography in detecting early sacroiliitis, radioisotope imaging has been advocated for early diagnosis. However, though it is sensitive, radionuclide imaging is not specific enough for effective diagnosis of sacroiliitis. Subtle focal bone erosions, joint-space irregularity, and subarticular sclerosis may be evident only on CT cross-sectional images (88,185,194,300) (Figs. 86–88).

Osteoarthritis of the SIJ, characterized by osteophytes, is commonly encountered, most often as an incidental

FIG. 87. Ankylosing spondylitis. Symmetric bilateral involvement of the sacroiliac joints, as manifested by fusion across the articulations, is present in this 45-year-old man. Ossification of the annulus fibrosis (*arrow*) at the level of the disc space can be distinguished from the cortex of the vertebral body. (Courtesy of Dr. James B. Vogler III, Durham, North Carolina.)

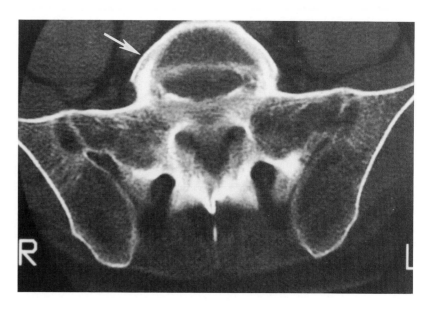

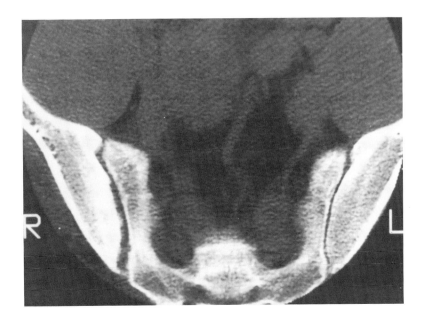

FIG. 88. Reiter's syndrome. CT section through the sacrum demonstrates pronounced erosion, widening, and iliac sclerosis on the right, whereas the left side shows only minor changes consistent with the asymmetric sacroiliitis of Reiter's syndrome. (Courtesy of Dr. James B. Vogler III, Durham, North Carolina.)

finding (Fig. 89). In a more advanced state, there may be focal or diffuse joint-space narrowing, with associated subchondral sclerosis. Patients with altered weight-bearing functions, whether secondary to trauma, neuromuscular disorder, or a developmental hip abnormality, may have unilateral osteoarthropathy. On occasion, this must be differentiated from sacroiliitis. The clinical context generally will resolve this problem.

Hips

The hip is a ball-and-socket joint, with a complex origin of the socket involving contributions of three bones joined at the triradiate cartilage. The acetabular roof is contributed by the ilium, the small anteromedial portion by the pubic bone, and the major posteromedial portion by the

ischium. These separate contributions to the acetabulum are seen in pediatric patients. CT and MRI contribute to an appreciation of the spatial relationships of many pediatric hip disorders, including congenital hip dislocation, Legg-Calvé-Perthes disease, proximal femoral focal deficiency, other dysplasias, and trauma (336). MRI is particularly effective because it can demonstrate the relationship of the unossified femoral head within the acetabulum without the need for an intraarticular contrast agent.

In adults, CT of the hip has been useful because of its display of cross-sectional bony anatomy (Fig. 90). CT shows that the acetabulum is not merely a socket, but rather is a focal concavity supported at the apex of an arch derived from two substantial columns of bone. The posterior or ilioischial column is large and descends from the sciatic notch to the ischial tuberosity. The anterior or

FIG. 89. Anterior osteophyte. CT section through the superior aspect of the sacrum demonstrates an anterior osteophyte bridging the anterosuperior aspect of the SIJ.

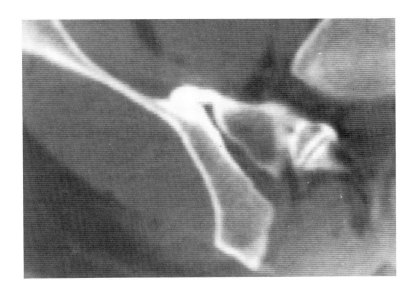

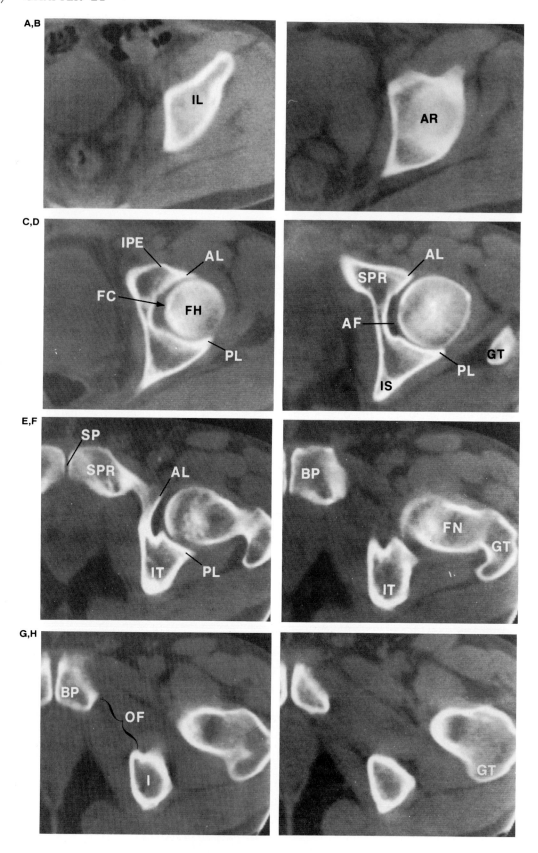

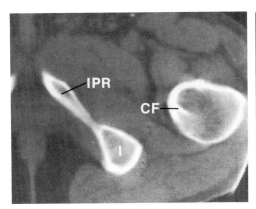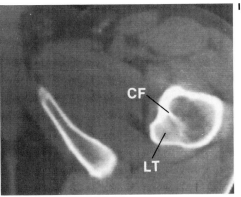

FIG. 90. Normal adult hip. Parts **A–H** on *facing page*. **A:** Supraacetabular ilium. **B:** Ilium broadens into roof of acetabulum. **C:** Cranial aspect of femoral head, maximally surrounded by acetabulum, with its anterior and posterior labra. Adjacent to the anterior acetabular rim is the iliopubic eminence, the result of fusion of the triradiate cartilage in this region. The fovea capitis, a shallow depression in the femoral head for the femoral ligament, is just visible. **D:** At midsection through the femoral head, the lateral aspect of the superior pubic ramus and ischial spine are seen. The fat-filled acetabular fossa is maximum size. **E:** Caudal section of the femoral head shows the cranial aspect of the femoral neck, the complete pubic ramus, and the ischial tuberosity. **F:** A section through the femoral neck shows cortical and medullary continuity of the femoral head, neck, and greater trochanter. The pubic body and symphysis are optimally shown. **G:** Section through the central portion of the obturator foramen between the pubis and ischium. **H:** The greater trochanter is almost incorporated into the femoral shaft. **I:** Just caudal to the greater trochanter, the origin of the calcar femoris from the anteromedial cortex is shown. The inferior pubic ramus joins the ischium. **J:** The calcar femoris is still present adjacent to the lesser trochanter. The ischial tuberosity is now shown. Note that the rim of the acetabulum constantly changes contour. Cranially (**C**), the acetabulum is deepest, and the labra longest. Caudally (**E**), the acetabulum is most shallow, and the labra smallest. Throughout, the anterior labrum is always shorter than the posterior, and the ischium makes up the medial and posterior portions of the acetabulum. Also note that when cortices are perpendicular to the cross-sectional tomogram, they are imaged as sharp lines. However, if they pass obliquely through the section, the partial-volume effect will cause cortical regions to be represented as broad and unsharp; (AF) acetabular fossa; (AL) anterior labrum; (AR) acetabular roof; (BP) body of pubis; (CF) calcar femoris; (FC) fovea capitis; (FH) femoral head; (FN) femoral neck; (GT) greater trochanter; (I) ischium; (IL) ilium; (IPE) iliopubic (iliopectineal) eminence; (IPR) inferior pubic ramus; (IS) ischial spine; (IT) ischial tuberosity; (LT) lesser trochanter; (OF) obturator foramen; (PL) posterior labrum; (SP) symphysis pubis; (SPR) superior pubic ramus.

iliopubic column runs downward, inward, and forward from the iliac crest to the pubic symphysis. The periphery of the acetabulum narrows into a labrum that is complete, except inferiorly, where it meets the acetabular fossa. The posterior acetabular rim is more substantial and extends farther laterally than the anterior rim. The femoral head is seated centrally in the acetabulum, but may not be shown with a constant width of cartilage space around it. When supine and relaxed, the patient, assisted by gravity, will permit the leg to rotate externally. This will cause minimal subluxation of the femoral head, so that the anterior joint space is slightly wider than the posterior.

CT and MRI can help elucidate the cause of hip pain due to a bone or soft-tissue abnormality. In addition to showing tumor and infections, both methods have helped show iliopsoas bursa abnormalities (262,326). Because the bursa crosses anterior to the hip joint, sectional imaging of iliopsoas bursitis will show a fluid-filled mass that displaces the femoral vessels just anterior to the joint. If necessary, the distended bursa can be aspirated, or a hip arthrogram can be performed for confirmation (Fig. 91).

Trauma

CT of the hip has made its greatest contribution in evaluation of hip fracture dislocations (25,38,188, 274,301,306,317). Standard radiography requires moving the patient into various positions and may be limited to a frontal projection. Movement of the patient into various positions can be painful, and there is always concern that further displacement may result. When optimal radiographs are obtained, they still provide only two-dimensional information. CT is accomplished without moving the patient's leg or pelvis into various positions and provides the third dimension. CT sections can be reformatted such that multiple additional planes are created (96,215), and three-dimensional renderings are available (95,339, 345); these may provide additional useful information in selected circumstances.

Recognition of the fracture-dislocation pattern and the complications associated with each hip injury is important because it dictates whether the particular injury will be treated closed or be subjected to surgery (198). For a hip

A,B

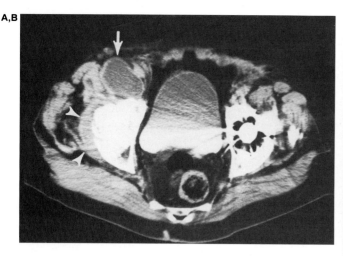

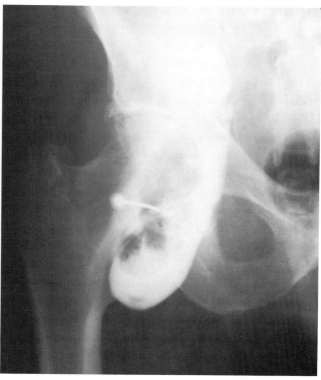

FIG. 91. Iliopsoas bursitis in a 71-year-old man. **A:** CT section shows large, fluid-filled bursa (*arrow*) anterior to right hip joint, causing displacement of femoral vessels. Note the associated hip joint effusion (*arrowheads*). Also note the presence of a left total hip replacement. **B:** Contrast bursogram confirms the nature of this cystic mass.

to function well following acetabular fracture, there must be no major intraarticular fragments, the posterior acetabular labrum must be stable, and the fracture fragments must be anatomically reduced so that there is minimal incongruity between the femur and acetabulum (198). In the past, the decision to operate because of intraarticular fragments was based on physical examination and on radiologic documentation of an ossified intraarticular fragment or joint-space widening. However, neither method was accurate, and care of such patients was difficult. CT has helped resolve these difficult therapeutic decisions (188) (Fig. 92). It readily confirms and accurately localizes intraarticular fragments first shown radiographically. More important, CT can show intraarticular fragments not suspected clinically and not shown on radiographs (Fig. 93). However, CT cannot show an intraarticular cartilage fragment if it has no associated ossified component. CT may be similarly valuable following reduction of posterior hip dislocations to solve any clinical or plain radiographic problem. It can show the relationships of fracture fragments, locate intraarticular osseous fragments, and help estimate stability and congruity, in addition to showing associated soft-tissue changes. It may also be useful for follow-up of these patients (214).

CT may be helpful for certain other orthopedic hip problems. It can show the anatomic orientation of posttraumatic hips prior to total hip replacement (Fig. 94). Such information helps the surgeon plan the procedure for hip replacement by showing the amount of bone stock available to seat the acetabular component. Following

gunshot wounds, CT may show the radial spread of bullet fragments better than radiographs. The information derived from CT may help the surgeon decide whether or not to explore the hip (Fig. 95).

Long-Bone Torsion

Rotational deformities of lower-extremity long bones occur developmentally, with certain metabolic bone diseases, and following trauma. These may require surgical correction. Measurement of the rotational deformity has always been rather complicated. CT provides cross-sectional images of the lower extremities that permit direct measurement of the amount of femoral anteversion (152,217,352) or tibial torsion (169,358). Preliminary CT digital radiographs also have proved useful for quantitation of leg length discrepancies (3,111,146,184).

Knee

The knee is a complex biomechanical structure that often is injured, commonly is a source of pain and disability, and frequently is subjected to surgery. The patellofemoral articulation is a source of mechanical instability and pain for patients of all ages. CT can provide new information regarding the normal anatomic relationships of the patellofemoral joint and variations that cause orthopedic problems (168,228,229).

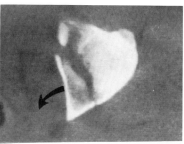

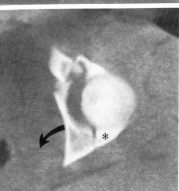

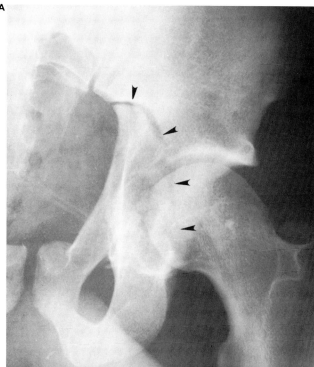

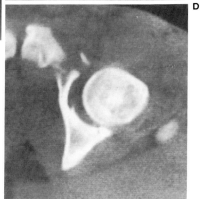

FIG. 92. Acetabular fracture. **A:** This 25-year-old man sustained an acetabular fracture in an automobile accident. The frontal radiograph shows a fracture of the supraacetabular ilium, which extends through the posterior acetabulum (*arrowheads*). The pubic rami are also fractured. **B–D:** CT sections confirm the iliac fracture, but also show rotation of the posteromedial fragment (*arrows* indicate direction of rotation). CT sections show that the posterior acetabular fragment (∗) is sufficiently large to permit hip instability (i.e., predispose to posterior femoral dislocation). The comminution of the anterior rim of the acetabulum (**C,D**) was greater than expected. The femoral head is subluxed laterally (**D**).

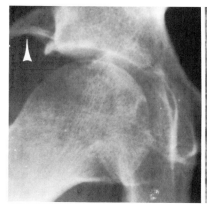

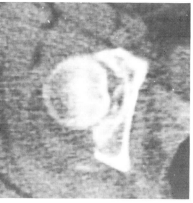

A,B FIG. 93. Intraarticular fracture fragments. **A:** This 30-year-old woman sustained a posterior dislocation of the femoral head in an automobile accident. Postreduction radiograph shows centric position of the femoral head and a large posterior acetabular fragment displaced cranially (*arrowhead*). **B:** CT section through the fovea capitis shows two unsuspected fracture fragments in the acetabular fossa. At surgery, these were in contact with the femoral articular cartilage. Note that absence of the posterior acetabulum, as shown by CT, could predispose the femoral head to recurrent posterior dislocation.

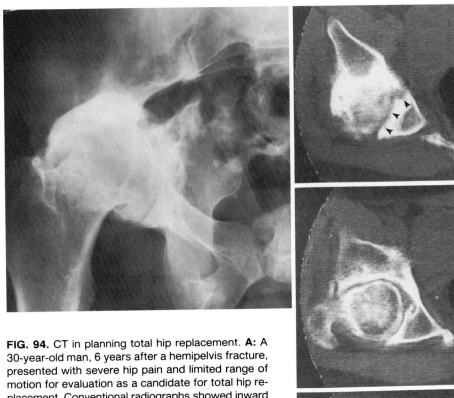

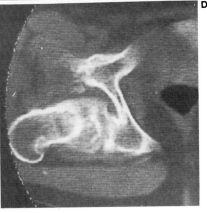

FIG. 94. CT in planning total hip replacement. **A:** A 30-year-old man, 6 years after a hemipelvis fracture, presented with severe hip pain and limited range of motion for evaluation as a candidate for total hip replacement. Conventional radiographs showed inward rotation of the ischium and advanced secondary osteoarthritis of the hip. **B:** CT section through the ilium showed incomplete bony bridging of the acetabular roof fracture (*arrowheads*). **C:** CT section through the hip confirmed osteoarthritis, with deformity of the femoral head and acetabulum. **D:** CT section more distally revealed that the inward rotation of the ischium was so severe that there was insufficient posterior bone stock to provide normal anatomic stability for the acetabular component of a total hip replacement. Therefore, the surgical plan would have to include a method to provide posterior stabilization.

Sectional imaging of the knees has proved effective for evaluation of bone tumors, soft-tissue masses (195), internal derangements, and trauma (272). Joint effusions are commonly discovered (14) (Fig. 96). Masses about the knee commonly originate from a variety of structures, including muscle, fascia, nerve, artery, synovium, and bone (310) (Fig. 97). The site of origin is readily determined by CT and MRI (328). Concurrent with localization of origin, sectional imaging usually will establish the character of the condition, including tumor, cyst, or aneurysm. Finally, if the problem does not arise from the joint, involvement of the joint can be determined, because surgical management of tumors depends on this information. If a tumor has violated the joint, the treatment decisions are more difficult, and more extensive surgery may be indicated.

Internal derangements

Both CT and MRI have been adapted for detection of cruciate ligament injury (113,261) and meniscal tears (16,37,100,175,209,256,280,281). CT evaluation of cruciate ligaments can be accomplished, but it tends to be cumbersome for patients. MRI is proving effective for demonstration of both anterior and posterior cruciate tears (Fig. 98). Its major advantages are that the patient can assume a comfortable neutral position, and the parasag-

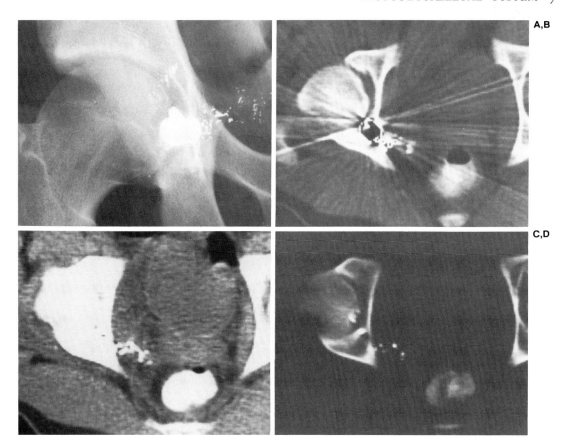

FIG. 95. Localization of intraarticular foreign bodies. **A:** This 20-year-old man had been shot through the left buttock, leaving a bullet lodged near the right hip. Conventional radiographs did not provide precise localization of the bullet or its fragments. Positions of the fragments would determine whether or not surgery was necessary. **B:** CT section through the main bullet fragment showed that it had perforated the acetabulum, but had not contacted the femoral head. **C:** CT section slightly more cephalad at a soft-tissue window showed several small metallic fragments in the soft tissues. **D:** The same section at a bone window showed one fragment in the ischium and another in the fovea capitis, but none in the joint. Thus, no surgery was done.

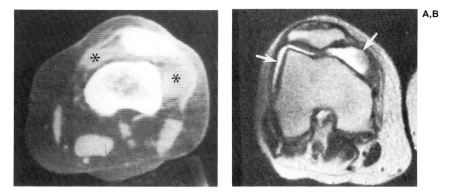

FIG. 96. Knee joint effusions. **A:** CT section shows distension of the medial and lateral recesses (∗) by effusion. **B:** T2-weighted (TR = 1,500 msec, TE = 90 msec) MR image in another person shows bright signal of the fluid in the joint (*arrows*).

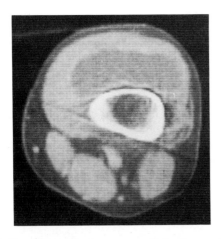

FIG. 97. Noncommunicating suprapatellar bursa. Contrast-enhanced CT through a thigh mass just above the knee shows an encapsulated, near-water-density collection that wraps around the anterior femur, but is separated from it by a thin layer of fat. The mass displaces the quadriceps femoris muscle.

ittal images can display the ligaments bordered by fat, which enhances their visibility.

Thin-section, high-resolution CT has effectively demonstrated meniscal tears, cysts, and deformities (106,218, 219,258,282,283,325) (Fig. 99). However, MRI is rapidly becoming the sectional imaging method of choice for demonstration of meniscal abnormalities (15,17,220,327) (Fig. 100). Specialized surface coils, high-field-strength systems, and pulse sequences that emphasize the water content of meniscal tears and meniscal degeneration have provided results that compare favorably with those from arthrography and arthroscopy. Meniscal tears are detected as morphologic changes and signal alterations in the substance of the cartilage (Fig. 100). MRI likely will supplant other methods as the preferred way to image internal derangements of the knee.

Trauma

CT aids characterization of fractures of the tibial plateau by determining the amount of impaction and displace-

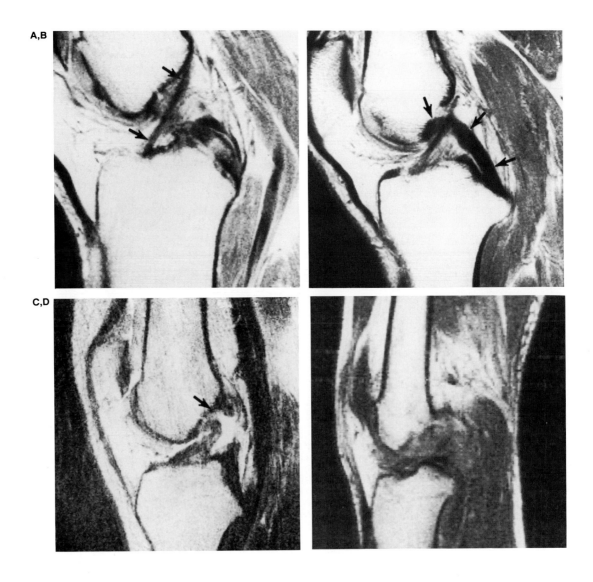

A,B

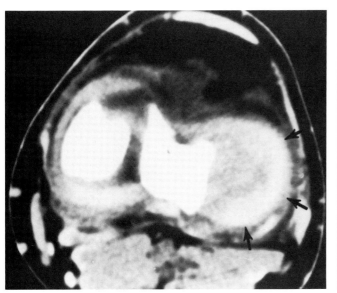 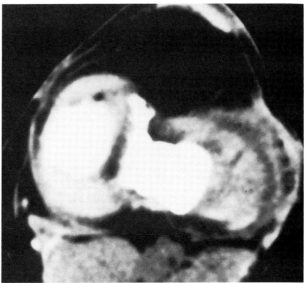

FIG. 99. CT of menisci. **A:** Normal menisci shown in thin section as curved, high-density structures. Note particularly the lateral meniscus (*arrows*) in this normal knee. **B:** Extensively torn lateral meniscus (shown in thin section). (Courtesy of Dr. Lawrence G. Manco, Albany, New York.)

ment of the fragments (105). CT and MRI have also proved useful for detection, localization, and staging of femoral condyle osteochondral injury (osteochondritis dissecans) (123,133,266).

Ankle and Foot

CT and MRI are both effective for analysis of ankle and foot problems (125,138,211,315,316,320,321,322) (Figs. 101–104). In general, CT has greatest effectiveness for demonstration and characterization of osseous abnormalities such as tarsal coalitions (71,225,265,302) (Fig. 101), other congenital abnormalities, arthropathies, fractures (calcaneus and talus) (122,139,293,312), fracture dislocations, bone tumors, and osteomyelitis. MRI is effective for most soft-tissue conditions, including soft-tissue masses, abscesses, and ligament or tendon abnormalities.

Unlike the situation for many other parts of the body, it is relatively easy to obtain CT images of the foot in a variety of planes using combinations of patient positioning and gantry angulation. Thin (4-mm) contiguous sections generally are desirable, and specific planes should be

adapted for certain disorders. For example, talocalcaneal coalition is best studied using the coronal plane, whereas imaging of fractures of the calcaneus benefits from a plane parallel to the long axis of the foot. For complex fractures, two or more planes are helpful, but transverse sections may be all the patient can tolerate. Under these circumstances, 1- to 2-mm sections should be obtained, and reformatted images in other planes should be produced.

Calcaneal fractures are well characterized by CT study (Fig. 102). The assessment includes specification of the number and type of principal fragments, the position of any sustentacular fragment, and involvement of anterior, middle, or posterior articular facets. Likewise, CT aids the detection and evaluation of tarsometatarsal fracture dislocations, as well as other fractures of the hindfoot and midfoot. CT is useful for detection of complicating features of tarsal fracture, including intraarticular bone fragments and trapped soft-tissue structures. Finally, CT is effective for assessment of postreduction fracture position.

Ankle injuries are readily evaluated on CT images. In addition to disclosing specific features of tibial, fibular, and talar fractures, CT provides details concerning the integrity of the distal tibiofibular joint and the congruity

◄────────────────────────────

FIG. 98. Cruciate ligaments. **A:** Parasagittal MR image (TR = 3,000 msec, TE = 28 msec) of knee shows normal anterior cruciate ligament (*arrows*). Note that the ligament appears composed of multiple fibers and is stretched between femoral and tibial attachments. **B:** Parasagittal MR image (TR = 3,000 msec, TE = 28 msec) of knee shows normal posterior cruciate ligament (*arrows*), as well as a portion of a normal anterior cruciate ligament. Note that the posterior cruciate ligament is thicker and of homogeneous low signal intensity, as compared with the anterior cruciate ligament. **C:** Parasagittal MR image (TR = 3,000 msec, TE = 28 msec) of knee shows rupture of the anterior cruciate ligament at its femoral attachment (*arrow*). **D:** Parasagittal MR image (TR = 300 msec, TE = 30 msec) of knee of a young man with surgically proven tears of both cruciate ligaments shows absence of the ligaments and the presence of a joint effusion. (From ref. 247.)

A,B

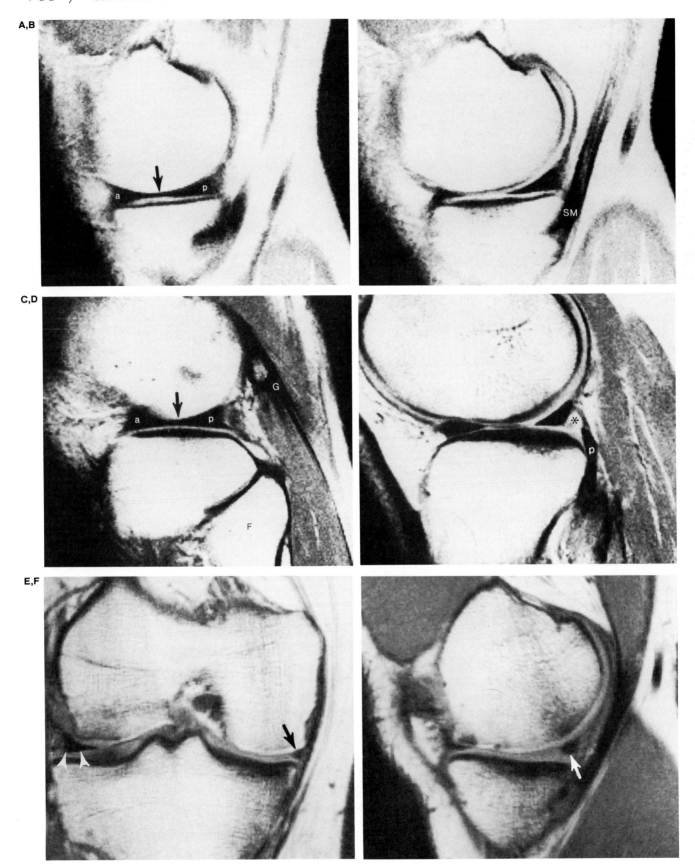

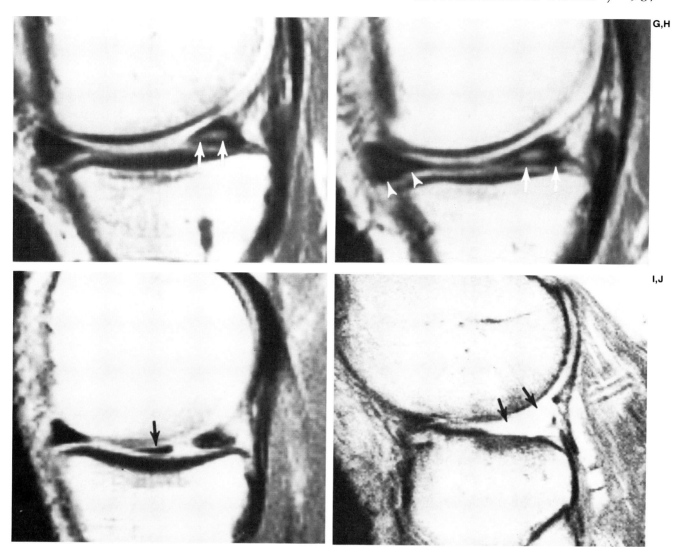

G,H

I,J

FIG. 100. MRI of menisci. Parts **A–F** on *facing page*. **A:** Parasagittal MR image (TR = 3,000 msec, TE = 28 msec) through medial side of knee shows anterior (a) and posterior (p) horns of medial meniscus at level of mid-zone connection (*arrow*) through middle third of meniscus. Note homogeneous absence of signal of meniscal cartilage. **B:** Parasagittal MR image (TR = 3,000 msec, TE = 28 msec) through a more central zone of knee medial compartment shows individual sections of anterior and posterior horns. Note that posterior horn is larger and longer than anterior horn; (SM) semimembranosus tendon. **C:** Parasagittal MR image (TR = 3,000 msec, TE = 28 msec) through lateral side of knee shows anterior (a) and posterior (p) horns of lateral meniscus at level of mid-zone connection (*arrow*) through middle third of meniscus. Note homogeneous absence of signal of lateral meniscus; (F) fibula; (G) lateral head of gastrocnemius. **D:** Parasagittal MR image (TR = 3,000 msec, TE = 28 msec) through more central zone of knee lateral compartment shows individual sections of anterior and posterior horns. Note popliteal tendon bursa (∗) and popliteal tendon (p). **E:** Coronal MR image (TR = 900 msec, TE= 21 msec) through knee shows normal lateral meniscus (*arrowheads*) and a short, degenerated medial meniscus (*arrow*). **F:** Parasagittal MR image (TR = 900 msec, TE = 21 msec) confirms the tear extending to involve the posterior horn of the medial meniscus (*arrow*). **G:** Parasagittal MR image (TR = 3,000 msec, TE = 28 msec) through the knee of another person shows a torn meniscus posteriorly (*arrows*), characterized by linear high signal intensity extending from the center of the meniscus to its inner tibial margin. Note that the anterior portion shows normal homogeneous low signal (*arrowheads*). **H:** Adjacent MR image (TR = 3,000 msec, TE = 28 msec) shows a short, frayed tip of the torn posterior horn of meniscus. Again, note the linear high signal intensity extending to the tip (*arrows*). **I:** Parasagittal MR image (TR = 3,000 msec, TE = 28 msec) through medial compartment shows a torn posterior horn, with a separated free fragment (*arrow*). **J:** Parasagittal MR image (TR = 3,000 msec, TE = 28 msec) through lateral compartment shows absence of posterior horn (*arrows*) because of prior injury. The high signal in the joint space results from joint effusion.

A,B

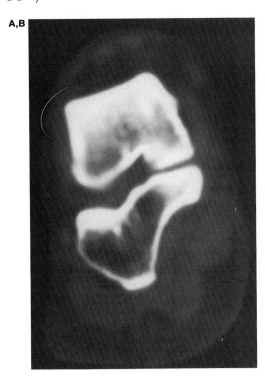

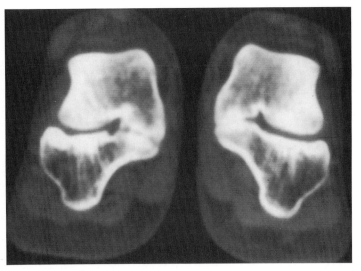

FIG. 101. Subtalar joints. **A:** CT of normal subtalar joint. **B:** CT of bilateral subtalar coalition shows narrow subtalar joints, with sclerosis of the apposed articular surfaces, consistent with fibrous ankylosis.

A,B

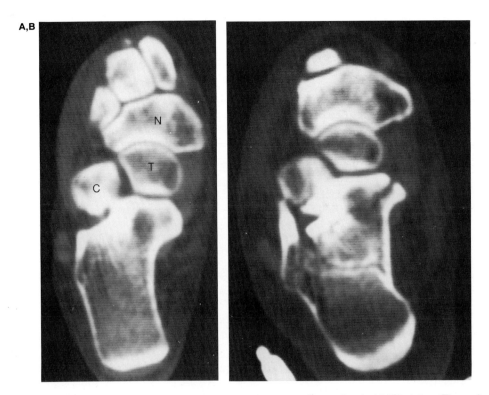

FIG. 102. Calcaneus. **A:** CT of normal calcaneus in long axis shows portions of cuboid (C), talus (T), navicular (N), and three cuneiform bones. **B:** CT in similar position shows comminuted fracture of calcaneus and relationships of fracture fragments to one another and to other major bones.

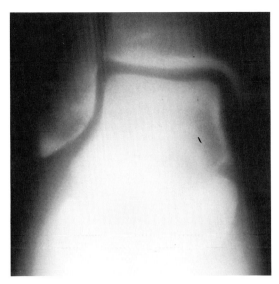
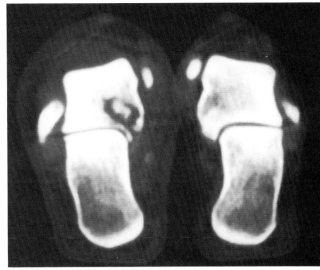

A,B

FIG. 103. Osteomyelitis of talus in a 59-year-old man 2 weeks following steroid injection into the subtalar joint. **A:** Conventional tomogram in the anterior projection shows vague osteopenia of the medial aspect of the talus. **B:** CT section through the talus and subtalar joint demonstrates osteomyelitis of the talus and discloses a sequestrum.

of the fit of the ankle mortise. Ankle tendon injuries, including tendinitis, rupture, and dislocation, usually are evident on CT images. Normal tendons generally show densities of 75 to 95 HU, and ruptured or degenerated tendons usually show densities of 30 to 50 HU. Abnormal tendons are identified because of their fusiform enlargement, irregular borders, heterogeneous appearance, and decreased attenuation.

Osteomyelitis and soft-tissue abscesses of the foot, particularly in diabetics, are well demonstrated by CT (Figs. 103 and 104). Early infections tend to be confined to compartments adjacent to skin ulcerations. Later, the inflammatory mass extends to involve other compartments. CT overestimates the soft-tissue extent of infection by a small amount because secondary edematous changes

cannot be differentiated from the actual abscess. This problem tends to be of little clinical importance.

MRI has proved a sensitive and effective method for evaluation of bone marrow and soft-tissue structures of the ankle and foot. It is particularly useful for delineation of osteonecrosis, osteomyelitis, soft-tissue abscesses, and tumors, as well as acute and chronic tendon abnormalities. A combination of planes is chosen to complement the specific anatomy and condition undergoing evaluation. In general, T1-weighted images are best for detection of the abnormality, and T2-weighted images are best for characterizing the amounts of fibrous tissue, blood, and extracellular water. Together, these features help determine the chronicity of the problem and limit the differential diagnostic possibilities.

Shoulder Girdle

A number of muscles unite the scapula and clavicle to the thorax, forming a scapulothoracic articulation. This articulation, along with the sternoclavicular, acromioclavicular, and glenohumeral joints, moves in a synchronized fashion to provide upper-extremity mobility. Thus, the shoulder girdle, the most mobile region of the body, is a coordinated balance of muscular function provided by muscles of the neck, back, anterior thorax, and arm. Those muscles directly related to the glenohumeral joint include the supraspinatus, infraspinatus, subscapularis, teres minor, and deltoid (Fig. 105).

Double-contrast shoulder arthrography has been widely used to evaluate the cartilage surfaces and the integrity of the rotator cuff. The use of CT immediately following standard arthrography is the ideal method for evaluating

FIG. 104. Osteomyelitis of first metatarsal in 50-year-old diabetic man. CT, following a normal plain film, shows destruction of the right metatarsal head and of the articulating plantar sesamoids. By comparison, the opposite side is normal.

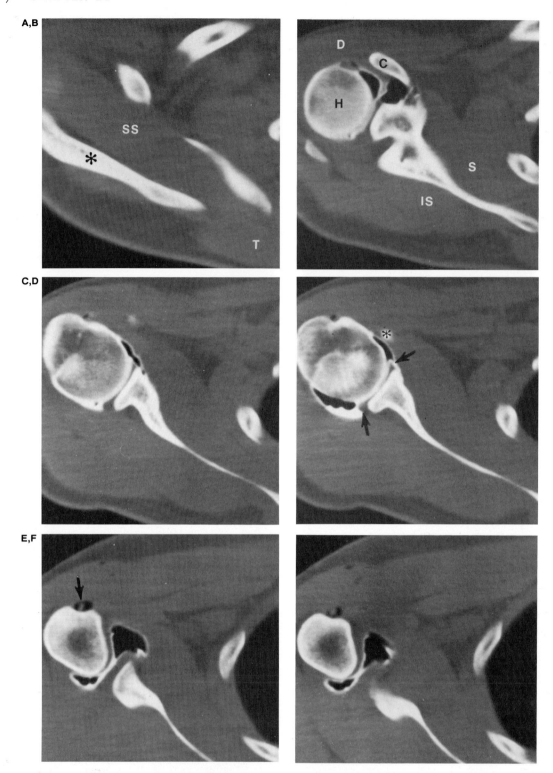

FIG. 105. Normal CT arthrotomogram of shoulder joint. **A:** Level cranial to joint shows supraspinatus muscle (SS), trapezius muscle (T), and spine of scapula (∗). **B:** Level at cranial margin of glenoid shows apex of humeral head (H), coracoid process (C), deltoid muscle (D), subscapularis muscle (S), infraspinatus muscle (IS), and superior glenohumeral ligament (*arrowhead*). **C:** Level cranial to middle glenoid shows anterior and posterior capsular boundaries. **D:** Level at middle glenoid shows anterior and posterior glenoid labra (*arrows*) and tendon of subscapularis muscle (∗). **E:** Level caudal to middle glenoid shows inferior glenoid cartilage and bicipital tendon bursa, with central long head of the biceps muscle tendon (*arrow*). **F:** Level at caudal margin of glenoid shows axillary recess of joint.

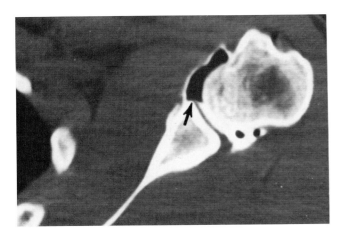

FIG. 106. Glenoid cartilaginous deficiency. CT arthrotomographic section shows deficiency of the anterior cartilaginous rim of the glenoid labrum (*arrow*) (compare with Fig. 105C,D).

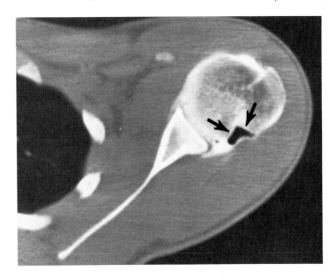

FIG. 107. Humeral head (Hill-Sachs) fracture. CT arthrotomographic section shows deep, V-shaped fracture (*arrows*) resulting from prior impaction of the humeral head against the anterior rim of the glenoid labrum during anterior dislocation.

the glenoid labrum, as well as the general structure of the shoulder, the scapula, the humeral head, and the muscles about the glenohumeral joint (72,73). No significant changes are made in routine arthrographic technique, except that slightly less air is instilled, about 6 to 10 ml. Iodinated contrast material (1 ml) is injected, and cross-sectional CT images are obtained from the acromioclavicular joint inferiorly to below the axillary recess. Some 15 to 20 contiguous 4-mm sections are obtained using a high mas and small field of view.

The normal joint capsule is smooth and regular (311) (Fig. 105). Posteriorly and inferiorly the capsule attaches directly to the glenoid edge. Anteriorly and superiorly the attachment is less regular, being separated from the bone edge by the biceps tendon insertion and the subscapularis tendon bursa. Depending on arm position, the capsule is redundant either anteriorly or posteriorly. One can select anterior redundancy and thus better visualization of the anterior labrum by rotating the humerus internally. External rotation makes the posterior labrum more easily seen. Coated by contrast material, the anterior labrum is relatively sharp (318). Its margins are smooth and regular. Posteriorly, the labrum is more rounded and thicker.

Abnormalities of the capsular attachments and of the labrum can be easily recognized (273,277). Anterior humeral dislocations tear the capsule away from the bone margin. The labrum may be blunted, frayed, or torn free (Fig. 106). Similar findings are present posteriorly in patients who have experienced posterior humeral dislocation. CT arthrography is very accurate in identifying such labral abnormalities (135,270,314). In addition to labrum evaluation, CT arthrography is ideal for identification of Hill-Sachs fractures of the humerus (Fig. 107) and Bankart fractures of the glenoid (Fig. 108). Cystic joint extensions, joint bodies, and biceps tendon abnormalities are similarly well demonstrated (116,179,288).

Both CT and MRI are being evaluated as methods for detection of rotator cuff tears (11). Coronal and transverse MR images probably will prove most effective for evaluation of glenoid and rotator cuff abnormalities (154,177,178,180,232).

Elbow and Wrist

Although anatomic delineation of the structures of the elbow and wrist (8,21,354) is excellent using CT and MRI, clinical applications for these parts have been limited. Both the elbow and wrist are complex, small articulations; as a result, positioning of the part and interpretation of images may be difficult. Special coronal, sagittal, or even three-dimensional protocols may be valuable for exami-

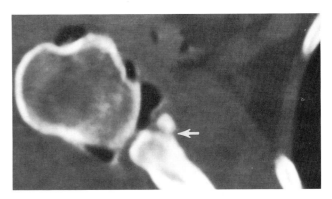

FIG. 108. Glenoid osteochondral (Bankart) fracture. CT arthrotomographic section shows osteochondral fracture of the anterior glenoid labrum (*arrow*).

A,B

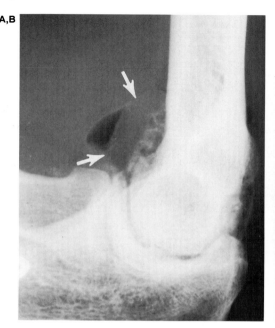
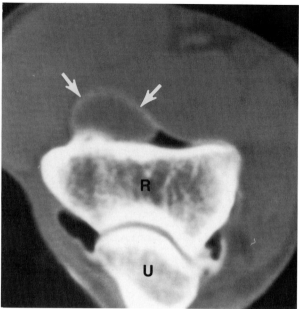

FIG. 109. CT arthrotomography of elbow joint xanthoma. A: Lateral radiograph of elbow arthrogram shows intraarticular mass (*arrows*). B: CT section through the joint confirms the intraarticular location of the mass (*arrows*); (U) ulna; (R) radius.

nation of these joints (260,351). CT and MRI may be used to diagnose osteochondritis dissecans and intraarticular tumors involving the elbow (Fig. 109).

The major application of CT about the wrist has been for diagnosis of distal radioulnar joint disruption (59,234,235,307). Plain film diagnosis of subluxation or dislocation of this joint may be difficult despite strong clinical suspicion. CT provides an accurate cross-sectional

display of distal radioulnar joint anatomy, greatly facilitating the diagnosis.

CT and MRI have also been used for diagnosis of carpal tunnel syndrome because they provide excellent anatomic detail of the carpal tunnel and its contents (60,183,233,369). CT and MRI may be able to identify patients with carpal tunnel stenosis (171). Signs used include a reduced cross-sectional area at the level of the

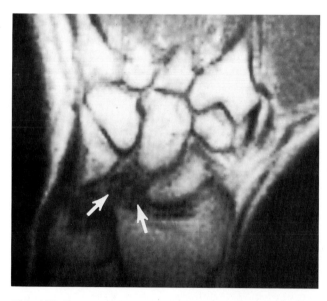

FIG. 110. Devascularization of lunate. T1-weighted (TR = 600 msec, TE = 30 msec) coronal section of wrist shows very low signal intensity from lunate (*arrows*) as compared with the other carpal bones, a finding consistent with lunate malacia.

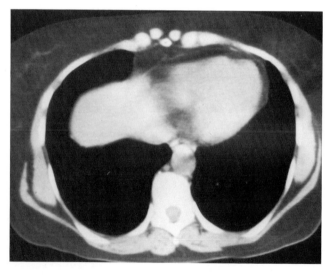

FIG. 111. Developmental incomplete ossification. A routine chest radiograph showed a questionable area of lytic destruction involving the lower sternum, with possible soft-tissue swelling. CT section of the lower sternum showed multiple separate ossicles forming a multipartite sternum, a normal variant.

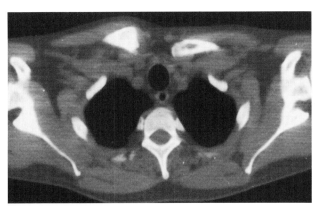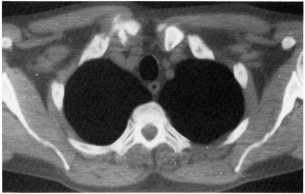

A,B

FIG. 112. Anterosuperior dislocation of the right clavicle in a 45-year-old man following right-shoulder injury. **A:** CT section through the medial ends of the clavicles confirms the anterior position of the right clavicle. **B:** A more caudal CT section shows dystrophic mineralization about the right clavicle and an associated SCJ effusion.

hamate hook to less than 0.1 cm^2 (normal = 0.18 (R) and 0.16 (L) cm^2), thickening of the flexor retinaculum, and increased density of the carpal tunnel tissues. Carpal CT has also proved to be of occasional use as a problem-solving tool for diagnosis of subtle fracture (134,260,268,351) and evaluation of tumor and of joint-space abnormalities (353).

MRI has been employed to evaluate a spectrum of carpal abnormalities, including confirmation of devascularization of the lunate (lunate malacia) or a scaphoid fragment following fracture (avascular necrosis) (285) (Fig. 110).

Sternum, Sternoclavicular Joint, and Ribs

Because of the complex anatomy of the thoracic cage, radiographic evaluation of the sternum, sternoclavicular joint (SCJ), and ribs often is suboptimal. When standard radiography is inconclusive in confirming clinical or scintigraphic findings, CT is the preferred method for further evaluation (70,80,115,324).

The sternum is a flat cancellous bone that measures 15 to 20 cm in length and consists of a manubrium, body, and xiphoid process. The SCJ usually is divided into two articular components by a fibrocartilaginous disc that may be visible on CT when a normal vacuum phenomenon is present (see Chapter 7, Figs. 28–30). The body of the sternum is longer and narrower than the manubrium, and it ossifies in segments that fuse together (see Chapter 7, Fig. 115). Sometimes, incomplete or irregular ossification occurs and persists in the adult (Fig. 111).

There are 12 pairs of ribs. Each rib consists of two parts: the costocartilage anteriorly and the long, thin, curved osseous portion posteriorly. The first seven ribs are attached to the manubrium and sternum, whereas each of the lower five ribs is attached to the rib above by costo-cartilages.

Trauma

Anterior dislocation of the SCJ is much more common than posterior dislocation because the sternoclavicular ligament is stronger posteriorly (251). Anterior dislocations are easier to diagnose clinically because of the obvious deformity of the anterior chest wall (Fig. 112). By comparison, posterior dislocation is difficult to diagnose both clinically and radiologically. Because of the proximity of the great vessels, trachea, and esophagus to the medial end of the clavicle, posterior dislocation of the SCJ can be fatal. The cross-sectional display of CT enables more accurate demonstration of sternoclavicular dislocation, with less discomfort and inconvenience for the patient, than does conventional tomography (70,206).

Fractures of the ribs may cause diagnostic problems in any patient who has had an abnormal radionuclide study and a history of carcinoma. Conventional radiographs may not reveal a corresponding abnormality, and the question of a subtle metastasis presents a diagnostic problem. CT can demonstrate callus formation and rib deformity characteristic of a healed fracture (Fig. 113), confirm that an acute rib fracture is not pathologic, show that the rib does contain a focus of metastatic tumor (80), or help assess the cause of otherwise unexplained chest-wall or rib pain (79).

Infection

Infection of the sternum and SCJ usually occurs following surgery (114) or radiation therapy. Drug addiction, infective endocarditis, and adjacent mediastinal infections are other causes of SCJ septic arthritis and osteomyelitis.

Radiographic findings of periosteal reaction and focal erosion can be subtle and difficult to detect because of osteopenia and the complex bony anatomy. In postoperative patients, radionuclide imaging usually is not beneficial, because the isotope normally concentrates in sur-

A,B

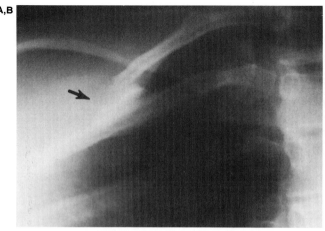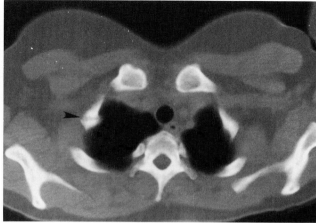

FIG. 113. Healing fracture of right first rib in a 25-year-old woman. **A:** Coned-down view from a chest radiograph shows what appears to be a destructive lesion of the first rib (*arrow*). A radionuclide bone scan confirmed a focal abnormality of the rib. **B:** CT through the abnormal area clearly documented a healing fracture (*arrowhead*).

gical sites. CT can effectively demonstrate small areas of bone destruction, periosteal reaction, and the presence of soft-tissue abscess (Fig. 114).

Neoplasia

Metastatic disease to the sternum and ribs due to hematogenous spread or contiguous involvement by a neoplasm is common, whereas primary neoplasms of these structures, such as multiple myeloma, lymphoma, Ewing tumor, or chondrosarcoma, are rare. Except for multiple myeloma, these lesions usually demonstrate increased radionuclide accumulation. In patients known to have neoplasms and unexplained chest-wall pain, CT may demonstrate abnormalities not evident on conventional radiographs (80) (Fig. 115). A major advantage of CT is the ability to image bone and soft tissues of the mediastinum simultaneously.

Arthropathy

The SCJ frequently is involved with osteoarthritis, rheumatoid arthritis, scleroderma, ankylosing spondylitis, and other collagen vascular diseases. Sternocostoclavicular hyperostosis is characterized by periosteal and endosteal hyperossification of the sternum, clavicles, and upper ribs, as well as ossification of the surrounding soft tissues (50,289,305) (Fig. 116). Patients with SCJ arthropathy may present with focal tenderness and soft-tissue swelling over the involved joint, clinically indistinguishable from infection. When plain radiographs are equivocal, CT is very useful in assessing bony reaction, joint effusion, and soft-tissue involvement.

Accessory Vertebral Joints

Costotransverse and costovertebral joints are imaged each time a CT study is performed on the thorax or spine; CT provides a much better image of these joints than does conventional radiography and can be relied on to solve an occasional imaging problem related to them (Fig. 117).

Temporomandibular Joint

CT can make important contributions to the diagnosis and management of temporomandibular joint (TMJ) disorders. In general, cross-sectional images of the TMJ have not been useful. Instead, sagittal images have been obtained either by reformatting data from a stack of transaxial images (51) (Fig. 118) or by positioning the patient so that direct sagittal images are possible (221,224,304)

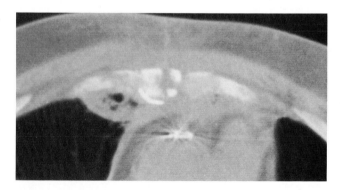

FIG. 114. Infection of the postoperative sternum. Conventional radiographs of this 55-year-old man with cellulitis were suggestive, but not diagnostic, of osteomyelitis. CT section clearly shows destruction of the sternum, soft-tissue swelling, and retrosternal gas.

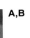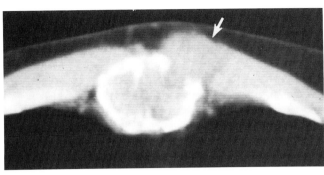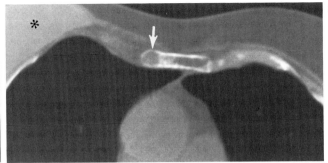

FIG. 115. Tumors of the sternum. **A:** Plasmacytoma of the sternum has expanded the bone, fragmented the cortex, and invaded the adjacent soft tissues (*arrow*). **B:** Metastatic breast cancer of the manubrium is manifested as permeative destruction associated with thinning of the cortex and focal expansion on the right side (*arrow*). Note the breast prosthesis (*).

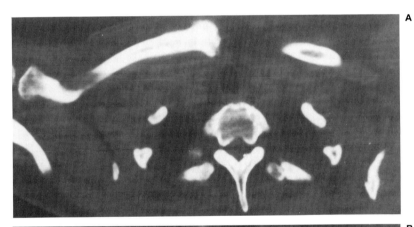

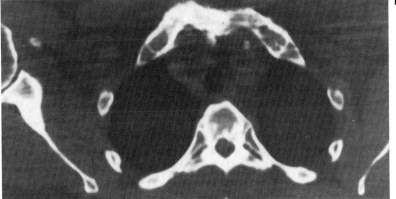

FIG. 116. Sternocostoclavicular hyperostosis in a 49-year-old man with ankylosing spondylitis. **A:** CT through the long axis of the right clavicle shows enlargement, sclerosis, and hyperostosis. **B:** CT section through the sternoclavicular articulation shows hyperostosis, with fusion of the rib to the sternum. Note also ankylosis of the costovertebral and costotransverse articulations.

A,B

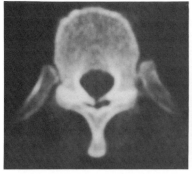
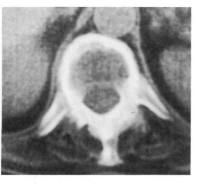

FIG. 117. Costovertebral joints. A: CT section of a lower thoracic vertebra shows articulation of the ribs with the vertebra at the body-pedicle junction. B: Ankylosing spondylitis. CT section of a lower thoracic vertebra shows ankylosis of the left costovertebral joint.

(Fig. 119). Reformatted sagittal images often are degraded by small amounts of motion and may lack sharp anatomic edges. Direct sagittal images are much sharper, but may be awkward for the patient owing to positioning constraints.

CT is very useful for evaluation of osseous anatomy, including detection and staging of tumors, arthritic changes, and fractures (221,224,335). Detection of internal derangement of the disc can be accomplished because of its inherent difference in density from surrounding structures. CT generally performs as well as arthrography for demonstration of disc position (147,335).

The disc or meniscus normally sits between the condyle and the mandibular fossa. When the disc is in normal position, the anterior angle between the condylar head and the fossa contains the two bellies of the lateral pterygoid muscle, separated by the lateral pterygoid fat pad. The combined density of these structures is lower than that of the disc, usually less than 65 HU (221). With the disc dislocated anteriorly, this angle fills with tissue of higher density than the adjacent muscle and soft tissue. The normal lateral pterygoid fat pad is distorted or obliterated. Return to the normal meniscocondylar relationship (recapture of the disc) is recognized by a return of the normal appearance of the condyloglenoid angle, with the condyle translated anteriorly.

The advantages of CT are its sectional display of osseous and soft-tissue anatomy and its noninvasive nature. Its disadvantages are that it is technically demanding to perform CT well, it fails to delineate the condition of the disc itself, and it provides no dynamic functional information.

MRI provides greater inherent soft-tissue contrast than any other imaging method. For TMJ imaging, the sagittal plane is preferred (131,132,144,286). Surface coils have been employed to improve the signal-to-noise ratio, increase the spatial resolution, and decrease the section thickness (174). Proton-density or balanced images (intermediate TR, short TE) obtained with a high-field-strength unit (1.5 T) seem to provide optimal contrast and signal for TMJ imaging.

The normal disc can be seen on MR images as a biconcave structure of relatively low signal located between the condyle and the mandibular fossa (Fig. 120). Using a

plane parallel to the mandibular ramus as a standard, the posterior aspect of the disc rests at or near the apex of the head of the condyle. Medial to that plane, the disc is more anterior in position, whereas lateral to the ramus, the disc tends to be more posterior. Lower-signal cortical bone defines the condyle, eminence, and fossa. Both the bone and the disc are surrounded by high-signal fat. Thin, linear, intermediate-signal structures are visible posterior to the disc in many patients, depicting the retrodiscal bilaminar zone.

Abnormal discs are recognized by a signal lower than normal and an abnormal position (131,132,144) (Figs. 121 and 122). When displaced, the disc is seen anterior to the condyle, often folded on itself. If recapture occurs, the disc is seen in normal position on the open-mouth

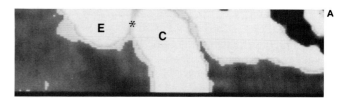

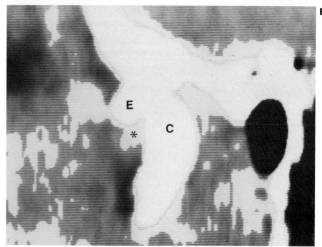

FIG. 118. Sagittally reformatted CT section of temporomandibular joint. A: Closed-mouth position shows normal position of disc (*) between condyle (C) and temporal eminence (E). B: Partially open mouth position of another person shows anterior dislocation of disc (*), as demonstrated by computer highlighting of pixels with defined attenuation values (blink mode).

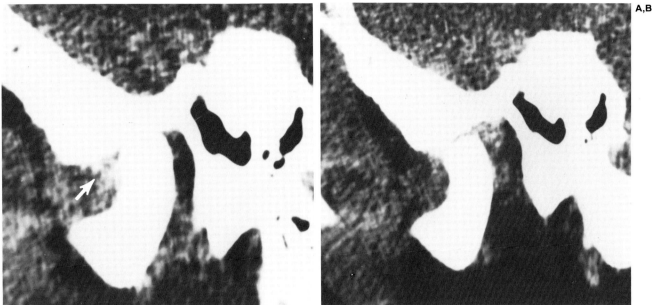

FIG. 119. Direct sagittal CT sections of TMJ. **A:** Disc is anteriorly dislocated (*arrow*) in jaw-relaxed position. **B:** Disc returns to normal position (recaptured) in partially open mouth position.

images. MRI may also be of help in evaluating meniscal prostheses (181).

Like CT, MRI is an excellent method for demonstration of disc position. MRI yields better soft-tissue contrast than does CT, but it provides inferior osseous detail compared with CT. MRI performs as well as arthrography in the demonstration of disc position, but less well in the demonstration of disc condition or dynamic function (132,174,355). At present, MRI is the best noninvasive method for determination of disc location.

Ligaments and Tendons

Until the development of sectional imaging, ligaments and tendons were best evaluated by physical examination (250). Ultrasonography contributed to ligament and tendon analysis, but never became routine. CT provided the first major advance in the investigation of these problems, but its use has been limited because it generally shows these structures in cross section, whereas a longitudinal image would be more desirable. Nonetheless, CT has been effective for showing soft-tissue edema associated with tenosynovitis or tendon injury (292).

MRI has developed into a useful method for imaging ligaments and tendons (13,64,247). These structures are primarily collagenous and therefore of low signal intensity on both T1-weighted and T2-weighted images because of their low proton density and short T2 relaxation values (99). Because they are invariably surrounded by fat, normal tendons are easily demonstrated as structures of very low signal outlined by high-signal fat. Also, the imaging

plane can be oriented along the long axis of any ligament or tendon.

Abnormal ligaments and tendons are detected because of alterations within the structures themselves or in the surrounding tissues. A rupture may be seen as the anatomic disruption of the structure, with associated signal changes due to hemorrhage and edema. Infiltration of surrounding fat is common. Among the commonly imaged ligaments are those about the knee (208,257,340) and ankle (16). Quadriceps, patellar, and Achilles tendon ruptures (284) are easily documented (Fig. 123). MRI is

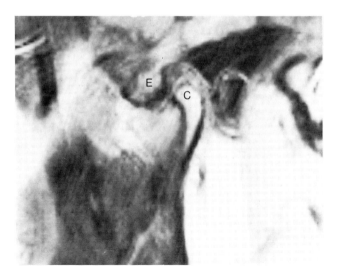

FIG. 120. MRI of normal TMJ. T1-weighted (TR = 900 msec, TE = 17 msec) sagittal image shows disc interposed between condyle (C) and temporal eminence (E).

A,B

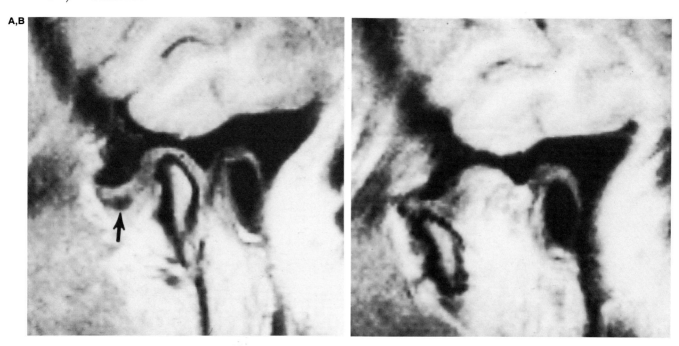

FIG. 121. MRI of dislocated disc, with recapture. **A:** T1-weighted (TR = 900 msec, TE = 17 msec) sagittal image shows low-signal-intensity disc (*arrow*) anterior to condyle. Note also the small spur on the anterior aspect of the condyle. **B:** In the maximally open position, the disc is shown in its normal position interposed between the condyle and the apex of the eminence.

A,B

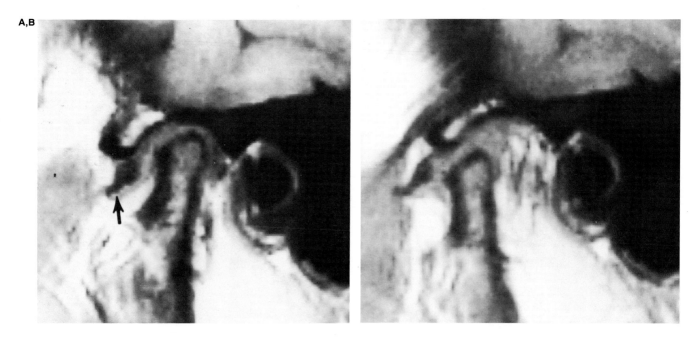

FIG. 122. MRI of dislocated disc, without recapture. **A:** T1-weighted (TR = 900 msec, TE = 17 msec) sagittal image shows low-signal-intensity disc (*arrow*) anterior to condyle. Note also the flattening and irregularity of the condyle, indicating osteoarthritis. **B:** In the maximally open position, the disc remains anterior to the condyle. Note that the range of condyle mobility is less than that shown in Fig. 121B because of restriction caused by the nonreducing disc.

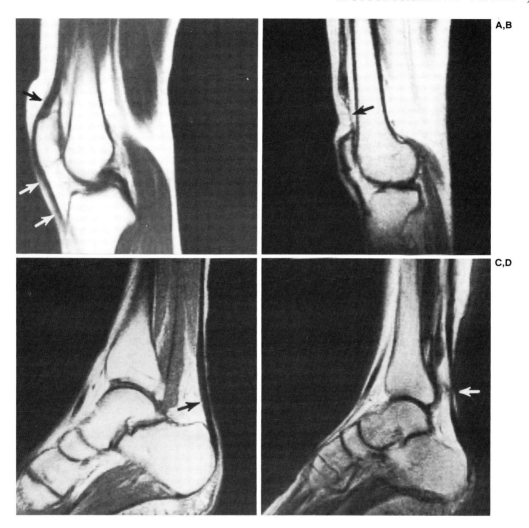

FIG. 123. Tendon imaging. **A:** Parasagittal MRI (TR = 300 msec, TE = 30 msec) of normal volunteer's knee showing normal quadriceps and patellar tendons (*arrows*). **B:** Parasagittal MRI (TR = 500 msec, TE = 30 msec) of patient with rheumatoid arthritis whose quadriceps tendon has ruptured (*arrow*) at the junction with the patella. Note that the patellar tendon is lax. **C:** Parasagittal MRI (TR = 1,500 msec, TE = 30 msec) of normal ankle showing normal Achilles tendon (*arrow*). **D:** Parasagittal MRI (TR = 500 msec, TE = 30 msec) of Achilles tendon rupture, showing disruption of the tendon (*arrow*) and signal-intensity changes in adjacent fat, probably due to hemorrhage and edema. (From ref. 247.)

also effective for analysis of reinjured tendons following surgical repair.

CONFIRMATION OF SCINTIGRAPHIC ABNORMALITIES

Many times it is necessary to confirm and decide the importance of a skeletal abnormality detected when a patient is surveyed by a radionuclide study. Conventional or coned-down radiographs of the region of interest are then obtained and in most cases answer these questions. In the past, when there was no good roentgenographic correlate for a scintigraphic abnormality, there were limited options: (a) to ignore the image, (b) to obtain follow-up films at a later date, or (c) to perform "blind" biopsy. Now, if a scintigraphic abnormality appears important, but cannot be confirmed by radiographic techniques, CT and MRI are available for further assessment. When used in carefully selected cases, these methods have been very

rewarding (175) (Fig. 124). CT has proved much more sensitive than radiography for detecting bone density changes, and MRI for detecting marrow alterations. In many cases, CT has shown convincingly that a focal radionuclide accumulation was caused by a benign osseous process (e.g., dystrophic or degenerative changes).

CT AND PERCUTANEOUS MUSCULOSKELETAL BIOPSY

Percutaneous biopsy of lesions of the musculoskeletal system can be a very valuable diagnostic procedure (6,231,245,246,333). CT and MRI may affect decision making and biopsy performance in several ways (129). First, CT or MRI may localize and characterize a lesion, helping to decide whether or not to perform a biopsy (Fig. 125). Second, sectional imaging may show the peripheral

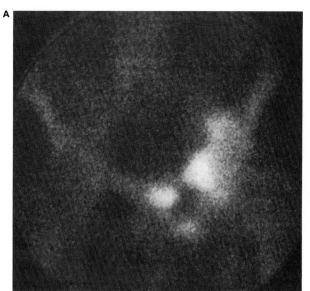

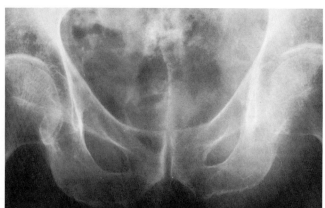

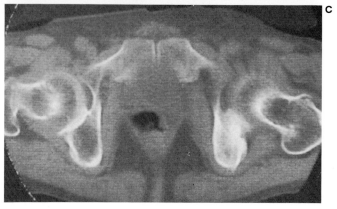

FIG. 124. Confirmation of abnormality shown by bone scan. **A:** ^{99m}Tc bone scan in this 79-year-old man, now 13 years after the diagnosis of prostate cancer, shows focal radionuclide accumulation in the acetabulum. **B:** Although, in retrospect, the left ''teardrop'' is denser than the right, initially the conventional radiographs did not seem to confirm a focal osseous abnormality. **C:** CT sections clearly showed diffuse osteosclerosis of the acetabulum, here seen as sclerosis of the ischial tuberosity and posterior acetabulum.

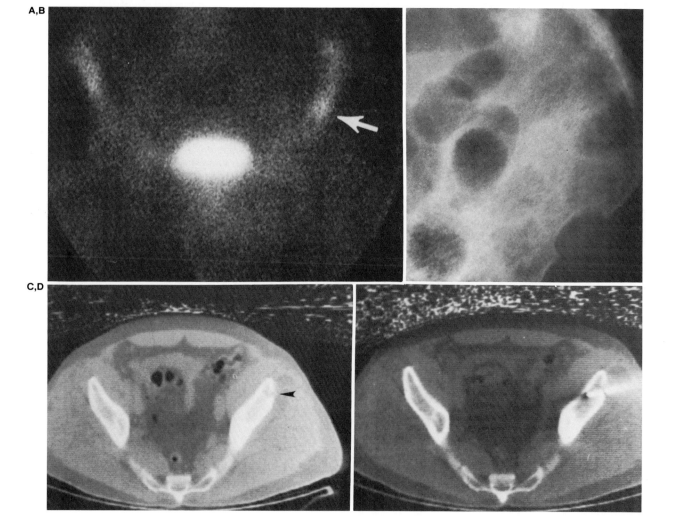

REFERENCES

1. Aisen AM, Glazer GM. Diagnosis of osteoid osteoma using computed tomography. *J Comput Tomogr* 1984;8:175–178.
2. Aisen AM, Martel W, Braunstein EM, McMillin KI, Phillips WA, Kling TF. MRI and CT evaluation of primary bone and soft-tissue tumors. *AJR* 1986;146:749–756.
3. Aitken AG, Flodmark O, Newman DE, Kilcoyne RF, Shuman WP, Mack LA. Leg length determination by CT digital radiography. *AJR* 1985;144:613–615.
4. Amendola MA, Glazer GM, Agha FP, Francis IR, Weatherbee L, Martel W. Myositis ossificans circumscripta: computed tomographic diagnosis. *Radiology* 1983;149:775–779.
5. Amendola MA, Shirazi K, Amendola BE, Kuhns LR, Tisnado J, Yaghmai I. Computed tomography of malignant tumors of the osseous pelvis. *Comput Radiol* 1983;7:107–117.
6. Ayala AG, Zornosa J. Primary bone tumors: percutaneous needle biopsy, radiologic-pathologic study of 222 biopsies. *Radiology* 1983;149:675–679.
7. Baker HL Jr, Berquist TH, Kispert DB, et al. Magnetic resonance imaging in a routine clinical setting. *Mayo Clin Proc* 1985;60:75–90.
8. Baker LL, Hajek PC, Bjorkengren A, et al. High-resolution magnetic resonance imaging of the wrist: normal anatomy. *Skeletal Radiol* 1987;16:128–132.
9. Bankoff MS, Sarno RC, Carter BL. CT scanning in septic sacroiliac arthritis or periarticular osteomyelitis. *Comput Radiol* 1984;8:165–170.
10. Bassett LW, Gold RH, Reicher M, Bennett LR, Tooke SM. Magnetic resonance imaging in the early diagnosis of ischemic necrosis of the femoral head: preliminary results. *Clin Orthop* 1987;214:237–248.
11. Beltran J, Gray LA, Bools JC, Zuelzer W, Weis LD, Unverferth LJ. Rotator cuff lesions of the shoulder: evaluation by direct sagittal CT arthrography. *Radiology* 1986;160:161–165.
12. Beltran J, Noto AM, Chakeres DW, Christoforidis AJ. Tumors of the osseous spine: staging with MR imaging versus CT. *Radiology* 1987;162:565–569.
13. Beltran J, Noto AM, Herman LJ, Lubbers LM. Tendons: high-field-strength, surface coil MR imaging. *Radiology* 1987;162:735–740.
14. Beltran J, Noto AM, Herman LJ, Mosure JC, Burk JM, Christoforidis AJ. Joint effusions: MR imaging. *Radiology* 1986;158:133–137.
15. Beltran J, Noto AM, Mosure JC, Bools JC, Zuelzer W, Christoforidis AJ. Meniscal tears: MR demonstration of experimentally produced injuries. *Radiology* 1986;158:691–693.
16. Beltran J, Noto AM, Mosure JC, Shamam OM, Weiss KL, Zuelzer WA. Ankle: surface coil MR imaging at 1.5T. *Radiology* 1986;161:203–209.
17. Beltran J, Noto AM, Mosure JC, Weiss KL, Zuelzer W, Christoforidis AJ. The knee: surface-coil MR imaging at 1.5T. *Radiology* 1986;159:747–751.
18. Beltran J, Simon DC, Levy M, Herman L, Weis L, Mueller CF. Aneurysmal bone cysts: MR imaging at 1.5T. *Radiology* 1986;158:689–690.
19. Bernardino ME, Jing BS, Thomas JL, Lindell MM, Zornoza J. The extremity soft-tissue lesion: a comparative study of ultrasound, computed tomography, and xeroradiography. *Radiology* 1981;139:53–59.
20. Berquist TH, Brown ML, Fitzgerald RH, May GR. Magnetic resonance imaging: application in musculoskeletal infection. *Magn Reson Imaging* 1985;3:219–230.
21. Biondetti PR, Vannier MW, Gilula LA, Knapp R. Wrist: coronal and transaxial CT scanning. *Radiology* 1987;163:149–151.
22. Bloem JL, Bluemm RG, Taminiau AHM, van Oosterom AT, Stolk J, Doornbos J. Magnetic resonance imaging of primary malignant bone tumors. *RadioGraphics* 1987;7:425–445.
23. Bloem JL, Mulder JD. Chondroblastoma: a clinical and radiological study of 104 cases. *Skeletal Radiol* 1985;14:1–9.
24. Bluemm RG, Falke THM, Ziedes des Plantes BG, Steiner RM. Early Legg-Perthes disease (ischemic necrosis of the femoral head) demonstrated by magnetic resonance imaging. *Skeletal Radiol* 1985;14:95–98.
25. Blumberg ML. Computed tomography and acetabular trauma. *Comput Tomogr* 1980;4:47–53.
26. Bohndorf K, Reiser M, Lochner B, Feaux de Lacroix W, Steinbrich W. Magnetic resonance imaging of primary tumours and tumour-like lesions of bone. *Skeletal Radiol* 1986;15:511–517.
27. Borlaza GS, Seigel R, Kuhns LR, Good AE, Rapp R, Martel W. Computed tomography in the evaluation of sacroiliac arthritis. *Radiology* 1981;139:437–440.
28. Bouras A, Larde D, Mathieu D, Delepine G, Benameur C, Ferrane J. The value of computed tomography in osseous hydatid disease (echinococcosis). *Skeletal Radiol* 1984;12:192–195.
29. Boyko OB, Cory DA, Cohen MD, Provisor A, Mirkin D, DeRosa GP. MR imaging of osteogenic and Ewing's sarcoma. *AJR* 1987;148:317–322.
30. Braithwaite PA, Lees RF. Vertebral hydatid disease: radiological assessment. *Radiology* 1981;140:763–766.
31. Braunstein EM, Silver TM, Martel W, Jaffe M. Ultrasonographic diagnosis of extremity masses. *Skeletal Radiol* 1981;6:157–163.
32. Braunstein EM, Weissman BN, Seltzer SE, Sosman JL, Wang A-M, Zamani A. Computed tomography and conventional radiographs of the craniocervical region in rheumatoid arthritis: a comparison. *Arthritis Rheum* 1984;27:26–31.
33. Breatnach E, Robinson PJ. Repositioning errors in measurement of vertebral attenuation values by computed tomography. *Br J Radiol* 1983;56:299–305.
34. Brooks RA. A quantitative theory of the Hounsfield unit and its application to dual energy scanning. *J Comput Assist Tomogr* 1977;1:487–493.
35. Brooks RA, Di Chiro G. Beam-hardening in x-ray reconstructive tomography. *Phys Med Biol* 1976;21:390–398.
36. Bulcke JA, Termote JL, Palmers Y, Crolla D. Computed tomography of the human skeletal muscular system. *Neuroradiology* 1979;17:127–136.
37. Burk DL Jr, Kanal E, Brunberg JA, Johnstone GF, Swensen HE, Wolf GL. 1.5-T surface-coil MRI of the knee. *AJR* 1986;147:293–300.
38. Burk DL Jr, Mears DC, Herbert DL, Straub WH, Cooperstein LA, Beck EA. Pelvic and acetabular fractures: examination by angled CT scanning. *Radiology* 1984;153:548.
39. Burk DL Jr, Mears DC, Kennedy WH, Cooperstein LA, Herbert DL. Three-dimensional computed tomography of acetabular fractures. *Radiology* 1985;155:183–186.
40. Campanacci M, Picci P, Gherlinzoni F, Guerra A, Bertoni F, Neff JR. Parosteal osteosarcoma. *J Bone Joint Surg* 1984;66(B):313–321.
41. Cann CE. Low-dose CT scanning for quantitative spinal mineral analysis. *Radiology* 1981;140:813–815.
42. Cann CE, Genant HK. Precise measurement of vertebral mineral content using computed tomography. *J Comput Assist Tomogr* 1980;4:493–500.
43. Cann CE, Genant HK. Cross-sectional studies of vertebral mineral using quantitative computed tomography. *J Comput Assist Tomogr* 1982;6:216.
44. Cann CE, Genant HK, Ettinger B. Quantitative computed tomography for prediction of vertebral fracture risk. *Bone* 1985;6:1–7.
45. Cann CE, Genant HK, Ettinger B, Gordan GS. Spinal mineral loss in oophorectomized women. *JAMA* 1980;244:2056–2059.
46. Cann CE, Martin MC, Genant HK, Jaffe RB. Decreased spinal mineral content in amenorrheic women. *JAMA* 1984;251:626.
47. Carrera GF. Computed tomography in sacroiliitis. *Clin Rheum Dis* 1983;9:403–415.
48. Carrera GF, Foley WD, Kozin F, Ryan L, Lawson TL. CT of sacroiliitis. *AJR* 1981;136:41–46.
49. Castor WR, Miller JDR, Russell AS, Chiu PL, Grace M, Hanson J. Computed tomography of the craniocervical junction in rheumatoid arthritis. *J Comput Assist Tomogr* 1983;7:31–36.
50. Chigira M, Maehara S, Nagase M, Ogimi T, Udagawa E. Sternocostoclavicular hyperostosis. A report of nineteen cases, with special reference to etiology and treatment. *J Bone Joint Surg* 1986;68(A):103–112.
51. Christiansen EL, Thompson JR, Hasso AN, Hinshaw DB Jr. Correlative thin section temporomandibular joint anatomy. *RadioGraphics* 1986;6:703–723.

52. Clark M, Gosnell M, Hager M, Doherty S. The calcium craze. *Newsweek* 1986 Jan 27:48–52.

53. Coffre C, Vanel D, Contesso G, et al. Problems and pitfalls in the use of computed tomography for the local evaluation of long bone osteosarcoma: report on 30 cases. *Skeletal Radiol* 1985;13:147–153.

54. Cohen JM, Weinreb JC, Redman HC. Arteriovenous malformations of the extremities: MR imaging. *Radiology* 1986;158:475–479.

55. Cohen MD, Klatte EC, Baehner R, et al. Magnetic resonance imaging of bone marrow disease in children. *Radiology* 1984;151:715–718.

56. Cohen MD, McGuire W, Cory DA, Smith JA. MR appearance of blood and blood products: an in vitro study. *AJR* 1986;146:1293–1297.

57. Cohen MD, Weetman RM, Provisor AJ, et al. Efficacy of magnetic resonance imaging in 139 children with tumors. *Arch Surg* 1986;121:522–529.

58. Coleman BG, Mulhern CB, Arger PH, et al. New observations of soft tissue sarcomas with contrast medium-enhanced computed tomography. *J Comput Tomogr* 1985;9:187–193.

59. Cone RO, Szabo R, Resnick D, Gelberman R, Taleisnik J, Gilula LA. Computed tomography of the normal radioulnar joints. *Invest Radiol* 1983;18:541–545.

60. Cone RO, Szabo R, Resnick D, Gelberman R, Taleisnik J, Gilula LA. Computed tomography of the normal soft tissues of the wrist. *Invest Radiol* 1983;18:546–551.

61. Consensus conference. Limb-sparing treatment of adult soft-tissue sarcomas and osteosarcomas. *JAMA* 1985;254:1791–1794.

62. Custer RP. Studies on the structure and function of bone marrow. I. Variability of the hematopoietic pattern and consideration of method for examination. *J Lab Clin* 1932;17:951–959.

63. Daffner RH, Lupetin AR, Dash N, Deeb ZL, Sefczek RJ, Schapiro RL. MRI in the detection of malignant infiltration of bone marrow. *AJR* 1986;146:353–358.

64. Daffner RH, Reimer BL, Lupetin AR, Dash N. Magnetic resonance imaging in acute tendon ruptures. *Skeletal Radiol* 1986;15:619–621.

65. de Santos LA, Edeiken B. Purely lytic osteosarcoma. *Skeletal Radiol* 1982;9:1–7.

66. de Santos LA, Ginaldi S, Wallace S. Computed tomography in liposarcoma. *Cancer* 1981;47:46–54.

67. de Santos LA, Goldstein HM, Murray JA, Wallace S. Computed tomography in the evaluation of musculoskeletal neoplasms. *Radiology* 1978;128:89–94.

68. de Santos LA, Murray JA. Evaluation of giant cell tumor by computerized tomography. *Skeletal Radiol* 1978;2:205–212.

69. Destouet JM, Gilula LA, Murphy WA. Computed tomography of long-bone osteosarcoma. *Radiology* 1979;131:439–445.

70. Destouet JM, Gilula LA, Murphy WA, Sagel SS. Computed tomography of the sternoclavicular joint and sternum. *Radiology* 1981;138:123–128.

71. Deutsch AL, Resnick D, Campbell G. Computed tomography and bone scintigraphy in the evaluation of tarsal coalition. *Radiology* 1982;144:137–140.

72. Deutsch AL, Resnick D, Mink JH. Computed tomography of the glenohumeral and sternoclavicular joints. *Orthop Clin* 1985;16:497–511.

73. Deutsch AL, Resnick D, Mink JH, et al. Computed and conventional arthrotomography of the glenohumeral joint: normal anatomy and clinical experience. *Radiology* 1984;153:603–609.

74. Dooms GC, Fisher MR, Hricak H, Higgins CB. MR imaging of intramuscular hemorrhage. *J Comput Assist Tomogr* 1985;9:908–913.

75. Dooms GC, Fisher MR, Hricak H, Richardson M, Crooks LE, Genant HK. Bone marrow imaging: magnetic resonance studies related to age and sex. *Radiology* 1985;155:429–432.

76. Dooms GC, Hricak H, Sollitto RA, Higgins CB. Lipomatous tumors and tumors with fatty component: MR imaging potential and comparison of MR and CT results. *Radiology* 1985;157:479–483.

77. Dorfman HD, Bhagavan BS. Malignant fibrous histiocytoma of soft tissue with metaplastic bone and cartilage formation: a new radiologic sign. *Skeletal Radiol* 1982;8:145–150.

78. Dunnill MS, Anderson JA, Whitehead R. Quantitative histological studies on age changes in bone. *J Pathol* 1967;94:275–291.

79. Edelstein G, Levitt RG, Slaker DP, Murphy WA. Computed tomography of Tietze syndrome. *J Comput Assist Tomogr* 1984;8:20–23.

80. Edelstein G, Levitt RG, Slaker DP, Murphy WA. CT observation of rib abnormalities: spectrum of findings. *J Comput Assist Tomogr* 1985;9:65–72.

81. Ekelund L, Herrlin K, Rydholm A. Comparison of computed tomography and angiography in the evaluation of soft tissue tumors of the extremities. *Acta Radiol* [*Diagn*] *(Stockh)* 1982;23:15–28.

82. Elsasser U, Ruegsegger P, Anliker M, Exner GU, Prader A. Loss and recovery of trabecular bone in the distal radius following fracture—immobilization of the upper limb in children. *Klin Wochenschr* 1979;57:763–767.

83. Engelstad BL, Gilula LA, Kyriakos M. Ossified skeletal muscle hemangioma: radiologic and pathologic features. *Skeletal Radiol* 1980;5:35–40.

84. Enneking WF. Staging of musculoskeletal neoplasms. *Skeletal Radiol* 1985;13:183–194.

85. Enneking WF, Chew FS, Springfield DS, Hudson TM, Spanier SS. The role of radionuclide bone-scanning in determining the resectability of soft-tissue sarcomas. *J Bone Joint Surg* 1981;63(A):249–257.

86. Exner GU, Prader A, Elsasser U, Anliker M. Bone densitometry using computed tomography. Part II: Increased trabecular bone density in children with chronic renal failure. *Br J Radiol* 1979;52:24–28.

87. Exner GU, Prader A, Elsasser U, Ruegsegger P, Anliker M. Bone densitometry using computed tomography. Part I: Selective determination of trabecular bone density and other bone mineral parameters. Normal values in children and adults. *Br J Radiol* 1979;52:14–23.

88. Fam AG, Rubenstein JD, Chin-Sang H, Leung FYK. Computed tomography in the diagnosis of early ankylosing spondylitis. *Arthritis Rheum* 1985;28:930–937.

89. Firooznia H, Golimbu C, Rafii M, Schwartz MS, Alterman ER. Quantitative computed tomography assessment of spinal trabecular bone. I. Age-related regression in normal men and women. *J Comput Tomogr* 1984;8:91–97.

90. Firooznia H, Golimbu C, Rafii M, Schwartz MS, Alterman ER. Quantitative computed tomography assessment of spinal trabecular bone. II. In osteoporotic women with and without vertebral fractures. *J Comput Tomogr* 1984;8:99–103.

91. Firooznia H, Rafii M, Golimbu C. Computed tomography of osteoid osteoma. *J Comput Tomogr* 1985;9:265–268.

92. Firooznia H, Rafii M, Golimbu C, Lam S, Sokolow J, Kung JS. Computed tomography of pressure sores, pelvic abscess, and osteomyelitis in patients with spinal cord injury. *Arch Phys Med Rehabil* 1982;63:545–548.

93. Fischer HJ, Lois JF, Gomes AS, Mirra JM, Deutsch L-S. Radiology and pathology of malignant fibrous histiocytomas of the soft tissues: a report of ten cases. *Skeletal Radiol* 1985;13:202–206.

94. Fisher MR, Dooms GC, Hricak H, Reinhold C, Higgins CB. Magnetic resonance imaging of the normal and pathologic muscular system. *Magn Reson Imaging* 1986;4:491–496.

95. Fishman EK, Drebin B, Magid D, et al. Volumetric rendering techniques: applications for three-dimensional imaging of the hip. *Radiology* 1987;163:737–738.

96. Fishman EK, Magid D, Mandelbaum BR, et al. Multiplanar (MPR) imaging of the hip. *RadioGraphics* 1986;6:7–54.

97. Fletcher BD, Scoles PV, Nelson AD. Osteomyelitis in children: detection by magnetic resonance (work in progress). *Radiology* 1984;150:57–60.

98. Frame B, Marel GM. Paget disease: a review of current knowledge. *Radiology* 1981;141:21–24.

99. Fullerton GD, Cameron IL, Ord VA. Orientation of tendons in the magnetic field and its effect on T2 relaxation times. *Radiology* 1985;155:433–435.

100. Gallimore GW Jr, Harms SE. Knee injuries: high-resolution MR imaging. *Radiology* 1986;160:457–461.

101. Gatenby RA, Mulhern CB Jr, Moldofsky PJ. Computed tomography guided thin needle biopsy of small lytic bone lesions. *Skeletal Radiol* 1984;11:289–291.

102. Genant HK, Boyd D. Quantitative bone mineral analysis using dual energy computed tomography. *Invest Radiol* 1977;12:545–551.

103. Genant HK, Boyd D, Rosenfeld D, Abols Y, Cann CE. Computed tomography. In: Cohn SH, ed. *Non-invasive measurements of bone*

mass and their clinical application. Boca Raton, FL: CRC Press, 1981:121–149.

104. Genant HK, Cann CE, Ettinger B, Gordan GS. Quantitative computed tomography of vertebral spongiosa: a sensitive method for detecting early bone loss after oophorectomy. *Ann Intern Med* 1982;97:699–705.

105. Gershuni DH, Skyhar MJ, Thompson B, Resnick D, Donald G, Akeson WH. A comparison of conventional radiography and computed tomography in the evaluation of spiral fractures of the tibia. *J Bone Joint Surg* 1985;76(A):1388–1395.

106. Ghelman B. Mensical tears of the knee: evaluation of high-resolution CT combined with arthrography. *Radiology* 1985;157:23–27.

107. Gill K, Bucholz RW. The role of computerized tomographic scanning in the evaluation of major pelvic fractures. *J Bone Joint Surg* 1984;66(A):34–39.

108. Gillespy T III, Genant HK, Helms CA. Magnetic resonance imaging of osteonecrosis. *Radiol Clin North Am* 1986;24:193–208.

109. Gilula LA, Murphy WA, Tailor CC, Patel RB. Computed tomography of the osseous pelvis. *Radiology* 1979;132:107–114.

110. Ginaldi S, de Santos LA. Computed tomography in the evaluation of small round cell tumors of bone. *Radiology* 1980;134:441–446.

111. Glass RBJ, Poznanski AK. Leg-length determination with biplanar CT scanograms. *Radiology* 1985;156:833–834.

112. Glass RBJ, Poznanski AK, Fisher MR, Shkolnik A, Dias L. Case report. MR imaging of osteoid osteoma. *J Comput Assist Tomogr* 1986;10:1065–1067.

113. Golimbu C, Firooznia H, Rafii M, Beranbaum E. Computerized tomography of the posterior cruciate ligament. *Comput Radiol* 1982;6:233–238.

114. Goodman LR, Kay HR, Teplick SK, Mundth ED. Complications of median sternotomy: computed tomographic evaluation. *AJR* 1983;141:225–230.

115. Goodman LR, Teplick SK, Kay H. Computed tomography of the normal sternum. *AJR* 1983;141:219–223.

116. Gould R, Rosenfield AT, Friedlander GE. Loose body within the glenohumeral joint in recurrent anterior dislocation: CT demonstration. *J Comput Assist Tomogr* 1985;9:404–406.

117. Graves VB, Wimmer R. Long-term reproducibility of quantitative computed tomography vertebral mineral measurements. *J Comput Tomogr* 1985;9:73–76.

118. Griffiths HJ, Hamlin DJ, Kiss S, Lovelock J. Efficacy of CT scanning in a group of 174 patients with orthopedic and musculoskeletal problems. *Skeletal Radiol* 1981;7:87–98.

119. Grindrod S, Tofts P, Edwards R. Investigation of human skeletal muscle structure and composition by x-ray computerised tomography. *Eur J Clin Invest* 1983;13:465–468.

120. Gross AE, McKee NH, Farine I, et al. A biological approach to the restoration of skeletal continuity following en bloc excision of bone tumors. *Orthopedics* 1985;8:586–591.

121. Guilford WB, Mintz PD, Blatt PM, Staab EV. CT of hemophilic pseudotumors of the pelvis. *AJR* 1980;135:167–169.

122. Guyer BH, Levinsohn EM, Fredrickson BE, Bailey GL, Formikell M. Computed tomography of calcaneal fractures: anatomy, pathology, dosimetry, and clinical relevance. *AJR* 1985;145:911–919.

123. Gylys-Morin VM, Hajek PC, Sartoris DJ, Resnick D. Articular cartilage defects: detectability in cadaver knees with MR. *AJR* 1987;148:1153–1157.

124. Haggmark T, Jansson E, Svane B. Cross-sectional area of the thigh muscle in man measured by computed tomography. *Scand J Clin Lab Invest* 1978;38:355–360.

125. Hajek PC, Baker LL, Bjorkengren A, Sartoris DJ, Neumann CH, Resnick D. High-resolution magnetic resonance imaging of the ankle: normal anatomy. *Skeletal Radiol* 1986;15:536–540.

126. Hajek PC, Baker LL, Goobar JE, et al. Focal fat deposition in axial bone marrow: MR characteristics. *Radiology* 1987;162:245–249.

127. Hall RB, Robinson LH, Malawar MM, Dunham WK. Periosteal osteosarcoma. *Cancer* 1985;55:165–171.

128. Harbin WP. Metastatic disease and the nonspecific bone scan: value of spinal computed tomography. *Radiology* 1982;145:105–107.

129. Hardy DC, Murphy WA, Gilula LA. Computed tomography in planning percutaneous bone biopsy. *Radiology* 1980;134:447–450.

130. Harms SE, Muschler G. Three-dimensional MR imaging of the knee using surface coils. *J Comput Assist Tomogr* 1986;10:773–777.

131. Harms SE, Wilk RM. Magnetic resonance imaging of the temporomandibular joint. *RadioGraphics* 1987;7:521–542.

132. Harms SE, Wilk RM, Wolford LM, Chiles DG, Milam SB. The temporomandibular joint: magnetic resonance imaging using surface coils. *Radiology* 1985;157:133–136.

133. Hartzman S, Reicher MA, Bassett LW, Duckwiler GR, Mandelbaum B, Gold RH. MR imaging of the knee. Part II. Chronic disorders. *Radiology* 1987;162:553–557.

134. Hauser H, Rheiner P. Computed tomography of the hand. II: Pathological conditions. *Medicamundi* 1983;28:128–134.

135. Haynor DR, Shuman WP. Double contrast CT arthrography of the glenoid labrum and shoulder girdle. *RadioGraphics* 1984;4:411–421.

136. Healey JH, Ghelman B. Osteoid osteoma and osteoblastoma. Current concepts and recent advances. *Clin Orthop* 1986;204:76–85.

137. Healey JH, Lane JM. Chondrosarcoma. *Clin Orthop* 1986;204:119–129.

138. Heger L, Wulff K. Computed tomography of the calcaneus: normal anatomy. *AJR* 1985;145:123–129.

139. Heger L, Wulff K, Seddiqi MSA. Computed tomography of calcaneal fractures. *AJR* 1985;145:131–137.

140. Heiken JP, Lee JKT, Smathers RL, Totty WG, Murphy WA. CT of benign soft-tissue masses of the extremities. *AJR* 1984;142:575–580.

141. Heller M, Jend H-H, Bucheler E, Hueck E, Viehweger G. The role of CT in diagnosis and follow-up of osteosarcoma. *J Cancer Res Clin Oncol* 1983;106(suppl):43–48.

142. Helms CA, Cann CE, Brunelle FO, Gilula LA, Chafetz N, Genant HK. Detection of bone-marrow metastases using quantitative computed tomography. *Radiology* 1981;140:745–750.

143. Helms CA, Genant HK. Computed tomography in the early detection of skeletal involvement with multiple myeloma. *JAMA* 1982;248:2886–2887.

144. Helms CA, Gillespy T III, Sims RE, Richardson ML. Magnetic resonance imaging of internal derangement of the temporomandibular joint. *Radiol Clin North Am* 1986;24:189–192.

145. Helms CA, Jeffrey RB, Wing VW. Computed tomography and plain film appearance of a bony sequestration: significance and differential diagnosis. *Skeletal Radiol* 1987;16:117–120.

146. Helms CA, McCarthy S. CT scanograms for measuring leg length discrepancy. *Radiology* 1984;151:802.

147. Helms CA, Vogler JB III, Morrish RB Jr, Goldman SM, Capra RE, Proctor E. Temporomandibular joint internal derangements: CT diagnosis. *Radiology* 1984;152:459–462.

148. Herman GT, Vose WF, Gomori JM, Gefter WB. Stereoscopic computed three-dimensional surface displays. *RadioGraphics* 1985;5:825–852.

149. Hermann G, Yeh H-C, Gilbert MS. Computed tomography and ultrasonography of the hemophilic pseudotumor and their use in surgical planning. *Skeletal Radiol* 1986;15:123–128.

150. Hermann G, Yeh H-C, Schwartz I. Computed tomography of soft-tissue lesions of the extremities, pelvic and shoulder girdles: sonographic and pathological correlations. *Clin Radiol* 1984;35:193–202.

151. Hernandez RJ, Conway JJ, Poznanski AK, Tachdjian MO, Dias LS, Kelikian AS. The role of computed tomography and radionuclide scintigraphy in the localization of osteomyelitis in flat bones. *J Pediatr Orthop* 1985;5:151–154.

152. Hernandez RJ, Tachdjian MO, Poznanski AK, Dias LS. CT determination of femoral torsion. *AJR* 1981;137:97–101.

153. Hertzanu Y, Glass RBJ, Mendelsohn DB. Sacrococcygeal chordoma in young adults. *Clin Radiol* 1983;34:327–329.

154. Huber DJ, Sauter R, Mueller E, Requardt H, Weber H. MR imaging of the normal shoulder. *Radiology* 1986;158:405–408.

155. Hudson TM. Fluid levels in aneurysmal bone cysts: a CT feature. *AJR* 1984;141:1001–1004.

156. Hudson TM, Galceran M. Radiology of sacrococcygeal chordoma—difficulties in detecting soft tissue extension. *Clin Orthop* 1983;175:237–242.

157. Hudson TM, Hamlin DJ, Fitzsimmons JR. Magnetic resonance imaging of fluid levels in an aneurysmal bone cyst and in anticoagulated human blood. *Skeletal Radiol* 1985;13:267–270.

158. Hudson TM, Hawkins IF. Radiological evaluation of chondroblastoma. *Radiology* 1981;139:1–10.

159. Hudson TM, Manaster BJ, Springfield DS, Spanier SS, Enneking WF, Hawkins IF Jr. Radiology of medullary chondrosarcoma: preoperative treatment planning. *Skeletal Radiol* 1983;10:69–78.

160. Hudson TM, Schakel M II, Springfield DS. Limitations of computed

tomography following excisional biopsy of soft tissue sarcomas. *Skeletal Radiol* 1985;13:49–54.

161. Hudson TM, Schakel M II, Springfield DS, Spanier SS, Enneking WF. The comparative value of bone scintigraphy and computed tomography in determining bone involvement by soft-tissue sarcomas. *J Bone Joint Surg* 1984;66(A):1400–1407.

162. Hudson TM, Schiebler M, Springfield DS, Enneking WF, Hawkins IF Jr, Spanier SS. Radiology of giant cell tumors of bone: computed tomography, arthro-tomography, and scintigraphy. *Skeletal Radiol* 1984;11:85–95.

163. Hudson TM, Schiebler M, Springfield DS, Hawkins IF Jr, Enneking WF, Spanier SS. Radiologic imaging of osteosarcoma: role in planning surgical treatment. *Skeletal Radiol* 1983;10:137–146.

164. Hudson TM, Springfield DS, Benjamin M, Bertoni F, Present DA. Computed tomography of parosteal osteosarcoma. *AJR* 1985;144:961–965.

165. Hudson TM, Springfield DS, Spanier SS, Enneking WF, Hamlin DJ. Benign exostoses and exostotic chondrosarcomas: evaluation of cartilage thickness by CT. *Radiology* 1984;152:595–599.

166. Hudson TM, Vandergriend RA, Springfield DS, et al. Aggressive fibromatosis: evaluation by computed tomography and angiography. *Radiology* 1984;150:495–501.

167. Hunter JC, Johnston WH, Genant HK. Computed tomography evaluation of fatty tumors of the somatic soft tissues: clinical utility and radiologic-pathologic correlation. *Skeletal Radiol* 1979;4:79–91.

168. Ihara H. Double-contrast CT arthrography of the cartilage of the patellofemoral joint. *Clin Orthop* 1985;188:50–55.

169. Jakob RP, Haertel M, Stussi E. Tibial torsion calculated by computerised tomography and compared to other methods of measurement. *J Bone Joint Surg* 1980;62(B):238–242.

170. Jensen PS, Orphanoudakis SC, Rauschkolb EN, Baron R, Lang R, Rasmussen H. Assessment of bone mass in the radius by computed tomography. *AJR* 1980;134:285–292.

171. Jetzer T, Erickson D, Webb A, Heithoff K. Computed tomography of the carpal tunnel with clinical and surgical correlation. *CT Clinical Symposium* 1984;7(4).

172. Kangarloo H, Dietrich RB, Taira RT, et al. MR imaging of bone marrow in children. *J Comput Assist Tomogr* 1986;10:205–209.

173. Kaplan PA, Williams SM. Mucocutaneous and peripheral soft-tissue hemangiomas: MR imaging. *Radiology* 1987;163:163–166.

174. Katzberg RW, Bessette RW, Tallents RH, et al. Normal and abnormal temporomandibular joint: MR imaging with surface coil. *Radiology* 1986;158:183–189.

175. Kean DM, Worthington BS, Preston BJ, et al. Nuclear magnetic resonance imaging of the knee: examples of normal anatomy and pathology. *Br J Radiol* 1983;56:355–364.

176. Kenney PJ, Gilula LA, Murphy WA. The use of computed tomography to distinguish osteochondroma and chondrosarcoma. *Radiology* 1981;139:129–137.

177. Kieft GJ, Bloem JL, Obermann WR, Verbout AJ, Rozing PM, Doornbos J. Normal shoulder: MR imaging. *Radiology* 1986;159:741–745.

178. Kieft GJ, Sartoris DJ, Bloem JL, et al. Magnetic resonance imaging of glenohumeral joint diseases. *Skeletal Radiol* 1987;16:285–290.

179. Kinnard P, Tricoire J, Levesque R, Bergeron D. Assessment of the unstable shoulder by computed arthrography: a preliminary report. *Am J Sports Med* 1983;11:157–159.

180. Kneeland JB, Carrera GF, Middleton WD, et al. Rotator cuff tears: preliminary application of high-resolution MR imaging with counter rotating current loop-gap resonators. *Radiology* 1986;160:695–699.

181. Kneeland JB, Carrera GF, Ryan DL, Jesmanowicz A, Froncisz W, Hyde JS. MR imaging of a fractured temporomandibular disk prosthesis. *J Comput Assist Tomogr* 1987;11:199–200.

182. Kneeland JB, Jesmanowicz A, Froncisz W, Grist TM, Hyde JS. High-resolution MR imaging using loop-gap resonators. *Radiology* 1986;158:247–250.

183. Koenig H, Lucas D, Meissner R. The wrist: a preliminary report on high-resolution MR imaging. *Radiology* 1986;160:463–467.

184. Kogutt MS. Computed radiographic imaging: use in low-dose leg length radiography. *AJR* 1987;148:1205–1206.

185. Kozin F, Carrera GF, Ryan LM, Foley D, Lawson T. Computed tomography in the diagnosis of sacroiliitis. *Arthritis Rheum* 1981;24:1479–1485.

186. Kuhn JP, Berger PE. Computed tomographic diagnosis of osteomyelitis. *Radiology* 1979;130:503–506.

187. Kulkarni MV, Drolshagen LF, Kaye JJ, et al. MR imaging of hemophiliac arthropathy. *J Comput Assist Tomogr* 1986;10:445–449.

188. Lange TA, Alter AJ. Evaluation of complex acetabular fractures by computed tomography. *J Comput Assist Tomogr* 1980;6:849–852.

189. Lange TA, Austin CW, Seibert JJ, Angtuaco TL, Yandow DR. Ultrasound imaging as a screening study for malignant soft-tissue tumors. *J Bone Joint Surg* 1987;69(A):100–115.

190. Lanir A, Aghai E, Simon JS, Lee RGL, Clouse ME. MR imaging in myelofibrosis. *J Comput Assist Tomogr* 1986;10:634–636.

191. Lanir A, Hadar H, Cohen I, et al. Gaucher disease: assessment with MR imaging. *Radiology* 1986;161:239–244.

192. Laval-Jeantet AM, Cann CE, Roger CB, Dallant P. A postprocessing dual energy technique for vertebral CT densitometry. *J Comput Assist Tomogr* 1984;8:1164–1167.

193. Laval-Jeantet AM, Roger B, Bouysee S, Bergot C, Mazess RA. Influence of vertebral fat content on quantitative CT density. *Radiology* 1986;159:463–466.

194. Lawson TL, Foley WD, Carrera GF, Berland LL. The sacroiliac joints: anatomic, plain roentgenographic, and computed tomographic analysis. *J Comput Assist Tomogr* 1982;6:307–314.

195. Lee KR, Cox GG, Neff JR, Arnett GR, Murphey MD. Cystic masses of the knee: arthrographic and CT evaluation. *AJR* 1987;148:329–334.

196. Lee KR, Tines SC, Yoon JW. CT findings of suprapatellar synovial cysts. *J Comput Assist Tomogr* 1984;8:296–299.

197. Leeson MC, Kay D, Smith BS. Intraosseous lipoma. *Clin Orthop* 1983;181:186–190.

198. Letournel E. Acetabulum fractures: classification and management. *Clin Orthop* 1980;151:81–106.

199. Levi C, Gray JE, McCullough EC, Hattery RR. The unreliability of CT numbers as absolute values. *AJR* 1982;139:443–447.

200. Levin DN, Herrmann A, Spraggins T, et al. Musculoskeletal tumors: improved depiction with linear combinations of MR images. *Radiology* 1987;163:545–549.

201. Levine E, Batnitzky S. Computed tomography of sacral and perisacral lesions. *Crit Rev Diagn Imaging* 1984;21:307–374.

202. Levine E, De Smet AA, Neff JR. Role of radiologic imaging in management planning of giant cell tumor of bone. *Skeletal Radiol* 1984;12:79–89.

203. Levine E, Lee KR, Neff JR, Maklad NF, Robinson RG, Preston DF. Comparison of computed tomography and other imaging modalities in the evaluation of musculoskeletal tumors. *Radiology* 1979;131:431–437.

204. Levine E, Neff JR. Dynamic computed tomography scanning of benign bone lesions: preliminary results. *Skeletal Radiol* 1983;9:238–245.

205. Levine E, Wetzel LH, Neff JR. MR imaging and CT of extrahepatic cavernous hemangiomas. *AJR* 1986;147:1299–1304.

206. Levinsohn EM, Bunnell WP, Yuan HA. Computed tomography in the diagnosis of dislocations of the sternoclavicular joint. *Clin Orthop* 1979;140:12–16.

207. Levitt RG, Sagel SS, Stanley RJ, Evens RG. Computed tomography of the pelvis. *Semin Roentgenol* 1978;13:193–200.

208. Li DKB, Adams ME, McConkey JP. Magnetic resonance imaging of the ligaments and menisci of the knee. *Radiol Clin North Am* 1986;24:209–227.

209. Li KC, Henkelman RM, Poon PY, Rubenstein J. MR imaging of the normal knee. *J Comput Assist Tomogr* 1984;8:1147–1154.

210. Lindell MM Jr, Shirkhoda A, Raymond AK, Murray JA, Harle TS. Parosteal osteosarcoma: radiologic–pathologic correlation with emphasis on CT. *AJR* 1987;148:323–328.

211. Lindsjo U, Hemmingsson A, Sahlstedt B, Danckwardt-Lilliestrom G. Computed tomography of the ankle. *Acta Orthop Scand* 1979;50:797–801.

212. Littrup PJ, Aisen AM, Braunstein EM, Martel W. Magnetic resonance imaging of femoral head development in roentgenographically normal patients. *Skeletal Radiol* 1985;14:159–163.

213. Lopez M, Sauerbrei E. Septic arthritis of the hip joint: sonographic and CT findings. *J Can Assoc Radiol* 1985;36:322–324.

214. Mack LA, Duesdieker GA, Harley JD, Bach AW, Winquist RA. CT of acetabular fractures: postoperative appearances. *AJR* 1983;141:891–894.

215. Magid D, Fishman EK, Brooker AF, Mandelbaum BR, Siegelman SS. Multiplanar computed tomography of acetabular fractures. *J Comput Assist Tomogr* 1986;10:778–783.

216. Magid D, Fishman EK, Scott WW Jr, et al. Femoral head avascular necrosis: CT assessment with multiplanar reconstruction. *Radiology* 1985;157:751–756.

217. Mahboubi S, Horstmann H. Femoral torsion: CT measurement. *Radiology* 1986;160:843–844.

218. Manco LG, Kavanaugh JH, Fay JJ, Bilfield BS. Mensicus tears of the knee: prospective evaluation with CT. *Radiology* 1986;159:147–151.

219. Manco LG, Kavanaugh JH. Lozman J, Colman ND, Bilfield BS, Fay JJ. Diagnosis of meniscal tears using high-resolution computed tomography. Correlation with arthroscopy. *J Bone Joint Surg* 1987;69(A):498–502.

220. Manco LG, Lozman J, Coleman ND, Kavanaugh JH, Bilfield BS, Dougherty J. Noninvasive evaluation of knee mensical tears: preliminary comparison of MR imaging and CT. *Radiology* 1987;163:727–730.

221. Manco LG, Messing SG, Busino LJ, Fasulo CP, Sordill WC. Internal derangements of the temporomandibular joint evaluated with direct sagittal CT: a prospective study. *Radiology* 1985;157:407–412.

222. Mankin HJ, Gebhardt MC. Advances in the management of bone tumors. *Clin Orthop* 1985;200:73–84.

223. Mantravadi RVP, Trippon MJ, Patel MK, Walker MJ, Das Gupta TK. Limb salvage in extremity soft-tissue sarcoma: combined modality therapy. *Radiology* 1984;152:523–526.

224. Manzione JV, Katzberg RW, Brodsky GL, Seltzer SE, Mellins HZ. Internal derangements of the temporomandibular joint: diagnosis by direct sagittal computed tomography. *Radiology* 1984;150:111–115.

225. Marchisello PJ. The use of computerized axial tomography for the evaluation of talocalcaneal coalition. A case report. *J Bone Joint Surg* 1987;69(A):609–611.

226. Markisz JA, Knowles RJR, Altchek DW, Schneider R, Whalen JP, Cahill PT. Segmental patterns of avascular necrosis of the femoral heads: early detection with MR imaging. *Radiology* 1987;162:717–720.

227. Marshall WH, Alvarez RE, Macovski A. Initial results with prereconstruction dual-energy computed tomography (PREDECT). *Radiology* 1981;140:421–430.

228. Martinez S, Korobkin M, Fondren FB, Hedlund LW, Goldner JL. Computed tomography of the normal patellofemoral joint. *Invest Radiol* 1983;18:249–253.

229. Martinez S, Korobkin M, Fondren FB, Hedlund LW, Goldner JL. Diagnosis of patellofemoral malalignment by computed tomography. *J Comput Assist Tomogr* 1983;7:1050–1053.

230. McKinstry CS, Steiner RE, Young AT, Jones L, Swirsky D, Aber V. Bone marrow in leukemia and aplastic anemia: MR imaging before, during, and after treatment. *Radiology* 1987;162:701–707.

231. Mick CA, Zinreich J. Percutaneous trephine bone biopsy of the thoracic spine. *Spine* 1985;10:737–740.

232. Middleton WD, Kneeland JB, Carrera GF, et al. High-resolution MR imaging of the normal rotator cuff. *AJR* 1987;148:559–564.

233. Middleton WD, Kneeland JB, Kellman GM, et al. MR imaging of the carpal tunnel: normal anatomy and preliminary findings in the carpal tunnel syndrome. *AJR* 1987;148:307–316.

234. Mino DE, Palmer AK, Levinsohn M. Radiography and computerized tomography in the diagnosis of incongruity of the distal radioulnar joint. *J Bone Joint Surg* 1985;67(A):247–252.

235. Mino DE, Palmer AK, Levinsohn M. The role of radiography and computerized tomography in the diagnosis of subluxation and dislocation of the distal radioulnar joint. *J Hand Surg* 1983;8:23–31.

236. Mitchell DG, Kressel HY, Arger PH, Dalinka M, Spritzer CE, Steinberg ME. Avascular necrosis of the femoral head: morphologic assessment by MR imaging with CT correlation. *Radiology* 1986;161:739–742.

237. Mitchell DG, Rao VM, Dalinka MK, et al. Femoral head vascular necrosis: correlation of MR imaging, radiographic staging, radionuclide imaging, and clinical findings. *Radiology* 1987;162:709–715.

238. Mitchell DG, Rao VM, Dalinka M, et al. Hematopoietic and fatty bone marrow distribution in the normal and ischemic hip: new observations with 1.5-T MR imaging. *Radiology* 1986;161:199–202.

239. Mitchell MD, Kundel HL, Steinberg ME, Kressel HY, Alavi A, Axel L. Avascular necrosis of the hip: comparison of MR, CT, and scintigraphy. *AJR* 1986;147:67–71.

240. Modic MT, Feiglin DH, Piraino DW, et al. Vertebral osteomyelitis: assessment using MR. *Radiology* 1985;157:157–166.

241. Modic MT, Pflanze W, Feiglin DHI, Behlobek G. Magnetic resonance imaging of musculoskeletal infections. *Radiol Clin North Am* 1986;24:247–258.

242. Montana MA, Richardson ML, Kilcoyne RF, Harley JD, Shuman WP, Mack LA. CT of sacral injury. *Radiology* 1986;161:499–503.

243. Moore SG, Gooding CA, Brasch RC, et al. Bone marrow in children with acute lymphocytic leukemia: MR relaxation times. *Radiology* 1986;160:237–240.

244. Morgan GJ, Schlegelmilch JG, Spiegel PK. Early diagnosis of septic arthritis of the sacroiliac joint by use of computed tomography. *J Rheumatol* 1981;8:979–982.

245. Murphy WA. Radiologically guided percutaneous musculoskeletal biopsy. *Orthop Clin North Am* 1983;14:233–241.

246. Murphy WA, Destouet JM, Gilula LA. Percutaneous skeletal biopsy 1981: a procedure for radiologists—results, review, and recommendations. *Radiology* 1981;139:545–549.

247. Murphy WA, Totty WG. Musculoskeletal magnetic resonance imaging. In: Kressel HY, ed. *Magnetic resonance annual 1986.* New York: Raven Press, 1985:1–35.

248. Murphy WA, Totty WG, Carroll JE. MRI of normal and pathological skeletal muscle. *AJR* 1986;146:565–574.

249. Naidich DP, Freedman MT, Bowerman JW, Siegelman SS. Computerized tomography in the evaluation of the soft tissue component of bony lesions of the pelvis. *Skeletal Radiol* 1978;3:144–148.

250. Nance EP Jr, Kaye JJ. Injuries of the quadriceps mechanism. *Radiology* 1982;142:301–307.

251. Nettles JL, Linscheid RL. Sternoclavicular dislocations. *J Trauma* 1968;8:158–164.

252. O'Doherty DS, Schellinger D, Raptopoulos V. Computed tomographic patterns of pseudohypertrophic muscular dystrophy: preliminary results. *J Comput Assist Tomogr* 1977;1:482–486.

253. Olson DO, Shields AF, Scheurich CJ, Porter BA, Moss AA. Magnetic resonance imaging of the bone marrow in patients with leukemia, aplastic anemia, and lymphoma. *Invest Radiol* 1986;21:540–546.

254. Osborn AG, Koehler PR, Gibbs FA, et al. Direct sagittal computed tomographic scans in the radiographic evaluation of the pelvis. *Radiology* 1980;134:255–257.

255. Ott SM, Kilcoyne RF, Chestnut CH III. Ability of four different techniques of measuring bone mass to diagnose vertebral fractures in postmenopausal women. *J Bone Min Res* 1987;2:201–210.

256. Passariello R, Trecco F, De Paulis F, Bonanni G, Masciocchi C, Zobel BB. Computed tomography of the knee joint: technique of study and normal anatomy. *J Comput Assist Tomogr* 1983;7:1035–1042.

257. Passariello R, Trecco F, De Paulis F, Masciocchi C, Bonanni G, Zobel BB. CT demonstration of capsuloligamentous lesions of the knee joint. *J Comput Assist Tomogr* 1986;10:450–456.

258. Passariello R, Trecco F, de Paulis F, Masciocchi C, Bonanni G, Zobel BB. Meniscal lesions of the knee joint: CT diagnosis. *Radiology* 1985;157:29–34.

259. Pate D, Resnick D, Andre M, et al. Perspective: three-dimensional imaging of the musculoskeletal system. *AJR* 1986;147:545–551.

260. Patel RB. Evaluation of complex carpal trauma: thin-section direct longitudinal computed tomography scanning through a plaster cast. *J Comput Tomogr* 1985;9:107–109.

261. Pavlov H, Hirschy JC, Torg JS. Computed tomography of the cruciate ligaments. *Radiology* 1979;132:389–393.

262. Penkava RR. Iliopsoas bursitis demonstrated by computed tomography. *AJR* 1980;135:175–176.

263. Petasnick JP, Turner DA, Charters JR, Gitelis S, Zacharias CE. Soft-tissue masses of the locomotor system: comparison of MR imaging with CT. *Radiology* 1986;160:125–133.

264. Pettersson H, Gillespy T III, Hamlin DJ, et al. Primary musculoskeletal tumors: examination with MR imaging compared with conventional modalities. *Radiology* 1987;164:237–241.

265. Pineda C, Resnick D, Greenway G. Diagnosis of tarsal coalition with computed tomography. *Clin Orthop* 1986;208:282–288.

266. Pollack MS, Dalinka MK, Kressel HY, Lotke PA, Spritzer CE.

Magnetic resonance imaging in the evaluation of suspected osteonecrosis of the knee. *Skeletal Radiol* 1987;16:121–127.

267. Porter BA, Shields AF, Olson DO. Magnetic resonance imaging of bone marrow disorders. *Radiol Clin North Am* 1986;24:269–289.

268. Quinn SF, Murray W, Watkins T, Kloss J. CT for determining the results of treatment of fractures of the wrist. *AJR* 1987;149:109–111.

269. Quint LE, Gross BH, Glazer GM, Braunstein EM, White SJ. CT evaluation of chondroblastoma. *J Comput Assist Tomogr* 1984;8:907–910.

270. Rafii M, Firooznia H, Bonamo JJ, Minkoff J, Golimbu C. Athlete shoulder injuries: CT arthrographic findings. *Radiology* 1987;162:559–564.

271. Rafii M, Firooznia H, Golimbu C. Computed tomography of septic joints. *J Comput Tomogr* 1985;9:51–60.

272. Rafii M, Firooznia H, Golimbu C, Bonamo J. Computed tomography of tibial plateau fractures. *AJR* 1984;142:1181–1186.

273. Rafii M, Firooznia H, Golimbu C, Minkoff J, Bonamo J. CT arthrography of capsular structures of the shoulder. *AJR* 1986;146:361–367.

274. Rafii M, Firooznia H, Golimbu C, Waugh T Jr, Naidich D. The impact of CT in clinical management of pelvic and acetabular fractures. *Clin Orthop* 1983;178:228–235.

275. Ram PC, Martinez S, Korobkin M, Breiman RS, Gallis HR, Harrelson JM. CT detection of intraosseous gas: a new sign of osteomyelitis. *AJR* 1981;137:721–723.

276. Ramos A, Castello J, Sartoris DJ, Greenway GD, Resnick D, Haghighi P. Osseous lipoma: CT appearance. *Radiology* 1985;157:615–619.

277. Randelli M, Gambrioli PL. Glenohumeral osteometry by computed tomography in normal and unstable shoulders. *Clin Orthop* 1986;208:151–156.

278. Rao VM, Fishman M, Mitchell DG, et al. Painful sickle cell crisis: bone marrow patterns observed with MR imaging. *Radiology* 1986;161:211–215.

279. Raskin RJ, Schnapf DJ, Wolf CR, Killian PJ, Lawless OJ. Computerized tomography in evaluation of atlantoaxial subluxation in rheumatoid arthritis. *J Rheumatol* 1983;10:33–41.

280. Reicher MA, Bassett LW, Gold RH. High-resolution magnetic resonance imaging of the knee joint: pathologic correlations. *AJR* 1985;145:903–909.

281. Reicher MA, Hartzman S, Bassett LW, Mandelbaum B, Duckwiler G, Gold RH. MR imaging of the knee. Part I. Traumatic disorders. *Radiology* 1987;162:547–551.

282. Reicher MA, Hartzman S, Duckwiler GR, Bassett LW, Anderson LJ, Gold RH. Mensical injuries: detection using MR imaging. *Radiology* 1986;159:753–757.

283. Reicher MA, Rauschning W, Gold RH, Bassett LW, Lufkin RB, Glen W. High-resolution magnetic resonance imaging of the knee joint: normal anatomy. *AJR* 1985;145:895–902.

284. Reinig JW, Dorwart RH, Roden WC. MR imaging of a ruptured Achilles tendon. *J Comput Assist Tomogr* 1985;9:1131–1134.

285. Reinus WR, Conway WF, Totty WG, et al. Carpal avascular necrosis: MR imaging. *Radiology* 1986;160:689–693.

286. Reiser M, Rupp N, Biehl TH, et al. MR in diagnosis of bone tumors. *Eur J Radiol* 1985;5:1–7.

287. Reiser M, Rupp N, Heller HJ, et al. MR-tomography in the diagnosis of malignant soft-tissue tumours. *Eur J Radiol* 1984;4:288–293.

288. Resnik CS, Deutsch AL, Resnick D, et al. Arthrotomography of the shoulder. *RadioGraphics* 1984;4:963–976.

289. Resnick D. Sternoclavicular hyperostosis. *AJR* 1980;135:1278–1280.

290. Rosen RA, Morehouse HT, Karp HJ, Yu GSM. Intracortical fissuring in osteomyelitis. *Radiology* 1981;141:17–20.

291. Rosenberg D, Baskies AM, Deckers PJ, Leiter BE, Ordia JI, Jablon IG. Pyogenic sacroiliitis: an absolute indication for computerized tomographic scanning. *Clin Orthop* 1984;184:128–132.

292. Rosenberg ZS, Feldman F, Singson RD. Peroneal tendon injuries: CT analysis. *Radiology* 1986;161:743–748.

293. Rosenberg ZS, Feldman F, Singson RD. Intra-articular calcaneal fractures: computed tomographic analysis. *Skeletal Radiol* 1987;16:105–113.

294. Rosenthal DI. Computed tomography in bone and soft tissue neoplasm: application and pathologic correlation. *CRC Crit Rev Diagn Imaging* 1982;18:243–278.

295. Rosenthal DI, Ganott MA, Wyshak G, Slovik DM, Doppelt SH, Neer RM. Quantitative computed tomography for spinal density measurement factors affecting precision. *Invest Radiol* 1985;20:306–310.

296. Rosenthal DI, Schiller AL, Mankin HJ. Chondrosarcoma: correlation of radiological and histological grade. *Radiology* 1984;150:21–26.

297. Rosenthal DI, Scott JA, Barranger J, et al. Evaluation of Gaucher disease using magnetic resonance imaging. *J Bone Joint Surg* 1986;68(A):802–808.

298. Rosenthal DI, Scott JA, Mankin HJ, Wismer GL, Brady TJ. Sacrococcygeal chordoma: magnetic resonance imaging and computed tomography. *AJR* 1985;145:143–147.

299. Rubin JI, Gomori JM, Grossman RI, Gefter WB, Kressel HY. High-field MR imaging of extracranial hematomas. *AJR* 1987;148:813–817.

300. Ryan LM, Carrera GF, Lightfoot RW Jr, Hoffman RG, Kozin F. The radiographic diagnosis of sacroiliitis. A comparison of different views with computed tomograms of the sacroiliac joint. *Arthritis Rheum* 1983;26:760–763.

301. Saks BJ. Normal acetabular anatomy for acetabular fracture assessment: CT and plain film correlation. *Radiology* 1986;159:139–145.

302. Sarno RC, Carter BL, Bankoff MS, Semine MC. Computed tomography in tarsal coalition. *J Comput Assist Tomogr* 1984;8:1155–1160.

303. Sartoris DJ, Devine S, Resnick D, et al. Plantar compartmental infection in the diabetic foot. The role of computed tomography. *Invest Radiol* 1985;20:772–784.

304. Sartoris DJ, Neumann CH, Riley RW. The temporomandibular joint: true sagittal computed tomography with meniscus visualization. *Radiology* 1984;150:250–254.

305. Sartoris DJ, Schreiman JS, Kerr R, Resnik CS, Resnick D. Sternocostoclavicular hyperostosis: a review and report of 11 cases. *Radiology* 1986;158:125–128.

306. Sauser DD, Billimoria PE, Rouse GA, Mudge K. CT evaluation of hip trauma. *AJR* 1980;135:269–274.

307. Scheffler R, Armstrong D, Hutton L. Computed tomographic diagnosis of distal radio-ulanar joint disruption. *J Can Assoc Radiol* 1984;35:212–213.

308. Schreiman JS, Crass JR, Wick MR, Maile CW, Thompson RC. Osteosarcoma: role of CT in limb-sparing treatment. *Radiology* 1986;161:485–488.

309. Schreiman JS, McLeod RA, Kyle RA, Beabout JW. Multiple myeloma: evaluation by CT. *Radiology* 1985;154:483–486.

310. Schwimmer M, Edelstein G, Heiken JP, Gilula LA. Synovial cysts of the knee: CT evaluation. *Radiology* 1985;154:175–177.

311. Seeger LL, Ruszkowski JT, Bassett LW, Kay SP, Kahmann RD, Ellman H. MR imaging of the normal shoulder: anatomic correlation. *AJR* 1987;148:83–91.

312. Segal D, Marsh JL, Leiter B. Clinical application of computerized axial tomography (CAT) scanning of calcaneus fractures. *Clin Orthop* 1985;199:114–123.

313. Seltzer SE. Value of computed tomography in planning medical and surgical treatment of chronic osteomyelitis. *J Comput Assist Tomogr* 1984;8:482–487.

314. Seltzer SE, Weissman BN. CT findings in normal and dislocating shoulders. *J Can Assoc Radiol* 1985;36:41–46.

315. Seltzer SE, Weissman BN, Braunstein EM, Adams DF, Thomas WH. Computed tomography of the hindfoot. *J Comput Assist Tomogr* 1984;8:488–497.

316. Seltzer SE, Weissman BN, Braunstein EM, Adams DF, Thomas WH. Computed tomography of the hindfoot with rheumatoid arthritis. *Arthritis Rheum* 1985;28:1234–1242.

317. Shirkhoda A, Brashear HR, Staab EV. Computed tomography of acetabular fractures. *Radiology* 1980;134:683–688.

318. Shuman WP, Kilcoyne RF, Matsen FA, Rogers JV, Mack LA. Double contrast computed tomography of the glenoid labrum. *AJR* 1983;141:581–584.

319. Sierra A, Potchen EJ, Moore J, Smith HG. High-field magnetic resonance imaging of aseptic necrosis of the talus. *J Bone Joint Surg* 1986;68(A):927–928.

320. Smith RW, Staple TW. Computerized tomography (CT) scanning technique for the hindfoot. *Clin Orthop* 1983;177:34–38.

321. Solomon MA, Gilula LA, Oloff LM, Oloff J. CT scanning of the

foot and ankle: 2. Clinical applications and review of the literature. *AJR* 1986;146:1204–1214.

322. Solomon MA, Gilula LA, Oloff LM, Oloff J, Compton T. CT scanning of the foot and ankle: 1. Normal anatomy. *AJR* 1986;146:1192–1203.

323. Soye I, Levine E, De Smet AA, Neff JR. Computed tomography in the preoperative evaluation of masses arising in or near the joints of the extremities. *Radiology* 1982;143:727–732.

324. Stark P, Jaramillo D. CT of the sternum. *AJR* 1986;147:72–77.

325. Steinbach LS, Helms CA, Sims RE, Gillespy T III, Genant HK. High resolution computed tomography of knee menisci. *Skeletal Radiol* 1987;16:11–16.

326. Steinbach LS, Schneider R, Goldman AB, Kazam E, Ranawat CS, Ghelman B. Bursae and abscess cavities communicating with the hip. Diagnosis using arthrography and CT. *Radiology* 1985;156:303–307.

327. Stoller DW, Martin C, Crues JV III, Kaplan L, Mink JH. Meniscal tears: pathologic correlation with MR imaging. *Radiology* 1987;163:731–735.

328. Sundaram M, McGuire MH, Fletcher J, Wolverson MK, Heiberg E, Shields JB. Magnetic resonance imaging of lesions of synovial origin. *Skeletal Radiol* 1986;15:110–116.

329. Sundaram M, McGuire MH, Herbold DR. Magnetic resonance imaging of osteosarcoma. *Skeletal Radiol* 1987;16:23–29.

330. Sundaram M, McGuire MH, Herbold DR, Wolverson MK, Heiberg E. Magnetic resonance imaging in planning limb-salvage surgery for primary malignant tumors of bone. *J Bone Joint Surg* 1986;68(A):809–819.

331. Swensen SJ, Keller PL, Berquist TH, McLeod RA, Stephens DH. Magnetic resonance imaging of hemorrhage. *AJR* 1985;145:921–927.

332. Taconis WK, Mulder JD. Fibrosarcoma and malignant fibrous histiocytoma of long bones: radiographic features and grading. *Skeletal Radiol* 1984;11:237–245.

333. Tehranzadeh J, Freiberger RH, Ghelman B. Closed skeletal needle biopsy: review of 120 cases. *AJR* 1983;140:113–115.

334. Termote JL, Baert A, Crolla D, Palmers Y, Bulcke JA. Computed tomography of the normal and pathologic muscular system. *Radiology* 1980;137:439–444.

335. Thompson JR, Christiansen E, Hasso AN, Hinshaw DB Jr. Temporomandibular joints: high-resolution computed tomographic evaluation. *Radiology* 1984;150:105–110.

336. Toby EB, Koman LA, Bechtold RE. Magnetic resonance imaging of pediatric hip disease. *J Pediatr Orthop* 1985;5:665–671.

337. Totty WG, Murphy WA, Ganz WI, Kumar B, Daum WJ, Siegel BA. Magnetic resonance imaging of the normal and ischemic femoral head. *AJR* 1984;143:1273–1280.

338. Totty WG, Murphy WA, Lee JKT. Soft-tissue tumors: MR imaging. *Radiology* 1986;160:135–141.

339. Totty WG, Vannier MW. Complex musculoskeletal anatomy: analysis using three dimensional surface reconstruction. *Radiology* 1984;150:173–177.

340. Turner DA, Prodromos CC, Petasnick JP, Clark JW. Acute injury of the ligaments of the knee: magnetic resonance evaluation. *Radiology* 1985;154:717–722.

341. Unger EC, Glazer HS, Lee JKT, Ling D. MRI of extracranial hematomas: preliminary observations. *AJR* 1986;146:403–407.

342. Unni KK, Dahlin DC, Beabout JW. Periosteal osteogenic sarcoma. *Cancer* 1976;37:2476–2485.

343. Unni KK, Dahlin DC, Beabout JW, Ivins JC. Parosteal osteogenic sarcoma. *Cancer* 1976;37:2466–2475.

344. Vanel D, Contesso G, Couanet D, Piekarski JD, Sarrazin D, Masselot J. Computed tomography in the evaluation of 41 cases of Ewing's sarcoma. *Skeletal Radiol* 1982;9:8–13.

345. Vannier MW, Totty WG, Stevens WG, et al. Musculoskeletal applications of three-dimensional surface reconstructions. *Orthop Clin North Am* 1985;16:543–555.

346. Vogelzang RL, Matalon TA, Neiman HL, Sakowicz BA. Lateral scout radiograph in CT-guided aspiration biopsy. *AJR* 1983;140:164.

347. Vogler JB III, Brown WH, Helms CA, Genant HK. The normal sacroiliac joint: a CT study of asymptomatic patients. *Radiology* 1984;151:433–437.

348. Wall SD, Fisher MR, Amparo EG, Hricak H, Higgins CB. Magnetic resonance imaging in the evaluation of abscesses. *AJR* 1985;144:1217–1221.

349. Weekes RG, Berquist TH, McLeod RA, Zimmer WD. Magnetic resonance imaging of soft-tissue tumors: comparison with computed tomography. *Magn Reson Imaging* 1985;3:345–352.

350. Weekes RG, McLeod RA, Reiman HM, Pritchard DJ. CT of soft-tissue neoplasms. *AJR* 1985;144:355–360.

351. Weeks PM, Vannier MW, Stevens WG, Gayou D, Gilula LA. Three-dimensional imaging of the wrist. *J Hand Surg* 1985;10(A):32–39.

352. Weiner DS, Cook AJ. Practical considerations in the use of computed tomography in the measurement of femoral anteversion. *Isr J Med Sci* 1980;16:288–294.

353. Weiss KL, Beltran J, Lubbers LM. High-field MR surface-coil imaging of the hand and wrist. Part II. Pathologic correlations and clinical relevance. *Radiology* 1986;160:147–152.

354. Weiss KL, Beltran J, Shamam OM, Stilla RF, Levey M. High-field MR surface-coil imaging of the hand and wrist. Part I. Normal anatomy. *Radiology* 1986;160:143–146.

355. Westesson P-L, Katzberg RW, Tallents RH, Woodworth-Sanchez RE, Svensson SA. CT and MR of the temporomandibular joint: comparison with autopsy specimens. *AJR* 1987;148:1165–1171.

356. Whelan MA, Gold RP. Computed tomography of the sacrum: 1. Normal anatomy. *AJR* 1982;139:1183–1190.

357. Whelan MA, Hilal SK, Gold RP, Luken MG, Michelson WJ. Computed tomography of the sacrum: 2. Pathology. *AJR* 1982;139:1191–1195.

358. Widjaja PM, Ermers JWLM, Sijbrandij S, Damsma H, Klinkhamer AC. Technique of torsion measurement of the lower extremity using computed tomography. *J Comput Assist Tomogr* 1985;9:466–470.

359. Wing VW, Jeffrey RB Jr, Federle MP, Helms CA, Trafton P. Chronic osteomyelitis examined by CT. *Radiology* 1985;154:171–174.

360. Wittenberg J, Fineberg HV, Ferrucci JT, et al. Clinical efficacy of computed body tomography. II. *AJR* 1980;134:1111–1120.

361. Woolson ST, Dev P, Fellingham LL, Vassiliadis A. Three-dimensional imaging of bone from computerized tomography. *Clin Orthop* 1986;202:239–248.

362. Yiu-Chiu VS, Chiu LC. Complementary values of ultrasound and computed tomography in the evaluation of musculoskeletal masses. *RadioGraphics* 1983;3:46–82.

363. Yulish BS, Mulopulos GP, Goodfellow DB, Bryan PJ, Modic MT, Dollinger BM. MR imaging of osteochondral lesions of talus. *J Comput Assist Tomogr* 1987;11:296–301.

364. Zagoria RJ, Karstaedt N, Koubek TD. MR imaging of rhabdomyolysis. *J Comput Assist Tomogr* 1986;10:268–270.

365. Zimmer WD, Berquist TH, McLeod RA, et al. Bone tumors: magnetic resonance imaging versus computed tomography. *Radiology* 1985;155:709–718.

366. Zimmer WD, Berquist TH, McLeod RA, et al. Magnetic resonance imaging of osteosarcomas. Comparison with computed tomography. *Clin Orthop* 1986;208:289–299.

367. Zlatkin MB, Lander PH, Begin LR, Hadjipavlou A. Soft-tissue chondromas. *AJR* 1985;144:1263–1267.

368. Zornoza J, Bernardino ME, Ordonez NG, Thomas JL, Cohen MA. Percutaneous needle biopsy of soft tissue tumors guided by ultrasound and computed tomography. *Skeletal Radiol* 1982;9:33–36.

369. Zucker-Pinchoff B, Hermann G, Srinivasan R. Computed tomography of the carpal tunnel: a radioanatomical study. *J Comput Assist Tomogr* 1981;5:525–528.

CHAPTER 22

The Spine

Mokhtar Gado, Klaus Sartor, and Fred J. Hodges III

The inherently high soft-tissue contrast achieved with computed tomography (CT), as compared with conventional radiography, allowed, for the first time, direct imaging of soft-tissue structures such as intervertebral discs, ligaments, muscles, and vessels, as well as adequate imaging of bone detail (61). However, demonstration of intradural structures by CT often requires intrathecal administration of water-soluble contrast material. Postmyelography CT may also be used to enhance or clarify myelographic findings of intradural as well as extradural abnormalities. Following the introduction of magnetic resonance imaging (MRI) as a clinically useful imaging modality for the brain in 1980 (65), it soon became obvious that the technique had even higher soft-tissue contrast sensitivity than CT, but its spatial resolution was limited. Only 5 years later (34), improvements in the spatial resolution of MR images and in the speed of data acquisition were made possible by a gain in the signal-to-noise ratio made possible by developments in surface-coil technology (103,111). Thus, intradural structures are demonstrated on MRI and in some cases may be differentiated on the basis of their inherent tissue contrast. On the other hand, the greatest topographic detail is provided by intrathecal-contrast-enhanced CT.

TECHNICAL CONSIDERATIONS

Whereas conventional radiographic examination of the entire spinal column is practical, CT and MRI examinations ordinarily are confined to certain regions. The limitation is imposed by the number of axial sections required and, in the case of MRI, by the length of spine that can be imaged at one time by a surface coil.

Computed Tomography

1. Image localization is essential. This is achieved by obtaining a digital radiograph (topogram) of the region in a lateral projection (Fig. 1). By interaction with software, the operator determines on the digital radiograph the upper and lower limits and the orientation of a set of parallel sections. At the end of the imaging procedure, a set of parallel lines corresponding to the imaging levels and orientation is generated by computer software, superimposed on the digital radiograph. These are valid, assuming that no patient motion has taken place during the examination and assuming correct registration of table increments between sections.

2. The raw data of the image should be processed in a small field of view (e.g., 125 × 125 mm) such that the total number of picture elements (pixels) of the matrix is condensed in a small area, allowing improvement of spatial resolution in the plane of the section, with a pixel size of 0.8 mm or better. Spatial resolution in the plane perpendicular to the plane of the section, i.e., in the longitudinal axis, is determined by slice thickness.

3. Slice orientation is in the axial plane. Images can also be obtained at an angle determined by the degree to which the scanner gantry can be tilted. This allows orientation of the sections to be modified to match the curvature of the spine (Fig. 1).

4. A slice thickness of 4 or 5 mm yields adequate spatial resolution in the longitudinal axis and acceptable signal-to-noise ratio in the image. Reformatting of sets of axial images is required to generate images in sagittal, coronal, or oblique planes, at a significant loss of spatial resolution. This loss may be reduced by using thinner sections (e.g., 1.5–2 mm) or by overlapping.

On the basis of the foregoing considerations, protocols for CT examination may be designed. One protocol we recommend consists of 4- to 5-mm-thick parallel sections oriented parallel to the intervertebral disc space, with as many sections as are required to include the pedicles of the vertebrae on both sides of the disc space.

5. The use of intravenous contrast agents may be required. We prefer to give a 4-min infusion containing

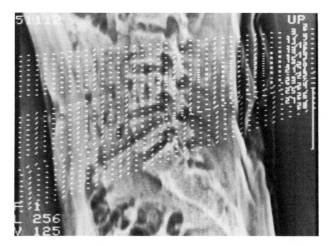

FIG. 1. CT: A scout lateral view of the lumbosacral spine. The dotted lines are entered on the digital radiograph (topogram, scout view, or scannogram) by software interaction between the operator and the computer of the CT scanner. These lines determine the level and plane of orientation of each individual slice. Note that this examination consisted of three groups or subsets of parallel slices. Each subset covers one intervertebral disc space and extends from one pedicle to the other. The change in orientation from one subset to the other is dictated by the lordosis of the lumbosacral spine.

42 g of iodine (e.g., 150 ml of a solution containing 282 mg of iodine per milliliter), followed by a "fast drip" of a similar volume and concentration as the imaging procedure is initiated. This provides opacification of both the intravascular and extravascular compartments of the tissues.

6. CT often is performed following a lumbar myelogram. It has been suggested that a delay period of several hours should be allowed between the intrathecal injection and CT examination (48) to avoid masking of intradural structures by excessive density of the contrast material. We have found, however, that the duration of the myelographic procedure and an additional 30-min interval before imaging are adequate if particular attention has been given to spread the contrast material to the upper lumbar spinal canal. Furthermore, as the patient is transferred to the scanning table, a rolling-over maneuver should be carried out to allow mixing of contrast material and cerebrospinal fluid (CSF) to prevent separation in layers.

Magnetic Resonance Imaging

MRI examination consists primarily of sagittal images with slice thickness of 5 mm or less. These are followed by axial images. Two spin-echo sequences generate three sets of images at the same anatomic levels, as follows: A short-TR/short-TE sequence (e.g., TR = 500 msec, TE = 15 msec) generates a set of T1-weighted images (T1-WI). A long-TR/short- and long-TE sequence (e.g., TR = 2,000 msec, TE = 30 msec and 120 msec) generates two more sets of images, balanced images (Bal-I) and T2-weighted images (T2-WI), respectively. Artifacts and loss of signal caused by pulsatile motion of CSF can be markedly reduced by cardiac or pulse gating and by motion-suppression (gradient-refocused) sequences.

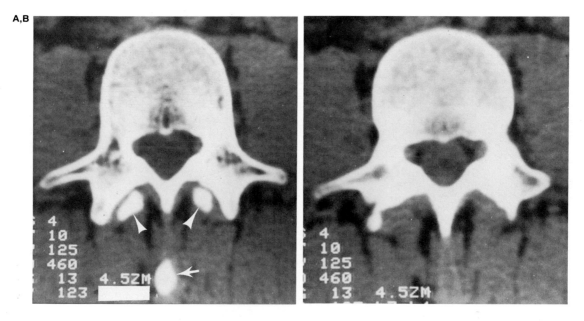

FIG. 2. CT: Normal anatomy through the pedicle of the superior vertebra. **A:** The vertebral body, pedicle, and laminae form a complete bony ring at this level. The tips of the inferior articular processes (*arrowheads*) and spinous process (*arrow*) of the preceding vertebra also can be seen. **B:** Four millimeters caudal, only the bony structures that belong to this vertebra are shown.

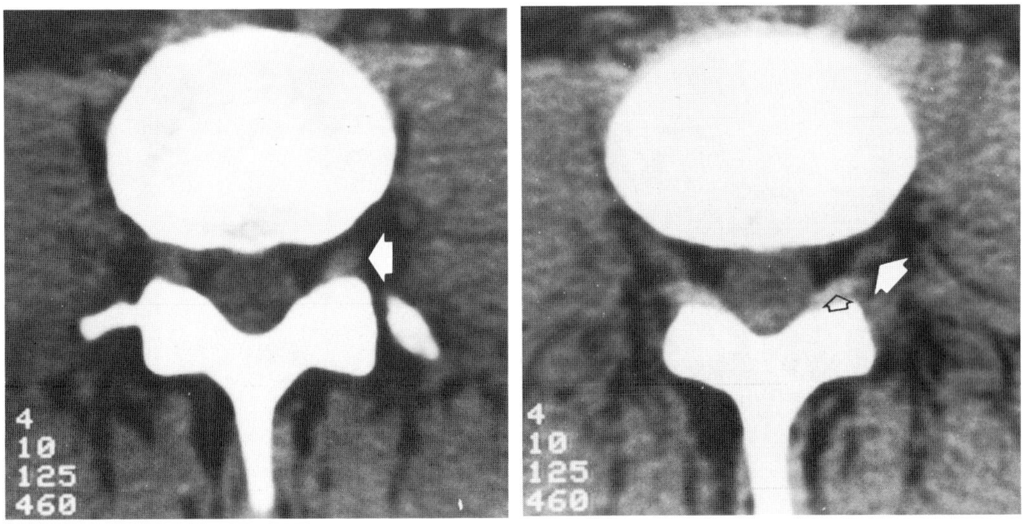

A,B

FIG. 3. CT: Normal anatomy through the upper part of the intervertebral foramen. **A:** The nerve ganglion (*arrow*) occupies the intervertebral foramen, which appears as a gap in the bony ring on each side. A portion of the transverse process also can be seen at this level. **B:** Four millimeters caudal, the nerve (*closed arrow*) distal to the ganglion can be identified. Posteromedial to the nerve root lies the capsule for the posterior articular joint (*open arrow*), an attachment site for the ligamentum flavum.

NORMAL ANATOMY—LUMBAR SPINE

Computed Tomography

The axial anatomy of an intervertebral articulation can be described in 4 selected planes (Figs. 2–4) spanning the pedicles of the vertebrae on both sides of the disc, referred to here as the superior and inferior vertebrae, respectively: (a) The superior pedicle (Fig. 2). At this level, the vertebral body, pedicle, and laminae of the superior vertebra form a complete bony ring. When a lordotic angle exists between two vertebrae, the most cephalad slice of the series

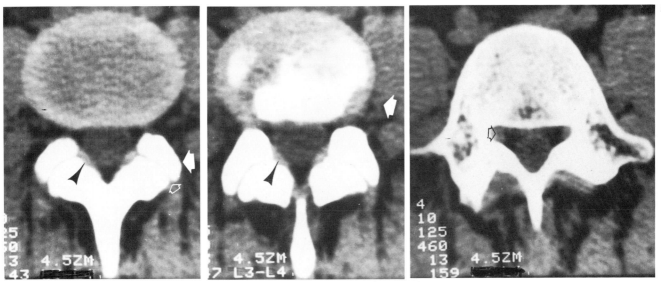

A–C

FIG. 4. CT: Normal anatomy through the lower part of the intervertebral foramen. **A:** At this level, the posterior aspect of the intervertebral disc, which has a higher density than the adjacent dural sac, forms the anterior border of the foramen. The superior articular process of the inferior vertebra (*closed arrow*) lies anterior to, and articulates with, the inferior articular process of the superior vertebra (*open arrow*). The laminae of the superior vertebra are continuous with the inferior articular process and the spinous process of the same vertebra. The ligamentum flavum (*arrowhead*) lies anteromedial to the lamina and the joint. **B:** Four millimeters caudal, the upper disc plate of the inferior vertebra and the intervertebral disc form the anterior border of the foramen. The foramen appears smaller in size; the nerve (*arrow*) has migrated farther lateral to the foramen. The superior articular process of the inferior vertebra is larger in size than in the previous slice, and the laminae of the superior vertebra are no longer in continuity with the spinous process. The ligamentum flavum (*arrowhead*) can again be seen. **C:** Twelve millimeters caudal, a complete bony ring of the inferior vertebra is established. The upper border of the laminae and the superior articular process of the inferior vertebra are now seen. The nerve root sheath (*arrow*) for the next intervertebral foramen lies medial to the pedicle.

A,B

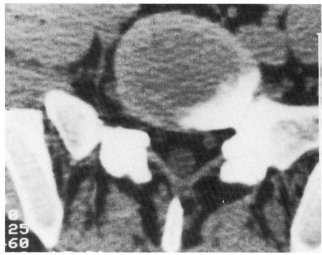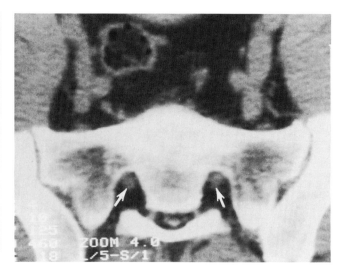

FIG. 5. CT: Normal anatomy. **A:** At the level of the lumbosacral junction, the dural sac is small and is surrounded by a large amount of the epidural fat. **B:** Inferior to the lower end of the cul-de-sac, the sacral and coccygeal root sheaths appear as rounded soft-tissue structures surrounded by fat (*arrows*).

may run through the interlaminar space above the upper vertebra. The next lower slice, however, will then demonstrate the complete bony ring. The configuration of the bony ring is more or less triangular, and the dural sac occupies the entire contained space in the upper lumbar region. More caudad, particularly at the lumbosacral junction, the dural sac is significantly smaller in size, occupying only a fraction of the area of the bony spinal canal (Fig. 5A), and is surrounded by epidural fat. (b) The upper part of the intervertebral foramen (Fig. 3). Just below the pedicle of the superior vertebra, the intervertebral

foramen appears as a "gap" separating the posterior border of the body and the laminae of that vertebra. The ganglion of the lumbar nerve root and its surrounding fat occupy the gap (foramen), with no encroachment by the superior articular process of the inferior vertebra. (c) The lower part of the intervertebral foramen (Fig. 4). At this level, the intervertebral disc replaces the vertebral body if the slice is oriented exactly in the plane of the disc and if the thickness of the slice is less than the thickness of the disc. Behind the disc and separated from it by the intervertebral foramen is the posterior articular joint. Both the inferior

A–C

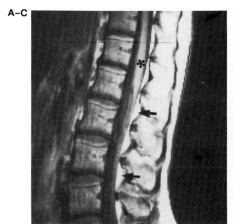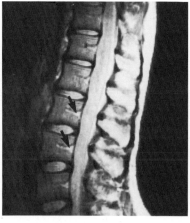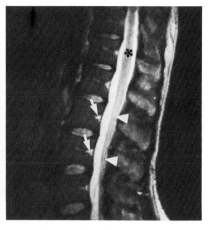

FIG. 6. MRI, 1.5 T: Normal anatomy in the midsagittal plane. **A:** T1-WI (SE, TR = 500 msec, TE = 21 msec). Low signal intensity of CSF contrasts well with the conus of the spinal cord (*asterisk*). The intervertebral discs show low signal intensity. There is no demonstrable contrast between the nucleus pulposus and the annulus fibrosus. Epidural fat between the laminae of the vertebrae on the dorsal aspect of the dural sac has high signal intensity (*arrows*). **B:** Balanced image (SE, TR = 2,600 msec, TE = 35 msec). At each level of intervertebral disc, the posterior part of the annulus fibrosus and the adjoining posterior longitudinal ligament have low signal intensity and stand out in comparison with the high signal of the nucleus pulposus and the CSF. Thus, the posterior border of the disc is well defined, and its integrity is ascertained. High signal in the middle of the vertebral body is due to slow-flowing blood in the basivertebral veins (*arrows*). **C:** T2-WI (SE, TR = 2,600 msec, TE = 90 msec). CSF has remarkably high signal intensity compared with other components of the image, giving a myelographic effect. The conus of the spinal cord (*asterisk*) and the cauda equina (*arrowheads*) appear as negative shadows within the dural sac. There is high signal intensity in the basivertebral veins (*arrows*), as in part **B.**

articular process of the superior vertebra and the superior process of the inferior vertebra are seen in this slice. As a result, the foramen itself may appear small in its antero-posterior diameter; this should not be considered a pathologic finding, because the nerve at this level is already lateral to the foramen, which is occupied only by fat (Fig. 4A). The capsule of the posterior articular joint gives origin to the ligamentum flavum, which is also attached to the anterior border of the lamina. Because the lamina is slanting downward and posteriorly, the thickness of the ligamentum flavum increases cephalocaudad in successive slices.

The nerve that has crossed the intervertebral foramen lies close to the lateral border of the disc. On the other hand, the nerve root and sheath that originate from the dural sac close to the posterior disc border leave the spinal canal below the lower border of the pedicle of the inferior vertebra (i.e., exit in the next foramen below).

The superior articular process of the inferior vertebra increases gradually in size on sequential slices, whereas the inferior aspects of the laminae and the spinous process of the superior vertebra diminish in size and finally disappear. (d) Eventually, at the lowest slice of the set, the base of the superior articular process of the lower vertebra connects with the upper border of its pedicle, the upper disc plate, and the laminae (Fig. 4B). The complete bony ring of the inferior vertebra below is thus formed (Fig. 4C). At this level, the root sheath, which ultimately will exit in the foramen below, appears close to the medial aspect of the pedicle (Fig. 4C). Because the amount of epidural fat at the level of the pedicle is much less than that at the level of the foramen, visualization of the root sheath at the level of the pedicle may be difficult. At the lumbosacral junction, sufficient fat is present to render the sheaths easily visible (Fig. 5A).

Magnetic Resonance Imaging

Sectional anatomy in the sagittal plane may be described in three separate planes on either side of the midline:

1. Near the midline (Fig. 6), the dural sac separates the vertebral bodies in front from the spinous processes in the back. In the T1-WI (Fig. 6A) and in the Bal-I (Fig. 6B), the higher signal from the marrow-containing cancellous bone contrasts with the very low signal (or virtual signal void) of the enveloping compact bone. Epidural fat, which has the highest signal intensity of any structure in the T1-WI (Fig. 6A) and the Bal-I (Fig. 6B), may be seen dorsal to the dural sac in the interlaminal spaces between the neighboring vertebrae (Fig. 6A). Anteriorly, epidural fat is seen in the lower part of the spinal canal, e.g., at the level L5-S1. In the T2-WI (Fig. 6C), signal intensity for marrow-containing structures drops dramatically.

The dural sac and contents in the lumbar region have the signal-intensity pattern of CSF. Therefore, in the T1-WI (Fig. 6A), they appear darker than the vertebral bodies. In the Bal-I (Fig. 6B), CSF signal intensity may be equal to or higher than that of the vertebral body, depending on the TR. In the T2-WI (Fig. 6C), CSF shows the highest intensity of all tissues. This is particularly true with the use of cardiac-gating and/or gradient-motion-refocusing pulse sequences.

The MRI appearance of the intervertebral disc is more detailed than that from CT because of the ability of MRI to distinguish the peripheral and central components (113). This distinction is best appreciated in the Bal-I (Fig. 6B), in which the central component of the disc shows high signal and the peripheral collagenous component appears as signal void, in contrast to both the CSF and the central disc material. The higher signal intensity of the nucleus, presumed to reflect its higher water content, is more obvious in the T2-WI (113) (Fig. 6C). But the signal-to-noise ratio is poor compared with that of the Bal-I. The latter therefore is ideal for evaluating the status of the posterior border of the intervertebral disc.

2. At the plane of the lateral recess (Fig. 7A), the anteroposterior diameter of the spinal canal is narrow and is occupied by epidural fat. The medium-intensity nerve roots in the lateral recess are contrasted against high-intensity epidural fat.

3. Further laterally, the sagittal plane runs through the intervertebral foramina (Fig. 7B). At each intervertebral level, the foramen is delimited superiorly and inferiorly by the pedicles of the vertebrae above and below, respectively. Posteriorly, the foramen is delimited by the posterior articular joint and anteriorly by the posterolateral

FIG. 7. Normal lumbar spine, MRI, 1.5 T, T1-WI, same case as in Fig. 6, but at different sagittal planes. **A:** At a plane lying 12 mm lateral to Fig. 6A. The roots (*arrows*) are seen in the lateral recess of the spinal canal, surrounded with epidural fat. **B:** At a plane 18 mm lateral to Fig. 6A. This plane shows the intervertebral foramina. The nerve roots (*arrows*) and accompanying vessels (*small arrows*) appear as low-signal-intensity structures contrasted against the high signal of the surrounding fat within the foramina.

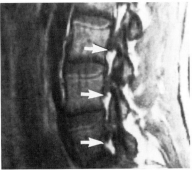
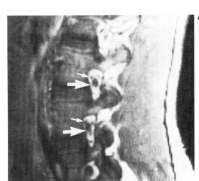

A,B

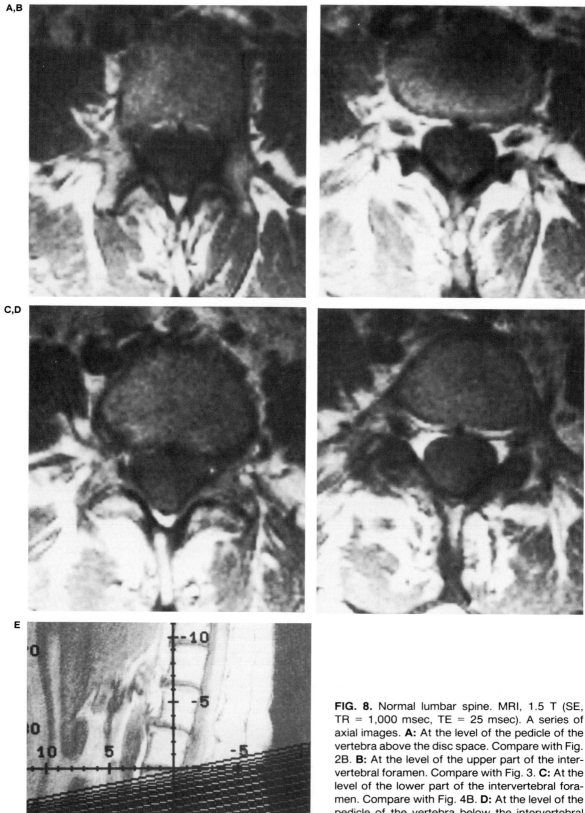

FIG. 8. Normal lumbar spine. MRI, 1.5 T (SE, TR = 1,000 msec, TE = 25 msec). A series of axial images. **A:** At the level of the pedicle of the vertebra above the disc space. Compare with Fig. 2B. **B:** At the level of the upper part of the intervertebral foramen. Compare with Fig. 3. **C:** At the level of the lower part of the intervertebral foramen. Compare with Fig. 4B. **D:** At the level of the pedicle of the vertebra below the intervertebral disc. Compare with Fig. 4C. **E:** A midsagittal image serves as a scout view on which the planes of the axial images are projected. Compare with Fig. 1.

portions of the vertebral bodies and intervertebral disc (Fig. 7B). The upper part of foramen contains the nerve root and accompanying vascular structures; the lower part is occupied by fat. The posterior border of the disc lies at a lower level than the nerve root and does not encroach upon the nerve root.

Axial sectional anatomy seen by MRI is similar to that seen by CT and is shown in Fig. 8.

Comparison of CT and MRI

The data provided by CT and MRI are largely comparable. The high density of bone on CT stands out in contrast to the densities of all other tissues. Therefore, hypertrophic bony changes, small subarticular erosions in the posterior articular facets, defects in the pars interarticularis, and calcifications of soft tissues, including displaced disc material, may be more easily appreciated by CT. Also, on CT, the high density of disc material where it abuts on the dural sac and epidural fat in the axial projection allows excellent delineation of the entire disc border.

In contradistinction, sagittal MR images provide an excellent overview of the entire lumbar region. The inherent high soft-tissue contrast discrimination allows direct imaging of intradural soft-tissue structures, such as the conus (Fig. 6A). Furthermore, the ability to differentiate central and peripheral components of the disc (Fig. 6B) is another advantage of MRI. Lastly, the quality of MR images is not degraded when imaging patients of large size.

DEGENERATIVE DISEASES—LUMBAR SPINE

The intervertebral articulation is a three-joint complex consisting of the intervertebral disc and the two posterior articular joints. Degeneration of the intervertebral disc may predispose to changes in the posterior articular joints, and vice versa. Patients may therefore present with manifestations of disease in the intervertebral disc or the posterior articular joints or both.

Degenerative *intervertebral disc disease* includes degenerative bulge, disc protrusion, and herniation of the nucleus pulposus. These commonly involve the L5-S1 and L4-L5 levels, but occasionally involve higher levels. The manifestations of *posterior articular joint disease* are those of osteoarthritis. Hypertrophic bone and soft-tissue changes resulting from disease at both sites constitute the picture of *spondylosis* and may lead to *spinal stenosis.* Another sequela of the degenerative process is subluxation, i.e., *spondylolisthesis* that may result from laxity of the ligaments and loss of height of the disc space. Each of these entities can be a cause of low-back pain and/or sciatica. In many cases, compression of a nerve root or of the cauda equina, shown on CT or MRI, explains the clinical findings, but in some cases it does not. It is therefore essential to interpret the significance of radiologic findings in the light of the symptoms, clinical signs, and results of paraclinical tests in order to establish a cause-and-effect relationship prior to the planning of management.

Desiccation of the Intervertebral Disc

A decrease in water content in the nucleus has been described as an early manifestation of degenerative change or part of the aging process. The disc becomes brittle, fibrous, and inelastic (149). When enough internal disruption of the disc has taken place, accumulation of gas in the disc space leads to the so-called vacuum phenomenon seen on plain radiographs (41). Changes in water content are not reflected on the CT image, but the vacuum phenomenon (55) can be demonstrated. Associated reduction in the height of the disc space is also difficult to detect in axially oriented images. The high signal of the nucleus normally seen in T2-WI is drastically reduced in the case of a degenerated disc (102) (Fig. 9C).

A,B

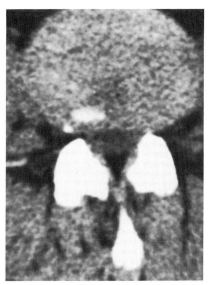 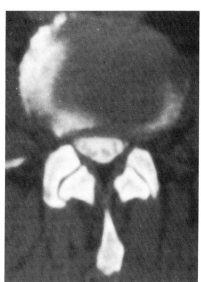

FIG. 9. Degenerative disc bulge at L3-L4. A: Plain CT. There is uniform expansion of the disc border in all directions, with no focal deformity. B: CT after myelogram with water-soluble contrast material. The bulging disc impinges slightly on the anterior border of the contrast column.

A–C

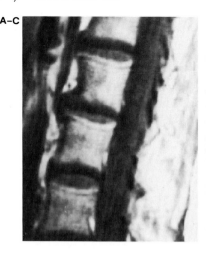
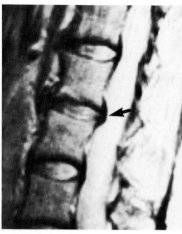
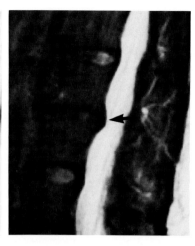

FIG. 10. Degenerative bulge at L2-L3. MRI, 1.5 T. **A:** T1-WI (SE, TR = 500 msec, TE = 21 msec). The bulge is not well appreciated because there is lack of contrast between the low density of the disc and CSF in this pulse sequence. **B,C:** Balanced image and T2-WI (SE, TR = 3,000 msec, TE = 35 msec and 90 msec). The posterior border of the disc contrasts well with the signal intensity of CSF in these images and can be well identified. Note bulging of the posterior border of the degenerated disc (*arrow*), with no disruption of the disc border. There is, however, low signal within the disc space at that level, particularly noticeable in **C.** Compare the disc spaces above and below.

Degenerative Disc Bulge

At an early stage in the degenerative process, small circumferential cracks occur in the annulus. Some of these may coalesce to form a radial crack. As they become confluent, the nucleus expands into them and permeates the annulus, which has become thinner and weaker. As a result, the circumference of the disc is uniformly expanded beyond the margin of the disc plate, but its configuration remains parallel to it, a condition called degenerative disc

bulge (150). Diffuse uniform bulging of the disc border is easily seen in axial CT images (Fig. 9A) and is further confirmed by reformatting in the sagittal plane. Although by definition a disc bulge is diffuse and uniform in all directions, bulging in the posterior direction only is likely to cause symptoms by encroachment on the anterior border of the dural sac. Sagittal MR images have a definite advantage in showing the degree of bulging at a given level by comparison with other levels (Fig. 10B). The dark line forming the posterior disc border appears intact in the case of degenerative bulge.

A–C

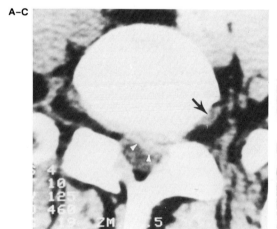
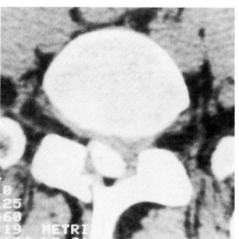
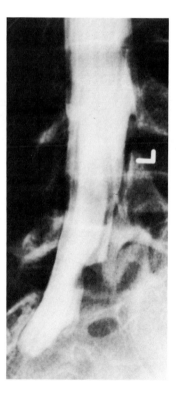

FIG. 11. Herniated disc at L5-S1 level. **A:** Plain CT. There is loss of parallelism between the posterior border of the high-density disc and the disc plate on the left. The herniated disc fragment (*arrowheads*) has completely replaced the epidural fat and deformed the anterior aspect of the dural sac. Because the nerve root (*arrow*) that exits at this level lies farther laterally to the intervertebral foramen, it may not be affected by the disc herniation. **B:** Repeat image after a water-soluble myelogram again demonstrates the distorted dural sac. Notice that the herniated disc material intimately contacts the origin of the root sheath of the nerve at the corner of the contrast column; this nerve root eventually exits at the foramen below the level of the disc. **C:** Oblique view of the water-soluble myelogram confirms the CT findings, but offers no additional information.

Herniation of the Nucleus Pulposus

When coalescent tears extend through the whole thickness of the annulus, the substance of the nucleus pulposus presents outside the confinement of the annulus. This extrusion or herniation of the nucleus material implies rupture or tear of the annulus and causes deformity of the border of the disc at the site of the tear. Because the annulus is thinner posteriorly than anteriorly, herniation of the nucleus pulposus (HNP) occurs posteriorly and is more likely to occur posterolaterally than in the midline. Less commonly, HNP may occur far laterally in the intervertebral foramen. The clinical signs of radiculopathy caused by rupture of a given disc depend on the site of the rupture.

A brief review of the anatomic relationships of the nerve roots and the intervertebral disc spaces in the lumbar region will explain the differing symptoms produced by medial and lateral disc herniations. The nerve roots are designated by the levels of individual vertebrae and thus are referred to as L1 root, L2 root, etc. There are two pairs of nerve roots in relation to each disc space: One pair exits through the foramina at the level of the disc, and these are designated by the vertebra above the disc; the other pair exits through the foramina below the disc level, and they are designated by the level of the vertebra below the disc. When disc rupture occurs at a posterolateral location, the herniated nucleus material contacts the nerve root designated by the lower vertebral level (i.e., L5 root in case of rupture of the L4-L5 disc) on that side. If the same disc is ruptured in a more lateral location, the herniated disc material encounters the nerve root designated by the vertebra above the disc (i.e., L4 root in case of rupture of the L4-L5 disc).

The term "protrusion" refers to the situation of severe focal thinning and weakening of the annulus, which becomes displaced by the nucleus, causing discrete deformity of the disc border. The displaced nucleus material is thus contained by the remaining superficial fibers of the annulus (25,82). Although it is conceivable that disc protrusion and HNP may be differentiated at surgical exploration, they are radiologically indistinguishable. The term

A–C

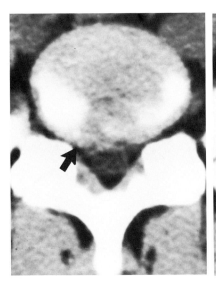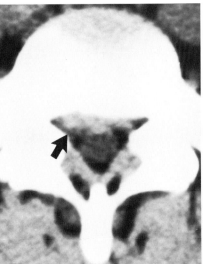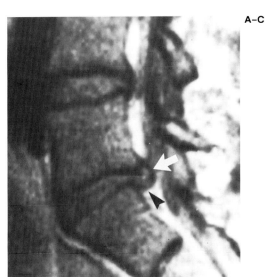

D

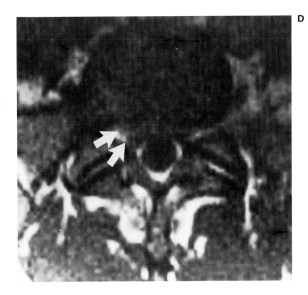

FIG. 12. Posterolateral HNP at L5-S1. **A,B:** Plain CT. Note the herniated fragment on the right side compressing the first sacral root and displacing it posteriorly (*arrow*). Because of the wide epidural space, there is little deformity of the dural sac. **C,D:** MRI, 0.5 T. The sagittal Bal-I (SE, TR = 1,500 msec, TE = 35 msec) in **C** shows the black line of the posterior border of the disc disrupted at L5-S1. It is attached to the posterior inferior angle of the body of L5 vertebra (*arrow*), but detached from the superior posterior corner of S1 (*arrowhead*). The herniated material has lifted the black line away from S1 segment. The axial T1-WI (SE, TR = 500 msec, TE = 25 msec) in **D** shows the same information as in **B**.

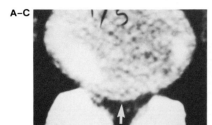
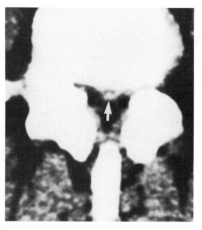
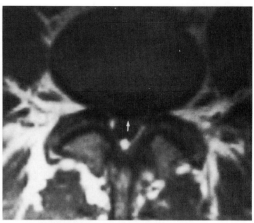

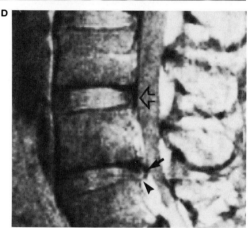

FIG. 13. Central HNP at L4-L5. **A,B:** CT shows the posterior border of the centrally herniated fragment (*arrow*) beyond the border of the vertebral end plate. The dorsal elements are massive and cause some degree of spinal stenosis. **C:** Axial MRI, 1.5 T. T1-WI (SE, TR = 700 msec, TE = 25 msec) at the level L4-L5 shows the same information (*arrow*) as in **A** and **B. D:** Sagittal MRI, 1.5 T. Bal-I (SE, TR = 1,800 msec, TE = 35 msec) shows disruption of the black line forming the posterior border of the disc (*arrow*). The black line is seen attached to the posterior inferior corner of L4 (*arrow*), but is detached from the posterior superior corner of L5 (*arrowhead*). The herniated fragment (*arrowhead*) lifts the black line away from the 5th lumbar vertebra. Compare the intact posterior border of the disc at L3-L4 (*open arrow*).

A,B

C,D

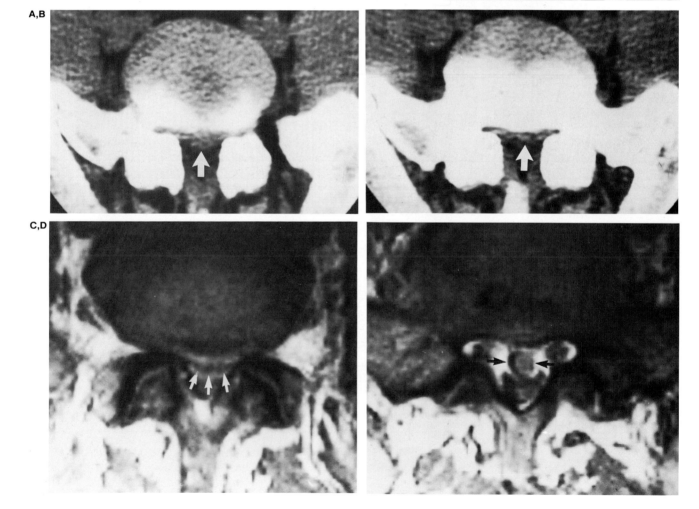

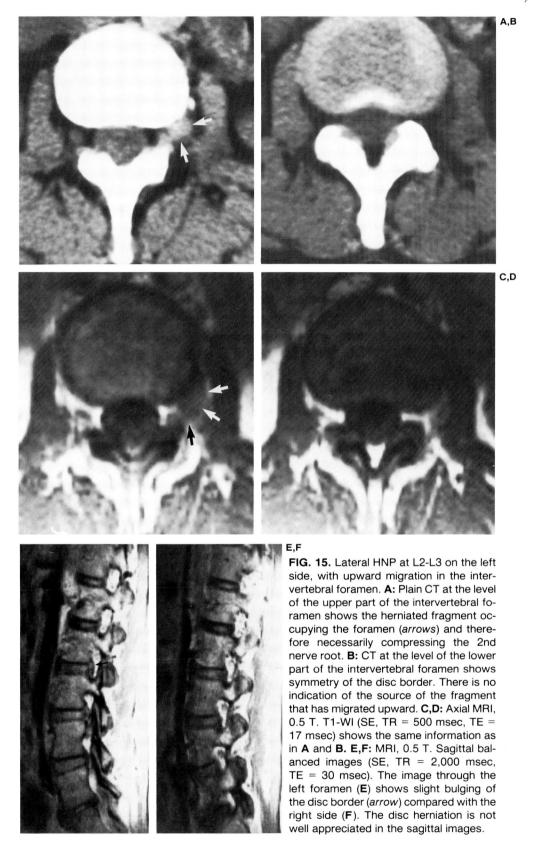

A,B

C,D

E,F

FIG. 15. Lateral HNP at L2-L3 on the left side, with upward migration in the intervertebral foramen. **A:** Plain CT at the level of the upper part of the intervertebral foramen shows the herniated fragment occupying the foramen (*arrows*) and therefore necessarily compressing the 2nd nerve root. **B:** CT at the level of the lower part of the intervertebral foramen shows symmetry of the disc border. There is no indication of the source of the fragment that has migrated upward. **C,D:** Axial MRI, 0.5 T. T1-WI (SE, TR = 500 msec, TE = 17 msec) shows the same information as in **A** and **B. E,F:** MRI, 0.5 T. Sagittal balanced images (SE, TR = 2,000 msec, TE = 30 msec). The image through the left foramen (**E**) shows slight bulging of the disc border (*arrow*) compared with the right side (**F**). The disc herniation is not well appreciated in the sagittal images.

FIG. 14. Central HNP at L5-S1. **A,B:** Plain CT shows disc herniation, with downward migration of the fragment (*arrow*) behind the upper border of the first sacral segment. **C,D:** MRI, 1.5 T. Bal-I (SE, TR = 1,600 msec, TE = 28 msec) shows the same information as **A** and **B,** but to better advantage. The downward migration of the fragment behind the first sacral segment is well illustrated in **D** (*arrows*).

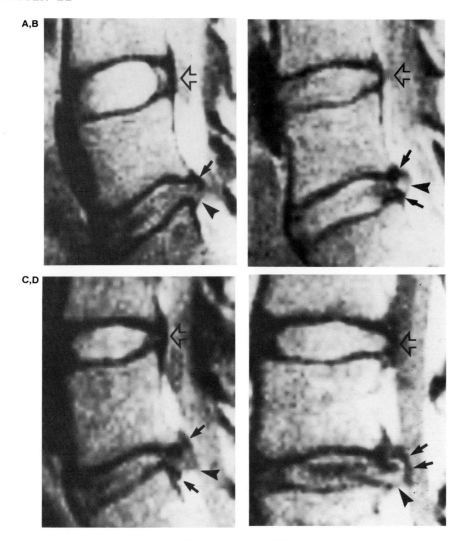

FIG. 16. Herniation of the nucleus pulposus in four different cases. MRI, 0.5 T. Balanced images (SE, TR = 1,500 msec, TE = 35 msec). Sagittal images show loss of continuity of the black line forming the posterior border of the disc (*arrows*). Compare the continuous black line at the normal level (*open arrow*). Disruption of the border of the disc allows the herniated material of the nucleus pulposus to extrude out of the confinement of the disc and lie in contact with the epidural fat (*arrowhead*).

"protrusion" should therefore not be used in radiologic interpretation.

On CT, the appearance of HNP reflects the description just presented (152). These same criteria can be easily applied to MRI (96,101), with slight modifications imposed by the effects of different pulse sequences on tissue contrast.

1. With focal deformity of the posterior border of the disc, the displacement is most often posterolateral in location (Figs. 11 and 12), but may be central (Figs. 13 and 14) or lateral (Fig. 15) depending on the site of rupture of the annulus. Lateral disc herniation in the intervertebral foramen needs a special note, because myelography findings often are negative (44), and the radiologic diagnosis then depends entirely on CT and/or MRI.

2. As the posterior border of the disc is displaced, it displaces and deforms the anterior border of the dural sac (Fig. 11).

3. Deformity of the anterior border of the dural sac by the herniated material depends on the relative sizes of the dural sac and bony canal. Therefore, at the level L5-S1, where the bony canal may be large relative to the dural sac, an insensitive space filled with epidural fat separates the dural sac and the disc border. In this situation, a large HNP may be present with no deformity of the dural sac (Fig. 12). The criterion for diagnosis in this case is replacement of epidural fat by a soft-tissue mass, the herniated nucleus material.

The foregoing criteria are also applicable to MRI (Figs. 14–17).

4. Furthermore, MRI often reveals the defect in the posterior disc border, thus offering a pathognomonic sign of the process (Figs. 12, 16, and 17).

5. Figure 18B shows the presence of gas within the bony spinal canal. As previously mentioned, gas within the disc space is a sign of disc degeneration, not HNP (Fig. 18A).

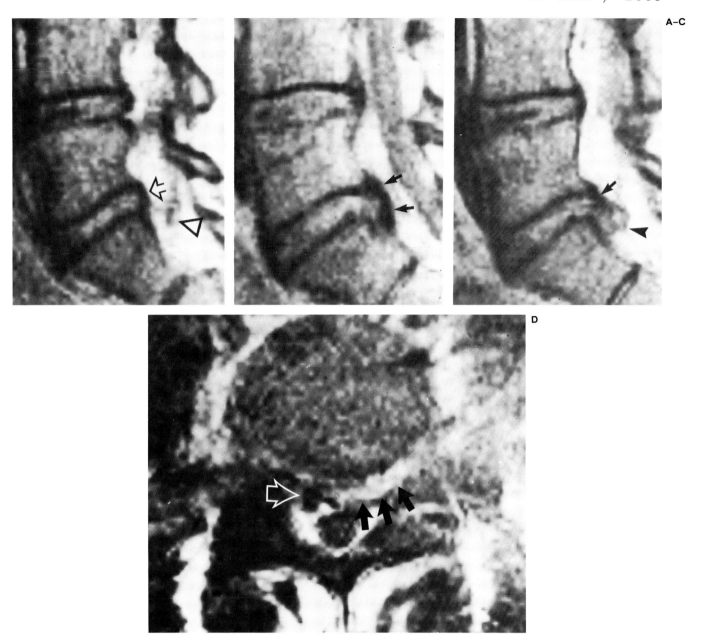

FIG. 17. Lateral disc herniation at L5-S1 on the left side. MRI, 0.5 T. Balanced images (SE, TR = 1,500 msec, TE = 35 msec). **A:** Sagittal section through the right lateral recess shows normal appearance of the posterior border of the disc (*open arrow*) and the nerve root (*open arrowhead*) in the vicinity. **B:** Sagittal section through the midline shows degenerative bulging of the disc border, without disruption (*arrows*). **C:** Sagittal section through the left lateral recess shows disruption of the posterior border of the disc (*arrows*). A large amount of material of the nucleus pulposus is extruded in the epidural space (*arrowheads*) and lies in contact with the first sacral root. Note the focality of the abnormal findings seen in one sagittal plane (**C**), but not **A** or **B. D:** This focality can also be demonstrated in the axial image. The right S1 root (*open arrow*) is in its normal place, surrounded with clear fatty space. On the left side, the herniated disc material (*arrows*) fills the space, and the nerve root is not visualized.

However, when a gas-containing fragment is displaced from the disc space into the bony spinal canal, gas becomes a marker indicating the location of a fragment. Gas may be visible by MRI as an area of signal void, but it may be overlooked (52) if it lies close to the vertebral end plate, because the latter also appears as signal void.

6. As the disc degenerates, calcification may occur in the disc space, presumably because of invasion of the disc space by osteoblasts migrating together with connective-tissue cells that replace cartilage (149). Calcification occurring in the disc space, like gas formation, is therefore a sign of degeneration, not herniation. Furthermore, it is

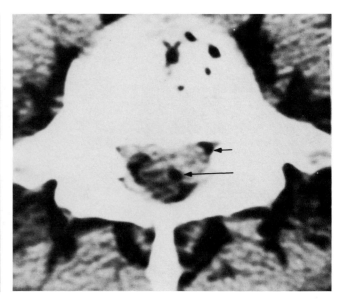

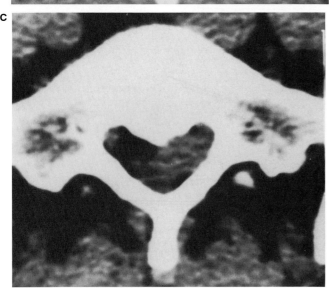

FIG. 18. Gas associated with herniated disc. **A:** CT image at the level of the disc space. Gas appears as a lucency within the intervertebral disc. The presence of gas in this location alone is not a sign of disc herniation. Also of note is a herniated soft-tissue fragment (*arrowheads*) encroaching on the dural sac. **B:** CT image below the level of the disc space demonstrates collections of gas bubbles within the herniated disc fragment (*arrows*). The fragment is denser than the dural sac. The nerve root is indistinct from the herniated fragment, a sign of nerve root compression. **C:** The lower border of the herniated fragment is still present on this image obtained more than 2 cm below the disc space. This is seen when the herniated material is large in size or when part of the herniated material has been sequestered from the disc.

rare in the lumbar region as compared with the thoracic region. A more common type of calcification associated with lumbar HNP is an osteophyte-like lesion, thought to be caused by displacement of periosteum secondary to a tear in the annulus, compounded by a decrease in the height of the disc, increased movement between the two neighboring vertebrae, and displacement of disc material. It is the same mechanism responsible for the more familiar anterolateral osteophytes often seen on radiographs. On CT (Fig. 19), such calcification tends to have a curvilinear, linear, or speck-like appearance. It is seen in the periphery of the herniated fragment, but when large enough, it can be traced in consecutive sections to the point where it is attached to the border of the vertebral end plate (Fig. 19A). On MRI, calcification may produce a signal void or may go undetected.

7. The term "sequestration" implies that the herniated fragment has lost continuity with the disc material in the intervertebral space (25). Lying free in the epidural space, it may migrate away from the disc border. On CT or MRI, the migrant fragment appears as a soft-tissue mass in the epidural space behind the vertebral body (Fig. 20), above or below the disc space. To determine the disc level from which the migrant fragment has originated, one has to take into consideration signs of disc degeneration and the proximity of a disc space to the soft-tissue mass.

8. Intraspongy herniation (Schmorl's node) denotes herniation through a breach in a degenerated disc plate into the spongy bone of the vertebral body, although its presence may be an incidental finding (149). The lesion appears on CT as a lucent area at the upper or lower border of the vertebral body, surrounded with a dense margin representing the displaced rim of disc plate. The lesions often are multiple. The dense margin and the location away from the center of the vertebral body help differentiate this condition from metastases. On MRI, the

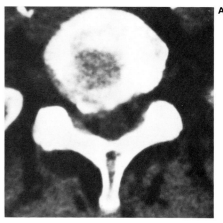
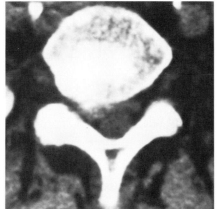

FIG. 19. Posterolateral disc herniation at L5-S1, with calcification. CT images. **A:** At the level of the lower end plate of L5 vertebra. **B:** At the level of the L5-S1 intervertebral disc. Calcification in the herniated disc fragment is shown to blend with the lower end plate of L5 vertebra in **A.**

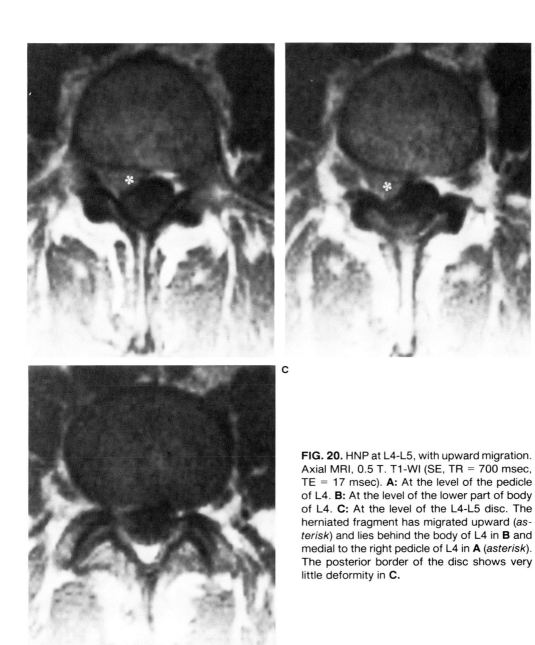

FIG. 20. HNP at L4-L5, with upward migration. Axial MRI, 0.5 T. T1-WI (SE, TR = 700 msec, TE = 17 msec). **A:** At the level of the pedicle of L4. **B:** At the level of the lower part of body of L4. **C:** At the level of the L4-L5 disc. The herniated fragment has migrated upward (*asterisk*) and lies behind the body of L4 in **B** and medial to the right pedicle of L4 in **A** (*asterisk*). The posterior border of the disc shows very little deformity in **C.**

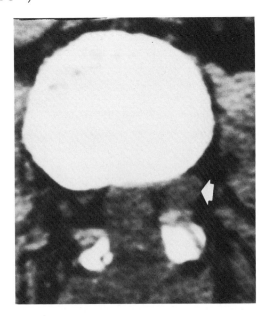

FIG. 21. Neurofibroma of the nerve root sheath within the foramen. A soft-tissue mass (*arrow*) is present in the left intervertebral foramen in a patient with a prior laminectomy for removal of an intradural neurofibroma in the cauda equina. Although slightly lower in density than a disc fragment, this mass can easily be confused with a lateral herniated disc.

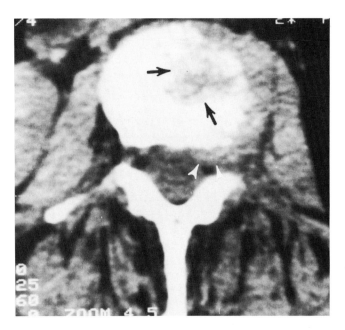

FIG. 22. Metastases from a renal cell carcinoma. A soft-tissue mass (*arrowheads*) is present in the left intervertebral foramen. In addition, there is a left paraspinal soft-tissue mass associated with vertebral destruction (*arrows*). These findings are most compatible with metastatic bone disease, with intraspinal extension.

A,B

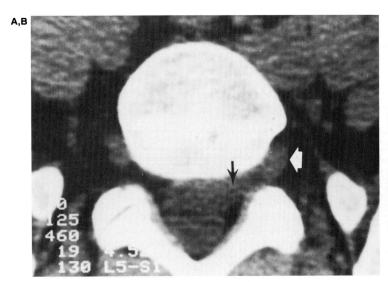

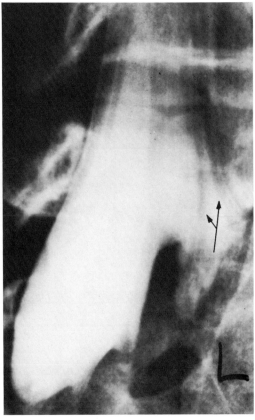

FIG. 23. Conjoint root sheath of L5 and S1 on the left side. **A:** Plain CT. The conjoint root sheath (*black arrow*), which has a density identical with that of the dural sac, obliterates the epidural fat. The nerve ganglion (*white arrow*) is continuous with, and to the lateral side of, the conjoint sheath. **B:** Myelogram of the same case shows the two roots to appear within a large conjoint sheath (*arrows*), thus firmly establishing the diagnosis.

sagittal orientation is particularly suited for demonstrating this abnormality.

Differential diagnosis of HNP

Pathologic conditions that lead to the formation of a soft-tissue mass in the epidural space may mimic the appearance of HNP on CT (44).

1. Primary neoplasm. A neurofibroma of the nerve root or ganglion can present as a soft-tissue mass in the lateral gutter of the bony spinal canal medial to the pedicle or in the intervertebral foramen just below the pedicle (82) (Fig. 21). Generally, such a mass appears less dense than disc herniation. CT, after intravenous injection of contrast material, often shows enhancement of the neoplasm. When long-standing, the neoplasm may cause enlargement of the intervertebral foramen. In neurofibromatosis, the lesions may be multiple, a feature that should suggest the correct diagnosis.

2. Metastatic neoplasm. A metastatic neoplasm may appear as a soft-tissue mass in the epidural space, sometimes extending to the intervertebral foramen (Fig. 22). Unlike a neurofibroma, a metastatic lesion usually has an ill-defined margin and infiltrates the paravertebral fat, causing an increase in the thickness of the normal paravertebral tissue (44). The presence of bony destruction, which usually is recognizable on CT, and the clinical history of a known primary or metastatic neoplasm elsewhere often aid in its correct diagnosis.

3. Conjoined-sheath anomaly. This anomaly usually is unilateral and involves the fifth lumbar and first sacral roots. The anomaly consists of a common origin of two root sheaths. Although each root sheath has its own arachnoid space, they share the same dural sheath. Consequently, this results in an asymmetric appearance of the root sheaths on CT (Fig. 23). On the side of the conjoint sheath, the root sheath is large and may resemble a soft-tissue mass in the lateral gutter medial to the pedicle (44). The clue to the diagnosis is that the "mass" has a uniform density similar to that of the dural sac. The mass does not show enhancement after intravenous injection of contrast material. A definitive diagnosis can be made by myelography, but often this is unnecessary. Failure to recognize this anomaly, occurring in association with disc rupture and spinal stenosis, prior to surgery may result in inadvertent damage to the nerve roots and contribute to poor surgical results.

4. A synovial cyst may resemble an HNP fragment in the lateral recess, but should be differentiated (22) by its location adjacent to the facet joint, which shows degenerative changes (Fig. 24).

5. Epidural and subdural collections of blood and pus will be discussed in the section under intraspinal tumors.

Posterior Joint Disease

Degenerative changes in the posterior articular joints (facet joints) may occur secondary to degeneration of the intervertebral disc, because loss of the disc height and turgidity may cause increases in the stresses on the facet joints. The term "arthrosis" has been used to describe these secondary changes, reserving the term "osteoarthritis" for the primary changes of the facet joints similar to those occurring in synovial joints elsewhere in the body.

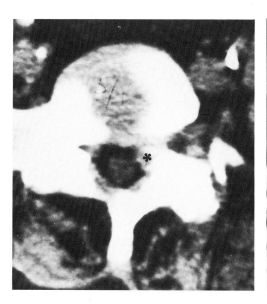 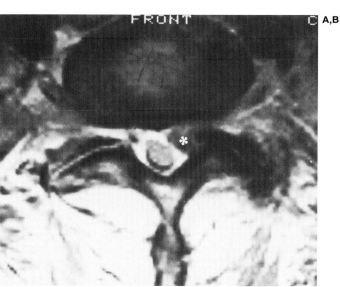

FIG. 24. Synovial cyst. **A:** CT. **B:** MRI, 1.5 T. Bal-I (SE, TR = 2,400 msec, TE = 34 msec). The soft-tissue mass (*asterisk*) is more closely related to the medial border of the facet joint than to the posterior border of the intervertebral disc. The facet joint on the left side shows advanced degenerative disease, which is the underlying process for synovial cyst formation.

The presence of degenerative changes in the intervertebral disc in association with changes in the posterior articular joints is a frequent occurrence. In these cases it is not possible to determine which of the two is primary and which is secondary, because osteoarthritis of the posterior articular joints may also predispose to degeneration of the intervertebral disc (82).

The pathologic changes due to osteoarthritis are reflected in CT (22) and MRI (53) findings (Figs. 25 and 27–29). There is narrowing of the joint space due to cartilage loss. The articular surfaces appear irregular as a result of subchondral bone erosions, and an intraarticular vacuum phenomenon may be seen. Lucent cyst-like lesions in the bone may be demonstrated close to the articular surface, with increased density of the surrounding bone. In advanced cases there is fragmentation of the articular process with intraarticular loose fragments or actual fracture of the articular process.

Eventually, hypertrophic bone formation takes place, with increases in the sizes of the articular processes, capsular and ligamentous calcification, and formation of large osteophytes that may extend in various directions. The effects of these depend on their locations in relation to the spinal canal and intervertebral foramen, and spinal stenosis may result.

Increased stresses on the posterior articular joints lead to further degeneration, with increased laxity of the capsule and surrounding ligaments. This, together with erosive changes in the articular facets, results in forward slipping of a vertebra over the vertebra below, i.e., spondylolisthesis. Retrolisthesis may also occur secondary to degeneration of the disc and laxity of the posterior articular joint capsule.

Spinal Stenosis

Reduction in the size of the spinal canal or regions thereof to a pathologic degree may result from a variety of causes. If one excludes encroachment caused by disease processes of the skeletal system (e.g., achondroplasia, Paget disease, infection, neoplasia), uncomplicated HNP, surgery, or displaced bone fragments in cases of trauma, the entity of spinal stenosis under discussion is defined.

Spinal stenosis is most commonly the result of spondylosis (defined earlier as degeneration of all components of the three-joint complex) superimposed on a developmentally abnormal vertebral configuration. Manifestations of compression of the cauda equina or a particular root or roots may result from degenerative changes that otherwise would have been insufficient to cause symptoms. Less commonly, the abnormal configuration alone or spondylosis alone may be sufficient to cause compression of the cauda equina or an individual root; hence the terms "developmental stenosis" and "degenerative stenosis" (82). The morbid anatomic components of developmental and degenerative stenoses will be discussed sep-

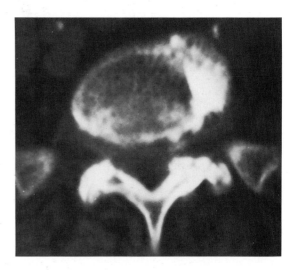

FIG. 25. Osteoarthritis of the facet joints. There is narrowing of the joint space, erosion, and hypertrophic bone formation. The changes are more pronounced on the left side.

arately, although the example cases presented may have concomitant manifestations of both, as is more commonly the case in clinical practice.

The descriptive names central, lateral, and foraminal stenoses refer to the sites of compression (entrapment) of the neural elements, although more than one site may be involved by a given pathologic process. Thus, central stenosis refers to compression of the cauda equina as a whole and is likely to be seen when there is reduction of the anteroposterior and/or transverse diameters of the canal by anterior or posterior elements. Lateral stenosis refers to narrowing of the lateral recess of the spinal canal. This is the space between the posterior border of the vertebral end plate or vertebral body anteriorly, the base of the superior articular process posteriorly, and the medial and inferomedial aspects of the pedicle laterally. Lateral stenosis may result from changes involving the posterior articular facet or the base of the superior articular process. Foraminal stenosis refers to narrowing of the intervertebral foramen, particularly the upper part of the foramen where the nerve root lies. This is therefore likely to result from changes involving the superior aspect of the facet joint.

Developmental Stenosis

This condition may involve the entire lumbar spine, the lower half, a segment of contiguous vertebrae, or rarely an individual vertebral level. The involved vertebra shows narrowing of the mid-sagittal diameter (Fig. 26). Based on intraoperative observations, the figures of 12 mm (147) and 15 mm (37) have been cited as the lower limit of normal. These figures can be applied to images of CT and MRI, because these do not suffer from distortion by photographic magnification. The interpedicular distance may be less than 20 mm (148). The lamina is thickened above a limit of 14 mm (43). Because of their location on each

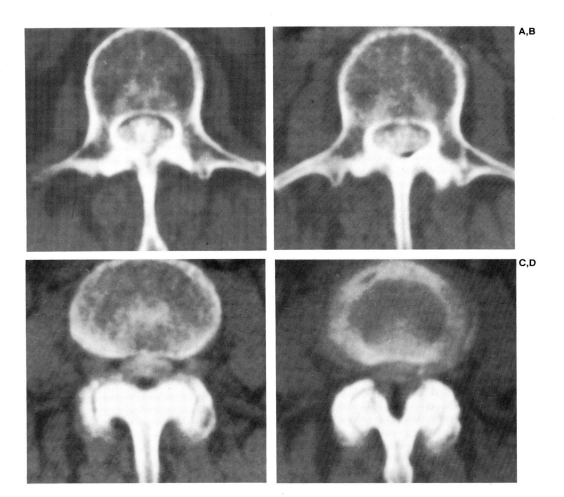

FIG. 26. Central spinal stenosis due to developmental features compounded by hypertrophic changes at the facet joints. CT after water-soluble myelography. **A:** At the level L2, the bony spinal canal shows the normal triangular configuration allowed by an adequate anteroposterior diameter. **B:** At the level L3, the bony spinal canal has an oval configuration caused by a shortened anteroposterior diameter. **C:** At the level of the L3-L4 foramen, the laminae are thick and short. The approximation of the laminae to the posterior border of the body of L3 resulted in compression of the dural sac. The contrast material has very low density, as a result of compression. **D:** At the level of the L3-L4 intervertebral disc, there is severe compression of the cauda equina. Thickening of ligamentum flavum has obliterated the greater part of the anteroposterior diameter of the spinal canal. The dural sac is squeezed against the posterior disc border. No contrast material is seen at this level, indicating a complete block.

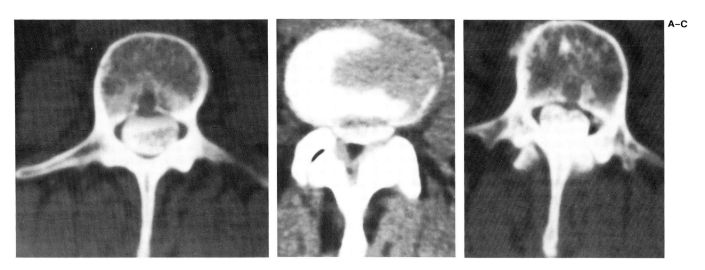

FIG. 27. Central stenosis caused by development abnormalities complicated by degenerative bulging of the disc at L3-L4. CT after water-soluble myelography. **A:** At the level of L3. **B:** At the disc L3-L4. **C:** At the level L4. Notice the normal configuration of the bony spinal canal in **A** and **C**. The unfavorable configuration in **B** is caused by narrowing of the angle between the lower borders of the laminae and the large size of the inferior articular processes and is compounded by bulging of the disc and thickening of the ligamenta flava. As a result, the dural sac is squeezed forward and occupies a fraction of the anteroposterior diameter of the spinal canal. The contrast column is oval in shape because of a decrease in the anteroposterior diameter compared with **A** and **C,** indicating compression of the cauda equina. The right facet joint shows the vacuum phenomenon.

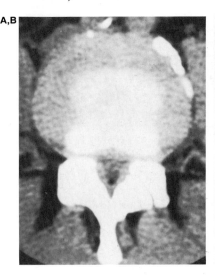
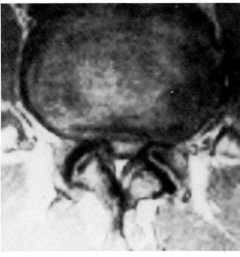

FIG. 28. Central stenosis at L4-L5 (same case in Fig. 15). **A:** CT. **B:** MRI, 1.5 T. Bal-I (SE, TR = 1,600 msec, TE = 28 msec). The laminae are short, the ligamenta flava are thick, and there is degenerative disc bulging.

side of the midline, the thickened laminae may cause encroachment on the canal while measurement of the midsagittal diameter may be within normal limits (Fig. 27B). Other features of developmental stenosis include short, thick pedicles (Fig. 26C), and inferior articular processes also may be developmentally bulky.

Degenerative Stenosis

This condition results from hypertrophic changes at the three-joint complex, constituting the picture of spondylosis, and in some cases compounded by degenerative spondylolisthesis. Intervertebral disc bulging associated with spur formation at the border of the vertebral end plate encroaches on the anterior aspect of the bony spinal canal. Thickening of the laminae, although described in developmental stenosis, may also result from or be in-

creased in spondylosis (Figs. 26 and 28–30). The ligamentum flavum normally measures 2 to 3 mm in thickness (148). Diffuse thickening of the ligamentum flavum (Figs. 28 and 30) in spondylosis is a common component of the overall degenerative process, but it may be seen in the absence of other manifestations of spondylosis.

Hypertrophy of the articular facets in spondylosis plays an important role in spinal stenosis. The enlarged facets may extend toward the midline, encroaching on the posterior aspect of the dural sac, thus contributing to central stenosis (Figs. 26D, 27B, and 30B). On the other hand, the large facets may compress the lateral aspects of the dural sac, causing the subarticular type of lateral stenosis (Fig. 29). Furthermore, the base of the superior articular process forms the dorsal boundary of the lateral recess, and when hypertrophied, it may compress the nerve against the posterior border of the vertebral end plate (Fig.

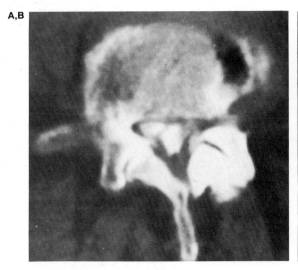
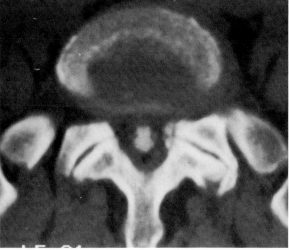

FIG. 29. Lateral spinal stenosis of the subarticular type caused by massive facets in two different patients. CT after water-soluble myelography. **A:** Indentation of the contrast column by the medial aspect of the facets gives the contrast column the "trefoil" configuration. **B:** Indentation of the dural sac by the medial aspect of the facets obliterates the lateral angles of the contrast column completely.

A,B

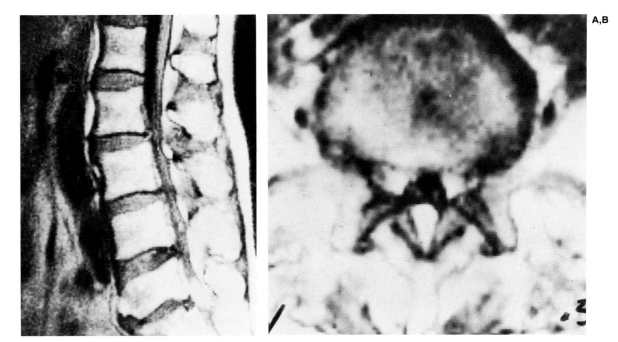

FIG. 30. Spinal stenosis due to a combination of developmental and degenerative changes. MRI, 0.5 T. T1-WI. **A:** Sagittal T1-WI (SE, TR = 500 msec, TE = 17 msec) shows marked narrowing of the anteroposterior diameter of the bony spinal canal. **B:** Axial T1-WI (SE, TR = 500 msec, TE = 25 msec) shows massive facets, thickened ligamenta flava, and narrowing of the angle between the laminae. As a result, the "effective" anteroposterior diameter of the bony spinal canal is greatly reduced, and the dural sac is squeezed in the anterior part of the bony spinal canal.

31). This entrapment involves the nerve root designated by the same vertebral level as the articular process. Finally, hypertrophy and upward elongation of the tip of the superior articular process result in foraminal stenosis and compression of the nerve root in the foramen (Fig. 32).

Spondylolisthesis

In spondylolisthesis there is anterior displacement of a vertebra on the adjacent vertebra below. The type of spinal stenosis that results depends on the changes that have

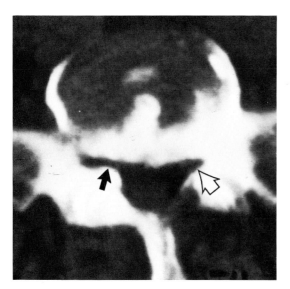

FIG. 31. Lateral stenosis of the lateral recess caused by the base of the superior articular process. CT at the level of the upper part of the lateral mass of S1. There is bony prominence at the base of the superior articular process of S1 on the right side, causing narrowing of the right lateral recess (*arrow*) for the right S1 root. Compare with the normal appearance of the opposite side (*open arrow*).

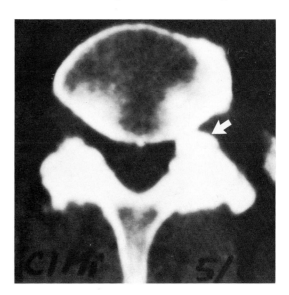

FIG. 32. Foraminal stenosis at L5-S1 on the left side. CT at the level of the end plate of L5. The right foramen accommodates the fifth nerve root and ganglion without encroachment. On the left side, there is a bony lesion (*arrow*), an osteophyte arising from the superior articular process of S1 and occupying the foramen, causing compression of the left 5th lumbar nerve root and ganglion.

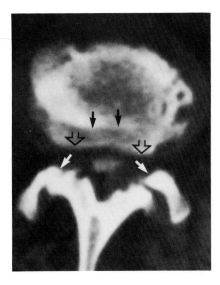

FIG. 33. Degenerative spondylolisthesis. CT at the L3-L4 level after water-soluble myelogram. There are advanced degenerative changes involving the posterior articular joints, with marked erosion resulting in forward slipping of L3 over L4. The posterior border of the lower end plate of L3 (*black arrows*) lies anterior to the border of the upper end plate of L4 (*open arrows*). The neural arch of L3 has moved forward and lies close to the posterior border of the upper end plate of L4, causing compression of the dural sac. The forward movement is made possible by erosion of the medial aspects of the superior articular processes of L4 (*white arrows*). Degenerative spondylolisthesis has resulted in a severe degree of spinal stenosis.

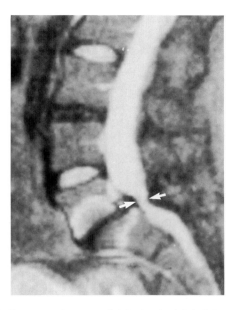

FIG. 34. Degenerative spondylolisthesis. MRI, 0.5 T, sagittal T2-WI (SE, TR = 2,000 msec, TE = 120 msec). Forward slipping of the body and the dorsal elements of L5 over S1. The dorsal elements of L5 close on the upper border of S1, causing severe spinal stenosis, with narrowing of the anteroposterior dimension of the CSF column at that level (*arrows*).

A,B

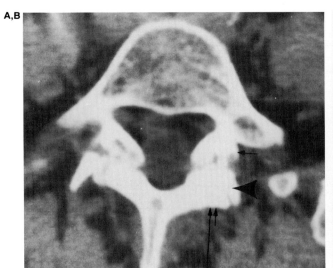
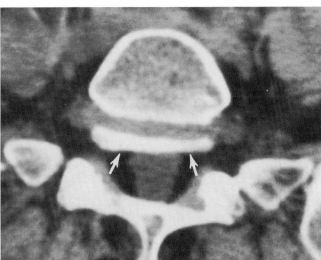

FIG. 35. Lytic spondylolisthesis at L5-S1. CT. **A:** Bilateral defects in the pars interarticularis of L5 are seen between the base of the superior articular process anteriorly (*arrow*) and the inferior articular process (*double arrow*). In the gap between the two components of the neural arch of L5, the tip of the superior articular process of S1 (*arrowhead*) can be seen. **B:** The posterior borders of the bodies of S1 (*arrows*) and L5 are seen on the same slice, creating the so-called double-margin sign.

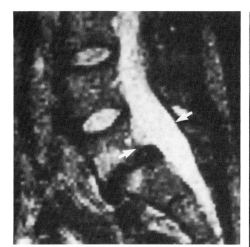

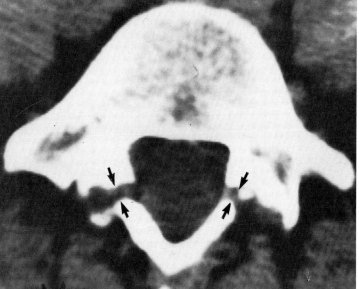

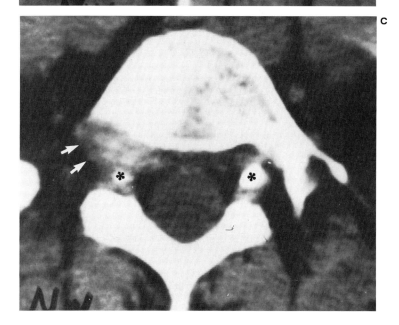

FIG. 36. Lytic spondylolisthesis of L5. **A:** MRI, 0.5 T. Sagittal T2-WI (SE, TR = 2,000 msec, TE = 120 msec). The body of L5 has moved forward in relation to S1, but the posterior elements of L5 have remained in place. As a result, there is an increase in the anteroposterior dimension of the CSF column, at L5 (*arrows*). **B:** CT at the level of the pedicles of L5. **C:** CT at the level of the intervertebral foramina. The defect in the pars interarticularis of L5 (*black arrows*) is shown in **B.** The stenosis in this condition is of the lateral type and is caused by the prominent bone formation at the inferior aspect of the defect in the pars interarticularis (*asterisks*) shown in **C.** In addition, there is in this case associated herniation of the nucleus pulposus of the L5-S1 disc in the right foramen (*white arrows*), shown also in **C.**

predisposed to the displacement (22,82). Spondylolisthesis that occurs as a manifestation of spinal instability due to advanced degenerative changes in all components of the three-joint complex is called degenerative spondylolisthesis. Anterior displacement of a vertebral body may also occur as a result of a congenital or traumatic bone defect in the pars interarticularis, while the posterior articular joints are intact. This type is called lytic spondylolisthesis.

In degenerative spondylolisthesis, axial CT (Fig. 33) shows erosion and loss of the medial aspect of the superior articular facet and forward displacement of the inferior articular facet (and neural arch) toward the posterior aspect of the upper border of the vertebral body below. The posterior borders of the two vertebral bodies appear in the same axial plane (Fig. 33).

Forward movement of the neural arch of the upper vertebra closer to the body of the lower vertebra results

in narrowing of the anteroposterior diameter of the bony spinal canal, i.e., central stenosis, with compression of the cauda equina. This is readily shown by CT (Fig. 33) and MRI (Fig. 34). Furthermore, forward movement of the inferior articular facet toward the posterior border of the disc plate impinges on the nerve root in the lateral recess.

In lytic spondylolisthesis, CT (Figs. 35, 36B, and 36C) shows bilateral defects in the pars interarticularis. The body of the involved vertebra slips forward, while the posterior joints and the rest of the neural arch remain aligned with the neural arch of the vertebra below. Therefore, the anteroposterior diameter of the spinal canal usually is elongated rather than shortened (Figs. 35A, 36A, and 36B). However, the lateral recess is compromised by hypertrophic bone formation at the "proximal" side of the defect (Fig. 36C), causing compression of the nerve against the lateral part of the end plate of the vertebra below. The

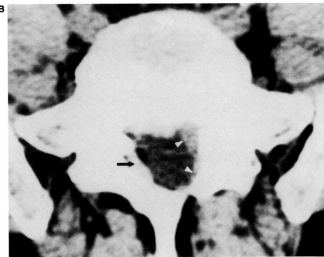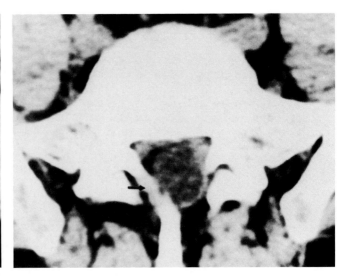

FIG. 37. Normal postoperative changes after left partial hemilaminectomy for removal of a herniated disc at L5-S1 level. **A:** There is a small bony defect in the left lamina associated with absence of the left ligamentum flavum. In addition, a soft-tissue band (*arrowheads*), believed to represent postoperative scar, can be seen extending along the left lateral aspect of the spinal canal. The normal right ligamentum flavum is clearly seen (*arrow*). **B:** Four millimeters caudal, the ligamentum flavum is again seen on the right side (*arrow*), but not on the left. Note the eccentric position of the dural sac, which has extended into the space created by removal of bone and ligamentum flavum, and the replacement of epidural fat by a band of soft tissue (scar) on the left. Asymmetric epidural fat is a normal postoperative finding and should not be interpreted as a sign of recurrent disc herniation.

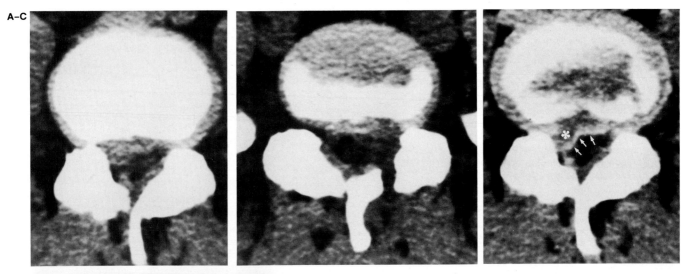

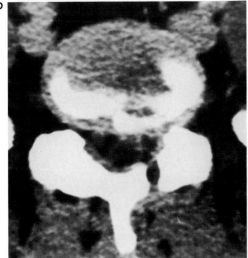

FIG. 38. Recurrent disc herniation at L4-L5 on the right side and postoperative scar at L5-S1 on the left side. **A,B:** Plain CT. **C,D:** CT after intravenous contrast injection. **A:** Plain CT at L4-L5. There is soft-tissue density at the right posterolateral border of the disc. **B:** Plain CT at the level L5-S1 shows a similar density at the left posterolateral border of the disc. **C:** CT at same level as **A,** after intravenous contrast injection. The recurrent disc herniation appears as a defect (*asterisk*) within a thin rim of contrast-enhancing scar (*arrows*). The defect caused by the disc fragment is continuous with the substance of the disc in the disc space. **D:** CT at same level as **B,** after intravenous contrast injection. The soft-tissue density is caused by contrast-enhancing scar tissue surrounding the root sheath. Compare with the root sheath on the right side. No evidence of recurrent disc herniation.

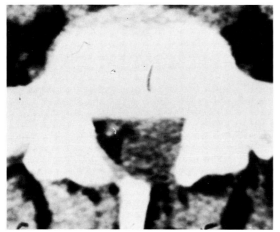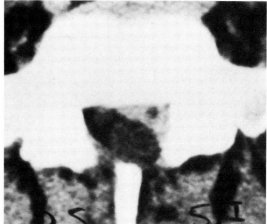

A,B

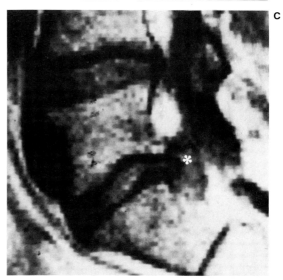

C

FIG. 39. Postoperative scar confirmed by reexploration. **A:** Plain CT shows soft-tissue density obliterating the epidural fat on the left side and encroaching on the left anterolateral aspect of the dural sac at the level of the first sacral segment. **B:** CT after intravenous contrast injection shows uniform enhancement of the soft-tissue density typical of scar tissue. The defect seen in the left lateral recess is due to the nerve root sheath of S1, compare with the normal root on the right side. **C:** MRI, 0.5 T. Sagittal T1-WI (SE, TR = 500 msec, TE = 17 msec) through the left lateral recess shows a soft-tissue mass (*asterisk*) resembling recurrent disc herniation. Reexploration confirmed the CT findings of scar tissue. There was no recurrent disc herniation.

effect is compounded if the end plate carries a degenerative spur. In some cases there may also be associated HNP, with further root compression (Fig. 36C). On axial CT, the posterior border of the disc has a characteristic appearance (Fig. 35B) as a result of the malalignment of the end plates of the two vertebrae. In some cases the defect in the pars interarticularis is shown close to the posterior articular joint and may indeed resemble a double-joint line (Fig. 35A). However, the presence of sclerosis and/or fragmentation of the neighboring bone will be helpful in making a correct interpretation.

THE POSTOPERATIVE SPINE

Recurrent symptoms after hemilaminectomy and discectomy represent a common diagnostic problem that often requires evaluation by multiple diagnostic techniques. The presence of postoperative scar (40,127) that obliterates the normal epidural fat and obscures the borders of the disc and dural sac makes the diagnosis of recurrent disc herniation difficult.

Although nondiagnostic, some features are useful to distinguish between recurrent disc herniation and postoperative scar formation (40,127). On noncontrast CT, scar tissue frequently appears as a linear band or curvilinear rim of density anterior, anterolateral, and lateral to the dural sac (Fig. 37A) and following its contour. The dural sac is retracted toward the side of surgery. In some instances, scar tissue appears nodular (Figs. 38B and 39A). The density of the scar usually is higher than that of the dural sac and lower than that of the intervertebral disc. The extent of postoperative scar is best shown on postcontrast CT study. After contrast injection, there is uniform enhancement of the rim (Fig. 37B) or nodule (Fig. 39B) of scar tissue in more than two-thirds of cases. The whole circumference of the annulus may also be enhanced, presumably because of the presence of a venous plexus. The nerve root sheath appears as a smooth rounded defect within the enhanced scar in the lateral recess (Figs. 38D, 39B, and 40D). In contradistinction, recurrent HNP appears in an unenhanced image as a nodular or mass-like lesion, with attenuation values similar to that of the disc, and causes a mass effect, distorting

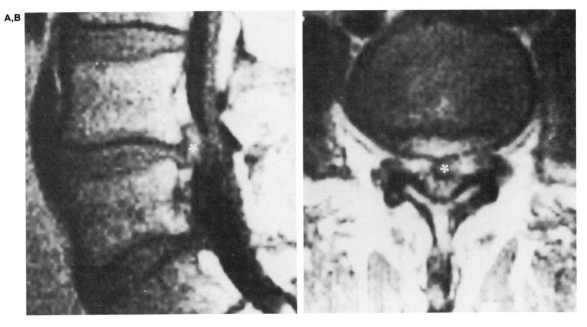

FIG. 40. Recurrent herniation of the disc at L4-L5. MRI, 0.5 T. **A:** Sagittal T1-WI (SE, TR = 700 msec, TE = 15 msec). **B:** Bal-I (SE, TR = 1,500 msec, TE = 45 msec) in the axial projection at the level L4-L5. Both MR images show convincing evidence of recurrence of L4-L5 disc herniation (*asterisk*), which appears as a well-defined mass displacing the dural sac away. The MRI findings were confirmed at surgery.

the dural sac (Fig. 38A). After contrast enhancement, HNP appears as a nodular defect within the enhanced scar, with no resemblance to a nerve root sheath (Fig. 38C). Using these criteria, it was reported that a correct diagnosis of recurrent HNP or scar was possible in 60% of cases on the basis of noncontrast CT alone, and 83% when both noncontrast and postcontrast CT findings were used for interpretation (40). Using MRI, it may be possible to diagnose recurrent HNP by its mass effect (Fig. 40). It also was reported (18) that the scar, relative to the annulus, was hypointense or isointense in T1-WI and hyperintense on T2-WI, whereas recurrent HNP was hypointense or isointense in all images. The exception was in the case of sequestered free fragments, which were slightly hyperintense in all images. Based on the currently available data, it is expected that MRI with contrast enhancement by gadolinium-DTPA will be more helpful than myelography and CT in differentiating recurrent HNP and postoperative scar (60).

Accumulation of cerebrospinal fluid (CSF) in the epidural and deep subcutaneous spaces at the site of surgery, often called a false meningocele, may occur due to inadvertent opening of the dural sac or a dural sheath. It is easily diagnosed by CT with intrathecal contrast material (41). In some cases, actual continuity with the dural sac may be demonstrated.

Arachnoiditis and disc-space infection are two complications of spinal surgery, but they also may occur in nonoperated cases. Changes associated with arachnoiditis can be demonstrated by myelography and postmyelography CT, but not by noncontrast CT (Fig. 42). There

may be clumping of the roots to form thickened, irregular elements of the cauda equina. The roots may appear adherent to the inner aspect of the arachnoid membrane or may be virtually absent, probably being walled off by arachnoid adhesions. For the same reason, the contrast-filled subarachnoid space may appear small and irregular. Finally, there may be complete block (Fig. 43). Similar findings can be demonstrated with heavily T2-weighted MRI without the need for intrathecal contrast injection (124).

Discitis may resemble degeneration of the intervertebral disc on CT. There is irregularity of the vertebral end plate, narrowing of the intervertebral space, and expansion of the disc borders. However, a paravertebral or epidural

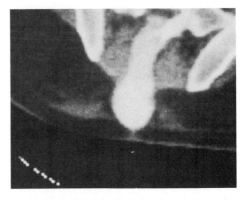

FIG. 41. Postoperative meningocele. CT after water-soluble myelogram. Contrast material fills the postoperative meningocele, which extends from the dural sac to the subcutaneous fat.

A,B

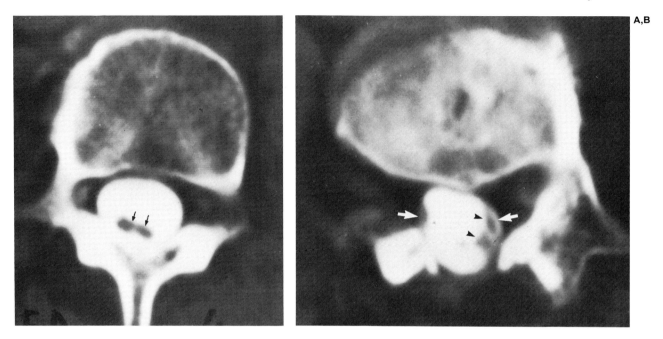

FIG. 42. Arachnoiditis: different patterns on postmyelography CT. **A:** At the level L4, there is clumping of the roots in an oval irregular mass (*arrows*). **B:** At the level L5, the roots (*arrows*) appear as if they are "plastered" against the inner aspect of the wall of the dural sac, and there are septa (*arrowheads*) formed within the dural sac.

A,B

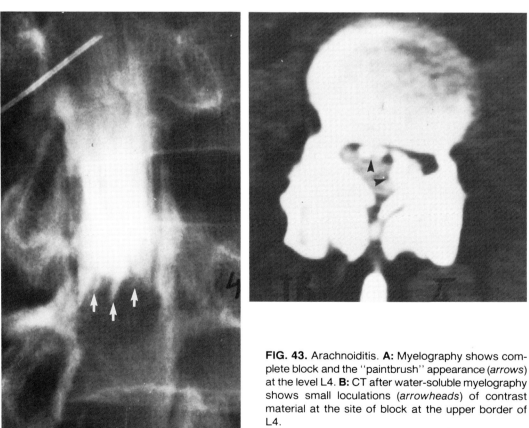

FIG. 43. Arachnoiditis. **A:** Myelography shows complete block and the "paintbrush" appearance (*arrows*) at the level L4. **B:** CT after water-soluble myelography shows small loculations (*arrowheads*) of contrast material at the site of block at the upper border of L4.

A,B

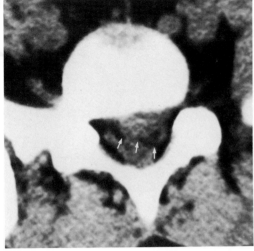

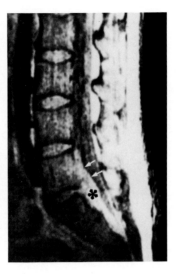

FIG. 44. Epidural abscess at L5-S1. A: Plain CT shows an epidural mass (*arrows*) anterior to the dural sac, which is pushed against the laminae of L5. The lesion is indistinguishable from HNP of L5-S1. B: MRI, 0.5 T. Bal-I (SE, TR = 1,500 msec, TE = 35 msec) shows the anteriorly located epidural mass (*asterisk*) stripping the dural sac (*arrows*) away from the posterior borders of the L5, S1, and S2 vertebrae.

soft-tissue mass (Fig. 44A), coupled with a high sedimentation rate and clinical evidence of infection, often can aid in the correct diagnosis. MRI is most helpful in making the diagnosis of disc-space infection. In balanced images and T2-WI there is high signal in the disc space and the epidural space (Fig. 44B).

ROLES OF DIFFERENT TECHNIQUES

In addition to plain radiographs, either CT or MRI may be used as the primary modality for evaluation of degenerative disease of the spine. Given equal accessibility, we prefer to use MRI as the primary procedure for suspected HNP, and CT for suspected spondylosis and spinal stenosis.

If the primary examination adequately reveals a lesion that satisfactorily explains the clinical picture, no further evaluation is needed, and effective treatment may be instituted. If the primary examination is equivocal or does not satisfactorily account for the clinical symptoms, examination with the alternative modality should be performed.

At the present time, myelography and postmyelography CT are still being used in a significant number of cases of HNP, spondylosis, suspected disc recurrence, arachnoiditis, and intradural neoplasm. However, the use of myelography will continue to diminish with increased experience in MRI interpretation, the availability of MRI contrast material, and better definition of the complementary roles of MRI and CT.

SPINAL TRAUMA

In spinal trauma, patient management depends on detailed knowledge of the pathoanatomic features of the injury, including its exact level. Careful radiologic eval-

uation is important, because failure to recognize a lesion or a specific type of injury may result in chronic disability of the patient, even permanent neurologic deficit.

Satisfactory plain radiographs often are impossible to obtain in acutely traumatized patients, who may have multiple injuries and thus cannot or should not be moved into positions that would be necessary for typical radiographic projections of the spine. Certain regions of the spine, such as the craniocervical and cervicothoracic junctions, are notoriously difficult to evaluate because of superimposition of overlying structures. In the cervical spine, as well as in other parts of the vertebral column, findings on plain radiographs may appear normal, despite the presence of a fracture (95).

CT, with equipment capable of thin-section imaging and image reformatting in nonaxial planes, has markedly changed the approach to evaluation of spinal trauma (14,15,38,58). Since 1982, MRI has become available and is being increasingly used in the diagnostic evaluation of patients with spinal injury, especially chronic injury to the spinal cord with new symptoms and signs (46,98,99,119), but also recent trauma (23,72,100,144).

Advantages of CT

Patients with acute spinal trauma, notably those with unstable fractures or fracture dislocations, are at risk of developing permanent neurologic deficits or worsening of already existing deficits whenever they are physically moved, as would be necessary for satisfactory conventional tomography. CT can be performed with the patient remaining in the stable supine position throughout the study, although the patient will have to be moved from the stretcher onto the scanner couch and back. The actual CT examination requires relatively little time, because imaging is done in only one plane (axial). In the cervical spine, contiguous 2-mm sections are optimal, and 4-mm sections can be used in the thoracic, lumbar, and sacral regions. Reformatted images in sagittal, coronal, or oblique planes can be computer-generated without any further radiation exposure or manipulation of the patient.

Axial images are optimal for determining spinal-canal size and possible cord compression, as well as for searching for intraspinal bony fragments (38). Unlike conventional radiography, CT has relatively high contrast resolution, permitting (limited) direct evaluation of the contents of the spinal canal. The intervertebral discs, ligaments, and spinal cord can all be demonstrated by noncontrast CT, although the quality of visualization of ligaments and spinal cord varies and may be diagnostically insufficient in a given case. Similarly, epidural, subdural, and intramedullary hematomas, inaccessible to conventional radiography, may be detected by CT (62,117). In penetrating injuries, such as gunshot wounds, the positions of foreign bodies relative to the vertebral column, spinal canal, and neural foramina can be easily determined (115). Fresh or healing fractures that have a "vertical" (i.e., sagittal, coronal, or oblique) course are effectively demonstrated by axial images. Fractures involving a demineralized spine may be difficult to detect by conventional radiography, including tomography, but often they are easily demonstrated by CT (58). Image reformatting in nonaxial planes facilitates the diagnosis of dislocation and facet locking; it also improves visualization of fractures with a more "horizontal" course. Intrathecal administration of water-soluble contrast material considerably improves the demonstration of spinal cord abnormalities, such as swelling from edema or hematoma, and is also necessary for the demonstration of dural tears (14).

Limitations of CT

Nondisplaced "horizontal" fractures, i.e., fractures oriented in the transverse plane, may be missed on standard CT images. Image reformatting may help, but the clarity of the computer-generated nonaxial views depends on the thickness of the original CT sections. A change in the position of the patient between two consecutive images may lead to missing even a vertically oriented fracture. Conversely, the well-known partial-volume phenomenon may produce CT appearances simulating fractures. Narrowing or widening of disc spaces and minor degrees of vertebral malalignment also may be overlooked on axial images. To rule out instability of the spine, radiologic examination is required in both extension and flexion of the spinal region of interest. This is difficult to accomplish with CT and preferably is done with conventional radiography or fluoroscopy. Artifacts caused by metallic surgical clips, Harrington rods, or external fixation devices may compromise CT evaluation in the postoperative stage.

Survey of the entire spinal column by CT is time-consuming and thus not practical. The region of the spine likely to yield abnormal findings on CT should be determined first by obtaining a limited number of plain films as part of the primary evaluation of the patient. Alternatively, in a given case, a digital radiograph obtained with the CT scanner can help to limit the area subsequently to be studied in detail (14). In fact, such a "topogram" (scanogram, scout view) usually is indispensable for level determination. A thorough CT study of the predetermined portion of the spine then greatly enhances the information on the type and extent of the injury and generally obviates thin-section conventional tomography.

Role of MRI

With the advent and improvement of surface coils, MRI, despite certain shortcomings in the demonstration of cortical bone, may be used to diagnose fractures and dislocations. At least in the thoracolumbar spine, MRI seems capable of demonstrating most, if not all, major fractures. MRI is superior to CT in demonstrating ligamentous injury and damage to intervertebral discs (98,100,143). With CT, rupture of ligaments often can be inferred only on the basis of significant vertebral malalignment, whereas with MRI, detachment and breaks in continuity of ligaments can be shown directly.

Within the spinal canal, MRI reveals traumatic effects that previously could be detected only by invasive methods such as myelography or CT-myelography. Compression of the thecal sac and spinal cord by dislocated vertebrae or bony fragments can be easily recognized; swelling of the cord likewise can be demonstrated. MRI not only shows the intramedullary mass effect but also may aid in differentiating between hemorrhagic damage to the cord and potentially reversible cord edema (23,56). Whereas subacute and chronic intramedullary hematomas exhibit a signal intensity higher than that of other intraspinal structures on both T1-WI and T2-WI, spinal cord edema appears as an area of high signal intensity extending above and below the site of injury into the neural substance on T2-WI (50,56). In patients with chronic spinal cord injuries, MRI may be used to distinguish between cord atrophy, myelomalacia, and posttraumatic spinal cord cysts. This is of great importance whenever new neurologic symptoms occur or existing symptoms worsen, because expanding cord cysts can be successfully decompressed (119).

Evaluation of acute or chronic spinal injury by MRI usually requires thin-section techniques, with slice thicknesses of 5 mm or less. Sagittal images provide the best overall information on the injury (including level localization), but additional transaxial images are necessary in most cases. Ideally, T1-WI, Bal-I, and T2-WI should be obtained. T1-WI probably are more important in chronic injury and less important in the acute situation. The introduction of MRI for imaging of the spine has drastically

A,B

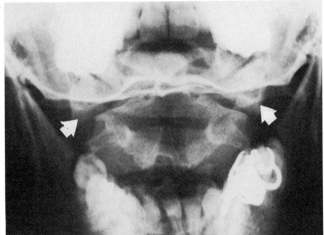

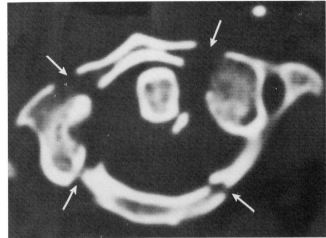

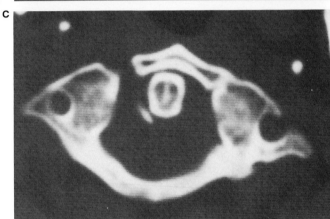

C

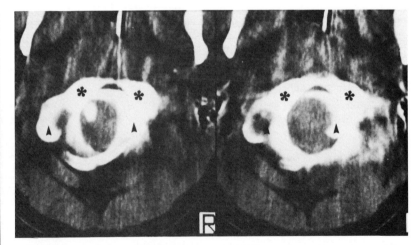

FIG. 45. Jefferson fracture. A: Open-mouth anteroposterior radiograph of the craniocervical junction shows lateral displacement of the lateral masses of the atlas (*arrows*). B: CT demonstrates fractures of the anterior and posterior arches (*arrows*) of the atlas. C: Follow-up CT image of the same patient 8 months later shows healing, with bony fusion at three of the four fracture sites.

reduced the need for myelography and postmyelography CT. With further improvement of MRI technology, as well as more experience in its use in spinal trauma, even plain CT may be obviated, at least for injuries of the thoracolumbar region (98). In patients with penetrating injury

of the spine, the possibility of ferromagnetic foreign bodies that may become dislodged, producing further cord damage, must be ruled out before a patient undergoes MRI. If the patient is dependent on life-support systems, these should be such that they are suitable for use inside the

A,B

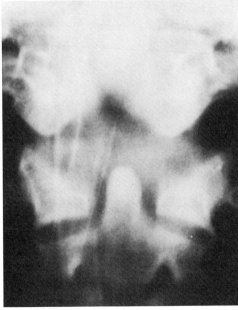

FIG. 46. Atlantooccipital dislocation. A: Anteroposterior tomogram of the cranial-cervical junction demonstrates wide gap between occipital condyles and atlas. B: CT (13-mm slice thickness) shows abnormal relationship between occipital condyles (*asterisks*) and superior articular facets (*arrowheads*) of atlas. Patient survived, with marked neurologic deficit.

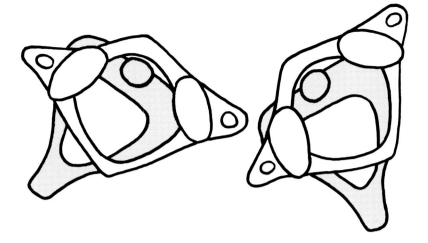

FIG. 47. Atlantoaxial rotary fixation. Schematic representation of atlas (*white*) and axis (*gray*) shows unilateral subluxation and lack of change in relative position between the two vertebrae on maximal head rotation to the right and left. Axis (which normally participates only very little in head rotation) rotates as much as atlas. (Drawing based on actual CT images, modified after ref. 122.)

magnet (99). Artifacts from nonferromagnetic foreign bodies or surgical implants usually are less troublesome with MRI than with CT.

Cervical Spine Injury

Craniocervical Junction and Upper Cervical Spine

Fractures of the atlas are relatively rare compared with fractures of the remainder of the cervical vertebrae. Most commonly they are the result of hyperextension or axial-compression injury. In the classic Jefferson fracture, the atlantal ring breaks at two points of the anterior arch, usually in front of the lateral masses, and at two additional points posteriorly, usually in the region of the sulcus for the vertebral artery (Fig. 45). Because the resulting fragments tend to move sideways, and because there may be additional injury to the transverse ligament, lateral as well as anterior atlantoaxial subluxation is common. Most of these features are easily recognized on CT images, provided the plane of section is appropriate, i.e., parallel to the injured atlas (77,79). The same applies to fractures that involve only the posterior arch. Differentiation from congenital clefts or partial agenesis of the anterior and/ or posterior arches of the atlas is based on the absence of prevertebral soft-tissue swelling and the presence of bony tapering, local bony deformity, and a cortical line at the site of bony discontinuity in the congenital abnormalities. Neurologic deficits are uncommon in fractures of the atlas. Using plain-film radiography, and even using thin-section tomography, these lesions are much more difficult to evaluate than with CT, although the occasional "horizontal" fractures of the anterior arch of the atlas still are recognized best on plain lateral radiographs or tomograms.

Traumatic atlantooccipital dislocation usually is fatal, but survival has been reported in some instances (12). The diagnosis usually is possible on conventional radiographs, though not easily. CT may be helpful in assessing associated soft-tissue abnormalities at the craniocervical

junction. The diagnosis can be made by CT alone by noting the relative positions of the occipital condyles and atlantal facets on axial images (12,89) (Fig. 46). Because of its direct multiplanar imaging capability and superior soft-tissue contrast sensitivity, MRI is superior to CT for evaluating the craniocervical junction.

Traumatic atlantoaxial subluxation is more easily evaluated by CT than by plain-film radiography (39). This is particularly true of the so-called atlantoaxial rotary fixation, which may require "functional" CT techniques. In this entity, images obtained with the head maximally rotated to the left, and then toward the right, show that the axis rotates as much as the subluxed atlas. Normally, the second cervical vertebra does not participate significantly in head rotation (122) (Fig. 47).

Fractures of the axis may affect the odontoid process (dens), body, or arch. Horizontally oriented, nondisplaced fractures of the midportion or base of the odontoid may be difficult to evaluate by CT, although reformatted images often are diagnostic (Figs. 48 and 49). Generally,

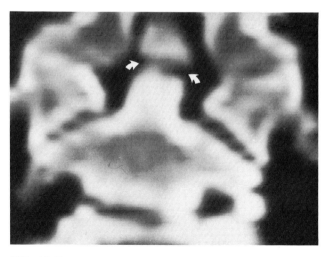

FIG. 48. Fracture at the midportion of the dens. Reformatted coronal CT image. Despite its transverse orientation, the fracture (*arrows*) is easily seen.

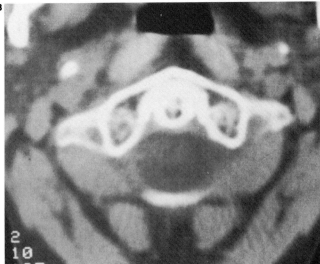
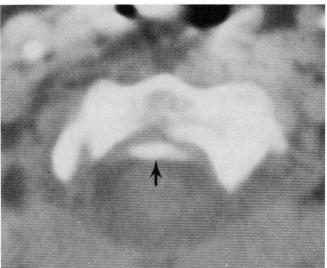
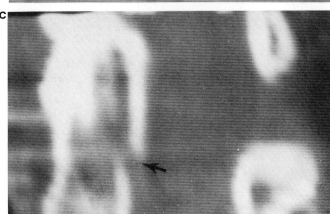

FIG. 49. Fracture at the base of the dens. CT images. A: At the level of the anterior arch of the atlas, there is normal relationship of the odontoid and anterior arch. B: At the level of the body of the axis, the inferior posterior border of the fractured dens (arrow) is seen posterior to the body of C2. C: Reformatted image in the sagittal plane provides better demonstration of the fracture (arrow).

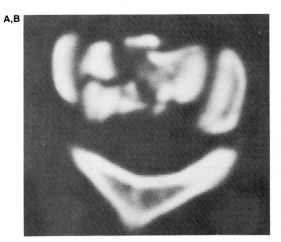
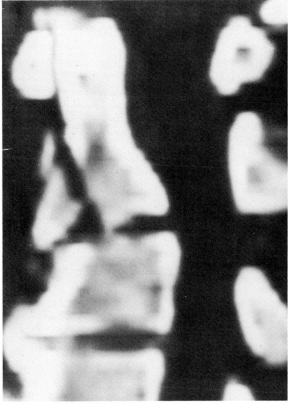

FIG. 50. Fractures of the body of the axis. A: Comminuted fracture as demonstrated on CT image at level of atlantoaxial joint. B: Vertical fracture, with anterior displacement of main fragment, suggesting additional injury to anterior longitudinal ligament (different patient). Fracture is best demonstrated on this reformatted midsagittal CT image, but was also easily identifiable on axial image (not shown).

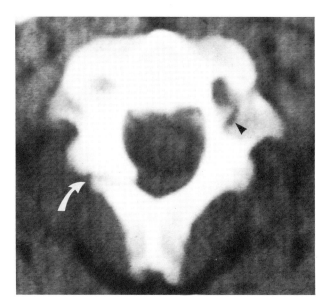

FIG. 51. Bilateral fracture of vertebral arch of C2, with corresponding widening of sagittal diameter of spinal canal. On this CT image, fracture is seen to involve lamina on right (*arrow*) and pedicle on left (*arrowhead*), thus representing an atypical hangman's fracture.

bilateral, although unilateral fractures occur. In the classic "hangman's fracture," the breaks extend through both pedicles. Injuries of this kind generally are the result of extreme hyperextension, and frequently there is additional trauma to the intervertebral disc C2-C3, including damage to the longitudinal ligaments. Anterior subluxation of C2 on C3 is almost the rule, and the posterior fragment tends to become slightly displaced backward. Consequently, the sagittal diameter of the spinal canal usually is widened. Neurologic symptoms and signs are therefore uncommon, and residual deficit is rare. In atypical "hangman's fracture," the fracture line passes through more posterior portions of the arch of C2, such as the articular pillars or laminae. The majority of these fractures have a more-or-less "vertical" course and thus are easily demonstrated by transaxial CT (Fig. 51). Most arch fractures of the axis are detectable by conventional radiography if carefully looked for. "Pseudo-hangman's fractures" affect posterior parts of the body of the axis rather than the arch (Fig. 52). Injuries with unilateral or bilateral locked facets are known to occur at the C2-C3 level, but are much less common than at the lower cervical spine.

conventional radiography provides the most convincing evidence of such injuries and thus should not be omitted. In the rare vertical fracture of the odontoid, the diagnosis may be possible only by CT (70). MRI provides excellent evaluation of the neural structures at the craniocervical junction and upper cervical cord. MRI, however, is not as good in demonstrating bony traumatic abnormalities, although nondisplaced fracture of the dens has been seen on T1-WI (88). Fractures of the body of the axis usually are well seen on plain radiographs, particularly lateral views and tomograms, but sometimes are best demonstrated by CT (Fig. 50). Fractures of the arch typically are

Lower Cervical Spine

About two-thirds of all major injuries to the cervical spine involve C5, C6, and C7, but C4 and especially C3 are infrequently involved. Trauma to the lower cervical spine deserves particular attention, because the subarachnoid space is narrow, and any substantial bony encroachment on the spinal canal is likely to produce cord compression. In this region, injuries may be caused by hyperflexion, hyperextension, distraction, hyperrotation, axial compression, or various combinations thereof. In the common wedge fractures, the prevailing causative

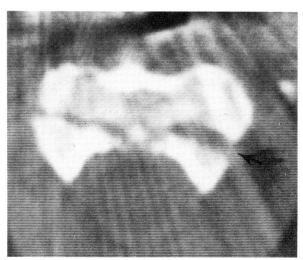

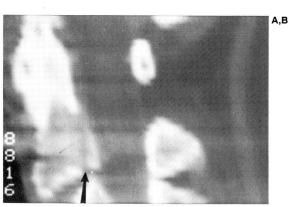

FIG. 52. Pseudo-hangman's fracture. **A:** The transverse fracture through the body of axis (*arrow*) is oriented in the craniocaudal plane and easy to demonstrate by CT. **B:** Reformatted image in the sagittal plane shows the craniocaudal orientation of the fracture line (*arrow*).

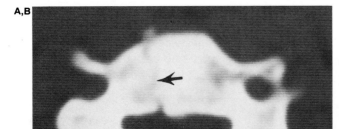

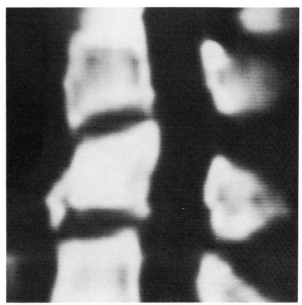

FIG. 53. Compression fracture of fourth cervical vertebra. **A:** Transaxial CT shows fracture through the body (*arrow*) and the right lamina (*arrowhead*) of C4. There is no encroachment on the spinal canal by bony fragments. **B:** Sagittally reformatted image demonstrates the wedge-like compression deformity and a small chip fracture at the anterior inferior border of the vertebral body. The spinal canal is intact.

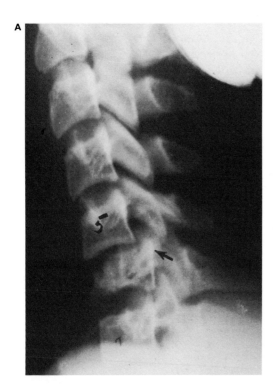

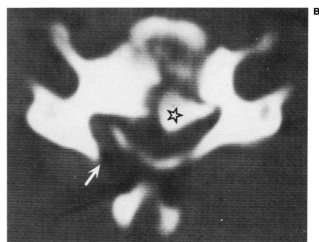

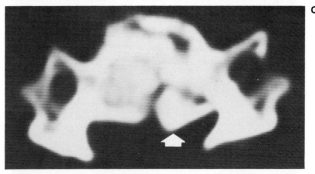

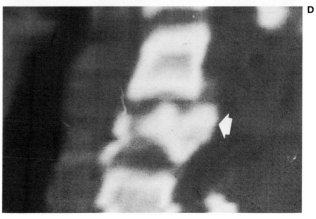

FIG. 54. Burst fracture of the sixth cervical vertebra, with posterior subluxation. **A:** Lateral radiograph demonstrates that the posterior border of the body of C6 is displaced into the spinal canal (*arrow*). **B:** Transaxial CT shows a comminuted fracture. A large fragment (*star*) impinges on the spinal canal. There is also a fracture of the right lamina (*arrow*). **C, D:** Postoperative axial CT (**C**) and sagittally reformatted image (**D**) show marked posterior displacement of the fractured body (*arrow*). The neural arch has been removed.

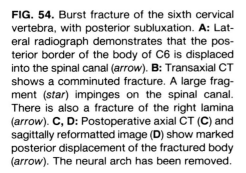

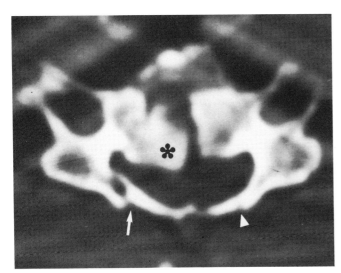

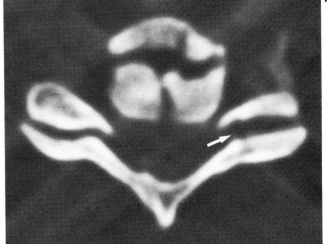

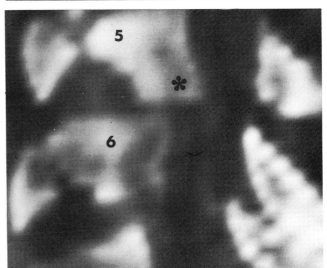

FIG. 55. Burst fractures of the fifth and sixth cervical vertebrae. **A:** Axial CT image at level of C5 shows a midsagittal fracture line through the vertebral body, posterior displacement of a large fragment (*asterisk*), a fracture of the right lamina (*arrow*), and a possible fracture of the left lamina (*arrowhead*). The sagittal diameter of the spinal canal is markedly narrowed. **B:** Image at the level of C6 reveals a comminuted fracture of the vertebral body, without significant retropulsion of fragments, as well as gaping of the left facet joint C6-C7 (*arrow*), suggesting severe damage to the joint capsule. The artifacts crossing these images result from an external fixation device. Note that the quality of the CT study has not suffered much from the presence of this device. **C:** A midsagittal reformatted image corroborates the severe deformation of the C5 and C6 vertebral bodies. The C5-C6 intervertebral disc protrudes into the comminuted vertebral body of C5. The *asterisk* marks the posteriorly displaced fragment of C5.

force is hyperflexion, whereas burst fractures result from a combination of hyperflexion and axial compression; neurologic deficits may occur in both, but are more likely in the latter. In wedge fractures, the spinal canal may be compromised by subluxation, whereas the narrowing of the canal in burst fractures typically results from retropulsion of bony fragments. Fragments encroaching on the dural sac and spinal cord are easily detected on axial CT images (26), although a more detailed evaluation of the lesion, including determination of the exact origin of the fragment, may require sagittal reformatted images (Figs. 53–55). Compared with conventional radiography, CT is clearly superior for assessment of complex trauma to the vertebral body, provided the course of the fracture line is more or less vertical.

For evaluation of the posterior vertebral elements, such as pedicles, articular pillars, articular processes, laminae, and spinous processes, CT is unsurpassed (26,38,153) (Figs. 53, 54, and 56). This is of particular significance because more than half of all major injuries to the cervical spine are accompanied by some damage to these structures, and satisfactory demonstration of many of these lesions by conventional radiographic methods is difficult

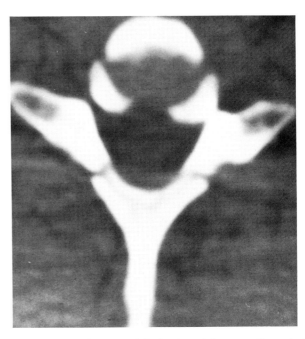

FIG. 56. Bilateral fracture of the lamina of the seventh cervical vertebra, without significant widening of the spinal canal. CT image at level of C7-T1 interspace.

A,B

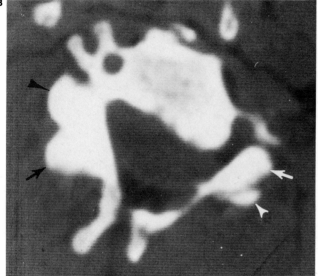

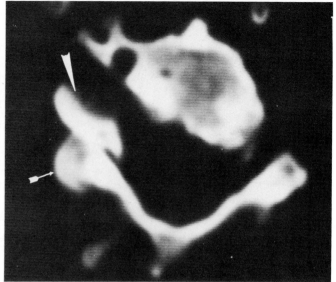

C

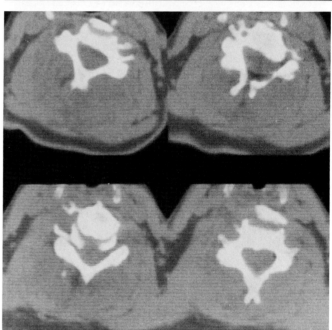

FIG. 57. Fracture dislocation at C5-C6, with locked facet on the right side. **A:** CT image through the articulation between C5 and C6 shows that the superior articular process of C6 (*white arrow*) lies in front of the inferior articular process of C5 (*white arrowhead*) on the normal left side. On the right side, the superior articular process of C5 (*black arrow*) lies behind the inferior articular process of C5 (*black arrowhead*). **B:** Same level, at bone window setting. Note the concave anterior surface of the inferior articular process of C5 on the right side (*arrowhead*), which is supposed to articulate with the posterior surface of the superior articular process of C6 (*arrow*). In addition, a fracture of the right superior articular process is present. **C:** Composite illustration of four slices through C5, C5-C6 articulation, and C6 in the same patient. Compare the orientation of the midsagittal plane of C5 (*upper left corner*) with that of C6 (*lower right corner*). This malalignment is an expression of the rotatory nature of the injury and is maintained by the locking of the facets.

or impossible in the acute situation. Unfortunately, as mentioned earlier, damage to the ligaments and compressive effects on the dural sac often can be assessed only by inference, rather than direct visualization. Although relatively minor subluxation can be recognized on the basis of a change in appearance of the uncovertebral or facet joints (153), routine image reformatting in nonaxial planes is advisable whenever clinically significant vertebral malalignment is suspected.

Certain hyperflexion injuries result in subluxation or dislocation of facet joints, usually at C5-C6 or C6-C7. In the extreme case, the inferior articular facet of the higher vertebra becomes "locked" anterior to the superior facet of the next lower vertebra. If this happens only on one side, the degree of narrowing of the spinal canal is moderate, but there may be marked encroachment on the

neural foramen, causing nerve root compression. In cases of bilaterally "locked" facets, the degree of narrowing of the spinal canal usually is severe (most patients with this type of injury are paraplegic) unless there is an associated fracture of the posterior arch of the dislocated vertebra, sparing the spinal cord from permanent damage. Dislocation with bilaterally "locked" facets is easily recognized on lateral plain radiographs, whereas unilateral facet locking may be difficult to see, even on multiple views. Also, associated articular-process (facet) or pillar fractures, which usually require open reduction, may be difficult to detect. CT images, on the other hand, usually permit diagnosis of the locked facet and the presence or absence of a fracture (Figs. 57 and 58). Again, image reformatting in sagittal, coronal, or oblique planes may be necessary to demonstrate less pronounced degrees of vertebral mal-

A,B

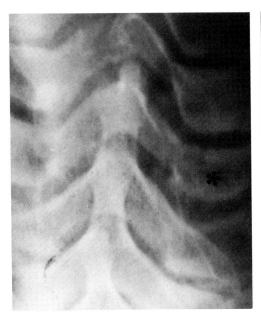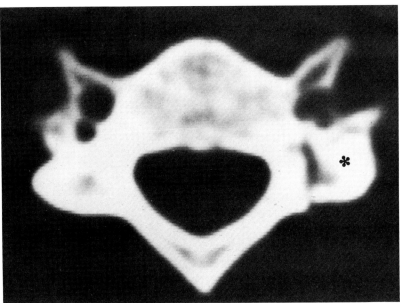

FIG. 58. Fracture of the articular pillar of the sixth cervical vertebra. **A:** Anteroposterior radiograph of the cervical spine (pillar view) shows deformation of the articular pillar of C6 (*asterisk*); there is a possible vertical fracture through the medial portion of the pillar. **B:** Axial CT image corroborates the deformity of the lateral portion of the pillar (*asterisk*) and additionally shows beyond doubt a sagittal fracture through the medial portion of the pillar.

alignment, "perched facets," and smaller fragments. Additionally, differentiation between normal joint spaces and fracture lines is facilitated (153).

Despite being a definite improvement over conventional radiographic techniques, plain CT is limited with respect to evaluation of most spinal soft-tissue structures. CT demonstration of extradural, subdural, subarachnoid, and intramedullary spinal hematomas of traumatic or nontraumatic origin has been described (117,142) (Fig. 59), but has not been consistent enough for routine di-

agnostic purposes. Less conspicuous traumatic abnormalities of intraspinal soft-tissue structures may entirely escape detection. With MRI, such changes may be demonstrated much more consistently (72,98,100,143). Disc abnormalities, including traumatic disc herniation, disc fragmentation, and intradiscal hemorrhage, can all be diagnosed on the basis of altered disc morphology and signal (Fig. 60). Discontinuity of the normally dark-appearing

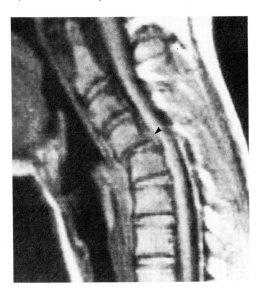

FIG. 60. Traumatic disc herniation at level of C4-C5 secondary to hyperflexion injury, with anterior subluxation. MRI, 0.5 T. sagittal T1-WI (SE, TR = 500 msec, TE = 30 msec) shows angular kyphosis at level of injury, with soft-tissue mass (*arrowhead*) anterior to slightly compressed-appearing spinal cord. Despite these findings, the patient had no neurologic deficits.

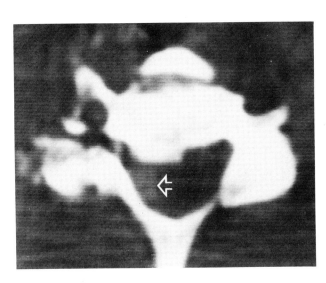

FIG. 59. Fracture of a vertebra complicated by hematoma. Fracture of the body of a cervical vertebra (C6), as well as fracture of the right articular pillar, can be seen. An intraspinal hematoma (*arrow*) is present medial to the right lamina.

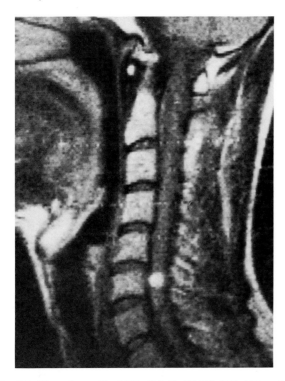

FIG. 61. Hematomyelia. MRI, 0.5 T. T1-WI (SE, TR = 300 msec, TE = 30 msec) demonstrates a focal high-signal cord abnormality consistent with subacute hematoma. The lesion occurred spontaneously; its cause could not be established at surgery. Axial images (not shown) corroborated the intramedullary location of the lesion.

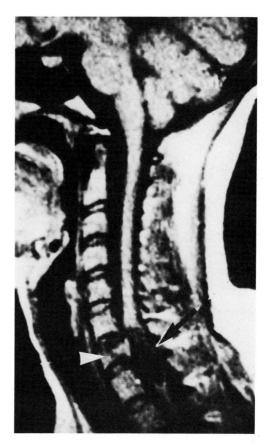

FIG. 62. Posttraumatic syringomyelia, MRI. T1-WI shows a cyst-like cavity (*arrow*) expanding the cord at the C7-T1 level. There is evidence of a burst fracture of the seventh cervical vertebra, with retropulsion of fragments (*arrowhead*). At surgery, a cyst was found, and decompression was achieved by placing a shunt catheter through a myelotomy on the dorsal cord surface at T1. (From ref. 119, with permission.)

ligaments suggests rupture. Ligaments, such as the longitudinal ligaments, that are normally indistinguishable from the cortical bone of the vertebral bodies may become visible when they are stripped away from bone because of hemorrhage or subluxation. Intraspinal hemorrhage may be difficult to detect in acute trauma, but is readily recognized in the subacute stage, at which time its signal is high on T1-WI and T2-WI (Fig. 61). Changes in size and shape of the cord can be clearly delineated on MR images, and there is little need for myelography or CT-myelography (Fig. 61). In one study (98), sagittal MRI sections were found to be almost as informative as conventional tomograms and more useful than lateral plain films of the spine in demonstrating fractures or subluxations. Furthermore, most fractures shown by axial CT, including fractures of the posterior elements, also can be detected on axial MR images. "Locked" facets are identified on parasagittal images. However, with regard to the evaluation of traumatic effects on the vertebral column, MRI is not as effective in the cervical region as it is in the thoracolumbar region. MRI of patients with unstable cervical spine injuries in skull traction is difficult, but is possible with some modifications of head positioning and if certain precautions are observed (99).

MRI may also be used in the chronic stage of cervical spinal cord injury to evaluate progressive myelopathy

(46,119). Although most major posttraumatic cord abnormalities can be demonstrated by CT-myelography with water-soluble contrast material combining early and delayed imaging, multiplanar MRI is more accurate, often permitting differentiation between syringomyelic cysts and myelomalacia (Fig. 62). On CT, both myelomalacia and cysts may show accumulation of contrast material on delayed images and thus become indistinguishable. On MRI, cysts show a signal behavior identical with that for CSF; i.e., they appear hypointense compared with the cord parenchyma on T1-WI, and hyperintense on T2-WI. Myelomalacia, though similar in appearance to cysts on T1-WI, exhibits essentially the same signal intensity as the cord parenchyma on T2-WI (119). Large cysts expanding the cord may be surgically shunted, with subsequent clinical improvement. After treatment, verification of cyst decompression is easy by MRI. MRI may thus replace CT-myelography for preoperative evaluation of posttraumatic progressive myelopathy, whereas patients with radiculopathy may require a detailed myelographic study, including CT (46).

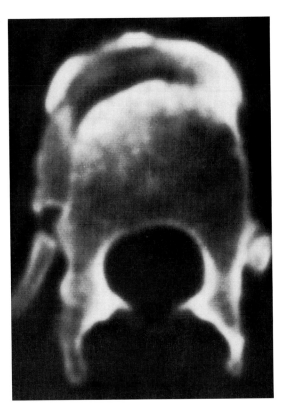

FIG. 63. Old compression fracture of the twelfth vertebra. As this axial CT image shows, the posttraumatic changes are confined to the anterior and right lateral portions of the vertebral body, and there is no evidence of involvement of the posterior elements. The spinal canal is intact.

Thoracolumbar Spine Injury

Traumatic fractures of the upper and middle thoracic spine are less common than fractures at the thoracolumbar junction. Pure hyperflexion injuries causing simple "wedge" fractures due to anterior compression of the vertebral body usually do not lead to permanent neurologic deficits. In hyperflexion injuries combined with increased axial load (vertical compression), more complex spine fractures are common, and permanent neurologic deficit is the rule (80,123). Absence of significant retropulsion of posterior fragments of the vertebral body and absence of a fracture of the vertebral arch ordinarily presage a more favorable prognosis. In the detection of neural-arch fractures, plain radiographs are of limited value because the ribs cause confusing superimpositions. CT is thus clearly superior to conventional radiography for evaluation of patients who have suffered acute trauma to the upper and middle thoracic spine.

Fractures and fracture dislocations of the lower thoracic spine and thoracolumbar junction, particularly at levels T12–L2, are among the most common spine injuries and typically occur as a result of severe hyperflexion. Again, with moderate axial load, i.e., forces developing on the concave side of the flexed spine that tend to compress the

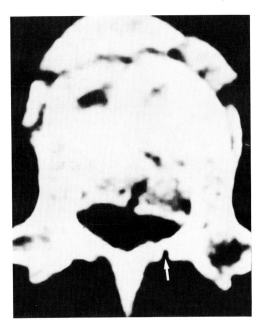

FIG. 64. Burst fracture of the first lumbar vertebra, with centrifugal displacement of fragments. Axial CT image shows, in addition to anterior and lateral displacement of fragments of the vertebral body, retropulsion of fragments, with corresponding narrowing of the spinal canal. There is also a fracture of the left lamina (arrow). Despite the considerable narrowing of the spinal canal, the patient was neurologically intact.

vertebrae, simple wedge fractures of the vertebral bodies result, and the neural arches remain undisturbed. With increased axial load, burst fractures, with centrifugal displacement of fragments, as well as fractures involving posterior vertebral elements, become more likely. Correspondingly, neurologic disturbances are present in about 40% of patients with such injuries. Although plain radiographs generally are more informative at the thoracolumbar junction than in higher parts of the thoracic spine, they markedly underestimate the damage to the spine and soft tissues. Until further experience is gained with MRI in thoracolumbar trauma, CT remains the imaging method of choice (Figs. 63–65), and this technique may have significant influence on patient management (14,54,80). The decision concerning which fractures are stable and which are not, necessitating immobilization and possible internal fixation or fusion, usually can best be made on the basis of CT. Scrutiny of plain anteroposterior and lateral radiographs of the thoracic and lumbar spine remains an integral part of the initial radiologic evaluation of patients with possible thoracolumbar spine injuries. They often provide a fairly detailed picture of the bony damage, but CT displays most trauma features better. However, as in other parts of the spine, recognition of lateral displacement of a vertebra or fragment may be difficult on axial images alone, and therefore image reformatting is needed. This is particularly important if retropulsed fragments encroaching on the spinal canal are to be recognized (27,54,112) (Figs. 64 and 65). The origin

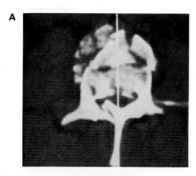

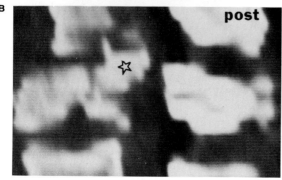

FIG. 65. Burst fracture of the second lumbar vertebra, with encroachment on the spinal cord. **A:** Severe comminution of the body. The size of the spinal canal has been greatly reduced by displacement of fragments into the spinal canal. **B:** Sagittal reformatted image shows marked reduction of the anteroposterior diameter of the spinal canal by a retropulsed fragment (*star*).

of such fragments usually is the posterosuperior portion of the vertebral body, and the most common location of a neural-arch fracture is the lamina just lateral to the midline.

Dislocations of the thoracolumbar facets, with or without associated fractures, usually result from severe deceleration injuries causing distraction of the dorsal elements, with translational shifts of vertebrae; rotational forces may contribute to the damage. If the resultant vector of the traumatic impact passes through the vertebral body, more or less "horizontal" fractures will occur, sometimes extending through the entire vertebra, including the neural arch (Fig. 66). If the vector passes through the disc space, there is disruption of the intervertebral joints, with "splaying" of dorsal elements, in addition to anterior subluxation. Whereas nondisplaced fractures of the former type may be less conspicuous on CT, the appearance of thoracolumbar flexion-distraction injuries, with joint disruption and bilateral facet dislocation, is characteristic in both axial images and sagittal reformations. The most prominent finding on axial images is the "naked" facet; i.e., the inferior facets of the anteriorly displaced superior vertebra are not in direct contact with the superior facets of the lower vertebra (27,47,94) (Fig. 67). Anterior subluxation, with facet "locking," may also occur in thoracolumbar fracture dislocation, but not nearly as often as in the cervical spine. Occasionally, even lateral subluxation with laterally locked facets may be seen. Flexion-distraction injuries with superiorly dislocated facets, resulting in the naked-facet sign, usually are accompanied by acute kyphosis at the level of the injury (94). In radiographically less conspicuous injuries, a detailed evaluation of the relationship between superior and inferior facets is

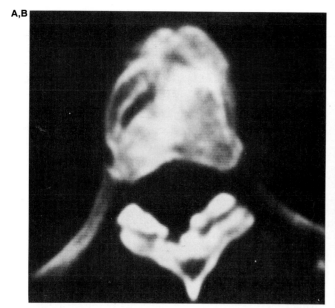

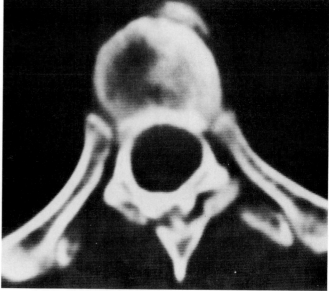

FIG. 66. Chance fracture of a lower thoracic vertebra. **A:** An oblique fracture through the vertebral body is noted on this image. **B:** Four millimeters caudal, a transverse fracture of the neural arch is present.

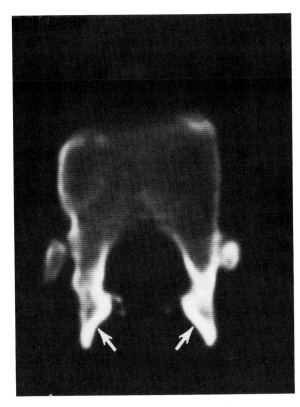

FIG. 67. The naked facet. The superior articular processes of the twelfth thoracic vertebra (*arrows*) are not in contact with any articular process of T11. There has been soft-tissue disruption that caused wide separation of the elements of the posterior articulation.

necessary to detect minor joint abnormalities (subluxation) and facet fractures.

In the absence of detectable fractures after severe spinal trauma, neurologic symptoms and signs usually are the result of an intraspinal hematoma or cord edema (62). Nonenhanced CT may be sufficient to diagnose an intraspinal hematoma, but CT-myelography usually is necessary to diagnose cord swelling (Fig. 68) if MRI is not available. Because MRI is also capable of showing fractures and traumatic deformities of the vertebrae (Figs. 69 and 70), surface-coil studies combined with plain-film radiography will become the primary method of investigation in acute thoracolumbar trauma. CT will still be used to rule out epidural mass effect from acute hematoma (which is poorly shown by MRI) or evaluate fractures with extensive comminution and displacement of fragments. CT will remain the primary modality for evaluation of gunshot injuries and other penetrating trauma (Fig. 71). Chronic cord damage is again best evaluated by MRI (Fig. 70).

Sacral Injury

Most injuries of the sacrum occur in conjunction with severe blunt abdominal trauma resulting in rupture of the pelvic ring. Sacral injuries have been classified as follows: (a) sacroiliac joint diastasis, (b) sacral lip fracture, with avulsion of the most lateral portion of sacrum, (c) vertical shear fracture, with the fracture line passing through the sacral foramina, and (d) comminuted fracture (105). Because these lesions may lead to pelvic instability as well as neurologic disturbances (nerve root compression), and because they are frequently associated with trauma to the

A,B

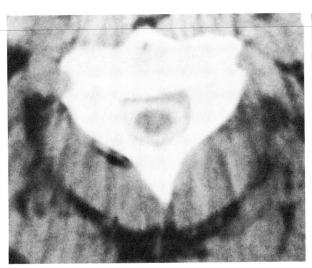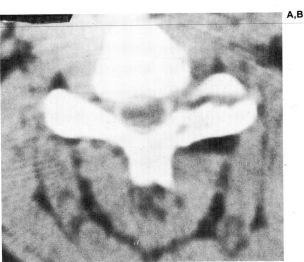

FIG. 68. Traumatic swelling of the cord. CT image of the cervical region after intrathecal injection of metrizamide. **A:** Metrizamide outlines the normal size of the cord at the level of the second cervical vertebra. **B:** At the level of the third cervical vertebra, the contrast material around the cord is reduced because of encroachment on the subarachnoid space by the swollen cord. Note asymmetry in the configuration of the cord due to uneven swelling.

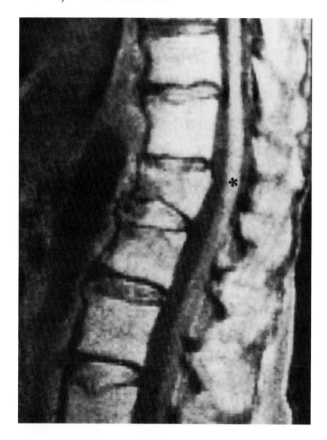

FIG. 69. Compression fracture of the twelfth thoracic vertebra. MRI, midsagittal T1-WI (SE, TR = 500 msec, TE = 15 msec) shows deformity of vertebral body, with mild retropulsion of fragments, but no significant narrowing of the spinal canal and no encroachment on the conus medullaris (*asterisk*).

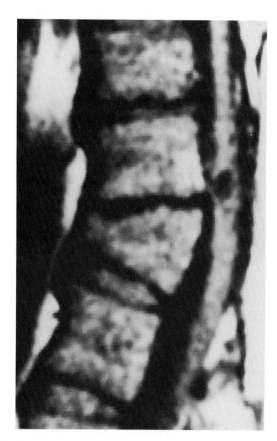

FIG. 70. Compression deformity of the twelfth thoracic vertebral body and posttraumatic intramedullary cavity (syringomyelia). MRI, 0.5 T. T1-WI (SE, TR = 500 msec, TE = 30 msec) reveals cavity to slightly expand the cord.

intrapelvic soft tissues, a detailed radiologic evaluation is very important. Plain-film radiography is known to vastly underestimate both the frequency and degree of sacral injury in pelvic or direct sacral trauma. Moreover, it provides little information regarding the status of the intrapelvic structures. In contradistinction, CT is an excellent means for evaluating simultaneously the sacrum and the intrapelvic organs. Most sacral fractures have a longitudinal (vertical) course, making transaxial views quite satisfactory (Fig. 72). However, in direct trauma to the sacrum, fracture lines may have a transverse (horizontal) course, and then they are easier to detect on sagittal reformatted images or lateral plain films. Theoretically, MRI should be similarly useful in sacral trauma as it is in trauma to the thoracolumbar or cervical spine, and it could be tried first whenever myelography is contemplated to evaluate the status of the dural sac or root sleeves.

MALFORMATIONS OF THE SPINE AND SPINAL CORD

Developmental anomalies of the spinal cord and its surrounding structures range from minor, clinically in-

significant bony abnormalities to major, severely disabling malformations that may involve derivatives of all three germ layers. The term "spinal dysraphism" refers to those disorders that are characterized by an incomplete fusion of midline structures or absence of fusion. For practical reasons, these disorders are described according to their primary abnormalities, but there is considerable overlap between the various entities. Because corrective surgery often is necessary to alleviate symptoms and signs or at least halt the progression of neurologic dysfunction, an exact morphologic analysis of the malformation usually is indispensable. Ultrasonography can be used in newborns and whenever there is an acoustic window providing access to the intraspinal component of the abnormality. In all other cases, conventional radiography and modern imaging techniques such as CT and MRI have to be used.

Role of CT

Most developmental anomalies involving the vertebral column and paraspinal soft tissues, even some of the malformations of the cord and dural sac, can be well demonstrated by nonenhanced high-resolution CT. However,

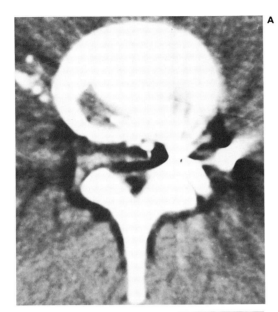

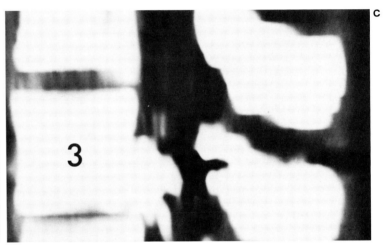

FIG. 71. Gunshot injury of the lumbar spine. A: CT image at the level of the lower end plate of L3 shows missile fragments within the right psoas muscle, disc space, end-plate region, spinal canal, as well as lateral to left neural foramen. B: Image at the level of the L3-L4 interspace reveals fragments anterior in the spinal canal. C: On a mid-sagittal reformatted image it becomes clear that the bulk of the intraspinal missile fragments is at the level of the L3 vertebral body. The dark area posterior to these fragments represents computer artifact. The positions of all these fragments suggest considerable damage to nerve roots and possibly the peripheral nerve L3 on the left. The patient had lower-motor-neuron dysfunction.

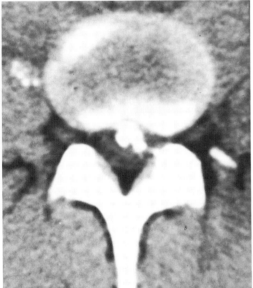

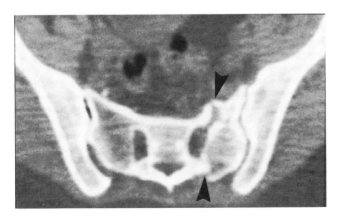

FIG. 72. Fracture of the sacral bone. The fracture line has a vertical (longitudinal) course and involves the sacral foramina on the left (arrows). There is mild posterior displacement of the lateral mass. The sacroiliac joints are intact.

precise definition of the abnormal intraspinal anatomy frequently requires intrathecal administration of a water-soluble contrast material. Myelography with water-soluble contrast material, followed by CT (CT-myelography), is still unsurpassed in its ability to demonstrate nerve root and root sleeve anomalies. In small children, *direct* sagittal CT images providing much better spatial resolution than reformatted images may be obtained to show the extension of lesions in the anteroposterior direction (2).

Role of MRI

MRI depicts bony malformations less well than CT. However, MRI is noninvasive, does not use ionizing radiation, and has direct multiplanar imaging capability and superior soft-tissue contrast. MRI, in conjunction with

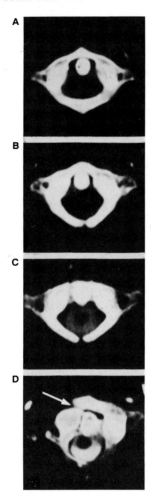

FIG. 73. Anomalies of atlas and axis. **A:** CT at level of anterior atlantoaxial joint shows normal atlas, with well-formed anterior and posterior tubercles. **B:** Atlas with normal anterior arch, but notch instead of tubercle at posterior arch. **C:** True cleft of posterior arch (spina bifida). **D:** Irregular segmentation of atlas and axis, with cleft in anterior arch of atlas (*arrow*). Both **C** and **D** performed after intrathecal contrast administration.

plain-film radiography, may be diagnostically sufficient in many spinal malformations that are sonographically inaccessible. Myelography and CT-myelography are necessary only in cases in which the information provided by MRI is incomplete or equivocal (7). Myelographic techniques may also be preferable if severe kyphoscoliosis accompanies the malformation, although many MRI problems then encountered can be solved by meticulous technique, if necessary, by sectioning in "paraxial" planes. In one report (110) it was possible to completely visualize the spinal cord, including associated abnormalities, in all of 28 scoliosis patients studied with MRI. Thin-section surface-coil imaging with T1-WI usually gives the best result, though head-coil or body-coil imaging with slices thicker than 5 mm may be satisfactory in some cases. T2-WI may be necessary to increase specificity. The optimal section plane or combination of planes depends on the type of lesion suspected. Generally, sagittal images provide

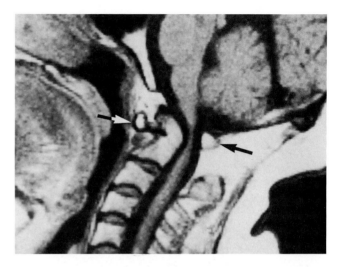

FIG. 74. Os odontoideum and dens hypoplasia causing chronic atlantoaxial subluxation. MRI, 0.5 T. Midsagittal T1-WI (SE, TR = 500 msec, TE = 35 msec) shows marked narrowing of the spinal canal at the level of the atlas (*arrows*). Long-standing cord compression has resulted in severe focal cord atrophy.

the best overview of spine and intraspinal soft tissues and often are obtained first. Supplementary axial images are necessary in many cases to corroborate findings or add information. Coronal images are occasionally helpful, e.g., to evaluate the extent of the cleft of the cord in diastematomyelia.

Malformations of the Craniocervical Junction

Malformations of the occipital skull base, with associated anomalies of the upper cervical spine, may cause neurologic dysfunction by compression or distortion of lower cranial nerves, medulla oblongata, or upper cervical cord. A coexisting Chiari malformation, a fairly common occurrence, compounds the problem. The most accurate definition of the bony features of anomalies such as basilar impression, assimilation of the atlas, os odontoideum, dens hypoplasia and aplasia, atlantoaxial fusion, or irregular segmentation of C1 and C2 probably is still provided by conventional radiography. However, some features, as well as the various congenital defects of the atlas and axis, are better demonstrated by CT (33) (Fig. 73). The relatively wide subarachnoid space surrounding the lower medulla and upper cervical cord permits a limited study of the latter structures by plain CT, but any detailed evaluation, including precise determination of the position of the cerebellar tonsils, requires intrathecal enhancement, i.e., CT-myelography. By comparison, MRI provides excellent delineation of the craniovertebral neural structures together with a satisfactory depiction of the skull base and cervical spine (88) (Fig. 74). Compression or distortion of the brain and cord is easily recognized on sagittal T1-WI, but cranial nerve deformity is not routinely seen. The Chiari I malformation (tonsillar ectopia, Fig. 75), as well

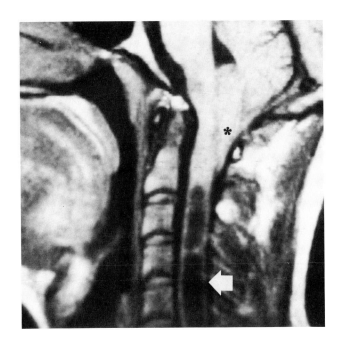

FIG. 75. Chiari type I malformation, with syringohydromyelia of the cervical cord. T1-WI demonstrates the hindbrain anomaly (tonsillar ectopia, *asterisk*) as well as the dark-appearing intramedullary cavity (*arrow*). The appearance of the occipital skull base is unremarkable, and segmentation of the cervical spine is normal. Note mild hydrocephalus secondary to distortion of the neural structures below the fourth ventricle, causing obstruction to CSF flow.

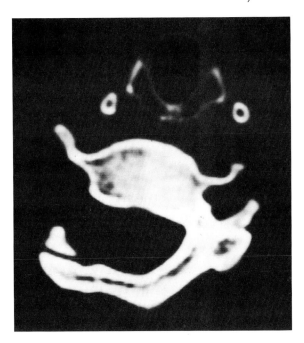

FIG. 76. Congenital absence of the right pedicle of the sixth cervical vertebra. Axial CT image shows the vertebral body to be corticated at the location where the pedicle would normally originate. There is distortion of the right half of the neural arch, which is displaced posteriorly. Adjacent images revealed widening of the neural foramen C6-C7. The appearance of the soft tissue in the region of the anomaly suggests a lateral outpouching of the dural sac, which extends through the bony defect into the paravertebral space. The patient had no neurological symptoms referable to this level.

as the Z-shaped kink of the medullocervical cord junction occurring in Chiari II malformation, can also be identified without difficulty. Bal-I and T1-WI may be necessary to further evaluate associated anomalies of the lower cervical cord and exclude other pathologic processes, e.g., tumors.

Spinal Dysraphism

Anomalies mainly or exclusively involving the vertebral bodies, such as "butterfly" vertebrae, hemivertebrae, and block vertebrae, can be identified with CT and MRI, but are most efficiently demonstrated by plain-film radiography. Anomalies of the neural arch, specifically lateral clefts and partial aplasias, usually can be better evaluated by CT (17,87). This includes congenital or acquired defects in the pars interarticularis (spondylolysis), which are, if present bilaterally, the cause of most nondegenerative cases of spondylolisthesis (145). Congenital absence of a pedicle usually is a unilateral phenomenon, most commonly occurring in the lower cervical spine, particularly at C6. CT, with intravenous contrast material, if necessary, can differentiate between this condition and foraminal widening due to a "dumbbell" tumor (usually neurofibroma) or a vascular anomaly, neoplastic destruction, or

trauma by demonstrating a distorted and posteriorly displaced articular pillar, an abnormal transverse process, an intact cortex at the site of the missing pedicle, and a normal enhancement pattern of the soft tissue in the foramen (Fig. 76). Knowledge of this anomaly can prevent misinterpretation and unnecessary invasive diagnostic procedures such as myelography (28).

In diastematomyelia, the spinal cord is focally divided into two "hemicords," usually by a midline septum or spur arising from the back of a vertebral body. Association with other anomalies of the spine is the rule rather than the exception. The diastomatomyelic cleft is most frequently located below the level of T9, commonly in the lumbar region. In addition, the conus medullaris has an abnormally low position (106). CT findings include the presence of a fibrous or osteocartilaginous septum and splitting of the cord (Fig. 77). Although the usually capacious lumbar subarachnoid space tends to allow identification of these abnormalities on plain CT images, their visualization is greatly enhanced by intrathecal administration of water-soluble contrast material (3). Studies have suggested that MRI may become the method of choice in diastomatomyelia, obviating invasive procedures such as myelography and CT-myelography (57). However,

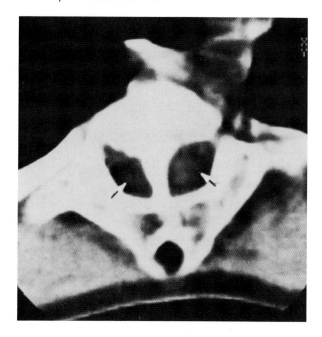

FIG. 77. Diastematomyelia. Plain CT shows the midline osseous spur. The hemicords (*arrows*) can be identified on either side of the spur. (From ref. 64, with permission.)

although the divided cord is well visualized on MR images, plain-film radiography may still be necessary for a detailed evaluation of the associated bony abnormalities. Osteocartilaginous spurs or septa, especially when large, are adequately seen with T1-WI because of the bright signal of their marrow space. Partitions that have a different tissue composition may be better demonstrated using sequences with more T2 weighting. Above and below the abnormality, the spinal cord may appear normal.

Neurenteric cysts are rare malformations belonging to a group of anomalies referred to as the "split-notocord syndrome." These disorders are characterized by various degrees of persistent connection between the intestinal tract and the dorsal skin, passing through the spinal structures (106). Whereas posterior or posterovertebral (dorsal) neurenteric cysts and fistulae usually are detected in the newborn period, the less obvious anterior ones that commonly involve the cervical or upper thoracic region may manifest later in childhood (cord compression). A prevertebral (mediastinal) cyst, a circular defect in the vertebral body containing the fistulous duct, and the local widening of the spinal canal characteristic of these lesions can all be demonstrated by noncontrast CT (59). However, an intraspinal cyst may be indistinguishable from a displaced and distorted cord without use of intrathecal contrast enhancement. As has recently been shown, MRI allows clear delineation of all components of a neurenteric cyst, including its relationship to the spinal cord, obviating the need for invasive procedures in most cases (76).

Congenital dermal sinuses, another rare manifestation of spinal dysraphism, are characterized by a small fistulous

tract that in full-blown cases extends from the skin into the spinal canal (128). Dermal sinuses are most common in the lumbosacral region, but may be encountered at higher levels. Usually there is some degree of posterior spina bifida at the level of the fistulous tract. The tract tends to have a slightly superior course from the dimple toward the spinal canal. Because of the danger of meningeal infection, early diagnosis is important. Physical examination will reveal a small midline dimple that may discharge CSF. CT-myelography can be used to confirm or exclude a communication between the subarachnoid space and the skin. At the same time, it helps by showing the full extent of the abnormality and its relationship to surrounding muscles, vertebrae, dura, subarachnoid space, and spinal cord or cauda equina (128). MRI is similarly helpful, although it may not assist in establishing the presence or absence of a communication between the skin and neural structures. Associated hamartomatous masses, such as dermoid and epidermoid cysts, have a fairly characteristic appearance on both CT and MRI, with fat often being the most conspicuous tissue element.

In the tethered-cord or tight-filum-terminale syndrome, the conus medullaris is abnormally low in position, abuts the posterior wall of the lower lumbosacral spine, and continues into a particularly thick (greater than 2 mm) filum terminale. As a result of the low position of the conus, the lumbar and sacral nerve roots course more horizontally instead of obliquely through the subarachnoid space. Symptoms and signs such as progressive lower motor neuron dysfunction, sensory disturbances, and sphincter disturbances are presumed to be due to stretching of the cord. The disorder usually manifests in childhood, but may remain asymptomatic or relatively asymptomatic until adulthood. A tethered cord may be associated with the Chiari I malformation, and bony abnormalities (spina bifida occulta) of the lumbosacral spine are common. On plain CT images, the abnormal cord is readily seen, but the root abnormalities and the exact level of transition between conus and filum usually are less evident. This limitation of CT may be overcome by intrathecal enhancement, although the overall best information is afforded by a combination of conventional myelography followed by CT (Fig. 78); for sensitivity, MRI compares favorably with this technique (1,7) (Fig. 79). Sagittal T1-WI provide the most efficient way of verifying a normal position of the conus medullaris or delineating an abnormally low conus. Occasionally, however, volume averaging of the cauda equina makes it difficult to determine exactly where the conus ends. In such cases, additional coronal images may be warranted. Although a reduced diameter of the cord is most easily recognized on axial CT-myelographic images, cord "atrophy" can be seen on sagittal MRI as well. After surgical "untethering," the cord may become visibly thicker.

Congenital herniations of intraspinal soft tissues through defects in the spinal column are called menin-

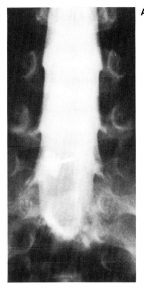

A

FIG. 78. "Tethered cord" associated with a lipoma. A: Metrizamide myelogram shows a defect in the lower end of the dural sac. The exact location of the cord cannot be determined. B–E: Postmyelography CT. B: At the L3 level, the conus medullaris is visible. C: The tip of the conus is seen at the level of the lower disc plate of L3, with several nerve roots around it. D: A lipoma, which has a much lower density than the conus, is present in the subarachnoid space, below the tip of the conus, lying among the roots of the cauda equina. E: The bulk of the lipoma lies at the level of the sacral segments.

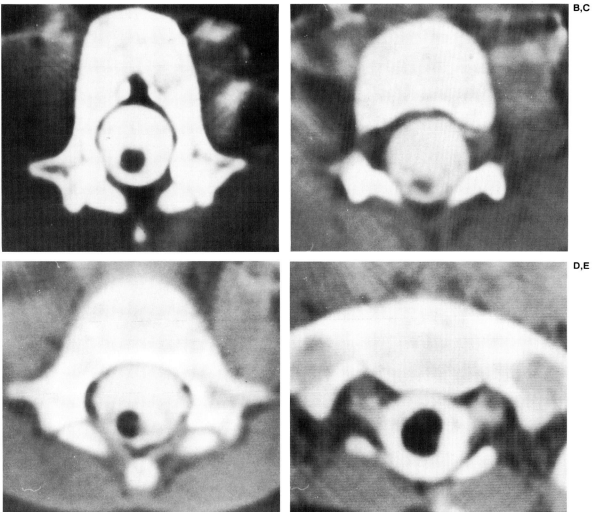

B,C

D,E

goceles when the protruding sac contains only CSF and its walls are formed by the meninges. When portions of malformed spinal cord are included in the herniation, the abnormality is called a myelomeningocele. In lipomyelomeningoceles, accumulations of fatty tissue are asso-

ciated with the malformation, usually forming an amorphous mass at the posterior aspect of the distorted part of the cord (placode), and often extending into the subcutaneous fat. Meningoceles are most common in the lumbosacral region, but also occur in the upper cervical

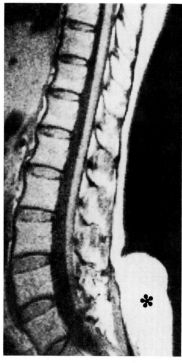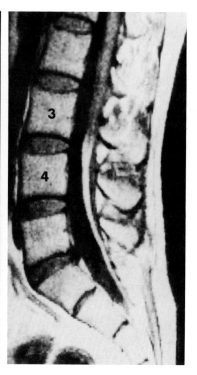

FIG. 79. "Tethered cord" associated with lipomas. MRI, 0.5 T. **A:** Midsagittal T1-WI (SE, TR = 500 msec, TE = 30 msec) demonstrates abnormally low position of lumbosacral spinal cord. The cord abuts the posterior aspect of the spinal canal. On multiple parasagittal sections it appeared to extend to the level of at least L5. Note that the lumbosacral sac is unusually wide. A subcutaneous lipoma, apparently without connection to the spinal structures, is noted at the same level (*asterisk*). **B:** In another patient, sagittal T1-WI (SE, TR = 500 msec, TE = 30 msec) shows an abnormal position of the conus medullaris, which at the level of L3-L4 continues into a lipomatous structure. This intradural formation adheres to the posterior wall of the lumbosacral spinal canal and extends inferiorly to at least the level of S2. Again, the lumbosacral dural sac is unusually wide. The posterior spinal and subcutaneous structures are unremarkable.

region. Lateral meningoceles, a form of dural ectasia, may be seen in neurofibromatosis, usually at thoracic levels. Occasionally an anterior sacral meningocele will present as a pelvic mass (5) (Fig. 80). As mentioned earlier, sonography is an effective screening method for infants suspected of having spinal dysraphism. Normal findings on examination usually will obviate more expensive and invasive procedures, but abnormal findings often imply the need for further investigation (73). Although MRI allows better tissue differentiation and can be used to determine the presence or absence of additional hind-brain anomalies (Chiari II) and cord anomalies (hydromyelia), plain CT is superior for demonstration of the bony abnormalities associated with meningoceles and meningomyelo-

celes. Although CT-myelography provides the most detailed information about the intradural structures (7), improvements in MRI technology may modify the diagnostic approach. Meningoceles may or may not be associated with cord tethering. In the lipomyelomeningoceles, the herniated tissue forms a dorsal subcutaneous mass composed of fat, fibrous tissue, neural tissue, and protruding meninges (106,147) (Fig. 81). The rare intradural lipomas predominantly involve the cervical and thoracic region and may be intramedullary or extramedullary in location; dysraphic abnormalities of the spine may be minimal or absent. In these less complex lesions, the ideal technique to demonstrate the relationship between abnormal tissue and spinal cord or cauda equina is MRI.

Syringohydromyelia

Hydromyelia is a developmental anomaly of the spinal cord characterized by abnormal distension of the central canal. It is usually, although not invariably, associated with a Chiari I malformation (Fig. 76). Syringomyelia represents formation of intramedullary cavities that are primarily independent of the central canal. In some cases the cause of syringomyelia is not known; in others the abnormality is associated with and presumably caused by intramedullary or intradural-extramedullary mass lesions, or it may have developed after a trauma (Figs. 62 and 71). Because the two conditions, hydromyelia and syringomyelia, may be difficult to differentiate even at autopsy (67), the name syringohydromyelia is commonly used to encompass both. In developmental syringohydromyelia, the cord typically is expanded over many segments, whereas in tumor-related and posttraumatic cavitations,

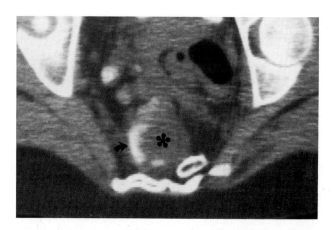

FIG. 80. Anterior sacral meningocele. Axial CT image following lumbar myelography with water-soluble contrast material shows deformity of the lower portion of the sacrum, with partial filling of a roundish, presacral soft-tissue mass (*asterisk*) with contrast (*arrow*).

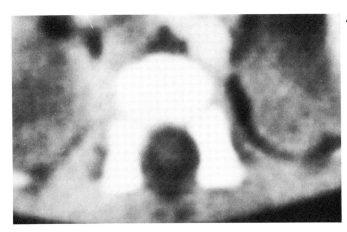

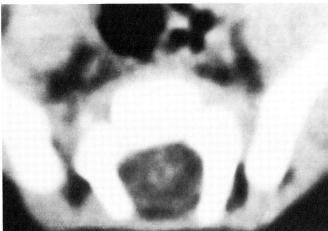

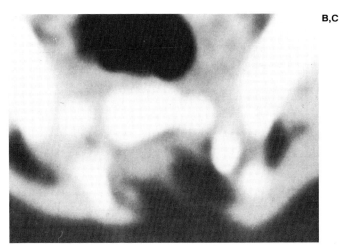

FIG. 81. Lipomeningocele with "tethered cord." **A,B:** The tethered cord is surrounded by CSF and demonstrated on plain CT at the level of L3 and S1. There are defects in the neural arch at both levels. **C:** A larger defect in the neural arch is seen at the level of the upper sacral segments. A lipoma fills the spinal canal at this level.

abnormal changes tend to be more localized. There may be widening of the spinal canal due to chronic pressure erosion, most commonly in the cervical region. Flattening and atrophy of the cord, rather than expansion, may be present in cases in which the cavity has become decompressed through a spontaneously occurring or surgically created communication with the subarachnoid space. Al-

though plain CT is capable of showing the abnormality without the use of intrathecal enhancement, especially if the cervical cord is involved (11) (Fig. 82), it is not sufficiently reliable (4). In fact, below the cervical region, plain CT is rarely useful. Opacification of the CSF-containing intramedullary cavity may occur shortly after intrathecal introduction of water-soluble contrast material

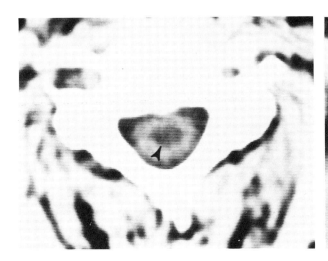

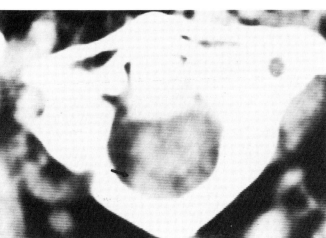

FIG. 82. Syringohydromyelia with associated Chiari type I malformation. **A:** At the C2 level, an enlarged cord is seen surrounded by CSF. There is a central low-density area within the cord (*arrowhead*) representing cord cavitation. **B:** At the C1 level, the cerebellar tonsils (*arrow*) are seen behind the cord.

A,B

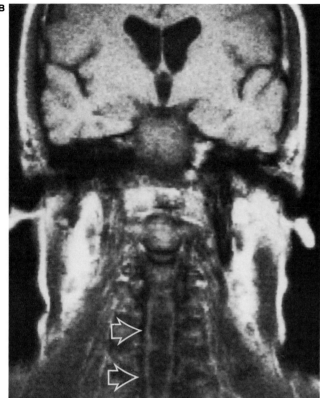

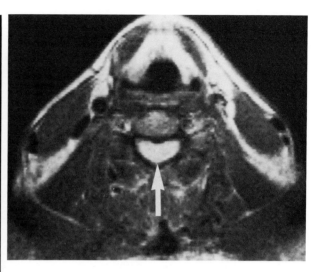

FIG. 83. Syringohydromyelia. **A:** MRI, 0.5 T. Coronal T1-WI (SE, TR = 500 msec, TE = 30 msec) shows a partially septated cord cavitation at lower cervical levels (*arrows*). **B:** T2-WI (SE, TR = 1,500 msec, TE = 120 msec) demonstrates reversal of signal intensity of fluid inside the syrinx from low (**A**) to high (**B**, *arrows*).

via rents in the cord or via the fourth ventricle, but in most cases only delayed CT images obtained later (4–8 hr or more) will show this effect. Intrathecal enhancement is also necessary for reliable demonstration of the presence or absence of a Chiari malformation by CT.

Meanwhile, MRI has become the screening method of choice for suspected syringohydromyelia, obviating CT-myelography in most cases (90,116,126,132) (Figs. 75 and 83). Although the diagnosis is usually easy, occasional difficulties may be encountered (116,132). Sagittal T1-WI should be obtained first, because they provide excellent morphologic information; axial T1-WI may be necessary if cord cavitation is doubtful. The presence of a Chiari I malformation usually is indicative of hydromyelia, but does not preclude a tumor as the cause of the intramedullary cavitation (132). T2-WI may lend more specificity to the diagnosis and help differentiate true hydromyelia from the syringomyelia associated with tumors (by showing absence of soft tissue with abnormal signal). Increased

signal intensity of the cord adjacent to or above or below an intramedullary cavity may, however, be seen in both developmental and neoplastic syringomyelia. Cord biopsy of these areas in patients with proven developmental syringomyelia has revealed gliosis (132). In tumors, the areas of increased signal represent either parenchymal infiltration by abnormal cells or tumor-induced perifocal edema. In such cases, differentiation between nonneoplastic and neoplastic cord cavitation largely depends on history and clinical findings, though careful attention to the anatomic characteristics of the lesion may also help. In contrast to what one might expect, the CSF-like fluid within the intramedullary cavities often remains low in signal intensity on T2-WI. This phenomenon is more common in developmental syringohydromyelia than in posttraumatic or tumor-related cavities. It is believed to be analogous to the flow-void sign associated with pulsatile turbulent or jet-stream-like movements of CSF within the intracranial cavity (132).

TABLE 1. *Primary intraspinal tumors*

Anatomic compartment	Tissue or cell	Tumor
Intramedullary	Glial	Astrocytoma, ependymoma
	Neuron	Neuroblastoma, ganglioma
	Sheath of Schwann	Neurilemmoma, neurofibroma
	Vascular	Hemangioblastoma, angioma
	Ectopic	Neurenteric cyst
		Lipoma
		Epidermoid, dermoid, teratoma
Intradural extramedullary	Arachnoid-dura	Meningioma (Arachnoid cyst)
	Sheath of Schwann	Neurilemoma neurofibroma
	Filum terminale	Glioma
	Vascular	Hemangioblastoma, angioma
		Epidermoid, dermoid, teratoma
		Lipoma
		Neurenteric cyst
Extradural intraspinal	Fibrous	Sarcoma, Fibroma
	Vascular	Hemangioblastoma
	Lymphoid	Lymphoma, chloroma
	Adipose	Lipoma, liposarcoma
	Nerve root	Neurofibroma, schwannoma
		Neuroblastoma
		Paraganglioma
		Bone and cartilage
	Ectopic	Neurenteric cyst
		Ependymoma
		Chordoma
		Chondroma, chondrosarcoma
		Osteoblastoma, etc.

INTRASPINAL TUMORS

Intraspinal disorders classically are divided into three groups according to the anatomic compartments they occupy (extradural, intradural-extramedullary, and intramedullary). The tissues within each compartment determine the type of neoplasm or other abnormality that can originate within it (Table 1). Tumors that invade the spinal canal, as well as metastases, are true neoplasms that occur within the canal but do not originate there and therefore are not determined by the tissues native to the canal. Some tumors and abnormalities, though not acting as masses to deform the normal anatomic components of the canal, nevertheless are recognizable by CT or MRI.

Role of CT

Most intraspinal tumors have X-ray attenuation values not notably different from those for the spinal cord, nerve roots, meninges, or the combined effect of the cauda equina and its surrounding CSF bath (Fig. 84). Numerical

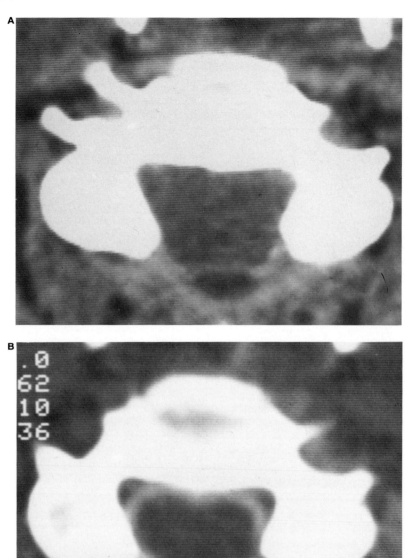

FIG. 84. Recurrent astrocytoma. **A:** The entire spinal canal is filled with a homogeneous soft tissue mass. Neither the spinal cord nor the subarachnoid space can be distinguished from the tumor mass. **B:** After the administration of metrizamide. CT scan demonstrates marked narrowing of the subarachnoid space by the tumor.

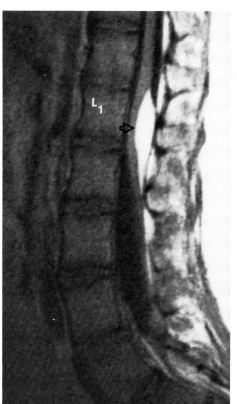

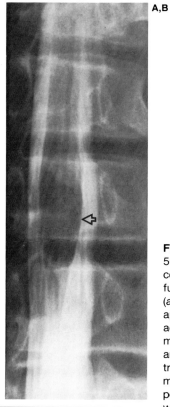

A,B

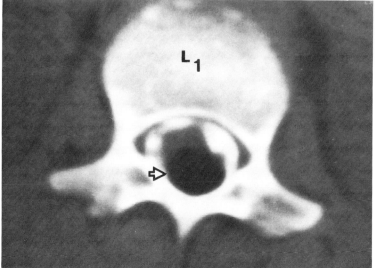

C

FIG. 85. Lipoma. **A:** MRI, 0.5 T. T1-WI (SE, TR = 500 msec, TE = 17 msec). The lower cord and conus are outlined by the low signal of CSF. The fusiform lipoma is bright with high signal intensity (*arrow*), similar to epidural and subcutaneous fat. It appears that the lipoma is intramedullary, although actually it is extramedullary, but beneath the pia mater, and blends with the contour of the conus and cord. **B:** Myelography shows an apparent intramedullary conus mass. The low density of fat might be suspected, but is easily confused with superimposed shadows. **C:** CT after myelography with water-soluble contrast material shows the displaced and deformed cord (*arrow*), as well as the low-density (−120 HU) lipoma.

determinations of attenuation (Hounsfield units, HU) are of limited additional value because of statistical variation and artifactual alteration. They are of use to confirm gross differences, as between fat, CSF, and gas, when simple inspection is not convincing. A few tumors are of visibly lower or higher density: Lipoma is significantly lower (Fig. 85); meningioma containing calcium may be higher (Fig. 86); tumors containing or associated with cystic cavities may be lower in density than the cord. Simple syrinx usually is recognizable (Fig. 87). Neurilemmoma or neuro-

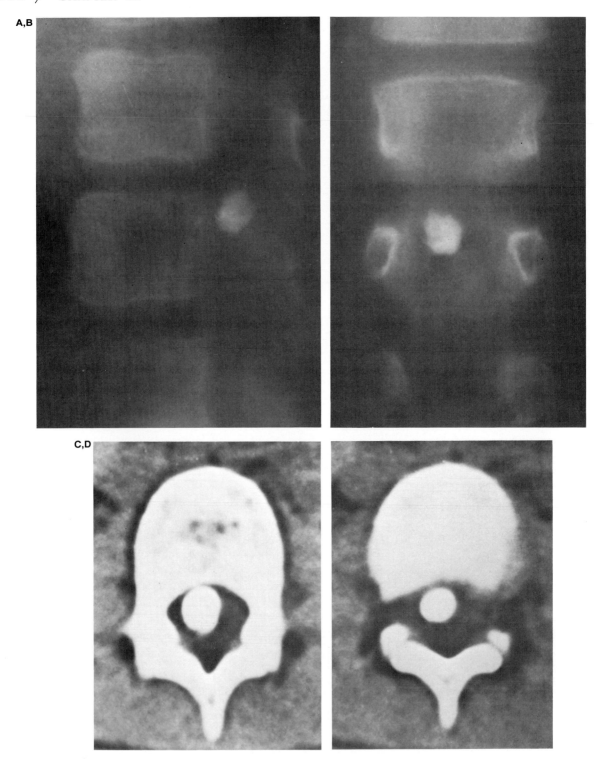

FIG. 86. Meningioma. Dense calcification is shown within the spinal canal by AP and lateral tomograms (**A,B**) and also by the transverse CT images (**C,D**) in a 10-year-old girl. At operation, an intradural meningioma was removed from within the filaments of the cauda equina.

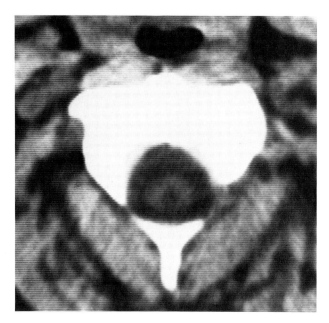

FIG. 87. Syrinx. A low-density (the same as CSF) cavity is seen in the center of the normal-diameter cervical cord at C2.

fibroma within the intervertebral canal or spinal canal may have a slightly higher density than the CSF and the cauda-equina-filled lumbar subarachnoid canal (Fig. 88). Secondary changes in bone are important features in detection and identification of various intraspinal masses (Fig. 89). Intraspinal fat is an important natural contrast agent, particularly in the lumbar region and in lipoma. Myelography and postmyelography CT provide the best outlining of the subarachnoid fluid compartment and those structures within it or deforming it (Figs. 84 and 90–92). Communication within the subarachnoid canal or between various compartments can be studied reliably only in this way, and real-time phenomena such as tumor

movement (30), pulsation, and flow patterns, although seldom clinically important, are detectable only by myelography under fluoroscopic control. Intravenous contrast material, contrary to its tremendous value for intracranial CT, has limited usefulness for intraspinal CT, although one group noted enhancement in 18 of 23 intraspinal tumors (85). Certain hypervascular lesions, such as arteriovenous malformations and hemangioblastoma (Fig. 93), as well as some other tumors and conditions, may undergo selective enhancement. Intravenous contrast material, by enhancing vascularized structures such as dura, arachnoid, and blood vessels, but not avascular tissues such as intervertebral disc, fat, and CSF, may provide improved anatomic separation, but intravenous contrast material is not regularly used when intraspinal tumor is suspected.

Role of MRI

Since 1983, MRI has rapidly become the clear choice for the initial screening examination in suspected intraspinal tumor. Its relatively high cost usually is equal to that of detailed CT, but much less than the combined cost of hospitalization and myelography. It is not available everywhere and may be contraindicated or impossible in some circumstances.

The use of MRI to survey or screen the entire spine for suspected tumor necessitates using short time sequences and limited plane selections. Fortunately, restricted portions usually can be preselected on the basis of clinical findings, plain radiographs, or radionuclide bone scintigraphy. With this limitation, MRI, without the need for intrathecal invasion, with its markedly increased ability to display tissue differences, and its easy selection of tomographic-plane orientation, is the first choice for diag-

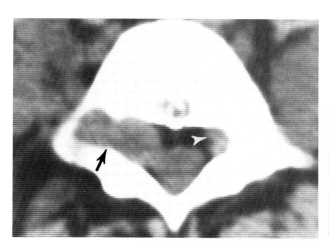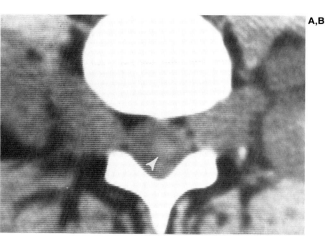

A,B

FIG. 88. Neurofibromatosis. Image at the L5-S1 level in a 13-year-old boy demonstrates multiple intraspinal and paraspinal tumors. The large tumor on the right has resulted in a markedly enlarged intervertebral foramen (*arrow*). A smaller lesion fills the left lateral recess (*arrowhead*). At the L4-L5 level, large tumors fill the foramina bilaterally. In addition, an intradural lesion is also seen (*arrowhead*), outlined by CSF.

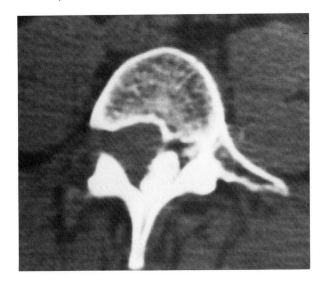

FIG. 89. Fibrolipoma. A homogeneous low-density extradural mass markedly deforms the metrizamide-filled canal and accounts for smooth focal excavation along the right posterior surface of L4. The smooth bony deformity, with a cortical margin that appears normal, usually implies a slow-growing lesion of benign nature.

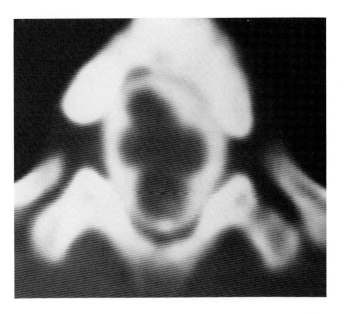

FIG. 90. Neurenteric cyst. The metrizamide-outlined cord is shaped like a four-leaf clover in the high dorsal region of a 2-year-old boy. The attenuation values were the same for all four lobes. At the time of surgery, the posterior and anterior lobes were composed of a large, thin-walled cyst, filled with jelly-like contents, covered by the pia mater of the cord (therefore intramedullary), splitting the spinal cord, represented by the two lateral lobules.

A,B

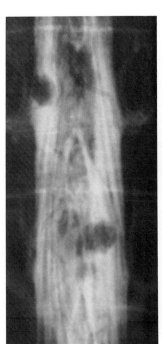 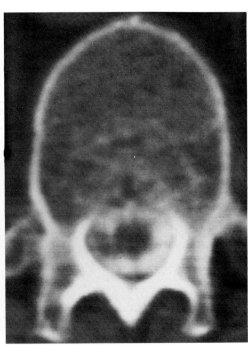

FIG. 91. Metastatic melanoma to the roots of the cauda equina. These multiple nodular lesions shown by the metrizamide lumbar myelogram are also recognized on the transerve CT examination.

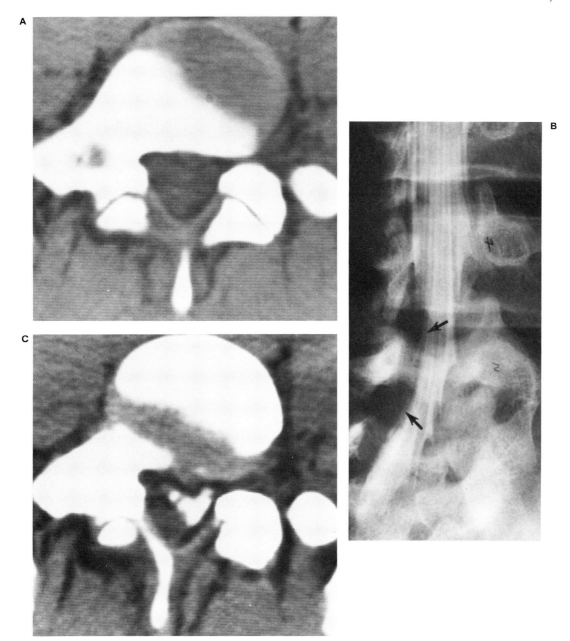

FIG. 92. Epidural abscess in a 12-year-old boy with back pain, 1 month after treatment for an abdominal infection. **A:** Plain Ct study was prospectively interpreted as normal. In retrospect, blurring of the epidural fat can be seen on the right side, presumably due to infiltration of the fat by inflammatory cells. No diagnosis was made. **B:** Metrizamide myelogram shows a posterolateral extradural defect on the right (*arrows*). **C:** Postmyelogram CT through the level of the myelographic abnormality demonstrates a soft-tissue mass deviating the contrast-filled subarachnoid space to the left. An extradural abscess was drained surgically.

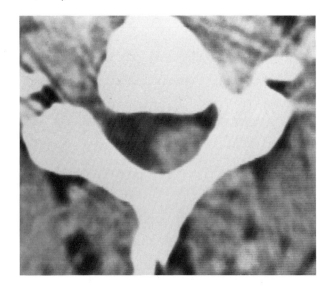

FIG. 93. Hemangioblastoma. The cord itself at the C3 level is not seen in this image after intravenous contrast injection. An eccentric intramedullary hemangioblastoma is readily shown.

nostic evaluation of suspected intraspinal tumor, if not contraindicated, technically impossible, or unavailable. CT may still be necessary when bone abnormality affecting intraspinal structures is suspected but is not adequately shown by MRI. The rare need to employ CT and intravenous contrast material will likely be supplanted by the availability and use of gadolinium as an intravenous contrast agent with MRI. Myelography may still be the logical choice in the search for metastatic seeding, multiple neurofibromas, arachnoiditis, or vascular malformation.

Role of Angiography

Angiography remains the definitive examination for demonstrating the blood vessels in vascular malformation and perhaps other lesions, but only after these have been diagnosed or suggested by MRI, CT, or myelography. Also, MRI may be the only conclusive way to demonstrate the intramedullary location of the nidus of an arteriovenous malformation (31).

A real, but unlikely, source of difficulty and potential for serious oversight is the presence of extensive neoplasm completely filling the canal. Diffuse tumor, such as ependymoma, astrocytoma, or sarcoma, filling the lumbar canal may be completely unrecognizable because of a lack of contrasting CT densities. Tumor filling the canal may be unrecognizable by MRI as well. Overall density within the canal on CT will be slight, and there is no readily available way to assess diffuse MR signal in an absolute sense. It is likely that the use of gadolinium with MRI will greatly reduce or eliminate this problem. Myelography usually will clarify the situation, but it can be frustrating and complicated.

Intramedullary Tumors

Neoplasm and assorted other intramedullary lesions usually result in enlargement of the spinal cord, whereas atrophy and collapsed cavities lead to reduction in cord size. Some abnormalities, such as multiple sclerosis, syrinx, and myelomalacia, can be detected even when the cord is neither enlarged nor shrunken, because of differences in density, enhancement, or signal intensity (51).

The adult spinal cord is only slightly variable in its anteroposterior diameter from foramen magnum to conus medullaris, measuring 7 to 9 mm. Its transverse diameter, on the other hand, varies from 8 to 12 mm at the level of C1 to a maximum width at C5-C6 of 12 to 15 mm. It then narrows to about 9 mm at C7 and reaches a minimum in the middle or lower thoracic region. At the level of the conus medullaris, it again widens in a bulbous fashion at T11-T12 before narrowing abruptly to form the filum terminale at L1-L2, which continues caudally in the midline as a 1- to 2-mm structure to the end of the canal in the upper sacrum.

These measurements are derived from CT and MR images, but cannot be used as absolute indicators of enlargement or narrowing. Actual measurements are affected by slice orientation and the window center of the image (121,130). Fortunately, most tumors produce focal or obvious enlargement. When the cord is deformed by extrinsic pressure, as, for example, by an osteophyte or an extramedullary mass, it is difficult to assess size by diameters, and cross-sectional area measurements are seldom employed (35,155).

In order to assess cord size, it is necessary to visualize it separate from the other contents of the spinal canal. In the upper cervical region, and to a varying extent in the thoracic region, the cord can be recognized by plain CT because of the surrounding CSF. When CSF is not reliably depicted, it can be made clearly visible by subarachnoid injection of a water-soluble contrast agent. MRI circumvents that limitation and also provides the more informative sagittal plane (lateral view). Images in axial and coronal planes are easily obtained, though limited by time. The most desirable examination for suspected cord tumor, therefore, is MRI, specifically the midline sagittal view.

In addition to enlarging the cord, some tumors and most cavities are sufficiently different in density to be shown on CT, such as lipoma (152), syrinx, and calcified lesions. Intrathecal water-soluble contrast material may intensify intramedullary cavities (4,74), and intravenous contrast material will enhance some tumors and vascular lesions (85). However, MRI, even without added contrast agent, will show most tumors and cystic cavities (90).

The most common intramedullary tumors are astrocytoma and ependymoma (Fig. 94). Oligodendroglioma and glioblastoma multiforme are uncommon. Hemangioblastomas are also rare except in patients with a family history of these tumors or established von Hippel-Lindau

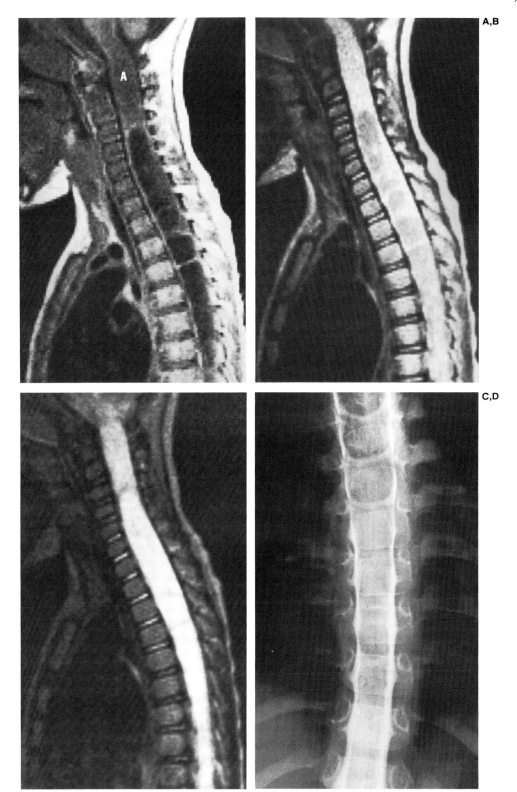

FIG. 94. Astrocytoma, cystic and solid. **A–C:** MRI, 0.5 T. **D:** Myelogram. **A:** T1-WI (SE, TR = 500 msec, TE = 17 msec) shows multiloculated syrinx of the cervicothoracic cord C3-T12, but the curved spinal canal bends out of the MRI plane in the region of T6. The cord and medulla appear enlarged (**A**) and of slightly lower signal than the pons and cerebellar tonsil. **B:** Balanced image (SE, TR = 1,500 msec, TE = 35 msec). The cystic portion is less obvious, and the difference between tumor and normal pons and cerebellum is inapparent. **C:** T2-WI (SE, TR = 1,500 msec, TE = 120 msec). Both tumor and syrinx (cyst) are of increased signal, apparently higher than CSF, although the swollen cord has replaced CSF in the canal. **D:** Myelogram shows swollen cord extending to T11 and the curvature that precluded a midsagittal section of the entire tumor.

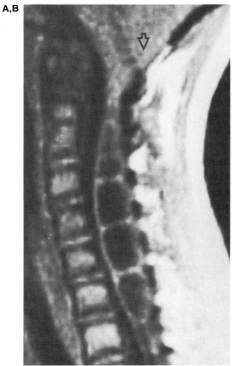
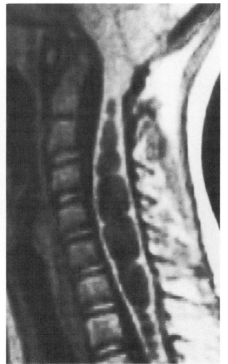

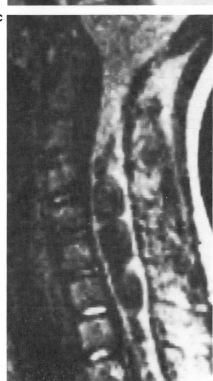

FIG. 95. Syrinx and Arnold-Chiari malformation. MRI, 0.5 T. **A:** T1-WI (SE, TR = 700 msec, TE = 15 msec). Multilobulated cavities are shown, but the spine is slightly oblique to the MRI plane, causing the upper and lower regions to the paramidline. One cerebellar tonsil is well shown below the plane of the foramen magnum (*open arrow*). The lower extent of the syrinx was shown on adjacent slices. **B:** Bal-I (SE, TR = 1,500 msec, TE = 35 msec). The syrinx is of low signal intensity. **C:** T2-WI (SE, TR = 1,500 msec, TE = 120 msec). They syrinx remains dark (i.e., has low signal intensity), apparently because of CSF pulsation (nongated image), although CSF surrounding the cord at C2 is essentially isointense with parenchyma. Simple syrinx tends to display this paradoxic signal, whereas tumor cysts are more likely to have high signal intensity on T2-WI.

disease. All of these tumors may be associated with cysts or syrinx formation, and the differentiation between simple syrinx or hydromyelia and neoplasm associated with cyst is sometimes impossible (90,125,132). Primary intramedullary tumor commonly cannot be differentiated from surrounding or adjacent spinal cord by CT and, in fact, may be difficult or impossible to differentiate from cystic fluid. Intravenous and intrathecal contrast material may provide differentiation, but MRI usually is better

and more direct. Tumor usually has a higher signal intensity than normal cord on T2-WI, and a similar signal intensity on T1-WI.

A syrinx should have signal intensities similar to or identical with those for CSF. Transmitted cardiac pulsation and respiratory movement, however, frequently result in flow or motion void in the syrinx and a low signal on T2-WI (Fig. 95). This paradoxical appearance is largely eliminated by the use of motion-compensating measures,

A–C

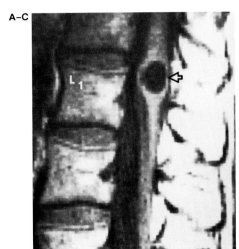
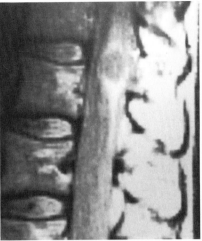
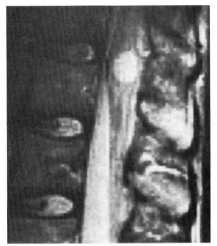

D

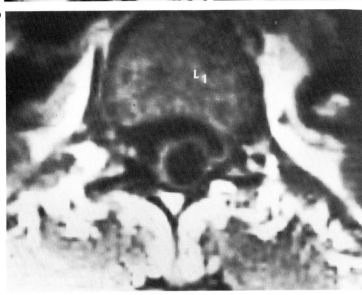

FIG. 96. Simple cyst, presumably posttraumatic. MRI, 1.5 T, performed for clinically suspected herniated disk. **A:** T1-WI (SE, TR = 500 msec, TE = 17 msec) discloses an intraconal cyst (*open arrow*), with signal intensity similar to that of CSF. **B:** Bal-I (SE, TR = 1,900 msec, TE = 28 msec) shows the cyst and no evidence of midline disk protrusion. **C:** T2-WI (SE, TR = 1,900 msec, TE = 70 msec) demonstrates the cyst in the conus to have signal characteristics identical with those of CSF, without any adjacent tumor. **D:** Axial T1-WI (SE, TR = 500 msec, TE = 17 msec) shows the intramedullary cyst.

such as cardiac gating and gradient refocusing. Very short sequences utilizing narrow flip angles also reduce the effects of CSF motion. Cysts associated with tumor and small, simple, or benign cavities usually do not exhibit the effects of motion, probably because of the noncompliant nature of the tumor or more abundant surrounding cord tissue. In the search for syrinx or cyst, it is unnecessary to resort to delayed CT imaging after intrathecal contrast injection unless MRI cannot be accomplished. CT may, however, be useful in distinguishing between communicating and noncommunicating syrinx and in assessing the effect of surgical treatment for syrinx. Recently, attention has been drawn to posttraumatic or compressive cystic degeneration of the cord (69,119) (Fig. 96). We observed one case in which a nonspecific intramedullary conus cyst was drained elsewhere, resulting in atrophy of the conus, and another case of a simple-appearing "cyst" in the conus by MRI (Fig. 96) not yet operated on. Both of these cases are thought to be the result of prior trauma. Other causes of cyst-like intramedullary lesions are distinctly uncommon, at least in North Amer-

ica. They include neurenteric cysts (84) (Fig. 24), dermoid or teratoma cyst, and parasitic cyst (91,109).

The mass effect of tumor generally is easily detectable on mid-sagittal MRI using T1-WI, but less reliably by CT, except in the upper cervical region or when the cord is surrounded by an adequate amount of CSF.

Lipoma is relatively uncommon, but is readily demonstrated by CT, and even more convincingly by MRI (Fig. 85). Although lipoma appears to be and is classified as an intramedullary tumor, it usually is subpial in location and characteristically is located on the posterior aspect of the cord (71). By CT, lipoma is clearly demarcated and is of lower density than cord (−30 to −120 HU) (Fig. 85). With MRI, only fat and subacute or chronic blood-containing lesions are known to produce such high signal intensity on T1-WI of the spine. Subacute or chronic blood collection also results in very high signal on T2-WI (Fig. 97), but fat is isointense with cord on T2-WI (50,71). Subpial lipoma of the cord ordinarily is not associated with tethering of the cord or a dysraphic state.

Sporadic and unusual intramedullary lesions include

A,B

C,D

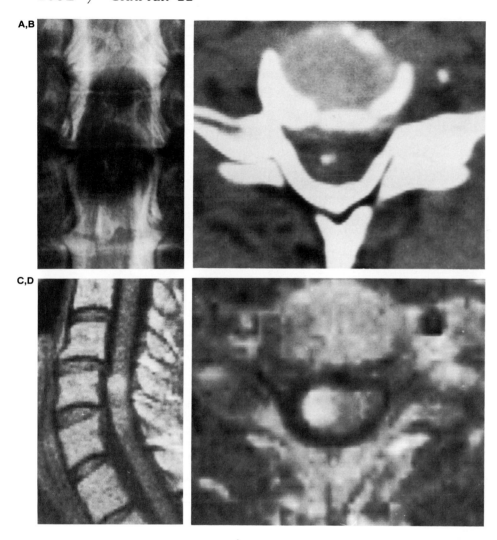

FIG. 97. Hematoma of the spinal cord. **A:** Cervical myelogram shows focal intramedullary swelling (lateral view excluded a prolapsed disc). **B:** CT before myelogram shows a high-density focus within the cord, compatible with a recent blood clot. **C:** MRI, 0.5 T. T1-WI (SE, TR = 300 msec, TE = 30 msec) demonstrates the intramedullary lesion to have elevated signal intensity and focal cord enlargement. There is some extradural abnormality in front of the cord at this level, but no clear-cut disc protrusion. **D:** Axial T1-WI (SE, TR = 300 msec, TE = 30 msec) confirms a high-signal-intensity intramedullary lesion on the right side.

intramedullary neurilemmoma (154), ganglioneuroma, sarcoid (6,133) and other granulomas, primary melanoma, and metastatic tumor (86,104) (Fig. 98). These lesions cannot be distinguished from one another on CT or MRI. Trauma (contusion) and transverse myelitis presumably due to infarct or virus can cause focal enlargement of the cord, and multiple sclerosis involving the spinal cord may cause swelling and simulate tumor (Fig. 99).

Intramedullary metastatic neoplasm is quite uncommon, but should be considered when primary neoplasm elsewhere is present, including the central nervous system (8,127). The appearance of primary neoplasm is similar to that of metastasis by MRI or CT.

Calcification and blood vessels usually produce a signal void (blackening) on MRI. Calcification is most reliably detected by CT. Larger vessels can be seen on MRI, for example, in highly vascular neoplasm or vascular malformations. They can also be seen on CT, but are nonspecific (Fig. 100).

The vascular malformations or hamartomas may involve any or all of the intraspinal compartments. When they are on the surface of the cord or within it, they are best considered as intramedullary lesions. They can be

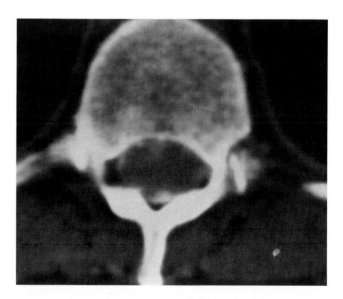

FIG. 98. Intramedullary metastasis from bronchogenic carcinoma. The cord in the conus region is markedly enlarged, and metrizamide is barely visible surrounding it. There was a total block by myelography.

A–C

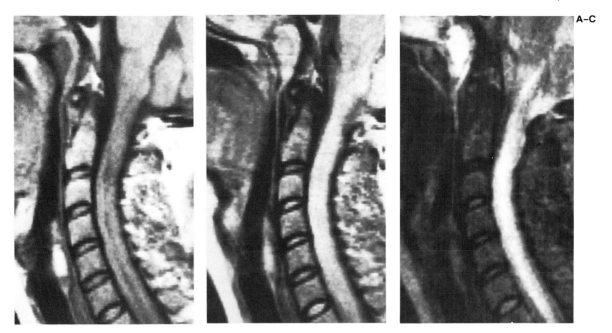

FIG. 99. Multiple sclerosis, Devic's type (biopsy-proven). MRI, 0.5 T. **A:** T1-WI (SE, TR = 500 msec, TE = 35 msec) shows diffusely enlarged cervical cord, with a central, irregular lower signal intensity, suggesting syrinx. **B:** Bal-I (SE, TR = 1,500 msec, TE = 35 msec) shows uniform increased signal intensity in the spinal cord. No central lucent band is seen in this image. **C:** T2-WI (SE, TR = 1,500 msec, TE = 120 msec). Increased cord signal is clearly evident, higher than that for surrounding CSF or fluid in fourth ventricle.

detected by MRI and CT (83) when individual vessels are large enough to be resolved (about 1 mm or larger) and tortuous, or when they have aneurysmal components or larger draining veins. The use of CT and intravenous contrast material would seem a logical approach, but probably not for small vessels or for investigation of the entire cord. Angiography is the definitive way to display these lesions, although it is not acceptable as a screening examination. Myelography is still the most sensitive way to detect or exclude a surface vascular malformation, but some, at

A–C

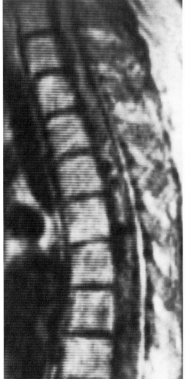
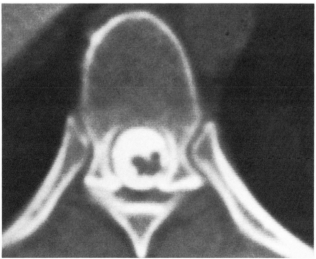
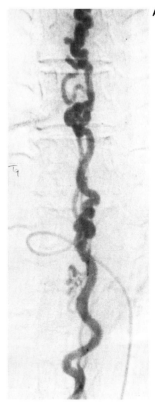

FIG. 100. Vascular malformation. **A:** MRI, 0.5 T (SE, TR = 500 msec, TE = 30 msec), nongated. Large tortuous vessels are shown as signal voids. Some of the vessels appear as areas of slightly decreased signal, believed to be due to effect of partial volume of the vessel and cord parenchyma. **B:** CT after intrathecal contrast injection shows cross sections of several vessels and the atrophic thoracic cord. **C:** Subtracted spinal angiogram delineates the extent of the malformation.

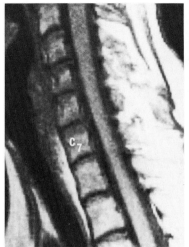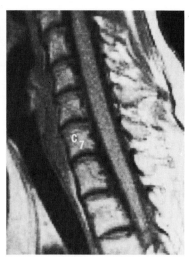

A,B

FIG. 101. Apparent cord abnormality due to scoliosis. **A:** MRI, 1.5 T, T1-WI (SE, TR = 500 msec, TE = 17 msec). A midsagittal section suggests atrophy of the cervical cord at C6 and C7. **B:** A contiguous section shows normal dimensions at C6 and C7. It might be misinterpreted as a cord swelling. This case clearly demonstrates the need for contiguous or interleaved sections. Axial sections might be necessary to definitely evaluate shape and size.

least, will be found by MRI, and the intramedullary portions or the nidus are more likely to be detected by MRI (31). The signal voids produced by the dense cortical bone bordering the spinal canal, such as the pedicles, laminae, and facets, may simulate the undulating or serpiginous pattern of abnormal vessels. On T2-WI, the dentate ligaments and intraarachnoid nerve roots may also be outlined by the increased signal from CSF or produce swirling CSF flow patterns in such a way as to simulate tortuous vessels on a para-midline sagittal section.

Although most intramedullary tumors are detected easily by sagittal MRI, it may be desirable to obtain axial cross-sectional images or coronal images in selected planes. The increased time needed for these images should be weighed against the possibility of interleaving images, other sequences, and the actual need for such images. When the cord is not longitudinally centered in the sagittal plane because of poor position or patient motion or spinal curvature, a fusiform configuration or apparent reduced diameter of the cord may be shown, simulating tumor or atrophy (Fig. 101). Axial sections perpendicular to the long axis of the cord can be useful in establishing the true diameters under these circumstances.

Extramedullary-Intradural Compartment

The spinal cord ends at about the first lumbar vertebral segment; therefore, there is no true intramedullary compartment in the lumbar region. The filum terminale gives rise to gliomas, especially in children and young adults, but these can be considered as extramedullary masses in the lumbar canal. In the cord-bearing regions, the most common intradural-extramedullary tumors are meningioma and schwannoma. The latter arise from the sheath of Schwann, which envelops the extramedullary axons of the nerve roots. They occur in all sections of the spinal canal, whereas meningioma is quite uncommon in the

lumbar canal (Fig. 86). The Schwann cell tumors have several different names that frequently are used indiscriminately: schwannoma, neuroma, neurinoma, neurilemmoma, neurolemoma, and neurofibroma. The histologic differences are somewhat confusing to a nonpathologist, and these tumors generally are indistinguishable radiologically, although central low signals on T2-WI may be characteristic of neurofibromas (19). In the syndrome of neurofibromatosis, the tumors are neurofibromas and frequently are multiple, whereas schwannomas are otherwise nearly always solitary.

Meningioma and solitary schwannoma differ mainly in regard to gender incidences, age, location in the spinal canal, and the presence of bony changes or calcification. Schwannomas commonly involve the bone by smooth erosion and are particularly prone to enlarge the intervertebral foramen or canal (Fig. 102). Meningioma may contain enough calcium to be detected by CT or even by radiography (Fig. 86), but this is an uncommon finding. Usually there are no reliable density or magnetic-relaxation-time differences between these two tumors, and in fact, both of these tumors usually appear similar (nearly isointense) to spinal cord or nerve roots (Figs. 103 and 104). Some nerve-sheath tumors yield significantly elevated signals, and meningiomas commonly produce slightly elevated signal on Bal-I and T2-WI, but both tumors are recognized chiefly by virtue of partial outlining by CSF and by the extramedullary deformity or displacement of the cord. Small lesions can escape detection because they do not have sufficient size or contrast differences to be resolved by CT or MRI. Axial sections through a tumor will indicate its relationship to the cord or canal and possible erosion of bone or extension into the neural foramen or beyond. Tumor replacement of the normal fat in the intervertebral canal is an important feature in both CT and MRI. CT is a more nearly definitive way to assess bone erosion, but it also can be recognized by MRI.

The uncommon neoplasms occurring in the extramedullary-intradural compartment include metastases

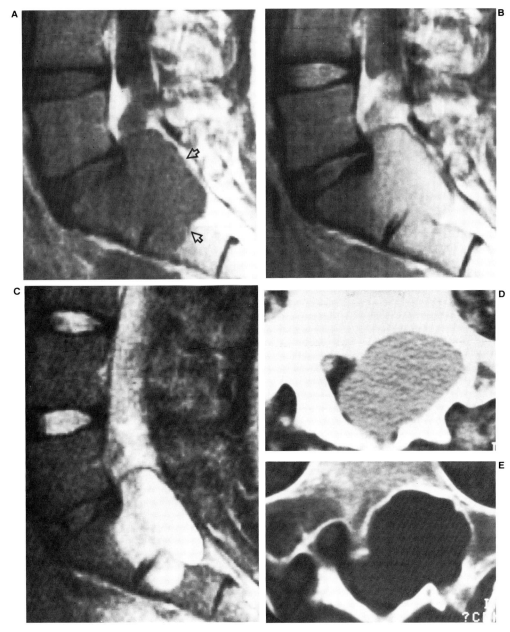

FIG. 102. Neurofibroma. **A–C:** MRI, 0.5 T. **D:** CT (soft-tissue window). **E:** CT (bone windows). **A:** T1-WI (SE, TR = 500 msec, TE = 30 msec) just to the left of midline demonstrates a low-signal lesion (*arrows*), slightly higher than CSF and slightly less than bone marrow, involving the spinal canal and the bony sacrum, displacing the surrounding high-signal-intensity fat. **B:** Bal-I (SE, TR = 1,500 msec, TE = 30 msec) shows the lesion to have a higher signal than bone marrow and CSF. **C:** WI (SE, TR = 1,500 msec, TE = 120 msec) demonstrates the lesion still has a higher signal intensity than CSF. **D, E:** CT shows the bony erosion more clearly. The lesion is of greater density than fat, but isodense with nerve root. A giant sacral cyst might contain sufficient protein to mimic the MRI characteristics of this lesion, but the bony changes are typical of a neurofibroma.

FIG. 103. Neurilemoma. MRI, 0.5 T. **A:** Bal-I (SE, TR = 1,500 msec, TE = 35 msec). A midsagittal section shows the thoracic cord inseparable from an isointense mass at T11-L1. The CSF space is of lower signal intensity. The tortuous outline of the cord above the tumor suggests that partially obstructed and congested vessels are present (*open arrow*). **B:** T2-WI (SE, TR = 1,500 msec, TE = 120 msec). The CSF is of higher signal than the cord, but not as high as the mass. Note the displaced cauda equina at the margin of the mass (*white arrow*).

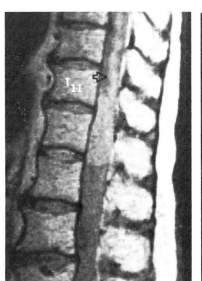
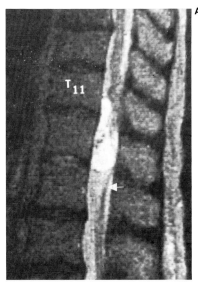

A–C

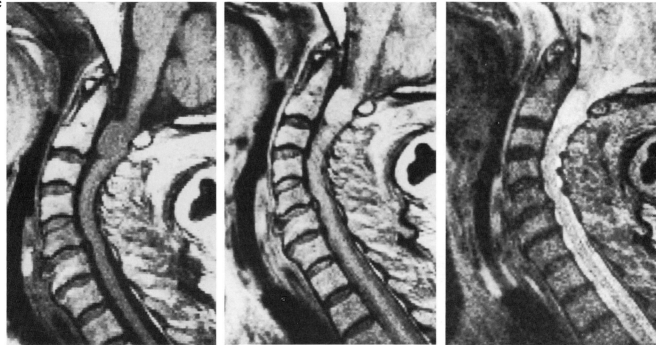

FIG. 104. Meningioma. MRI, 0.5 T. **A:** T1-WI (SE, TR = 500 msec, TE = 35 msec). A mass is easily identified at C2 that is nearly isointense with the cord. It lies in front and slightly to one side of the greatly compressed cervical cord. Degenerative disease of the cervical spine is present, slightly displacing the cord at C5-C6. **B:** Bal-I (SE, TR = 1,500 msec, TE = 35 msec). In this sequence, the tumor signal is greater than that for the cord or the medulla. CSF is of low signal and more accurately outlines the signal void of the vertebral cortical bone and ligaments, but less clearly outlines the cord itself. **C:** T2-WI (SE, TR = 1,500 msec, TE = 120 msec). In this sequence, CSF has a relatively high signal. The tumor signal is between those for spinal cord and CSF.

dropped from intradural-intracranial lesions (medulloblastoma, germinoma, pinealoma, brain metastases, and occasional gliomas) (Fig. 91) or, much less commonly, by hematogenous spread. The condition frequently is called metastatic seeding, and although larger deposits can be seen, some are surely too small to be detected by MRI. Myelography is still a more accurate method for detecting these lesions and may be required in the treatment planning of intracranial medulloblastoma or in the evaluation of spinal neurologic symptoms in a patient with a known primary cancer or intracranial neoplasm (140). However, the noninvasive capabilities of MRI make it an attractive initial examination, and usually it is sufficient when findings are positive (Fig. 105). CT, without intrathecal or intravenous injection of contrast material, is an insensitive modality for intradural-extramedullary lesions. As an adjunct to water-soluble myelography, however, CT may be indispensable. The hazard of not recognizing extensive intrathecal lumbar neoplasm should be reemphasized (Fig. 106).

A number of nonneoplastic abnormalities occur in the intradural-extramedullary compartment. Some are relatively common, such as the redundant root or roots in severe spinal stenosis (120). Some are uncommon, such as arachnoid cyst and epidermoid, dermoid, or teratoma cyst (93). Some are rare conditions, such as hypertrophic neuritis (Dejerine-Sottas disease, neurofibromatosis, lym-

phoma, Charcot-Marie-Tooth and Refsum diseases) (Fig. 107), neurenteric cyst, parasitic cyst (68,84), and granuloma (sarcoid, etc.) (21). Blood clot, as opposed to mixed subarachnoid blood and CSF, is uncommon (42,136). The various manifestations of dysraphism and the tethered-

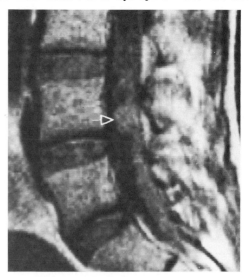

FIG. 105. Melanoma, drop metastases. MRI, 0.5 T. T1-WI (SE, TR = 500 msec, TE = 30 msec). The normal signal void of CSF is interrupted by a mass (*open arrow*) and suggested amorphous filling defects in the lumbar region. The conus medullaris is normal.

cord syndrome, disc herniation, spinal stenosis, arachnoiditis, and syringohydromyelia are discussed elsewhere.

Extradural Compartment

The most common disorders of this compartment fall into the degenerative, traumatic, and developmental categories and are discussed elsewhere. The next most common causes of extradural deformity or compression are metastatic neoplasm and lymphoma (9,66). The tissues in this compartment potentially can give rise to a wide spectrum of primary neoplasms and diseases, including those of lymphoid, vascular, adipose, neural, fibrous, osseous, and primitive-notochord origin (Table 1). Neuren-

teric cyst has been reported. Bony disease such as primary or metastatic neoplasm (92), hemangioma, or Paget disease may expand or extend to compress or deform the spinal canal. Infection arising in the intervertebral disc or bone may affect this compartment, and, of course, infection can arise within the canal as epidural abscess (Fig. 92), granuloma (75), and parasitic cyst (49). Metastatic neoplasms occurring outside the spinal canal itself in the paravertebral tissues may extend into the bony canal by way of the neural foramen or through direct destruction, extension, or expansion (Fig. 108).

Hematoma, though mainly traumatic and postoperative, can occur as a result of disease or anticoagulation (117), as well as idiopathically. The vascular malformations, as mentioned earlier, can occur primarily as epidural

A–C

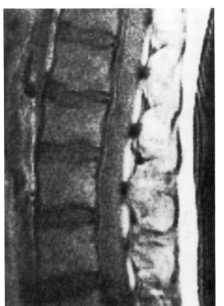 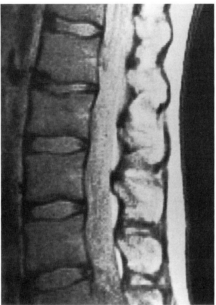 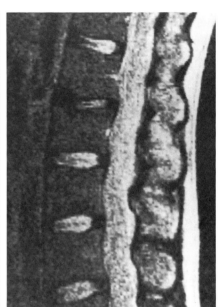

D,E

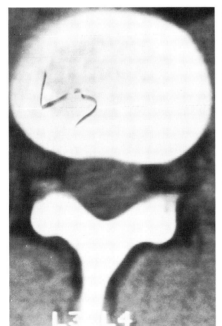 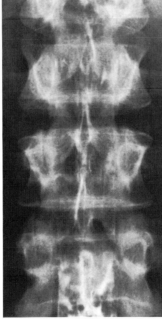

FIG. 106. Diffuse tumor filling the subarachnoid space. A–C: MRI, 0.5 T. A: T1-WI (SE, TR = 700 msec, TE = 15 msec). B: Bal-I (SE, TR = 1,500 msec, TE = 35 msec). C: T2-WI (SE, TR = 1,500 msec, TE = 120 msec). No obvious abnormality is detected in any of the three MR images. D: Plain CT is also normal. E: Myelogram, initially suspected to indicate subdural injection, shows extensive filling defect of the lumbar canal (and involvement of thoracic and cervical regions) by tumor. Surgical exploration revealed an extensive, poorly differentiated tumor believed to be of dural origin.

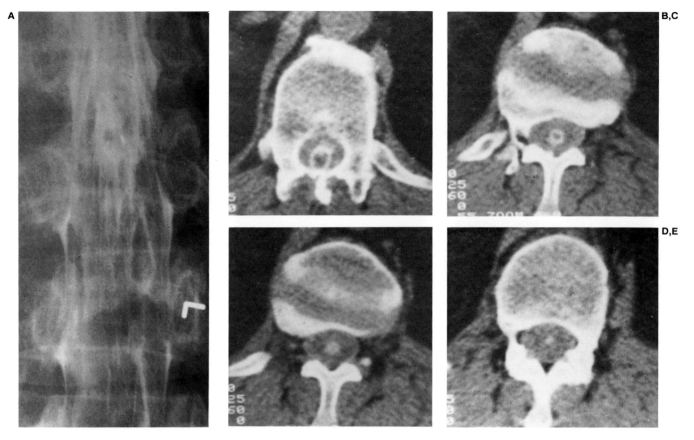

FIG. 107. Hypertrophic neuritis. The individual roots of the cauda equina are markedly enlarged, as seen by metrizamide myelography. Four images from a CT study taken after administration of metrizamide demonstrate that the contrast-filled subarachnoid space can be seen only around the conus and filum terminale. At the more inferior levels, the subarachnoid space is obliterated by the thickened roots of the cauda.

conditions (13) and in fact may be more common than strictly intradural malformations (141). Conditions such as pachymeningitis (81), the dural or extradural thickening in mucopolysaccharidosis (78,138), increased fibrous tissue of obscure origin (141) (Fig. 89), and excessive fat (lipomatosis) in patients with morbid obesity or patients undergoing steroid therapy are distinctly uncommon (24,114). Neurofibroma and, rarely, meningioma may arise outside the dural canal, but otherwise are no different than the intradural variety. Extradural ependymoma has been described (131). In general, except for blood, blood vessels, and fat, there is little or no MRI or CT difference among the various tumors occurring in this compartment.

CT is the best way to demonstrate the osseous spine, but MRI is perhaps more dramatic in showing tumor or disease that replaces the fatty or hematopoietic marrow of the vertebral bodies, or tumor extending from the epidural space into surrounding bone. The presence of epidural soft-tissue abnormality is also more easily recognized by MRI, especially when it lies anteriorly, where it deforms the CSF-filled canal in the sagittal plane. Lateral deformity is similarly appreciated on coronal planes (45). CT depends on fat or CSF to demonstrate epidural disease, except for bone, and is therefore much more useful after intrathecal contrast injection. Both CT and MRI depend to a large extent on clinical findings or results of prior radiologic studies (e.g., radionuclide bone scintigraphy or myelography) to direct attention and to limit examination to a reasonable length of spine. Although examination of the entire spine may not be practical, survey of the spine when seeking gross disease, such as spinal block due to

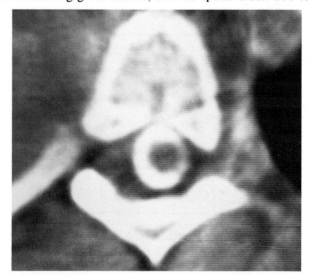

FIG. 108. Neuroblastoma in a 10-year-old boy. The tumor mass enters the dorsal spinal canal through an intervertebral foramen and displaces the metrizamide-filled subarachnoid canal and spinal cord to the left.

metastatic neoplasm, may be practical, because relatively fast sequences and sagittal planes alone will suffice without the necessity for long sequences and axial planes. Repositioning of the patient on the surface coil in order to examine different segments of the spine results in prolongation of examination time. Curvature and motion jeopardize the examination, and the result may be that myelography is a more reliable and quicker procedure in an emergency setting, especially because CT can be added to verify or expand on the findings.

Postoperative Evaluation

After laminectomy, the existence of various stages and forms of scar tissue and blood clot, as well as alterations in normal anatomic features, makes assessment by CT, MRI, myelography, and postmyelographic CT difficult and complex. The use of intravenous contrast material for both CT and MRI is of some help. At the present time, however, attempts at differentiation between tumors (new or recurrent) and postoperative alterations have been disappointing.

REFERENCES

1. Altman N, Altman D. MR imaging of spinal dysraphism. *AJNR* 1987;8:533–538.
2. Altman N, Harwood-Nash DC, Fitz CR, Chuang SH, Armstrong D. Evaluation of the infant spine by direct sagittal computed tomography. *AJNR* 1985;6:65–69.
3. Arredondo F, Haughton VM, Hemmy DC, Zelaya B, Williams AL. Computed tomographic appearance of spinal cord in diastematomyelia. *Radiology* 1980;136:685–688.
4. Aubin ML, Vignaud J, Jardin C, Bar D. Computed tomography in 75 clinical cases of syringomyelia. *AJNR* 1981;2:199–204.
5. Baleriaux-Waha D, Osteaux M, Terwinghe G, de Meeus A, Jeanmart L. The management of anterior sacral meningocele with CT. *Neuroradiology* 1977;14:45–46.
6. Banerjee T, Hunt WE. Spinal cord sarcoidosis. Case report. *J Neurosurg* 1972;36:490–493.
7. Barnes PD, Lester PD, Yamanashi WS, Prince JR. Magnetic resonance imaging in infants and children with spinal dysraphism. *AJNR* 1986;7:465–472.
8. Barnwell SL, Edwards MSB. Spinal intramedullary spread of medulloblastoma. Case report. *J Neurosurg* 1986;65:253–255.
9. Beres J, Pech P, Daniels DL, Williams AL, Haughton VM. Spinal epidural lymphomas: CT features in seven patients. *AJNR* 1986;7: 327–328.
10. Berger PE, Atkinson D, Wilson WJ, Wiltse L. High resolution surface coil magnetic resonance imaging of the spine: normal and pathologic anatomy. *RadioGraphics* 1986;6:573–602.
11. Bonafe A, Ethier R, Melancon D, Belanger G, Peters T. High resolution computed tomography in cervical syringomyelia. *J Comput Assist Tomogr* 1980;4:42–47.
12. Bools JC, Rose BS. Traumatic atlantooccipital dislocation: two cases with survival. *AJNR* 1986;7:901–904.
13. Bradac FB, Simori RS, Schramm J. Cervical spidural AVM. Report of a case of uncommon location. *Neuroradiology* 1977;14:97–100.
14. Brant-Zawadzki M, Jeffrey RB, Minagi H, Pitts LH. High resolution CT of thoracolumbar fractures. *AJNR* 1982;3:69–74.
15. Brant-Zawadzki M, Miller EM, Federle MP. CT in the evaluation of spine trauma. *AJR* 1981;136:369–375.
16. Braun IF, Hoffman JC Jr, Davis PC, et al. Contrast enhancement in CT differentiation between recurrent disc herniation and postoperative scar. *AJNR* 1985;6:607–612.
17. Brugman E, Palmer Y, Staelens B. Congenital absence of a pedicle in the cervical spine: a new approach with CT scan. *Neuroradiology* 1979;17:121–125.
18. Bundschuh CV, Modic MT, Ross JS, Masaryk TJ, Bohlman H. Epidural fibrosis and recurrent disc herniation in the lumbar spine: MR imaging assessment. *AJNR* 1988;9:169.
19. Burk DL, Brunberg JA, Kanal E, Latchaw RE, Wolf GL. Spinal and paraspinal neurofibromatosis: surface MR imaging at 1.5 T. *Radiology* 1987;162:797–801.
20. Bydder GM, Brown J, Niendorf HP, Young IR. Enhancement of central intraspinal tumors in MR imaging with intravenous gadolinium DTPA. *J Comput Assist Tomogr* 1985;9:847–851.
21. Cambell JN, Black P, Ostrow PT. Sarcoid of the cauda equina. *J Neurosurg* 1977;47:109–112.
22. Carrerra GF, Haughton VM, Syvertsen A, Williams AL. Computed tomography of the lumbar facet joints. *Radiology* 1980;134:145.
23. Chakeres DW, Flickinger F, Bresnahan JC, et al. MR imaging of acute spinal cord trauma. *AJNR* 1987;8:5–10.
24. Chapman PH, Matuza RL, Poletti CF, Karchmer AW. Symptomatic spinal epidural lipomatosis associated with Cushing's syndrome. *Neurosurgery* 1981;8:724–727.
25. Committee on the Spine, American Academy of Orthopedic Surgeons. *A glossary on spinal terminology* (Document 675-80), 1980.
26. Coin CG, Pennick M, Ahmad WD, Keranen VJ. Diving-type injury of the cervical spine: contribution of computed tomography to management. *J Comput Assist Tomogr* 1979;3:362–372.
27. Colley DP, Dunsker SB. Traumatic narrowing of the dorsolumbar spinal canal demonstrated by computed tomography. *Radiology* 1978;129:95–98.
28. Cox HE, Bennett WF. Computed tomography of absent cervical pedicle. Case report. *J Comput Assist Tomogr* 1984;8:537–539.
29. Dake MD, Dillon WP, Dowart RH. CT of extraarachnoid metrizamide instillation. *AJR* 1986;147:583–586.
30. Denes LJ, et al. Ellusive tumors of the cauda equina. Case report. *J Neurosurg* 1987;66:131–133.
31. Di Chiro G, et al. Tumors and arteriovenous malformations of the spinal cord: assessment using MR. *Radiology* 1985;156:689–697.
32. Di Chiro G, et al. MR cisternography and myelography with Gd-DTPA in monkeys. *Radiology* 1985;157:373–377.
33. Dorne HL, Just N, Lander PH. CT recognition of anomalies of the posterior arch of the atlas vertebra: differentiation from fracture. *AJNR* 1986;7:176–177.
34. Edelman RR, Shoukimas GM, Stark DD, et al. High resolution surface coil imaging of lumbar disc disease. *AJNR* 1985;5:479–485.
35. Elliott HC. Cross-sectional diameters and areas of the human spinal cord. *Anat Rec* 1945;93:287–293.
36. Enzman DR, Rubin JB, Wright A. Use of cerebrospinal fluid gating to improve T2-weighted images. Part I. The spinal cord. *Radiology* 1987;162:763–773.
37. Epstein BS, Epstein JA, Lavine L. The effect of anatomic variations on the lumbar vertebrae and spinal canal on cauda equina nerve root syndromes. *AJR* 1964;91:105.
38. Faerber EN, Wolpert SM, Scott RM, Belkin SC, Carter BL. Computed tomography of spinal fracture. *J Comput Assist Tomogr* 1979;3:657–661.
39. Fielding JW, Stillwell WT, Chynn KY, Spyropoulos EC. Use of computed tomography for the diagnosis of atlanto-axial rotatory fixation. A case report. *J Bone Joint Surg* 1978;6A:1102–1104.
40. Firooznia H, Krichesff II, Rafii M, Colimba C. Lumbar spine after surgery: examination with intravenous contrast-enhanced CT. *Radiology* 1987;163:221.
41. Ford LT, Gilula LA, Murphy WA, Gado M. Analysis of gas in vacuum lumbar disc. *AJR* 1977;126:1056–1057.
42. Frager D, Zimmerman RD, Wisoff HS, Leeds NE. Spinal subarachnoid hematoma. *AJNR* 1982;3:77–79.
43. Friedman E. Narrowing of the spinal canal due to thickened lamina. *Clin Orthop* 1961;21:190.
44. Gado MH, Patel J, Hodges FJ III. Lateral disc herniation into the lumbart intervertebral foramen: differential diagnosis. *AJNR* 1983;4:598–600.
45. Gawehn J, Schroth G, Thron A. The value of paraxial slices in MR imaging of spinal cord disease. *Neuroradiology* 1986;28:347–350.
46. Gebarski SS, Maynard FW, Gabrielsen TO, Knake JE, Latach JT,

Hoff JT. Posttraumatic progressive myelopathy. *Radiology* 1985;157:379–385.

47. Gellad FE, Levine AM, Joslyn JN, Edwards CC, Bosse M. Pure thoracolumbar facet dislocation: clinical features and CT appearance. *Radiology* 1986;161:505–508.

48. Genant H. Technical considerations. In: Newton TH, Potts DG, eds. *Computed tomography of the spine and spinal cord.* Clavadel, San Anselmo, CA: Clavadel Press, 1983.

49. Giordono GB, Cerisoli M, Bernardi B. Hydatic cysts of the spine. *J Comput Assist Tomogr* 1982;6:488–509.

50. Gomori JM, Grossman RI, Goldberg HI, Zimmerman RA, Bilaniuk LT. Intracranial hematomas: imaging by high-field MR. *Radiology* 1985;157:87–93.

51. Goy AMC, Pinto RS, Raghavendra BN, Epstein FJ, Kricheff II. Intramedullary spinal cord tumors: MR imaging, with emphasis on associated cysts. *Radiology* 1986;161:381–386.

52. Grenier N, Grossman RI, Schiebler ML, et al. Degenerative lumbar disc disease: pitfalls and usefulness of MR imaging in detection of vacuum phenomenon. *Radiology* 1987;164:861.

53. Grenier N, Kressel HY, Schiebler ML, et al. Normal and degenerative posterior spinal structures: MR imaging. *Radiology* 1987;165:517.

54. Guerra J, Garfin SR, Resnick D. Vertebral burst fractures: CT analysis of the retropulsed fragment. *Radiology* 1984;153:769–772.

55. Gulati AN, Weinstein PR. Gas in the spinal canal in association with the lumbosacral vacuum phenomenon: CT findings. *Neuroradiology* 1980;20:191.

56. Hackney DB, Asato R, Joseph PM, et al. Hemorrhage and edema in acute spinal cord compression: demonstration by MR imaging. *Radiology* 1986;161:387–390.

57. Han JS, Benson JE, Kaufman B, et al. Demonstration of diastematomyelia and associated abnormalities with MR imaging. *AJNR* 1985;6:215–219.

58. Handel SF, Lee Y. Computed tomography of spinal fractures. *Radiol Clin North Am* 1981;19:69–89.

59. Harwood-Nash DCF, Fitz CR, Resjo IM, Chuang S. Congenital spinal and cord lesions in children and computed tomographic metrizamide myelography. *Neuroradiology* 1978;16:69–70.

60. Haughton VM. MR imaging of the spine. *Radiology* 1988;166:297.

61. Haughton VM, Syverisen A, Williams AL. Soft tissue anatomy within the spinal canal as seen on computed tomography. *Radiology* 1980;123:649–655.

62. Haughton VM, Williams AL. *Computed tomography of the spine.* St Louis: CV Mosby, 1982.

63. Heithoff KB, Ray CD. Principles of the computed tomographic assessment of lateral spinal stenosis. In: *Spine update 1984.*

64. Hirschy JC, Leue WM, Berninger WH, Hamilton RH, Abbott GF. CT of the lumbosacral spine: importance of tomographic planes parallel to vertebral end plate. *AJR* 1981;136:47–52.

65. Holland GN, Moore WS, Hawkes RC. Nuclear magnetic resonance tomography of the brain. *J Comput Assist Tomogr* 1980;4:1–3.

66. Holtas SL, Kido DK, Simon JH. MR imaging of spinal lymphoma. Case report. *J Comput Assist Tomogr* 1986;10:111–115.

67. Hughes JT. Diseases of the spine and spinal cord. In: Blackwood W, Corsellis J, eds. *Greenfield's neuropathology.* 3rd ed. London: Edward Arnold, 1976:668–670.

68. Hyman AD, Gray CE, Lanzieri C, Belman AS. Tapework cysts of the equina. *AJNR* 1986;7:977–978.

69. Jenkins JR, Bashir R, Al-Mefty O, Al-Kawi MZ, Fox JL. Cystic necrosis of the spinal cord in compressive cervical myelopathy: demonstration by iopamidol CT-myelography. *AJR* 1986;147:767–775.

70. Johnson JE, Yang PJ, Seeger JF, Iacono RP. Vertical fracture of the odontoid: CT diagnosis. Case report. *J Comput Assist Tomogr* 1986;10:311–312.

71. Johnson RE, Roberson GH. Subpial lipoma of the spinal cord. *Radiology* 1974;111:121–126.

72. Kadoya S, Nakamura T, Kobayashi S, Yamamoto H. Magnetic resonance imaging of acute spinal cord injury. *Neuroradiology* 1987;29:252–255.

73. Kangarloo H, Gold RH, Diament MJ, Boechat MI, Barrett C. High resolution spinal sonography in infants. *AJNR* 1984;5:191–195.

74. Kan S, Fox AJ, Vinuela F. Delayed metrizamide CT enhancement of syringomyelia: post-operative observation. *AJNR* 1985;6:613–616.

75. Kanoff RB, Rubert RL. Sarcoidosis presenting as a dorsal spinal cord tumor: report of a case. *J Am Osteopathic Assoc* 1980;79:765–767.

76. Kantrowitz CR, Pais JM, Burnett K, Choi B, Fritz MB. Intraspinal neurenteric cyst containing gastric mucosa: CT and MRI findings. *Pediatr Radiol* 1986;16:324–327.

77. Keene GCR, Hone MR, Sage MR. Atlas fracture: demonstration using computerized tomography. A case report. *J Bone Joint Surg* 1978;60A:1106–1107.

78. Kennedy P, Swash M, Dean MF. Cervical cord compression in mucophysacharidosis. Case report. *Dev Med Child Neurol* 1973;15:194–198.

79. Kershner MS, Goodman GA, Perlmutter GS. Computed tomography in the diagnosis of an atlas fracture. *AJR* 1977;128:688–689.

80. Kilcoyne RF, Mack LA, King HA, Ratcliffe SS, Loop JW. Thoracolumbar spine injuries associated with vertical plunges: reappraisal with computed tomography. *Radiology* 1983;146:137–140.

81. Kim KS, Weinberg PE, Hemmati M. Spinal pachymeningeal carcinomatosis: myelographic features. *AJNR* 1980;1:199–200.

82. Kirkaldy-Willis WH, Heithof KB, Tchang S, et al. Lumbar spondylosis and stenosis: correlation of pathologic anatomy with high resolution computed tomography scanning. In: Post JD, ed. *Computed tomography of the spine.* Baltimore: Williams & Wilkins, 1984:546–569.

83. Kulkarni M, Burks DD, Price AC, Cobb C, Allen JH. Diagnosis of spinal arteriovenous malformation in a pregnant patient by MR imaging. *J Comput Assist Tomogr* 1985;9:171–173.

84. Kwok DMF, Jeffreys RV. Intramedullary enterogenous cyst of the spinal cord. Case report. *J Neurosurg* 1982;56:270–274.

85. Lapointe JS, Grach DA, Nugent RD, Robertson WD. Value of intravenous contrast enhancement in the CT evaluation of intraspinal tumors. *AJNR* 1985;6:939–943.

86. Larson TC, Hauser OW, Onofrio BM, Piepgras DG. Primary spinal melanoma. *J Neurosurg* 1987;66:47–49.

87. Lauten GJ, Wehunt WP. Computed tomography in absent cervical pedicle. *AJNR* 1980;1:201–203.

88. Lee BCP, Deck MDF, Kneeland JB, Cahill PT. MR imaging of the craniocervical junction. *AJNR* 1985;6:209–213.

89. Lee C, Woodring JH, Goldstein SJ, Daniel TL, Young AB, Tibbs PA. Evaluation of traumatic atlantooccipital dislocations. *AJNR* 1987;8:19–26.

90. Lee BCP, Zimmerman RD, Manning JJ, Deck MDF. MR imaging of syringomyelia and hydromyelia. *AJNR* 1985;6:221–228.

91. Ley JA, Marti A. Intramedullary hydatid cyst. Case report. *J Neurosurg* 1970;33:457–459.

92. Lozes G, et al. Chondroma of the cervical spine. Case report. *J Neurosurg* 1987;66:128–130.

93. Manasati A, Spitzer RM, Wiley JL, Heggeness L. MR imaging of a spinal teratoma. *J Comput Assist Tomogr* 1986;10:307–310.

94. Manaster BJ, Osborn AG. CT patterns of facet fracture dislocations in the thoracolumbar region. *AJNR* 1986;7:1007–1012.

95. Maravilla KR, Cooper PR, Sklar FH. The influence of thin-section tomography on the treatment of cervical spine injuries. *Radiology* 1978;127:131–139.

96. Maravilla KR, Lesh P, Weinreb JC, et al. Magnetic resonance imaging of the lumbar spine with CT correlation. *AJNR* 1985;6:237–245.

97. Maravilla KR, Weinreb JC, Suss R, Nunnally RL. Magnetic resonance demonstration of multiple sclerosis: plaques in the cervical cord. *AJNR* 1984;5:685–689.

98. McArdle CB, Crofford MJ, Mirfakhraee M, Amparo EG, Calhous JS. Surface coil MR of spinal trauma: preliminary experience. *AJNR* 1986;7:885–893.

99. McArdle CB, Wright JW, Prevost WJ, Dornfest DJ, Amparo EG. MR imaging of the acutely injured patient with cervical traction. *Radiology* 1986;159:273–274.

100. Mirvis SE, Geisler FH, Jelinek JJ, Joslyn JN, Gellaud F. Acute cervical spine trauma: evaluation with 1.5-T MR imaging. *Radiology* 1988;166:807–816.

101. Modic MT, Masaryk TJ, Paushter DM. Magnetic resonance imaging of the spine. *Radiol Clin North Am* 1986;24:229.

102. Modic MT, Pavlicek W, Weinstein MA, et al. Magnetic resonance

imaging of intervertebral disc disease. *Radiology* 1984;152:102–111.

103. Modic MT, Weinstein MA, Pavlicek W, et al. Nuclear magnetic resonance imaging of the spine. *Radiology* 1983;148:757–762.

104. Moffie D, Stefanko SZ. Intramedullary metastasis. *Clin Neurol Neurosurg* 1980;82:199–202.

105. Montana MA, Richardson ML, Kilcoyne RF, Harley JD, Shuman WP, Mack LA. CT of sacral injury. *Radiology* 1983;148:757–762.

106. Naidich TP, McLone DG, Harwood-Nash DC. Spinal dysraphism. In: Newton TH, Potts DG, eds. *Modern neuroradiology: computed tomography of the spine and spinal cord* (vol 1). San Anselmo, CA: Clavadel Press, 1983.

107. Naidich TP, Pudlowski RM, Moran CJ, Gilula LA, Murphy W, Naidich JB. Computed tomography of spinal fractures. *Adv Neurol* 1979;22:207–252.

108. Nayashima C, Yamaguchi T, Reizo T. Arteriovenous malformation on the spinal cord: computed tomography with intraarterial enhancement. *J Comput Assist Tomogr* 1981;5:586–587.

109. Naseem M, Zachariah SB, Stone J, Russell E. Cervicomedullary hematoma: diagnosis by MR. *AJNR* 1986;7:1096–1098.

110. Nokes SR, Murtaugh FR, Jones DJ, et al. Childhood scoliosis: MR imaging. *Radiology* 1987;164:791–797.

111. Norman D, Mills CM, Brant-Zawadzki M, Yeates A, Crooks LE, Kaufman L. Magnetic resonance imaging of the spinal cord and canal: potentials and limitations. *AJNR* 1984;5:9–14.

112. Nykamp PW, Levy JM, Christensen F, Dunn R, Hubbard J. Computed tomography for a bursting fracture of the lumbar spine. Report of a case. *J Bone Joint Surg* 1978;60A:1108–1109.

113. Pech P, Haughton VM. Lumbar intervertebral disc: correlative MR and anatomic study. *Radiology* 1985;156:699–701.

114. Pennisi AK, Meisler WS, Dina TS. Lymphomatous meningitis and steroid-induced epidural lipomatosis: CT evaluation. *J Comput Assist Tomogr* 1985;9:595–598.

115. Plumley TF, Kilcoyne RF, Mack LA. Computed tomography in the evaluation of gunshot wounds of the spine. *J Comput Assist Tomogr* 1983;7:310–312.

116. Pojunas K, Williams AL, Daniels DL, Haughton VM. Syringomyelia and hydromyelia: magnetic resonance evaluation. *Radiology* 1984;153:679–683.

117. Post MJD, Seminer DS, Quencer RM. CT diagnosis of spinal epidural hematoma. *AJNR* 1982;3:190–192.

118. Quencer RM, El Gammal T, Cohen G. Syringomyelia associated with extramedullary masses of the spinal canal. *AJNR* 1986;7:143–148.

119. Quencer RM, Sheldon JJ, Donovan Post MJ, et al. Magnetic resonance imaging of the chronically injured cervical spinal cord. *AJNR* 1986;7:457–464.

120. Rengachary SS, McGregor DH, Watanabe I, Arjunan K, Kepes JJ. Suggested pathologic basis of "redundant nerve root syndrome" of the cauda equina. *Neurosurgery* 1980;7:400–411.

121. Resjo IM, Harwood-Nash DC, Fitz CR, Chuang S. Normal cord in infants and children examined with computed tomographic metrizamide myelography. *Radiology* 1971;130:692–696.

122. Rinaldi I, Mullins WJ, Delaney WF, Fitzer PM, Tornberg DN. Computerized tomographic demonstration of rotational atlanto-axial fixation. Case report. *J Neurosurg* 1979;50:115–119.

123. Rogers LF, Thayer C, Weinberg PE, Kim KS. Acute injuries of the upper thoracic spine associated with paraplegia. *AJR* 1980;134:67–73.

124. Ross JS, Masaryk TJ, Modic MT, et al. Lumbar spine: post-operative assessment with surface coil MR imaging. *Radiology* 1987;164:851.

125. Rubin JM, Aisen AM, DiPietro MA. Ambiguities in MR imaging of tumoral cysts in the spinal cord. *J Comput Assist Tomogr* 1986;10:395–398.

126. Samuelsson L, Bergstron K, Thuomas K-A, Hemmingsson A, Wallensten R. MR imaging of syringohydromyelia and Chiari malformations in myelomeningocele patients with scoliosis.

127. Schubiger O, Valvanis A. CT differentiation between recurrent disc herniation and post-operative scar formation. *Neuroradiology* 1982;22:251.

128. Scotti G, Harwood-Nash DC, Hoffman JH. Congenital thoracic dermal sinus: diagnosis by computer assisted metrizamide myelography. *J Comput Assist Tomogr* 1980;4:675–677.

129. Scotti G, Scialfa G, Columbo N, Landon L. MR imaging of intradural extramedullary tumors of the cervical spine. *J Comput Assist Tomogr* 1985;9:1037–1041.

130. Seibert CE, Barnes JE, Dreisbach JN, Swanson WB, Heck RJ. Accurate CT measurements of the spinal cord using metrizamide: physical factors. *AJNR* 1981;2:75–78.

131. Seigel RS, Williams AG, Metter FA, Wicks JD. Intraspinal extradural ependymoma. *J Comput Assist Tomogr* 1982;5:189–192.

132. Sherman JL, Barkovich AJ, Citrin CM. The MR appearance of syringomyelia: new observations. *AJNR* 1986;7:985–995.

133. Semins H, Nugent GR, Chou SM. Intramedullary spinal cord sarcoidosis. Case report. *J Neurosurg* 1972;37:233–236.

134. Sherman JL, Citrin CM, Gangarosa RE, Bowen BJ. The MR appearance of CSF pulsations in the spinal canal. *AJNR* 1986;7:879–884.

135. Shinsuke U, Saito A, Inomori S, Kin I. Cavernous angioma, the cauda equina producing subarachnoid hemorrhage. *J Neurosurg* 1987;66:134–136.

136. Smaltino F, Bernini FP, Santoro S. Computerized tomography in the diagnosis of intramedullary metastasis. *Acta Neurochirgica* 1980;52:299–303.

137. Smoker WRK, Biller J, Moore SA, Beck DW, Hart MN. Intradural spinal teratoma: case report and review of the literature. *AJNR* 1986;7:905–910.

138. Sostrin RD, Hasso AN, Peterson DI, Thompson JR. Myelographic features of mucopolysacchraidoses: a new sign. *Radiology* 1977;125:421–424.

139. Stanley P, Senac MO Jr, Segall HD. Intraspinal seeding from intracranial tumors in children. *AJNR* 1984;5:805–809.

140. Symon L, Kuyama H, Kendall B. Dural arteriovenous malformation of the spine: clinical features and surgical results in 55 cases. *J Neurosurg* 1984;60:238–247.

141. Sze G, Brant-Zawadzki MKI, Wilson CR, Norman D, Newton TH. Pseudotumor of the craniovertebral junction associated with chronic subluxation: MR imaging studies. *Radiology* 1986;161:391–394.

142. Tantana S, Pilla TJ, Luisiri A. Computed tomography of acute spinal subdural hematoma. *J Comput Assist Tomogr* 1986;19:891–892.

143. Tarr RW, Drolshager LF, Kerner TC, Allen JH, Partain CL, James AE Jr. MR imaging of recent spinal trauma. *J Comput Assist Tomogr* 1987;11:412–417.

144. Thijssen H, Keyser A, Horstink MWM, Meiser E. Morphology of the cervical spinal cord on computed myelography. *Neuroradiology* 1979;18:57–62.

145. Teplick JG, Laffey PA, Berman A, Haskin ME. Diagnosis and evaluation of spondylolisthesis and/or spondylolysis on axial CT. *AJNR* 1986;7:479–491.

146. Vade A, Kennard D. Lipomeningomyelocystocele. *AJNR* 1987;8:375–377.

147. Verbiest H. Further experiences on the pathological influence of a developmental narrowness of the bony lumbar vertebral canal. *J Bone Joint Surg* 1955;37B:576.

148. Wedge JH, Kirkaldy-Willis WH, Kinnard P. Lumbar spinal stenosis. In: Helfet AJ, Lee DMG, eds. *Disorders of the lumbar spine.* Philadelphia: Lippincott, 1978:51–68.

149. Weinstein PR. Pathology of lumbar stenosis and spondylosis. In: Weinstein PR, Ehni G, Wilson C, eds. *Lumbar spondylosis.* Chicago: Year Book 1977:43–91.

150. Williams AL, Haughton VM, Meyer GA, Hok C. Computed tomographic appearance of the bulging annulus. *Radiology* 1982;142:403.

151. Williams AL, Haughton VM, Syvertsen A. Computed tomography in the diagnosis of herniated nucleus pulposus. *Radiology* 1980;135:95–99.

152. Wood BP, Harwood-Nash DC, Berger P, Goske M. Intradural spinal lipoma of the cervical cord. *AJNR* 1985;6:452–454.

153. Yetkin Z, Osborn AG, Giles DS, Haughton VM. Uncovertebral and facet joint dislocations in cervical articular pillar fractures: CT evaluation. *AJNR* 1985;6:633–637.

154. Young HA, Robb P, Hardy DG. Large intramedullary neurofibroma of the conus medullaris: case report. *Neurosurgery* 1983;13:48–51.

155. Yu YL, du Boulay GH, Stevens JM, Kendall BE. Morphology and measurements of the cervical spinal cord in computer assisted myelography. *Neuroradiology* 1985;27:399–402.

156. Zee C-S, Segall HD, Ahmadi J, Tsai FY, Apuzzo M. CT myelography in spinal cysticercosis. *J Comput Assist Tomogr* 1986;10:195–198.

CHAPTER 23

Pediatric Applications

Marilyn J. Siegel

Pediatric diseases frequently are different in type and presentation from those in adults. But, as in the older population, valuable diagnostic information can be gained from computed tomography (CT) of the body, and CT is accepted as an important method for diagnosis of extracranial disease in children (38,125). Using CT and, more recently, magnetic resonance imaging (MRI), the diagnosis, extent, and progress of disease can be evaluated more accurately than was possible a decade ago.

The contribution of CT to diagnostic imaging is based on two unique properties: its ability to distinguish small differences in tissue densities and its ability to provide three-dimensional, cross-sectional delineation of anatomic relationships unobscured by overlying structures. However, extracranial CT in children presents unique problems not encountered in adults. The most important of these problems is the relative paucity of perivisceral fat, making delineation of the borders of organs and structures more difficult in pediatric patients; another problem is the small size of these patients. Furthermore, small children frequently are unable to cooperate, and sedation may be needed. The radiation doses from CT in children are also different from those in adults. The skin dose and organ dose in the directly irradiated area, as well as the exposure of organs outside the area examined, are higher in children because of their smaller body diameter. However, the absorbed dose is lower in children than in adults because of their smaller volume (82). Newer-generation CT scanners, especially, have reduced the radiation dose while improving image quality (21,23).

MRI also is a safe and effective method for diagnosing pediatric disease, and like CT it has advantages and disadvantages. The advantages of MRI are its direct multiplanar imaging capability, absence of ionizing radiation, and superior soft-tissue resolution compared with CT. Blood vessels, the heart, and intraspinal contents can be well visualized without the need for injection of contrast material. Unlike CT, MRI does not produce artifacts from bone or implanted metal objects. The advantages, how-

ever, must be weighed against the disadvantages of MRI. These include a relatively long image acquisition time in comparison with CT, requiring prolonged sedation and increasing the potential for motion degradation of images. Patients with pacemakers and ferrous metallic clips cannot be examined by MRI. Another disadvantage is that patients on life-support systems cannot be readily examined. The relative insensitivity of MRI to calcification is also a drawback, because some common pediatric tumors, such as neuroblastoma, have calcifications, whose recognition is important for differential diagnosis. Finally, the cost of an MRI examination is currently greater than that for CT, whereas its spatial resolution is poorer. The exact role of MRI in pediatric disease is uncertain and will require further investigation, including comparative studies of MRI and CT. At present, there is little doubt that in some disorders, such as abnormalities in the posterior mediastinum and musculoskeletal system, MRI can provide unique information. But in most other areas, it provides information that can also be obtained with CT or other imaging studies.

TECHNIQUE

Special Preparation for Pediatric Patients

Sedation

Generally, no sedation is necessary for newborns and infants less than 1 month old if they are securely wrapped in blankets and restrained on a board. However, children from 1 month to 5 years of age often require sedation. A popular regimen is intramuscular secobarbital (Seconal®), 5 mg/kg (to a maximum dose of 100 mg), or intramuscular pentobarbital (Nembutal®), 6 mg/kg for a body weight up to 15 kg, or 5 mg/kg for children weighing more than 15 kg (to a maximum dose of 120 mg). The injection of either drug is given 20 min before scanning. If adequate

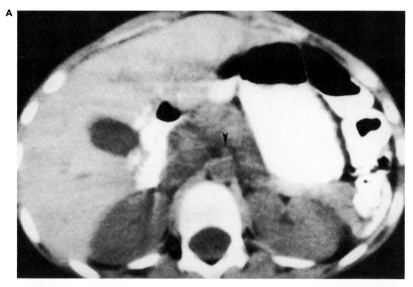

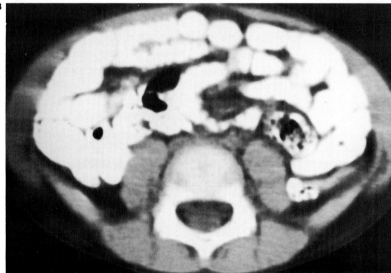

FIG. 1. Normal CT scans in a 7-year-old boy after oral administration of contrast material. **A:** Upper abdomen. Pancreatic body and tail are well profiled by contrast material in the surrounding antrum of the stomach and the descending duodenum. A small amount of fat surrounds the superior mesenteric artery (*arrowhead*). **B:** Lower abdomen. Abundant contrast material fills both the large bowel and small bowel completely, thereby excluding a retroperitoneal or mesenteric mass.

sedation is not achieved in 1 hr, a second dose of 2 mg/kg may be given intramuscularly. Sedation failure occurs in about 3% of patients, and supplemental sedation is required in about 15% (139). Most children are sufficiently alert to be discharged within 60 to 90 min after administration of these drugs. Recently, intravenous sedation with pentobarbital, 2 to 6 mg/kg (to a maximum dose of 100 mg), has been advocated. It is injected slowly in fractions of one-fourth to one-half the total dose and is titrated against the patient's response. Initial experience has shown intravenous barbiturate to be a safe, efficient, and effective form of sedation, with a failure rate of 0.5% and supplemental sedation necessary in only 4% of patients. The major advantages of intravenous barbiturate are its rapid action and the relatively short recovery time. The mean duration of drug activity, from injection to the time that it is safe to release the patient, is 55 min.

Other methods of sedation include chloral hydrate, rectal barbiturate, and a combination of meperidine, chlorpromazine, and promethazine, commonly referred to as a "cardiac cocktail." Chloral hydrate and rectal barbiturate have proved ineffective in sedating approximately 13% and 20% of patients, respectively (139). The prolonged duration of action for these drugs also is a major disadvantage. Moreover, the risks of apnea and respiratory and cardiac depression from narcotic analgesics (e.g., meperidine) are significantly greater than the risks from barbiturate sedation.

Because barbiturate sedation has fewer failures and a shorter mean duration of sedation, it is preferred by most examiners. Regardless of the choice of drug, the use of parenteral sedation requires the facility and ability to resuscitate and maintain adequate cardiorespiratory support during and after the examination.

Immobilization

Immobilization of young children frequently is required and may be accomplished by using a blanket and light sandbags. The child is snuggly wrapped in the blanket and secured to a board or pad on the CT table by velcro straps or adhesive tape. A light sandbag is placed on the lower extremities for restraint. The arms routinely are extended above the head to avoid streak artifacts and to provide an easily accessible route for intravenous injection. The upper extremities can be restrained with sandbags, adhesive tape, or velcro straps. Children 5 years of age or older generally will cooperate after verbal reassurance and explanation and will not need immobilization or sedation.

Temperature Regulation

Newborn infants must be kept warm to prevent complications associated with hypothermia. These include metabolic acidosis, hypoxemia, apnea, and disruption of coagulation, which can lead to intracranial hemorrhage. The safest and most effective technique for thermoregulation is to wrap the infant in several blankets that are secured with adhesive tape or velcro straps.

Intravenous Contrast Material

Scanning after intravenous administration of iodinated contrast material is helpful in confirming a lesion thought to be of vascular origin or closely related to vascular structures, in addition to improving differentiation between normal and pathologic parenchyma, especially in the liver and kidneys. If intravenous contrast material is to be administered, it is helpful to have an intravenous line in place when the child arrives in the department. Clearly, this reduces patient agitation that otherwise would be associated with venipuncture performed prior to administration of contrast material. The largest butterfly needle or plastic cannula that can be placed is recommended. For most pediatric chest and abdominal CT examinations, a 50% to 60% solution of iodinated contrast material at a dose of 2 ml/kg (not to exceed 4 ml/kg) is administered intravenously as a bolus injection. In the pelvis, a smaller amount of contrast material, usually 1 ml/kg, is given, because dense contrast material in the bladder sometimes results in scan artifact and obscures adjacent structures. Generally, scanning is begun after half the bolus has been injected and is continued during the remainder of the injection and until the desired images have been obtained. Delayed scans may be required to delineate the ureters and bladder.

Bowel Opacification

For most examinations of the abdomen, opacification of the small bowel and large bowel with contrast material

(dilute Gastrografin or E-Z Cat) given orally or through a nasogastric tube is necessary. The only exception is when the CT scan is performed as part of an evaluation for subtle calcifications or foreign bodies. The oral contrast agents usually can be given without additional flavoring, but they may be mixed with fruit juice and supplemented with water if needed. If the contrast agent is given 45 to 60 min before the examination and again 15 min prior to scanning, the small bowel usually is fairly well opacified (Fig. 1). Giving contrast agent 3 to 4 hr before CT or the evening before the examination will opacify the colon and is helpful in examining the pelvis, especially in older children. Streak artifacts from dessication of barium in the colon are seen occasionally when contrast medium is given several hours prior to scanning, but the advantage of this method is total bowel opacification, eliminating the possibility of unopacified bowel loops simulating a mass. The amount of oral contrast material given depends on body weight, but it generally approximates that of an average feeding. Sedation can be given approximately 10 min after the last dose of oral contrast material has been given. With this approach, we have had no problems with aspiration.

Imaging Techniques

For optimal examination of children, rapid scanners are necessary, because patient motion can cause significant degradation of the CT image. In patients who can cooperate, scans generally are performed with 4- or 5-sec timing. Uncooperative or sedated patients are scanned with 3-sec exposures. More recently, ultrafast CT with data acquisition times of 0.05 to 0.1 sec have been demonstrated to be useful for evaluating pediatric diseases (21). Slice thickness and interval will vary with the age of the patient, the area of interest, and the clinical indication for the examination. Generally, in chest examinations in older children, 1-cm collimated sections at 1-cm intervals are obtained from the thoracic inlet to the subdiaphragmatic region. In abdominal examinations, 1-cm collimated sections at 1- or 2-cm intervals are obtained from the xiphoid to the symphysis pubis. Decreased collimation (2–5 mm) and decreased scanning intervals (5 mm to 1 cm) are reserved for areas of maximum interest, for detailed examinations such as evaluation of pulmonary nodules or the adrenal, and for very small children. If the patient is cooperative, sections are obtained with breath holding at suspended inspiration. CT sections are obtained at resting lung volume if the patient is sedated.

Larger images that are more easily interpreted may be obtained either by magnification of the scan prior to filming or by using a limited circle of reconstruction. The latter technique offers the possibility of reconstructing, from the raw data, selected areas of the object scanned in order to reduce the pixel size to optimal values. Ideally, a pixel should be much smaller than the minimal distance

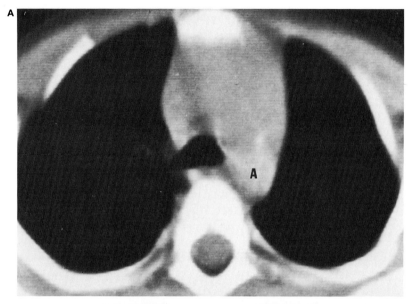

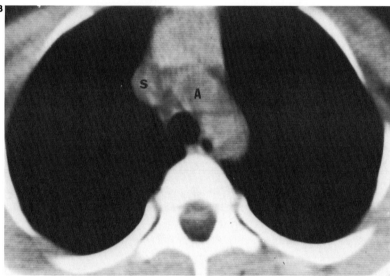

FIG. 2. A: Normal thymus in a 2-year-old girl. The thymus is quadrilateral in shape, with slightly convex lateral margins. Lack of mediastinal fat precludes clear separation from the aorta (A). **B:** Normal thymus in a 5-year-old boy. A quadrilateral shaped thymus is seen separated by fat from the aortic arch (A) and superior vena cava (S). The density of the thymus is equal to that of chest wall musculature.

resolvable by the scanner. The small circle of reconstruction results in improved spatial resolution and sharper, larger images. Because limited-field reconstruction scans do not require additional radiation, they should be obtained routinely in pediatric patients.

CHEST

Mediastinum

As in adults, CT is able to identify some normal mediastinal structures not seen on conventional chest radiographs, but the lack of fat in the mediastinum frequently precludes identification of each separate vessel. In the pediatric population, the normal thymus will be seen in virtually every patient. One must be aware that the appearance of the thymus changes with age, and in individuals under age 20 there are wide variations in size and shape

of the normal thymus (9,39,48,56,119). Recognition of the various appearances of the normal thymus is important if errors in diagnosis are to be avoided.

In patients under the age of 5 years, the thymus has a quadrilateral shape and is homogeneous in appearance, with convex lateral margins, although occasionally these may be straight (Fig. 2). As the thymus enlarges in the first decade and until puberty, it remains homogeneous, while assuming a more triangular appearance (Fig. 3). After puberty, areas of inhomogeneity may be visible on CT because of fatty infiltration. In general, in the first two decades of life the thymus abuts the sternum, separating the two lungs; a distinct anterior junction line between the lungs is rare. Rarely, thymic tissue can extend into the posterior mediastinum. On CT, this appears as a soft-tissue mass with a smooth margin extending from the anterior to posterior chest wall (33).

Mean values and standard deviations (SD) for thymic thickness, anteroposterior dimension, craniocaudad ex-

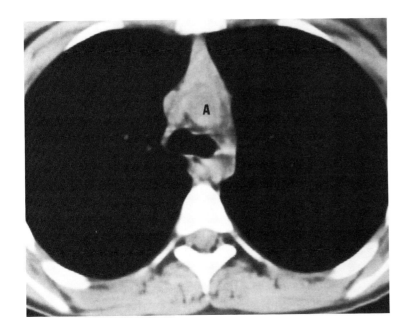

FIG. 3. Normal thymus in a 13-year-old girl. The thymus has assumed a more triangular appearance and is separated by fat from the aortic arch (A). The anterior junction line separating the two lungs is poorly developed at this age. Thus the thymus abuts the sternum.

tent, and transverse dimension vary with age (48,119). The craniocaudad measurements correlate directly with increasing age and appear to account for most of the increase in thymic size as imaged on CT. Anteroposterior and transverse dimensions show little change. Thymic thickness (the largest dimension perpendicular to the long axis of the lobe) correlates inversely with age, decreasing from 1.50 (0.46 SD) for patients 0 to 10 years of age to 1.05 (0.36 SD) for patients between 10 and 20 years. For infiltrative diseases of the thymus, thickness is a fairly sensitive indicator of an abnormality (8,9,48,119).

Indications for CT of the mediastinum include (a) characterization of mediastinal widening or a mass of uncertain origin suspected or clearly detected on chest radiography, (b) determination of the extent of a proven mediastinal tumor associated with an abnormal radiograph, and (c) evaluation of a mediastinum that appears normal on plain chest radiography in a patient with an underlying disease or radiographic signs that may be associated with a mediastinal mass. In these clinical settings, CT frequently supplies additional diagnostic information beyond that provided by conventional chest radiography (39,71,133).

Mediastinal Mass of Undetermined Cause Seen on Chest Radiograph

An abnormal mediastinum in infants and children often is due to a mass lesion, most commonly a neurogenic tumor, teratoma, lymphoma, or cyst of foregut origin (20,64,111). Abundant mediastinal fat and aneurysms or tortuosity of the mediastinal vessels are rare in children. CT confers the capability of differentiating among lesions composed predominantly of fat, water, or soft tissues, and therefore it often can permit a more accurate diagnosis

than can conventional techniques (10). Localized fatty masses in children usually are due to herniation of omental fat through the foramen of Morgagni and are easily recognized on CT scans (Fig. 4). Lesions that can present with attenuation values near that of water include pericardial cysts, thymic cysts, lymphangiomas, and the duplication cysts of foregut origin (77,102,103) (Fig. 5). Rarely, bronchogenic cysts or duplication cysts can have a density equal to that of soft tissue, because they contain thick viscid contents, not simple serous fluid (77,94,102). Vascular causes of mediastinal widening, such as an aortic aneurysm or a congenital anomaly of the thoracic vascular system, usually can be identified with confidence on CT

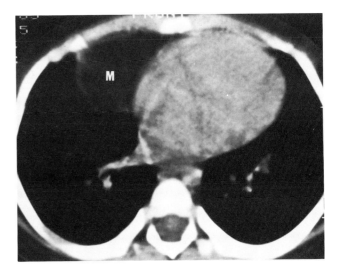

FIG. 4. Morgagni hernia in a 4-year-old girl with a right-cardiophrenic-angle mass on chest radiograph. Findings on chest radiograph 1 year previously had been normal. CT scan shows that the mass (M) has an attenuation value characteristic of fat. The primary consideration was a Morgagni hernia containing omentum, which was proved surgically.

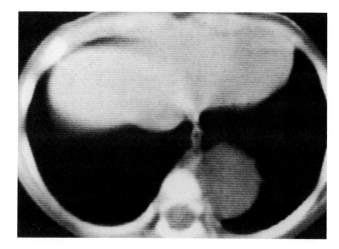

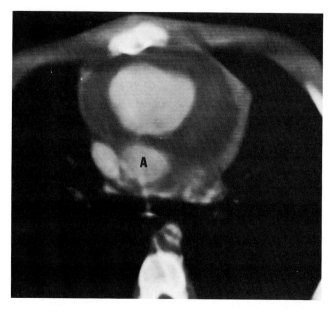

FIG. 5. Bronchogenic cyst in a 2-year-old boy. CT scan shows a well circumscribed homogeneous mass in the middle posterior mediastinum. The mass has an attenuation value slightly above that of water, consistent with a benign duplication cyst.

FIG. 6. Pseudoaneurysm of the aorta following prior surgery. Contrast-enhanced CT scan shows an enhancing pseudoaneurysm anterior to the ascending aorta (A). Lower-density thrombus surrounds the pseudoaneurysm.

scans after bolus injection of contrast material (7,151) (Fig. 6).

When a mass has an attenuation value equal to that of soft tissue, CT may be valuable in determining the extent or origin of the soft tissue density, but a specific pathologic diagnosis generally is not possible. The differential diagnosis, however, can be narrowed by determining the location of the mass in the mediastinum.

Anterior mediastinal masses

Germ cell tumors and lymphomas are the most common masses in the anterior mediastinum. Nearly all germ cell neoplasms are benign and dermoid cysts or teratomas. These lesions typically arise in the thymus or occur near the base of the great vessels. On CT, they are well-defined, thick wall cystic masses containing a variable admixture of densities: fat, water, soft tissue, and calcium (85). When calcifications or fat are present, the diagnosis of a germ cell neoplasm can be strongly suspected, but only half demonstrate these components (140). Malignant teratoma seems to be distinguishable from its benign counterpart

in most cases; it is poorly defined, of soft tissue density and invades and compresses surrounding structures. Hodgkin lymphoma is the other common cause of an anterior mediastinal mass in children and frequently infiltrates the thymus, producing relatively symmetric enlargement and lobulated, convex borders (Fig. 7). Associated mediastinal lymph node enlargement and displacement of vascular structures and airway are frequent.

Thymic hyperplasia, thymic cysts, and thymomas are more unusual anterior mediastinal masses. On CT, the hyperplastic thymus may be of normal size or diffusely enlarged, especially in thickness, with maintenance of its normal shape (Fig. 8). Thymic hyperplasia rarely may present as a dominant nodule (119). Thymoma is a rare solid neoplasm that originates from thymic epithelium. The CT appearance of thymomas varies from a focal soft tissue mass bulging the lateral thymic contour to a large lobulated mass totally replacing the organ. Calcifications have been reported in about one-third of thymomas. Ap-

FIG. 7. Lymphoma involving the thymus in a 17-year-old girl. CT scan demonstrates a large soft-tissue mass filling the anterior mediastinum and compressing and displacing the trachea. The planes around the great vessels are obscured. Axillary adenopathy and a left pleural effusion also are noted.

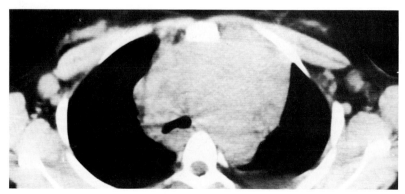

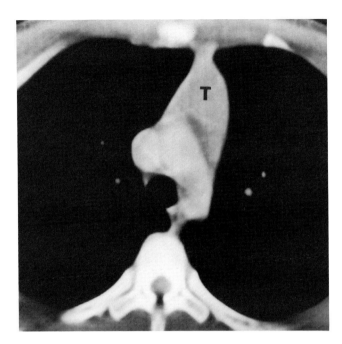

FIG. 8. Thymic hyperplasia in a 17-year-old boy with myasthenia gravis. The thymus (T), especially the left lobe, is too large for the patients age. Normal mediastinal fat separates the thymus from the aorta.

proximately 15% of thymomas are malignant. Malignant or invasive thymoma is associated with pulmonary metastases and mediastinal, pleural, or pericardial invasion. Thymic cyst can be encountered incidentally on a chest radiograph or can result from prior radiation treatment for mediastinal Hodgkin disease. On CT, a benign thymic cyst appears as a homogeneous, near water density mass with an imperceptible wall and no soft tissue elements. Although some teratomas or lymphomas may be predominantly cystic, they nearly always have a thick wall or soft tissue elements.

Middle mediastinal masses

Lymph node enlargement and bronchopulmonary foregut cysts are common causes of a soft tissue mass in the middle mediastinum or hilar regions. The former is usually due to lymphoma or granulomatous disease. On CT, adenopathy may appear as discrete, nonenhanced, round soft tissue densities or a single, solid mass with a poorly defined margin. If calcification is present, a diagnosis of granulomatous disease can be suggested (Fig. 9). In the absence of calcification, CT is valuable in predicting whether mediastinoscopy or thoracotomy would be better to yield a diagnosis. Foregut cysts are classified as bronchogenic, duplication, or neurenteric depending on their histology and most often are located near the carina or in the middle-posterior mediastinum. The CT appearance of a foregut cyst is usually that of a well circumscribed, round nonenhancing mass. As discussed previously, the attenuation values are often near water because they con-

tain serous fluid, but some have a density equal to soft tissue because their contents are viscus. Air-fluid levels may be present when a communication between the cysts and bronchial tree or gastrointestinal tract develops. Occasionally the cyst may have peripheral linear calcifications.

Posterior mediastinal masses

Posterior mediastinal tumors are of neural origin in approximately 95% of cases and may originate from ganglion cells (neuroblastoma, ganglioneuroblastoma, and ganglioneuroma) or nerve sheaths (neurofibromas). Nerve sheath tumors are rarely malignant, whereas ganglion cell tumors have varying degrees of malignancy. On CT, neural tumors are paraspinal in location and usually of soft tissue density, but they may be of lower density if the neural tissue contains a high amount of lipids. Benign tumors typically are elliptical or round, sharply marginated and homogeneous, while malignant lesions tend to be lobulated, have ill-defined borders and contain calcifications in up to 50% of cases (Figs. 10, 11). Because of their origin from neural tissue, neurogenic tumors have a tendency to invade the spinal canal. Recognition of intraspinal invasion is important because such involvement necessitates a laminectomy prior to tumor debulking. CT in conjunction with metrizamide myelography or MR imaging are particularly useful in depicting intraspinal tumor extension (6,113,114,130).

Malignant Mediastinal Neoplasms and Abnormal Chest Radiograph

Lymphoma and neuroblastoma are the commonest malignant mediastinal tumors in childhood. CT may contribute diagnostic information by demonstrating more extensive disease, including intraspinal or chest-wall ex-

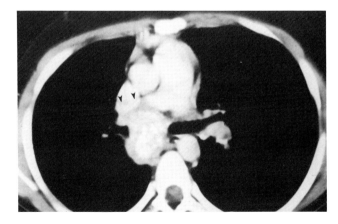

FIG. 9. Histoplasmosis in an 11-year-old boy. CT scan demonstrates a large, partially calcified subcarinal mass displacing the right pulmonary artery (*arrowheads*) anteriorly. Calcifications also are seen in the left hilum.

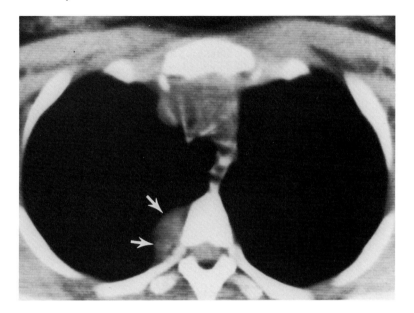

FIG. 10. Benign ganglioneuroma in a 15-year-old girl. CT scan at the level of the aortic arch shows a homogeneous, well-circumscribed soft-tissue mass (*arrows*) in the right paraspinal area, accounting for mediastinal widening noted on a chest radiograph.

tension, than expected from plain chest radiography. This information is helpful in providing a base line for follow-up examinations, but it appears to have little beneficial effect in regard to altering radiation or surgical management at the time of diagnosis in a patient with a known radiographic abnormality. Extrinsic tracheal compression also can be documented by CT; this does not lead to any alteration in therapy, but pretreatment knowledge may be important, because airway compression correlates with the presence of, or potential for, respiratory distress during radiation therapy (70). The use of CT to establish norms for tracheal cross-sectional areas in children of various ages has facilitated recognition of tracheal compression by mediastinal masses (42,53). In some patients, CT can be helpful in distinguishing between a mediastinal process and disease in the adjacent pulmonary parenchyma or pleura.

Underlying Disease and Normal Chest Radiograph

Computed tomography is useful in demonstrating thymic size and shape in patients with myasthenia gravis (8,133). In general, CT is not indicated in a child with myasthenia gravis and a normal chest radiograph, because of the extremely low incidence of thymoma in this age population. However, this type of investigation is rewarding in children with suspicious or abnormal chest radiographs. Delineation of a focal thymic mass can prompt surgery, whereas demonstration of a normal-size thymus, in conjunction with the knowledge that thymomas are rare in juvenile myasthenia gravis, can lead to medical management. Symmetric enlargement of the thymus suggests hyperplasia rather than thymoma (8). Demonstration of a hyperplastic thymus on CT, however, is not generally relevant to clinical decision making, be-

A,B

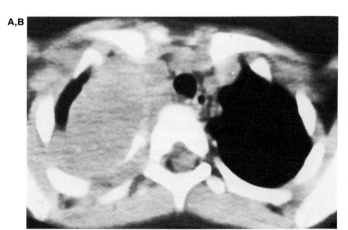
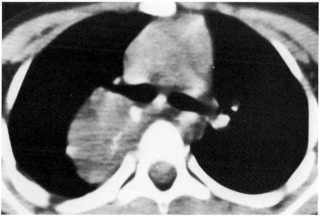

FIG. 11. Neuroblastoma in a 7-year-old boy. **A:** CT scan through the superior mediastinum shows a huge soft-tissue mass filling the right pulmonary apex. **B:** A section through the level of the carina shows the mass with calcification extending paraspinally. The posterior location of the tumor suggested a neuroblastoma, confirmed by surgical exploration.

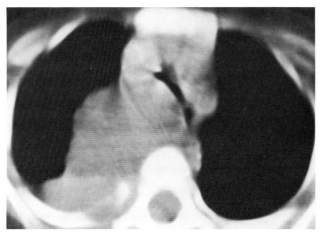
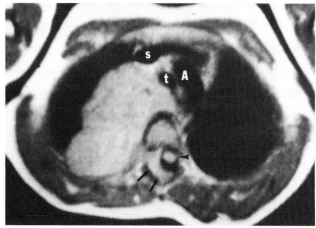

FIG. 12. Neuroblastoma in a 4-year-old girl. **A:** A CT scan through the superior mediastinum demonstrates a large paraspinal soft-tissue mass eroding the rib posteriorly and displacing and compressing the trachea. **B:** On a MR image (TR = 500 msec, TE = 30 msec) there is a high signal intensity paraspinal mass extending into the spinal canal and causing displacement of the spinal cord to the left. S = superior vena cava; A = aorta; t = trachea; arrows = intraspinal tumor; arrowhead = spinal cord.

cause there are no convincing data to suggest that removal of hyperplastic tissue is beneficial.

Enlarged lymph nodes in the paratracheal region, due to lymphoma, metastatic carcinoma, or infectious disease, may be recognized with CT and may prompt mediastinoscopy or thoracotomy. Additionally, the intrapericardial portions of the great vessels are well delineated, and anomalies such as aneurysm of the aorta in patients with Marfan syndrome can be diagnosed in a noninvasive fashion (7).

Comparative Imaging and Clinical Applications

Computed tomography can provide diagnostic information supplemental to that from conventional chest radiography in as many as 80% of patients known to have or suspected of having mediastinal abnormalities (133). CT is most useful in documenting a benign process, often

terminating the radiologic evaluation, and in demonstrating the full extent of a malignant neoplasm.

In comparison, MRI and CT are both sensitive for detection of mediastinal masses and provide comparable information on the presence and size of a lesion (24,131). MRI better discriminates a mediastinal mass and enlarged nodes from vascular structures and is more sensitive than CT in detecting intraspinal extension, whereas CT is better for demonstrating calcification and bronchial abnormalities (Figs. 12 and 13). Detection of airway or vascular compression usually does not indicate an alteration in therapy or prognosis, but demonstration of direct intraspinal extension is generally of therapeutic significance, because such affected patients usually undergo decompressive laminectomy prior to tumor debulking. Presently, however, the long examination time and additional expense combine to militate against MRI as the imaging technique to supplement the plain chest radiograph in a

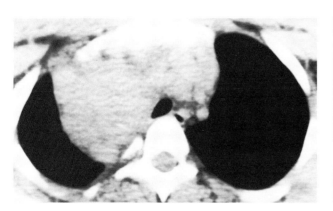
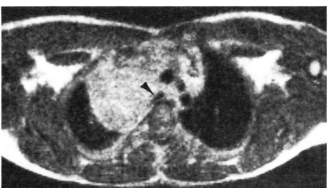

FIG. 13. Hodgkin disease in a 16-year-old boy. **A:** CT scan shows a mediastinal mass anterior to and slightly compressing the trachea. **B:** A T1 weighted MR image (TR = 500 msec, TE = 30 msec) demonstrates the mediastinal mass and more severe narrowing of the trachea (*arrowhead*) compared to CT. The patient, however, was asymptomatic and the narrowing was thought to be artifactual, due to respiratory motion and partial volume averaging. On MR the mass is easily separable from vessels.

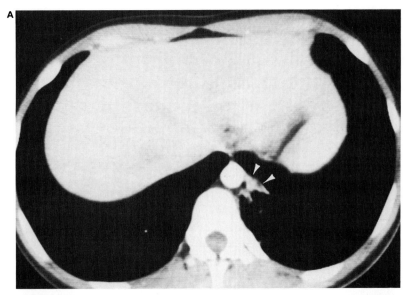

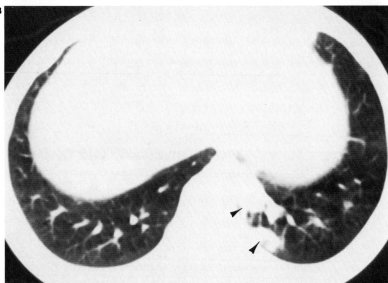

FIG. 14. Pulmonary sequestration in a 15-year-old girl with a chronic left lower lobe opacity on chest radiographs. **A:** CT scan through the lower thorax after intravenous administration of contrast material shows an anomalous vessel (*arrowheads*) extending to the left lower lobe. **B:** CT scan viewed at lung window settings demonstrates the anomolous vessel coursing posteriorly to areas of opacification (*arrowheads*) in the left lower lobe.

patient known to have or suspected of having mediastinal tumor. The two major advantages of MRI—that it does not involve ionizing radiation and does not require intravenous contrast material—are not important enough to overcome its disadvantages. We believe that CT still is the examination of choice for assessing the mediastinum, but MRI is the method of choice for evaluating patients with posterior mediastinal masses, because of the high likelihood of intraspinal extension.

Lungs

Pulmonary Metastases

Computed tomography is a valuable technique in searching for pulmonary metastases in patients with known malignancies with a high propensity for lung dissemination, such as Wilms tumor, osteogenic sarcoma, and rhabdomyosarcoma. Demonstration of a pulmonary nodule or nodules in such a patient, as well as additional nodules in a patient with an apparent solitary metastasis for whom surgery is planned, may be critical to treatment planning. In the first instance, such detection may lead to additional treatment (surgery, chemotherapy, or radiation), whereas in the latter setting, demonstration of several metastatic nodules may negate surgical plans. Our own experience and that of others comparing CT, plain chest radiography, and conventional tomography in children and adults support the contention that CT is able to demonstrate larger numbers of metastases, especially those located peripherally (pleural or subpleural) (31,40,72,100,121). More nodules are detected by CT, than by other examinations in up to 45% of patients. Confusion with benign granulomas does not appear to be as significant a clinical problem in children as it is in adults; almost all noncalcified nodules depicted by CT are due to metastases rather than granulomatous disease.

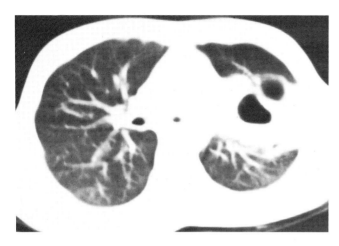

FIG. 15. Cystic adenomatoid malformation in a 10-year-old boy with recurrent lingular pneumonia and cystic areas on plain chest radiographs. CT scan with lung window settings demonstrates a large thick-walled mass containing two air-filled cavities.

Congenital Lesions

Chronic or recurrent segmental or subsegmental pneumonitis in children, especially at a lung base, is a finding suggestive of sequestration. Pathologically, a sequestered portion of lung has no normal connection with the tracheobronchial tree and is supplied by an anomalous artery, usually arising from the aorta. When the sequestered lung is confined within the normal visceral pleura and has venous drainage to the pulmonary veins, it is termed "intralobar." When the sequestered lung has its own pleura and venous drainage to systemic veins, it is referred to as "extralobar." Although demonstration of an anomalous vessel occasionally may be achieved by plain chest radiography or conventional tomography, CT is more sensitive for identifying such a vessel and may obviate aortography (96,105). Dynamic CT scanning after a bolus injection of contrast material demonstrates opacification of the anomalous vessel immediately following the enhancement of the descending thoracic aorta. The anom-

alous vessel often can be traced to the sequestered lung. The CT appearance of the pulmonary sequestration depends on whether or not the sequestered lung is aerated. When the sequestration communicates with the remainder of the lung, usually after being infected, it appears cystic; a sequestration that does not communicate appears as a homogeneous density, usually in the posterior portion of the lower lobe (Fig. 14).

Congenital lobar emphysema, cystic adenomatoid malformation; and bronchial atresia are other congenital lung anomalies resulting from abnormal bronchial development that can also be demonstrated by CT. In congenital lobar emphysema the affected lobe is severely hyperinflated with attenuated vascularity and causes compression of adjacent lung. Cystic adenomatoid malformation appears as a parenchymal mass that may be predominantly solid or cystic or contain an admixture of solid and cystic components (Fig. 15). The radiographic features of bronchial atresia include overaerated lung distal to the atresia and a round or ovoid density, representing mucoid impaction, just beyond the atretic bronchus (29,110). Although CT can evaluate these conditions, it is usually not required for the diagnosis. However, it may be performed to determine the extent of abnormality in patients in whom surgery is contemplated or to exclude other anomalies, such as bronchogenic cyst or pulmonary sling, which may cause aeration abnormalities.

An additional congenital lung abnormality with vascular anomalies that can be diagnosed by CT is the hypogenetic lung or scimitar syndrome (3). The diagnosis usually can be provided by conventional radiographs, but when these are equivocal, dynamic CT scanning is a convenient noninvasive method of establishing the diagnosis. This anomaly consists of partial hypoplasia of the right lung, ipsilateral displacement of the mediastinum, absence or hypoplasia of the corresponding pulmonary artery and occasionally partial anomalous pulmonary venous return from the right lung to the inferior vena cava (Figs. 16, 17). The hypogenetic lung may be supplied by systemic

FIG. 16. Congenital absence of the right pulmonary artery in a 6-month-old girl with decreased volume in the right lung and a small right hilum on chest radiography. A CT scan after intravenous contrast medium administration shows a normal left pulmonary artery (LPA) coursing over the left mainstem bronchus and no right pulmonary artery. Fibrofatty tissue (arrow) and small nodes fill the space anterior to the bronchus intermedius, normally filled by the main right pulmonary artery.

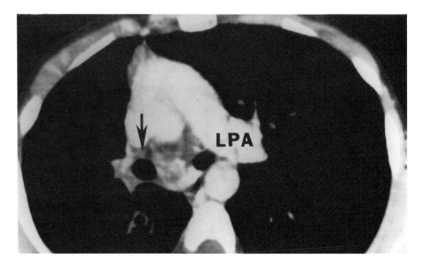

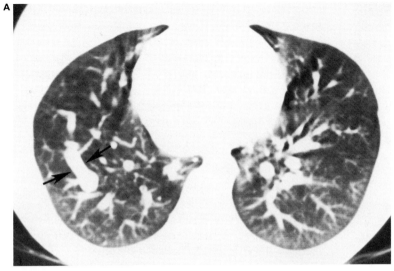

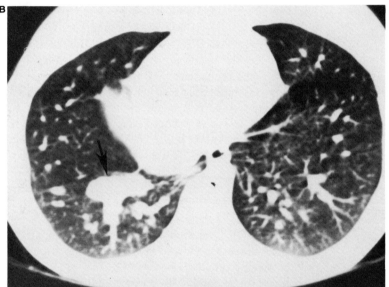

FIG. 17. A: Hypogenetic lung syndrome in an 18-year-old girl with a small right hemithorax, dextrocardia and a tubular density in the right lower lobe on chest radiography. CT scan at the level of the cardiac ventricles shows a smaller right hemithorax and an anomalous pulmonary vein (*arrows*). **B,C:** Several centimeters lower, the anomalous vessel (*arrow*) courses medially and inferiorly before entering the inferior vena cava (IVC).

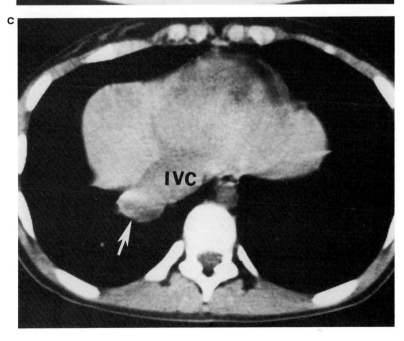

arteries, thus producing a left to right shunt. Several anomalies associated with hypogenetic lung syndrome can occur and be seen on CT scans. These include the accessory diaphragm and horseshoe lung. Horseshoe lung is a rare anomaly in which the posterobasal segments of both lungs are fused behind the pericardial sac. CT scanning can demonstrate the aerated isthmus as well as the other malformations of the scimitar syndrome. Cardiac anomalies also are common with pulmonary hypoplasia.

Parenchymal or Pleural Disease

In some patients, CT can be helpful in distinguishing between a parenchymal process and a pleural or extrapleural process. Lung abscess, pleural thickening, a mass, or a large effusion, as well as extension of a pleural process into the chest wall, may be detected by CT scans. On CT, the features of parenchymal lesions are a rounded or oval shape, acute or abrupt angles at the interface with the chest wall, and poorly defined margins with the adjacent lung. The CT features of pleural disease are a lenticular or crescentic shape, obtuse or tapering angles at the interface with the chest wall, and well-defined margins with adjacent lung, bone, and soft tissues. Extrapleural lesions are lenticular in shape, have poorly defined margins, and have obtuse or tapering angles at the interface with the pleura.

MRI currently has a limited role in evaluating pulmonary disease, including pleural processes. Although it is sensitive for detection of a wide variety of disorders of the lungs and pleura, it adds little clinically significant information over that gained with CT (118). For identification of small pulmonary nodules, it appears that MRI may even be less sensitive than CT (101).

ABDOMEN

The appearances of the abdomen on CT examinations are comparable in adults and children, except for the limitations imposed by the small sizes of the structures being examined and the relative paucity of perivisceral fat. Four major categories usually prompt CT examination of the abdomen: (a) determination of site of origin, extent, or character of an abdominal mass; (b) determination of the extent of a proven lymphoma; (c) determination of the presence or absence of abscess when it is suspected; (d) evaluation of the extent of injury from blunt abdominal trauma. Less often, CT is used to evaluate parenchymal disease of the kidney, liver, and pancreas, as well as abnormalities of the major abdominal vessels.

Abdominal Masses

Abdominal masses in the pediatric population are predominantly retroperitoneal in location, with the kidney

being the source in more than half of the cases (52,73). Beyond the neonatal period, the percentage of malignant neoplasms increases, and there is a decreased incidence of benign cystic masses (66). CT, with its superior demonstration of anatomy, has an increasingly important role in older infants and children in determining the site and extent of a mass, as well as the presence or absence of metastatic disease (30,81,128,136).

Renal Masses

Hydronephrosis and multicystic dysplastic kidneys are the causes of most abdominal masses in neonates, although any form of renal cystic disease may present as nephromegaly and be misdiagnosed as a solid tumor. Although CT can be used to detect and diagnose these conditions, usually it is unnecessary if the diagnosis can be established with urography or ultrasonography (US). If the cause or level of obstruction is uncertain, CT may provide the diagnosis (Fig. 18). On non-contrast-enhanced CT scans, the dilated collecting system of a hydronephrotic kidney appears as an area of low attenuation value within an enlarged renal silhouette. After contrast material is injected intravenously, delayed function on the affected side may be seen. In less severely affected kidneys, the entire collecting system usually is opacified on delayed CT scans, whereas in chronic obstruction, function usually is very poor or absent.

Wilms Tumor

Wilms tumor is the most common primary malignant renal tumor of childhood and accounts for approximately 20% of all abdominal masses (66,73). Affected children present most often under 4 years of age with a palpable abdominal mass, and less frequently with abdominal pain, fever, and microscopic or gross hematuria. Metastases are characteristically to the lungs and less frequently to the liver. On CT, a Wilms tumor usually appears as a large, spherical, and at least partially intrarenal mass, usually with a central density slightly lower than that of normal renal parenchyma (30,45,87,106,112). The periphery of the neoplasm, often referred to as a pseudocapsule, usually approximates the density of normal kidney and generally can be enhanced by the use of iodinated contrast material, although not to the same degree as functioning normal renal parenchyma. Frequently, the most central portion of the tumor is not enhanced after administration of contrast material, corresponding to areas of necrosis or hemorrhage, which occur in up to 80% of cases (112) (Fig. 19). Fewer than 15% of Wilms tumors contain calcifications or fat as a minor component (45,104). The fat may be focal and central or diffuse throughout the mass. Poor or absent function of the involved kidney occurs in about 10% of patients, resulting from either invasion or compression of hilar vessels or the collecting system or extensive infiltration of tumor throughout the kidney.

A,B

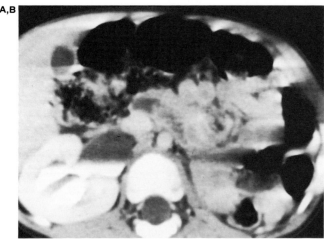

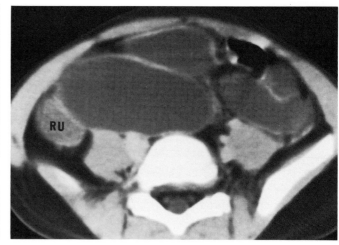

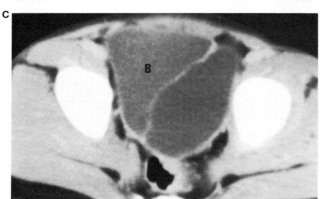

C

FIG. 18. Marked right hydroureter secondary to reflux and left hydroureter secondary to a ureterocele. **A:** A contrast enhanced CT scan through the upper abdomen shows a dilated right collecting system with a urine-contrast level in the renal pelvis. **B:** A CT scan at the pelvic inlet demonstrates several fluid-filled loops of a markedly dilated left ureter occupying almost the entire abdomen. A smaller tubular structure with a slightly higher density is noted in the right abdomen and corresponds to a dilated right ureter (RU). **C:** At a lower level the large fluid-filled distal left ureter is posterolateral to the displaced bladder (B). Surgical findings included a dysplastic left kidney with a huge ureter and a distal ureterocele.

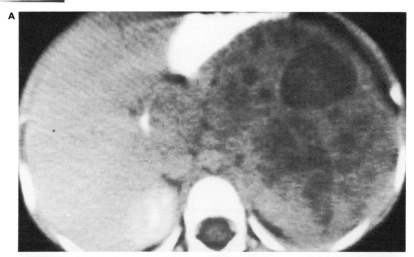

FIG. 19. Wilms tumor in a 4-year-old boy with a palpable abdominal mass. **A:** Contrast enhanced CT reveals a large soft-tissue mass with areas of necrosis in the area of the upper pole of the left kidney. The mass is lower in attenuation value than the liver. **B:** Caudad 4 cm, the mass is shown to be intrarenal, distorting the calices (c). The planes around the inferior vena cava and aorta are obscured, indicating extrarenal extension of tumor.

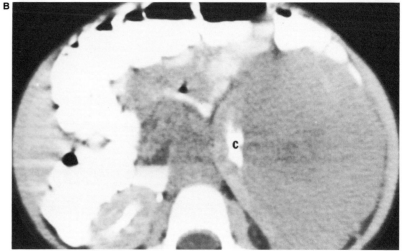

Intraabdominal extension may take the form of contiguous extension through the capsule, retroperitoneal lymphadenopathy, renal vein or inferior vena cava thrombosis, and hematogenous hepatic metastases. Perinephric tumor extension thickens the renal capsule and obliterates the perinephric fat. Lymph node involvement is demonstrated by enlarged perirenal, paracaval, para-aortic, or retrocrural lymph nodes. Renal vein thrombosis or tumor extension, which occurs in 4% to 10% of cases, may be demonstrated best after a bolus injection of contrast material. The thrombus may be seen as a low-density intraluminal defect or suggested by renal vein or inferior vena caval enlargement Fig. 20. Additionally, CT may identify bilateral tumors, present in as many as 5% to 10% of patients, and pulmonary or hepatic metastases. Besides being used for initial diagnosis, CT can be used to detect local recurrence in the renal fossa following nephrectomy.

Renal cell carcinoma

The mean age of presentation of children with renal cell carcinoma is approximately 9 years, in contrast to Wilms tumor with a mean age at presentation of 3 years. Presenting signs and symptoms are nonspecific and include mass (60%), pain (50%), and hematuria (30%). On CT, renal carcinoma is indistinguishable from Wilms tu-

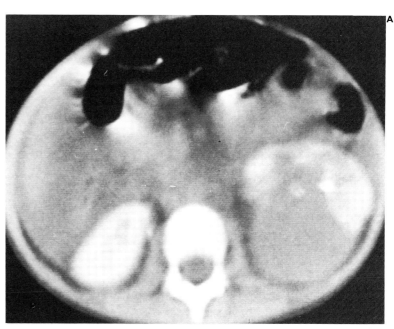

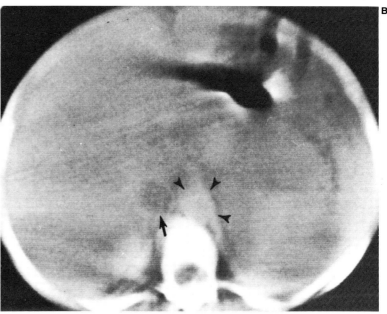

FIG. 20. Wilms tumor in an 18-month-old girl. **A:** CT scan after intravenous contrast medium administration shows a large, round, low-density intrarenal mass that distorts and displaces the calyces. The interface with the enhanced renal parenchyma is indistinct. **B:** At a higher level, the inferior vena cava (*arrows*) is noted to be of lower density than the aorta (*arrowheads*). A Wilms tumor with renal vein and inferior venal caval extension was confirmed at autopsy.

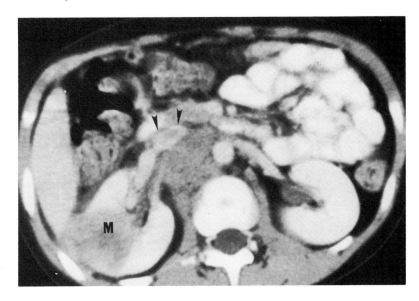

FIG. 21. Renal carcinoma in an 11-year-old boy with flank pain. Contrast-enhanced CT scan demonstrates a soft-tissue mass (M) in the mid-pole of the right kidney and multiple enlarged lymph nodes at the renal hilum. The inferior vena cava (*arrowheads*) containing tumor thrombus is displaced anteriorly.

mor, appearing as a solid intrarenal mass with ill-defined margins, often distorting the renal contour (Fig. 21). After intravenous administration of contrast medium, the mass enhances, but always less than that of the surrounding normal renal parenchyma. Calcification occurs in approximately 25% of tumors and is usually central (28). Like Wilms tumor, renal carcinoma may spread locally to retroperitoneal lymph nodes or may invade the renal vein and metastasize to lung or liver.

Lymphoma

Renal involvement by lymphoma is rare during the course of disease, but is not uncommon at autopsy. When present, it is more often associated with the non-Hodgkin rather than the Hodgkin form of disease (Fig. 22). The most common CT appearance is that of multiple bilateral nodules; these have been found in 28 to 43% of kidneys. Other manifestations include direct invasion from contiguous lymph node masses (10–25% of cases), solitary nodules (12–15% of cases) and diffuse infiltration (5% of cases) (30). Typically, the intrarenal tumors are hypodense relative to normal renal parenchyma and enhance less than normal renal tissue enhances after intravenous contrast medium administration. The CT appearance of renal lymphoma is indistinguishable from other solid intrarenal masses, but the diagnosis is possible when there is coexisting splenomegaly or widespread lymph node enlargement.

Mesoblastic nephroma

Mesoblastic nephroma, also termed fetal renal hamartoma, is a benign neoplasm that presents in the first year of life as an abdominal mass (16). On CT, the neoplasm appears as a fairly uniform intrarenal mass that enhances following intravenous contrast medium injection although not to the extent of normal renal paren-

chyma. Occasionally areas of cystic degeneration and necrosis are seen as low-density areas within the tumor. Invasion of the vascular pedicle or extension into the renal pelvis is rare, although the tumor may penetrate the renal capsule and invade the perinephritic space. Differentiation between Wilms tumor and mesoblastic nephroma is usually not possible without a biopsy.

Multilocular cystic nephroma

Multilocular cystic nephroma, also termed benign cystic nephroma, cystic hamartoma, cystic lymphangioma, and partial polycystic kidney, is a rare, nonhereditary cystic mass. Affected males are usually less than 4 years of age, while most females with the tumor are over 4 years of age. On CT, the lesion appears as a well-defined intrarenal mass with multiple cysts separated by septae (92). The

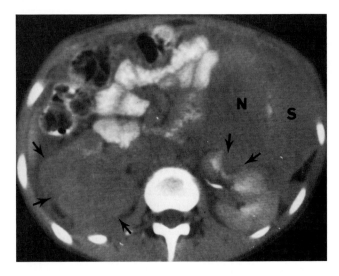

FIG. 22. Renal lymphoma in an 18-year-old girl. Soft tissue masses (*arrows*) are seen arising from both kidneys. Enlarged mesenteric lymph nodes (N) and splenomegaly (S) are also present.

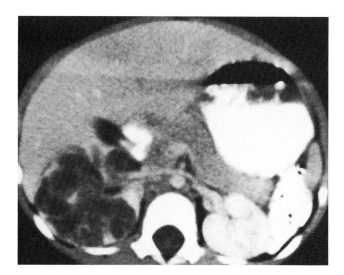

FIG. 23. Multilocular cystic nephroma in a 3-year-old boy. CT scan obtained after a bolus injection of intravenous contrast material shows a complex near-water density mass arising from the upper pole of the right kidney; internal septations, which enhance, are seen in this lesion.

cystic spaces do not enhance when contrast medium is given, but the septae are vascular and enhance after intravenous administration of contrast medium (Fig. 23). Curvilinear calcifications may be present within the wall or septae. When the cysts are small or filled with thick mucoid material, the multilocular nature may not be apparent and differentiation from Wilms tumor requires tissue sampling.

Angiomyolipoma

Renal angiomyolipoma is rare as an isolated lesion in the pediatric population, but is present in as many as 80% of children with tuberous sclerosis. These tumors most often are small, asymptomatic, and bilateral. Frequently they coexist with cystic renal disease, suggesting adult polycystic kidney disease on urography or US (97). Differentiation with CT usually is possible on the basis of differences in the attenuation values of cystic and lipomatous tissues (Fig. 24).

Inflammatory masses

Focal renal inflammatory masses may occur in the kidney and may represent either acute focal bacterial nephritis, if suppuration is absent, or an abscess, in the presence of liquefaction. Distinguishing between the two conditions is important, because acute focal nephritis responds well to antibacterial therapy, whereas an abscess may require surgical or percutaneous drainage. On CT, acute focal bacterial nephritis appears as a focal area or areas of diminished density without a well-defined wall. After intravenous administration of contrast material, inhomogeneous enhancement is seen in the involved area.

In contradistinction, an abscess often appears as a well-defined mass with a nonenhancing low-density center and a thick irregular wall exhibiting variable degrees of contrast enhancement (51,62,83). In most instances, the relative decreased density is apparent only after administration of contrast material. Perinephric extension and thickening of the renal fascia are more common with renal abscess than with acute focal nephritis.

Adrenal Masses

Neuroblastoma

Neuroblastoma is the most common solid malignant abdominal tumor in children under the age of 4 years. More than half of all neuroblastomas originate in the abdomen, with two-thirds of these arising in the adrenal gland. The extraadrenal tumors originate in the sympathetic ganglion cells or paraaortic bodies and may be found anywhere from the cervical region to the pelvis. Neuroblastoma tends to metastasize early, and more than half of all patients have bone marrow, skeletal, liver, or skin metastases when initially diagnosed. Lung metastases are rare and usually occur late in the course of disease.

The diagnosis of neuroblastoma can be rendered with confidence following CT, even when the lesion is small and escapes detection on urography or US (17,132). On CT, the tumor is recognized as an irregular, pararenal soft-tissue mass with lobulations, but no definable rim or pseudocapsule. On non-contrast-enhanced scans, the mass usually has a density lower than that of surrounding tissues (17,18,19,87,106,138). Intravenous administration of contrast material accentuates this difference. Calcifications

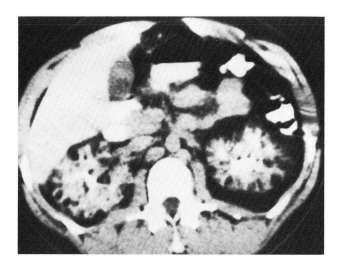

FIG. 24. Angiomyolipomas in a 16-year-old retarded boy with tuberous sclerosis. CT scan after intravenous administration of contrast material shows bilateral renal enlargement, distortion of the collecting systems, and multiple small renal masses of low attenuation value approaching fat density, consistent with angiomyolipomatosis.

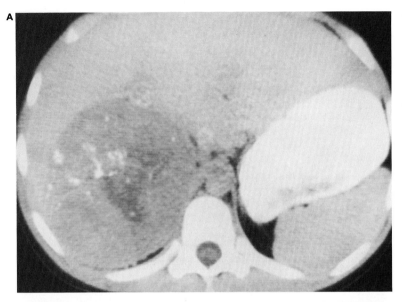

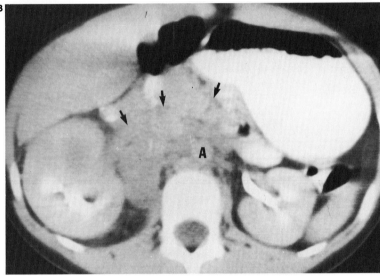

FIG. 25. Neuroblastoma in a 7-year-old boy with a palpable mass. **A:** CT scan through the upper abdomen demonstrates a low density mass with calcification in the right side of the abdomen behind the liver. **B:** At a lower level, the mass (*arrows*) is shown to extend across the midline in the retroperitoneum and surround the aorta (A). The planes around the vena cava are obscured.

within the tumor, which may be coarse, mottled, solid, or ring-shaped (4), can be observed in almost 85% of neuroblastomas on CT, whereas plain radiographs identify calcifications in only approximately 50% of patients (Fig. 25). Encasement and displacement of the aorta and inferior vena cava by the tumor, prevertebral extension across the midline, which occurs in up to 60% of patients, hepatic metastases and renal invasion can also be delineated (117). Intraspinal extension of tumor through intervertebral foramina occurs in about 15% of patients and is best seen on CT with metrizamide myelography or MRI (6,114,130). Following therapy, CT is valuable for monitoring the response to therapy and detecting recurrent disease (137).

Adrenocortical neoplasms

Adrenal lesions, other than neuroblastomas, are rare, accounting for 5% or less of all adrenal tumors. Of these the commonest are carcinomas; adenomas are next most frequent; and pheochromocytomas are the rarest adrenal tumors. The mean age of presentation for carcinoma is approximately 6 years and for adenomas 3 years (37). Adrenal carcinomas usually are hormonally active, producing virilization in girls and pseudoprecocious puberty in boys in about two-thirds of cases. Cushing syndrome, the overproduction of cortisol, is present in most of the remaining children with adrenal neoplasms. Approximately 60 to 80% of cases of Cushing syndrome in infants and young children are caused by adrenal carcinomas, whereas older children more often have adrenal adenomas or adrenal hyperplasia due to overproduction of pituitary ACTH. Primary aldosteronism is extremely rare in children and usually is caused by bilateral adrenocortical hyperplasia rather than an aldosterone secreting tumor. The latter when present usually are benign adenomas. Nonfunctioning adrenocortical tumors are extremely rare in childhood.

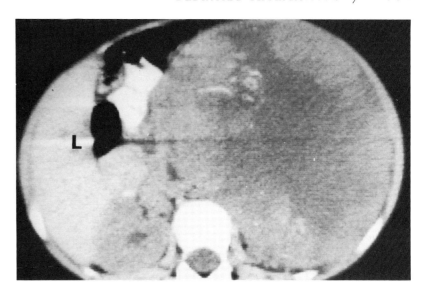

FIG. 26. Adrenal carcinoma in a 9-year-old girl with a palpable abdominal mass. A left upper quadrant mass is demonstrated by CT displacing the right lobe of the liver (L) laterally. Low density areas of necrosis as well as coarse central calcifications are present within the tumor.

Computed tomography has proved to be reliable in diagnosing adrenal masses with a reported accuracy of about 90%. Although the CT findings are not specific, a histologic diagnosis can be suggested when the CT findings are combined with biochemical tests. Adrenal carcinomas are typically large masses at the time of diagnosis, often greater than 4 cm in diameter. Many carcinomas contain low density areas from necrosis or prior hemorrhage and sometimes calcifications (Fig. 26). Local invasion occurs in about half of the cases of adrenal cancer (37). Adenomas are usually solitary, 2 to 5 cm in diameter, and may have low attenuation values because of their high lipid content. The rare aldosteronoma usually measures less than 2 cm in diameter, and like adenomas may be low density lesions because of a high fat content. In contradistinction to focal mass lesions, hyperplastic glands often demonstrate thickening of the limbs, but usually maintain a normal shape. Moreover, hyperplasia is bilateral, whereas primary mass lesions are generally unilateral with a normal appearing contralateral adrenal gland by CT.

Pheochromocytoma

Pheochromocytoma is a rare adrenal tumor in children. Approximately 70% to 75% of pheochromocytomas are located in the adrenal medulla, and the remainder are in extraadrenal locations, usually originating in the sympathetic ganglia adjacent to the vena cava or aorta, near the organ of Zuckerkandl, or in the wall of the urinary bladder (Fig. 27). Up to 70% of tumors are bilateral, and about 5% are malignant in children. The CT findings in pheochromocytomas are not specific, but with appropriate clinical findings the diagnosis usually is apparent. On CT, these tumors usually are larger than 2 cm in diameter and may be entirely solid, may contain both cystic and solid components, or may be almost entirely cystic (43). Calcifications within the tumor are rare.

Retroperitoneal Soft Tissue Masses

Although rare, both benign and malignant primary tumors may occur in the soft tissues of the retroperitoneum. Benign tumors usually are teratomas, lipomas, lymphangiomas, and neurofibromas. Teratomas most often arise in the sacrococcygeal region, but they can occur high in the retroperitoneal space. On CT, retroperitoneal teratoma appears as a well-defined mass with cystic and solid components and a variable amount of fat or calcium. A definitive diagnosis can be made if calcific and fatty com-

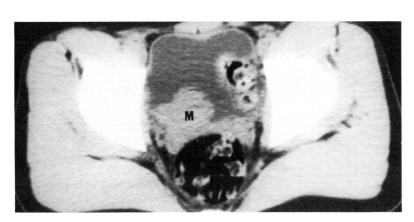

FIG. 27. Bladder pheochromocytoma in a 15-year-old boy with hypertension. A noncontrast CT scan shows a lobulated soft-tissue mass (M) projecting into the bladder lumen from the posterior wall.

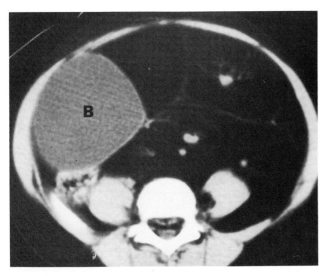

FIG. 28. Diffuse infiltrating lipomatosis in a 4-year-old girl with abdominal distention. Fatty density mass fills almost the entire abdomen displacing the bladder (B) superiorly and to the right. At surgery the tumor originated from the retroperitoneum and encased the major abdominal vessels.

usually homogeneous, well-defined cylindrical lesions with a characteristic location in the neurovascular bundle.

Rhabdomyosarcoma is the most common malignant tumor of the retroperitoneum, followed by liposarcoma, fibrosarcoma and extragonadal testicular tumors. Except for liposarcoma, all of these tumors produce bulky, solid retroperitoneal masses with attenuation values similar to muscle tissue. Liposarcomas usually are inhomogeneous, poorly marginated, or infiltrative and vary in density depending on the amount and distribution of fat to solid connective tissue.

Hepatic Tumors

Primary hepatic tumor is the third most frequent solid abdominal mass in children, following Wilms tumor and neuroblastoma. The majority of hepatic tumors are malignant, with hepatoblastoma and hepatoma being the most commonly encountered (149). The former occurs in children under the age of 3 years, whereas hepatocellular carcinoma is more frequent after 5 years of age. Usually these tumors are discovered as asymptomatic upper abdominal masses, occasionally associated with anorexia and weight loss. The CT appearances of hepatoblastoma and hepatocellular carcinoma are similar. The tumor usually is confined to a single lobe, with the right lobe affected twice as often as the left, but the lesion may involve both lobes or be multicentric. On non-contrast-enhanced CT scans both tumors appear as single or multiple solid masses that are of lower density than normal hepatic parenchyma, although occasionally the tumors are isodense and undetected on non-contrast-enhanced scans (2,14,76,126). Calcifications are seen by CT in up to 50% of cases. Malignant tumors usually become less dense than normal

ponents can be identified. If calcifications are absent and the teratoma has a high lipid content, it will be indistinguishable from a lipoma. Lipomas are seen on CT as sharply marginated homogeneous masses with attenuation values equal to normal fat. Rarely these masses are more diffuse and infiltrative, growing along fascial planes, and in places, invading musculature (148) (Fig. 28). The CT appearance of a lymphangioma is that of a well-circumscribed, multiloculated mass. The attenuation values within the loculi vary from that of fluid to that of fat, correlating with the variable nature of the cystic contents: chylous, serous, or hemorrhagic fluid. Neurofibromas are

FIG. 29. Hepatoblastoma in a 4-year-old girl with a right upper quadrant mass. Contrast enhanced CT scan demonstrates a large soft-tissue mass, slightly lower in density than the surrounding normal hepatic parenchyma, occupying the right lobe of the liver. A second smaller focus of tumor lies beneath the capsule of the left lateral segment (*arrowheads*).

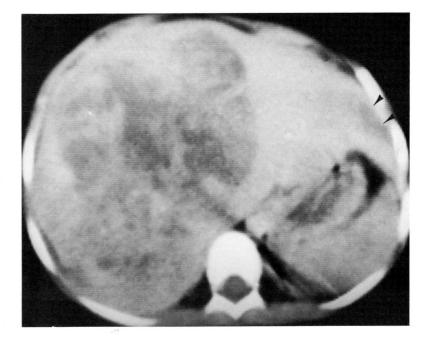

hepatic parenchyma following intravenous use of iodinated contrast material, but occasionally they may be isodense or hyperdense relative to the adjacent hepatic tissue (Fig. 29).

Benign hepatic tumors typically are of vascular origin, usually cavernous hemangiomas or hemangioendotheliomas; the latter are relatively more common in the newborn. Those tumors with significant arterial-venous shunting present early in the neonatal period with high-output cardiac failure, whereas tumors with less vascular shunting present later with hepatomegaly or are discovered incidentally. On non-contrast-enhanced CT scans, these lesions appear as well-circumscribed areas of low density that cannot readily be differentiated from any other non-vascular lesion. However, serial scans after bolus intravenous injection of contrast material demonstrate early peripheral enhancement and variably delayed central enhancement (36,88). In occasional cases, small tumors may rapidly become totally hyperdense and not show initial enhancement limited to the periphery.

After the vascular lesions, mesenchymal hamartoma is the next most common benign hepatic tumor of childhood. Most frequently this tumor is found as an asymptomatic mass in boys under 2 years of age. Rarely, the hamartoma has a large vascular component and produces arteriovenous shunting and congestive heart failure. On CT the tumor appears as a well-circumscribed mass containing multiple low-density cysts separated by solid septae. Following intravenous administration of contrast material, the central contents are not enhanced, but the thicker septae may appear more dense (14,50,115).

Biliary Masses

Choledochal cyst is the most common mass of the biliary ductal system. Patients with this condition classically present with jaundice, pain, and a palpable abdominal mass, although the complete triad is present in only about one-third of patients. CT can be used to detect and diagnose a choledochal cyst, but usually it is unnecessary if the diagnosis can be made by US supplemented by radionuclide studies using hepatobiliary agents. If the diagnosis remains in doubt, CT can suggest the diagnosis by demonstrating cystic dilatation of both intrahepatic and extrahepatic biliary ducts. The intrahepatic dilatation is limited to the central portions of the left and right hepatic ducts (5). Generalized ductal dilatation, with gradual tapering to the periphery, characteristic of acquired obstruction, is absent.

Comparative Imaging

Several series have shown that CT is the single most useful procedure for detecting and staging pediatric ab-

dominal tumors. Diagnostic accuracies of 95% and 71% for CT and US, respectively, have been reported in a variety of abdominal tumors (22). In a study comparing CT, US, skeletal scintigraphy, and urography in neuroblastoma, it was found that CT detected 100% of primary tumors and correctly staged the extent of disease in 82% of cases. US, scintigraphy, and urography alone correctly detected the tumors in 91%, 59%, and 45%, respectively, and defined the stage of the disease in 55%, 53%, and 15% of cases. CT understaged neuroblastoma in cases with distant skeletal metastases; when complemented by bone scintigraphy or marrow aspiration, the staging accuracy of CT was 97% (138). In our experience, CT is as sensitive (100%) as US for detecting Wilms tumor, but is superior to US for staging the extent of tumor (77% versus 23%, respectively). US is less accurate than CT in its ability to detect local extension and retroperitoneal spread of tumor (112).

Clinical Applications

The choice of examination for evaluation of a patient suspected of having an abdominal mass varies with the age of the patient, the available equipment and expertise at a given institution, and the relative advantages and disadvantages of each imaging method. An overview of the various diagnostic techniques follows.

Plain film radiography usually is performed prior to evaluation of an abdominal mass in any pediatric patient. The plain abdominal radiograph is simple, readily available, and inexpensive and can serve to confirm the presence, size, and position of a mass. Although such information may be helpful in planning other investigative procedures, the plain radiograph usually is not diagnostic.

Excretory urography with total-body opacification traditionally has provided the most useful and direct information about intraabdominal masses. However, urography at times not only fails to detect disease but also may underestimate its extent. Moreover, excretion of contrast material by the neonatal kidney is poor, and adequate delineation of the kidney often cannot be achieved. Nonetheless, excretory urography can be used to detect functioning tissue in obstructive or cystic renal disease and often is performed after the first week of life if information about renal function is required.

For the most part, radionuclide imaging has its greatest application in evaluating the degree of function of renal or hepatobiliary masses. Renal scintigraphy is superior to urography for detecting functioning renal tissue in severely obstructed kidneys and has the additional advantage of permitting quantitation of total and individual renal functions. Because radionuclide imaging is relatively organ-specific and has poor anatomic resolution, it has a limited role in diagnosing most abdominal masses, with the exception of utilizing a hepatobiliary agent to confirm the diagnosis of a choledochal cyst. Recently, ^{131}I-MIBG (metaiodobenzylguanidine), an adrenergic-tissue-localizing radiopharmaceutical, has been used to diagnose pheochromocytoma. The role of ^{131}I-MIBG in other tumors of the adrenal medulla, including neuroblastoma, is also under investigation.

Ultrasonography and CT are procedures that are excellent for revealing cross-sectional anatomy and usually provide more detailed information than the aforementioned radiologic techniques. US can be performed in multiple planes, does not require patient sedation, and does not involve ionizing radiation. It can clearly reveal the location, extent, and solid or cystic nature of a mass. It is especially important in evaluating neonatal abdominal masses, because the majority of these are benign. However, it provides no information concerning the function or vascularity of the mass. In addition, gas-filled viscera, normally found in young children, can impair sound transmission. The advantage of CT over the other imaging techniques lies in its ability to distinguish small differences in tissue densities (blood, fat, calcium) as well as to provide images unobscured by overlying structures, such as bowel gas or bone. Thus, it is ideal in assessing tumor extent in the retroperitoneum, because artifacts from gas-filled viscera do not arise with CT as with ultrasound. However, CT is not without certain drawbacks.

These include exposure to ionizing radiation, the necessity for sedation in most children under 5 years of age, and the need to use an oral contrast agent, because infants and children have little perivisceral fat, making anatomic delineation difficult in many cases.

Because of these limitations, US usually is considered the screening technique of choice for evaluation of a pediatric abdominal mass. If the US study is normal, further radiographic evaluation generally is not required. If US cannot yield adequate information or if it suggests a malignant mass, CT generally should be considered, particularly in the latter instances to better delineate the tumor extent. CT is recommended in preference to US if clinical findings or plain radiographs suggest a malignant neoplasm.

The exact role of MRI for evaluation of abdominal masses presently is uncertain, but preliminary reports suggest that this technique can effectively demonstrate primary and metastatic disease and aid in predicting tumor resectability (11,34,46). It is especially well-suited for displaying vascular encasement and intraspinal extension of tumor. At this moment, however, MRI has no proven advantage over CT in the diagnosis and management of renal tumors. In contrast, MRI is the preferred imaging technique in patients with a paraspinal neoplasm, since these tumors have a likelihood of intraspinal extension

A,B

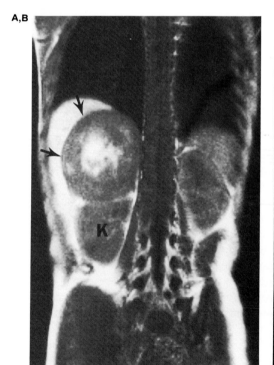
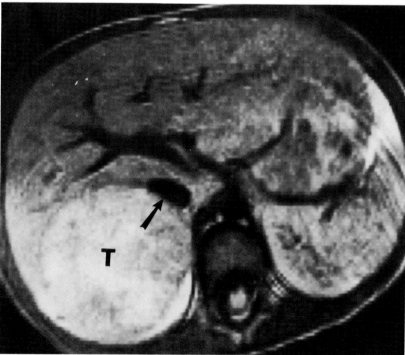

FIG. 30. Neuroblastoma in a 2-year-old girl. MR imaging was performed to exclude spinal involvement. **A:** On a coronal T1-weighted image (TR = 300 msec, TE = 15 msec) the tumor of the right adrenal gland (*arrows*) has an intensity similar to that of kidney (K). High signal intensity within the neoplasm reflects hemorrhage. The interface with the kidney and spine are well-defined. **B:** On an axial T2-weighted image (TR = 2100 msec, TE = 30 msec) the signal intensity of the tumor increases and is easily differentiated from adjacent liver. The inferior vena cava (*arrow*) is displaced anteriorly by the tumor (T).

A,B

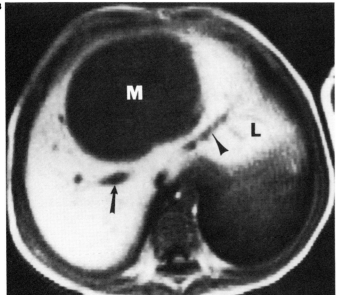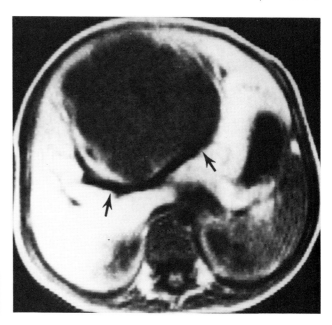

FIG. 31. Hepatoblastoma in a 10-month-old girl with abdominal distention. The lateral segment of the left lobe was obscured by streak artifacts on CT so MR imaging was obtained to determine precisely the extent of tumor involvement. **A:** A T1-weighted image (TR = 300 msec, TE = 15 msec) demonstrates a mass (M) of decreased signal intensity in the anterior segment of the right lobe and the medial segment of the left lobe. Particularly well-defined are the right (*arrows*) and left (*arrowheads*) hepatic veins. The middle hepatic vein is not visualized reflecting tumor encasement. The lateral segment (L) of the left lobe is normal. **B:** Three centimeters caudad, the tumor displaces the portal vein branches (*arrows*) posteriorly.

(Fig. 30). It also has an important role in determining the extent of hepatic neoplasms, particularly the relationship of a lesion to adjacent hepatic vascular structures (152) (Fig. 31).

Lymphoma

Although CT commonly demonstrates normal-size lymph nodes in the retroperitoneum and pelvis in the adult, these are rarely recognized in children. However, lymphoma and metastatic disease of any cause may produce sufficient lymph node enlargement to be demonstrable on CT. The appearance of such adenopathy varies from individually enlarged lymph nodes to a large homogeneous mass obscuring normal structures (78,144). In addition, CT may demonstrate lymphomatous involvement of solid organs such as the liver, spleen, or kidneys that is unsuspected. As in the adult, CT cannot differentiate normal lymph nodes and nodes that are of normal size but are replaced with tumor. In addition, it is impossible to distinguish between mild enlargement of lymph nodes due to inflammatory conditions and enlargement due to neoplastic involvement.

Clearly, CT is the initial radiologic procedure of choice for evaluating the abdomen in patients with lymphoma, especially because masses in childhood lymphoma can appear in the mesentery and range in size from small to bulky (Fig. 32). US is not as reliable as CT for detecting the smaller mesenteric masses, and lymphangiography can

study only a limited nodal area and is unable to evaluate mesenteric, high paraaortic, and internal iliac nodes.

Abdominal Abscess

Most abdominal abscesses in children are caused by appendicitis with perforation, Crohn disease, and/or postoperative complications. The CT appearance of an abscess most commonly consists of a mass of relatively low density, with or without a rim that often is enhanced after intravenous administration of contrast material. The internal contents of the mass may be only fluid or may be mixed with gas (1,80). Gas is found in slightly more than one-third of abscesses and may appear as multiple small bubbles or as a large collection with an air–fluid level (26) (Fig. 33). The size and shape are affected by location, because abscesses usually are confined to various fascial or intraperitoneal compartments, expanding the spaces and displacing contiguous structures. Abscesses commonly produce obliteration of adjacent fat planes and thickening of surrounding muscles, mesentery, or bowel wall.

Plain radiographs of the abdomen usually are obtained in patients suspected of having abscesses and often are helpful by demonstrating unusual gas collections, but if the findings on the abdominal radiograph are normal or nondiagnostic, additional imaging examinations are required. Radionuclide imaging, US, and CT are all accurate methods for confirming the presence of intraabdominal

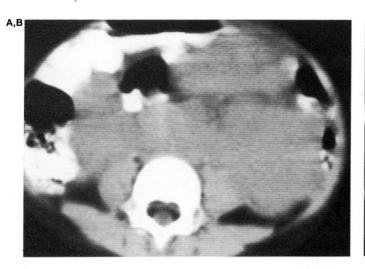
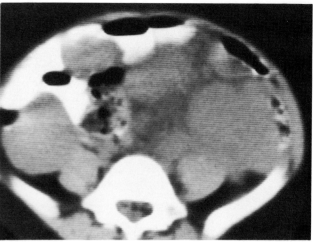

FIG. 32. Burkitt lymphoma in a 5-year-old boy with palpable lower abdominal masses. **A:** Multiple soft-tissue masses extend from the anterior abdominal wall to the retroperitoneum, displacing the contrast-filled small bowel to the right. **B:** CT scan 3 cm lower shows well circumscribed soft-tissue-density masses filling the upper pelvis.

abscesses (15,26,75,80,109). In children who are not acutely ill and have fever of unknown origin without localizing signs or symptoms, the use of ^{67}Ga-citrate or ^{111}In-leukocyte scanning is recommended as the primary screening test because of its ease of performance and ability to offer a view of the entire body in a single image. Generally, if the findings on the scan are normal, no further evaluation is needed. If the results on radionuclide scan are abnormal, CT or US is required for further documentation and to determine the full extent of the lesion. Conversely, a patient with localizing signs of disease usually is best studied initially with CT or US. In acutely ill patients who are without localizing signs and who are clinically suspected of having abdominal abscess, CT or US is the procedure of choice, particularly because imaging with gallium requires a delay of 24 hr or more.

The choice of examination between CT and US depends on the individual clinical situation. US examination often is hampered by a large amount of bowel gas; it can also be suboptimal in the immediate postoperative period because of the difficulty in imaging the area directly beneath the surgical wound, drainage tubes, and ostomy appliances. Moreover, the left subphrenic area and the lesser sac may be difficult to evaluate by US because of a gas-filled stomach. This is especially true in patients who have had prior splenectomy. Because these areas are readily studied by CT examination, CT is our preferred method. The right subphrenic and subhepatic areas are at least as well studied by US as by CT, and US is the initial procedure of choice. CT is considered the method of choice when a retroperitoneal abscess is suspected. In most instances, the relationship of an abscess to surrounding structures is best displayed by CT. If an abscess is detected, CT permits planning of the most appropriate approach for percutaneous or surgical drainage (135).

Blunt Abdominal Trauma

Computed tomographic imaging provides a radiologic display of the entire abdomen following nonpenetrating injuries and can document parenchymal injury to the liver, spleen, pancreas, kidney, and duodenum, as well as the presence of a subcapsular hematoma and intraperitoneal or retroperitoneal hemorrhage (13,65,67,68,69, 99,134) (Fig. 34). Fractures and lacerations often appear on CT as irregular linear or wedge-shaped areas of low density within an organ. Fresh hemorrhages show a density greater than those of surrounding tissues, whereas chronic hematomas are lower in attenuation value. Subcapsular hematomas usually are lenticular or oval in configuration and flatten or indent the underlying paren-

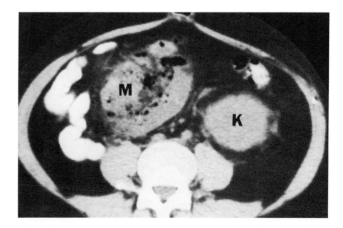

FIG. 33. Mesenteric abscess in an 18-year-old boy on steroid therapy following a renal transplant. A large soft-tissue-density mass (M) containing multiple gas bubbles occupies the right mid-abdomen and displaces adjacent bowel loops. At surgery perforation of the transverse colon was found. (K) renal transplant.

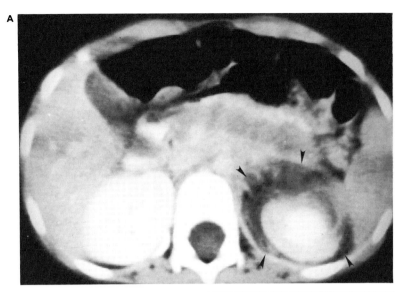

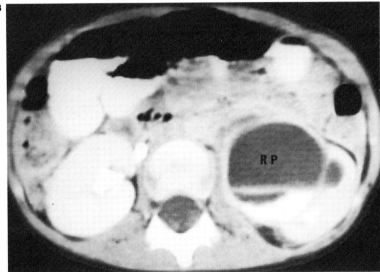

FIG. 34. Renal laceration and perirenal hematoma in a 10-year-old girl following abdominal trauma. **A:** A CT scan through the upper abdomen after contrast medium administration reveals a low density fluid collection (*arrowheads*) in the left perirenal space. **B:** CT scan at a lower level demonstrates dilated contrast-medium-urine filled calyces and a large dilated renal pelvis (RP). The CT diagnosis of a perirenal hematoma/urinoma complicating a ureteropelvic junction obstruction was confirmed at surgery.

chyma. CT also can identify blood in the paracolic gutter or Morison's pouch.

In a study comparing CT, US, and radionuclide imaging for abdominal trauma in children, CT was the most sensitive examination, detecting 96% of traumatic lesions (69). US and scintigraphy correctly detected 89% and 67% of lesions, respectively. Additionally, CT was shown to be superior to the other examinations in defining the extent and severity of injury. An advantage of CT compared with US is that it can be used to assess organ function and vascularity as well as anatomy. No transducer contact is necessary, and the ileus that is often associated with trauma is not a deterrent to CT. Unlike excretory urography and radionuclide scanning, CT is not organ-specific.

CT is employed as the initial imaging procedure for severely traumatized children whose vital signs are stable enough to permit the examination. Unstable pediatric patients generally proceed directly to surgery without imaging examinations. If the injury is mild and an isolated renal injury is suspected, an intravenous urogram may be the only examination required. When only hepatic or splenic injury is suspected, radionuclide imaging, because of its ease of performance and its ability to permit assessment of function, may be the screening procedure of choice. When an abnormality is suggested on the urogram or radionuclide scan, US or CT can provide more precise definition of the extent of injury if this information is required. Knowledge of the extent of injury is important because it affects the decision either to treat conservatively or to operate (25). Because most traumatized patients will be treated conservatively, CT also can have a role in follow-up evaluation.

Pancreatic Disorders

Acute pancreatitis is uncommon in children, but can follow trauma, viral infections, or chemotherapy. On CT, pancreatitis usually appears as diffuse enlargement of the gland, with a lower density than normal. The decreased

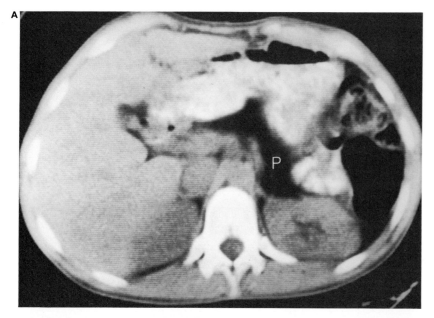

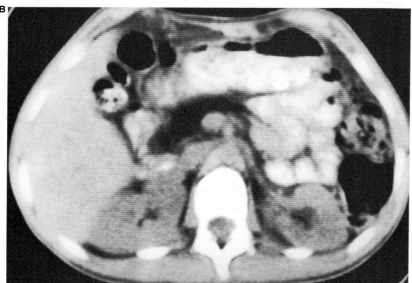

FIG. 35. Fatty pancreas in an 18-year-old girl with cystic fibrosis. Serial CT scans show the pancreas to be completely replaced by fatty tissue. **A:** Body and tail of pancreas (P). **B:** Head and neck of pancreas. **C:** Head and uncinate process of pancreas with visible duct (*arrowhead*).

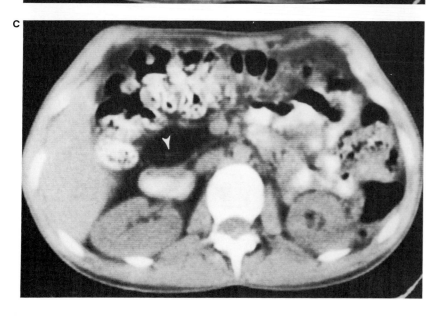

attenuation presumably corresponds to edema and/or necrosis. Frequently the normal peripancreatic fat planes are thickened or obliterated. Pancreatic and extrapancreatic fluid collections, resulting from escape of pancreatic secretions, may be present and usually are well demonstrated with CT and displayed as well-defined near-water-density masses that distend an already existing space in the retroperitoneal or intraperitoneal compartment. The configuration is variable, and the collections may be unilocular or multilocular. Common sites of involvement include the anterior pararenal space, lesser sac, and mesenteric root.

In children, recurrent or chronic pancreatitis usually is due to hereditary pancreatitis. The pancreas and ducts are of normal size, but multiple parenchymal calcifications can be identified by CT. Chronic pancreatitis also may result from cystic fibrosis; parenchymal calcification and ductal dilatation, as well as total replacement of the gland by fat or multiple macroscopic cysts, may be observed (61) (Fig. 35). Pancreatic neoplasms in children are extremely rare and usually are suspected when they are hormonally active or produce biliary tract obstruction. In these instances, CT can demonstrate a solid pancreatic mass, as well as provide information about the extent of tumor (55).

In general, US and CT are competitive methods for evaluating pancreatic disease. In patients with good clinical evidence supporting the diagnosis of uncomplicated acute pancreatitis, neither imaging method is necessary. Diagnostic evaluation is reserved for patients suspected of having complications. US is preferred as the screening examination because it does not require ionizing radiation. In cases where US is suboptimal because of bowel gas, commonly present in patients with acute pancreatitis, CT may be used to provide valuable information. CT is considered the procedure of choice for displaying calcification in patients suspected of having hereditary pancreatitis when findings on plain abdominal radiographs are negative or equivocal.

Diseases of the Liver

Diagnosis of infiltrative diseases of the liver can be made with CT because of its ability to measure tissue densities (126). Fatty infiltration, often associated with severe malnutrition and cystic fibrosis in children, is clearly recognizable by its diminished density (35). The decrease in hepatic attenuation value may be focal or diffuse and directly corresponds to the amount of fat deposited in the liver. With diffuse fatty infiltration, the portal veins appear as high-density structures against the background of low density caused by hepatic fat. Attenuation values higher than normal can occur with hemochromatosis and glycogen storage disease (41,86). As a result of the increased CT density, the hepatic vessels appear as low-density

branching structures surrounded by the background of the hyperdense liver. In addition, increased iron deposition may be present in the lymph nodes, spleen, pancreas, adrenal glands, and bowel wall (86). Dual-energy CT scanning is particularly helpful for assessing and quantitating hepatic iron content. Scanning at the same level at 80 and 120 kV will result in a large change in the CT number of the liver if there is excessive iron deposition. Dual-energy CT techniques, however, are not as precise for quantitating hepatic glycogen. When the liver is scanned at 80 kV, compared with 120 kV, there is a much smaller change in attenuation value compared with the great increase in hepatic CT numbers observed in hemochromatosis. As in adults, CT often does not detect differences in hepatic densities in children with cirrhosis, but it will demonstrate changes in liver contour or size. A small liver with a nodular contour resulting from focal atrophy and/or regenerating nodules is seen in advanced cirrhosis, often associated with chronic hepatitis, biliary atresia, metabolic disorders, congenital hepatic fibrosis, or autosomal-recessive polycystic kidney disease (Fig. 36). Other findings include dilated collateral vessels that produce numerous round, soft-tissue densities in the porta hepatis and umbilical and splenic regions, splenomegaly, ascites, and enlargement of the caudate and left lobes. In patients with cystic fibrosis who have biliary cirrhosis, multiple cyst-like lesions may be seen, suggesting polycystic disease. Pathologically this corresponds to a combination of diffuse fatty infiltration and bile duct fibrosis and proliferation. Differentiation with CT is possible based on demonstration of attenuation values of lipomatous tissue (122).

In jaundiced patients, US is the preliminary imaging procedure of choice to detect intrahepatic ductal dilatation associated with obstruction, as well as a choledochal cyst. This can be supplemented by radionuclide studies using hepatobiliary imaging agents (95). Although the ability of CT to document the presence of dilated bile ducts is well known, CT should be reserved for cases in which the level or cause of obstruction cannot be determined by other radiologic methods. The most frequent lesions producing obstructive jaundice in children are biliary duct calculi, acute pancreatitis, and rhabdomyosarcoma of the biliary duct.

Renal Parenchymal Disease

Most renal calcifications in children are associated with obstruction and infection, and less frequently are due to metabolic disorders, cortical necrosis, glomerulonephritis, or ACTH therapy. In rare instances, CT may be of value in detecting lithiasis or nephrocalcinosis before it appears on conventional radiographs (89).

Acute pyelonephritis can present as uniform enlargement of the kidney. Findings on non-contrast-enhanced

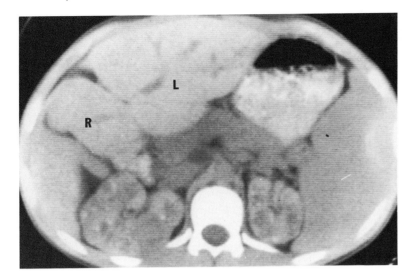

FIG. 36. Cirrhosis in a 13-year-old boy with congenital hepatic fibrosis and renal cystic disease. The liver is abnormally increased in density, accentuating the portal venous structures. Also noted is irregularity of the right lobe (R), an enlarged left lobe (L), splenomegaly, and multiple small renal cysts, some of which have areas of high attenuation, believed to represent inspissated mucoid material.

scans often are normal, but on contrast-enhanced CT scans, single or multiple areas of lower density, presumably related to inflammatory hypovascularity, vasoconstriction, or microabscesses, frequently are seen (63). More severe renal infection may extend into the perirenal space or produce a focal inflammatory mass or an abscess. A CT diagnosis of chronic pyelonephritis is based on recognition of a small kidney with cortical scars overlying clubbed calices. Unilateral renal hypoplasia or renal artery stenosis, in contradistinction, is associated with a small smooth kidney.

A voiding cystourethrogram (VCUG) is the initial imaging examination in a child with a first-time urinary tract infection to investigate the possibility of reflux. If reflux is present, an excretory urogram is performed to visualize the renal parenchyma. If the VCUG is normal, US is preferable to determine if there is coexistent obstruction predisposing to infection. CT may be a valuable ancillary examination in patients with acute pyelonephritis suspected of having perinephric extension, because it provides a better topographic display of the kidney and its adjacent structures than urography or US (62).

Vascular Structures

Aneurysms are rare in children and occur most frequently in association with Marfan syndrome, collagen vascular diseases, sepsis, or trauma. Thrombosis also is uncommon and usually is the result of severe illness associated with intense dehydration, tumor extension, or trauma (Fig. 37). In addition, various developmental anomalies of the venous system can occur, and their recognition is important lest they be misinterpreted as pathologic. CT can be used to diagnose congenital anomalies of the abdominal vascular structures as well as acquired lesions (74,93,145). Frequently this has been an unexpected discovery in patients studied for other clinical concerns.

Ultrasonography is the preferred examination for confirming a suspected aneurysm or venous thrombosis, because it has the advantage of easily being able to reveal the dimensions and the effective lumina of the aorta or cava and their branches in longitudinal and transverse sections. However, if the abdomen is obscured by bowel gas, CT can provide the necessary information.

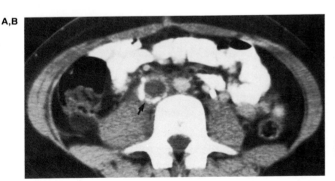
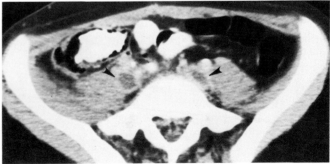

A,B

FIG. 37. Traumatic inferior vena caval thrombus in a 14-year-old girl following a gunshot wound and graft repair of the inferior vena cava. **A, B:** Serial CT scans through the abdomen and pelvis show low-density thrombus within a dilated inferior vena cava (*arrow*) and common iliac veins (*arrowheads*).

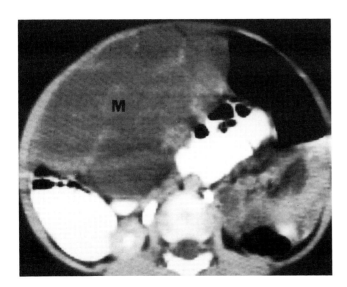

FIG. 38. Mesenteric cyst. An enhanced CT scan reveals a well-circumscribed water density mass (M) without a discernible wall occupying the anterior abdomen and displacing adjacent bowel loops to the left. The anterior location suggests a mesenteric origin of the mass. Streaky densities in the mass represent septations.

PELVIS

The great value of CT of the pelvis in children is for evaluation of a pelvic mass detected clinically or visible on a urogram, barium enema, or US examination. In addition to facilitating evaluation of patients suspected of having masses, CT can be useful in diagnosing pelvic abscesses, localizing nonpalpable testes, and evaluating the musculoskeletal structures of the pelvis (127).

Pelvic Masses

Pelvic masses in the pediatric population may arise in either the anterior or posterior pelvic compartment. In the anterior pelvis, masses may be of genital, gastrointestinal, or lower urinary tract origin, whereas in the posterior pelvis they usually are of neurogenic or teratomatous origin. Genital masses occur more often in females, usually are benign, and represent hydrometrocolpos or ovarian cysts or teratomas. An ovarian cyst appears as a near-water-density mass that has a thin or nearly imperceptible wall, whereas hydrometrocolpos is recognized as a near-water-density mass with a thick wall that may be enhanced after intravenous administration of contrast material. Teratomas can be diagnosed by identification of fatty tissue, calcification or ossification, or teeth. The usefulness of CT in benign disease is most often related to definitive characterization of a lesion based on the ability to distinguish different tissue densities, rather than establishment of the extent of disease (129).

Gastrointestinal masses in children are not as common

as those that arise from the genital structures. Enteric duplications and mesenteric cysts account for most benign gastrointestinal masses, while lymphoma is the most common malignant mass of bowel. Although CT can detect the former conditions, it is usually unnecessary if the diagnosis can be established with ultrasonography. If the extent or location of the cyst is uncertain, CT may provide the diagnosis (116). On CT, a mesenteric cyst is usually a near-water density mass that is extrinsic to the bowel and shows no discernible wall, while an enteric duplication appears as a cystic mass with a thick, enhancing wall (Fig. 38). The CT features of lymphoma include: single or multiple soft tissue nodules, mural infiltration, an endo-exoenteric mass with necrosis, and mesenteric invasion with extraluminal mass (Fig. 39). Mesenteric extension and other intraabdominal spread of tumor usually can be shown better by CT than by other imaging examinations.

Rhabdomyosarcoma (sarcoma botryoides) is the commonest neoplasm of the lower urinary tract in children. It most often affects children between 2 and 5 years of age, involving the vagina and bladder in girls and the prostate, bladder, and urethra in boys. The tumor tends to metastasize early by direct invasion and hematogenous and lymphatic dissemination. On CT, rhabdomyosarcoma appears as a soft-tissue mass with a density approaching that of muscle (Fig. 40). When it arises in the bladder or vagina, it often produces a polypoid appearance. Calcification may be present occasionally, along with variable enhancement after intravenous administration of contrast material. Metastases to pelvic lymph nodes can be seen on CT if the nodes are enlarged. Although less common, pheochromocytoma, neurofibroma, hemangioma, and, rarely, transitional cell carcinoma and leiomyosarcoma of the bladder may occur, whereas in the

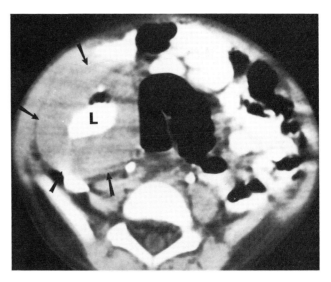

FIG. 39. Non-Hodgkin lymphoma of the distal ileum. There is circumferential thickening of the ileal wall (arrows), measuring 3 cm, associated with a distorted, excavated lumen (L).

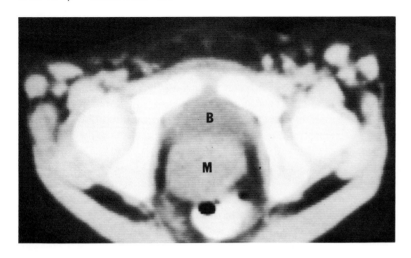

FIG. 40. Vaginal rhabdomyosarcoma in a 2-year-old girl with vaginal bleeding. CT scan obtained 2 months after surgical exploration and incomplete tumor resection shows residual soft-tissue mass (M) in the vagina. The soft tissues in the right pelvic wall posterolaterally are thickened secondary to prior surgery; (B) urinary bladder.

vagina and cervix, squamous cell carcinoma and adenocarcinoma are rarely encountered.

Sacrococcygeal teratomas, anterior meningoceles, and neuroblastomas are the most frequent presacral masses. Sacrococcygeal teratoma can be confirmed by identification of fatty tissue and calcific densities with or without associated bony anomalies (Fig. 41). Meningoceles or myelomeningoceles are recognized by their relatively low attenuation values (cerebrospinal fluid or fat), their position anterior to the sacrum, and the associated sacral defects. The soft-tissue contents of the herniated spinal sac can be seen best on CT in combination with metrizamide myelography or on MRI. Neuroblastomas appear as poorly circumscribed soft-tissue-density masses, often with amorphous calcifications. Rare presacral masses include neurofibromas, neurofibrosarcomas, lymphomas, and chordomas; precise identification usually requires tissue sampling.

Clinical Application

When a pelvic mass is detected on physical examination or another radiologic study (e.g., excretory urogram, barium enema), further characterization of the mass and a

suggestion of its cause are possible with US, CT, and MRI. US should be used for the initial evaluation of most suspected gynecological masses because it does not involve ionizing radiation. However, US often is suboptimal in the posterior pelvic compartment and the presacral space; CT is useful in these areas for confirming the presence of a suspected pelvic mass and for detecting possible bony involvement. When US suggests a malignant mass, or if a pelvic malignancy has been diagnosed, CT may be warranted to detect the extent of pelvic invasion prior to surgery, chemotherapy, or radiation therapy (27,127,129). The exact role of MRI in the pelvis in children has not been clarified. Its potential role is likely to be that of staging known malignancies and characterizing pelvic masses (Figs. 42, 43).

Impalpable Testes

Identification of an undescended testis or cryptorchidism is important because of the increased risk of infertility if the testis remains undescended and because of the increased incidence of malignancy, particularly with an intraabdominal testis. Early surgery, either orchiopexy in younger patients or orchiectomy in patients past puberty,

FIG. 41. Malignant presacral teratoma in a 12-year-old girl with chronic constipation. A low-density soft-tissue mass displaces the rectum (*arrowhead*) anteriorly. The tumor extends into the perirectal and presacral fat and abuts the pyriformis muscle.

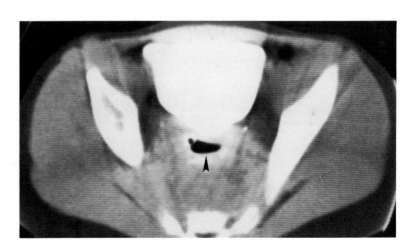

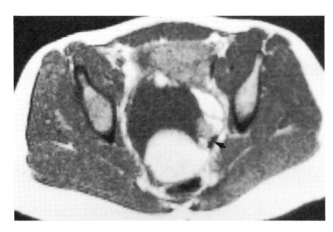

FIG. 42. Ovarian dermoid in a 18-year-old girl. MR image (TR = 500 msec, TE = 30 msec) shows an irregular mass containing areas of low and high signal intensities, characteristic of fluid and fatty components, posterior to the uterus. An area with absence of signal (*arrow*) in the left aspect of the mass corresponds to teeth seen on the plain radiograph.

can overcome these risks. Preoperative localization of a nonpalpable testis by CT is helpful in expediting surgical management and shortening the anesthesia time. CT diagnosis of an undescended testis is based on detection of a soft-tissue mass, often oval in shape, in the expected course of testicular descent (Fig. 44). The more normal the testis is in size and shape, the lower is its attenuation value. A very atropic testis appears as a small focus of soft tissue with a density similar to that of abdominal wall musculature. The diagnosis of an undescended testis is

easier if the testis is in the inguinal canal or lower pelvis, where structures usually are symmetrical. Differentiation of an undescended testis from adjacent structures, such as bowel loops, vascular structures, and lymph nodes, is more of a problem in the upper pelvis and lower abdomen. In fact, in young children, in whom there is little abdominal fat, scanning usually is not extended above the superior iliac spine. In spite of these problems, the accuracy of CT for localization of nonpalpable testes exceeds 90% (84,150).

Ultrasonography can detect an impalpable undescended testis when it is in a high scrotal or intracanalicular position, which occurs in about 90% of cases. Because it does not involve ionizing radiation, US is recommended as the initial imaging examination of choice for localizing impalpable testes. US, however, usually is not reliable for identifying undescended testes located higher in the pelvis or in the abdomen. Therefore, if US findings are equivocal or negative and preoperative localization of the testis is desired, CT is performed.

MUSCULOSKELETAL SYSTEM

Computed tomography is most valuable for delineating soft-tissue involvement in musculoskeletal tumors, for evaluating abnormalities of complex bony structures (pelvis and spine) and for assessing bone mineral content (49,59).

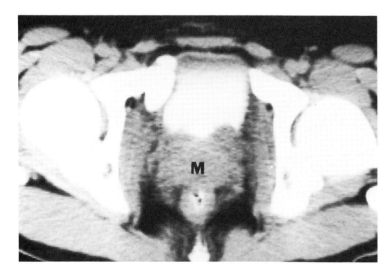

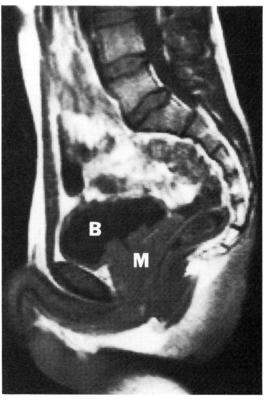

A,B

FIG. 43. Prostatic rhabdomyosarcoma in a 16-year-old boy with hematuria. **A:** CT scan demonstrates an irregular soft-tissue mass (M) between the bladder and rectum. The interface between the tumor and the bladder, rectum and periprostatic tissue is poorly defined. **B:** Sagittal MR image (TR = 500 msec, TE = 30 msec) shows the large prostatic mass (M) protruding into the bladder (B) but not the rectum. Cystoscopy confirmed bladder invasion.

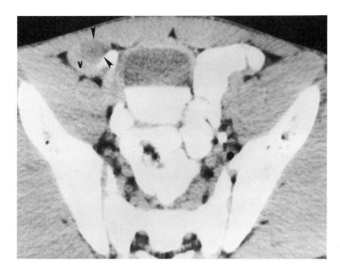

FIG. 44. Intraabdominal testes in a 17-year-old boy. CT scan through the lower pelvis demonstrates a round, low density mass (*arrowheads*), later shown to be the undescended testis, in the right side of the pelvis posterior to the abdominal wall. A loop of vas deferens (v) lies next to the testis.

Osseous Tumors

Routine radiographs are comparable or superior to CT in providing a specific diagnosis. When the lesion appears benign, but large, or appears malignant on plain radiographs, CT has been used to determine the extent of soft-tissue involvement, including information about adjacent blood vessels, nerves, and joints (90,146). Computed tomography also is useful in demonstrating very small cortical lesions such as osteoid osteomas when conventional radiographs are normal or equivocal. Such information often can affect the surgical or nonsurgical management of the patient and can be helpful in designing radiation ports.

Soft-Tissue Tumors

Although CT generally cannot lead to a specific histologic diagnosis unless lesions contain predominantly fatty components, it can delineate the anatomy prior to surgical extirpation. This is especially true around anatomically complex areas such as the spine and pelvis (Fig. 45). In the more distal extremities, where there is a paucity of fat and readily recognizable tissue planes exist, US or MRI is a superior method for delineating tumor extent.

Osteomyelitis

Computed tomography can display clearly the medullary portion of bone. Normally the marrow cavity of a long bone has a density equal to that of fat; when infected, the density increases to near that of water. In patients in whom the diagnosis of osteomyelitis is uncertain, CT may be helpful by showing this increased density in the abnormal extremity as compared with the normal side (79). Such an appearance, however, is not specific for osteomyelitis, but also can be observed in neoplasms, storage diseases, trauma, and primary bone marrow disorders. In some instances, CT may be helpful in demonstrating a sequestrum (58). This information may be useful in surgical planning.

Pelvis and Spine

The axial skeleton and pelvis frequently are difficult to evaluate with plain radiographs because of superimposition of bony parts. CT is especially useful in symptomatic patients with trauma or sacroiliitis and equivocal or normal findings on routine radiographs (91,147). Other indications for CT include orthopedic problems, especially the position of the femoral head in congenital hip dislocation and the angle of anteversion of the hip (57,59,60,108) (Fig. 46).

Appendicular Skeleton

The axial presentation provided by CT has made it valuable for assessing osseous and articular structures of the hindfoot and subtle tarsal coalitions (120,123) (Fig.

FIG. 45. Neurofibrosarcoma in an 11-year-old boy with neurofibromatosis and left-leg pain. CT scan through the lower pelvis demonstrates large soft-tissue masses (M) arising from the sacral plexus bilaterally. The planes between the left obturator internus and pyriformis muscles and the mass are obliterated. Also noted are multiple neurofibromas in the subcutaneous tissues. A neurofibrosarcoma of the left sacral nerve root plexus was found at surgery. The neurofibroma on the right side showed no evidence of malignant transformation.

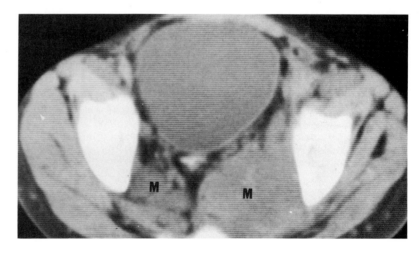

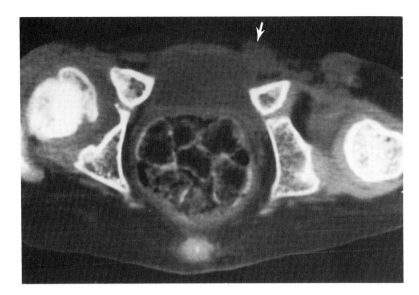

FIG. 46. A 9-year-old boy with bilateral dislocated hips. CT was used to evaluate the degree of dislocation and the position of the femur in relation to the acetabulum. CT demonstrates minimal anterior coverage of the right femoral head, with good posterior coverage. The left hip is dislocated laterally and has no anterior or posterior coverage. Incidentally noted is an undescended left testis (*arrow*).

47). CT may also be used to delineate fracture dislocations of the shoulder girdle and complex fractures of the foot and ankle (54).

Clinical Applications

Several studies have indicated that MRI is superior to CT for evaluating disorders of the musculoskeletal system (98,107,143,153). Because of its superb soft-tissue contrast and absence of streak artifacts from dense cortical bone, MRI can more reliably define the borders and extent of benign and malignant soft-tissue tumors, including disease in the bone marrow (Fig. 48). It can accurately detect the relationships of these neoplasms to surrounding blood

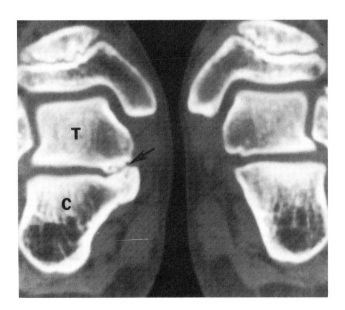

FIG. 47. Talocalcaneal coalition in an 11-year-old boy. A coronal CT scan reveals narrowing of the middle subtalar joint (*arrow*) between the talus (T) and calcaneus (C) on the right. The opposing cortical surfaces are sclerotic and irregular. A fibrous union was confirmed surgically.

vessels without intravenous administration of contrast material (Fig. 49). Cortical destruction and periosteal new bone production can be recognized by MRI, although these findings are demonstrated better by plain radiography or CT scans. MRI also is a sensitive method for evaluating bone marrow abnormality in disorders such as neuroblastoma or leukemia and osteomyelitis (32,47,141). The normal bone marrow has an intense, homogeneous signal intensity; infiltrative disease produces decreased signal intensity. Finally, it has been shown that MRI is sensitive for early diagnosis of ischemic necrosis of the femoral head and may provide a diagnosis when findings on radionuclide imaging are negative (12,142). On the basis of these observations, MRI is considered the imaging procedure of choice for evaluating many disorders of the musculoskeletal system.

RISKS OF CT SCANNING

The risks of CT scanning in children are those from administration of contrast material and radiation exposure. The overall incidence of adverse reactions to injection of contrast material in the general population is at or near 5%. In the pediatric age group, the incidence is similar, with adverse reactions, both major and minor, occurring in 3.8% to 5.2% of administrations of contrast material (124).

Exposure to ionizing radiation is the other major drawback of CT scanning. In CT scanning, the skin receives the highest dose of radiation, and skin-absorbed doses in children range from 1.1 to 2.4 rads for chest and abdominal examinations (44). By comparison, radiation exposures for examinations frequently used for diagnosis prior to CT are 0.05 to 0.07 rad for plain chest radiography, 0.8 to 2 rads for voiding cystourethrography, 0.2 to 0.75 rad for excretory urography, and 4 to 11 rads for abdominal angiography.

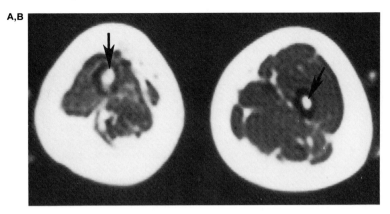

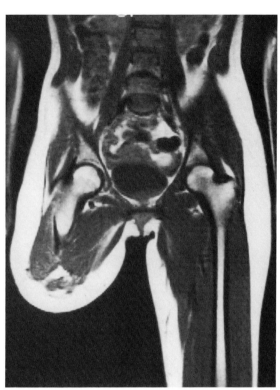

FIG. 48. Normal fatty marrow in an 18-year-old girl treated with above the knee amputation for osteosarcoma. Radionuclide bone scan had shown increased activity in the proximal femoral stump so MR imaging was performed to assess tumor involvement. **A:** Axial T1-weighted (TR = 500 msec, TE = 35 msec) and **B:** Coronal T2-weighted (TR = 1500 msec, TE = 35 msec) images show equally high signal intensities in the marrow cavities (*arrows*) of the proximal right femoral stump and entire left femur reflecting normal fatty marrow and not tumor.

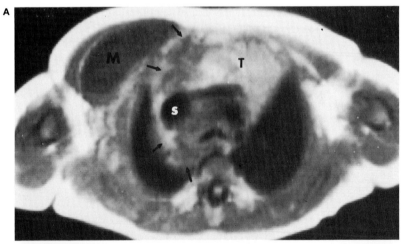

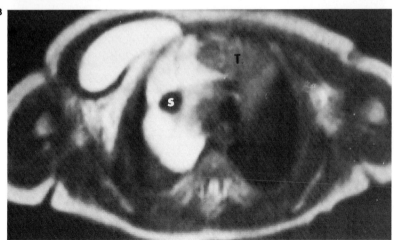

FIG. 49. A 2-month-old girl with chest-wall and mediastinal lymphangioma. **A:** On a T1-weighted axial MR image (TR = 500 msec; TE = 30 msec), the chest wall mass (M) has a homogeneous appearance and a signal intensity less than that of muscle. Note also a higher-signal-intensity superior mediastinal mass (*arrows*). **B:** On the T2-weighted image (TR = 1800 msec, TE = 120 msec) the lymphangioma has a very bright signal intensity and is easily differentiated from adjacent structures; (T) thymus; (S) superior vena cava.

REFERENCES

1. Afshani E. Computed tomography of abdominal abscesses in children. *Radiol Clin North Am* 1981;19:515–526.
2. Amendola MA, Blane CE, Amendola BE, Glazer GM. CT findings in hepatoblastoma. *J Comput Assist Tomogr* 1984;8:1105–1109.
3. Ang JGP, Proto AV. CT demonstration of congenital pulmonary venolobar syndrome. *J Comput Assist Tomogr* 1984;8:753–757.
4. Araki T, Itai Y, Iio M. CT features of calcification in abdominal neuroblastoma. *J Comput Assist Tomogr* 1982;6:789–791.
5. Araki T, Itai Y, Tasaka A. CT of choledochal cyst. *AJR* 1980;135:729–734.
6. Armstrong EA, Harwood-Nash DCF, Ritz CR, Chuang SH, Pettersson H, Martin DJ. CT of neuroblastomas and ganglioneuromas in children. *AJR* 1982;139:571–576.
7. Baron RL, Gutierrez FR, Sagel SS, Levitt RG, McKnight RC. CT of anomalies of the mediastinal vessels. *AJR* 1981;135:571–576.
8. Baron RL, Lee JKT, Sagel SS, Levitt RG. Computed tomography of the abnormal thymus. *Radiology* 1982;142:127–134.
9. Baron RL, Lee JKT, Sagel SS, Peterson RR. Computed tomography of the normal thymus. *Radiology* 1982;142:121–125.
10. Baron RL, Levitt RG, Sagel SS, Stanley RJ. Computed tomography in the evaluation of mediastinal widening. *Radiology* 1981;138:107–113.
11. Belt TG, Cohen MD, Smith JA, Cory DA, McKenna S, Weetman R. MRI of Wilms' tumor: promise as the primary imaging method. *AJR* 1986;146:955–961.
12. Beltran J, Herman LJ, Burk JM, et al. Femoral head avascular necrosis: MR imaging with clinical-pathologic and radionuclide correlation. *Radiology* 1988;166:215–220.
13. Berger PE, Kuhn JP. CT of blunt abdominal trauma in childhood. *AJR* 1981;136:105–110.
14. Berger PE, Kuhn JP. Computed tomography of the hepatobiliary system in infancy and childhood. *Radiol Clin North Am* 1981;19:431–444.
15. Biello DR, Levitt RG, Melson GL. The roles of gallium-67 scintigraphy, ultrasonography and computed tomography in the detection of abdominal abscesses. *Semin Nucl Med* 1979;9:58–65.
16. Bitter JJ, Harrison DA, Kaplan J, Irwin GA. Mesoblastic nephroma. *J Comput Assist Tomogr* 1982;6:180–183.
17. Boechat MI. Adrenal glands, pancreas, and retroperitoneal structures. In: Siegel MJ, ed. *Pediatric Body CT*. New York: Churchill Livingstone, 1988:177–217.
18. Boechat MI, Ortega J, Hoffman AD, Cleveland RH, Kangarloo H, Gilsanz V. Computed tomography in stage III neuroblastoma. *AJR* 1985;145:1283–1287.
19. Bousvaros A, Kirks DR, Grossman H. Imaging of neuroblastoma: an overview. *Pediatr Radiol* 1986;16:89–106.
20. Bower RJ, Kiesewetter WB. Mediastinal masses in infants and children. *Arch Surg* 1977;112:1003–1009.
21. Brasch RC. Ultrafast computed tomography and radiation considerations in children. In: Siegel MJ, ed. *Pediatric Body CT*. New York: Churchill Livingstone, 1988:371–388.
22. Brasch RC, Abols IB, Gooding CA, Filly RA. Abdominal disease in children: a comparison of computed tomography and ultrasound. *AJR* 1980;134:153–158.
23. Brasch RC, Cann CE. Computed tomographic scanning in children: II. An updated comparison of radiation dose and resolving power of commercial scanners. *AJR* 1982;138:127–133.
24. Brasch RC, Gooding CA, Lallemand DP, Wesbey GE. Magnetic resonance imaging of the thorax in childhood. *Radiology* 1984;150:463–467.
25. Brick SH, Taylor GA, Potter BA, Eichelberger MR. Hepatic and splenic injury in children: Role of CT in the decision for laparotomy. *Radiology* 1987;165:643–646.
26. Callen PW. Computed tomographic evaluation of abdominal and pelvic abscesses. *Radiology* 1979;131:171–175.
27. Carter BL, Kahn PC, Wolpert SM, Hammerschlag SB, Schwartz AM, Scott RM. Unusual pelvic masses: a comparison of computed tomographic scanning and ultrasonography. *Radiology* 1976;121:383–390.
28. Chan HSL, Daneman A, Gribbin M, Martin DJ. Renal cell carcinoma in first two decades of life. *Pediatr Radiol* 1983;13:324–328.
29. Cohen AM, Solomon EH, Alfidi RJ. Computed tomography in bronchial atresia. *AJR* 1980;135:1097–1099.
30. Cohen MD. Kidneys. In: Siegal MJ, ed. *Pediatric Body CT*. New York: Churchill Livingstone, 1988:135–175.
31. Cohen MD, Grosfeld J, Baehner R, Weetman R. Lung CT for detection of metastases: solid tissue neoplasms in children. *AJR* 1982;139:895–898.
32. Cohen MD, Klatte EC, Baehner R, et al. Magnetic resonance imaging of bone marrow disease in children. *Radiology* 1984;151:715–718.
33. Cohen MD, Weber TR, Sequeira FW, Vane DW, King H. The diagnostic dilemma of the posterior mediastinal thymus: CT manifestations. *Radiology* 1983;146:691–692.
34. Cohen MD, Weetman R, Provisor A, et al. Magnetic resonance imaging of neuroblastoma with a 0.15-T magnet. *AJR* 1984;143:1241–1248.
35. Cunningham DG, Churchill RJ, Reynes CJ. Computed tomography in the evaluation of liver disease in cystic fibrosis patients. *J Comput Assist Tomogr* 1980;4:151–154.
36. Dachman AH, Lichtenstein JE, Friedman AC, Hartman DS. Infantile hemangioendothelioma of the liver: a radiologic-pathologic clinical correlation. *AJR* 1983;140:1091–1096.
37. Daneman A, Chan HSL, Martin J. Adrenal carcinoma and adenoma in children: A review of 17 patients. *Pediatr Radiol* 13:11–18, 1983.
38. Daneman A. *Pediatric Body CT*. London: Springer-Verlag, 1987.
39. Donaldson JS. Mediastinum. In: Siegel MJ, ed. *Pediatric Body CT*. New York: Churchill Livingstone, 1988:29–79.
40. Donaldson JS, Siegel MJ. Lungs, pleura and chest wall. In: Siegel MJ, ed. *Pediatric Body CT*. New York: Churchill Livingstone, 1988:81–102.
41. Doppman JL, Cornblath M, Dwyer AJ, Adams AJ, Girton ME, Sidbury J. Computed tomography of the liver and kidneys in glycogen storage disease. *J Comput Assist Tomogr* 1982;6:67–71.
42. Effmann EL, Fram EK, Vock P, Kirks DR. Tracheal cross-sectional area in children: CT determination. *Radiology* 1983;149:137–140.
43. Farrelly CA, Daneman A, Martin DJ, Chan HSL. Pheochromocytoma in childhood: the important role of computed tomography in tumour localization. *Pediatr Radiol* 1984;14:210–214.
44. Fearon T, Vucich J. Pediatric patient exposure from CT examinations. *AJR* 1985;144:805–809.
45. Fishman EK, Hartman DS, Goldman SM, Siegelman SS. The CT appearance of Wilms tumor. *J Comput Assist Tomogr* 1983;7:659–665.
46. Fletcher BD, Kopiwoda ST, Strandjord SE, Nelson AD, Pickering SP. Abdominal neuroblastoma: magnetic resonance imaging and tissue characterization. *Radiology* 1985;155:699–703.
47. Fletcher BD, Scoles PV, Nelson AD. Osteomyelitis in children: detection by magnetic resonance. *Radiology* 1984;150:57–60.
48. Francis IR, Glazer GM, Bookstein FL, Gross BH. The thymus: reexamination of age-related changes in size and shape. *AJR* 1985;145:249–254.
49. Gilsanz V. Quantitative computed tomography. In: Siegel MJ, ed. *Pediatric Body CT*. New York: Churchill Livingstone, 1988:349–369.
50. Giyanani VL, Meyers PC, Wolfson JJ. Mesenchymal hamartoma of the liver: computed tomography and ultrasonography. *J Comput Assist Tomogr* 1986;10:51–54.
51. Gold RP, McClennan BL, Rottenberg RR. CT appearance of acute inflammatory disease of the renal interstitium. *AJR* 1983;141:343–349.
52. Griscom NT. The roentgenology of neonatal abdominal masses. *AJR* 1965;93:447–463.
53. Griscom NT, Wohl MEB. Dimensions of the growing trachea related to age and gender. *AJR* 1986;146:233–237.
54. Guyer BH, Levinsohn EM, Fredickson BE, Bailey GL, Formikell M. Computed tomography of calcaneal fractures: anatomy, pathology, dosimetry, and clinical relevance. *AJR* 1985;145:911–919.
55. Hecht ST, Brasch RC, Styne DM. CT localization of occult secretory tumors in children. *Pediatr Radiol* 1982;12:67–71.
56. Heiberg E, Wolverson MK, Sundaram M, Nouri S. Normal thymus: CT characteristics in subjects under 20. *AJR* 1982;138:491–494.
57. Hernandez RJ. Concentric reduction of the dislocated hip. Computed-tomographic evaluation. *Radiology* 1984;150:266–268.

58. Hernandez RJ. Visualization of small sequestra by computerized tomography. *Pediatr Radiol* 1985;15:238–241.
59. Hernandez RJ. Musculoskeletal system. In: Siegel MJ, ed. *Pediatric Body CT*. New York: Churchill Livingstone, 1988:253–291.
60. Hernandez RJ, Tachdjian MO, Poznanski AK, Dias LS. CT determination of femoral torsion. *AJR* 1981;137:97–101.
61. Hernanz-Schulman M, Teele RL, Perez-Atayde A, et al. Pancreatic cystosis in cystic fibrosis. *Radiology* 1986;158:629–631.
62. Hoddick W, Jeffrey RB, Goldberg HI, Federle MP, Laing FC. CT and sonography of severe renal and perirenal infections. *AJR* 1983;140:517–520.
63. Hoffman EP, Mindelzun RE, Anderson RU. Computed tomography in acute pyelonephritis associated with diabetes. *Radiology* 1980;135:691–695.
64. Hope JW, Borns PH, Koop CE. Radiologic diagnosis of mediastinal masses in infants and children. *Radiol Clin North Am* 1963;1:17–50.
65. Jeffrey RB, Laing FC, Federle MP, Goodman PC. Computed tomography of splenic trauma. *Radiology* 1981;141:729–732.
66. Kasper TE, Osborne RW Jr, Semerdjian HS, Miller HC. Urologic abdominal masses in infants and children. *J Urol* 1976;116:629–633.
67. Karp MP, Cooney DR, Berger PE, Kuhn JP, Jewett TC. The role of computed tomography in the evaluation of blunt abdominal trauma in children. *J Pediatr Surg* 1981;16:316–323.
68. Kaufman RA. CT of blunt abdominal trauma in children: A five-year experience. In: Siegel MJ, ed. *Pediatric Body CT*. New York: Churchill Livingstone, 1988:313–347.
69. Kaufman RA, Towbin R, Babcock DS, et al. Upper abdominal trauma in children: imaging evaluation. *AJR* 1984;142:449–460.
70. Kirks DR, Fram EK, Vock P, Effmann EL. Trachael compression by mediastinal masses in children: CT evaluation. *AJR* 1983;141:647–651.
71. Kirks DR, Korobkin M. Computed tomography of the chest in infants and children: techniques and mediastinal evaluation. *Radiol Clin North Am* 1981;19:409–419.
72. Kirks DR, Korobkin M. Computed tomography of the chest wall, pleura and pulmonary parenchyma in infants and children. *Radiol Clin North Am* 1981;19:421–429.
73. Kirks DR, Merten DF, Grossman H, Bowie JD. Diagnostic imaging of pediatric abdominal masses: an overview. *Radiol Clin North Am* 1981;19:527–545.
74. Kirks DR, Ponzi JW, Korobkin M. Computed tomographic diagnosis of calcified inferior vena cava thrombus in a child with Wilms' tumor. *Pediatr Radiol* 1980;10:110–112.
75. Knochel JW, Koehler RP, Lee TG, Welch DM. Diagnosis of abdominal abscesses with computed tomography, ultrasound, and ^{111}In leukocyte scans. *Radiology* 1980;137:425–432.
76. Korobkin M, Kirks DR, Sullivan DC, Mills SR, Bowie JD. Computed tomography of primary liver tumors in children. *Radiology* 1981;139:431–435.
77. Kramer SS, Blum EE. CT of bronchogenic cysts. In: Siegelman SS, ed. *Computed tomography of the chest*. New York: Churchill Livingstone, 1984:219–231.
78. Krudy AG, Dunnick NR, Magrath IT, Shawker TH, Doppman JL, Spiegel R. CT of American Burkitt lymphoma. *AJR* 1981;136:747–754.
79. Kuhn JP, Berger PE. Computed tomographic diagnosis of osteomyelitis. *Radiology* 1979;130:503–506.
80. Kuhn JP, Berger PE. Computed tomographic diagnosis of abdominal abscesses in children. *Ann Radiol (Paris)* 1980;23:153–158.
81. Kuhn JP, Berger PE. Computed tomography of the kidney in infancy and childhood. *Radiol Clin North Am* 1981;19:445–461.
82. Lassen MN. Dedicated CT technique for scanning neonates. *Radiology* 1986;161:363–366.
83. Lee JKT, McClennan BL, Melson GL, Stanley RJ. Acute focal bacterial nephritis: emphasis on grey scale ultrasonography and computed tomography. *AJR* 1980;135:87–92.
84. Lee JKT, McClennan BL, Stanley RJ, Sagel SS. Utility of computed tomography in the localization of the undescended testis. *Radiology* 1980;135:121–125.
85. Levitt RG, Husband JE, Glazer HS. CT of primary germ-cell tumors of the mediastinum. *AJR* 1984;142:73–78.
86. Long JA Jr, Doppmann JL, Nienhus AW, Mills SR. Computed

87. tomographic analysis of beta-thalassemic syndrome with hemochromatosis: pathologic findings with clinical and laboratory correlations. *J Comput Assist Tomogr* 1980;4:159–165.
87. Lowe RE, Cohen MD. Computed tomographic evaluation of Wilms' tumor and neuroblastoma. *Radiographics* 1984;4:915–928.
88. Lucaya J, Enriquez G, Amat L, Gonzalez-Rivero MA. Computed tomography of infantile hepatic hemangioendothelioma. *AJR* 1985;144:821–826.
89. Luers PR, Lester PD, Siegler RL. CT demonstration of cortical nephrocalcinosis in congenital oxalosis. *Pediatr Radiol* 1980;10:116–118.
90. Lukens JA, McLeod RA, Sim FH. Computed tomographic evaluation of primary osseous malignant neoplasms. *AJR* 1982;139:45–48.
91. Mack LA, Harley JD, Winquist RA. CT of acetabular fractures. Analysis of fracture patterns. *AJR* 1982;138:407–412.
92. Madewell JE, Goldman SM, Davis CJ, Hartman DS, Feigin DS, Lichtenstein JE. Multilocular cystic nephroma: a radiographic-pathologic correlation of 58 patients. *Radiology* 1983;146:309–321.
93. Mayo J, Gray R, St Louis E, Grosman H, McLoughlin M, Wise D. Anomalies of the inferior vena cava. *AJR* 1983;140:339–345.
94. Mendelson DS, Rose JS, Efremidis SC, Kirschner PA, Cohen BA. Bronchogenic cysts with high CT numbers. *AJR* 1983;140:463–465.
95. Miller JH, Sinatra FR, Thomas DW. Biliary excretion disorders in infants: evaluation using ^{99m}TcPIPIDA. *AJR* 1980;135:47–52.
96. Miller PA, Williamson BRJ, Minor GR, Buschi AJ. Pulmonary sequestration: visualization of the feeding artery by CT. *J Comput Assist Tomogr* 1982;6:828–830.
97. Mitnick JS, Bosniak MA, Hilton S, Raghavendra BN, Subramanyam BR, Genieser NB. Cystic renal disease in tuberous sclerosis. *Radiology* 1983;147:85–87.
98. Moon KL, Genant HK, Helms CA, Chafetz NI, Crooks LE, Kaufman L. Musculoskeletal applications of nuclear magnetic resonance. *Radiology* 1983;147:161–171.
99. Moon KL, Federle MP. Computed tomography in hepatic trauma. *AJR* 1983;141:309–314.
100. Muhm JR, Brown LR, Crowe JK, Sheedy PF, Hattery RR, Stephens DH. Comparison of whole lung tomography and computed tomography for detecting pulmonary nodules. *AJR* 1978;131:981–984.
101. Muller NL, Gamsu G, Webb WR. Pulmonary nodules: detection using magnetic resonance and computed tomography. *Radiology* 1985;155:687–690.
102. Nakata H, Nakayama C, Kimoto T, et al. Computed tomography of mediastinal bronchogenic cysts. *J Comput Assist Tomogr* 1982;6:733–738.
103. Pardes JG, LiPuma JP, Haaga JR, Petruschak MJ, Alfidi RJ. Lymphangioma of the thymus in a child. *J Comput Assist Tomogr* 1982;6:825–827.
104. Parvey LS, Warner RM, Callihan TR, Magill HL. CT demonstration of the fat tissue in malignant renal neoplasms: atypical Wilms' tumors. *J Comput Assist Tomogr* 1981;5:851–854.
105. Paul DJ, Mueller CF. Pulmonary sequestration. *J Comput Assist Tomogr* 1982;6:163–165.
106. Peretz GS, Lam AH. Distinguishing neuroblastoma from Wilms tumor by computed tomography. *J Comput Assist Tomogr* 1985;9:889–893.
107. Petasnick JP, Turner DA, Charters JR, Gitelis S, Zacharias CE. Soft-tissue masses of the locomotor system: comparison of MR imaging with CT. *Radiology* 1986;160:125–133.
108. Peterson HA, Klassen RA, McLeod RA, Hoffman AD. The use of computerised tomography in dislocation of the hip and femoral neck anteversion in children. *J Bone Joint Surg* 1981;63B:198–208.
109. Picus D, Siegel MJ, Balfe DM. Abdominal computed tomography in children with unexplained prolonged fever. *J Comput Assist Tomogr* 1984;8:851–856.
110. Pugatch RD, Gale ME. Obscure pulmonary masses: bronchial impaction revealed by CT. *AJR* 1983;141:909–914.
111. Ravitch MM, Sabiston DC. Mediastinal infections, cysts and tumors: In: Ravitch MM, Welch KJ, Benson CD, Aberdeen E, Randolph JG, eds. *Pediatric surgery*. Chicago: Year Book, 1979:499–512.

112. Reiman TAH, Siegel MJ, Shackelford GD. Abdominal CT and sonography in children with Wilms' tumor. *Radiology* 1986;160: 501–505.
113. Resjo IM, Harwood-Nash DC, Fitz CR, Chuang S. Normal cord in infants and children examined with computed tomographic metrizamide myelography. *Radiology* 1979;130:691–696.
114. Resjo IM, Harwood-Nash DC, Fitz CR, Chuang S. CT metrizamide myelography for intraspinal and paraspinal neoplasms in infants and children. *AJR* 1979;132:367–372.
115. Ros PR, Goodman ZD, Ishak KG, et al. Mesenchymal hamartoma of the liver: radiologic-pathologic correlation. *Radiology* 1986;158: 619–624.
116. Ros PR, Olmsted WW, Moser RP, et al. Mesenteric and omental cysts: Histologic classification with imaging correlation. *Radiology* 1987;164:327–332.
117. Rosenfield NS, Leonidas JC, Barwick KW. Aggressive neuroblastoma simulating Wilms tumor. *Radiology* 1988;166:165–167.
118. Ross JS, O'Donovan PB, Novoa R, et al. Magnetic resonance of the chest: initial experience with imaging in vivo T1 and T2 calculations. *Radiology* 1984;152:95–101.
119. St. Amour TE, Siegel MJ, Glazer HS, Nadel SN. CT appearances of the normal and abnormal thymus in childhood. *J Comput Assist Tomogr* 1987;11:645–650.
120. Sarno RC, Carter BL, Bankoff MS, Semine MC. Computed tomography in tarsal coalition. *J Comput Assist Tomogr* 1984;8:1155–1160.
121. Schaner EG, Chang AE, Doppman JL, Conkle DM, Flye MW, Rosenberg SA. Comparison of computed and conventional whole lung tomography in detecting pulmonary nodules: a prospective radiologic-pathologic study. *AJR* 1978;131:51–54.
122. Schwartz AM, Dorkin HL, Carter BL. CT appearance of the liver in a patient with biliary cirrhosis and cystic fibrosis. *J Comput Assist Tomogr* 1983;7:530–533.
123. Seltzer SE, Weissman BN, Braunstein EM, Adams DF, Thomas WH. Computed tomography of the hindfoot. *J Comput Assist Tomogr* 1984;8:488–497.
124. Shehadi WH, Toniolo G. Adverse reactions to contrast media. *Radiology* 1980;137:299–302.
125. Siegel MJ. *Pediatric Body CT.* New York, Churchill Livingstone, 1988.
126. Siegel MJ. Liver and biliary tract. In: Siegel MJ, ed. *Pediatric Body CT.* New York: Churchill Livingstone, 1988:103–134.
127. Siegel MJ. Pelvic organs and soft tissues. In: Siegel MJ, ed. *Pediatric Body CT.* New York: Churchill Livingstone, 1988:219–251.
128. Siegel MJ, Balfe DM, McClennan BL, Levitt RG. Clinical utility of CT in pediatric retroperitoneal disease: 5 years experience. *AJR* 1982;138:1011–1017.
129. Siegel MJ, Glasier CM, Sagel SS. CT of pelvic disorders in children. *AJR* 1981;137:1139–1143.
130. Siegel MJ, Jamroz GA, Glazer HS, Abramson CL. MR imaging of intraspinal extension of neuroblastoma. *J Comput Assist Tomogr* 1986;10:593–595.
131. Siegel MJ, Nadel SN, Glazer HS, Sagel SS. CT and MR of mediastinal lesions in children. *Radiology* 1986;160:241–244.
132. Siegel MJ, Sagel SS. Computed tomography as a supplement to urography in the evaluation of suspected neuroblastoma. *Radiology* 1982;142:435–438.
133. Siegel MJ, Sagel SS, Reed K. The value of computed tomography in the diagnosis and management of pediatric mediastinal abnormalities. *Radiology* 1982;142:149–155.
134. Stalker HP, Kaufman RA, Towbin R. Patterns of liver injury in childhood: CT analysis. *AJR* 1986;147:1199–1205.
135. Stanley P, Atkinson JB, Reid BS, Gilsanz V. Percutaneous drainage of abdominal fluid collections in children. *AJR* 1984;142:813–816.
136. Stanley P. Computed tomographic evaluation of the retroperitoneum in infants and children. *CT* 1983;7:63–75.
137. Stark DD, Brasch RC, Moss AA, et al. Recurrent neuroblastoma: the role of CT and alternative imaging tests. *Radiology* 1983;148: 107–112.
138. Stark DD, Moss AA, Brasch RC, et al. Neuroblastoma: diagnostic imaging and staging. *Radiology* 1983;148:101–105.
139. Strain JS, Harvey LA, Foley LC, Campbell JB. Intravenously administered pentobarbital sodium for sedation in pediatric CT. *Radiology* 1986;161:105–108.
140. Suzuki M, Takashima T, Itoh H, Choutoh S, Kawamura I, Watamabe Y. Computed tomography of mediastinal teratomas. *J Comput Assist Tomogr* 1983;7:74–76.
141. Tang JSH, Gold RH, Bassett LW, Seeger LL. Musculoskeletal infection of the extremities: Evaluation with MR imaging. *Radiology* 1988; 166:205–209.
142. Totty WG, Murphy WA, Ganz WI, Kumar B, Daum W, Siegel BA. Magnetic resonance imaging of the normal and ischemic femoral head. *AJR* 1984;143:1273–1280.
143. Totty WG, Murphy WA, Lee JKT. Soft-tissue tumors: MR imaging. *Radiology* 1986;160:135–141.
144. Tschappeler H. Computed tomography (CT) and lymphoma in children. *Ann Radiol (Paris)* 1980;23:87–91.
145. Vachon L, Gilsanz V. CT visualization of posterior vertebral veins: A sign of vena caval obstruction. *Pediatr Radiol* 1986;16:197.
146. Vanel D, Contesso G, Couanet D, Piekarski JD, Sarrazin D, Masselot J. Computed tomography in the evaluation of 41 cases of Ewing's sarcoma. *Skeletal Radiol* 1982;9:8–13.
147. Vas WG, Wolverson MK, Sundaram M, et al. The role of computed tomography in pelvic fractures. *J Comput Assist Tomogr* 1982;6: 796–801.
148. Walligore MP, Stephens DH, Soule EH, McLeod RA: Lipomatous tumors of the abdominal cavity. CT appearance and pathologic correlation. *AJR* 1981;137:539–545.
149. Weinberg AG, Finegold MJ. Primary hepatic tumors of childhood. *Hum Pathol* 1983;14:512–537.
150. Wolverson MK, Houttuin E, Heiberg E, Sundaram M, Shields JB. Comparison of computed tomography with high-resolution real-time ultrasound in the localization of the impalpable undescended testis. *Radiology* 1983;146:133–136.
151. Webb WR, Gamsu G, Speckman JM, Kaiser JA, Federle MP, Lipton MJ. Computed tomographic demonstration of mediastinal venous anomalies. *AJR* 1982;139:157–161.
152. Weinreb JC, Cohen JM, Armstrong E, Smith T. Imaging the pediatric liver: MR and CT. *AJR* 1986;147:785–790.
153. Zimmer WD, Berquist TH, McLeod RA, et al. Bone tumors: magnetic resonance imaging versus computed tomography. *Radiology* 1985;155:709–718.

CHAPTER 24

Radiation Oncology

Miljenko V. Pilepich, John Wong, and Todd H. Wasserman

Computed tomography (CT) has profoundly affected the management of a large proportion of cancer patients, including those treated with radiotherapy. The optimal applications of CT within the diversity of tumor sites and stages continue to emerge.

The strategy for diagnostic evaluation and treatment of cancer grows increasingly complex. Following the initial *diagnosis,* an accurate *staging* (definition of tumor extent) is required for most malignant neoplasms before a rational application of surgical, radiotherapeutic, and chemotherapeutic *treatment* can be planned. Of obvious importance is life-long *follow-up* for evaluation of the results of treatment and early detection of possible recurrences and complications of treatment. CT can play an important role in each of these four steps: diagnosis, staging, treatment, and follow-up.

A large percentage of cancer patients with localized or local-regional disease receive radiotherapy (either alone or in combination with other therapeutic modalities), with curative intent. Success of such treatment will depend on, among other factors, the radiotherapist's ability to deliver an adequate dose to the tumor in its entirety while preserving the normal structures included in the radiation field. There are several steps involved in achieving this rather complex goal. They include (a) accurate localization of tumor volume, with separation from surrounding normal structures, (b) prescription of a dose to be delivered to the tumor volume(s) and definition of limiting doses to normal tissues, (c) accurate computation of dose distribution within the treatment volume of the patient, and (d) precise delivery of the radiation dose over the entire course of treatment.

CT AND DETERMINATION OF TREATMENT VOLUME

Accurate localization of normal structures and tumor and their three-dimensional representation have long been

weak links in radiation treatment planning. Moreover, accurate computation of the absorbed-dose distribution within a patient requires precise knowledge of the patient's surface contour and the radiation-absorption properties of internal tissues. CT has become a vital tool in radiotherapy planning by providing this information with a precision that was not possible in the past.

Before making a rational decision on the choice of equipment, beam quality, position and shape of ports, use of accessories, doses, and fractionation pattern, the radiation therapist needs to define (a) the clinically and radiologically *detectable tumor volume,* (b) the *volume at risk for subclinical (microscopic) involvement,* although clinically and radiologically free of disease (in some instances, this volume of tissue will be defined by anatomical boundaries such as bony structures, fascias, organ capsules, and serosal surfaces), (c) the *locations of the critical normal structures* that are dose-limiting (e.g., spinal cord, bowel, kidney, lung), and (d) the *treatment volume* and the doses to be delivered within the volume. These terms are defined in some detail in Figs. 1 to 3.

Cross-sectional CT images delineating body contour, tumor, and internal structures are well suited for immediate application in radiotherapy (3,4,12,16,20,21,24, 28,34,38,45,48,52,55,56).

The important considerations to be reviewed during interpretation of CT images for radiotherapy by the diagnostic radiologist are (a) the anatomical and quantitative definition of tumor extent, (b) the relationship of tumor mass to bone structures as well as to key organs (i.e., heart, liver, kidney, spinal cord), and (c) identification of tumor in distinct anatomical compartments (e.g., mediastinum versus hilum, mesenteric versus retroperitoneal, or combinations thereof). It is important that the tumor extent be defined quantitatively in centimeters, and in all directions, as well as relative to key organs within the anatomical region. It also may be useful to represent the tumor extent in relation to vertebral-body positions. It is helpful

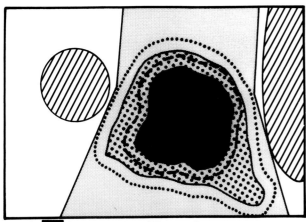

A) ■ (Detectable, Gross) Tumor volume
B) ⣿ Volume at risk for subclinical involvement
C) --- Target volume for full (tumoricidal) dose
D) ···· Target volume for moderate (prophylactic) dose
E) ▨ Dose limiting structures
F) ▢ Treated volume

FIG. 1. Schematic description of the frequently used terminology in radiotherapy treatment planning: (A) The gross tumor volume implies the radiographically and clinically detectable tumor. (B) The volume at risk for subclinical involvement is the volume of tissue in which the tumor is not clinically and radiographically detectable, but is at high risk for microscopic involvement. In defining this volume, the radiotherapist uses the known characteristics of the primary tumor, such as tendency toward lymphatic spread or permeation of tissues, as judged by the degree of histological differentiation. (C) The target volume, which needs to receive high tumoricidal doses to eradicate a tumor, is somewhat larger than the gross tumor volume. A safety margin has been added around the tumor to provide for the daily variation in positioning of the patient and the treatment beam. (D) The target volume that needs to be treated to lower (prophylactic) doses includes the volume at risk for subclinical involvement, with a safety margin to provide for variations in the positioning of the patient and the treatment beam. In most tumors, the prophylactic doses range between 4,000 and 5,000 rad. (E) Dose-limiting structures are important considerations in treatment planning. The spinal cord is an example, the dose to which is limited to 4,500 rad in 4 to 5 weeks. If a large area of the lung is to be treated, the dose usually is limited to 2,000 rad or less in 2 weeks or longer. The kidneys and the liver are also dose-limiting structures. The usually accepted level of tolerance for the kidneys, if the whole of the kidney parenchyma is to be treated, is 2,000 rad in 2 weeks or longer. For the liver, the accepted tolerance limit is 3,000 rad in 3 weeks. (F) The treated volume is composed of all tissues that get irradiated, including those that happen to be in the passage of the beam only incidentally.

A,B

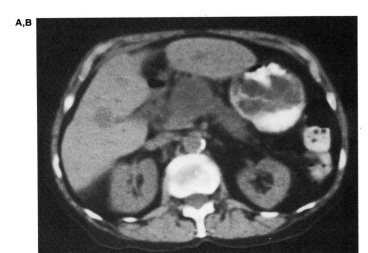

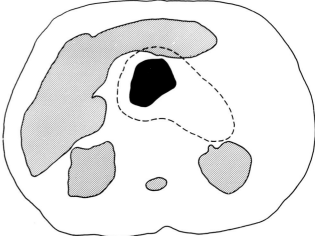

C

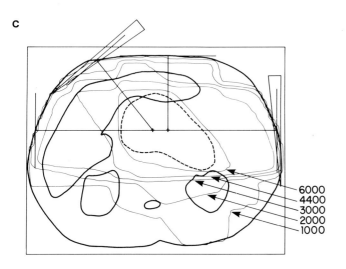

6000
4400
3000
2000
1000

FIG. 2. A 59-year-old man with carcinoma of the pancreas. A: The image delineates the tumor in the neck and body of the pancreas. B: The volume to receive the full tumoricidal doses has been delineated on the basis of several slices. Provision is made for inclusion of the tail. The dose-limiting structures are the spinal cord, kidneys, and liver. The delineation of the kidneys and the liver does not correspond exactly to Fig. 2A because other representative cuts above the slice shown in Fig. 2A are taken into account. C: Treatment plan delineating four-field arrangement. Fields 3 and 4 are wedged. The proximity of the tumor volume to critical structures (spinal cord, kidneys, and liver) makes irradiation of the pancreas particularly difficult. In this case, the tumor, with generous margins, receives a dose of approximately 6,000 rad. The major portion of the renal parenchyma remains outside the 2,000-rad isodose. A large portion of the hepatic parenchyma receives 3,000 rad or less. Isodose lines in this and subsequent figures refer to lines delineating areas within a treatment plan receiving the same dose.

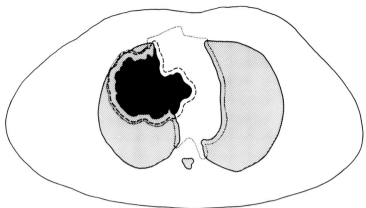

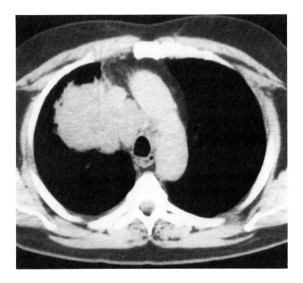

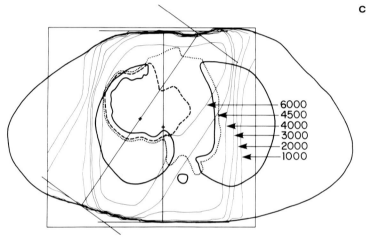

FIG. 3. A 65-year-old woman with bronchogenic carcinoma. **A:** The primary tumor is a relatively large right-upper-lobe lesion directly extending toward and invading the mediastinum. **B:** The blackened area is grossly detectable tumor. The areas to receive full tumoricidal doses (in this case, 6,000 rad) and the area to receive a prophylactic dose (in this case, 4,500 rad) are delineated. The shaded areas represent the dose-limiting structures, which are, in this case, the lungs and the spinal cord. **C:** Treatment plan that utilizes a complex set of four beams. Beams 1 and 2 are AP and PA; 3 and 4 are oblique opposed beams. A combination of 18- and 4-MV X-ray beams is used. A substantial portion of the lung parenchyma at the treated level is included in the treated volume. Even at this level, a substantial portion of the lung receives less than 2,000 rad. It should be stressed that in this patient, the bases of the lung need not be included in the treatment volume; the total volume of irradiated lung is therefore not excessive.

if the tumor mass can be defined on a supine conventional or computed (digital) radiograph.

There have been several attempts to quantitate the impact of CT on radiotherapy treatment planning. Munzenrider et al. (38) analyzed retrospectively one of the first sizable groups of patients for whom CT information had been used systematically in treatment planning. In that study, CT data were considered essential for therapeutic decision making in 55% of patients studied and prompted a change in treatment volume in 45% of cases.

Goitein et al. (20) reported the results of a prospective study designed to assess the value of CT in radiotherapy treatment planning for 77 patients. Conventional studies were performed first, and computer-generated treatment plans were drawn up. Subsequently, CT images were used to delineate the location of the tumor and adjacent normal tissues, and treatment plans were altered when necessary. In 31 patients (42%), techniques were changed because of inadequate tumor coverage. Considerations of normal tissue coverage were the only reasons for field changes in 4 patients. In 36 patients (47%), radiotherapy plans were changed as a result of CT examination.

The available literature indicates that, depending on tumor type, CT information has prompted changes in treatment planning in 34 to 61% of studied cases (9,16,20,21,38,41). Although there is no doubt that CT has a major influence on radiotherapy planning, the degree to which these CT-induced modifications alter the clinical course (tumor control and treatment-related morbidity) remains to be quantitated.

TECHNICAL CONSIDERATIONS

Certain technical problems associated with whole-body scanners must be eliminated before CT images can be used in treatment planning. For example, most scanner couches that support the patient are concave. The couches of radiotherapy treatment machines generally are flat. The difference in couch designs causes the patient's body contour and the locations of internal organs to be different during treatment than during imaging. In general, the position of a patient during CT should be identical with that used during radiation treatment. If a patient is to be treated in a position other than supine, the CT image should also be obtained in that position. With some of the early equipment, a small gantry aperture or small size of the field of image reconstruction results in edge cutoff of the patient's contour in many anatomical regions. This limitation poses a problem in treatment planning because lateral radiation beams often are employed for treatment. If it can be anticipated that the image will be used for radiotherapy treatment planning, an appropriate number of full-contour images should be obtained above, through, and below the tumor-bearing areas. To utilize the CT image for planning, one must properly register CT slices with respect to appropriate landmarks on a patient's skin surface or on computed or conventional radiographic film.

Most existing radiation therapy centers have dedicated computers for treatment planning. The information on patient contour and internal structures often is obtained from CT images. These data usually are entered into the computer by means of light-pen or tracing devices. Optically or photographically enlarged CT images also can be entered into a treatment-planning computer. Although this procedure can be used without any modifications of existing treatment-planning computers, the matrix of CT data should be transferred to the treatment-planning computer directly via a magnetic tape or a floppy disk for the sake of efficiency and accuracy of dose computation.

Based on our experience and that of others (13,18,26,47), the design features of a CT scanner that are most useful in radiation therapy are as follows: (a) large scanner aperture (60 cm or more); (b) flat couch surface; (c) capability of producing anteroposterior and lateral digital radiographs to reference imaging slices; (d) availability of patient-immobilization devices and alignment lasers; (e) fast scan time and capability of producing a large number of slices within a reasonable time period; (f) sagittal and coronal reconstruction capability; (g) data storage and transfer capability for treatment planning.

Almost all of the newer-generation CT scanners meet these specifications. These scanners have a large gantry aperture with a large reconstruction field of view available and may be used to obtain images containing the full contour of a patient. The locations of CT slices can be registered with respect to a digital radiograph obtained on the scanner. The concave couch on a CT scanner can be made flat by means of a hard-foam or wooden insert.

The patient positioning parameters (arms and legs appropriate; patient supine, prone, or lateral) should correspond to those used during radiotherapy. Therefore, prior to CT it is essential that the radiation therapist inform the diagnostic radiologist about the treatment position to be used. It is important that a CT study fully define the extreme dimensions of the tumor, with at least several levels of normal anatomy above and below the gross disease.

Table 1 lists the parameters of radiotherapy treatment that can be determined by CT information. Some of these

TABLE 1. *Parameters of radiotherapy treatment that can be determined by CT information*

Patient diameters—cross-sectional dimensions
Field size
Depth for dose specification
   From skin (depth dose)
   From skin to axis (distance for isocentric treatment)
Depth from surface of dose-limiting organs or structures
Portal or field angles for oblique and rotational fields
Absorption data (tissue density)
Isodose distribution

measurements can be determined accurately only by CT. These data provide not only for better tumor localization but also for better and truer physical representation of the effects of the radiation.

Radiation therapists often use a simulator, a machine that mimics the physical parameters of a radiation therapy machine, but is capable of producing X-rays of diagnostic energies only. The simulator is designed to test the options that may be available for treatment of a patient, to test the ability of a patient to maintain a reproducible position, and to provide clear X-ray images of the paths of the photon beam. Commercial units that integrate the CT scanner directly into the simulator currently are available. Most of these have a computer interface that allows for on-line treatment planning and control of the simulator to show the dose-delivery capability of such treatment planning.

CT AND DOSAGE COMPUTATION

At the present time, most radiotherapy treatments are delivered by cobalt 60 γ-rays or high-energy (megavoltage) X-rays produced by linear accelerators and betatrons. Electron beams produced by linear accelerators and betatrons are also gaining wider acceptance. In addition, a few specialized radiotherapy research centers are using charged particles such as protons, pions, and heavy ions (46).

In radiotherapy, accurate delivery of radiation doses to many anatomical sites within a patient is complicated by the presence of dose-perturbing inhomogeneities such as bone and air (e.g., lung). To take into account the effects of dose-perturbing tissues, the locations and absorption properties of tissues are determined primarily by the electron density (electrons per milliliter) or the physical density (grams per milliliter) of the tissue. Several investigators (10,22,23,39,40,44) have shown how these CT numbers, which are relative linear-attenuation coefficients at diagnostic energies, can be converted to show the electron or physical density of the tissue by an experimentally determined (computer-stored) curve. The absorbed dose is computed in two dimensions, where the difference in electron density of an individual pixel (picture element) relative to water is taken into account. The inhomogeneity corrections are important for dose calculations of photon beams and charged particles (4,10,17,22,28,44,45,53).

CT IN THE MANAGEMENT OF SELECTED TUMORS

Bronchogenic Carcinoma

Although the majority of intrapulmonary lesions can be easily identified on conventional radiographs, CT has proved invaluable in the definition of tumor extent. It is particularly useful for evaluation of the involvement of mediastinal lymph nodes and direct extension of the tumor to mediastinal structures and the chest wall. Invasion of any of these structures usually is considered a contraindication for surgical resection; therefore, this information is important in the selection of patients for radiotherapy. Documentation of the presence of gross tumor in the mediastinal lymph nodes or the chest wall indicates a need to increase the dosage and the field size substantially in these areas.

An example of the use of CT in treatment planning for carcinoma of the lung is shown in Fig. 3. Because patients breathe freely during radiation treatment, it is best to obtain the CT images during resting mid-expiration. In most instances, treatment is given with the arms positioned alongside the chest, rather than raised above the head. Obtaining the CT images with the arms in this same position prevents distortion of the patient contour and shifting of the internal structures. If accurate size determination of a pulmonary mass is required, the window level should be placed at the midpoint between the average CT number of the mass to be measured and the average CT number of the surrounding tissue (27).

Carcinoma of the Bladder

Determination of the depth of penetration of the primary tumor through the bladder wall is essential in the staging and choice of therapy for bladder carcinoma. The customary clinical staging procedures are cystoscopy, transurethral resection of the tumor, and bimanual examination under anesthesia. Clinical staging differs from pathological staging in a large percentage of cases. In most instances, the error is due to clinical understaging, which occurs in approximately one-third of cases (59). Because patients with deeply invasive tumors usually receive preoperative radiotherapy, identification of these patients prior to exploration-resection (cystectomy) is essential. Several reports indicate a high degree of correlation between CT staging and pathological staging in deeply invasive tumors (25,61); however, CT is not useful for as-

sessing the depth of penetration in more superficial tumors. Although CT can show grossly enlarged lymph node metastases, it will not indicate spread within normal-size lymph nodes, resulting in understaging.

CT has also been shown to be useful for optimization of radiotherapy treatment planning, primarily by providing better definition of the position and topographic relationships of the bladder. In the series of Schlager et al. (51), CT information led to revisions in 29% of treatment plans.

A potentially promising area for CT application in radiotherapy for bladder cancer is in the evaluation of tumor response following preoperative irradiation. In patients whose tumors regress significantly following a course of preoperative radiotherapy at moderate doses, cystectomy may be avoided if additional radiotherapy at full tumoricidal doses is given. Results from a study reported by Veenema et al. (58) support this approach.

Carcinoma of the Prostate

Radiotherapy is playing an increasingly important role in curative management for carcinoma of the prostate. Selection of treatment modality (surgery versus radiotherapy) and determination of the radiotherapy fields and doses usually are based on clinical staging. Clinical staging is largely dependent on the findings of rectal examination; the tumor extent often is underestimated.

The value of CT for definition of local and regional spread of prostatic carcinoma has been studied, but remains unresolved (54). Because most patients with more advanced tumors do not undergo exploration and prostatectomy, which would confirm or disprove the CT findings, it is difficult to compile a substantial number of cases with surgical-pathological correlation. The value of CT in the optimization of treatment planning, however, has been well documented (29,41,42). The target volume, which is to receive high tumoricidal doses and should include the primary tumor and its extension into the periprostatic tissue, is difficult to define with conventional radiographic techniques, which fail to demonstrate the lateral extent of the tumor and the position and shape of the seminal vesicles, a frequent site of involvement.

In one series of 82 patients treated with curative intent with external-beam radiotherapy (42), 7% of treatment plans drawn up without CT information were found inadequate in stage B and early stage C carcinoma of the prostate. Fifty-three percent (17 of 32) of patients with (clinically) involved seminal vesicles would not have had adequate treatment of the entire tumor volume without the CT information. Similar findings have been reported by other investigators (29,30).

CT has also been found useful for localization of radioactive-implant sources in patients so treated with carcinoma of the prostate (15).

Testicular Tumors

Management of testicular tumors depends to a great extent on accurate assessment of the retroperitoneal lymph nodes. The status of the periaortic and renal hilar lymph nodes in seminoma determines the extent of the radiation fields and the total dose. In testicular carcinomas, the nodal status determines the need for lymphadenectomy, radiotherapy, and chemotherapy. Although lymphangiography is superior to CT for detecting focal tumor deposits that do not cause enlargement of the lymph nodes, CT can assess the areas not visualized on lymphangiography, primarily those in the renal hilum and above the L2 level (30). In some institutions, lymphangiography is still performed in patients with equivocal or negative findings on CT study.

In terms of treatment planning, CT is particularly useful in patients with large retroperitoneal masses requiring enlargement of the routine radiotherapy fields and an increase in dosage. Massively involved lymph nodes frequently are not demonstrated with lymphangiography because of total replacement of the nodal tissue.

Lymphomas

Evaluation of intraabdominal lymphoid tissue is essential for adequate management of Hodgkin disease and non-Hodgkin lymphomas. The status of the retroperitoneal and mesenteric lymph nodes, among other factors, determines not only the need for irradiation, the extent of the abdominal fields, and the doses of irradiation but also the need for chemotherapy.

Hodgkin disease is characterized by orderly progression along the axial lymphatics. Periaortic lymph nodes are much more likely to be involved than celiac and mesenteric lymph nodes. The customary staging policies at most institutions include laparotomy in most lesser-stage clinical presentations.

Non-Hodgkin lymphomas tend to involve multiple intraabdominal sites and produce bulky enlargement of the celiac and mesenteric lymph nodes and also those in the splenic and hepatic hila. Staging laparotomy is not a customary procedure in non-Hodgkin lymphomas.

Major advantages of CT relative to lymphangiography and exploratory laparotomy are the simplicity and non-

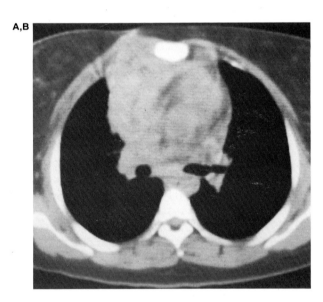

A,B

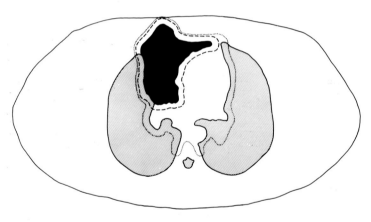

C

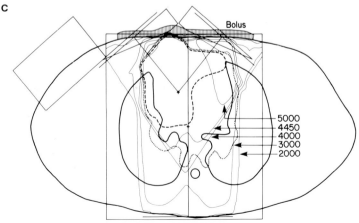

Bolus	
	—5000
	—4450
	—4000
	—3000
	—2000

FIG. 4. A 27-year-old man with locally advanced Hodgkin disease. **A:** A large tumor mass involves the region of the right lobe of the thymus in the anterior mediastinum and extends directly into the right chest wall. **B:** To the area containing the gross tumor, 4,400 rad is to be given. The prophylactic dose is 4,000 rad. **C:** Five beams have been utilized. Beams 1 and 2 are oblique-wedged 4-MV X-ray beams. Beams 3, 4, and 5 are parallel opposed. A block is added posteriorly to reduce the spinal cord dose. The spinal cord dose, according to the plan, is limited to 3,500 rad.

invasiveness of the procedure and its ability to assess nodes not ordinarily seen on a lymphangiogram (mesenteric, retrocrural, celiac, splenic, and hepatic hilar nodes). A major disadvantage of CT versus lymphangiography is its inability to detect abnormalities in intranodal architecture. CT can detect nodal disease only if the nodes are enlarged; CT is unable to identify an involved but normal-size lymph node as abnormal. However, in most cases of nodal involvement with lymphoma, in comparison with carcinoma, the nodes are enlarged enough to be detectable with CT. Several reports attest to a high degree of correlation between findings obtained by CT, lymphangiography, and laparotomy (2,6–8,14,31,33,49,62).

Abdominal CT is used as the primary radiologic staging method in non-Hodgkin lymphomas. Its use in Hodgkin disease varies considerably from institution to institution and depends largely on the institutional policies regarding laparotomy. We use CT as one of the first steps in the evaluation of patients with Hodgkin disease, lymphangiography being reserved for patients with equivocal CT findings and some patients with negative CT findings.

Chest CT can be of considerable usefulness for optimization of treatment planning in selected patients with Hodgkin disease and non-Hodgkin lymphomas. It is valuable in any radiation therapy candidate with a bulky mediastinal mass, which may be spreading along or invading the chest wall, and it can be used to assess lymph nodes difficult to evaluate by conventional radiographic methods (e.g., subcarinal, supradiaphragmatic). Such involvement may be an important cause of treatment failure (43). The use of CT for optimizing treatment planning in lymphomas is illustrated in Figs. 4 and 5.

Sarcomas

Soft-tissue malignant neoplasms show certain characteristics that make CT particularly valuable. These tumors generally are bulky at the time of diagnosis and frequently can be easily distinguished from the surrounding tissues. The attenuation values of these tumors usually are lower than those for surrounding normal tissues. This phenomenon is most prominent in well-differentiated liposarcomas (Fig. 6), where the attenuation value approaches that of normal fat.

Sarcomas permeate the surrounding tissues far beyond the grossly detectable tumor. The natural barriers to tumor spread are fasciae and aponeurotic membranes surrounding the muscle groups and forming the anatomical compartments. Recognition of the compartmental type of tu-

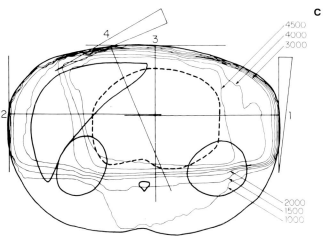

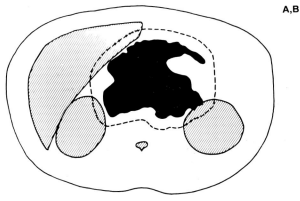

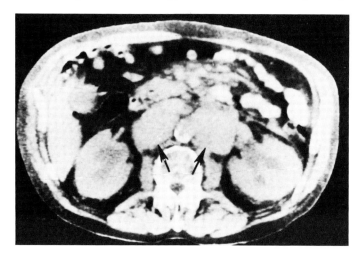

FIG. 5. A 60-year-old man with poorly differentiated nodular lymphocytic lymphoma presenting with massive retroperitoneal and mesenteric lymphadenopathy. Patient is to be treated with a combination of radiotherapy and chemotherapy. **A:** The retroperitoneal (periaortic and pericaval) lymphadenopathy (*arrows*) and mesenteric lymphadenopathy are shown. Bilateral moderate-degree hydronephrosis is caused by encasement of ureters at a lower level. **B:** The delineated volume is to receive 4,500 rad. Slices above the level shown in Fig. 5A have been utilized to delineate the liver. **C:** Treatment plan using four 18-MV X-ray beams. A large percentage of kidney parenchyma is in the treatment volume. A reduction of target volume during the treatment course is indicated and is often facilitated by the prompt shrinkage of tumor in patients with lymphoma.

A–C

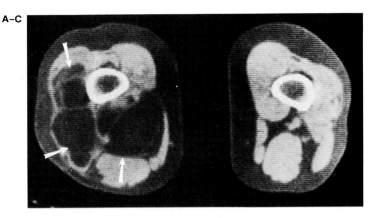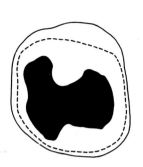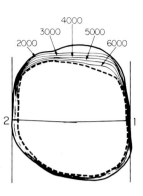

FIG. 6. A 62-year-old woman with myxoliposarcoma of the thigh. **A:** Tumor (*arrows*) is of strikingly low density and is clearly delineated in relation to the muscular groups involved. **B:** The delineated volume is to receive 6,000 rad. The patient will be treated with a combination of surgery and radiotherapy. **C:** A simple setup of two parallel-opposed 4-MV beams is used. CT has proved essential in choosing the site of the spared strip of tissue and its width. Because of the extent of the tumor, the width of the preserved tissue is minimal.

mor spread provides the basis for treatment of sarcomas, which, under optimal circumstances, should be directed not only toward the gross tumor but also toward the whole compartment within which the tumor arises. This therapeutic principle applies to both surgery and radiotherapy.

It has been shown that radiotherapy can consistently control subclinical (microscopic) extensions of sarcomas. Surgical removal of the gross tumor, preceded or followed by adjuvant radiotherapy directed to the sites of potential spread, can yield high control rates without the mutilation associated with radical surgery, such as amputation.

Radiotherapy for soft-tissue sarcomas (either adjuvant or definitive) poses a challenge to the radiation oncologist. The volumes that need to be treated generally are quite large, and the dosages required for tumor control are substantial. Highly sophisticated treatment techniques are needed to achieve adequate dose distribution and maximal preservation of normal tissues. It has been shown that a

A,B

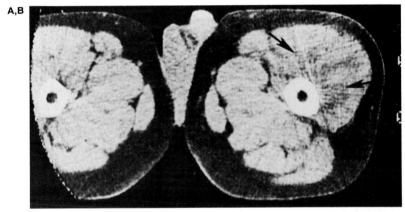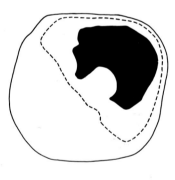

C

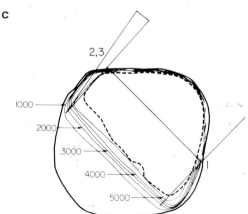

FIG. 7. A 37-year-old man with malignant fibrohistiocytoma of the anterolateral compartment of the left thigh. Patient is to be treated with a course of preoperative radiotherapy, chemotherapy, and limited resection. **A:** The tumor (*arrows*) is confined to the anterolateral muscle group. It extends to the femur, but does not appear to invade other compartments of the thigh. **B:** The delineated area is to receive approximately 5,000 rad. **C:** Parallel-opposed beams, one of which is wedged, are utilized, preserving posteromedial portion of the extremity to prevent lymphatic obstruction. CT imaging is essential in choosing the angle of the beams and the width of the preserved strip of normal tissue.

"strip" of normal tissues should be preserved when an extremity is irradiated, in order to spare lymphatic channels and prevent crippling extremity edema. Adequate coverage of all areas at risk, along with maximal preservation of normal tissues, frequently is a formidable task in patients with soft-tissue sarcomas. CT has proved invaluable in treatment planning for this group of patients. The compartments are easily identified, and the positioning of the beam and the choice of the spared tissue are greatly facilitated (Figs. 6 and 7). In patients to be treated postoperatively, CT images ideally should be obtained prior to surgical resection. In addition, CT is invaluable for follow-up of patients with deep-seated lesions, in whom early detection of recurrences may be lifesaving, with the application of further therapy. Ultrasound also may play a role (5) in defining the limits of these tumors, especially in areas where there is little or no perimuscular fat.

Recent studies have shown that magnetic resonance imaging (MRI) is superior to CT for delineating the extent of soft-tissue masses (57). Although there has been no report documenting the utility of MRI in radiation treatment planning for patients with soft-tissue sarcomas, the increased contrast sensitivity and the direct multiplanar imaging capability of MRI make it ideal for such use.

RECENT DEVELOPMENTS AND FUTURE APPLICATION OF CT IN RADIOTHERAPY

Application of CT data in three-dimensional treatment planning continues to be an area of major research inter-

est. With such a treatment plan, contiguous-image data are obtained for geometric optimization of therapy beams, dose calculations, and dose distribution.

Three-Dimensional Display for Geometric Optimization

The most noticeable development in three-dimensional treatment planning is the display of reconstructed three-dimensional images of CT data for the purpose of geometric optimization—a task that has been performed almost entirely on the simulator. The concept of "beam's-eye view" (BEV) has been most advocated in setting up a single beam (19,35). Another approach that transfers contour information from multiple CT images to a vector-graphics display device is also being tested when multiple beams are involved (36).

Besides application to external-beam radiotherapy, three-dimensional CT data also have been used for brachytherapy optimization, in particular brain implantation. With the aid of an immobilization device, the orientation of the tumor volume in space is determined by CT scanning and then can be used to guide the placement of implant sources in the operating room. An even more direct approach is to perform the actual placement of the "markers" in the CT scanner room as guided by repetitive CT scanning (1) (Fig. 8). These "markers" are then replaced with the radioactive source in a more appropriately shielded environment.

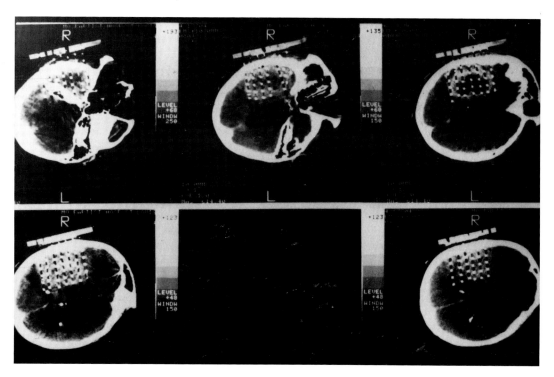

FIG. 8. CT images of "marker" seeds that have been guided for placement in the tumor volume of the brain. The CT information also allows definition of the distribution of the radioactive sources for dose calculation.

Three-Dimensional Dose Calculations

Tissue-density information necessary for accurate dose calculation in radiotherapy has become available through the use of CT. The images reveal the density variations of the human anatomy and allow direct dose calculation from individual-pixel information. At present, some commercial treatment-planning systems provide pixel-based calculations, and the rest employ contours assigned with uniform densities. Almost all available systems rely on methods that utilize only the two-dimensional information on each CT slice. Not surprisingly, large errors, as much as 10%, can occur. It has become apparent that in order to achieve the commonly recommended 3% accuracy, dose calculation would have to include scatter contributions from the distribution of all volume elements in three dimensions. Several potentially promising approaches to this complex task are currently being evaluated and are likely to be available for practical use within the next few years (32,37,50,60).

Three-Dimensional Display of Dose Distributions

The incorporation of a three-dimensional dose distribution onto a three-dimensional representation of anatomical structures remains a difficult problem. Several approaches are being studied. One of these is the "movie" display in which sequential reconstructed gray-scale anatomical images superimposed with colored isodose lines or shades are shown in rapid sequence, with the display of dose as a spectrum of colors superimposed on selected or "cutoff" solid-body anatomical structures. In addition, dose–volume histograms also appear useful in assessing rival treatment plans.

Additional potentially fruitful areas of investigation include the use of reconstructed "fluoroscopy" from three-dimensional CT data to assist in simulation (11), dynamic or conformal radiotherapy, and better verification of the actual treatment.

REFERENCES

1. Abrath FC, Henderson SD, Simpson JR, Moran CJ, Marchosky JA. Dosimetry of CT-guided volumentric Ir-192 brain implant. *Int J Radiat Oncol Biol Phys* 1986;12:359–363.
2. Alcorn FS, Mategrano VC, Petasnick JP, Clark JW. Contributions of computed tomography in the staging and management of malignant lymphoma. *Radiology* 1977;125:717–723.
3. Asbell SO, Schlager BA, Baker AS. Revision of treatment planning for carcinoma of the prostate. *Int J Radiat Oncol Biol Phys* 1980;6:861–865.
4. Battista JJ, Rider WD, Van Dyk J. Computed tomography for radiotherapy planning. *Int J Radiat Oncol Biol Phys* 1980;6:99–107.
5. Bernardino ME, Jing B-S, Thomas JL, Lindell MM, Zornoza J. The extremity soft-tissue lesion: a comparative study of ultrasound, computed tomography and xeroradiography. *Radiology* 1981;139:53–59.
6. Best JJK, Blackledge G, Forbes WSC, et al. Computed tomography of abdomen in staging and clinical management of lymphoma. *Br Med J* 1978;2:1675–1677.
7. Blackledge G, Best JJK, Crowther D, Isherwood I. Computed tomography in the staging of patients with Hodgkin's disease: a report on 136 patients. *Clin Radiol* 1980;31:143–147.
8. Breiman RS, Castellino RA, Harell GS, Marshall WH, Glatstein E, Kaplan HS. CT-pathologic correlations in Hodgkin's disease and non-Hodgkin's lymphoma. *Radiology* 1978;126:159–166.
9. Brizel HE, Livingston PA, Grayson EV. Radiotherapeutic applications of pelvic computed tomography. *J Comput Assist Tomogr* 1979;3:453–466.
10. Chen GTY, Singh RP, Castro JR, Lyman JT, Quivey JM. Treatment planning for heavy ion radiotherapy. *Int J Radiat Oncol Biol Phys* 1979;5:1809–1819.
11. Cheng CW, Chin LM, Kijewski PK. A technique for using anatomical information from CT during treatment simulation. *Med Phys* 1986;13:575.
12. Chernak ES, Rodriquez-Antunez A, Jelden GL, Dhaliwal RS, Lavik PS. The use of computed tomography for radiation therapy treatment planning. *Radiology* 1975;117:613–614.
13. de Winter J. Computed tomography and the radiotherapist. In: Kreel L, Steiner RE, eds. *Medical imaging.* Chicago: Year Book Medical Publishing, 1979:168–177.
14. Earl HM, Sutcliffe SBJ, Kelsey Fry I, et al. Computerized tomographic abdominal scanning in Hodgkin's disease. *Clin Radiol* 1980;31:149–153.
15. Elkon D, Kim JA, Constable WC. Anatomic localization of radioactive gold seeds of the prostate by computer-aided tomography. *Comput Tomogr* 1981;5:89–93.
16. Emami B, Melo A, Carter BL, Munzenrider JE, Piro AJ. Value of computed tomography in radiotherapy of lung cancer. *AJR* 1978;131:63–67.
17. Goitein M. Compensation for inhomogeneities in charged particle radiotherapy using computed tomography. *Int J Radiat Oncol Biol Phys* 1978;4:499–508.
18. Goitein M. Computed tomography in planning radiation therapy. *Int J Radiat Oncol Biol Phys* 1979;5:445–447.
19. Goitein M, Abrams M. Multi-dimensional treatment planning. II. Beam's eye-view, back projection, and projection through CT sections. *Int J Radiat Oncol Biol Phys* 1983;9:789–797.
20. Goitein M, Wittenberg J, Mendiondo M, et al. The value of CT scanning in radiation therapy treatment planning: a prospective study. *Int J Radiat Oncol Biol Phys* 1979;5:1787–1798.
21. Hobday P, Hodson NJ, Husband J, Parker RP, MacDonald JS. Computed tomography applied to radiotherapy treatment planning: techniques and results. *Radiology* 1979;133:477–482.
22. Hogstrom KR, Smith AR, Simon SL, et al. Stasis pion beam treatment planning of deep seated tumors using computed tomographic scans. *Int J Radiat Oncol Biol Phys* 1979;5:875–886.
23. Isherwood I, Pullan BR, Rutherford RA, Strang FA. Electron density and atomic number determination by computed tomography. Part I: Methods and limitation. Part II: A study of colloid cysts. *Br J Radiol* 1977;50:613–619.
24. Jelden GL, Chernak ES, Rodriquez-Antunez A, Haaga JR, Lavik PS, Dhaliwal RS. Further progress in CT scanning and computerized radiation therapy treatment planning. *AJR* 1976;127:179–185.
25. Kellett MJ, Oliver RTD, Husband JE, Fry IK. Computed tomography as an adjunct to bimanual examination for staging bladder tumors. *Br J Urol* 1980;52:101–106.
26. Kelsey CA, Berardo PA, Smith AR, Kligerman MM. CT scanner selection and specification for radiation therapy. *Med Phys* 1980;7:555–558.
27. Koehler PR, Anderson RE, Baxter B. The effect of computed tomography view controls on anatomical measurements. *Radiology* 1979;130:189–194.
28. Laughlin JS, Chu F, Simpson LD. Radiation treatment planning. *Cancer* 1977;39:719–728.
29. Lee D-J, Leibel S, Shiels R, Sanders R, Siegelman S, Order S. The value of ultrasonic imaging and CT scanning in planning the radiotherapy for prostatic carcinoma. *Cancer* 1980;45:724–727.
30. Lee JKT, McClennan BL, Stanley RJ, Sagel SS. Computed tomography in the staging of testicular neoplasms. *Radiology* 1979;130:387–390.

31. Lee JKT, Stanley RJ, Sagel SS, Levitt RG. Accuracy of computed tomography in detecting intraabdominal and pelvic adenopathy in lymphoma. *AJR* 1978;131:311–315.

32. Macki RT, Scimger JW, Battista JJ. A convolution method of calculating dose for 15 MV x-rays. *Med Phys* 1985;12:188–196.

33. Marshall WH Jr, Breiman RS, Harell GS, Glatstein E, Kaplan HS. Computed tomography of abdominal paraaortic lymph node disease: preliminary observations with a 6 second scanner. *AJR* 1977;128:759–764.

34. McCullough EC. Potential of CT in radiation therapy treatment planning. *Radiology* 1978;129:765–768.

35. McShan DL, Silverman A, Lanza DM, Reinstein LE, Glicksman AS. A computerized three-dimensional treatment planning system utilizing interactive color graphics. *Br J Radiol* 1979;52:478–481.

36. Molnar CE, Berry CD, Rosenberger FU. MMS-X molecular modeling system. Technical memorandum no. 229, Washington University, St. Louis, 1977.

37. Mohan R, Chui C, Lidofsky L. Differential pencil beam dose computation model for photons. *Med Phys* 1986;13:64–73.

38. Munzenrider JE, Pilepich M, Rene-Ferrero JB, Tchakarova I, Carter BL. Use of body scanner in radiotherapy treatment planning. *Cancer* 1977;40:170–179.

39. Parker RP, Hobday PA, Cassell KJ. The direct use of CT numbers in radiotherapy dosage calculation for inhomogeneous media. *Phys Med Biol* 1979;24:802–809.

40. Phelps ME, Gado MH, Hoffman EJ. Correlation of effective atomic number and electron density with attenuation coefficients measured with polychromatic x-rays. *Radiology* 1975;117:585–588.

41. Pilepich MV, Perez CA, Prasad S. Computed tomography in definitive radiotherapy of prostatic carcinoma. *Int J Radiat Oncol Biol Phys* 1980;6:923–926.

42. Pilepich MV, Prasad SC, Perez CA. Computed tomography in definitive radiotherapy of prostatic carcinoma. *Int J Radiat Oncol Biol Phys* 1980;6:923–926.

43. Pilepich MV, Rene JB, Munzenrider JE, Carter BL. Contribution of computed tomography to the treatment of lymphomas. *AJR* 1978;131:69–73.

44. Prasad SC, Glasgow GP, Purdy JA. Dosimetric evaluation of a computed tomography treatment system. *Radiology* 1979;130:777–781.

45. Prasad SC, Pilepich MV, Perez CA. Contribution of CT to quantitative radiation therapy planning. *AJR* 1981;136:123–128.

46. Proceedings of the Symposium on Particles and Radiation Therapy. Second International Conference. *Int J Radiat Oncol Biol Phys* 1977;3.

47. Purdy JA, Prasad SC. Computed tomography applied to radiation therapy treatment planning. In: Fullerton GD, Zagzebski JA, eds. *Medical physics of CT and ultrasound: tissue imaging and characteristics* (Medical physics monograph no. 6). New York: American Institute of Physics, 1980:221–250.

48. Ragan DP, Perez CA. Efficacy of CT-assisted two-dimensional treatment planning: analysis of 45 patients. *AJR* 1978;131:75–79.

49. Redman HC, Glatstein E, Castellino RA, Federal WA. Computed tomography as an adjunct in the staging of Hodgkin's disease and non-Hodgkin's lymphoma. *Radiology* 1977;124:381–385.

50. Rosenberger F, Krippner K, Stein D Jr, Wong J. Implementation of the delta-volume dose calculation algorithm. In: *Proceedings of the 8th International Conference on the Use of Computers in Radiotherapy.* New York: IEEE, Computer Society Press, 1984:78–82.

51. Schlager B, Asbell SO, Baker AS, Sklaroff DM, Seydel HG, Ostrum BJ. The use of computerized tomography scanning in treatment planning for bladder carcinoma. *Int J Radiat Oncol Biol Phys* 1979;5:99–103.

52. Seydel HG, Kutcher GJ, Steiner RM, Mohiuddin M, Goldberg B. Computed tomography in planning radiation therapy for bronchogenic carcinoma. *Int J Radiat Oncol Biol Phys* 1980;6:601–606.

53. Sontag MR, Cunningham JR. Clinical applications of a CT based treatment planning system. *Comput Tomogr* 1978;2:117–130.

54. Stanley RJ, Sagel SS, Fair WR. Computed tomography of the genitourinary tract. *J Urol* 1978;119:780–782.

55. Sternick ES, Lane FW, Curran B. Comparison of computed tomography and conventional transverse axial tomography in radiotherapy treatment planning. *Radiology* 1977;124:835–836.

56. Stewart JR, Hicks JA, Boone ML, Simpson LD. Computed tomography in radiation therapy. *Int J Radiat Oncol Biol Phys* 1978;4:313–324.

57. Totty WG, Murphy WA, Lee JKT. Soft-tissue tumors: MR imaging. *Radiology* 1986;160:135–141.

58. Veenema RJ, Harisiadis L, Chang C, et al. Bladder carcinoma: preliminary external radiotherapy used as a means for selecting complete treatment. In: Connolly JG, ed. *Progress in cancer research and therapy. Volume 18: Carcinoma of the bladder.* New York: Raven Press, 1981:183–191.

59. Whitmore WF. Bladder cancer. *Cancer* 1978;28:170–177.

60. Wong JW, Henkelman RM. A new approach to CT pixel-based photon dose calculations in heterogeneous media. *Med Phys* 1983;10:199–208.

61. Yu WS, Sagerman RH, King GA, Chung CT, Yu YW. The value of computed tomography in the management of bladder cancer. *Int J Radiat Oncol Biol Phys* 1979;5:135–142.

62. Zelch MG, Haaga JR. Clinical comparison of computed tomography and lymphangiography for detection of retroperitoneal lymphadenopathy. *Radiol Clin North Am* 1979;17:157–168.

CHAPTER 25

The History, Economics, and Politics of CT and MRI

Ronald G. Evens

Nearly everyone will agree that medical care in the United States has improved dramatically since World War II in almost every aspect. A series of major technological developments during the 1940s, 1950s, and 1960s having impact on every medical specialty resulted in greatly improved care for American citizens. This was an era of antibiotics, modern anesthetics, open-heart surgery, cobalt and linear-accelerator radiation therapy, specialty medicine, and substantive advances in our understanding of biology and pathophysiology. These medical advances were available to larger segments of the population as health care became "a right, not a privilege." Medical schools were scientifically based, the National Institutes of Health routinely obtained increased funding, and the modern hospital-based medical complex developed as a visible part of the landscape in most cities. Physicians, with the support of the biomedical sciences and hospitals, became more effective and more powerful.

At the same time, the costs of medical care were receiving increasing attention because of a combination of factors. Improved care and its accessibility made the total cost go up. Patients became more knowledgeable about health and demanded the best care. Insurance and other third-party programs became more widely available through employers and government. Most important, medical care became a political issue. A series of congressional actions resulted in programs to provide medical care for various segments of the population who were not covered by personal or employer-supported insurance programs. These included Title V (Maternal and Child Health), Title XVII (Medicare), and Title XIX (Medicaid). During the 1970s it was recognized by taxpayers, legislatures, and corporations that health care costs were rising faster than was growth in the other segments of the economy, and it was easy to predict that health care would

soon consume more than 10% of our gross national productivity. Political and societal attitudes changed during the 1970s, with increasing demands from politicians, big business, and the public to reduce or at least control costs. Computed tomography (CT) was born in this era.

CT was much more than a new diagnostic technique for medicine; it had significant political and economic ramifications for the specialty of radiology and for all of organized medicine, worldwide. It also provided the technological base for nuclear magnetic resonance (NMR) to become magnetic resonance imaging (MRI). Within a year after the introduction of CT in 1973, this invention was known throughout the world and became a major topic of discussion in Congress, in state legislatures, and at cocktail parties. Complete and total acclaim was not forthcoming, because CT became a symbol of extravagance to individuals concerned with mounting health care costs. Although most of these critics had no immediate responsibility in regard to caring for the ill, the early years of CT (1973–1978) saw the creation of as many enemies as friends, because of social and political concerns about rising medical costs.

EARLY INVESTIGATIONS IN CT

Exercises in reconstruction of images from individual data points have been of interest to mathematicians and physicists for many years. These investigators have included Radon (1917), Bracewell (1956), Oldendorf (1961), Kuhl (1963), and Cormack (1963) (20).

Allan M. Cormack, who shared the Nobel Prize in medicine with Godfrey Hounsfield in 1979, was relatively unknown to many radiologists and scientists who were closely involved with CT. Dr. Cormack was serving as a lecturer in physics to the University of Cape Town, South Africa, in 1955 when he was assigned as the hospital physicist to the Groote Schuur Hospital Department of Radiation Therapy for 1.5 days per week, because the full-time physicist had resigned. He quickly noted the problems, still present today, that arise from the inhomogeneity of normal body tissue that creates difficulties in treatment planning for radiation therapy. He developed a mathematical approach to this problem and intermittently performed experimental work over the next 6 years. Publications of his work appeared during 1963 and 1964 with "virtually no response" (21). Although the work of Cormack and others was fundamental, serious medical or commercial interest was not stimulated. It remained for Godfrey Hounsfield at the EMI Corporation to develop independently a practical system for clinical radiological studies.

In 1968, Mr. Hounsfield was completing a major project using large-scale computers for EMI and the government of the United Kingdom. He was at a transition time in his personal responsibilities and was asked by the Central Research Laboratory (CRL), the basic research organization of EMI, for his suggestions concerning his next project. He suggested that computers and mathematics could be used to reconstruct an image from sets of accurate X-ray measurements through the body from multiple angles. CRL and the management of EMI agreed to set aside resources to pursue this idea.

During the next several months, Mr. Hounsfield pursued this project in a laboratory located in Hayes, England, a short distance from Heathrow Airport. Early images were produced from an americium-isotope source of γ-rays using simple phantoms and an anatomical specimen of human brain. The initial results were highly encouraging, showing a computer-reconstructed image that was similar to the anatomical specimen, although it required 9 days to scan the object and 2.5 hr to process a single image (52).

Further investigations and the major decision to utilize an X-ray tube as a source of photons to replace the γ-ray source reduced the mechanical scanning time from 9 days to 9 hr. As is typical for research and development, many triumphs and catastrophes occurred during the early months. For example, the first experiments were performed with formalin-preserved cadaver specimens, and early apparent "anatomical observations" that confused the researchers were due to the formalin treatment. Finally, a prototype unit was prepared for clinical studies of the brain and placed in the Atkinson Morley Hospital near Wimbledon in 1972.

CLINICAL DEVELOPMENT OF CT

The early clinical results were reported at the April 1972 annual congress of the British Institute of Radiology and

were quickly recognized as providing a major improvement in neuroradiology (5). Essentially all early clinical research was performed in the United Kingdom and the United States with equipment from EMI. The clinical importance of this new radiologic technique was not initially recognized by the manufacturer, and the EMI Corporation projected the need for production of only 25 units. The first production model, called the Mark I, was limited to use on the head, because of the slow scanning time (4.5 min) and the need for a bag of water to be in close contact with the part of the anatomy scanned to eliminate any air gap. The first three production CT head units were installed at the Mayo Clinic, Massachusetts General Hospital, and the Presbyterian–St. Luke's Hospital in Chicago. The Mallinckrodt Institute of Radiology installed the 9th and 16th units built during 1973 and was the first institution to have two CT scanners.

The impact on neuroradiology was spectacular (8). Quickly, it was obvious that CT was a major advance. It was amazing to see the ventricles of the brain without having to instill air or contrast material. In a very few months, by the spring of 1974, CT was recognized as a major improvement by radiologists throughout the world, and the name CT was soon known to politicians, government regulators, and the general public. In the early years it was described as computerized axial tomography, or CAT scanning, and the acronym CAT became both famous and infamous.

During the years 1974 and 1975, the growth of the CT industry and the incorporation of CT into neuroradiologic practice were dynamic. Concern over uncontrolled expansion of this highly expensive new technology led to national controversy. CT became essential to modern neuroradiologic evaluation; many commercial corporations developed or announced plans to develop some form of CT unit (in 1976, at least 22 separate companies were advertising products), and serious concerns were voiced by politicians, health planners, and government regulators regarding the "dangers" (primarily economic) of this new technology.

Commercial competition was at a high level and generally was useful to the development of this new technology. An early commercial development from several manufacturers (1974) was a body scanner with scanning times of 2.5 min or longer that eliminated the water bag and had a larger gantry aperture so that the thorax or abdomen could be studied. Unfortunately, the contrast sensitivity and spatial resolution were poor because respiratory and other physiological motions caused severe degradation of the reconstructed images. Accordingly, diagnostic body CT was not initially viewed as providing clinically valuable information.

In the summer of 1975, EMI announced a CT unit (the 5000 series) with an 18-sec scanning time and no requirement for a water bag. It produced the first images of the chest and abdomen with reproducible and satisfactory resolution. The era of clinically useful body CT had finally arrived. The prototype EMI 5000 was initially located in London at Northwick Park, and two other units were soon installed, first at the Mallinckrodt Institute of Radiology and the Mayo Clinic in the United States. A series of important clinical evaluations at these and other medical centers demonstrated the importance of CT as a diagnostic method for use throughout the body (28,69,71,73).

Although CT development was very important for patients, it came at a time when considerations of cost for medical care were rapidly becoming a national concern. Questions of "cost control" and "efficacy" were especially prominent, not only in the United States but also throughout the world in the early 1970s. CT became the focus of questions about technology in medicine raised by politicians, regulators, and economists. Radiologists and clinicians had to evaluate critically the appropriate role for CT in regard to both medical and cost-conscious concerns.

HEALTH CARE PLANNING IN THE UNITED STATES

A system of health planning was first required by congressional legislation in 1966 (Public Law 89-749), which funded the development of local comprehensive health planning councils and established a certificate-of-need (CON) review process for new health care proposals. There were several objectives for local planning councils, including data gathering, long-range planning, and the approval or disapproval of capital-expenditure projects in each geographic region. In general, the local planning councils did little planning, and their primary role became the review and comment on specific projects.

The federal initiative for health planning was strengthened in 1972 when Section 1122 was added to the Social Security Act under Public Law 92-603. Section 1122 required prior approval by both local and state planning agencies for any capital expenditures exceeding $100,000 or for any significant change in clinical services if reimbursement was sought from federal funds through Medicare, Medicaid, Maternal and Child Health legislation, or federal employee insurance programs. Section 1122 gave "teeth" to the planning process, because denial of reimbursement was a major problem to most health care institutions. The responsibility for long-range planning and data collection in each local and state planning agency continued.

No one was particularly happy with the directives of Section 1122. Medical providers found them restrictive, highly bureaucratic, and inconsistent. Planning agencies were hampered by a lack of data and had difficulty in developing long-range plans. These agencies commonly stimulated considerable controversy when reviewing individual projects, particularly when a project was turned down. Congress was dissatisfied with progress toward the goals of cost containment and improving the accessibility of medical care.

Further revision of the planning activities was legislated by Congress in the National Health Planning and Resource Development Act of 1974 (Public Law 93-641). This law mandated extensive changes in the health planning system that included changing the geography of local planning areas and adding consumer representation to planning agencies (subsequently called Health Systems Agencies or HSAs) and their state counterparts. State planning agencies were required to develop a health systems plan to control costs and improve accessibility of care by defining criteria and standards for specific health service needs. To aid the HSAs in developing these plans, the secretary of the Department of Health, Education, and Welfare (HEW), which in 1981 was renamed the Department of Health and Human Services (HHS), was directed to develop a set of national goals "expressed where practicable in quantitative terms" (29) to guide the more than 200 local HSAs in their planning. The secretary of HEW did not actively pursue the development of such guidelines until 1977, when Secretary Califano saw the use of national guidelines as a mechanism to control health care costs, particularly to reduce the perceived inefficiency of hospitals (described by the secretary as "fat") and the growth of costly technologies.

On September 23, 1977, HEW published a set of guidelines and standards related to 11 specific areas. Of the 11 areas, 3 related to radiology: cardiac catheterization, megavoltage radiation therapy, and CT scanners. The guidelines stimulated a wave of protest as more than 50,000 individual comments were received by HEW. Most concerns were expressed regarding specific standards, including the impact of the guidelines on rural hospitals and teaching facilities, and the loss of local control or responsibility for health planning. This protest resulted in revised guidelines, published on January 20, 1978. The guidelines were considered reasonable by most radiologists, with the exception of those for CT.

CT BECOMES THE SYMBOL OF "TECHNOLOGY RUN WILD"

CT became the example politicians and planners used to symbolize the "inappropriate" use of medical technology, with its ultimate associated increase in cost. CT was in many respects a nearly perfect scapegoat: It was expensive, was of great interest to physicians, could easily be shown in a photograph, and even had an eponym, "CAT." It seemed that everyone from local planners to Secretary Califano to the president of the United States began to use the phrase "CAT scanner" and describe the dangers of "CAT fever" (9,12,48,70).

It was initially difficult to debate the opponents of CT

effectively because few data were available on the economics, utilization, and medical efficacy of CT—particularly for the body. Supportive documentation had not been published because of the limited time that prototype units had been in clinical use; yet most radiologists and other physicians were convinced of the importance of CT, not only for the head, but for the body as well. Although politicians and planners made CT a scapegoat because of its high cost, this approach clearly was a serious mistake, as CT has led to a major revolution in diagnostic imaging, so beneficial, in fact, that it could not be stopped by legislation and guidelines.

ECONOMICS AND UTILIZATION OF CT

Because of the need for data on CT economic utilization, studies (Table 1) were begun to obtain data from multiple CT users in the United States (35). With the cooperation of all known CT equipment manufacturers, a list of all operating CT installations as of January 1976 was compiled. At that time, the overwhelming experience was with head CT units, and the first understanding of the equipment's utilization, efficiency, and cost was limited to neuroradiology activity. The CT units were operated an average of 64 hr per week and examined 50 to 55 patients per week. Even at this early stage, radiologists were responsible for the performance and interpretation of CT images (92 of 98 facilities), and most equipment (90%) was installed in association with a hospital. Scheduling delays were lengthy, averaging 1.6 days for inpatients and 11.5 days for outpatients. An economic break-even analysis (27) was performed using data on equipment cost and its method of depreciation, equipment maintenance, space remodeling and upkeep, personnel, and the cost of iodinated contrast material and other supplies. The "typical" unit had an annual technical cost of $325,000 to $471,000, depending on patient volume. Data on charges indicated that the net technical revenue was $138 per patient, as compared with a net technical cost of $130 per patient. It was emphasized that this study obtained data on CT installations in order to satisfy interests and concerns about the use of this new imaging method, but most CT installations were not independent activities and should be considered as an integral part of a diagnostic radiology department or office.

This survey in 1976 became the first in a series of publications prompted by the continued need to justify the cost of utilization of CT to its opponents. A study in early 1979 (37) of the first CT installations capable of obtaining images with "breath holding" (18 sec or less scanning time) demonstrated different results. Even though 60% of studies were for evaluation of the head, only about 30 patients were studied per week on these early multipurpose scanners, and the units were operating at a significant financial loss.

A follow-up study (38,39) in November 1978 determined that dedicated head CT units were examining an average of 15% more patients per week than in the 1976 survey and were operating in the black, whereas body CT scanners averaged fewer patients and were operating at a loss. Most important, 73% of the head units were meeting the national guidelines of 1978, whereas only 17% of body CT scanners were meeting this level of activity.

The guidelines published by the Health Resource Administration for CT scanners were simple, but restrictive:

1. A CT scanner (head and body) should operate at a minimum of 2,500 medically necessary patient procedures per year, for the second year of its operation and thereafter.
2. There should be no additional scanners approved in a geographic region unless each existing scanner in the health service area is performing at a rate greater than 2,500 medically necessary patient procedures per year.
3. There should not be additional scanners approved unless the operators of the proposed equipment set in place data collection and utilization review systems.

The guidelines went on to define a "patient procedure" to include all diagnostic studies performed on the same visit, in the same area of anatomy, and with the same diagnostic interest—a definition specifically developed to count a patient examination with and without intravenous contrast material as a single procedure. The standard also stated that this level of activity should be possible in a 50- to 55-hr week, with a head-to-body ratio of 60/40, but no basis for possible adjustments was given. Data from our surveys demonstrated that 2,500 patient procedures per year was an impossible goal for most installations with body CT scanners of the technology available in 1978. Yet, the second guideline permitted no additional scanners within an HSA area unless all other scanners were performing more than 2,500 procedures per year. This essentially established a moratorium on the further purchase of CT scanners in most geographic regions.

Economic data on CT scanners were important for other reasons, in addition to demonstrating the moratorium effect of the national guidelines:

1. They were the first economic studies of a radiologic procedure or installation from national data that documented economic and utilization adjustments with time, experience, and improved technology (Table 1).
2. This approach demonstrated a model for analyzing costs based on standard utilization and expense data and suggested a method for establishing charges that would allow coverage of these costs (31).
3. The data and reports emphasized the critical importance of patient volume with most radiology procedures, where the vast majority of costs are fixed (unrelated to examination activity) and only a small

TABLE 1. *CT economic and utilization data from national surveys of experienced radiology facilities*

Parameter	Jan. 1976 (Head CT)	May 1977 (Body)	Nov. 1978 (Head)	Nov. 1978 (Body)
No. installations reporting	98	74	70	64
Operating hours/week	64	52	59	52
Patients/week	55	32	63	34
Percent head/body	100/0	60/40	100/0	55/45
Typical total charge ($)	258	286	247	273
Annual technical cost ($)	345,000	373,000	388,000	384,000
Annual technical profit (loss) ($)	22,880	(72,000)	123,000	(77,000)

portion of the cost is variable (related to examination activity). When most costs are fixed, patient volume is a critical component in evaluating the charge necessary to break even, because total costs vary little with examination volume, whereas the cost per patient changes dramatically (Table 2).

Other investigators reported on the cost of CT in their own departments, including studies on the effect of CT in reducing the numbers of other examinations or procedures. Cost-effectiveness in Canada (83), the reduction in radionuclide brain imaging in community hospital (5,78), and the beneficial impact of CT on multiple procedures in a large teaching hospital (81) were all reported during this period. These authors primarily were developing an analysis of CT cost. At the same time, and more importantly, an evaluation of the benefits of CT to patients (efficacy) was in progress.

EFFICACY STUDIES AND CT

While some criticized the lack of efficacy data in 1976–1978 (1), multiple studies were in progress from several medical centers, and results were beginning to be reported. These reports in the first 2 years of head and body CT experience were necessarily limited to clinical descriptions and studies of impact on diagnosis. Studies soon followed describing and documenting the effects of CT on treatment, clinical decision making, other diagnostic procedures, and, subsequently, mortality and morbidity.

One center reported dramatic decreases in the numbers of brain scans, arteriography, and air studies and a sig-

nificant reduction in exploratory surgery after the introduction of CT, but without a real change in mortality among patients following head injuries (4). Several authors (2,18,36) compared head CT to radionuclide brain scanning as a primary or screening test and showed CT to be slightly more accurate, but providing substantially more diagnostic data. In an early efficacy study, a marked decrease in the perceived need by clinicians for brain scans, angiograms, and pneumoencephalograms after CT was shown (42). Therapy was altered in 19% of those examined, including the abandonment of certain proposed treatments deemed worthless after CT findings. Another group showed a marked reduction in normal arteriograms following CT, no change in the length of hospital stay or treatment plans in patients with cerebrovascular disease, but a reduction in the time to diagnosis, with alteration of the therapeutic approach, in patients suspected of having hydrocephalus or brain tumors (54–56).

Efficacy studies of body CT began in 1978 and soon demonstrated improvement in diagnosis, reduction in the cost of clinical diagnostic evaluation, and alterations in treatment plans, but without definite evidence for reductions in morbidity and mortality. One study found that 16% of CT examinations of the chest and abdomen produced clinically important information that was otherwise not available and that altered patient diagnosis, prognosis, and therapy (66). Another demonstrated that CT improved diagnostic understanding in 41%, reassured physicians about planned therapy in 43%, and changed therapy in 17% (82). A third compared CT and arteriography in patients with renal cell carcinoma, demonstrating that arteriography can be obviated in most patients (80). In summary, data from multiple institutions, essentially all

TABLE 2. *Effect of patient volume on CT technical costs*

Costs	Patients/weeks			
	25	30	40	50
Fixed costs	$217,183	$217,183	$217,183	$217,183
Variable costs	22,230	26,676	35,568	44,460
Indirect costs	119,770	121,930	126,376	130,822
Total costs	359,183	365,789	379,127	392,465
Cost/patient	276	234	182	151

From ref. 35.

favorable, were being reported regarding the benefit to patients and overall efficacy of CT in both the head and extracranial portions of the body.

Several authors recommended more extensive efficacy studies (1,22,41) and indicated the need for multiinstitutional approaches. One such study on head CT (9) was funded by the National Cancer Institute, and data were obtained from five university centers. This study began in 1974 and collected data for several years (during the critical time of controversy), but was not reported until July 1980, when it was essentially out of date, the results contained being already widely accepted by all involved. Efficacy studies with new technology are critically important, but multiinstitutional projects are not timely. The responsibility for efficacy data rests primarily with the medical institutions that have early access to the equipment.

CT IS NATIONALLY ACCEPTED

For the United States, 1976 was a good year (our bicentennial celebration), but a bad year for CT. CT was a very expensive technology and a major challenge to medical cost control. Local HSAs became battlegrounds, with physicians and radiologists (and sometimes patients) against planners and politicians. Radiologists and others were advised to cooperate with planning agencies and to provide data to evaluate CT effectively, without emotion (19,29,61). Economic and efficacy data (as described earlier) were being reported.

Important institutions and societies, often coordinated by the American College of Radiology, were particularly effective in the formulation and publication of statements dealing with efficacy. In April 1977, radiologists from five institutions, the Cleveland Clinic Foundation, the Mallinckrodt Institute of Radiology at Washington University, the Mayo Clinic, New York Hospital–Cornell Medical Center, and the University of California at San Francisco, jointly stated their opinion that body CT was a clinically important and efficacious radiologic procedure (34). The Society of Computed Body Tomography soon reported on a list of indications for CT that it deemed appropriate based on its members' evaluation and experience and on published sources (3).

In 1979, the increasing amount of data demonstrating the efficacy of CT and the increasing number of patients who benefited from its use began to sway the opinion of the public and the planners. Economic data from several sources were used in an independently funded study that predicted that CT would not increase the overall cost of diagnostic procedures, because of reductions in other medical tests (45). This view was further supported by a study based on an analysis of operational CT units in 1980, which showed that improved diagnostic information was provided at essentially no cost to the medical public

(30). This study emphasized that CT equipment must be readily available to patients to prevent the use of less effective diagnostic procedures and associated lengthened hospital stay. The pendulum for CT swung farther with an interesting technology-assessment report demonstrating that expensive new technologies (CT) do not actually cost that much, but "little-ticket" (i.e., less expensive, but high volume) technologies result in very high costs (60).

Further studies confirmed the economic and medical necessity for CT in contemporary medical care. Sharing of CT scanners had not been effective for patient care in municipal health care facilities (i.e., city and state hospitals) that relied on other institutions for CT, because of difficulties in patient scheduling and patient transportation, often because the patients were too ill to be moved (17). A study from the congressional Office of Technology Assessment (OTA) reported major problems in health care due to lack of access to CT facilities for major segments of United States citizens (10).

A notable milestone for CT came with the announcement that the 1979 Nobel Prize in medicine was awarded to Hounsfield and Cormack for their pioneering efforts in the development of CT. CT was becoming accepted as an important diagnostic radiologic procedure. By 1981, a consensus conference at the National Institutes of Health reported on the major advances of head CT and encouraged its increased use and availability for neurologic studies.

THE DEVELOPMENT AND INTRODUCTION OF MRI

In a fashion similar to the development of CT and the entire specialty of radiology, MRI traces its beginning to the work of nonradiologists, primarily physicists and engineers. Spectroscopy with the visible and ultraviolet wavelengths was developed before 1900 and became useful in chemical analysis. Several observations about light patterns were not understood, even with a growing comprehension about the structure of the atom. For example, it had been observed by many scientists that each and every wavelength of emitted light divided into two separate wavelengths in the presence of a magnetic field, by an unknown mechanism; in 1924, Pauli recognized that this separation was due to magnetic interactions between the nucleus and the surrounding electrons of each atom.

Pauli's theoretical insight was the beginning of our understanding of the nuclear magnetic properties that allowed Bloch (11) and Purcell (64) in 1945 to independently measure the magnetic properties of the proton (and subsequently other nuclei) with great accuracy. NMR spectroscopy quickly became an important analytical technique, initially to chemists and subsequently to biochemists and physiologists. Bloch and Purcell were awarded the Nobel Prize in physics in 1952.

NMR uses rapidly expanded into a variety of scientific disciplines between 1945 and 1980, primarily in various subspecialties of chemistry. Almost every laboratory used the technique initially for quantitative analysis of non-organic materials, but with improved equipment and knowledge NMR spectroscopy could be used to examine biological materials and to measure time-dependent and rate-limiting biochemical processes.

NMR was not a major consideration in clinical medicine until the early 1970s, when several laboratories began to subject various pathologic tissues to NMR spectroscopy and suggested that clinical diagnosis could be made (24). Although these observations have not resulted in clinically useful pathologic diagnostic methods, the interest in NMR in medicine was established.

MRI was first suggested by Paul Lauterbur in 1973 (58), including the suggested name of "zeugmatography" (for the Greek word "zeugma," or "that which joins together"). Although the proposed term did not become popular, the imaging of complex anatomy using the principles of NMR quickly developed. In 1974, a proton image of a recently killed mouse was obtained (almost *"in vivo,"* but because the imaging required approximately 1 hr, respiration was stopped by a cervical spine fracture that was observed in the image) (53). The first human *in vivo* image was published in 1977 (25), and the development of MRI accelerated such that by 1985 more than 10 manufacturers had announced their entry into the competition to sell commercial units. Within a relatively short period of time, significant improvements in both software and hardware were made, resulting in high-resolution proton images of the human body requiring only a few minutes for scanning and image reconstruction. Although some of these advances originated at university center (23,51), most technical advances came from commercial corporations without scientific publication.

MRI was possible because of the successful blending of three specific technologies: NMR, large-bore magnets with homogeneous high magnetic fields (0.35–2.0 tesla), and computer-reconstruction techniques from CT. It is ironic that one of the key factors leading to the development of MRI (i.e., CT imaging) was also the greatest impediment to MRI's clinical acceptance.

CLINICAL AND EFFICACY EVALUATION OF MRI

The first clinical reports on MRI were published in 1981, initially from the United Kingdom (84) and subsequently from the United States, just as with CT. Also as with CT, early publications (1982–1985) came from institutions with prototype machines from commercial manufacturers.

Most of the early reports were very positive and emphasized the absence of ionizing radiation, the ability to directly obtain coronal and sagittal images, and the predicted high tissue specificity of MRI over currently available diagnostic procedures, specifically CT. Unfortunately, many of these reports were overly optimistic, and initial case reports showing the presumed ability of MRI to make a tissue-specific pathologic diagnosis have not been confirmed by subsequent larger series employing appropriate scientific methods.

The early 1980s proved that MRI was technically feasible, and high-quality images were obtained from several commercial units. This was also the time for radiologists to become familiar with imaging protocols and techniques (62,66) and to determine MRI's safety (63). Although MRI did not use ionizing radiation, the required strong magnetic fields created problems for patients and staff with cardiac pacemakers or implanted ferromagnetic clips and other devices.

Large clinical series allowing evaluation of MRI's clinical utility and efficacy, as well as the very important comparison with CT, began to appear in late 1984. The initial efficacy reports evaluated imaging of the head and spine and generally were *strongly* supportive of MRI becoming the dominant imaging technique (16,43,47,65,68). The results of some of these reports, in retrospect, were biased by faulty methods, such as preferential inclusion of patients with known malignant neoplasms, multiple sclerosis, or other large lesions, without sufficient numbers of normal controls or those with benign or previously undiagnosed diseases.

Likewise, some of the initial reports outlining the apparent advantages of MRI for extracranial organs (including tissue specificity) were not well-controlled scientific studies (7,26,44,72). With few exceptions, in which tissue characterization by MRI may prove to be useful (46), most of the initial claims (in other parts of the body) were not corroborated by subsequent studies of larger groups of patients.

In 1985 and 1986, interest in MRI efficacy continued with reports that included carefully controlled and prospective analyses of larger patient populations that were more conservative in their conclusions (49,57,59,67,79). At the end of 1986 it was generally concluded that MRI was often superior to CT for the brain and spine because of its ability to obtain coronal and sagittal views, the absence of bone artifact (especially important in regions near the base of the skull), and its ability to detect subtle tissue changes. CT remains superior for studying trauma and other clinical situations in which analysis of bone or calcium is important. At present, CT remains the initial diagnostic imaging procedure for the brain and spine in most hospitals solely because of the availability of CT and the lack of access to MRI. As MR imagers become more widely available, it is apparent that MRI will become the preferred method for imaging the central nervous system and will soon supplant myelography, plain films of the spine, CT, and angiography in most cases.

Regulation and legislation impacted MRI, but only at a state or local level. Some states (e.g., California) had completely dismantled the planning process. Although the political process often was not a barrier to the purchase and placement of MRI, other considerations were formidable. The cost of MRI equipment ranged from half a million to over $2 million, and new construction usually was necessary. The capital requirements sometimes reached $3 million. These were days of cost concerns for most hospitals, and a capital requirement in the millions made most institutions cautious about entering a "high-stakes" business with many unknowns. MRI had more questions than most new technologies. For example, a still unanswered question is the issue of magnet size, ranging from 0.35 to 2.0 tesla. Generally, each manufacturer selected a particular size magnet and promoted its selection as "the best."

Medical economics added another complicating factor. Although planning usually was not a factor, it was easy to predict that many important medical insurance providers (especially Medicare) would not pay for the examination until clinical efficacy was demonstrated, a difficult task with the availability of CT and other traditional diagnostic procedures. Consequently, in many instances, hospital administrators were nervous and timid, with resultant slow sales of MRI equipment. American capitalism had recently become a factor in medical care, and many of the first MRI units were purchased and put into operation by various combinations of venture capitalists, clinicians, and radiologists, outside of the hospital setting.

ECONOMICS OF MRI

The costs of establishing and operating an MRI facility have been examined by several health care providers and researchers interested in medical economics. Table 3 summarizes data regarding costs, charges, and utilization in 1985 (40). The data were confirmed by other studies in 1985 and 1986 (6,13–15,33,75–77).

The purchase cost of MRI equipment varied primarily with the type of magnet employed in the system. Even though resistive-magnet systems could be purchased for half of the cost of most superconducting-magnet systems, only 7% of the MR imagers installed in the United States by the end of 1985 were the less expensive resistive-magnet systems (74). Purchase costs of approximately $1.5 million to $2 million are typical of the MRI systems being installed in the United States in 1987.

Installation costs for MR imagers vary with the field strength of the magnet, the required site preparation, and the spaciousness and quality of furnishings in the MRI facility. We reported mean national installation costs of $380,000, with a range between $100,000 and $900,000.

Estimates of annualized capital (equipment and facility) costs depend on depreciation schedules and the cost of

TABLE 3. *MRI cost and utilization*

Parameter	Mean	Range
Equipment cost ($1,000)	1,362	750–1,900
Equipment maintenance ($1,000)	98	0–150
Construction cost ($1,000)	380	100–900
Variable cost/study ($)	27	5–75
Cryogen cost/month ($)	2,145	1,000–3,500
Electricity cost/month ($)	1,872	—
Downtime, maintenance (hr/week)	3	0–8
Downtime, breakdown (hr/week)	2	0–8
Space (gross ft^2)	2,747	500–7,500
Exams/month (head)	85	21–234
Exams/month (body)	43	5–123

capital (i.e., interest rates or opportunity costs), as well as the cost of equipment and construction. Most reported cost estimates have assumed a useful life for MRI equipment of 5 to 7 years, a useful life for an MRI facility of 10 to 30 years, and a relevant interest rate of 10 to 12%. Three reports (13,33,40) have annualized capital costs varying between $240,000 to $340,000. Capital costs for resistive- and permanent-magnet systems are lower than these values, whereas those for 1.5-T superconducting-magnet systems are higher.

There has been considerably more variability in reported operating costs than in capital costs. For example, reported annual personnel costs, exclusive of physician salaries, have varied from $70,000 for one shift (75) to $180,000 for two shifts (13), with typical personnel costs reported as being $89,000 (40). The variability in these estimates is primarily attributable to the number of technologists being employed and the assignment of physicists, engineers, and other professionals by some installations. Although the personnel costs reported by Bradley (13) were higher than most, he argued that using four technologists is cost-effective because of the increased patient throughput it permits. Supply costs for MRI are small. Estimates vary from $15 per procedure (33,75) to $27 per procedure (40). Similarly, the costs of cryogens or electricity have averaged about $20,000 per year and are not important economic factors. Estimates for maintenance costs are also variable, in part because some reports apply to maintenance contracts on equipment only, whereas others also include maintenance costs for the facility, and because maintenance-contract costs vary with manufacturer. We found that maintenance costs averaged $98,000 per year nationwide. Reported overhead costs vary considerably. We believe that overhead costs are best estimated at 50% of direct costs, and MRI overhead costs averaged $106,500 in 1985.

Total annualized operating costs will vary with patient throughput because of the direct relationship between supply costs and throughput and because of the higher level of personnel costs required to operate an MR imager for two shifts per day rather than one. Steinberg et al. (76)

estimated total annual costs at $490,000 to $590,000 for a 0.15-T resistive-magnet system, $659,000 to $759,000 for a 0.3-T permanent-magnet system, $832,000 to $932,000 for a 0.5-T superconducting system, and $1,015,000 to $1,115,000 for a 1.5-T superconducting system. These estimates are consistent with our analyses (33,40) and that of Bradley (13), even though the specific assumptions in each case varied.

Given these estimates of capital and operating costs, the estimated cost per MR image is strongly dependent on a given facility's annual patient throughput, as well as estimates for partial pay/bad debt, in a similar fashion as for CT and other newer radiologic procedures. In 1985, we found that MR images of the head averaged 60 min, whereas those of the body averaged 72 min, and typical throughput was six to seven patients per day, or just over 1,500 patients per year. Bradley reported shorter imaging times required for each examination (30 min for either head or body) (14) and an average throughput of 12 patients per day from a single institution after 2 years of experience.

Economic data that we gathered from a 1985 study (40) demonstrated that most MRI units were in serious economic difficulty. A "typical" MRI installation was losing about $440,000 each year. This was due to a combination of factors, notably the high fixed costs of equipment, space, and personnel, the low patient volumes in many units, the poor collection rates due to high diagnostic charges of $600 or more per examination, and the unwillingness of many insurance companies and Medicare to pay, because they considered MRI to be "experimental."

Patient volumes and partial-pay/bad-debt rates will vary with a facility's case mix and local insurers' coverage and payment policies. Given recent trends of increasing coverage for MRI and increasing patient throughput, an estimated rate of 20% partial pay/bad debt is probably reasonable. This improved rate and increasing patient volumes have certainly improved the financial positions of most MRI units.

COMPARISON OF MRI AND PREVIOUS CT DATA

Evens and Jost (35) performed a survey of CT in 1976, a time at which its development as a new diagnostic imaging technology was similar to that of MRI in 1985. At that time, CT technology had developed rapidly, but installations were performing only diagnostic head procedures. CT was introduced in 1973, and so the 1976 study was 3 years after initial clinical use, whereas the MRI study in 1985 was 3 years after the first clinical installation of November 1982. The data from the 1985 study and our previous studies (40) are shown in Table 4.

Note that MRI units are fewer in number and are op-

TABLE 4. Comparison of MRI and CT development

Parameter	CT: 1976 (Head)	CT: 1981	MRI: 1985
Units responding	98	153	47
Total patients/week/ unit	55	62	35
Operational hr/week	64	56	53
% Head	100	65	66
% Spine	. . .	4	11
Typical total charge ($)	280	335	638
Outpatient scheduling delay (days)	12	8	5
% Hospital location	90	. . .	52
Cost, equipment ($1,000)	387	. . .	1362
Space allocated (gross ft²)	537	. . .	2747
Remodel or building cost ($1,000)	20	. . .	384
Annual technical costs ($1,000)	337	. . .	1151
Radiologist responsible (%)	93	. . .	93
Average technical profit (loss) ($1,000)	21	. . .	(440)

erating fewer hours per week. We believe the difference in outpatient scheduling delay (12 days for CT and 5 days for MRI), along with fewer operational hours per week and fewer patients studied per week, indicates a much lower clinical demand for MRI than had been found for CT at a similar time in its development. There are many possible reasons for the apparent difference in clinical demand, including the higher costs for MRI, the availability of "competing" diagnostic procedures, especially CT, and a more conservative approach by referring clinicians.

Essentially all economic comparisons show MRI to be more costly than CT. The typical total charge is 2.5 times higher, and equipment costs are three times higher; the units require five times the space, annual technical costs are more than three times higher, and CT units operate above the technical-cost break-even point, whereas MRI units are operating at a considerable loss. Radiologists were responsible for more than 90% of CT installations in 1976 and were responsible for more than 90% of MRI installations in 1985.

Table 4 also compares utilization and charge data determined in 1981 (our most recent CT survey) (38,39) with CT in 1976 and MRI in 1985. Unfortunately, we did not perform an economic cost analysis in 1981. Between 1976 and 1981, CT became more clinically efficient, and more studies per week were performed in fewer operational hours; the number of body procedures increased; outpatient scheduling delay was reduced; and the total charge increased by only 20% during a 5-year period with several years of double-digit inflation.

THE DIFFUSION OF MRI IN THE UNITED STATES

As a demonstration of the interest in the growth of MRI, one journal (*AJR*) had three reports (August and December 1985, May 1986) in one year on the distribution of MRI equipment (40,50,74). Each report confirmed the results of the others. The number of MRI installations in the United States is growing rapidly, but the growth curve lags behind that of CT at a comparable time after the introduction of the new technology (Fig. 1). There is another difference in the diffusion of the two technologies. Nearly half of the installed MRI units are not in hospitals, with a large portion being owned by physicians.

Is the diffusion of MRI in the United States appropriate? Although there is no doubt that the installation of MRI units is moving quickly, the determination of "appropriateness" depends on the bias of the evaluator. I suggest that the diffusion curve for MRI is no different from that for any new technology in science, business, or medicine. There is always an S-shaped curve with useful technology, and the important questions are the magnitude and time scale of the curve. Similar curves describe the installation and diffusion of CT, image intensifiers, NMR spectrometers, word processors, electronic copiers, and so forth. With any technology, including MRI, the dimensions of the curve depend on the consumer's analysis of the advantages in the new technology, its costs, and the ability of the suppliers to get the product to market.

Why is the curve for MRI lower than that for CT? The analysis of this question in the three *AJR* papers was influenced by the interests of the authors. Hillman and Schwartz (50) and Steinberg (74) emphasized the importance of health policy issues (e.g., prospective payment, certificate of need, Medicare payment approval); Evens et al. (40) suggested that the important issues are related to medical and radiologic practice. MRI has important diagnostic utility, but CT is readily available and has ex-cellent diagnostic efficacy in most organ systems, making it difficult for MRI to demonstrate that its diagnostic supremacy is worth a considerable added cost. All authors agree that the current concern about medical costs is a major factor preventing more rapid diffusion of MRI. If MRI cost half as much to the radiologist and half as much to the patient, if MRI had no installation problems, and if CT were not available, then the MRI diffusion rate would be spectacular. But wishes are not reality.

What is the future of the MRI diffusion curve? How high will it go, and when will it plateau? These questions are important to many, including manufacturers, health care planners, and radiologists. The parameters for the dynamics of this curve include many unknowns. Does NMR spectroscopy have clinical importance? Can MRI units be installed in hospital and acute-care locations with new technology for shielding? Will the operational and capital costs stay at current levels? Will the current proposed advantages of MRI (e.g., direct sagittal and coronal imaging) be matched by new developments in CT? Are there useful, organ-specific MRI contrast agents? Until some of these questions are answered, no one can predict the total number of MRI units or when they will be in operation.

The paper by Steinberg (74) identified two bits of information worth watching. In 1986, he reported on 15 (or more) manufacturers of MRI equipment, more than double the 7 manufacturers identified in 1984. If the CT experience is an accurate predictor, less than 10 manufacturers will survive, and the battle for market shares will be fierce. Steinberg also reported that more than 70% of MRI units now installed are in the United States. The U.S. market is approximately 50% of the world radiology market. Either we are buying fast or the rest of the world is buying slow; I bet on the former.

CONCLUSIONS

Who would have thought that medicine and the specialty of radiology would be blessed by two exciting technologies in one decade? CT is no longer controversial; it is an established and often essential component of modern medical practice (32). There are more than 2,500 CT units in the United States and more than 6,000 worldwide. Its inventor, Sir Godfrey Hounsfield, shared the Nobel Prize with Allan Cormack in 1979. It is a mature commercial and technical market, served by a few large electronic/radiology corporations.

MRI is in the position that CT occupied in the late 1970s, with about 300 units in the United States and 500 worldwide. The technology is constantly changing, and the literature is growing. It is well established as an important diagnostic procedure for neuroradiology and some musculoskeletal applications, but its utility in the rest of the body is still evolving. A major factor is the ready avail-

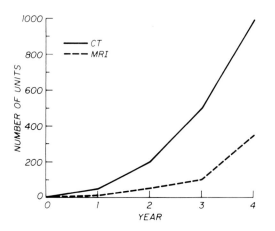

FIG. 1. Cumulative numbers of CT and MRI installations in the United States at comparable times. "Time zero" is 1973 for CT and 1981 for MRI.

ability and lesser cost of CT. MRI's promise remains, and we look forward to more thorough analyses.

MRI and CT have been important challenges, as well as advancements, to traditional radiology and our scientific evaluation of new technology. They made us aware of the increasing importance for medicine of economics, politics, and other social issues. As an example, how many textbooks of radiology that were written before 1980 would have a chapter on economics and politics?

REFERENCES

1. Abrams HL, McNeil BJ. Computed tomography: cost and efficacy implications. *AJR* 1978;131:81–87.
2. Alderson PO, Mikhacl M, Coleman R, Gado M. Optimal utilization of computerized cranial tomography and radionuclide brain imaging. *Neurology (Minneap)* 1976;26:803–807.
3. Alfidi RJ, Evens RG, Glenn W, et al. (Society for Computed Body Tomography). Special report: new indications for computed body tomography. *AJR* 1979;133:115–119.
4. Ambrose J, Gooding MR, Uttley D. EMI scan in the management of head injuries. *Lancet* 1976;1:847–848.
5. Ambrose J, Hounsfield G. Computerized transverse axial tomography. *Br J Radiol* 1973;46:148.
6. American Hospital Association. Hospital technology series guideline report. NMR issues for 1985 and beyond 4(3/4), 1985.
7. Axel L, Kressel HY, Thickman D, et al. NMR imaging of the chest at 0.12 T: initial clinical experience with a resistive magnet. *AJR* 1983;141:1157–1162.
8. Baker HL Jr. Computed tomography and neuroradiology: a fortunate primary union. *AJR* 1976;127:101–110.
9. Baker HL, Houser OW, Campbell JK. National Cancer Institute study: evaluation of computed tomography in the diagnosis of intracranial neoplasms. I. Overall results. *Radiology* 1980;136:91–96.
10. Banta D. Computed tomography: cost containment misdirected. *Am J Public Health* 1980;70:215–216.
11. Bloch F. The principle of nuclear induction. In: *Nobel lectures in physics: 1946–62.* New York: Elsevier, 1964.
12. Bogue T, Wolfe SM. *CAT scanners: is fancier technology worth a billion dollars of health consumer money?* Washington, DC: Health Resource Group, 1976.
13. Bradley WG Jr. Comparing costs and efficacy of MRI. *AJR* 1986;146:1307–1310.
14. Bradley WG Jr, Johnson KC. Hints for establishing a profitable MR practice. *Diagnostic Imaging* 1985;7(3):39–42.
15. Bradley WG, Opel W, Kassabian JP. Magnetic resonance installation: siting and economic considerations. *Radiology* 1984;151:719–721.
16. Bradley WG Jr, Walnuch V, Yadley RA, Wycoff RR. Comparison of CT and MR in 400 patients with suspected disease of the brain and cervical spinal cord. *Radiology* 1984;152:695–702.
17. Brust JMC, Dickinson PCT, Healton EB. Failure of CT sharing in a large municipal hospital. *N Engl J Med* 1981;304:1388–1393.
18. Clifford JR, Connolly ES, Vorhees RM. Comparison of radionuclide scans with computer assisted tomography in diagnosis of intracranial disease. *Neurology (Minneap)* 1976;26:1119–1123.
19. Cloe LE. Health planning for computed tomography: perspectives and problems. *AJR* 1976;128:187–190.
20. Cormack AM. Representation of a function by its line integrals, with some radiological application. *J Appl Physiol* 1963;34:2722–2727.
21. Cormack AM. Early two-dimensional reconstruction (CT scanning) and recent topic stemming from it. *J Comput Assist Tomogr* 1980;4:658–664.
22. Creditor MC, Garrett JB. The information base for diffusion of technology: computed tomography scanning. *N Engl J Med* 1977;297:49–52.
23. Crooks LE. Selective irradiation line scan techniques for NMR imaging. *IEEE Trans Nuc Sci* 1980;3:1239–1241.
24. Damadian R. Tumor detections by nuclear magnetic resonance. *Science* 1971;171:1151–1153.
25. Damadian R, Goldsmith M, Minkoff L. NMR in cancer, FONAR image of the live human body. *Physiol Chem Phys* 1977;9:97.
26. Doyle FH, Pennock JM, Banks LM, et al. Nuclear magnetic resonance imaging of the liver: initial experience. *AJR* 1982;138:193–200.
27. Evens RG. Cost accounting in radiology and nuclear medicine. *CRC Crit Rev Clin Radiol Nucl Med* 1975;6:67–80.
28. Evens RG. New frontier for radiology: computed tomography. *AJR* 1976;126:1117–1129.
29. Evens RG. National guidelines and standards for health planning: their relation to radiology. *AJR* 1978;131:1101–1104.
30. Evens RG. The economics of computed tomography: comparison with other health care costs. *Radiology* 1980;136:509–510.
31. Evens RG. Economic implications of a new technology installation: a CT model. *AJR* 1981;136:673–677.
32. Evens RG. Computed tomography—a controversy revisted. *N Engl J Med* 1984;310:1183–1185.
33. Evens RG. Economic costs of nuclear magnetic resonance imaging. *J Comput Assist Tomogr* 1984;8(2):200–203.
34. Evens RG, Alfidi RJ, Haaga JR, et al. Body computed tomography: a clinically important and efficacious radiologic procedure. *Radiology* 1977;123:239–240.
35. Evens RG, Jost RG. Economic analysis of computed tomography units. *AJR* 1976;127:191–198.
36. Evens RG, Jost RG. The clinical efficacy and cost analysis of cranial computed tomography and the radionuclide brain scan. *Semin Nucl Med* 1977;7:129–136.
37. Evens RG, Jost RG. Economic analysis of body computed tomography units including data on utilization. *Radiology* 1978;127:151–157.
38. Evens RG, Jost RG. Utilization of head computed tomography units in installations with greater than two-and-a-half years' experience. *Radiology* 1979;131:691–693.
39. Evens RG, Jost RG. Utilization of body computed tomography units in installations with greater than one-and-a-half years' experience. *Radiology* 1979;131:695–698.
40. Evens RG, Jost RG, Evens RG Jr. Economic and utilization analysis of magnetic resonance imaging units in the United States in 1985. *AJR* 1985;145:393–398.
41. Fineberg HV. Editorial: evaluation of computed tomography: achievement and challenge. *AJR* 1978;131:1–4.
42. Fineberg HV, Bauman R, Sosman M. Computerized cranial tomography: effect on diagnostic and therapeutic plans. *JAMA* 1977;238:224–227.
43. Franken EA, Berbaum KS, Dunn V, et al. Impact of MR imaging on clinical diagnosis and management: a prospective study. *Radiology* 1986;161:377–380.
44. Gamsu G, Webb WR, Sheldon P, et al. Nuclear magnetic resonance imaging of the thorax. *Radiology* 1982;147:473–480.
45. Gempel PA, Harris GH, Evens RG. *Comparative cost analysis: computed tomography versus alternative diagnostic procedures, 1977–1980.* Cambridge, Massachusetts: Arthur D. Little, Inc., 1977.
46. Glazer GM, Woolsey EJ, Borrello J, et al. Adrenal tissue characterization using MR imaging. *Radiology* 1986;158:73–79.
47. Han JS, Kaufman B, Alfidi RJ, et al. Head trauma evaluated by magnetic resonance and computed tomography: a comparison. *Radiology* 1984;150:71–77.
48. Harris JM. The hazards of bedside bays. *JAMA* 1981;246:2602–2605.
49. Haughton VM, Rimm AA, Sobocinski KA, et al. A blinded clinical comparison in MR imaging and CT in neuroradiology. *Radiology* 1986;160:751–755.
50. Hillman AL, Schwartz JS. The diffusion of MRI: patterns of siting and ownership in an era of changing incentives. *AJR* 1986;146:963–969.
51. Holland GN, Moore WS, Hawkes RC. Nuclear magnetic resonance tomography of the brain. *J Comput Assist Tomogr* 1980;4:1–3.
52. Hounsfield GN. Computed medical imaging. *Science* 1980;210:22–28.
53. Hutchinson JMS, Mallard JR, Goll CC. In-vivo imaging of body structures using proton resonance. In: Allen PS, Andres ER, Bates CA, eds. *Proceedings of the 18th Ampere Congress, University of Nottingham* 1974:283.

54. Larson EB, Omenn GS, Loop JW. Computed tomography in patients with cerebrovascular disease: impact of new technology on patient care. *AJR* 1978;131:35–40.

55. Larson EB, Omenn GS, Magno J. Impact of computed tomography on the care of patients with suspected hydrocephalus. *AJR* 1978;131: 41–44.

56. Larson EB, Omenn GS, Margolis MT, Loop JW. Impact of computed tomography on utilization of cerebral angiograms. *AJR* 1977;129: 1–3.

57. Latack JT, Abou-Khalil BW, Siegel GJ, Sackellares JC, Gabrielsen TO, Aisen AM. Patients with partial seizures: evaluation by MR, CT, and PET imaging. *Radiology* 1986;159:159–163.

58. Lauterbur PC. Image formation by induced local interactions: examples employing nuclear magnetic resonance. *Nature (London)* 1973;242:190–191.

59. Levitt RG, Glazer HS, Roper CL, Lee JKT, Murphy WA. Magnetic resonance imaging of mediastinal and hilar masses: comparison with CT. *AJR* 1985;145:9–14.

60. Maloney TW, Rogers DE. Medical technology: a different view of the contentious debate over costs. *N Engl J Med* 1979;301:1413–1419.

61. Meaney TF. CT and the planners. *AJR* 1976;126:1095–1097.

62. Murphy WA, Totty WG, Gado M, Levitt RG, Lee JKT, Evens RG. Utilization characteristics of a superconductive MR system undergoing initial clinical trial. *J Comput Assist Tomogr* 1985;9:258–262.

63. Pavlicek W, Geisinger M, Castle L, et al. The effect of nuclear magnetic resonance on patients with cardiac pacemakers. *Radiology* 1983;147:149–153.

64. Purcell EM. Research in nuclear magnetism. In: *Nobel lectures in physics: 1946–62*. New York: Elsevier Publishing, 1964.

65. Randell CP, Collins AG, Young IR, et al. Nuclear magnetic resonance imaging of posterior fossa tumors. *AJR* 1983;141:489–496.

66. Robbins AH, Pugatch RD, Gerzof SG, Faling LJ, Johnson WC, Sewell DH. Observations on the medical efficacy of computed tomography of the chest and abdomen. *AJR* 1978;131:15–19.

67. Ross JS, O'Donovan PB, Novoa R, et al. Magnetic resonance of the chest: initial experience with imaging and in vivo T1 and T2 calculations. *Radiology* 1984;152:95–101.

68. Runge VM, Price AC, Kirshner HS, Allen JH, Partain CL, James AE Jr. Magnetic resonance imaging of multiple sclerosis: a study of pulse-technique efficacy. *AJR* 1984;143:1015–1026.

69. Sagel SS, Stanley RJ, Evens RG. Early clinical experience with mo-tionless wholebody computed tomography. *Radiology* 1976;119: 321–330.

70. Shapiro SH, Wyman SM. CAT fever. *N Engl J Med* 1976;294:954–956.

71. Sheedy PF, Stephens DH, Hattery RR, Muhm JR, Hartman GW. Computed tomography of the body: initial clinical trial with the EMI prototype. *AJR* 1976;127:23–51.

72. Smith FW, Mallard JR, Reid A, Hutchinson JMS. Nuclear magnetic resonance tomographic imaging in liver disease. *Lancet* 1981;1:963–966.

73. Stanley RJ, Sagel SS, Levit RG. Computed tomography of the body: early trends in application and accuracy of the method. *AJR* 1976;127:56–67.

74. Steinberg EP. The status of MRI in 1986: rates of adoption in the United States and worldwide. *AJR* 1986;147:453–455.

75. Steinberg EP, Cohen AB. Health technology case study 27: nuclear magnetic resonance imaging technology: a clinical, industrial and policy analysis. US Congress, Office of Technology Assessment, OTA-HCS-27, September 1984.

76. Steinberg EP, Linton OW, Erickson JE. The economics and regulation of magnetic resonance imaging. In: Partain CL et al., eds. *Magnetic resonance imaging.* Philadelphia: WB Saunders, 1987.

77. Technical Appendices to the Report and Recommendations to the Secretary, Department of Health and Human Services. Washington, DC: Prospective Payment Assessment Commission, April 1, 1986.

78. Turcke DA, Gilmore GT. Computed tomography's impact on nuclear medicine service in two community hospitals. *Appl Radiol* 1977;6:149–151.

79. Webb WR, Jensen BG, Sollitto R, et al. Bronchogenic carcinoma: staging with MR compared with staging with CT and surgery. *Radiology* 1985;156:117–124.

80. Weyman PJ, McClennan BL, Stanley RJ, Levitt RG, Sagel SS. Comparison of computed tomography and angiography in the evaluation of renal cell carcinoma. *Radiology* 1980;137:417–424.

81. Whalen JP. Radiology of the abdomen: impact of new imaging methods. *AJR* 1979;133:587–618.

82. Wittenberg J, Fineberg HV, Black EB, et al. Clinical efficacy of computed body tomography. *AJR* 1978;131:5–14.

83. Wortzman G, Holgate RC, Morgan PP. Cranial computed tomography: an evaluation of cost effectiveness. *Radiology* 1975;117:75–77.

84. Young IR, Burl M, Clarke GJ, et al. Magnetic resonance properties of hydrogen: imaging the posterior fossa. *AJR* 1981;137:895–901.

Subject Index

Subject Index

A

Abdomen. *See also specific organ and*
Abdominal wall
  abscess in, in children, 1085–1086
  adrenal glands, normal anatomy of,
    439–442, 446
  alimentary tract, normal anatomy of,
    422–434, 435, 436
  anterior pararenal space, normal
    anatomy of, 443–445, 456
  aorta, 416, 436, 708–718, 719
    aneurysms of, 711–712, 713, 714,
      715
      in children, 1090
      CT depicting, 711–712, 713, 714
      CT imaging protocol for, 55
      MRI depicting, 712, 714, 715
      perirenal hemorrhage and, 816
    atherosclerosis affecting, 710, 711
      CT depicting, 710, 711
      MRI depicting, 710, 711
    and clinical application of imaging
      techniques, 717–718, 719
    dissection of, 712, 714
    normal anatomy of, 708–711
      CT depicting, 708
      MRI depicting, 708–711
    pathologic conditions affecting,
      711–712, 713, 714, 715. *See also*
      specific disorder
    postoperative complications and,
      712–717
      CT depicting, 712–717
      MRI depicting, 717
  ascending colon, normal anatomy of,
    452–455
  bile ducts, normal anatomy of, 430–
    431
  body wall muscles, normal anatomy
    of, 417, 418
  in children, 1075–1090
    abscess in, 1085–1086
    liver diseases and, 1089
    lymphoma in, 1085, 1086
    masses in, 1075–1085
    pancreatic disorders and, 1087–
      1089

    renal parenchymal disease and,
      1089–1090
    trauma to, 1086–1087
    vascular structures and, 1090
  descending colon, normal anatomy
    of, 452–455
  diaphragm, normal anatomy of, 417–
    419
  diaphragmatic crura, normal anat-
    omy of, 417–419, 420–421
  duodenum, normal anatomy of, 452,
    453
  esophageal hiatus, normal anatomy
    of, 417–419
  fascia of, normal anatomy of, 417
  gallbladder, normal anatomy of, 428–
    430
  gastroesophageal junction, normal
    anatomy of, 419–422
  gastrointestinal system
    embryogenesis of, 423–424
    normal adult anatomy of, 428–434,
      435, 436
  great vessels of, normal anatomy of,
    435–438, 439
  intramesenteric viscera, normal anat-
    omy of, 422–434
    adult, 428–434
    developmental, 423–424
  kidneys, normal anatomy of, 439–
    442, 444–445
  liver, normal anatomy of, 428–430
  lymphoma affecting, in children,
    1085, 1086
  mass of, in children
    clinical applications of imaging
      and, 1083–1085
    comparative imaging and, 1083
  mesenteric roots, normal anatomy of,
    443–452
  normal anatomy of, 415–455, 456
    CT versus MRI for imaging of,
      415–417
    MRI depicting, 416
  pancreas, normal anatomy of, 443–
    452

  perirenal spaces, normal anatomy of,
    439–442, 444–445, 446, 447
  peritoneal spaces, normal anatomy
    of, in adult, 424–428
  posterior pararenal space, normal
    anatomy of, 442–443, 448
  posterior recesses, normal anatomy
    of, 428
  psoas spaces, normal anatomy of,
    438–439, 441, 442, 443
  retroperitoneal spaces, normal anat-
    omy of, 435–455, 456
  small intestine, normal anatomy of,
    434, 435, 436
  spleen, normal anatomy of, 430–431,
    432
  stomach, normal anatomy of, 430–
    431, 432
  transverse colon, normal anatomy of,
    432–434
  trauma to. *See Abdominal trauma*
  ureters, normal anatomy of, 442, 447
  vascular structures of, in children,
    1090
Abdomen-pelvis, CT imaging protocol
  for survey of, 54
Abdominal fascia, 417
Abdominal trauma
  in children, 1086–1087
  CT imaging protocol for evaluation
    of, 55
  hemorrhage into juxtarenal spaces
    and, 816
  kidney affected in, 820–822
  pancreas affected in, 583, 584
  sacral injuries and, 1031–1032, 1033
  spleen affected in, 535, 536, 537
Abdominal wall, 417, 418, 661–666.
  See also Abdomen
  abscess in, 665
  desmoid tumor of, 665–666
  hematoma of, 661–664, 665
    CT depicting, 662, 664, 665
    MRI depicting, 662–664, 665
  hernias and, 661, 662, 663
  infection of, 664–665
  inflammation of, 664–665